Common Clinical Presentations in Dogs and Cats

Common Clinical Presentations in Dogs and Cats

Ryane E. Englar, DVM, DABVP (Canine and Feline Practice)
Assistant Professor and Clinical Education Coordinator
Kansas State University College of Veterinary Medicine
Manhattan, Kansas, USA

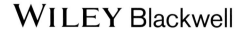

Registered Office
John Wiley & Sons, Inc., 111 River Street, Hoboken, NJ 07030, USA

Editorial Office
111 River Street, Hoboken, NJ 07030, USA

For details of our global editorial offices, customer services, and more information about Wiley products visit us at www.wiley.com.

Wiley also publishes its books in a variety of electronic formats and by print-on-demand. Some content that appears in standard print versions of this book may not be available in other formats.

Library of Congress Cataloging-in-Publication Data

Names: Englar, Ryane E., author.
Title: Common clinical presentations in dogs and cats / Ryane E. Englar.
Description: Hoboken, NJ : Wiley-Blackwell, 2019. | Includes bibliographical
   references and index. |
Identifiers: LCCN 2019003277 (print) | LCCN 2019004615 (ebook) | ISBN
   9781119414599 (Adobe PDF) | ISBN 9781119414605 (ePub) | ISBN 9781119414582
   (hardback)
Subjects: LCSH: Dogs–Diseases. | Cats–Diseases. | MESH: Dog Diseases | Cat
   Diseases | Handbook
Classification: LCC SF991 (ebook) | LCC SF991 .E54 2019 (print) | NLM SF 991
   | DDC 636.7089–dc23
LC record available at https://lccn.loc.gov/2019003277

Cover Design: Wiley
Cover Images: © Photo credit – Ryane E. Englar, © Photo credit – Daniel Foy,
© Photo credit – D.J. Haeussler, Jr., © Photo credit – Alexis Siler, © Photo credit – Aimee Wong

Set in 10/12pt Warnock by SPi Global, Pondicherry, India
Printed and bound in Singapore by Markono Print Media Pte Ltd

10 9 8 7 6 5 4 3 2 1

Dedication

Families come in all different shapes and sizes.

There is the family to whom we are born, that accepts us, as we are, from the moment we enter this world.

There is also the family that we grow into, the family that chooses to share with us days, moments, memories, and lifetimes.

There is a place in my heart for both of my families, but this book is dedicated to the latter, to honor my mother's greatest life lesson. Mom raised me to widen my circle of loved ones. It was she who taught me to accept others into my life as intricate threads that, when woven together, created one whole version, the better version, of me. She still speaks this truth today and reminds me of it when I lose my way.

I may not have understood it then, as a child, but I now see the power behind those words. I now see how the wings of others have lifted me in my journey through life, and how my life today would be incomplete those supporting my flight.

My Arizona *dance* family came into my life when I least expected it. I had moved to the desert to pursue a professional dream. Chance, laced with luck, caused me to stumble upon the oasis that was built by franchisee Mychael James Wooten, Arrowhead Arthur Murray Dance Studio.

When I introduced myself to Arrowhead, I initially saw the studio as a way to get involved in the community, to reach out and become more social. Little did I know then that dance would rise up to become a part of me, that it would inspire me, and that, three years later, when it came time to leave Arizona, I would do everything in my power to package it up and take it with me to the next leg of my journey.

It is hard to describe the magic of dance to those who have never experienced it. What I discovered, through dance, was how it changed me. It became a sanctuary of reason and perspective amidst the curveballs that life tossed my way.

Dance became a second home, and within those sacred walls, I found a family that I grew to love and trust. For three years, this family was ever-present. We trained hard together. We supported each other, and challenged each other to achieve new personal bests.

When it came time for me to move to Kansas, I feared that I would lose my dance friends forever. Yet despite being miles apart, our friendships grew.

My Arizona dance friends continue to be there when I need them most. They are a testament to the fact that life may change directions and paths may take us off-course, but those we love are never far from thought.

After all, as Richard Bach once said:

> Can miles truly separate you from friends …
> If you want to be with someone you love, aren't you already there?

This textbook is devoted to my dance friends who became family somewhere along the way:

To Lowell E. Fox, my dance instructor, a true artist, and a brilliant mind:

Thank you for coaching me through life, both on and off the dance floor.

Thank you for indulging in my science facts, and linking dance to veterinary medicine in a way that made sense to me. You taught me not to walk plantigrade like a diabetic cat, and you lit up neuronal connections to the tune of West Coast Animal Charades.

You made dance a part of my life by taking the time to really get to know me.

You looked beyond the awkward stages of my dance and refined the rough edges. You taught me that I could do anything I put my mind to, if only I just believed in myself the way that you did.

You were the first dance instructor to believe in me, and to see me for who I am. That faith in a student is priceless. It has driven me to dream in spite of barriers and to persevere against all odds.

You represent HOPE.

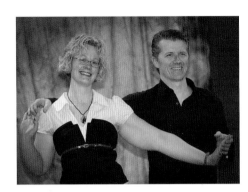

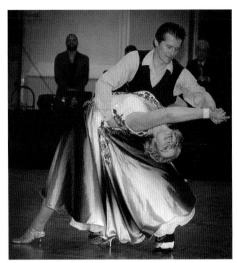

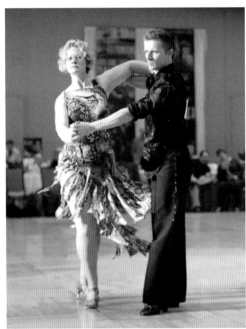

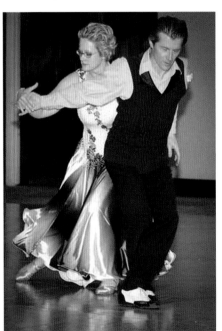

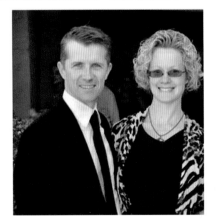

To Gail Nason, my Arizona "grandmother" and very dear friend:

Thank you for welcoming me into your home and heart, repeatedly.

Your kindness and generosity are refreshing in a world that sometimes comes across as drafty or cold. From day one, you have embraced me.

Thank you for being someone who is willing to sacrifice for others so that they might take flight. Your strength helps me to soar. Thanks to you, my compass always points me in the direction of home: your house.

You represent LOVE.

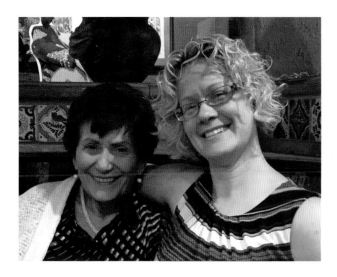

To Carolyn and Brad Vining, my Arizona dance "mom" and "dad":

Thank you for taking me under your wing. In the same way that you have transported me to and from dance events, you've carried my heart.

Thank you for being my "Captain" and my guide to the dance world.

Thank you for taking the baby dancer in me and showing me the ropes, so that I felt comfortable, confident, and poised.

You represent COMFORT.

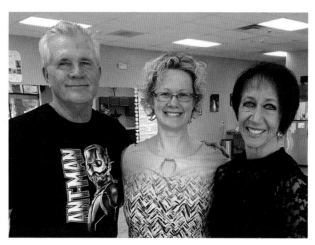

To Andy and Kristina Burch:

Thank you for finding a way to keep the memory of "Ryane the Lion" alive and well at the studio and beyond. On those days when I find myself missing the studio the most, you manage to find your way to me in thought and prayer, photographs, and videos. You manage to capture those moments that I would never want to miss. Because of you, I never have to. I can live them and relive them again and again.

Thank you for your selflessness, which is of comfort, particularly on those occasions when my heart is missing home.

You represent GENEROSITY.

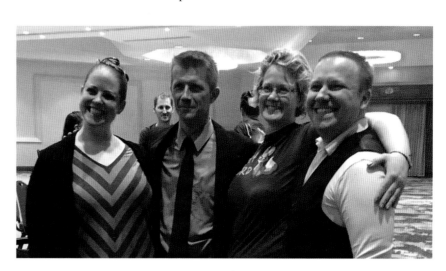

To Meghan Teixeira and Matt Stait:

Thank you for being like a sister to me, Meghan, and to Matt, for completing her as her Other Half. As a couple, you serve as a constant reminder that we are never as good alone as we can be together. You both challenge me to step outside of my comfort zone, yet not be afraid to lean on others so that collectively we can build a bridge to higher ground.

You represent CONNECTIVITY.

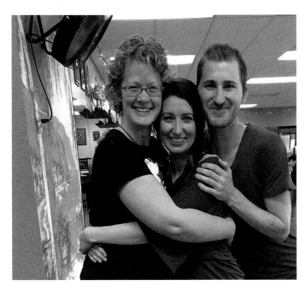

To Justine and Greg Cox:

Thank you for being the face of warmth and genuine energy, the kind of friends that I can be real with and that I can trust. Your perspective reminds me that life is not always easy, but we survive the rough spots by being true to our inner selves.

You represent FRIENDSHIP.

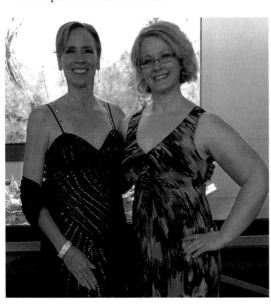

To Riley Haveman:

Growing up with you at the studio has been a privilege. You light up any room with your smile. You remind me that age is only a number: true wisdom knows no limits, and in you, I see an old soul, someone who is wise beyond her years, and is going to, no doubt, go on to do great things in life.

You represent the FUTURE.

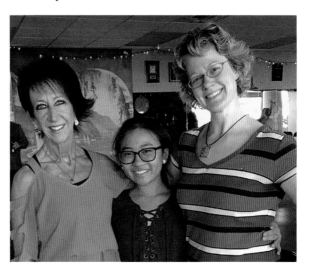

To Diana Smith:

Our dance journey started at around the same time, so in that way we have grown together in the ballroom. As we have together moved through the syllabi, as we have together explored the nuances of advanced dancing, you remind me that nothing worthwhile comes without its challenges. At times, our steps – and lives – may seem impossible, but the only true impossibility is the barrier we create for ourselves. If we allow fear and insecurities to get in the way, then we risk missing the view from the mountaintop, so climb we must.

You represent the JOURNEY.

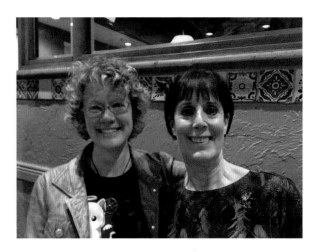

To Huddleston Photography and Steven Stringham Photography:

You manage to capture the emotional spark of energy that we bring to our dance, not just once, but for as long as I have known you. As beginners, we fear that first photo because of the rawness that it captures. As we improve our steps so that we might one day belong out there in a sea of other dancers, we treasure your snapshots for what they represent. Your photographs are slivers of insight into a dancer's world, mind, and heart. They make time stand still as we silently, ever so peacefully recall That Moment, The Move, The Dance, or That Smile.

You represent MEMORIES.

Contents

Author Bio

Ryane E. Englar, DVM, DABVP (Canine and Feline Practice), is a 2008 graduate of Cornell University College of Veterinary Medicine. Following graduation, she spent five years as an associate veterinarian in small animal practice, split between her home state of Maryland and her home away from home, upstate New York. She then became a Clinical Instructor of the Community Practice Service at Cornell's Companion Animal Hospital and a Consultant for the Louis J. Camuti Hotline in association with Cornell's Feline Health Center.

In February 2014, Dr. Englar relocated to Arizona, where she was privileged to be founding faculty for Midwestern University College of Veterinary Medicine. As an Assistant Professor of Small Animal Primary Care, she designed and debuted the communications coursework for the inaugural class of 2018. By developing 27 standardized client encounters over eight preclinical quarters, she was able to expand the breadth and depth of standardized client encounters in the veterinary curriculum. Her experiences in simulation-based education have been detailed in her active publication history with the *Journal of Veterinary Medical Education*.

Dr. Englar joined the faculty at Kansas State University in May 2017 to build the clinical skills curriculum for first and second year veterinary students. Her coursework emphasizes hands-on training with the opportunity for practice and repetition to build those clinical and professional skills that promote Day-One-Ready graduates. Her interests in the design and development of non-animal teaching models have led her and her team to create novel learning opportunities for her students.

When she is not teaching or brainstorming new approaches to learning, she is a competitive ballroom dancer and artist.

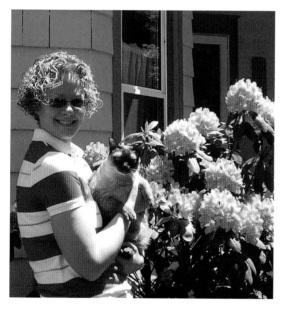
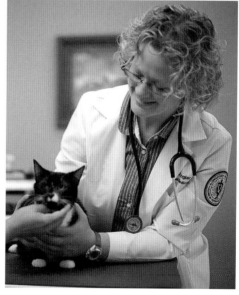

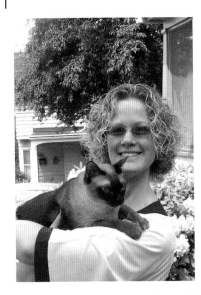

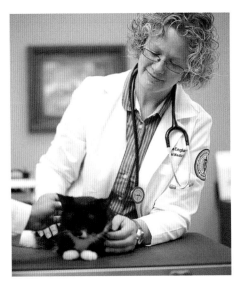

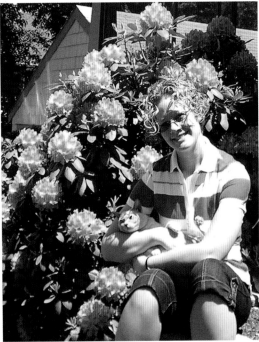

Preface

As an educator with a background in and passion for primary care, I am invested in training veterinary students to be "career-ready." Being "career-ready" requires veterinary students to rise to a level of proficiency and efficiency, confidence and competence that did not exist when I graduated in 2008. At that time, the expectation fell upon the employer to transform the often-panicky graduate from a static database of knowledge into a full-fledged, functional, and adaptable member of the profession. The transition from university to clinical practice was fraught with challenges, and the learning curve was steep.

Since then, educational theory and our improved understanding of how we learn best have reshaped the way in which we train veterinary students. Experiential opportunities are now prioritized as rote memorization takes a backseat to active learning. Students are entering the clinic sooner, and are encouraged to participate in experiences that reinforce clinical skills. Curricular revision has also led to the development of clinical skills coursework at a number of North American colleges of veterinary medicine, as well as the use of task trainers to simulate procedural medicine. These opportunities for learning integrate knowledge with clinically relevant tasks to facilitate the professional journey from student to doctor. As students explore clinical experiences, each is challenged to not just act like a doctor, but to think like one, too.

One challenge associated with this approach to learning is that students are novices in clinical practice. They have foundational knowledge, but they do not always know how to apply knowledge to clinical experiences. They also lack bridges between textbook content and real-life cases. For instance, we teach our students how to perform a comprehensive physical examination, yet they may not know what to do with the information that is gained.

The early learner thus experiences gaps in his or her professional journey. The student may want to learn more about a topic, yet because diagnoses, rather than clinical signs, define most textbook chapters, the student is powerless to do so.

Students who learn to recognize clinical signs build context into the growing library of cases that they are likely to experience in clinical practice. Context allows students to apply knowledge to cases and expand their understanding of case presentations. Patients will not present, for instance, as persistent right aortic arch (PRAA), but patients will present for regurgitation, of which PRAA is a cause.

Learning how to think through cases by considering each contributing problem facilitates decision making. It also models how to think like a clinician before one has acquired a functional library of illness scripts.

This textbook is an attempt, on my part, to provide students with the missing links they may need before they experience coursework in pathology and small animal medicine.

This textbook allows students to explore physical exam findings, regardless of whether the diagnosis is known. For example, the student that is concerned about skin fragility on physical examination can turn to Chapter 7 for additional details. The student that identifies abnormal lung sounds can turn to Chapter 37.

In total, this textbook offers 78 chapters, grouped by body system and outlined by presenting complaint. This problem-oriented approach allows students to work through case presentations that may not be familiar to them. It provides a foundation for problem solving *now* that can translate into pattern recognition *later*.

Acknowledgments

I fell in love with the profession of veterinary medicine in the usual way. As a child, I was captivated by all creatures great and small. I read James Herriot and even wrote him a letter, telling him that his tales of life in the trenches had in fact solidified my desire to become a veterinarian. I didn't know it at the time – those were the days *before* the Internet had taken off – but he had already passed away. His son wrote back, and expressed gratitude that I remembered his father. How could I not? His father had lived and breathed in a world in which I so very desperately wanted to belong.

Fast-forward to the present day: I am living my dream. I still love the profession today as I did then. However, my love for it has deepened in a way that is, at times, indescribable. It is hard to capture the compassionate determination that I see in my colleagues, and their fierceness, yet vulnerability, as they struggle with life-and-death decisions each day.

It is hard to relay to others that what makes this profession so life-giving is also what makes it disheartening sometimes, too. We doctors are all too familiar with the game of odds called Life. We expect to win, and it is hard to lose.

It doesn't help that, at times, our training assumes that we are infallible. We often sacrifice our wellness for others. We devote weekends and holidays to patient care. We run on autopilot, at times, fueled only by coffee and adrenaline. We spend our days putting out fires, and often our nights, too. Those under our care come first, and we are proud of this. We often define ourselves by how much we are willing to give up and for whom.

In the midst of being everyone else's hero, we, forget, sometimes, that we need a hero, too.

By *hero*, I don't mean the kind that fairy tales are full of, with the knight riding in to save the day on a white horse.

I mean the kind of person who is giving of time and space; the kind of person who accepts others as they are, and challenges them to rise above the obstacles that life has placed in their way.

I mean the kind of person who recognizes an emptiness inside of someone and rather than filling up the hole with arbitrary words, sits in the uncomfortable silence for as long as it takes the individual to realize s/he is not alone.

I mean the kind of person who helps you to find yourself again at any crossroads.

How blessed I am to have found that person many years ago in Dr. Ken Cohen.

Ken came to me when I needed him most.

Call it luck, call it coincidence, call it fate – I found him in the Counseling Department of the Student Health Center at Cornell University. It was the Fall Semester of my second year as a veterinary student.

What most of my classmates didn't know at the time – and what I hid from everyone that I could – was that I was falling apart inside. Between the summer of my first and second year, my grandmother died in an automobile accident. I witnessed the traumatic event. Not only that, I was a passenger inside of the vehicle.

My grandmother's death was an event that would later define the way I saw the world. It shook me up. I grappled with the usual questions, the normal questions, the whys and the what-ifs. I thought that if the Logical Me could just wrap itself around the Emotional Me, then I would survive.

The harder things got, the harder I dug into my studies. But post-traumatic stress is difficult to shake. You can only push the "snooze" button on the alarm for so long before the interior cracks exteriorize.

Ken came into my life when I was one crack short of fracturing. I'd been tasked to lead a Pet Loss Support group, and I had reached out to Ken to provide volunteer training. Ken trained the group, as promised, but what he really did was save me.

Something about Ken made him seem safe. Perhaps it was that he represented the world of the living at a time when I felt like my heart was dying.

For whatever reason, I reached out to him that day. I started to meet with Ken shortly after that. I met with Ken once a week for the remainder of vet school.

My experiences with Ken were powerful. They were not easy sessions. Ken didn't have all the answers, and I had to work hard to find answers of my own.

Ken couldn't take away the images that I had seen. Ken couldn't bring my loved one back to life. Ken couldn't do the impossible. But he was the face of humanity during a time when I needed it most.

They say that time heals wounds. What they don't say is that scars run deep.

Sometimes we need people like Ken to experience life with because they make us whole and more human, too.

Ken helped me to adapt my perspective. He reshaped me. He taught me the life skills that I needed to cope with the past. Ken gave me the courage to find the New Me.

But Ken's most powerful lesson was bigger than me and is in fact what our profession needs to hear today.

It's okay to need people. It's okay to ask for help. It isn't easy. Sometimes it's downright hard and scary. But asking for help isn't weak.

It's a sign of strength to find your inner voice.

Ken's greatest gift was giving me back mine, so that now I can encourage others to find theirs.

Thank you, Ken, for everything.

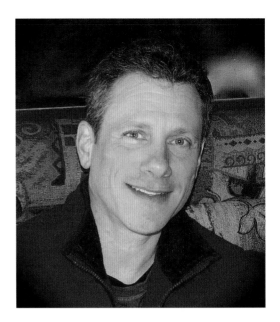

Part One

Introducing the Problem-Oriented Approach

1

The Problem-Oriented Approach to Clinical Medicine

1.1 The Role of Clinical Reasoning in Diagnosis Making

In an ideal world, every patient would display unambiguous signs of disease conforming to classical textbook descriptions, and the clinician's pharmacy would be an assembly of rational and efficacious therapeutic agents that would collectively address all the diseases of the animal kingdom. Unfortunately, the ideal world is not the real world, and a series of limitations relating to all aspects of diagnosis and therapy make veterinary medicine (as with human medicine) "a science of uncertainty." Arriving at the most likely diagnosis, "best" treatment, and most informed prognosis is a higher-order skill. *(Ref. [1], p. 200)*

To be successful veterinarians, students must diagnose and treat their patients. To do so adequately and accurately, they must think like clinicians. They must consider, for every patient, the odds that disease "x" is most likely, and balance these odds against clinical unknowns and uncertainties [2, 3]. They must develop and fine-tune the skill of clinical reasoning.

Clinical reasoning refers to "the practitioner's ability to assess patient problems or needs and analyze data to accurately identify and frame problems within the context of the individual patient's environment" [4]. This skill allows clinicians to initiate, evaluate, and adapt case management to the patient as patient needs change and/or as diagnostic test results provide additional insight into the root of the patient's problem [4].

Clinical reasoning is thus intimately tied to critical thinking, and both are dynamic processes. They do not begin and end with diagnosis [5]. They evolve as external factors and internal inputs are considered. Internal inputs include prior experiences with the same set of clinical signs. These so-called "illness scripts" generate context as well as a working memory of which

treatments have been historically effective at managing the presenting complaint [6, 7].

Over time, the experienced clinician develops a library of patterns to assist with clinical decision making [8]. Associations are made between new patient presentations and past events in such a way as to guide diagnostic approaches and therapeutic plans [1, 8]. Eventually, these associations become automatic as the clinician unconsciously draws from these reserves to approach and manage new cases [9].

To become effective at clinical reasoning, clinicians have to master critical thinking and develop the ability to acquire, define, and compare key pieces of patient data [10]. Probing questions that may assist with this process include [9, 11] the following:

- What do I ask to gather the information that I need from the history?
- Which findings from the history and physical examination are pertinent to case management?
- What additional data are needed to clarify, support, or refute these findings?
- How do I best obtain that additional data?
- What are the differential diagnoses?
- Which differential diagnosis is most likely for this patient?
- If the diagnosis is "x," then how will I proceed?
- If the diagnosis is not "x," then where do I go from here?

History taking begins the process by which clinicians gather data. Physical examination findings add to the collection of data and allow for further characterization of the data as being "normal" or "abnormal." Clinicians must be able to interpret data to form and test hypotheses about which diagnosis is most consistent with case presentation [10, 11].

Pattern recognition speeds this process for clinicians because, by virtue of their experience, they already have an established library of data against which to compare new findings. Even then, when faced with clinical cases that they have not experienced before, clinicians are

Common Clinical Presentations in Dogs and Cats, First Edition. Ryane E. Englar.
© 2019 John Wiley & Sons, Inc. Published 2019 by John Wiley & Sons, Inc.

able to sift through their memory bank to draw upon similarities to past events. These links to the past trigger the clinician's recall of pathophysiology that is relevant to the current case [12].

Students lack this memory bank. They are slow to find patterns because there is much that they have yet to experience. As learners, they must overcome these gaps in knowledge and experience, and channel what they do know into viable approaches to patient care and solutions to patient problems. Mastering the possibilities and probabilities of disease, and applying these to the individual patient are major steps in the evolution of student to clinician.

The "preclinical/clinical divide" is a milestone in that professional journey [13]. As the student transitions from the classroom into the clinic and assumes the professional role of clinician, he starts to think like one. Yet, waiting until the clinical year to practice this skill may contribute to graduates who do not feel competent or confident to engage in clinical reasoning on their own [8]. It takes time to develop clinical reasoning as is the case with any other skill, and one clinical year of rotations may be insufficient [8].

In an effort to deliver "Day One Ready" graduates, accrediting bodies have established a set of core competencies that veterinary educators must infuse into the curriculum. Both the American Veterinary Medical Association (AVMA) and the Royal College of Veterinary Surgeons (RCVS) now consider clinical reasoning a core competency. Both expect graduates to be well versed in problem-solving skills so that they are primed for success in clinical practice [8, 14].

In response to demands by accrediting bodies, many veterinary educators are actively reshaping curricula to encourage critical thinking as early as the first year of veterinary college [15]. Educators have experimented with problem-based learning (PBL), self-reflection and experiential learning exercises, concept mapping, and integrative curricula [4, 16–22].

The most effective approach to teaching clinical reasoning in veterinary medicine is unclear [8, 14]. As veterinary educators, we just know that we need to do better. Simply exposing students to the clinic floor is not sufficient to develop clinical reasoning [8]. Learning to imitate mentors and learning to reason are not one and the same.

Students are often shielded from the responsibility of decision making in teaching hospitals. The intern, resident, or attending clinician makes case management decisions. This takes away the opportunity for students to make decisions on their own and learn from the consequences of each decision [14].

An added complication is that veterinary educators tend to encourage rote memorization. This often occurs at the expense of clinical reasoning. Teaching to the test and asking students to retain information without context proves challenging for students, who are easily overwhelmed by the vastness of medical knowledge and clinical theory [1].

Memorizing lists of differential diagnoses also encourages a backward approach to case management [1]. Students stamp what they know onto a clinical case and try to make it fit when, in fact, most patients stray from the classic textbook case [1].

If students do not know that a particular differential diagnosis exists, they are limited in terms of the resources that they turn to. For example, if gastric dilatation-volvulus (GDV) does not exist in their vocabulary, then how might students learn about it? Most reference guides outline content by diagnosis, and students do not know how to research a medical condition that is foreign to them.

It is true that students ultimately need to be able to make the diagnosis. They need to be able to diagnose GDV to manage the patient effectively. However, a student with no previous association with or knowledge of GDV is unlikely to come to that diagnosis on his own. On the other hand, a student who works forward from the presenting complaints, abdominal distension and nonproductive retching, may find greater success.

1.2 The Evolution of the Problem-Oriented Approach

The problem-oriented approach allows students to work their way through case presentations that may not be familiar to them. It provides a foundation for problem solving *now* that can translate into pattern recognition *later* [8].

Students who learn to recognize clinical signs and apply these to clinical algorithms actively build context into their library of cases that they are likely to experience in clinical practice [8, 23]. Context allows students to develop, structure, and apply knowledge methodically in a way that fits how cases will present to them. Cases will not present, for instance, as the diagnosis of persistent right fourth aortic arch (PRAA), but they will present for regurgitation.

Learning how to think through cases by considering each contributing problem, one at a time, facilitates decision making. It also models how to think like a clinician before one has acquired a functional library of illness scripts.

The problem-oriented approach is relatively new to clinical medicine. It was adopted by the veterinary teaching hospital at the University of Georgia in the early 1970s [24]. Most North American colleges of veterinary medicine have since adapted it for their use in teaching, as has the Royal Veterinary College (RVC) [24, 25].

Rather than jumping straight to diagnosis, which requires clinical experience and pattern recognition, the problem-oriented approach concentrates on clinical signs. These so-called "problems" reflect the patient's underlying disease and can be studied both in isolation and collectively to build a case for a particular disease process [24, 26].

Because this approach emphasizes patient problems, the clinician must devote time and resources to gathering information. This patient-specific information constitutes the database.

1.3 The Database

A minimum patient database includes a comprehensive history and physical examination [24]. For more information on history-taking, refer to Chapter 2. For additional guidance with the examination of canine or feline patients, consult the textbook *Performing the Small Animal Physical Examination* [27].

The goal of the database is to gather enough information to identify all patient problems [24]. Some of these problems may pertain to the presenting complaint.

Other problems may be incidental findings, meaning that they were unearthed by history taking or through the physical examination, but are unrelated to the presenting complaint. Incidental findings need to be addressed at some point. However, they may not be prioritized at that office visit if they are not urgent matters that must be tended to right away. For example, consider a patient that presents with a hemoabdomen and dyspnea after automobile trauma. On physical examination, this patient may also have aural discharge. Both hemoabdomen and aural discharge are problems for the patient. The former is the reason for presenting to the clinic, and the latter is incidental. The aural discharge should be evaluated to determine if there is underlying otitis externa. However, stabilizing the patient is more important during the patient's initial assessment than addressing the aural discharge. Therefore, the aural discharge must take a back seat to the hemoabdomen, which could result in patient fatality.

In addition to history and physical examination findings, patient databases may include other details [28]. Database contents often vary from practice to practice and between clinicians. Some databases include bloodwork, such as a complete blood count (CBC), chemistry panel, and urinalysis (UA). Others include diagnostic imaging, such as three-view thoracic radiographs or abdominal ultrasound.

Increasingly, there is a push in healthcare to tailor the database as well as diagnostic test recommendations to the patient rather than to pursue a universal database [29–32].

1.4 The Problem List

From the database, a collection of problems emerges. These accumulated problems form the basis of the problem list. The problem list is a collection of ailments, clinical signs, presenting complaints, or diagnostic findings that the clinician has identified [24].

Problems are listed with only as much detail as can be provided at the time of documentation [26]. For instance, a patient that presents for diarrhea will have *diarrhea* listed as a problem until that problem can be further refined. It would be inaccurate for the initial entry in the medical record to list *large bowel diarrhea* unless this degree of specificity is accurate. Doing so would cause the clinician to rule out causes of *small bowel diarrhea* prematurely, unless the patient's *large bowel diarrhea* truly has been confirmed.

The problem list is thus dynamic: it changes as the case evolves. Listed problems are often initially vague or poorly defined [33, 34]. As the work-up proceeds, clinicians update problems to their current level of understanding [26, 33, 34]. *Right hind limb lameness* may be refined to *right stifle pain and right cranial drawer* following orthopedic examination. Subsequent radiography may reveal additional problems, such as *right stifle* and *right tarsal osteoarthritis*.

This process of refining the problem list reflects the appropriate and methodical funneling of information toward a diagnosis. Refining the problem list as the case evolves also guards against tunnel vision. Consider a patient that presents for owner-witnessed "seizures." History taking reveals that these episodes may or may not be seizures and would be more appropriately labeled as collapse. A problem of *collapse* allows the clinician to consider seizures as well as cardiovascular events until diagnostic test results prove otherwise. This prevents the clinician from inappropriately ruling out syncope at the start of the work-up.

The same could be same of the "coughing" cat: is it really coughing or is it wheezing? Is it dyspneic or it is trying to bring up a hairball?

A broad problem list at the start of a work-up keeps options open. It allows the clinician to consider each option as being possible until there is sufficient evidence to suggest otherwise.

As clinicians acquire more information about each case through diagnostic investigation, problem lists grow. The discovery of one problem may unearth several more. Problems may be interrelated or they may be stand-alone. The burden falls upon the clinician to discover if, when, and how they intersect.

1.5 Prioritizing the Problem List

Patients often present with more than one problem. Not all problems are of equal concern to the client and clinician. The client may be most concerned about problem "x"; the clinician may be more concerned about problem "y." This disparity in perceived value demonstrates the importance of establishing priorities and communicating these to the client so that clinician and client are on the same page. In order to move forward with case management, both parties need to find common ground concerning the following questions:

- Which problem(s) need(s) to be addressed now?
- Which problem(s) can be addressed later?
- Which problem(s) should be addressed now, but have been tabled for later?
- When will tabled problems be reconsidered?

Prioritizing the problem list is an important aspect of case management [8, 23]. Patient outcomes rely upon the clinician being able to effectively distinguish problems that require immediate action from those that do not [8, 23].

Let us revisit the patient that presented on emergency with hemoabdomen and dyspnea. Physical examination reveals conjunctivitis and brittle nails in addition to aural discharge. In total, this patient has five problems. However, not all five carry equal value at the time of presentation. Whether the patient lives or dies depends upon whether or not the hemoabdomen and dyspnea can be medically or surgically managed and resolved. Thus, hemoabdomen and dyspnea become the patient's primary problems.

By contrast, the resolution of aural discharge, conjunctivitis, and brittle nails does not affect patient survival. Although aural discharge, conjunctivitis, and brittle nails appear on the problem list, they do not require immediate attention. Their presence on the problem list is a reminder that they can and will be addressed at a later point in time, when doing so is in the best interest of the patient.

To reflect this prioritization, the problem list is often written in order from most to least pressing concerns:

- Hemoabdomen
- Dyspnea
- Aural discharge
- Conjunctivitis
- Brittle nails

This reminds the novice to focus on what is most important first. Sometimes this organization is inherently obvious. Sometimes the case presentation makes it difficult to discern what the primary problem is and how best to address it.

Another organizational tool may assist novices as they gain additional clinical experience: the lumping of "like problems" together. Consider again the aforementioned case of the patient with hemoabdomen. Physical examination also reveals pallor, tachycardia, and thready femoral pulses. Packed cell volume (PCV) is well below the normal reference range. The evolving problem list may now read as follows:

- Hemoabdomen
- Pallor
- Anemia
- Tachycardia
- Thready pulses
- Dyspnea
- Aural discharge
- Conjunctivitis
- Brittle nails

This organization reflects a higher level of thinking and data processing. The clinician has moved beyond simply listing data. Instead, the clinician is making use of critical thinking to interpret the data and consider how the underlying pathophysiology may in fact link one or more problems to each other.

1.6 Moving Beyond the Problem List to Consider the Cause of Disease

Anyone can be trained to scan through a patient file, take a patient history, examine a patient, and list problems. However, knowing how to use the problem list is what makes a clinician successful at managing patient care. An experienced clinician moves beyond the basics of problem identification to consider the source(s) of the problem(s).

Problems may stem from local or systemic disease. For example, epistaxis could result from embedded foxtails in the nasal cavity or from ingested rodenticide that triggers coagulopathy. Retinal detachments could result from trauma sustained by one or both eyes, or from systemic hypertension. Coughing may be due to upper airway irritation or cardiac chamber enlargement secondary to cardiomyopathy that displaces the trachea. Lameness may be due to thermal burns on paw pads, or secondary to immune-mediated polyarthropathy.

For the novice, the possibilities may seem endless. Consider, for example, the problem of *weight loss*. Weight loss is a vague problem, of which there are many causes. Weight loss could stem from anorexia: a patient that is not consuming calories will lose body condition. But anorexia is not the only cause of weight loss in companion animals. What if the patient is eating, but is incapable of keeping food down? A vomiting patient may take in sufficient calories, but lose them via emesis before they can be absorbed.

The gastrointestinal tract may seem the most obvious source of the problem, *weight loss*, but is it the only source? Weight loss may also result from disease outside of the gastrointestinal tract. Consider, for example, feline hyperthyroidism. In this case, endocrinopathy rather than gastrointestinal disease causes loss of body condition. Similarly, consider cachexia due to chronic kidney disease (CKD), congestive heart failure (CHF), or neoplasia. None of these conditions directly target the gastrointestinal tract, yet weight loss is a clinical sign that may be attributed to each.

Because the novice is still learning about pathology and pathophysiology, he may struggle to consider all possible causes or sources of disease. Considering these potential sources *broadly* may facilitate the novice's approach. Rather than deducing a list of differential diagnoses with which he may or may not be familiar, the novice may start with an outline of broad categories of disease that may apply to the patient. These broad categories have been integrated into acronyms for ease of recall by veterinary students and new graduates alike. Consider, for example, the acronyms of NITSCOMP DH [35] and DAMN-IT [26, 36, 37] (see Tables 1.1 and 1.2).

Note that there is overlap between the NITSCOMP DH and DAMN-IT schemes. Both acronyms include infectious disease as well as developmental and toxicity-induced disease. The categories for disease are simply worded differently, depending upon the acronym.

Neither acronym is perfect. Neither represents the "best" approach. Instead, both are diagnostic tools to keep clinicians from developing tunnel vision. They are reminders that every problem has a multitude of potential causes. These include causes that are *iatrogenic*, induced by either the examination or medical treatment, and causes that are *idiopathic*, that is, still unknown.

Not all categories of the acronym may apply to every patient. Additionally, some categories may be more likely than others, depending upon the patient's signalment and geographical zone of residence.

Consider how age may lead the clinician to prioritize one cause of the patient's problem over others. A congenital defect such as patent ductus arteriosus (PDA) is unlikely to be diagnosed in a 16-year-old Newfoundland dog whose primary problem is collapse. PDA typically causes heart failure and death at a young age [38]. This patient would not likely have survived to age 16 with an undiagnosed and untreated PDA.

Consider how geography may also influence a clinician's assessment of the patient's presenting complaint. Visceral leishmaniasis may be considered in a tropical region such as Brazil [39], but would be unlikely as a

Table 1.1 The NITSCOMP DH acronym as a practical diagnostic aid.

First Initial	What the First Initial Stands for
N	Neoplasia
I	Infectious
T	Toxic
S	Structural
C	Congenital
O	Other
M	Metabolic
P	Parasitic
D	Diet
H	Husbandry

This acronym prevents students from making a premature diagnosis by encouraging them to consider all options.

Table 1.2 The DAMN-IT acronym is a second example of a practical diagnostic aid.

First Initial	What the First Initial Stands for
D	Degenerative
D	Developmental
A	Anomalous
A	Accident
A	Autoimmune
M	Metabolic
M	Mechanical
M	Mental
N	Nutritional
N	Neoplastic
I	Inflammatory
I	Infectious
I	Ischemic
I	Iatrogenic
I	Idiopathic
T	Traumatic
T	Toxic

It is a reminder that most problems on the problem list have more than one potential cause, and that all potential causes ought to be considered until they have been ruled out.

cause of lymphadenopathy and weight loss in a United-States-born dog that has never traveled outside of the state of Maryland.

The burden falls upon the clinician to assimilate and interpret the data in a way that makes the most sense in that it fits the clinical picture.

Much as the problem list is the starting point for considering the source of the problem, these acronyms provide a starting point for making patient-specific plans that take into account the probable diagnoses.

1.7 The Patient-Specific Plan

Although it is possible that the diagnosis is obvious without further investigation – for example, a urinary tract obstruction in a cat – the clinician most often has to formulate a patient-specific plan before making the diagnosis. Decisions for the patient must be made in spite of uncertainty, and potential benefits and risks to the patient must be considered [40–42]. Cost of care is weighed against the cost of benign neglect, and proceeding with case management requires buy-in from the client.

Ultimately, a tripartite plan is implemented by the clinician and includes [24]

- The diagnostic plan
- The therapeutic plan
- The plan for client education.

In the problem-oriented approach, there is a set of plans for each problem [24]. These plans may overlap into one master plan, particularly if there is overlap in the problems.

The diagnostic plan outlines the tests that the clinician has selected to get to the root of the problem [24]. For example, an appropriate diagnostic plan for acute vomiting in a two-month-old Golden Retriever puppy may include a CBC, chemistry panel, fecal analysis, a tabletop parvovirus antigen test, and abdominal radiographs.

All tests may be performed at once, or the tests may be performed sequentially. In the case of the latter, shared decision making between the clinician and the client dictates which test(s) will be performed first. In the example provided, consider that the client only wants to test for parvovirus. If that test is negative, then the client may proceed with additional diagnostic tests.

The diagnostic plan also tests clinical reasoning skills. The clinician must consider which tests are indicated and why, based upon the problem list for that particular patient, rather than testing for everything because every tool is available [24].

The therapeutic plan addresses specific care measures that the clinician will take, relative to the patient, in an attempt to diminish, if not resolve, the problem [24]. In the aforementioned example of the vomiting puppy, the therapeutic plan might include hospitalization for monitoring, placement of an intravenous catheter, and the administration of intravenous fluids and an injectable antiemetic.

The therapeutic plan also challenges the clinician to reason through which treatments may be initiated before

diagnostic testing and which may need to wait until after diagnostic test results have been finalized [24]. For example, the administration of maropitant citrate to halt emesis is contraindicated in those patients with gastrointestinal obstruction [43]. Clinicians must rule out gastrointestinal obstruction first before this arm of the therapeutic plan can be initiated, for the safety of the patient.

The client education plan outlines any discussions with the pet owner relative to the patient's condition, apparent prognosis, and care options including, but not limited to, the patient's diagnostic and therapeutic plans [24]. This section challenges the clinician to document the exact nature of these conversations: what was actually discussed rather than what the clinician assumes the client knows. The clinical reasoning component here is deciding what needs to be said, when it needs to be said, and how it needs to be said.

Just as the problem list evolves over time as case management progresses, so, too, does the set of patient-specific plans. As results trickle in from diagnostic testing, the clinician must constantly pool, assess, and interpret data. At any given point in time, the clinician should consider

- What is the test result?
- What does this test result mean for this patient?
- What does it mean for the patient if my interpretation is wrong?
- Where do we go from here?

The clinician must ask a similar set of questions as the patient endures therapeutic management:

- Is the patient responding to therapy?
- If so, which therapy?
- How did the patient respond?
- Should we continue treatment as is?
- Should we modify treatment?
- If so, why and how?

As plans evolve, their reason for doing so should be clear. Case management is facilitated by having logical decision making outlined in the medical record, and recognizing that care should be adapted to the patient rather than the other way around.

1.8 How does the Problem-Oriented Approach "Fit" this Textbook?

Most textbooks are outlined by diagnosis. In order to research diagnostic and therapeutic plans for a given problem, students are required to know the diagnosis. This is an effective approach to learning when the diagnosis is known, or when the learner has successfully developed the art of pattern recognition. Past experiences with similar cases trigger recall that leads to reasonably accurate diagnosis making even in the face of uncertainty.

However, students' lack of experience and exposure to clinical cases makes them particularly weak when it comes to pattern recognition. They are less likely to arrive at the correct diagnosis [8, 26]. They may or may not stumble upon the condition of interest; they may or may not be able to research the topic from which their patient would directly benefit.

Students are, however, more reliably able to identify clinical signs or presenting complaints. These problems provide them with a foundation to embark upon a journey of critical reasoning. They allow students to work

though the thought process, as would a clinician. In this way, students learn a problem-oriented approach that is more likely to lead them to the answer.

Because of its approach, this textbook is not intended to be comprehensive. Those details are best left up to a diagnosis-based resource.

What this textbook aims to provide is a new perspective on approaching medicine based upon the presenting complaint. The hope is that over time, the process will become automatic, and students may begin to develop subconscious rules and patterns that fit various clinical situations. As students evolve into clinicians, their ability to work through this process facilitates diagnosis making. Learning how to process data using this approach should make even the most complex cases approachable, one problem at a time.

References

1 May, S.A. (2013). Clinical reasoning and case-based decision making: the fundamental challenge to veterinary educators. *J. Vet. Med. Educ.* 40 (3): 200–209.

2 Osler, W. (1910). *Teacher and Student. Aequanimitas, with Other Addresses to Medical Students, Nurses, and Practitioners of Medicine.* Philadephia, PA: P. Blakiston.

3 Bean, W.B. (1968). *Sir William Osler: Aphorisms From his Bedside Teachings and Writings*, 3e. Springfield, IL: Charles C Thomas.

4 Murphy, J.I. (2004). Using focused reflection and articulation to promote clinical reasoning: an evidence-based teaching strategy. *Nurs. Educ. Perspect.* 25 (5): 226–231.

5 Leblanc, V.R., Brooks, L.R., and Norman, G.R. (2002). Believing is seeing: the influence of a diagnostic hypothesis on the interpretation of clinical features. *Acad. Med.* 77 (10 Suppl): S67–S69.

6 Norman, G.R. and Schmidt, H.G. (1992). The psychological basis of problem-based learning: a review of the evidence. *Acad. Med.* 67 (9): 557–565.

7 Norman, G. (2006). Building on experience – the development of clinical reasoning. *N. Engl. J. Med.* 355 (21): 2251–2252.

8 Maddison, J. (2017). Clinical reasoning skills. In: *Veterinary Medical Education: A Practical Guide* (ed. J.L. Hodgson and J.M. Pelzer). Hoboken, N.J.: Wiley.

9 Bowen, J.L. (2006). Educational strategies to promote clinical diagnostic reasoning. *N. Engl. J. Med.* 355 (21): 2217–2225.

10 Elstein, A.S. and Schwartz, A. (2002). Clinical problem solving and diagnostic decision making: selective review of the cognitive literature. *BMJ* 324 (7339): 729–732.

11 Elizondo-Omana, R.E., Morales-Gomez, J.A., Morquecho-Espinoza, O. et al. (2010). Teaching skills to promote clinical reasoning in early basic science courses. *Anat. Sci. Educ.* 3 (5): 267–271.

12 Norman, G. (2005). Research in clinical reasoning: past history and current trends. *Med. Educ.* 39 (4): 418–427.

13 Parsell, G.J. and Bligh, J. (1995). The changing context of undergraduate medical education. *Postgrad. Med. J.* 71 (837): 397–403.

14 Vinten, C.E., Cobb, K.A., Freeman, S.L., and Mossop, L.H. An Investigation into the clinical reasoning development of veterinary students. *J. Vet. Med. Educ.* 43 (4): 398–405.

15 Ferguson, D.C., McNeil, L.K., Schaeffe, D.J., and Mills, E.M. (2017). Encouraging critical clinical thinking (CCT) skills in first-year veterinary students. *J. Vet. Med. Educ.* 44 (3): 531–541.

16 Rochmawati, E. and Wiechula, R. (2010). Education strategies to foster health professional students' clinical reasoning skills. *Nurs. Health Sci.* 12 (2): 244–250.

17 Davis, M.H. (1999). AMEE Medical Education Guide No. 15: Problem-based learning: a practical guide. *Med. Teach.* 21 (2): 130–140.

18 Gul, R.B. and Boman, J.A. (2006). Concept mapping: a strategy for teaching and evaluation in nursing education. *Nurse Educ. Pract.* 6 (4): 199–206.

19 Levett-Jones, T.L. (2007). Facilitating reflective practice and self-assessment of competence through the use of narratives. *Nurse Educ. Pract.* 7 (2): 112–119.

20 Wheeler, L.A. and Collins, S.K. (2003). The influence of concept mapping on critical thinking in baccalaureate nursing students. *J. Prof. Nurs.* 19 (6): 339–346.

21 Windish, D.M., Price, E.G., Clever, S.L. et al. (2005). Teaching medical students the important connection

between communication and clinical reasoning. *J. Gen. Intern. Med.* 20 (12): 1108–1113.

22 Lane, E.A. (2008). Problem-based learning in veterinary education. *J. Vet. Med. Educ.* 35 (4): 631–636.

23 Maddison, J.E., Volk, V.A., and Church, D.B. (2015). *Clinical Reasoning in Small Animal Practice*. Oxford: Wiley Blackwell.

24 Lorenz, M.D. (2009). The problem-oriented approach. In: *Small Animal Medical Diagnosis* (ed. M.D. Lorenz, T.M. Neer and P. DeMars), 3–12. Ames, IA: Blackwell Publishing.

25 Maddison, J. (2014). Encouraging a problem-based approach to diagnosis. Veterinary Record [Internet]. [i–ii pp.]. http://veterinaryrecord.bmj.com/content/175/3/i.

26 Rand, J. (2006). How to make a problem-based diagnosis. In: *Problem-Based Feline Medicine* (ed. J. Rand), 1–4. Philadelphia: Elsevier Limited.

27 Englar, R.E. (2017). *Performing the Small Animal Physical Examination*. Hoboken, NJ: Wiley.

28 Kipperman, B.S. (2014). The demise of the minimum database. *J. Am. Vet. Med. Assoc.* 244 (12): 1368–1370.

29 Bartges, J., Boynton, B., Vogt, A.H. et al. (2012). AAHA canine life stage guidelines. *J. Am. Anim. Hosp. Assoc.* 48 (1): 1–11.

30 Hoyumpa Vogt, A., Rodan, I., Brown, M. et al. (2010). AAFP-AAHA: feline life stage guidelines. *J. Feline Med. Surg.* 12 (1): 43–54.

31 Pittari, J., Rodan, I., Beekman, G. et al. (2009). American association of feline practitioners. Senior care guidelines. *J. Feline Med. Surg.* 11 (9): 763–778.

32 Senior Care Guidelines Task Force A, Epstein, M., Kuehn, N.F. et al. (2005). AAHA senior care guidelines for dogs and cats. *J. Am. Anim. Hosp. Assoc.* 41 (2): 81–91.

33 Weed, L.L. (1968). Medical records that guide and teach. *N. Engl. J. Med.* 278 (11): 593–600.

34 Lane, I. The problem oriented medical approach. http://libguides.utk.edu/ld.php?content_id=7167021.

35 Riegger, M.H. (2011). Using S.O.A.P. is good medicine. DVM 360.

36 Osborne, C.A. (2005). 'DAMN-IT' acronym offers practical diagnostic aid. DVM360 [Internet]. http://veterinarynews.dvm360.com/damn-it-acronym-offers-practical-diagnostic-aid.

37 Lorenz, M.D., Neer, T.M., and Demars, P.L. (2009). *Small Animal Medical Diagnosis*, 3e, vol. xv, 502. Ames, Iowa: Wiley-Blackwell.

38 Buchanan, J.W. and Patterson, D.F. (2003). Etiology of patent ductus arteriosus in dogs. *J. Vet. Intern. Med.* 17 (2): 167–171.

39 Pimentel Dde, S., Ramos, R.A., Santana Mde, A. et al. (2015). Prevalence of zoonotic visceral leishmaniasis in dogs in an endemic area of Brazil. *Rev. Soc. Bras. Med. Trop.* 48 (4): 491–493.

40 Vandeweerd, J.M., Vandeweerd, S., Gustin, C. et al. (2012). Understanding veterinary practitioners' decision-making process: implications for veterinary medical education. *J. Vet. Med. Educ.* 39 (2): 142–151.

41 Del Mar, C., Doust, J., and Glasziou, P. (2006). *Clinical Thinking: Evidence, Communication and Decision Making*. Oxford, U.K.: Blackwell.

42 Cockcroft, P.D. and Holmes, M.A. (2003). Decision analysis, models and economics as evidence. In: *Handbook of Evidence-Based Veterinary Medicine* (ed. P.D. Cockcroft and M.A. Holmes), 154–181. Oxford, U.K.: Blackwell.

43 Trepanier, L.A. (2015). Maropitant: Novel Antiemetic. Clinician's Brief. 75–77.

2

The Role of the Comprehensive Patient History in the Problem-Oriented Approach

2.1 Factors that Contribute to Diagnosis Making in Human Healthcare

> There is no more important field in medicine than diagnosis. Without it, we are charlatans or witch doctors treating in the dark with potion and prayers. [1]

To make an accurate diagnosis, the clinician must consider three pieces of medical data: the patient history, physical examination findings, and diagnostic test results [2–4]. The relative contributions of each have been debated since the mid-1900s.

In 1947, the Professor of Medicine at Manchester University, Dr. Robert Platt, claimed that history alone was responsible for the bulk of diagnosis making [5]. Although Platt recognized the importance of ancillary services such as laboratory diagnostics and diagnostic imaging, he believed that their results could be misleading and wasteful if patient history did not guide the clinician's decision to order testing [5].

History taking allowed for a provisional diagnosis to be made with a reasonably high degree of accuracy: 68% of Platt's patients were diagnosed correctly based upon history alone [5]. To confirm the diagnosis, Platt believed in following up the history with diagnostic investigation. To emphasize his perspective, he acknowledged that "one would not give insulin on a history of thirst and polyuria, nor liver extract upon breathlessness, pallor, and paresthesia [5]."

Multiple studies in human healthcare have supported Platt's claim that history taking leads to the diagnosis with frequency. Hampton et al., Sandler, Peterson et al., and Roshan et al. concluded that patient history made the diagnosis in 82, 56, 76, 78.6, and 77.8% of patients in 1975, 1979, 1992, 2000, and 2003, respectively [2, 4, 6–8]. By contrast, diagnoses due to physical examination findings were on the order of 8% [2], 9% [4], and 12% [6]. Laboratory testing contributed an additional 9% [4], 11% [6], and 13% [2] of diagnoses.

All three aspects of patient care have value. Peterson et al. found that, on a scale of 1–10, the confidence of clinicians regarding their ability to diagnose a patient accurately grew from 7.1 after the history, to 8.2 after the exam, to 9.3 after diagnostic testing [6].

Roshan and Rao reported similar findings: clinicians' confidence grew from 6.36 after the history, to 7.57 after the exam, and 9.84 after diagnostic testing [2]. Therefore, the physical examination and diagnostic testing provide additional security in diagnosis making.

However, the ability of a clinician to construct a history carries substantial weight [8]. History taking in most cases provides enough information for the clinician to both diagnose the patient and feel comfortable about initiating treatment. Laboratory test results may augment that comfort; however, their cost-effectiveness is low [4]. According to Hampton et al., 24% of follow-up diagnostic tests yielded abnormal results, yet in only 7 of 80 patients did those abnormal results yield a diagnosis other than what had been reported based upon the history [4].

2.2 The Evolution of the Patient History in Human Healthcare

As technology in healthcare grows, it is tempting to shift focus onto diagnostic testing [9]. This is not a new phenomenon. When the stethoscope was invented by Laennec in 1816 and became a staple of human healthcare in the United States in 1850, this tool "largely replaced the [previous] model constructed from the patient's subjective impressions and the physician's own visual observations of the patient" [10].

Prior to the introduction of the stethoscope, eighteenth-century clinicians emphasized the patient perspective: what clinical signs was the patient experiencing and how the patient felt about them [3]. Thereafter, physical examination findings and diagnostic results took priority [3, 11].

The invention of thermometry, ophthalmoscopy, laryngoscopy, and radiography furthered this trend toward the collection of *objective* data [3]. The patient's narrative was reduced to *subjective* dialogue, subject to interpretation [3].

In fact, attending physicians began to caution medical students against believing what patients shared because

> most persons ramble in describing their symptoms, and many insist on giving their own or other persons' opinions as to the nature of their disease, instead of confining themselves to the narration of facts. [12]

A patient-derived history was largely considered extraneous and flawed. The clinician was responsible for making sense of it by reconstructing a timeline of events that highlighted key facts [3].

Taking a history was not enough. Clinicians required skill to finesse the history out of the patient and obtain accurate details [3].

Patients described *symptoms* based upon feelings and ideas; physicians reconstructed these into factual *clinical signs* [3].

Patients often made reference to medical terms that were inappropriate or misunderstood; physicians-in-training were taught to ignore these references and come to their own conclusions about the source(s) of the presenting complaint [3, 13].

By the early to mid-1900s, history was seen as "all important" [13], yet requiring translation. The clinician who could not take a history well was likely to misdiagnose the patient:

> More errors in diagnosis are traceable to lack of acumen in eliciting of interpreting symptoms than have ever been caused by a failure to hear a murmur, feel a mass, or take an electrocardiogram. [14]

History taking was viewed as an art [3, 15–17]. If the history was to become a masterpiece, clinicians needed to understand the patient's perspective [3]. This required clinicians to develop rapport with the patient, and so the doctor–patient relationship was born [3].

This relationship was wrought with hurdles, primarily lack of trust. Physicians-in-training were taught to approach the patient narrative with skepticism because

> we are dealing with subjective manifestations filtered through the consciousness of individuals who vary in their capacity to observe and describe … whose accounts are coloured, consciously or unconsciously, by fears and misconceptions. [18]

Yet patient needs and expectations were real and required addressing, particularly since the patient had sought out the physician for assistance, not the other way around [3, 19].

As medicine evolved in the twentieth century, human healthcare began to consider the role of the patient. Physicians were expected to develop tact, patience, and diplomacy [3]. Although it was true that the patient may differ from the clinician by way of perspective, the physician had to understand where the patient was coming from to facilitate care [3]. Physician interest in the patient and allowing the patient to have a voice were considered appropriate demonstrations of empathy that paved the way for a successful consultation [18].

Today, the physician's ability to elicit and encourage patient contributions to medical care is valued. Patient care is not necessarily advanced by over-reliance on technology [2, 9]. By contrast, interpersonal skills correlate with and contribute to patient satisfaction and positive patient outcomes [20–28]. The ability to take a medical history not only facilitates the detection of health risks and underlying medical problems, it also contributes to patient compliance and physician satisfaction [20, 24–28].

Although history taking may still be seen as an art, it is also a teachable science [20]. Accordingly, history taking is paired with communication as cornerstones of present-day medical curricula [20, 23, 25, 29–34].

2.3 Pediatric Practice as a Model for Veterinary Medicine

Human healthcare professionals have been able to quantify the contributions of patient history, physical examination, and diagnostic testing to diagnosis-making. How these categories of patient data contribute to the diagnosis and medical management of veterinary patients remains to be determined. For example, the percentage of veterinary diagnoses that history alone is responsible for is unknown.

However, veterinary medicine is in many ways similar to the practice of pediatric medicine in human healthcare. Both the veterinarian and pediatrician are participants in a tripartite relationship [35]. These relationships, veterinarian–client–patient and pediatrician–parent–child, are unique. The veterinary client in many ways functions as the patient's parent: the veterinary client and the child's parent are both responsible for being the voice of the patient, the patient's advocate, and the patient's decision maker.

Both the veterinarian and the pediatrician must rely upon history from a third party in lieu of a direct patient history to initiate the work-up [3, 36]. It is therefore reasonable to compare the veterinarian–client–patient relationship to that of the pediatrician–parent–child [35–37].

Initially, human physicians were reluctant to take a child's history from an adult [36]. However, by the late nineteenth century, some credence was given to the parental history:

> It is well never entirely to discredit a statement without good reason, for many women … are excellent observers when their powers are guided by affection. Besides, being thoroughly acquainted with their children's habits and dispositions, they will often detect deviations from heath that the physician might overlook entirely. [38]

Over time, parental observations gained in clinical value. Today, history taking in pediatric medicine is of paramount importance to diagnosis-making. In pediatric neurology, for instance, effective critical case management relies upon patient history to cement the diagnosis [39].

The veterinary professional would do well to consider that history taking is likely to be of equal value when considering patient presentation.

2.4 Components of History Taking

History taking involves the gathering of historical data from the patient (in human healthcare) or the client (in veterinary medicine). It is a process of data mining, most typically through a combination of pre-consultation questionnaires as well as live, face-to-face, question-and-answer interactions. Over time, and with patience, personal, psychosocial, and symptomatic patient details are unearthed [20].

In addition, history taking involves observation on the part of the clinician. As was described in human healthcare by Dr. Platt:

> We do not take histories with our eyes shut. We know how old the patient is; how he walks into the room, whether he is pale or flushed, thin or fat, healthy looking or cachectic, and in some cases we may know a great deal more, that he has facial paralysis for instance or a tremor of the hands. All this is observed … [5]

So, too, is how veterinary professionals function in the consultation room. Veterinarians rely upon the case history as a melting pot of statements shared and observations made, long before laying a hand on the patient to initiate the physical examination. Although it is true that

this collective data may be subject to interpretation, the history provides critical insight into the circumstances surrounding the patient's presenting complaint [40, 41]. It also highlights the clinician's approach to treatment by emphasizing particular areas of interest that require further investigation.

What constitutes appropriate history taking in veterinary medicine depends upon the context of the case.

When a patient presents to a primary care clinic for the first time, it is essential that history taking be comprehensive [42]. The veterinarian must take the time to gather as much pertinent patient data as is possible to complete a comprehensive portrait of that patient's home life. This data includes, but is not limited to [40, 41, 43–50] the following:

- Patient demographic data
  - What is the patient's age/date of birth?
  - What is the patient's breed?
  - What is the patient's sex?
  - What is the patient's sexual status?
  - What are the patient's defining features, such as coat color and markings?
  - Does the patient have permanent identification such as a tattoo or microchip?
- Past pertinent history with regards to ownership
  - How did the patient come to be owned by the client?
  - For how long has the patient been owned?
- Past pertinent behavioral history?
  - Does the patient have any pre-existing behavioral issues?
  - Has the patient developed any new behavioral issues?
- Past pertinent patient history with regard to medical and surgical history
  - Has the patient been previously diagnosed with one or more medical conditions? If so, which conditions and how were they diagnosed?
  - Has the patient ever been anesthetized?
  - Has the patient ever had surgery?
  - Has the patient ever had any adverse reactions to medications, including anesthetic agents?
- Past pertinent reproductive history (if intact)
  - Has the patient been bred before?
  - Does the client have plans to breed the patient in the future?
  - What (if any) experience does the client have with regards to breeding?
- Patient function and client expectations
  - Is the patient a companion?
  - Is the patient a show or performance animal?
  - Is the patient a service animal or a working dog? If so, in what capacity?

– What are the client's expectations with regards to the patient's purpose?
– Are client expectations reasonable?
- Client perceptions of the patient's breed
  – Is the client familiar with the breed?
  – Is the client familiar with the breed's predispositions to disease?
- Patient serological status
- Patient home life
  – Is the patient indoor only, outdoor only, or indoor–outdoor?
  – What is the patient's home environment like?
  – Is the patient crated or does the patient have free rein?
  – Whom does the patient live with (in terms of human companions)?
  – Whom does the patient live with (in terms of conspecifics)?
  – Whom does the patient live with (in terms of other species)?
  – Who is primarily responsible for patient care?
- Patient activity level
  Which activities does the patient participate in and how often?
  – How active is the patient expected to be?
  – What (if any) problems has the client encountered with regards to exercise?
- Patient travel history
- Diet history
  – How often is the patient fed?
  – What is the patient fed for meals?
  – What is the patient fed for snacks?
  – What is the patient's body condition score?
  – Is the patient of the appropriate or expected weight for its size and breed?
- Vaccination history
  – For which core vaccines is the patient up-to-date?
  – For which elective vaccines is the patient up-to-date?
  – Has the patient ever had any acute or delayed-onset vaccine reactions?
- Pharmacologic history
  – Is the patient currently taking any prescription medication(s)?
  – Is the patient currently taking over-the-counter medications, including vitamins and supplements?
  – Is the patient currently taking any flea, tick, endoparasite, and/or heartworm preventative?
- Presenting complaint
  – What is the patient's current problem?
  – Onset of current problem?
    o Peracute
    o Acute
    o Chronic
    o Acute-on-chronic

– Duration and/or frequency of current problem?
– Are there any known inciting factors that played a role in the development of the problem?
– How, if at all, has the problem evolved?
- Client perspective
  – What has the client observed?
  – What does the client think the problem is?
  – What concerns the client most and why?
  – What past history (if any) contributes to the client's perspective and/or concerns?

Consider, on the other hand, an emergent situation: a canine patient presents to a clinic after being hit by a car. It would be inappropriate to take a comprehensive history as outlined above until the patient is stable.

In an emergency setting, the veterinarian may only require the following information right away:

- Who (if anyone) witnessed the event?
- What specifically was witnessed?
- When did the event take place?
- What was witnessed with regards to the patient's condition immediately after the event?
- How, if at all, has the problem evolved?
- What, if any, treatment has been provided?
- What are the client's wishes concerning cardiopulmonary resuscitation (CPR) in the event that the patient codes?

Emergency medicine requires prompt patient assessment and veterinary action in the face of the unknown. Details that are not relevant to the patient's survival are placed on hold until the patient has been stabilized. Only after stabilization is it appropriate to resume history taking to build a more complete picture of the patient and its overall health.

2.5 Role of Demographic Data in History Taking

Demographic data assists with pattern recognition by veterinarians. Although it is an imperfect science, learning breed predispositions to disease facilitates diagnosis-making [51].

Consider the following examples:

- Two-year-old, male castrated Maine Coon cat, presenting for acute onset of dyspnea
- Three-year-old, female intact Standard Poodle dog, presenting for intermittent diarrhea
- Seven-year-old, female spayed Miniature Schnauzer dog, presenting for acute abdomen and vomiting
- Nine-year-old, male intact Boxer dog, presenting for dyschezia

A veterinarian who has considered demographic data will recognize that hypertrophic cardiomyopathy (HCM) is possible in the Maine Coon cat [51–53]. That same veterinarian will likely prioritize the differential diagnosis of hypoadrenocorticism in the Standard Poodle [54–56], pancreatitis in the Miniature Schnauzer [57, 58], and benign prostatic hypertrophy in the Boxer [59, 60, 51]

2.6 Role of Clarifying Questions in History Taking

The history begins with the client's perceptions about the presenting complaint [41]. However, what the client considers important may differ from that which the veterinarian prioritizes. Therefore, clients may share only a limited narrative unless prompted by the veterinarian to expand upon their observations.

The veterinarian can facilitate this transfer of information by asking clarifying questions. Clarifying questions invite the client to share more about their observations, perceptions, and thought processes so that veterinarians are more likely to understand the presenting complaint.

It may help to consider that history taking is a treasure hunt. The clinician's primary task is to find buried treasure. On their own, clients may provide one or more coordinates on the map to that treasure. However, the clinician who digs deeper and engages the client in a dialogue is more apt to unearth the diagnosis.

To facilitate this dialogue, consider taking a journalist's approach to the medical interview. Invite the client to provide an answer for each of the five W's [61, 62]:

- Who?
- What?
- When?
- Where?
- Why?

In addition, the clinician may benefit from asking a sixth guiding question, *how?* [61, 62].

Consider, for example, the case of a three-month-old kitten that presents for sneezing and audible upper airway congestion. Using the journalist's approach, the veterinarian should take care to ask the following questions:

- Who?
  - Who (else) in the house (if anyone) is sneezing?
  - Who (else) in the house (if anyone) is experiencing congestion?
  - To whom has the kitten been exposed?
- What?
  - What has the owner observed?
  - Is the sneezing productive, and if so, what does the nasal discharge look like?

- Is there concurrent ocular discharge, and if so, what does it look like?
  - What is the kitten's activity level?
  - What is the kitten's appetite?
- When?
  - When was the kitten taken into the home?
  - When did the sneezing and congestion start relative to the adoption?
- Where?
  - Where has the kitten been within the past two weeks? (e.g. shelter, boarding, or grooming facility)
  - Where has the kitten traveled? (e.g. both in state and out of state)
  - From where was the kitten acquired? (e.g. a breeder, a pet store, the shelter)
- Why?
  - Why does the client think the kitten is sneezing?
  - Why does the client think the kitten is congested?
- How?
  - How does the kitten act before, during, and after each episode of sneezing?
  - How (if at all) has the kitten's appetite changed?
  - How (if at all) has the kitten's energy level changed?

2.7 History Taking and the Medical Record

There is no universal system of record keeping in veterinary medicine. However, one of the most common types of medical records in veterinary medicine is the SOAP note. A SOAP note is a structured summary of a patient encounter that consists of four components [44–48]:

- "S" for Subjective
- "O" for Objective
- "A" for Assessment
- "P" for Plan

The "S" in SOAP is where the patient history belongs because it is both subjective and historical [44–48]. The "S" relays the client's perspective in terms of what has been observed, to what degree, in what frequency, and for how long [44–48].

2.8 History Taking as Just One Piece of the Puzzle

The history provides the foundation for the veterinary consultation. It also provides clues regarding patient health that may not be apparent to the clinician. However, as much as the history can be clarified, the clinician still needs to perform a thorough and comprehensive physical examination of the patient. This data adds to the clinical picture and is documented in the "O" of the SOAP to demonstrate that it is *objective* in nature [44–48].

Together, the "S" and the "O" build the problem list. The problem list is the launchpad of diagnostic investigation. It is how the clinician knows where to begin, and anticipates where the investigation may lead.

The remainder of this text is constructed around clinical signs or presenting complaints as they may appear either in the "S" or the "O." The hope is that this guide will facilitate case management, particularly for novices who may be unclear about diagnostic investigations and may benefit from assistance concerning "next steps."

References

1 Cutler, P. (1979). *Problem Solving in Clinical Medicine: From Data to Diagnosis*. Baltimore, M.D.: The Williams and Wilkins Company.

2 Roshan, M. and Rao, A.P. (2000). A study on relative contributions of the history, physical examination and investigations in making medical diagnosis. *J. Assoc. Physicians India* 48 (8): 771–775.

3 Gillis, J. (2006). The history of the patient history since 1850. *Bull. Hist. Med.* 80 (3): 490–512.

4 Hampton, J.R., Harrison, M.J., Mitchell, J.R. et al. (1975). Relative contributions of history-taking, physical examination, and laboratory investigation to diagnosis and management of medical outpatients. *Br. Med. J.* 2 (5969): 486–489.

5 Platt, R. (1947). Two essays on the practice of medicine. *Lancet* 2 (6470): 305–307.

6 Peterson, M.C., Holbrook, J.H., Vonhales, D. et al. (1992). Contributions of the history, physical-examination, and laboratory investigation in making medical diagnoses. *West. J. Med.* 156 (2): 163–165.

7 Sandler, G. (1980). The importance of the history in the medical clinic and the cost of unnecessary tests. *Am. Heart J.* 100 (6): 928–931.

8 Bensenor, I.M. (2003). Do you believe in the power of clinical examination? The answer must be yes! *Sao Paulo Med. J.* 121 (6): 223.

9 Oyedokun, A., Adeloye, D., and Balogun, O. (2016). Clinical history-taking and physical examination in medical practice in Africa: still relevant? *Croat. Med. J.* 57 (6): 605–607.

10 Reiser, S. (1978). *Medicine and the Reign of Technology*. Cambridge: Cambridge University Press.

11 Newman, C. (1957). *The Evolution of Medical Education in the Nineteenth Century*. London: Oxford University Press.

12 Fenwick, S. (1873). *The Student's Guide to Medical Diagnosis*, 3e. London: J. & A. Churchill.

13 Horder, T. and Gow, A.E. (1928). *The Essentials of Medical Diagnosis*. London: Cassell.

14 Cabot, R.C. and Adams, F.D. (1938). *Physical Diagnosis*, 12e, 3 p. l., v–xxii, 846 p. Baltimore: W. Wood & Company.

15 MacBryde, C. (ed.) (1944). *The Analysis and Interpretation of Symptoms*. Philadelphia: Lippincott.

16 Pullen, R. (ed.) (1944). *Medical Diagnosis*. Philadelphia: Saunders.

17 Stokes, E.H. (1953). *Clinical Investigation*. Sydney: Angus and Robertson.

18 Harrison, T.R., Adams, R.D., and Bennett, I.L. (eds.) (1958). *Principles of Internal Medicine*, 3e. New York: McGraw-Hill.

19 Ryle, J. (1931). The Study of Symptoms. *Lancet* 1: 737–741.

20 Keifenheim, K.E., Teufel, M., Ip, J. et al. (2015). Teaching history taking to medical students: a systematic review. *BMC Med. Educ.* 15: 159.

21 Engel, G.L. (1973). Enduring attributes of medicine relevant for the education of the physician. *Ann. Intern. Med.* 78 (4): 587–593.

22 Lipkin, M. Jr. (1987). The medical interview and related skills. In: *Office Practice of Medicine* (ed. W. Branch), 1287–1306. Philadelphia: WB Saunders Co.

23 Novack, D.H., Volk, G., Drossman, D.A., and Lipkin, M. Jr. (1993). Medical interviewing and interpersonal skills teaching in US medical schools. Progress, problems, and promise. *JAMA* 269 (16): 2101–2105.

24 Fortin, A.H., Haeseler, F.D., Angoff, N. et al. (2002). Teaching pre-clinical medical students an integrated approach to medical interviewing: half-day workshops using actors. *J. Gen. Intern. Med.* 17 (9): 704–708.

25 Hatem, D.S., Barrett, S.V., Hewson, M. et al. (2007). Teaching the medical interview: methods and key learning issues in a faculty development course. *J. Gen. Intern. Med.* 22 (12): 1718–1724.

26 Novack, D.H., Dube, C., and Goldstein, M.G. (1992). Teaching medical interviewing. A basic course on interviewing and the physician-patient relationship. *Arch. Intern. Med.* 152 (9): 1814–1820.

27 Windish, D.M., Price, E.G., Clever, S.L. et al. (2005). Teaching medical students the important connection between communication and clinical reasoning. *J. Gen. Intern. Med.* 20 (12): 1108–1113.

28 Sanson-Fisher, R. and Maguire, P. (1980). Should skills in communicating with patients be taught in medical schools? *Lancet* 2 (8193): 523–526.

29 Rosenthal, J. and Ogden, J. (1998). Changes in Medical education: the beliefs of medical students. *Med. Educ.* 32 (2): 127–132.

30 Schildmann, J., Kampmann, M., and Schwantes, U. (2004). Teaching courses on aspects of medical history taking and communication skills in Germany: a survey among students of 12 medical faculties. *Z. Arztl. Fortbild. Qualitatssich.* 98 (4): 287–292.

31 Simpson, M., Buckman, R., Stewart, M. et al. (1991). Doctor-patient communication: the Toronto consensus statement. *BMJ* 303 (6814): 1385–1387.

32 Hargie, O., Dickson, D., Boohan, M., and Hughes, K. (1998). A survey of communication skills training in UK schools of medicine: present practices and prospective proposals. *Med. Educ.* 32 (1): 25–34.

33 Association of American Colleges (1998). *Learning Objectives for Medical Student Education: Guidelines for Medical Schools (MSOP Report).* Washington, D.C.: Association of American Colleges.

34 General Medical Council (1991). *Tomorrow's Doctors: Recommendations on Undergraduate Medical Education.* London: General Medical Council.

35 Shaw, J.R., Adams, C.L., Bonnett, B.N. et al. (2004). Use of the roter interaction analysis system to analyze veterinarian-client-patient communication in companion animal practice. *J. Am. Vet. Med. Assoc.* 225 (2): 222–229.

36 Gillis, J. (2005). Taking a medical history in childhood illness: representations of parents in pediatric texts since 1850. *Bull. Hist. Med.* 79 (3): 393–429.

37 Goodhart, J.F. (1885). *Diseases of Children.* London: Churchill.

38 Starr, L. and Westcott, T.S. (1898). *An American Text-Book of the Diseases of Children*, 2e, vol. xvi, 1244. Philadelphia: W. B. Saunders.

39 Dooley, J.M., Gordon, K.E., Wood, E.P. et al. (2003). The utility of the physical examination and investigations in the pediatric neurology consultation. *Pediatr. Neurol.* 28 (2): 96–99.

40 Johnson, S.W. (2016). Medical history and client communication. In: *Clinical Medicine of the Dog and Cat*, 3e (ed. M. Schaer and F. Gaschen), 3–9. Boca Raton, FL: Taylor & Francis Group.

41 Rijnberk, A. (2009). The history. In: *Medical History and Physical Examination in Companion Animals* (ed. A. Rijnberk and F.J. van Sluijs), 40–43. Philadelphia: Elsevier Limited.

42 Bickley, L.S., Szilagyi, P.G., and Bates, B. (2013). *Bates' Guide to Physical Examination and History-Taking*, 11e, vol. xxv, 994. Philadelphia: Wolters Kluwer Health/ Lippincott Williams & Wilkins.

43 Duguma, A. (2016). Practice manual on veterinary clinical diagnostic approach. *J. Vet. Sci. Technol.* 7 (4): 337. https://doi.org/10.4172/2157-7579.1000337.

44 Cameron, S. and Turtle-song, I. (2002). Learning to write case notes using the SOAP format. *J. Couns. Dev.* 80 (3): 286–292.

45 Rockett, J., Lattanzio, C., and Christensen, C. (2013). *The Veterinary Technician's Guide to Writing SOAPS: A Workbook for Critical Thinking.* Heyburn, Idaho: Rockett House Publishing LLC.

46 Borcherding, S. (2005). *Documentation Manual for Writing SOAP Notes in Occupational Therapy*, 2e. Thorofare, NJ: SLACK Incorporated.

47 Kettenbach, G. and Kettenbach, G. (2004). *Writing Patient/ Client Notes: Ensuring Accuracy in Documentation*, 4e, 248. Philadelphia: F.A. Davis Company.

48 Kettenbach, G. (2004). *Writing SOAP Notes: With Patient/Client Management Formats*, 3e. Philadelphia: F.A. Davis Company.

49 Rand, J. (2006). How to make a problem-based diagnosis. In: *Problem-Based Feline Medicine* (ed. J. Rand), 1–4. Philadelphia: Elsevier Limited.

50 Thayer, V. (2012). Deciphering the cat: the medical history and physical examination. In: *The Cat: Clinical Medicine and Management* (ed. S.E. Little), 26–39. St. Louis, Missouri: Saunders.

51 Gough, A. and Thomas, A. (2010). *Breed Predispositions to Disease in Dogs and Cats*, 2e, vol. xvii, 330. Chichester, West Sussex; Ames, Iowa: Wiley-Blackwell.

52 Camacho, P., Fan, H., Liu, Z., and He, J.Q. (2016). Small mammalian animal models of heart disease. *Am. J. Cardiovasc. Dis.* 6 (3): 70–80.

53 Godiksen, M.T., Granstrom, S., Koch, J., and Christiansen, M. (2011). Hypertrophic cardiomyopathy in young Maine Coon cats caused by the p.A31P cMyBP-C mutation – the clinical significance of having the mutation. *Acta Vet. Scand.* 53: 7.

54 Pedersen, N.C., Brucker, L., Tessier, N.G. et al. (2015). The effect of genetic bottlenecks and inbreeding on the incidence of two major autoimmune diseases in standard poodles, sebaceous adenitis and Addison's disease. *Canine Genet. Epidemiol.* 2: 14.

55 Klein, S.C. and Peterson, M.E. (2010). Canine hypoadrenocorticism: part I. *Can. Vet. J.* 51 (1): 63–69.

56 Famula, T.R., Belanger, J.M., and Oberbauer, A.M. (2003). Heritability and complex segregation analysis of hypoadrenocorticism in the standard poodle. *J. Small Anim. Pract.* 44 (1): 8–12.

57 Bishop, M.A., Steiner, J.M., Moore, L.E., and Williams, D.A. (2004). Evaluation of the cationic trypsinogen gene for potential mutations in miniature schnauzers with pancreatitis. *Can. J. Vet. Res.* 68 (4): 315–318.

58 Bishop, M.A., Xenoulis, P.G., Levinski, M.D. et al. (2010). Identification of variants of the SPINK1 gene and their association with pancreatitis in Miniature Schnauzers. *Am. J. Vet. Res.* 71 (5): 527–533.

59 Pinheiro, D., Machado, J., Viegas, C. et al. (2017). Evaluation of biomarker canine-prostate specific arginine esterase (CPSE) for the diagnosis of benign prostatic hyperplasia. *BMC Vet. Res.* 13 (1): 76.

60 Barsanti, J.A. and Finco, D.R. (1986). Canine prostatic diseases. *Vet. Clin. North Am. Small Anim. Pract.* 16 (3): 587–599.

61 Journalistic writing: Eastern Washington University (2016). http://research.ewu.edu/c.php?g=403887.

62 Arnold, C., Cook, T., Koyama, D., et al. (2013). How to write a lead: Purdue University. https://owl.english.purdue.edu/owl/resource/735/05.

Part Two

The Integumentary System

3

Claw and Claw Bed Pathology

3.1 Basic Anatomy of the Claw and Claw Bed

The nails or claws are extensions of the skin [1, 2]. The epidermal layer of each nail is highly keratinized to create a claw horn, which is curved [3]. The underlying dermal layer, the so-called quick, contains nerves and blood vessels (See Figure 3.1) [1, 3]. Deep to the dermis is the periosteum of the third phalanx [1, 3].

Nail growth is due to activity at the proximal end of the claw, at the proliferative claw matrix or the so-called coronary band [1, 3]. There is a fold of skin, the claw fold, which envelops this band [1, 3]. If the coronary band is damaged, then the resultant claw will be malformed [3].

Normal claw growth is faster along the dorsal margin of the nail to create the downward curve of a typical claw [4]. Abnormal claw growth may lead to misshapen nails without that characteristic curl.

Because claw growth is relatively slow, at a rate of 1.9 mm per week, malformations of claw anatomy take months to resolve [1, 5, 6].

3.2 Species Differences with Regard to the Structure and Function of the Claw

Dogs' claws are fixed compared to the retractable claws of cats (See Figures 3.2a and b) [7]. Nail pathology in dogs is therefore more readily apparent than in cats. The clinician must therefore take care to extend cats' claws for inspection by applying firm, yet gentle pressure to the base of each toe.

Dogs are more likely than cats to have rear dewclaws, that is, rudimentary digits on one or both hind paws (See Figure 3.3a).

These dewclaws may have bony attachments that anchor them rigidly in place or the attachments may be loose and floppy. Regardless of attachment type, dewclaws are non-weight-bearing. Because daily activity does not wear them down, they are likely to overgrow unless routinely trimmed (See Figure 3.3b) [7, 8].

Cats less commonly have dewclaws; however, cats are more likely to be polydactyl than dogs, meaning that they have more than the expected number of digits on one or more paws (See Figure 3.4) [7]. These cats are at increased risk of claws growing into the interdigital toe webs or digital pads [7, 8].

3.3 Claw and Claw Bed Terminology

Whereas onychology refers to the study of nails, onychopathy refers to the study of nails that are diseased. Claw and claw bed diseases take on a variety of presentations.

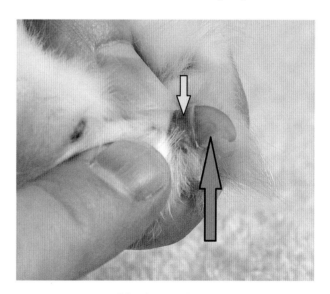

Figure 3.1 Anatomy of the claw and claw bed in a feline paw with a manually extended claw. Note the quick, highlighted by the blue arrow, and the claw bed, highlighted by the yellow arrow.

Common Clinical Presentations in Dogs and Cats, First Edition. Ryane E. Englar.
© 2019 John Wiley & Sons, Inc. Published 2019 by John Wiley & Sons, Inc.

(a)

(b)

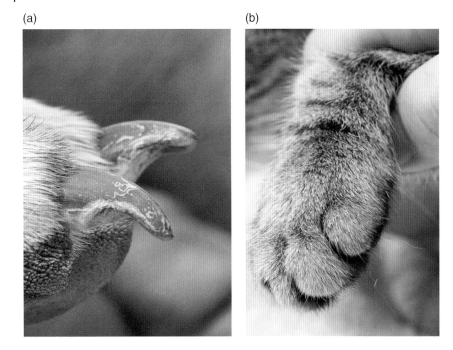

Figure 3.2 (a) Lateral view of canine forepaw with fixed claws evident. (b) Lateral view of feline forepaw with claws retracted. *Source:* (a & b) Courtesy of the Media Resources Department at Midwestern University.

(a)

(b)

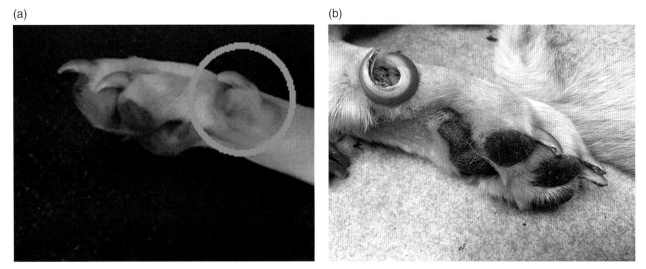

Figure 3.3 (a) This patient has a rear dewclaw associated with the right hind paw. Note how overgrown it is. *Source:* Courtesy of the Burches. (b) This patient has an overgrown nail associated with a rear dewclaw. *Source:* Courtesy of Stephanie Harris.

Each presentation has its own medical jargon that appears throughout the literature.

Table 3.1 summarizes the most common presentations.

Of these presentations, paronychia occurs with frequency, in up to 40% of canine patients that present for claw or claw-associated disease (See Figure 3.5) [5].

Figures 3.6a–e demonstrate additional clinical presentations that are routinely observed in companion animal practice.

Do not mistake brittleness for normal fraying of cat claws. Consider that cat claws are a lot like onions, that is, they are layered. When cats use their claws

to scratch, scratching removes the outermost layer to reveal a leaner, sharper inside layer. It can be normal to see flaking when examining cat claws (See Figures 3.7a, b).

3.4 Frequency of Claw and Claw Bed Disease in Dogs and Cats

As stand-alone medical complaints, claw and claw bed pathology are relatively rare in companion animal practice, affecting 1.3% of dogs and 2.2% of cats [1, 3, 5, 9–11].

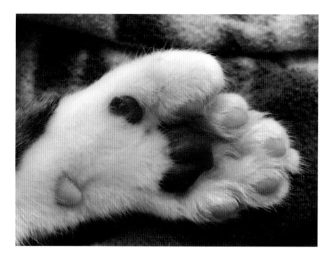

Figure 3.4 Plantar aspect of the hind paw of a polydactyl cat. *Source:* Courtesy of Karen Burks, DVM.

Table 3.1 Medical terminology associated with claw and claw bed pathology.

Terminology	Definition
Onychalgia	Painful claw
Onychia/Onychitis	Inflammation of the nail bed
Onychoclasis	Breaking of the claw(s)
Onychocryptosis	Ingrown claw(s)
Onychodystrophy	Abnormal claw growth that leads to claw deformity
Onychogryphosis	Abnormal claw hypertrophy or thickening
Onycholysis	Separation of the claw from the nail bed
Onychomadesis	Claw sloughing
Onychomalacia	Abnormal claw softening
Onychomycosis	Claw-associated fungal infection
Onychorrhexis	Brittleness of the nails leading to spontaneous breaking
Onychoschizia	Cracked and/or split nails
Paronychia	Infection of the nail bed

Claw and claw bed pathology are more likely to develop because of underlying, systemic disease [1, 2]. For example, immunosuppressive disorders commonly result in claw and claw bed pathologies [2]. For feline patients, these include feline leukemia virus (FeLV) and feline immunodeficiency virus (FIV) [2]. Canine patients may be immunosuppressed as a result of underlying endocrinopathies, such as hypothyroidism or hyperadrenocorticism [2].

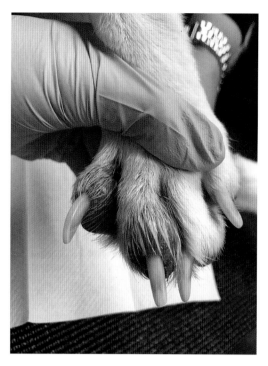

Figure 3.5 Overt paronychia in a canine patient. *Source:* Courtesy of Alexis Siler, DVM.

3.5 Clinical Approach to Claw and Claw Bed Disease

3.5.1 The History

Patients typically present for foot pain, as detected by lameness, excessive licking at one or more nail beds, pigmentary changes to the nails or nail beds, swelling, and/ or discharge at one or more nail beds [2].

Clients may have witnessed a traumatic event that led to acute injury, such as an avulsion of the claw. In this case, diagnosis is straightforward. Alternatively, clients may be in the dark in terms of what, if anything, led to the presenting complaint.

It is important that the clinician discern the following from history taking:

- Is this the first time that the patient has been diagnosed with claw or claw bed pathology?
- If this is a recurrent issue, what, if anything, has the patient been treated with in the past?
- If this is a recurrent issue, is there an apparent seasonality?
- Has the patient been diagnosed with any other form of skin disease previously?
- Has the patient ever been or is the patient currently immunosuppressed?
- What is the patient's travel history?

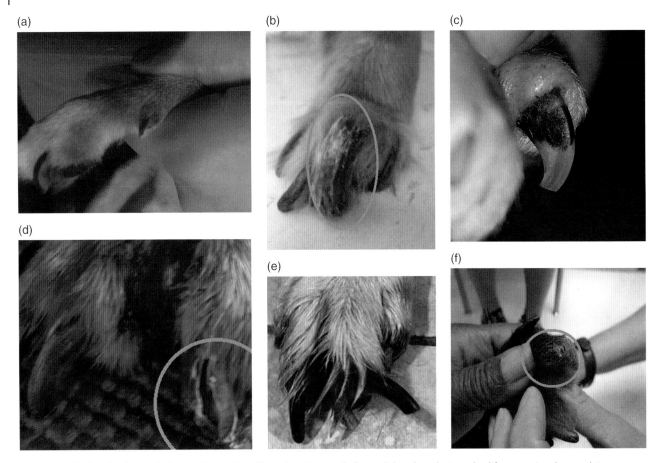

Figure 3.6 (a) Onychodystrophy in a canine patient. Note the abnormally formed dewclaw that resulted from a prior claw avulsion. The dewclaw is shorter and thinner than normal. *Source:* Courtesy of Lydia McDaniel, DVM. (b) Onychogryphosis in a canine patient. (c) Onychomycosis in a feline patient. *Source:* Courtesy of Kelli L. Crisfulli, RVT. (d) Onycholysis in a canine patient. *Source:* Courtesy of Patricia Bennett, DVM. (e) Onychomadesis of several claws in a canine patient. (f) Traumatic avulsion in this canine patient has caused a claw to break off entirely, demonstrating the aftermath of onychoclasis. *Source:* Courtesy of Patricia Bennett, DVM.

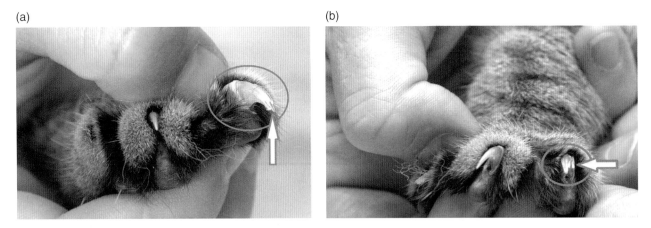

Figure 3.7 (a) Lateral view of a feline patient with normal flaking of the outer coat of the claw. (b) Head-on view of a feline patient with normal fraying of the outer coat of the claw.

Documenting the timeline of disease is critical. Chronicity of claw or claw bed disease is supportive of an underlying or predisposing disorder.

3.5.2 The Physical Examination

All patients that present for claw or claw bed pathology should receive a comprehensive physical examination given the possibility of underlying, systemic, concurrent disease. For example:

- Cats with pemphigus foliaceus often have facial dermatitis in addition to paronychia [2].
- Dogs with underlying hypothyroidism may also present with bilaterally symmetrical truncal alopecia, rat tail, and pyoderma [2].

Because there is the potential for infectious disease to trigger claw or claw bed pathology, regional and distant lymph nodes should be palpated and assessed for size and symmetry [1].

Given that immune-mediated disease may also cause claw or claw bed pathology, the integrity of the following structures should be evaluated: nasal planum, pinnae, footpads, and mucocutaneous junctions [1].

Only after thorough assessment of the whole dog should the clinician concentrate on the dermatological examination. The clinician should evaluate the patient's feet for

- the presence or absence of one or more claws
- claw integrity
- claw bed pain
- claw bed swelling
- claw bed exudate.

In particular, the clinician will want to establish whether a single claw is affected, or multiple claws. This detail carries weight concerning the patient's likely list of differential diagnoses (see Table 3.2).

Asymmetrical disease implies that only one foot is affected [12]. One or more claws may be involved, but these are confined to a single foot [1]. By contrast, symmetrical disease involves multiple claws on multiple feet [1, 12]. Having multiple claws affected is suggestive of a systemic condition such as parasitic, protozoal, or fungal infection, or autoimmune disease [1].

Table 3.2 Differential diagnoses for claw and claw bed pathology based upon whether it affects one or more claws, on one or more feet.

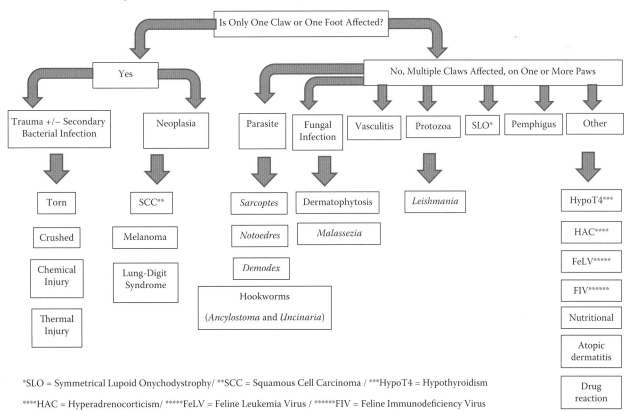

*SLO = Symmetrical Lupoid Onychodystrophy/ **SCC = Squamous Cell Carcinoma / ***HypoT4 = Hypothyroidism

****HAC = Hyperadrenocorticism/ *****FeLV = Feline Leukemia Virus / ******FIV = Feline Immunodeficiency Virus

3.6 Asymmetrical Claw or Claw Bed Disease

When the patient has asymmetrical disease, trauma is most likely in the dog, and second only to idiopathic claw deformity in the cat [13, 14].

3.6.1 Trauma and Asymmetrical Claw or Claw Bed Disease

Most typically, trauma is physical in nature, as from biting or crushing injuries that avulse the nail from the nail bed [13]. This is common in racing Greyhounds and working breeds [13]. However, thermal and chemical burns are also possible [13].

Treatment requires removal of the damaged portion of claw under sedation or anesthesia [13]. Doing so prevents further injury, irritation, inflammation, and pain that would be expected if fragments persisted and pinched the quick with each walking step. Antiseptic soaks, such as dilute chlorhexidine, and analgesia are often prescribed with or without protective bandaging depending upon the patient [13, 15].

When removing fragments of the claw, the clinician should preserve the quick at all costs. Normal regrowth of the claw is not possible without an intact quick. Furthermore, if the blood supply to the area is damaged, then the third phalanx (P3) is at risk of either osteomyelitis or avascular necrosis [13].

Secondary bacterial infection is commonly seen with traumatic claw or claw bed injury [2, 13]. These infections tend to be exudative and inflammatory [13].

Underlying systemic diseases, such as allergic dermatitis or endocrinopathies, can also predispose to secondary bacterial infection [13].

Staphylococcus intermedius is the most common isolate from the nail fold of dogs and cats with paronychia [2]. Positive cultures from dogs have also included growth of *Escherichia coli, Corynebacterium* spp., *Bacillus* spp., *Streptococcus* spp., and *Enterococcus* spp. [3].

Cytology facilitates a diagnosis of bacterial paronychia [2, 13]. Sample selection is critical. Swabbing the outer surface of the claw is unlikely to yield useful results, given the high likelihood of contamination [13, 15]. Similarly, swabbing the bleeding surface of a nail bed immediately after claw removal is of little value because blood contamination dilutes out the cells of interest in the sample [2].

In order to sample material that is more likely to be of diagnostic value, swab under a recently sloughed nail, separated nail plates, or within the claw fold itself [13, 15, 16]. Impression smears may also be performed on moist and/or eroded surfaces [2].

The finding of extracellular cocci alone does not confirm the diagnosis. Recall that cocci may be commensal organisms on the skin of companion animals. However, finding intracellular bacteria within neutrophils and/or degenerate neutrophils is supportive of a diagnosis of bacterial paronychia [2].

When the client does not wish to pursue a diagnostic work-up, clinicians may opt to treat the patient for presumptive disease. In this case, a positive patient response to antibiotic therapy is supportive of the initial diagnosis.

3.6.2 Neoplasia and Asymmetrical Claw or Claw Bed Disease in the Dog

Compared to trauma as a cause of asymmetrical claw or claw bed disease, neoplastic disease is less likely. The risk of neoplasia increases in aged, large-breed, canine patients [2]. These patients typically present for a painful swelling of a digit or claw fold with variable amounts of soft tissue erosion [13, 15]. Depending upon the presentation, the claw may be deformed or entirely absent [17]. These patients may also be lame [17].

The two most common types of claw, claw bed, and/or digital neoplasia are subungual squamous cell carcinoma (SCC) and malignant melanoma. Black-coated dogs are more likely to develop the former (see Figure 3.8). The Standard Poodle, Scottish Terrier, Bouvier de Flandres, Golden Retriever, Labrador Retriever, Giant Schnauzer, Gordon Setter, Kerry Blue Terrier, and Rottweiler are also overrepresented when it comes to nail bed neoplasia [2, 13, 15, 17, 18].

When nail bed SCC is caught early, prior to lysis of the P3, the prognosis is positive. Prior to metastasis, amputation at P3 is usually curative [17].

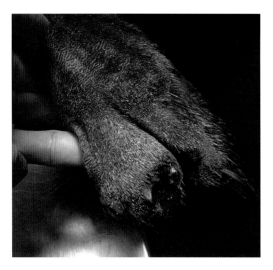

Figure 3.8 Canine patient with digital squamous cell carcinoma that eroded the claw and claw bed. *Source:* Courtesy of Amanda Maltese, DVM.

Contrary to popular thought, malignant melanoma is more likely to affect non-pigmented digits and is associated with a one-year survival rate in 43% of patients that undergo digital amputation at P3 [2, 19].

Other forms of claw neoplasia that have been reported in the dog include subungual keratinizing acanthoma and inverted squamous papilloma [3, 5, 13, 20].

Cytology may point the clinician toward a diagnosis of neoplasia if the cells are exfoliative [2]. However, more often than not, a biopsy is required to provide a definitive diagnosis [1]. Historically, this required amputation of the third phalanx in order to submit the entire intact claw. A phalanx-sparing technique was reported in 1999; however, its success is variable [1, 21].

Fine-needle aspiration of local lymph nodes and subsequent cytology is important for the staging of neoplastic disease. Suspicious cytology in the face of one or more enlarged lymph nodes indicates the need for lymph node biopsy [2].

The affected digit should be radiographed to evaluate the integrity of the distal phalanx [2, 17]. Three-view thoracic radiographs are also indicated to evaluate for metastatic disease [2].

3.6.3 Neoplasia and Asymmetrical Claw or Claw Bed Disease in the Cat

Compared to the dog, primary claw bed neoplasia is unlikely in the cat. Primary SCC, fibrosarcoma, and digital apocrine sweat gland carcinosarcoma have been reported in the cat [22, 23]. However, when claw bed neoplasia occurs in feline patients, it is more typically due to metastatic disease to the digit [2, 22, 24–26]. This phenomenon is referred to as the lung-digit syndrome. Cats with primary bronchial adenocarcinoma or bronchoalveolar carcinoma are often asymptomatic for pulmonary disease [2, 24, 27, 28].

Metastatic tumors may present in many different ways [26]. Some cases demonstrate relatively minor changes to the nail or nail bed, such as a deviated nail or a claw that will not retract [29].

More typically, digit lesions tend to be aggressive, ulcerative, or erosive (See Figures 3.9a, b) [2, 25, 26, 30–32].

Digits that bear weight are more commonly affected than those that do not [25].

Although infrequent, patients may also present with signs of systemic illness, such as inappetence, weight loss, fever, and general malaise [29].

(a)   (b)

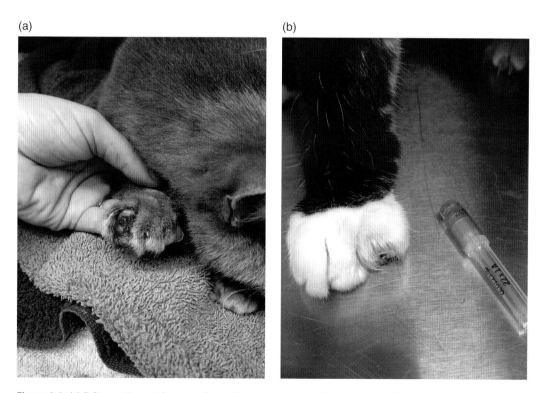

Figure 3.9 (a) Feline patient with erosive lung-digit syndrome that is associated with the forepaw. *Source:* Courtesy of Beki Cohen Regan, DVM, DACVIM (Oncology). (b) Feline patient with lung-digit syndrome that is associated with the hindpaw. *Source:* Courtesy of Beki Cohen Regan, DVM, DACVIM (Oncology).

There does not appear to be a breed or sex predilection; however, most afflicted cats average 12 years old at presentation [25, 26, 30, 32].

Baseline bloodwork, including complete blood count (CBC) and serum biochemistry panels, are routinely normal [25, 30]. Rarely is there evidence of hypercalcemia of malignancy [33, 34].

Radiographs of the affected digit demonstrate P3 osteolysis [26]. Occasionally there is involvement of the second phalanx, P2 [25].

Thoracic radiographs should be taken in any cat that presents with a digital, claw, or claw bed mass [26]. Imaging of patients with lung-digit syndrome is confirmatory for pulmonary neoplasia. Classically, there is a solitary, well-defined caudal lung lobe lesion [30, 35].

Pleural effusion is more likely to be present in patients that present with respiratory signs [24, 25, 35–37]. In these patients, it is possible to diagnose exfoliated carcinoma cells in pleural fluid that is obtained via thoracocentesis [24].

Cytology may be supportive of a diagnosis of lung-digit syndrome if the neoplastic cells are exfoliative. Incisional biopsies or avulsed nail submissions may or may not support the diagnosis [11, 25]. Histopathology of the amputated digit is required for a definitive diagnosis [22, 24, 31].

Prognosis is poor for patients with lung-digit syndrome: mean survival time is on the order of 58 days from the time of diagnosis [25]. Amputation of the affected digit may extend median survival time to 104 days; however, its primary benefit is removing the ulcerated source of the pain [24]. Patients are often euthanized for humane reasons, poor quality of life and the anticipated short survival time [24].

3.7 Diagnostic Approach to Asymmetrical Claw or Claw Bed Disease

The approach to asymmetrical claw or claw bed disease is straightforward. If the primary lesion is due to trauma, then addressing the trauma should resolve the presenting complaint.

If there is exudative discharge at the claw bed of the affected digit, or if there is swelling only at the affected digit, then diagnostic tests may be warranted.

Table 3.3 summarizes an appropriate diagnostic approach.

Table 3.3 A diagnostic approach to asymmetrical claw or claw bed disease.

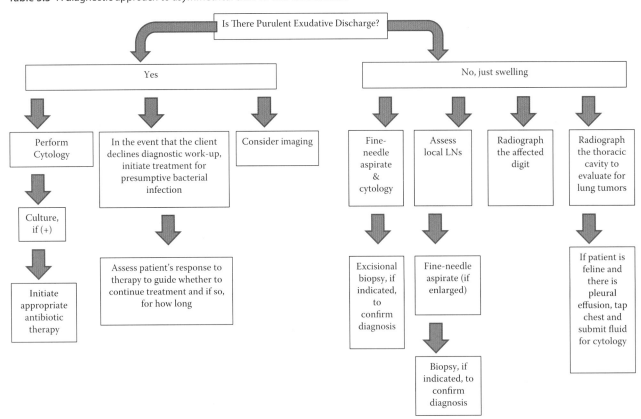

3.8 Symmetrical Claw or Claw Bed Disease

Patients that present with symmetrical claw or claw bed disease are more likely to have concurrent systemic disease [9]. These include underlying parasitic, protozoal, or fungal infection, vasculitis, nutritional imbalance, autoimmune disease, or endocrinopathy [1, 3, 5, 6, 9, 11].

3.8.1 Parasitic Infection and Symmetrical Claw or Claw Bed Disease

Both endo- and ectoparasites can cause claw or claw bed disease.

Of all endoparasites, hookworms such as *Ancylostoma* spp. and *Uncinaria* spp. have been known to induce onychopathy in dogs through unknown mechanisms [9]. Claw growth is rapidly enhanced through this parasitism: claws grow longer, faster [10]. The resulting misshapen claws have abnormal curvature [9]. Both puppies and adults can become parasitized.

In addition to onychopathy, these patients tend to present with malaise. Their owners may report unthriftiness, poor coat, weight loss or failure to gain weight, and diarrhea [10]. On physical examination, they may demonstrate pale mucous membranes (see Figure 3.10). This paleness stems from parasite-induced anemia.

Diagnosis of hookworm infestation is typically via fecal flotation to demonstrate ova (see Figure 3.11) [38, 39].

Note, however, that marked blood loss can take place before eggs are shed in the feces [38]. Therefore, a negative fecal analysis in a young, anemic, and shocky patient does not definitively rule out hookworm disease [38].

In addition to fecal flotation results, the patient's serum biochemistry profile may reveal hyponatremia and hyperkalemia. This classic electrolyte imbalance may be mistaken for hypoadrenocorticism [38–40].

Treatment for hookworm disease involves anthelmintic therapy such as pyrantel, fenbendazole, or ivermectin [38]. Resolution of hookworm infestation will not cure the current state of the claws. However, as the claws grow out, new growth will be as expected and consistent with normal claw curvature.

Paronychia may also result from infestation with ectoparasites such as *Demodex canis* [9]. *Demodex* spp. are considered to be part of the dog's normal cutaneous microfauna [41]. However, immunocompromised patients may experience mite overgrowth and proliferation of disease [41]. Poor nutritional planes and concurrent endoparasites may promote demodicosis in young patients [41, 42]. Older patients may also develop demodicosis if they are immunosuppressed from chemotherapy, neoplasia, or endocrinopathy [41, 43–45].

Demodicosis may result in localized or generalized disease. The former has a good prognosis, particularly in cases of juvenile onset. These cases tend to resolve spontaneously, whereas generalized demodicosis requires an investigation into the underlying disease [41].

Patients with generalized demodicosis present with paronychia in addition to one or more of the following signs: erythema, hypotrichosis or alopecic patches with or without a papulopustular rash, folliculitis or furunculosis, scaling and follicular casts, and pododermatitis [9, 41, 46]. The face and forelimbs are often affected first, before the disease spreads throughout the body. The patient may or may not exhibit

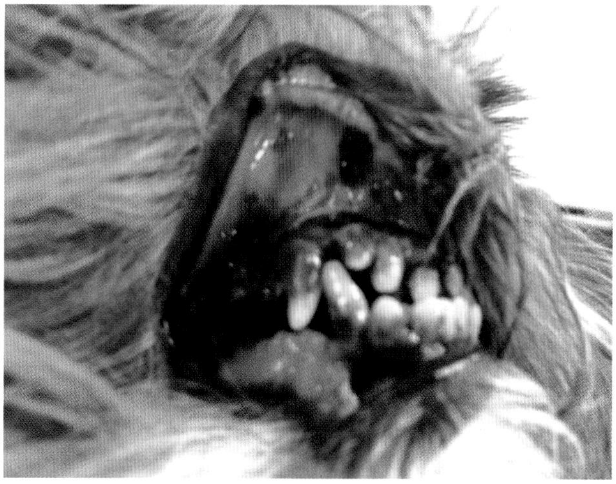

Figure 3.10 Pale mucous membranes in a canine patient. This patient had an underlying coagulopathy as opposed to hookworm infestation; however, the pale mucous membranes would appear similarly in a dog with hookworms.

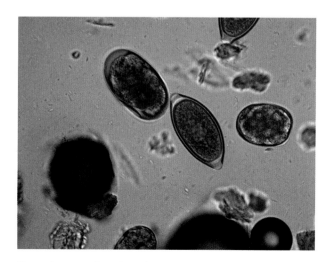

Figure 3.11 Fecal cytology demonstrating ova of several hookworm species. *Source:* Courtesy of Dr. Araceli Lucio-Forster, Cornell University College of Veterinary Medicine.

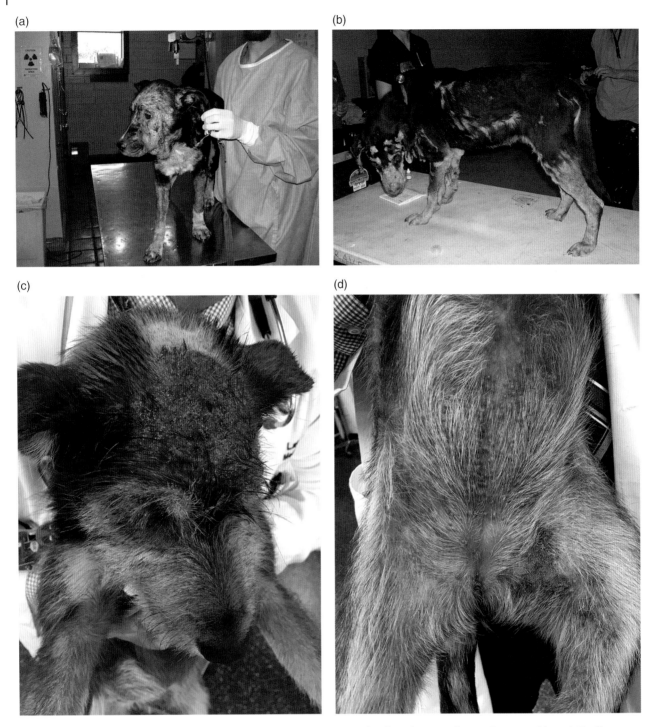

Figure 3.12 (a) Generalized demodicosis in a canine patient, demonstrating facial involvement. *Source:* Courtesy of Joseph Onello at Central Mesa Veterinary Hospital. (b) Generalized demodicosis in a canine patient, demonstrating facial and truncal involvement. *Source:* Courtesy of Laura Polerecky. (c) Generalized demodicosis in a canine patient, demonstrating severe lesions on the dorsal aspect of the head. *Source:* Courtesy of Dr. Elizabeth Robbins. (d) Generalized demodicosis in a canine patient, demonstrating secondary pyoderma along the ventrum. *Source:* Courtesy of Dr. Elizabeth Robbins.

lymphadenopathy. The patient may or may not be febrile (see Figures 3.12a–d).

Diagnosis of demodicosis is made via deep skin scrapings to the point of capillary bleeding [41, 47, 48]. Squeezing the skin at the time of scrapings increases the yield [47]. Mites can be visualized by light microscopy at low power magnification, using the 4× or 10× lens (see Figure 3.13) [41]. Note the classic cigar shape that is associated with *D. canis*.

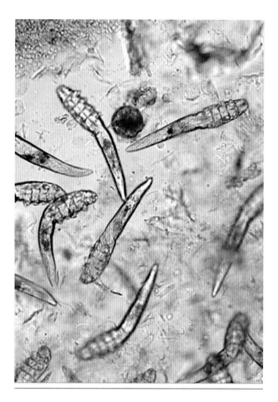

Figure 3.13 Adult *Demodex canis* as seen via light microscopy. *Source:* Courtesy of Dr. Elizabeth Robbins.

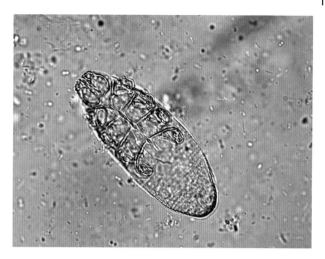

Figure 3.14 Adult *Demodex gatoi* as seen via light microscopy at 40×. *Source:* Courtesy of Dr. Araceli Lucio-Forster, Cornell University College of Veterinary Medicine.

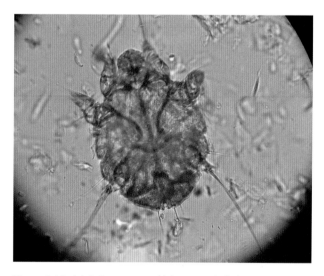

Figure 3.15 Adult *Sarcoptes scabiei* as seen via light microscopy. *Source:* Courtesy of Alexis Siler, DVM.

Treatment of generalized demodicosis is twofold: employ a miticidal agent, such as amitraz, ivermectin, or milbemycin oxime, and medically manage the secondary pyoderma [45, 46, 49].

Cats may also succumb to demodicosis; however, neither *Demodex cati* nor *Demodex gatoi* tends to affect the claws or claw bed. *D. cati* tends to cause focal crusting around the face, eyelids, and ears. Diagnosis is much the same as for *D. canis* [50].

By contrast, *D. gatoi* is more of a surface dweller. Rather than living within the hair follicle as is the case for *D. canis* and *D. cati*, *D. gatoi* resides within the stratum corneum. It causes alopecia of the limbs, flank, and ventrum, and is diagnosed via superficial skin scrapes. On cytology, *D. gatoi* is rounder than the classic cigar shape (see Figure 3.14) [50].

Cats that are afflicted with mange tend to exhibit extensive crusting. For example, an isolated case report of *Sarcoptes scabiei* in a cat documented yellow-gray exudative crusts along the caudal thighs, tail, and feet. In addition to these lesions, the cat presented with paronychia and dystrophic nails. The development of pruritic papules in the veterinary technician who had handled the patient prompted superficial skin scrapings of the cat, which supported the diagnosis. *S. scabiei* has a very round body on cytology with long limb pedicles (see Figure 3.15) [51].

Notoedres cati may also cause paronychia; however, more typical presentations involve crusting and eczema-like facial and pinnal lesions [52]. Like *Sarcoptes* spp., *N. cati* causes a zoonotic infestation that causes intense pruritus in cats and humans alike [52]. Skin scrapings confirm the diagnosis (see Figure 3.16). *N. cati* is a smaller mite than *S. scabiei*. Its limb pedicles are also shorter, and it has a dorsal rather than a terminal anus as is seen in *Sarcoptes* spp. [52].

3.8.2 Fungal Infection and Symmetrical Claw or Claw Bed Disease

Onychomycosis can result from superficial dermatophytosis, deep systemic mycoses, or overgrowth of the commensal skin organism, *Malassezia pachydermatis* [13, 53, 54].

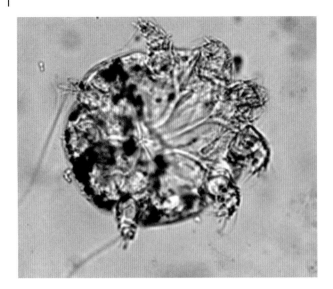

Figure 3.16 Adult *Notoedres cati* as seen via light microscopy.

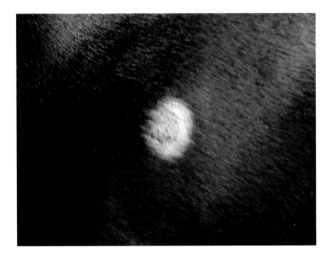

Figure 3.17 Circular alopecia in a canine patient with dermatophytosis.

Colloquially, superficial dermatophytosis is called ringworm. Ringworm in canine patients is typically due to *Trichophyton mentagrophytes*, *Microsporum gypseum*, and occasionally *Microsporum canis* [13, 53, 54]. *M. canis* predominates as the source of ringworm in cats [13, 53, 54].

Claw lesions result from the invasion of keratin by dermatophytes, leading to misshapen and often brittle nails [13]. In addition to claw lesions, dogs may present with circular alopecia, scale, and crust (see Figure 3.17).

Kerion formation is also common in dogs in response to *T. mentagrophytes* and *M. gypseum* (see Figure 3.18) [53]. Kerions are raised cutaneous nodules that typically arise on the face or feet as an inflammatory response to dermatophyte invasion of the host [53]. These may be mistaken for histiocytomas.

Feline lesions from dermatophytosis are more varied in presentation [53]. Partial alopecia and crusting on the face and limbs is typical (see Figure 3.19).

Kerions are atypical findings in cats with dermatophytosis; however, Persians and Himalayans may develop subcutaneous nodular lesions that develop draining tracts [53].

Diagnosis of dermatophytosis is supported by positive, apple green fluorescence of lesions with a Wood's lamp (see Figures 3.20a, b).

Only about 50% of *M. canis* fluoresce, and most other species do not. Therefore, a negative Wood's lamp does not rule out dermatophytosis.

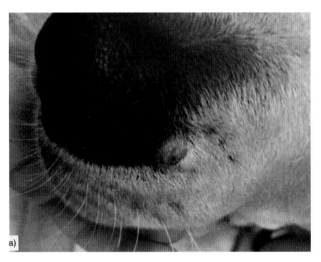

Figure 3.18 Kerion in a canine patient.

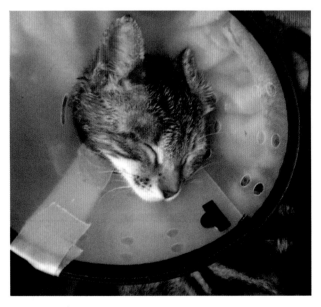

Figure 3.19 Gross lesions in a feline patient with dermatophytosis. *Source:* Courtesy of Colleen M. Cook, Midwestern University College of Veterinary Medicine, Class of 2019.

(a) (b)

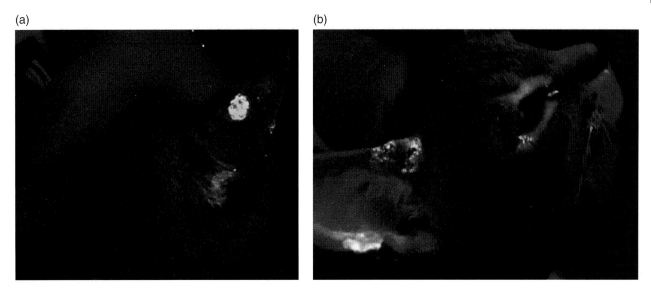

Figure 3.20 (a) Positive fluorescence of gross lesions in a feline patient with dermatophytosis. (b) Positive fluorescence of gross lesions in a feline patient with dermatophytosis. *Source:* (a & b) Courtesy of Colleen M. Cook, Midwestern University College of Veterinary Medicine, Class of 2019.

Fur can also be plucked at the periphery of suspicious lesions, treated with 10% potassium hydroxide, and examined under the microscope for fungal hyphae. However, false negatives are common [53].

Fungal culture is required to make a definitive diagnosis [53]. Suspicious fur is plucked and inoculated onto a dermatophyte test medium (DTM) plate. Media is examined daily for up to 21 days. Growth usually appears within seven to ten days. A result is said to be positive if there is white colony growth and the DTM plate color changes from yellow to red (see Figure 3.21a). If there is growth without the red color change, then dermatophytosis is unlikely.

To confirm the positive result that is demonstrated in Figure 3.21a, a tape mount preparation of the fungal colonies can be performed. Tape is placed over the colony to get the colony to adhere. The tape is then dipped into Diff-Quik solution II, the violet-colored thiazine dye, and placed on a slide. Fungal hyphae will be evident (see Figure 3.21b).

Treatment for dermatophytosis involves either topical antifungals, such as miconazole, in the case of focal disease, or systemic antifungal therapy with azoles when disease is generalized. It will take months for damaged nails to grow out. Treatment must continue until all of the damaged nails have been replaced with new, unaffected growth [13].

Malassezia dermatitis results from overgrowth of the commensal organism, *M. pachydermatis* [13, 53]. This organism is found on the skin's surface of normal dogs and cats [53]. *Malassezia* has also been isolated from ear canals and anal sacs of healthy dogs, and within nail folds of healthy cats [53, 54]. Devon Rex cats in particular have high numbers of *Malassezia* on cytological preparations of swabs taken from the nail base [54]. High numbers of yeast in nail folds are associated with the progressive accumulation of dark brown, greasy exudate at the nail base (see Figure 3.22) [54].

In addition to this waxy material at the nail bed, the nails themselves may become discolored (see Figure 3.23).

Patients with *Malassezia* dermatitis may become pruritic. This is often evident as brown discoloration of the fur associated with the paws due to excessive licking (see Figure 3.24).

When *Malassezia* dermatitis is chronic, affected skin in other regions of the body becomes hyperpigmented (see Figure 3.25).

Lichenification of the skin, such that the skin appears thick and elephant-like, is also common (see Figure 3.26).

Malassezia overgrowth may occur for a number of reasons including the environment, genetics, or changes in the host's immune system. For example, warm, humid environments increase the risk for *Malassezia* dermatitis [53, 55]. Veterinary patients with abundant skin folds are also predisposed because they have poor aeration of the skin. Consider, for instance, Pugs, English Bulldogs, Bloodhounds, and Shar-Pei dogs. Other breeds that are predisposed to *Malassezia* dermatitis include West Highland White Terriers, Basset Hounds, Cocker Spaniels, and Shih Tzus [56].

In addition to breed predispositions, there are a multitude of underlying conditions that increase the

(a)

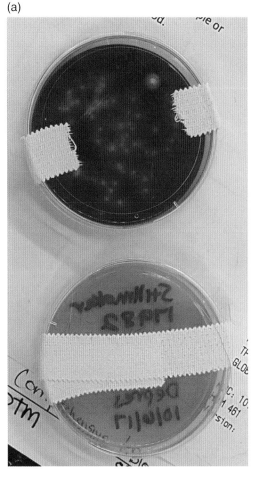

(b)

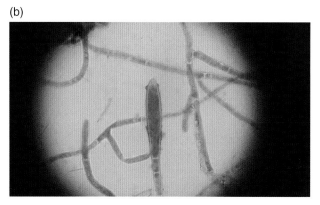

Figure 3.21 (a) The top DTM plate exhibits the classic white colony growth and red color change that would be expected to yield a positive (+) result for dermatophytosis. The bottom plate represents the negative (−) control. *Source:* Courtesy of Lori A. Stillmaker, DVM. (b) Fungal hyphae from *Microsporum canis*. *Source:* Courtesy of Lori A. Stillmaker, DVM.

likelihood that a patient will develop *Malassezia* dermatitis, including the following [56]:

- Allergic or atopic skin disease
- Endocrinopathies such as hypothyroidism and hyperadrenocorticism
- Recurrent bacterial pyoderma
- Ectoparasite infestation
- Immunosuppressive disease such as FeLV and FIV
- Immunosuppressive therapy
- Keratinization disorders

Diagnosis of *Malassezia* dermatitis is based upon swabbing affected skin and finding increased numbers of yeast on cytology (see Figure 3.27).

Impression smear or acetate tape preps may also increase the yield [56]. Treatment typically consists of a combination of topical and systemic antifungal products including the azoles.

Blastomycosis, cryptococcosis, and sporotrichosis are deep systemic mycoses that have been reported to cause claw and claw bed disease [13, 53]. However, given the infrequency with which they cause this presentation, they are beyond the scope of this chapter.

3.8.3 Pemphigus as a Cause of Symmetrical Claw or Claw Bed Disease

Pemphigus refers to a complex of autoimmune diseases that target the skin and mucous membranes [38, 57, 58]. A consequence of pemphigus is that keratinocytes lose their connections between one another and separate [9]. This leads to crusting and eventual ulceration of tissue. Of the various types of pemphigus, pemphigus foliaceus is the most likely in the cat to target the nail bed, causing paronychia [2].

In these feline patients, lesions typically start at the pinnae and muzzle before involving nail beds and foot pads. Lesions are characteristically crusty (see Figure 3.28). The patient may also be systemically unwell and present with fever [59]. It is estimated that paronychia occurs in 30% of feline patients with pemphigus foliaceus [9, 10].

Cytology that demonstrates acantholytic keratinocytes is supportive of a diagnosis of pemphigus. Treatment involves long-term immunosuppressive agents such as prednisolone and/or chlorambucil [2].

Drug reactions may also induce lesions that bear a striking resemblance to pemphigus foliaceus [13]. For example, an isolated case report describes paronychia, facial and pinnal dermatitis, and footpad lesions that developed in an 18-month-old Siamese cat following cimetidine therapy.

The lesions resolved with discontinuation of the medication, and recurred when therapy was reinitiated [60].

3.8.4 Symmetrical Lupoid Onychodystrophy (SLO) as a Cause of Symmetrical Claw or Claw Bed Disease

SLO is a less understood disease of dogs that some dermatologists consider to be autoimmune [13, 38, 61, 62]. The consequence of disease is that multiple nails on multiple paws exhibit onychomadesis over the course of weeks to months. This leads to claw bed pain and associated lameness [13, 38, 61]. When claws regrow, they are typically misshapen, soft, brittle, and discolored [13, 38, 61]. They are also likely to slough again.

Affected patients are typically young to middle-aged large-breed dogs [9]. German Shepherds are most often reported in the medical literature [3, 62, 63]. Other breeds

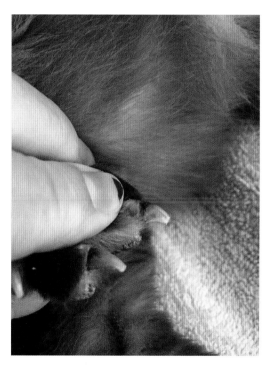

Figure 3.22 Brown exudate at the claw bed of a cat, associated with *Malassezia*.

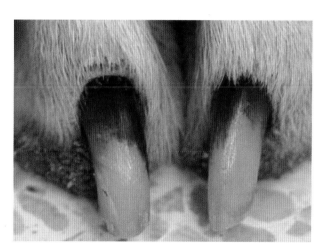

Figure 3.23 Brown discoloration of canine nails, associated with *Malassezia*.

(a)

(b)

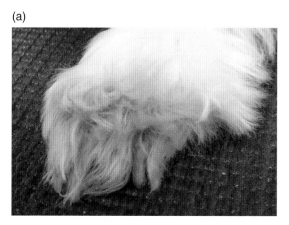 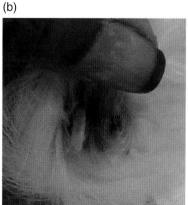

Figure 3.24 (a) Subtle discoloration of the fur, caused by excessive licking of the coat due to pruritus associated with *Malassezia*. (b) Overt discoloration of the fur, caused by excessive licking of the coat due to pruritus associated with *Malassezia*. *Source:* Courtesy of Patricia Bennett, DVM.

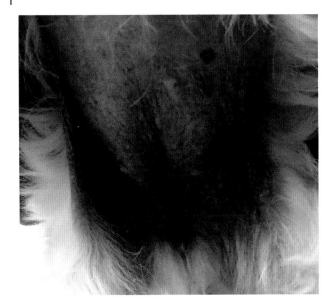

Figure 3.25 Hyperpigmentation of the ventrum, associated with *Malassezia*.

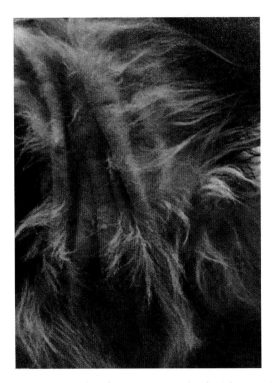

Figure 3.26 Lichenification associated with *Malassezia*. *Source:* Courtesy of Patricia Bennett, DVM.

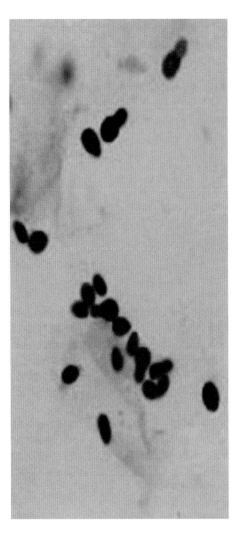

Figure 3.27 Cytological evidence of *Malassezia* overgrowth.

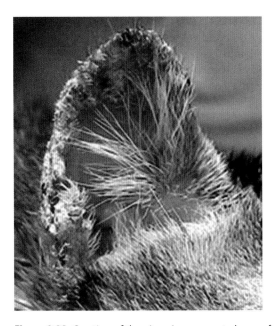

Figure 3.28 Crusting of the pinna in a suspected case of pemphigus foliaceus.

with an apparent predisposition include the Gordon and English Setters, and the Finnish Bearded Collie [63].

Diagnosis is made based upon histopathology following amputation of P3, including the claw bed [13].

Treatment is challenging and must be continued long-term. Various approaches have been tried, including immunosuppressive therapy with prednisolone, cyclosporine, or azathioprine; pentoxifylline; nicotinamide,

Table 3.4 A diagnostic approach to symmetrical claw or claw bed disease.

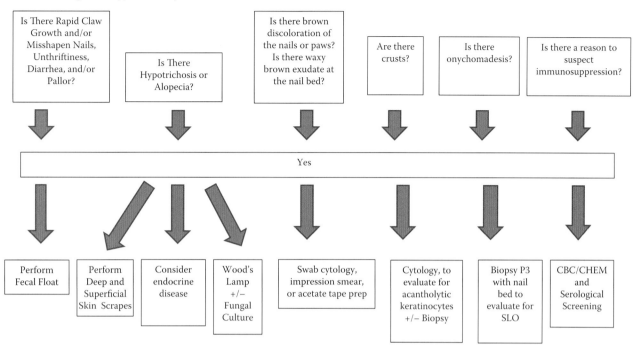

minocycline, oxytetracycline, or doxycycline, and high-dose essential fatty acid supplementation [9, 13, 51, 64].

3.8.5 Other Causes of Symmetrical Claw or Claw Bed Disease

Section 3.6.1 touched upon the fact that bacterial paronychia is often secondary to trauma. It may also result from endocrinopathies. Hypothyroidism and hyperadrenocorticism are the most likely culprits in canine patients [3, 5]. Hyperadrenocorticism in cats can also cause paronychia, but is more likely to present with papery, fragile skin that tears readily even during routine diagnostic and therapeutic interventions [65]. Feline hyperthyroidism is unlikely to cause paronychia. Instead, it is more likely to cause extremely thickened claws.

Protozoal infections with *Leishmania* spp. can also cause claw and claw bed disease. Patients with leishmaniasis typically present with onychogryphosis and overgrown, easily damaged nails [9, 66–68]. A patient that

originated from or traveled recently to Mediterranean Europe, Central Asia, and Latin America should raise a high index of suspicion. Leishmaniasis is rare in the United States; however, it has been reported sporadically, particularly in outdoor-housed foxhounds in regions where the vector, the sandfly, is endemic [38].

Diagnosis is typically made through serologic titers and/or through histopathology of skin lesions.

3.9 Diagnostic Approach to Symmetrical Claw or Claw Bed Disease

There are so many different causes of symmetrical claw or claw bed disease, and so many different presentations. It is easy to get lost in a sea of differential diagnoses. Table 3.4 summarizes one of many appropriate diagnostic approaches to take when trying to work up a case with symmetrical claw or claw bed disease.

References

1 Warren, S. (2013). Claw disease in dogs: part 1 – anatomy and diagnostic approach. *Companion Anim.* 18 (4): 165–170.

2 Scarff, D.H. (2004). Nail disease in the dog and cat. *Small Anim. Dermatol.* 9 (7): 1–4.

3 Mueller, R.S. (1999). Diagnosis and management of canine claw diseases. *Vet. Clin. North Am. Small Anim. Pract.* 29 (6): 1357–1371.

4 Harvey, R.G. and Markwell, P.J. (1996). The mineral composition of nails in normal dogs and comparison with shed nails in canine idiopathic onychomadesis. *Vet. Dermatol.* 7 (1): 29–33.

5 Scott, D.W. and Miller, W.H. (1992). Disorders of the claw and Clawbed in dogs. *Compend. Contin. Educ. Pract.* 14 (11): 1448–1458.

6 Rosychuk, R.A.W. (1995). Diseases of the claw and claw fold. In: *Kirk's Current Veterinary Therapy XII* (ed. J.D. Bonagura), 641. Philadelphia: WB Saunders.

7 Freiman, H.S. and Grubelich, L.S. (1994). Diseases of the foot and nails: humans, cats, and dogs. *Clin. Dermatol.* 12 (4): 573–577.

8 Carter, H.E. (1968). Pedal disorders in the dog and cat. *J. Small Anim. Pract.* 9 (7): 357–366.

9 Rouben, C. (2016). Claw and claw bed diseases. *Clinician's Brief* (April): 35–40.

10 Miller, W.H., Griffin, C.E., and Campbell, K.L. (2012). Diseases of eyelids, claws, anal sacs, and ears. In: *Muller and Kirk's Small Animal Dermatology*, 7e, 731–739. Philadelphia, P.A.: WB Saunders.

11 Scott, D.W. and Miller, W.H. (1992). Disorders of the claw and clawbed in cats. *Compend. Contin. Educ. Pract.* 14 (4): 449–457.

12 Boord, M.J., Griffin, C.E., and Rosenkrantz, W.S. (1997). Onychectomy as a therapy for symmetric claw and claw fold disease in the dog. *J. Am. Anim. Hosp. Assoc.* 33 (2): 131–138.

13 Warren, S. (2013). Claw disease in dogs: part 2 - diagnosis and management of specific claw diseases. *Companion Anim.* 18 (5): 226–231.

14 Foil, C.S. (1995). Facial, pedal, and other regional dermatoses. *Vet. Clin. North Am. Small Anim. Pract.* 25 (4): 923–944.

15 Neuber, A. (2009). Nail diseases in dogs. *Small Anim. Dermatol.* 14 (6): 1–6.

16 Stern, A.W. and Pieper, J. (2015). Pathology in practice. Symmetric lupoid onychodystrophy of the claw bed epithelium. *J. Am. Vet. Med. Assoc.* 246 (2): 197–199.

17 Duclos, D. (2013). Canine pododermatitis. *Vet. Clin. North Am. Small Anim. Pract.* 43 (1): 57–87.

18 Paradis, M., Scott, D.W., and Breton, L. (1989). Squamous cell carcinoma of the nail bed in three related giant schnauzers. *Vet. Rec.* 125 (12): 322–324.

19 Schultheiss, P.C. (2006). Histologic features and clinical outcomes of melanomas of lip, haired skin, and nail bed locations of dogs. *J. Vet. Diagn. Investig.* 18 (4): 422–425.

20 Yoo, C.B., Kim, D.H., Lee, A.J. et al. (2015). Canine nail bed keratoacanthoma diagnosed by immunohistochemical analysis. *Can. Vet. J.* 56 (11): 1181–1184.

21 Mueller, R.S. and Olivry, T. (1999). Onychobiopsy without onychectomy: description of a new biopsy technique for canine claws. *Vet. Dermatol.* 10 (1): 55–59.

22 Wobeser, B.K., Kidney, B.A., Powers, B.E. et al. (2007). Diagnoses and clinical outcomes associated with surgically amputated feline digits submitted to multiple veterinary diagnostic laboratories. *Vet. Pathol.* 44 (3): 362–365.

23 Herraez, P., Rodriguez, F., Ramirez, G. et al. (2005). Espinosa de Los Monteros A. Multiple primary digital apocrine sweat gland carcinosarcoma in a cat. *Vet. Rec.* 157 (12): 356–358.

24 Apple, S. (2015). Senior cat with front paw swelling and pain. *Today's Veterinary Practice* (September/October): 41–44.

25 Gottfried, S.D., Popovitch, C.A., Goldschmidt, M.H., and Schelling, C. (2000). Metastatic digital carcinoma in the cat: a retrospective study of 36 cats (1992–1998). *J. Am. Anim. Hosp. Assoc.* 36 (6): 501–509.

26 Goldfinch, N. and Argyle, D.J. (2012). Feline lung-digit syndrome: unusual metastatic patterns of primary lung tumours in cats. *J. Feline Med. Surg.* 14 (3): 202–208.

27 Maritato, K.C., Schertel, E.R., Kennedy, S.C. et al. (2014). Outcome and prognostic indicators in 20 cats with surgically treated primary lung tumors. *J. Feline Med. Surg.* 16 (12): 979–984.

28 Mehlhaff, C.J. and Mooney, S. (1985). Primary pulmonary neoplasia in the dog and cat. *Vet. Clin. North Am. Small Anim. Pract.* 15 (5): 1061–1067.

29 May, C. and Newsholme, S.J. (1989). Metastasis of feline pulmonary-carcinoma presenting as multiple digital swelling. *J. Small Anim. Pract.* 30 (5): 302–310.

30 Hanselman, B.A. and Hall, J.A. (2004). Digital metastasis from a primary bronchogenic carcinoma. *Can. Vet. J.* 45 (7): 614–616.

31 Jacobs, T.M. and Tomlinson, M.J. (1997). The lung-digit syndrome in a cat. *Feline Pract.* 25 (1): 31–36.

32 van der Linde-Sipman, J.S. and van den Ingh, T.S.G.A.M. (2000). Primary and metastatic carcinomas in the digits of cats. *Vet. Q.* 22 (3): 141–145.

33 Anderson, T.E., Legendre, A.M., and McEntee, M.M. (2000). Probable hypercalcemia of malignancy in a cat with bronchogenic adenocarcinoma. *J. Am. Anim. Hosp. Assoc.* 36 (1): 52–55.

34 Schoen, K., Block, G., Newell, S.M., and Coronado, G.S. (2010). Hypercalcemia of malignancy in a cat with bronchogenic adenocarcinoma. *J. Am. Anim. Hosp. Assoc.* 46 (4): 265–267.

35 Hahn, K.A. and McEntee, M.F. (1997). Primary lung tumors in cats: 86 cases (1979–1994). *J. Am. Vet. Med. Assoc.* 211 (10): 1257–1260.

36 Barr, F., Gruffyddjones, T.J., Brown, P.J., and Gibbs, C. (1987). Primary lung-tumors in the cat. *J. Small Anim. Pract.* 28 (12): 1115–1125.

37 Hahn, K.A. and McEntee, M.F. (1998). Prognosis factors for survival in cats after removal of a primary lung tumor: 21 cases (1979–1994). *Vet. Surg.* 27 (4): 307–311.

38 Côté, E. (2015). *Clinical Veterinary Advisor. Dogs and Cats*, 3e, xxxvii, 1642 p. St. Louis, Missouri: Elsevier Mosby.

39 Tilley, L.P. and Smith, F.W.K. (2016). *Blackwell's Five-Minute Veterinary Consult. Canine and Feline*, 6e, lxix, 1622 p. Ames, Iowa, USA: Wiley.

40 Venco, L., Valenti, V., Genchi, M., and Grandi, G. (2011). A dog with pseudo-Addison disease associated with Trichuris vulpis infection. *J Parasitol. Res.* 2011: 682039.

41 Mueller, R.S., Bensignor, E., Ferrer, L. et al. (2012). Treatment of demodicosis in dogs: 2011 clinical practice guidelines. *Vet. Dermatol.* 23 (2): 86–96, e20–1.

42 Plant, J.D., Lund, E.M., and Yang, M. (2011). A case-control study of the risk factors for canine juvenile-onset generalized demodicosis in the USA. *Vet. Dermatol.* 22 (1): 95–99.

43 Lemarie, S.L., Hosgood, G., and Foil, C.S. (1996). A retrospective study of juvenile- and adult-onset generalized demodicosis in dogs (1986–91). *Vet. Dermatol.* 7 (1): 3–10.

44 Miller, W.H., Scott, D.W., Wellington, J.R., and Panic, R. (1993). Clinical efficacy of Milbemycin Oxime in the treatment of generalized Demodicosis in adult dogs. *J. Am. Vet. Med. Assoc.* 203 (10): 1426–1429.

45 Duclos, D.D., Jeffers, J.G., and Shanley, K.J. (1994). Prognosis for treatment of adult-onset demodicosis in dogs: 34 cases (1979–1990). *J. Am. Vet. Med. Assoc.* 204 (4): 616–619.

46 Manning, T.O. (1983). Cutaneous diseases of the paw. *Clin. Dermatol.* 1 (1): 131–142.

47 Beco, L., Fontaine, F., and Bergvall, K. (2007). Comparison of skin scrapes and hair plucks for detecting Demodex mites in canine demodicosis, a multicentre, prospect study. *Vet. Dermatol.* 18: 381.

48 Mueller, R.S. and Bettenay, S.V. (2010). Skin scrapings and skin biopsies. In: *Skin Scrapings and Skin Biopsies* (ed. S.J. Ettinger and E.C. Feldman), 368–371. Philadelphia: W.B. Saunders.

49 Holm, B.R. (2003). Efficacy of milbemycin oxime in the treatment of canine generalized demodicosis: a retrospective study of 99 dogs (1995–2000). *Vet. Dermatol.* 14 (4): 189–195.

50 Young S. (2010). Feline demodicosis: prevalence, diagnostics, treatment. DVM360.

51 Hawkins, J.A., McDonald, R.K., and Woody, B.J. (1987). Sarcoptes scabiei infestation in a cat. *J. Am. Vet. Med. Assoc.* 190 (12): 1572–1573.

52 Sivajothi, S., Sudhakara Reddy, B., Rayulu, V.C., and Sreedevi, C. (2015). Notoedres cati in cats and its management. *J. Parasit. Dis.* 39 (2): 303–305.

53 Outerbridge, C.A. (2006). Mycologic disorders of the skin. *Clin. Tech. Small Anim. Pract.* 21 (3): 128–134.

54 Colombo, S., Nardoni, S., Cornegliani, L., and Mancianti, F. (2007). Prevalence of Malassezia spp. yeasts in feline nail folds: a cytological and mycological study. *Vet. Dermatol.* 18 (4): 278–283.

55 Chen, T.A. and Hill, P.B. (2005). The biology of Malassezia organisms and their ability to induce immune responses and skin disease. *Vet. Dermatol.* 16 (1): 4–26.

56 Schmidt, V. (2008). Malassezia in dogs and cats: part 1. *Small Anim. Dermatol.* 13 (4): 1–4.

57 Preziosi, D.E., Goldschmidt, M.H., Greek, J.S. et al. (2003). Feline pemphigus foliaceus: a retrospective analysis of 57 cases. *Vet. Dermatol.* 14 (6): 313–321.

58 Simpson, D.L. and Burton, G.G. (2013). Use of prednisolone as monotherapy in the treatment of feline pemphigus foliaceus: a retrospective study of 37 cats. *Vet. Dermatol.* 24 (6): 598–601, e143–4.

59 Peterson, A. and McKay, L. (2010). Crusty cats: feline pemphigus foliaceus. *Compend. Contin. Educ. Vet.* 32 (5): E1–E4.

60 McEwan, N.A., McNeil, P.E., Kirkham, D., and Sullivan, M. (1987). Drug eruption in a cat resembling pemphigus foliaceus. *J. Small Anim. Pract.* 28: 713–720.

61 Verde, M.T. and Basurco, A. (2000). Symmetrical lupoid onychodystrophy in a crossbred pointer dog: long-term observations. *Vet. Rec.* 146 (13): 376–378.

62 Scott, D.W., Rousselle, S., and Miller, W.H. Jr. (1995). Symmetrical lupoid onychodystrophy in dogs: a retrospective analysis of 18 cases (1989–1993). *J. Am. Anim. Hosp. Assoc.* 31 (3): 194–201.

63 Ziener, M.L. and Nodtvedt, A. (2014). A treatment study of canine symmetrical onychomadesis (symmetrical lupoid onychodystrophy) comparing fish oil and cyclosporine supplementation in addition to a diet rich in omega-3 fatty acids. *Acta Vet. Scand.* 56 (1): 66.

64 Barrand, K.R. (2006). What is your diagnosis? Symmetrical lupoid onychodystrophy. *J. Small Anim. Pract.* 47 (12): 757–759.

65 Boland, L.A. and Barrs, V.R. (2017). Peculiarities of feline hyperadrenocorticism: update on diagnosis and treatment. *J. Feline Med. Surg.* 19 (9): 933–947.

66 Koutinas, A.F., Carlotti, D.N., Koutinas, C. et al. (2010). Claw histopathology and parasitic load in natural cases of canine leishmaniosis associated with Leishmania infantum. *Vet. Dermatol.* 21 (6): 572–577.

67 Ciaramella, P., Oliva, G., Luna, R.D. et al. (1997). A retrospective clinical study of canine leishmaniasis in 150 dogs naturally infected by Leishmania infantum. *Vet. Rec.* 141 (21): 539–543.

68 Koutinas, A.F., Polizopoulou, Z.S., Saridomichelakis, M.N. et al. (1999). Clinical considerations on canine visceral leishmaniasis in Greece: a retrospective study of 158 cases (1989–1996). *J. Am. Anim. Hosp. Assoc.* 35 (5): 376–383.

4

Wounds

4.1 Overview of Wounds in Companion Animal Medicine

Wounds occur with frequency in companion animal medicine, both within the primary care and emergency settings [1]. Clients may witness the actual wounding event itself, or they may observe the impact of the wound on the patient after the fact. For example, a client may present a patient for acute onset of lameness. Physical examination discloses that the patient has an embedded foxtail in its paw.

Most wounds are created by external factors. These include physical altercations, both with conspecifics and members of other species [1–6]; automobile trauma, gunshot wounds and falls from great heights [5–14]; surgery and/or surgical complications [15–21]; thermal and chemical injuries, such as burns [11, 22]; pressure injuries that cause decubital ulcers [23–25]; aberrant migration of larvae, such as cuterebra [26, 27]; other foreign bodies [28–30]; and adverse reactions to topical medications (see Figures 4.1a–m).

Not all wounds are from external injury. Wounds may be self-induced [31, 32]. For example, patients with intense pruritus may scratch at their skin to the point that they create curvilinear excoriations (see Figures 4.2a–c) [32–34].

These excoriations may deepen over time with repeated trauma if the itch is not resolved. A history of pruritus, combined with a clinical presentation of scratch marks, should prompt the clinician to investigate the possibility that patient-specific pathology has caused self-mutilation.

Underlying allergic disease and atopic dermatitis are common causes of self-mutilation in companion animals [34]; so too are obsessive–compulsive disorders such as tail biting and flank sucking [35–38]. Anxiety and pain may exacerbate these behaviors.

Wounds may also occur as a result of underlying pathology, such as anal sac disease and neoplasia (see Figures 4.3a–e).

Underlying pathology may also potentiate wound formation. Consider, for example, Ehlers–Danlos syndrome [39, 40]. This syndrome is characterized by inherited defects in collagen that result in skin hyperextensibility and fragility [39–47] (see Figures 4.4a–c).

Patients with Ehlers–Danlos syndrome often present for significant gaping wounds without apparent cause [39, 44]. These "fish-mouth" wounds typically require primary closure [39, 44, 48]. Scars will appear sunken due to reduced collagen deposition [43, 44]. The fragility of the skin may also extend to the vasculature [43]. Pronounced bruising, bleeding, and hematoma formation is not atypical in affected patients following minor trauma [43]. Additionally, patients may present because of clinically abnormal ligaments, joints, eyes, and other organs [41, 43, 47].

A second example of pathology that typically results in wounds is feline skin fragility syndrome (FSFS). Unlike Ehlers–Danlos syndrome, FSFS is not characterized by hyperextensible skin [49, 50]. Patients with FSFS have exceptionally thin skin that tears readily. This is an acquired condition secondary to a primary disease state such as hyperadrenocorticism, which adversely impacts collagen synthesis [49, 51, 52].

4.2 Bite Wounds and Abscesses

The incidence of bite wounds in companion animals has been poorly studied as compared to the incidence of bite wounds in humans. However, isolated reports suggest that 10–15% of veterinary trauma cases in companion animal medicine involve bite wounds in dogs and cats [1, 4, 11, 53]. In all dogs, the head, neck, and limbs are most often affected [1, 4, 11, 54] (see Figures 4.5a–f).

Cats and small breed dogs are at increased risk of sustaining bites to the thoracic and abdominal cavities [2]. These are often extensive and may result in pneumothorax, diaphragmatic tears, and/or evisceration (see Figures 4.6a–c).

Common Clinical Presentations in Dogs and Cats, First Edition. Ryane E. Englar.
© 2019 John Wiley & Sons, Inc. Published 2019 by John Wiley & Sons, Inc.

(a)   (b)   (c)

(d)   (e)   (f)

(g)   (h)   (i)

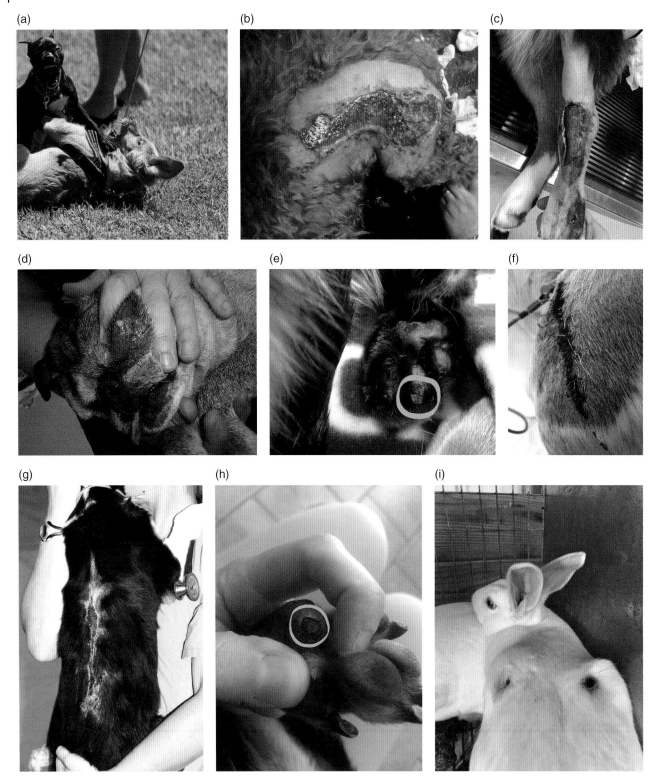

Figure 4.1 (a). Altercation between two dogs that could result in bite wounds. *Source:* Courtesy of Genevieve LaFerriere, DVM. (b). Hit-by-car injuries resulted in this canine lateral thigh laceration. *Source:* Courtesy of Pamela Mueller, DVM. (c). Degloving injury of the left cranial tarsus and metatarsus. *Source:* Courtesy of Sarah Bashaw, DVM. (d). Orbital abscess in a pug that had previously undergone unilateral enucleation. *Source:* Courtesy of Daniel Foy. (e). Scabs from healing surgical wounds created during an onychectomy procedure. (f). Wound dehiscence in a canine patient. *Source:* Courtesy of Dr. Stephanie Harris. (g). Burns along the dorsum of a canine patient. *Source:* Courtesy of Laura Polerecky. (h). Paw pad burn in a canine patient. *Source:* Courtesy of Jule Schweighoefer. (i). Cuterebriasis in a rabbit. *Source:* Courtesy of Monica Witt Meek. (j). A close-up of a cuterebra maggot. (k). Pharyngeal stick foreign body. *Source:* Courtesy of Victoria Jenkins, DVM. (l). Surgical removal of a pharyngeal stick foreign body. *Source:* Courtesy of Victoria Jenkins, DVM. (m). Cutaneous reaction to topical miconazole in a feline patient. *Source:* Courtesy of Colleen M. Cook, Midwestern University College of Veterinary Medicine, Class of 2019.

(j)

(l)

(k)

(m)

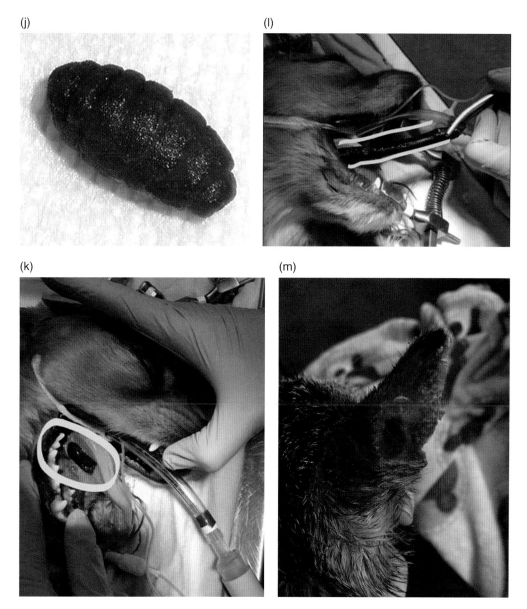

Figure 4.1 *(Continued)*

The perineum and the tail are less commonly reported as sites of bite wounds [11]. The tail is more often a site of degloving, for example, when cats get their tails snagged in slammed doors (see Figure 4.7).

Bite wounds caused by dogs and cats involve tensile, shearing, and/or compressive forces [1, 11].

When teeth strike at acute angles, they create tensile force that separates skin from underlying tissue [1, 55]. This creates empty pockets of so-called dead space. Muscle layers can also be avulsed, causing devitalization and hernias [1].

Incisors and canine teeth create puncture wounds through compression [1, 11]. They may also exert shearing force if they make perpendicular contact with the skin's surface [11]. When premolars and molars exert compressive forces, they cause crushing injuries [1, 11]. In severe cases, crushing results in necrosis secondary to ischemia [55].

Bite wound management in dogs and cats can be challenging, particularly because it is easy to underestimate the extent of damaged tissue. On the surface, many bite wounds appear to be innocuous. However, beneath the visible punctures, there is often extensive unseen damage [1, 11].

Certain breeds of dogs can exert a force of up to 450 pounds per square inch (psi) [11, 56–58]. Consider the impact of this on those patients who are overrepresented as victims of bite wounds in the veterinary medical

(a)   (b)

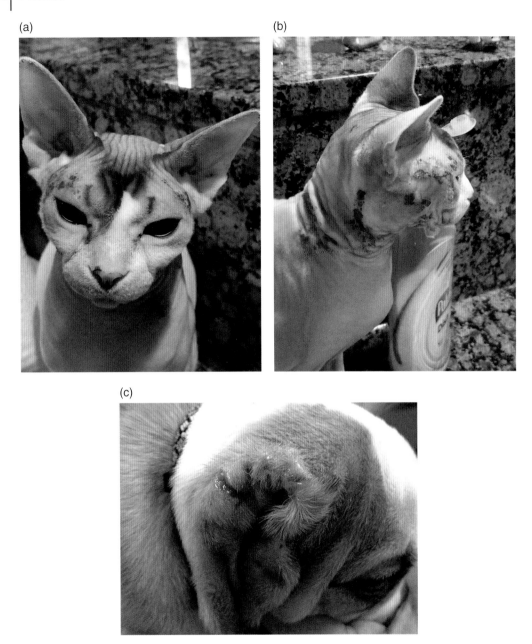

(c)

Figure 4.2 (a). Self-induced peri-aural excoriations in a Sphynx cat. *Source:* Courtesy of Kelli L. Crisfulli, RVT. (b). Side-view of peri-aural, facial, and cervical excoriations in a Sphynx cat. *Source:* Courtesy of Kelli L. Crisfulli, RVT. (c). External ear excoriations secondary to pruritus in a canine patient. *Source:* Courtesy of Kara Thomas, DVM, CVMA.

literature, those weighing 10 kg or less [2]. These "big dog/little dog" (BDLD) altercations may result in fractures, particularly involving the limbs and the chest wall [1]. The victims may also be picked up and shaken, resulting in significant avulsion injuries that complicate wound management due to the "iceberg effect," the presence of invisible damage beneath the skin's surface [11].

Small puncture wounds may also prematurely seal over as a result of the body's attempt to heal. However,

this traps one or more bacterial populations from the biter's mouth and teeth, the victim's skin, and the environment beneath the skin's surface [11, 59]. Bacteria are often a mix of aerobes and anaerobes [59]. The most common bacteria that is cultured from bite wounds of dogs and cats is *Pasteurella multocida* [56, 60].

The result of bacterial inoculation is a contaminated wound [1, 11, 61]. Cat bites are notorious for causing contamination because their sharp teeth effectively inoculate bacteria deep beneath the skin's surface [11, 56, 62].

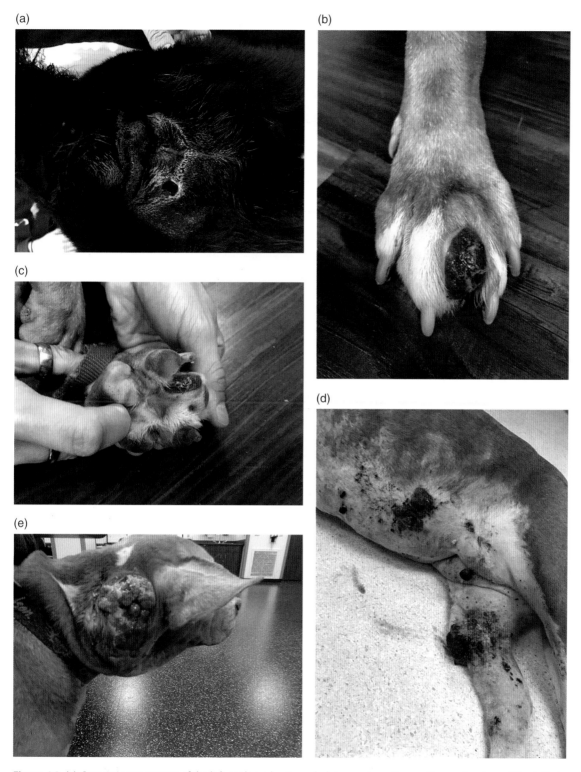

Figure 4.3 (a). Spontaneous rupture of the left anal sac due to underlying anal sac disease. *Source:* Courtesy of Sarah Bashaw, DVM. (b). Canine interdigital mass, dorsal view. *Source:* Courtesy of Samantha B. Thurman, DVM. (c). Canine interdigital mass, plantar view. *Source:* Courtesy of Samantha B. Thurman, DVM. (d). Solar-induced squamous cell carcinoma in a canine patient. *Source:* Courtesy of Beki Cohen Regan, DVM, DACVIM (Oncology). (e). Erosive wound in a canine patient caudal to the right pinna due to rapidly growing neoplasia. *Source:* Courtesy of Kara Thomas, DVM, CVMA.

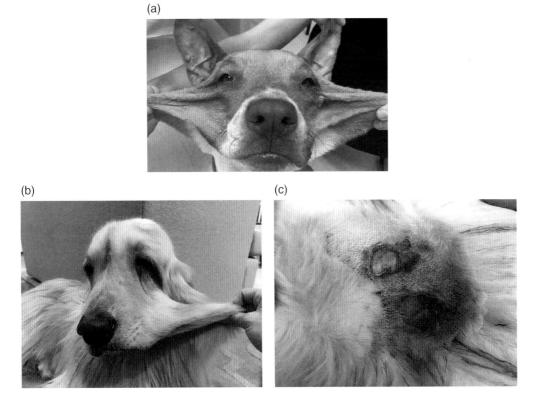

Figure 4.4 (a). Ehlers–Danlos syndrome in a canine patient. *Source:* Courtesy of the Small Animal Internal Medicine Service at the University of Missouri Veterinary Health Center. (b). Ehlers–Danlos syndrome in a canine patient. *Source:* Courtesy of Erika Sox Burns, DVM, DACVIM-SAIM. (c). Ventral neck wounds in a canine patient with Ehlers–Danlos syndrome. *Source:* Courtesy of Erika Sox Burns, DVM, DACVIM-SAIM.

Once inoculated, bacteria take advantage of an environment that is conducive to growth [1, 25]. Abscesses frequently form as localized accumulations of purulent discharge. These may become quite large, visible, and painful swellings (see Figure 4.8).

Abscesses complicate wound management because the pool of infected tissue potentiates the inflammatory response. Healing cannot progress until the purulent material has been drained and the infected tissue has been removed [1, 11, 25]. Moreover, care must be taken when repairing the wound to prevent dead space (see Figures 4.9a, b).

Dead space promotes seroma or hematoma formation, which will prevent the wound from healing and may allow infection to persist [11]. Persistent infection may trigger the development of systemic inflammatory response syndrome (SIRS) and/or sepsis [1, 11].

The placement of surgical drains is a means of preventing dead space [11, 63, 64]. The approach to drainage is determined on a case-by-case basis, and in large part depends upon the wound site. Drains may be as simple as a stab incision that allows fluid to exit the wound by gravity. Penrose drains also allow for passive drainage (see Figures 4.10a, b).

Active drainage may be achieved via vacuum-assisted closure (VAC), otherwise referred to as negative pressure wound therapy (NPWT). This facilitates wound healing through uniform, controlled removal of excessive fluid at the site of injury, and may be preferred for anatomically challenging locations such as the distal limb [65–68].

Refer to Section 4.6 for a brief discussion concerning wound management.

4.3 Other Important Considerations Regarding Bite Wounds

Bacterial contamination of bite wounds is just one important consideration from the standpoint of infectious disease. It is important to recall that disease transmission can also involve viruses.

In both dogs and cats, the transmission of rabies is possible when saliva from the attacker contaminates the wound of the victim [1, 11]. The American Veterinary Medical Association (AVMA) has prepared guidelines

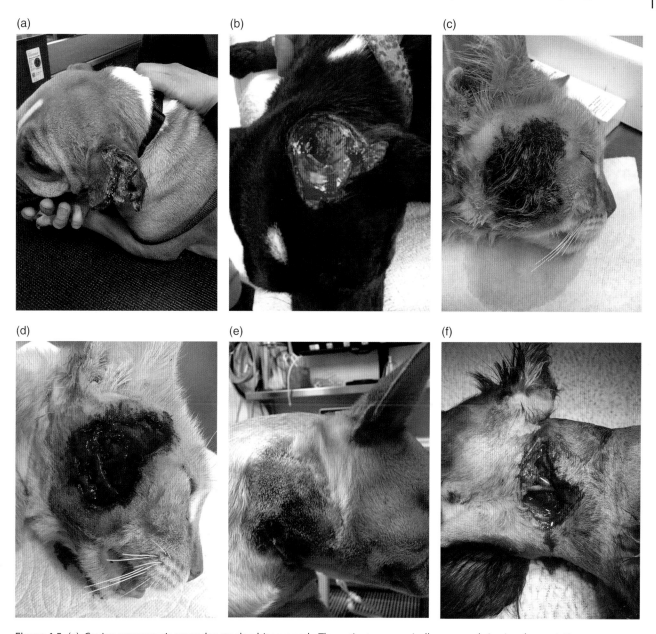

Figure 4.5 (a). Canine ear necrosis secondary to dog bite wounds. The patient was surgically managed via pinnal amputation. *Source:* Courtesy of Rachel Kinkade. (b). Bite wound sustained to the dorsum of a canine patient. *Source:* Courtesy of Dr. Stephanie Harris. (c). Necrotic skin over the right cheek of a feline patient secondary to bite wounds. *Source:* Courtesy of Aimee Wong. (d). The same feline patient as depicted in Figure 4.5c, following debridement of necrotic tissue. *Source:* Courtesy of Aimee Wong. (e). Canine patient that sustained bite wounds to the right cervical region. *Source:* Courtesy of Daniel Foy. (f). Canine patient that sustained deep bite wounds to the left cervical region, with exposure of the jugular vein. *Source:* Courtesy of Kimberly Wallitsch.

regarding bite management in vaccinated and unvaccinated dogs and cats [69].

Bite wound victims that are current on their rabies vaccination at the time of injury should be revaccinated immediately and observed for 45 days [1].

According to the AVMA, unvaccinated bite victims should be humanely euthanized and tested for rabies; however, clinicians should consult with local and state regulations [69]. Clients who do not elect to euthanize

may have the option of a six-month quarantine, with the bite victim vaccinated against rabies one month prior to release [1].

In addition to rabies, transmission of feline leukemia virus (FeLV) and feline immunodeficiency virus (FIV) are also concerns for cats. Feline victims of bite wounds from cats with unknown serological status should themselves be tested for FeLV and FIV both at the time of and six months after wounding [1, 11].

(a)

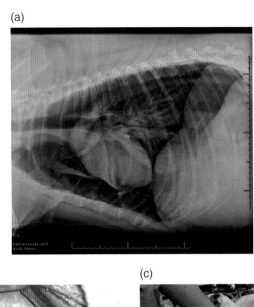

(b)

(c)

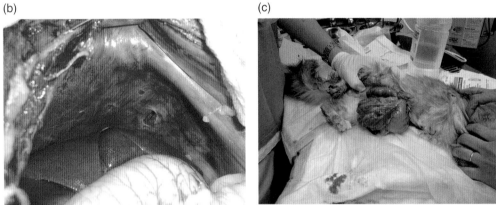

Figure 4.6 (a). Right lateral thoracic radiograph demonstrating pneumothorax. Note how the heart appears to float in space. *Source:* Courtesy of Daniel Foy. (b). Diaphragmatic tear secondary to a "big dog/little dog" (BDLD) altercation. *Source:* Courtesy of Daniel Foy. (c). Feline evisceration secondary to traumatic bite wounds. *Source:* Courtesy of Daniel Foy.

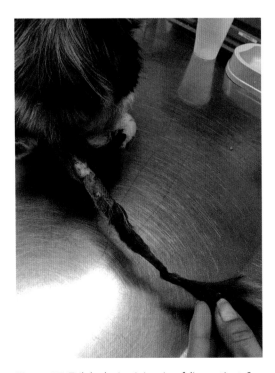

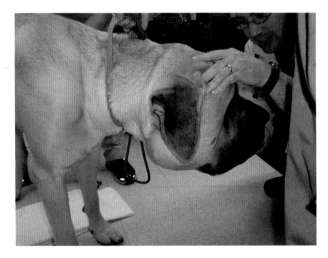

Figure 4.8 Right ventrolateral cervical abscess in a canine patient. *Source:* Courtesy of Daniel Foy.

Figure 4.7 Tail degloving injury in a feline patient. *Source:* Courtesy of Frank Isom.

(a) 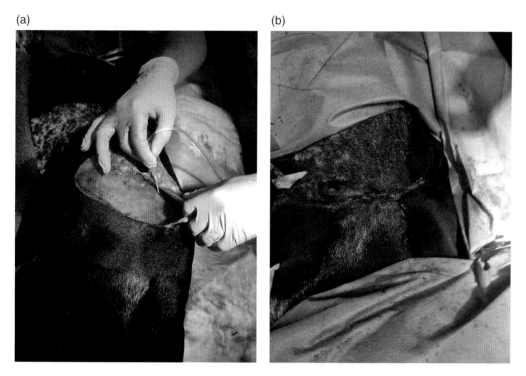 (b)

Figure 4.9 (a). Extensive lateral flank wound in a canine patient. Note the large amount of dead space between the skin and the underlying tissue. Source: Courtesy of Lori A. Stillmaker, DVM. (b). Tacking sutures have been placed in an attempt to reduce dead space. Source: Courtesy of Lori A. Stillmaker, DVM.

Figure 4.10 (a). Ventral cervical bite wound in a cat with Penrose drain placement to allow for passive drainage. *Source:* Courtesy of Daniel Foy. (b). Penrose drain placements in a canine patient with a right lateral flank wound. *Source:* Courtesy of Lori A. Stillmaker, DVM.

(a)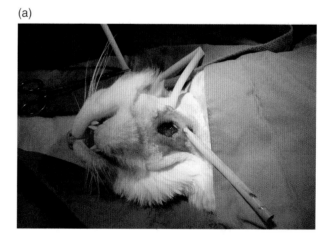

(b)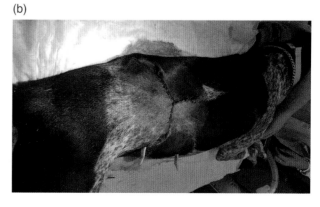

4.4 Non-Animal-Induced Puncture Wounds and Lacerations

Recall from Section 4.1 that not all wounds are the result of conflict between animals. Non-animal puncture wounds and lacerations are also seen frequently in companion animal practice and range the gamut from pinpoint foreign body penetration to extensive ulceration and full-thickness separation of skin from underlying tissue (see Figures 4.11a–c).

Unlike bite wounds, which are all considered contaminated, non-animal puncture wounds and lacerations may or may not be. Those that are not contaminated are typically managed by primary closure.

Refer to Section 4.6 for a brief discussion concerning wound management.

4.5 Degloving Wounds

Degloving in dogs and cats refers to the traumatic process by which skin tears free from underlying tissue. When moving vehicles drag veterinary patients, as is the case in automobile trauma, degloving is a typical

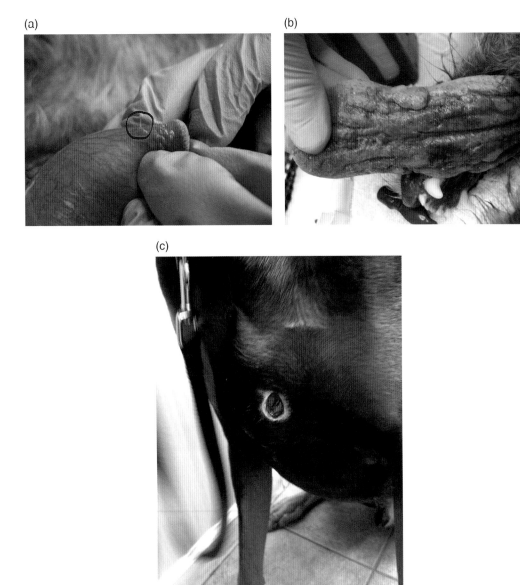

Figure 4.11 (a). Single cocklebur penetration of the dorsal aspect of a canine tongue. *Source:* Courtesy of Daniel Foy. (b). "Burr tongue" or "Burdock tongue," also known as granulomatous glossitis, in a canine patient. The hooked burrs from ingested burdock plants become embedded in the tongue and create an intense foreign body reaction. *Source:* Courtesy of Daniel Foy. (c). Laceration of the skin overlying the chest in a canine patient. *Source:* Courtesy of Jetta Schirmer.

(a)　　　　　　　　　　　　　　　　(b)

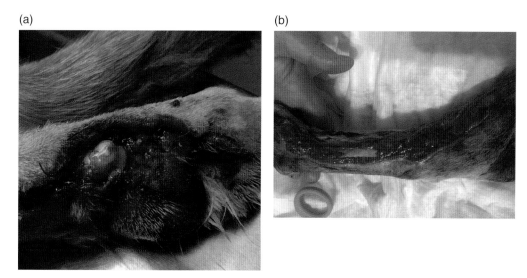

Figure 4.12 (a). Degloving injury of the canine paw. *Source:* Courtesy of Frank Isom. (b). Healing degloving injury of the distal hind limb of a one-year-old German Shepherd that had been hit by a car. *Source:* Courtesy of Jule Schweighoefer.

injury [70–74]. Degloving most often impacts the distal limbs, particularly the medial tarsus and metatarsus (see Figures 4.12a, b) [71, 72]. Degloving in cats also results when tails catch in shutting doors.

Because blood supply to underlying tissues is compromised as a result of trauma, these wounds prove difficult to heal [70]. Extremities do not have an excess of neighboring skin from which to create flaps, and there is little cushion to buffer what tissue remains from the immense crushing forces that force debris and bacteria deep down into open wounds. Joints may become unstable, with or without joint capsule penetration, and the patient may sustain one or more fractures.

Despite these complicating factors, the long-term prognosis for degloving wounds is favorable [70, 71]. Open wound management is often required, with or without grafting; however, these wounds can heal, and the patient can return to function.

4.6 An Introduction to Wound Management

The details of wound management are beyond the scope of this text. Wound care in veterinary medicine has evolved rapidly over the past 25 years, and continues to advance as new products, procedures, and techniques come under investigation [75]. For specific guidelines, surgical textbooks and current review articles should be consulted, and management considerations should always be tailored to patient care.

However, certain principles should be addressed at this time as these have broader implications for wound management in general.

The following factors broadly affect wound healing [75]:

- Motion
- Tension
- Nutrition
- Medications
- Infection

Motion delays healing. Proper bandaging helps to reduce motion's tug on the wound as it attempts to heal [75, 76].

Tension puts undue strain on the wound while it is healing. If the strain is sufficient, the result may be wound dehiscence (see Figure 4.13).

A good nutritional plane facilitates wound healing. Poor nutrition, particularly a diet that is deficient in protein, delays the patient's ability to heal [75, 77].

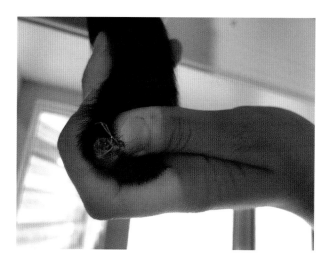

Figure 4.13 Dehiscence at the surgical site of a tail tip amputation in a feline patient. *Source:* Courtesy of Jule Schweighoefer.

Medications may impact wound healing. For example, the adverse effects of corticosteroids on wounds have been extensively researched. These drugs delay wound healing. They also reduce the strength of the replacement tissue [75, 78, 79]. Chemotherapeutic agents also antagonize wound healing. Because these drugs target rapidly dividing cells, they impact fibroblast proliferation and reduce wound strength [75, 80, 81].

4.6.1 Wound Preparation

Infection is distinct from contamination. All bite wounds are said to be contaminated. The attending clinician must take care to prevent contaminated wounds from becoming infected, that is, harboring 10^5 microorganisms per gram of tissue [82].

Careful wound preparation is one way to reduce the risk of infection. Adhering to "best practice" guidelines concerning clipping, scrubbing, and surgical preparation are of paramount importance in reducing surgical site infection (SSI) [75].

Upon initial presentation to the clinic, if not before, wounds should be covered with a dry, clean bandage [83]. This prevents further contamination of the open wound [83]. Similarly, when open wounds are clipped, as they are prior to surgical repair, they should be covered with a sterile, water-soluble gel during clipping to prevent further contamination [1]. Cleansing around the wound with chlorhexidine solution or povidone-iodine is standard protocol. However, the use of surgical scrubs at the site of the wound itself may impair wound healing by damaging healthy tissue and killing fibroblasts [1, 84, 85].

The patient's wound(s) should be thoroughly explored under anesthesia [1]. This allows for the identification of gross debris and pockets of dead space that will need to be eliminated to encourage healing.

Wounds may need to be debrided. Debridement refers to the removal of debris and/or damaged, devitalized tissue [83]. One or more methods of debridement are typically used to improve the success of efforts to transform contaminated wounds into clean wounds.

4.6.2 Nonselective Mechanical Debridement: Lavage

Irrigation of the wound, as through lavage, is often the first step [83]. Copious amounts of solution are flushed through the wound under pressure to reduce surface contaminants and debris [1].

Solutions that are appropriate for lavage include lactated Ringer's solution or sterile, physiologic saline [1]. *In vitro*, these do not appear to damage fibroblasts [1], whereas tap water may [86].

Other appropriate solutions include dilute (0.01–0.05%) chlorhexidine solution or 0.1% povidone-iodine [83]. More potent solutions may kill healthy tissue or delay the formation of a granulation bed, an essential step in wound healing [83]. One advantage of chlorhexidine solution is that organic matter such as blood and purulent debris does not inactivate it [83, 87, 88]. The same cannot be said of povidone-iodine [83, 87, 88]. Certain patients may also develop contact sensitivity to povidone-iodine [83].

Occasionally, mixtures of solutions are created. For example, tris-ethylenediaminetetraacetic acid (Tris-EDTA) may be added to a dilute chlorhexidine solution because it exerts some antimicrobial activity against gram-negative bacteria, such as *Pseudomonas aeruginosa* [83, 87].

Solutions that are inappropriate include those containing hydrogen peroxide or acetic acid [83]. These are relatively ineffective against bacteria, and the potential for cytotoxicity exceeds any benefit [89].

Much remains to be determined about the ideal pressure that should be used to flush acceptable solutions through wounds [83]. There is a fine balance between insufficient pressure, which does little to remove surface contaminants, and overwhelming pressure, which drives them deeper into tissues [83, 88].

Lavage with an 18-gauge needle and 35-ml syringe generates seven to eight pounds psi of pressure. This setup provides low-pressure irrigation that is thought to flush out bacteria as well as debris without damaging tissue [83, 90, 91].

Lavage under great pressure (70 psi or more) should be avoided. High-pressure irrigation only forces bacteria deeper into the wound and widens tissue planes, creating more dead space [1, 83, 88].

4.6.3 Nonselective Mechanical Debridement: Surgical Removal of Tissue

Following lavage, devitalized, or necrotic tissue, including fat and muscle, must be removed. If any remains, it will inhibit healing or promote bacterial growth [1, 83, 92, 93].

Aseptic technique is essential. Any break in sterility will contribute to, rather than reduce contamination [83]. Any remaining foreign material is removed via thumb forceps, followed by surgical excision of devitalized or necrotic tissue via sharp dissection. Necrotic tissue appears black [83]. Occasionally, its texture is leathery.

Sometimes it is difficult to assess for tissue health because lesions may or may not progress to necrosis. Some will recover on their own. It has been said that if the tissue bleeds, it is more likely to be viable; however, bleeding of tissue is not a guarantee that the tissue will remain healthy [83]. If there is any question as to the viability of tissue, the wound should remain open rather than closed and be re-examined daily [83]. For this reason, surgical debridement may require staging. Rushing debridement to close a wound prematurely does the patient no good if what tissue remains is not healthy enough to knit back together. It behooves the surgical team to be patient. Communication with the patient's family is critical so that all caretakers are on the same page as to why surgical closure of the wound may need to be delayed. It may take three to five days to yield a clean wound free of contamination that can then be successfully closed [1].

4.6.4 Nonselective Mechanical Debridement: Dry-To-Dry and Wet-To-Dry Bandaging

Historically, dry-to-dry and wet-to-dry bandaging were commonly used techniques to facilitate nonselective debridement of tissue [83].

In a dry-to-dry bandage, the wound is covered with dry gauze. Another dry covering is placed over the layer of dry gauze to hold the gauze in place. As the wound oozes discharge, the discharge is absorbed by the dry gauze. When the discharge dries, it essentially adheres the wound to the dry gauze like glue. When the bandage is removed, a layer of surface tissue is removed along with the bandage [83].

In a wet-to-dry bandage, the wound is covered with wet gauze. As the gauze dries, it adheres to the wound. When the bandage is removed, so too is surface tissue [83].

Both dry-to-dry and wet-to-dry bandages cause discomfort to the patient [94]. They also require an investment of care in that bandage changes must be frequent (once to three times a day) if debridement is to be most successful [83]. Dehydration of the wound may occur; if it does, wound healing will be delayed [83, 94, 95].

Because of these complications, newer methods of selective debridement have been developed in human medicine that result in both improved patient comfort and patient outcomes [95, 96]. These are applicable to veterinary patients and may be observed in clinical practice with increasing frequency as clinicians become more familiar with their use.

4.6.5 Selective Mechanical Debridement

Selective mechanical debridement refers to advanced techniques that promote the removal of non-viable tissue only. These include [83, 87, 97–99] the following:

- The use of enzymes to destroy necrotic tissue
- The use of sterile maggots to ingest necrotic tissue
- The maintenance of a moist wound surface to promote autolysis

Streptokinase, trypsin, protease, fibrinolysin, and/or collagenase can be incorporated into ointments or gels that can then be applied to damaged tissue [97]. These enzymes selectively destroy necrotic tissue and have demonstrated some success in the equine distal limb, where surgical wound repair is challenging. It is possible that these enzymes may be researched with regards to how one might manage equally difficult wounds in dogs and cats, or in those patients with surgical contraindications such as high anesthetic risk [83]. One advantage to this technique is that it does not appear to cause pain, and there is minimal to no bleeding [83].

Maggots are also being used to debride tissue without pain or discomfort [83]. Greenbottle flies (*Phaenicia sericata* or *Lucilia sericata*) are bred in the laboratory to create sterile maggots that are then applied directly to patient wounds. Maggots secrete enzymes that digest necrotic tissue or skin. They cause no damage to healthy dermis or subcutaneous tissue [83]. Five to eight maggots are placed every square centimeter, to allow each to feed on approximately 75 mg of necrotic tissue per day [83, 87, 98, 99]. Their requirements are minimal: other than a food source (the wound), they require oxygen and moisture [83].

Autolysis refers to self-destruction of body tissue. Whereas enzymes or maggots are external factors that can be applied to debride the wound, autolytic debridement requires the body to do its own work. Normal cellular processes are capable of cleaning up wounds, removing damaged tissue, and killing bacteria as long as a moist environment is maintained. Dry-to-dry and wet-to-dry bandages remove that moist environment, preventing autolysis from occurring. However, when moisture remains at the site of injury, endogenous enzymes, growth factors, and cytokines trigger formation of new blood vessels, granulation tissue, and skin regrowth. The body essentially heals itself. Special bandages or dressings are required to maintain wound moisture. A few examples include calcium alginate, polyurethane foam, hydrogel, and hydrocolloid. Semi-occlusive bandages are best because they allow oxygen to get to the wound. This expedites healing [83].

Unfortunately, autolysis only has the potential for success if there are not large areas of necrosis. Therefore, surgical debridement may still be indicated.

4.6.6 Antibiotic Use and Bite Wounds

The use of antibiotics to manage bite wounds in dogs and cats remains controversial, just as it is in human medicine [1]. As antibiotic resistance concerns abound, there is fear within the medical community and the general public about overusing antibiotics, particularly when their use may not be indicated or may not affect patient outcome. In human medicine, antibiotics are typically prescribed when bite wounds are considered high risk: full-thickness punctures; wounds at extremities or over joints, tendons, ligaments, and bones; wounds in immunocompromised patients; and wounds in those with orthopedic implants [1, 100, 101].

No similar risk analysis has been published in veterinary medicine; however, it is reasonable to assume that many if not all of the same risk factors apply. If antibiotics are used, it is important to recall that mixed aerobic and anaerobic bacterial populations are common in dog and cat bite wounds [1, 60].

Broad-spectrum antibiotics may provide the first line of defense when planning drug therapy; however, keep in mind that culturing wounds to establish the antibiotic sensitivities of the colonizers is ideal. Drug resistance is increasingly common: up to 30% of staphylococci in one study were resistant to penicillin, and multidrug resistance is common among the coliforms [3].

Antibiotics should be prescribed on a case-by-case basis rather than as part of a one-size-fits-all approach to wound management. Antibiotic use also does not obviate the need for aseptic technique.

4.6.7 Wound Healing "Enhancers"

Several topical "medications" have been used for decades to enhance wound healing. For example, wounds have been managed with topical applications of honey since 2000 BCE [102, 103]. Sugar, too, has been used for wound care globally for hundreds of years [102]. Research is only just beginning to shed light on how these products and others work.

Honey is advantageous for use in wound management for several reasons [103–110]. Honey absorbs inflammatory exudate from wounds, thereby reducing edema [102].

In addition, honey has antibacterial properties [105]. Honey produces hydrogen peroxide as a result of natural glucose oxidase enzyme activity [106–109, 111]. The resultant hydrogen peroxide serves as a natural antiseptic [109, 112]. In particular, honey is effective against *Staphylococcus, Streptococcus, Klebsiella, Pseudomonas, Escherichia coli, Salmonella typhimurium,* and *Serratia marcescens* [113, 114]. Furthermore, honey reduces growth of *Candida albicans* [115]. Manuka, kanuka, heather, and ling kamahi varieties of honey have the highest antibacterial activity [104].

Because not all types of honey share the same antimicrobial properties, honey has most recently been engineered in the laboratory to enhance its activity against microbes. One product, surgihoney, may even be more effective than natural honey against multidrug resistant bacteria [116].

The low levels of hydrogen peroxide that honey produces naturally also stimulate fibroblast growth and angiogenesis [112]. The creation of new blood vessels hastens oxygen delivery to wounded tissues, which need oxygen in order to regenerate [111].

Honey is also acidic. When wounded tissues are acidified, they experience accelerated rates of healing [117].

Unpasteurized honey is energy rich, containing 40% glucose, 40% fructose, 20% water, and trace amounts of essential and non-essential nutrients [104]. These energy sources fuel cellular regeneration, the formation of a granulation bed, and epithelialization [118]. Healing of burns in human patients is faster when honey is applied than when wounds are treated with silver sulfadiazine [119].

Sugar is similar to honey as a topical agent in that it absorbs exudate from wounds [102]. Healing is expedited because edema is reduced, facilitating the formation of a healthy granulation bed [120]. By virtue of dehydrating wounds and the microorganisms that they contain, sugar may also inhibit microbial growth [83, 87]. Less is known about sugar because it has primarily been used in remote and tropical regions of the country, where other medical staples are unavailable [113, 121]. Sugar is often mixed with glycerin to create a paste that can be packed into wounds.

Sugar is not often used in veterinary medicine to facilitate wound healing. More often, it is used as a saturated solution (50%) to reduce edema associated with emergency presentations such as paraphimosis, rectal, or uterine prolapse [122–125].

4.7 Differences in Wound Healing Between Dogs and Cats

Historically, cats have often been considered "small dogs" for the purpose of teaching companion animal medicine. However, this view is erroneous, particularly when considering wound healing. Recent reports in the veterinary literature suggest that cutaneous anatomy and healing are distinct in cats as compared to dogs [126, 127].

Cat skin is less perfused than dog skin [127, 128]. In particular, the trunk of a dog has greater vascular density. Because perfusion and rate of wound healing are related, cat skin heals slower than dog skin [126, 127, 129, 130].

In addition, it has been hypothesized that cats produce less collagen than dogs during wound healing [127]. This may account for the fact that it takes significantly less force in cats to break down sutured wounds, causing wound dehiscence [126, 127].

Cats also produce less granulation tissue than dogs during second-intention healing [127]. This contributes to a slower rate of healing in cats as compared to dogs.

The mechanism by which cats heal by second intention also differs from dogs. Cutaneous healing in cats requires wound edges to contract down. This reflects the so-called "picture frame" theory of wound contraction that was first proposed in human medicine in the 1950s to explain human wound healing [131]. The myofibroblasts at the wound edges contract the wound, pulling the inside out. By contrast, dogs adhere more to the "pull theory" [132]. Fibroblasts from within the bed of granulation tissue collectively contract, creating a centralized pull that draws the outer edges of the wound in [126].

Species-based differences in cutaneous healing impact wound management. Cats may benefit from having skin sutures remain in place longer than dogs [126]. This may

be of particular importance to wound repair at high-risk anatomical locations such as overlying joints, where motion and/or tension increase the risk of wound dehiscence. Surgeons may also need to prioritize skin grafts or flaps for cats, which may benefit from reconstruction earlier in the healing process than dogs [126]. Axillary wounds, for example, as caused by collar entrapment, are notoriously difficult to heal [133–135]. Dehiscence is common because of the high rate of motion at this site and poor vascular supply [133, 136]. Rather than risk delays in wound healing, omental pedicle grafts and thoracodorsal axial pattern flaps, combined with wound closure have proved effective [133–135]. These procedures are still largely experimental and not without complications, including incisional herniation and paracostal abscessation [134]. However, they reflect a need to promote healing in cats, recognizing that more aggressive approaches may be warranted to hasten recovery.

References

1 Holt, D.E. and Griffin, G. (2000). Bite wounds in dogs and cats. *Vet. Clin. North Am. Small Anim. Pract.* 30 (3): 669–679, viii.

2 Shamir, M.H., Leisner, S., Klement, E. et al. (2002). Dog bite wounds in dogs and cats: a retrospective study of 196 cases. *J. Vet. Med. A Physiol. Pathol. Clin. Med.* 49 (2): 107–112.

3 Kelly, P.J., Mason, P.R., Els, J., and Matthewman, L.A. (1992). Pathogens in dog bite wounds in dogs in Harare. *Zimbabwe. Vet. Rec.* 131 (20): 464–466.

4 Kolata, R.J., Kraut, N.H., and Johnston, D.E. (1974). Patterns of trauma in urban dogs and cats: a study of 1,000 cases. *J. Am. Vet. Med. Assoc.* 164 (5): 499–502.

5 Risselada, M., de Rooster, H., Taeymans, O., and van Bree, H. (2008). Penetrating injuries in dogs and cats. A study of 16 cases. *Vet. Comp. Orthop. Traumatol.* 21 (5): 434–439.

6 Shaw, S.R., Rozanski, E.A., and Rush, J.E. (2003). Traumatic body wall herniation in 36 dogs and cats. *J. Am. Anim. Hosp. Assoc.* 39 (1): 35–46.

7 Kolata, R.J. and Johnston, D.E. (1975). Motor vehicle accidents in urban dogs: a study of 600 cases. *J. Am. Vet. Med. Assoc.* 167 (10): 938–941.

8 Gordon, L.E., Thacher, C., and Kapatkin, A. (1993). High-rise syndrome in dogs: 81 cases (1985–1991). *J. Am. Vet. Med. Assoc.* 202 (1): 118–122.

9 Vnuk, D., Pirkic, B., Maticic, D. et al. (2004). Feline high-rise syndrome: 119 cases (1998–2001). *J. Feline Med. Surg.* 6 (5): 305–312.

10 Fullington, R.J. and Otto, C.M. (1997). Characteristics and management of gunshot wounds in dogs and cats: 84 cases (1986–1995). *J. Am. Vet. Med. Assoc.* 210 (5): 658–662.

11 Pavletic, M.M. and Trout, N.J. (2006). Bullet, bite, and burn wounds in dogs and cats. *Vet. Clin. North Am. Small Anim. Pract.* 36 (4): 873–893.

12 Bonner, S.E., Reiter, A.M., and Lewis, J.R. (2012). Orofacial manifestations of high-rise syndrome in cats: a retrospective study of 84 cases. *J. Vet. Dent.* 29 (1): 10–18.

13 Soukup, J.W. and Snyder, C.J. (2014). Traumatic Dentoalveolar and maxillofacial injuries in cats: overview of diagnosis and management. *J. Feline Med. Surg.* 16 (11): 915–927.

14 Soukup, J.W., Hetzel, S., and Paul, A. (2015). Classification and epidemiology of traumatic Dentoalveolar injuries in dogs and cats: 959 injuries in 660 patient visits (2004–2012). *J. Vet. Dent.* 32 (1): 6–14.

15 Eugster, S., Schawalder, P., Gaschen, F., and Boerlin, P. (2004). A prospective study of postoperative surgical site infections in dogs and cats. *Vet. Surg.* 33 (5): 542–550.

16 Nicholson, M., Beal, M., Shofer, F., and Brown, D.C. (2002). Epidemiologic evaluation of postoperative wound infection in clean-contaminated wounds: a retrospective study of 239 dogs and cats. *Vet. Surg.* 31 (6): 577–581.

17 Vasseur, P.B., Levy, J., Dowd, E., and Eliot, J. (1988). Surgical wound infection rates in dogs and cats. Data from a teaching hospital. *Vet. Surg.* 17 (2): 60–64.

18 Brown, D.C., Conzemius, M.G., Shofer, F., and Swann, H. (1997). Epidemiologic evaluation of postoperative wound infections in dogs and cats. *J. Am. Vet. Med. Assoc.* 210 (9): 1302–1306.

19 Beal, M.W., Brown, D.C., and Shofer, F.S. (2000). The effects of perioperative hypothermia and the duration of anesthesia on postoperative wound infection rate in clean wounds: a retrospective study. *Vet. Surg.* 29 (2): 123–127.

20 Frey, T.N., Hoelzler, M.G., Scavelli, T.D. et al. (2010). Risk factors for surgical site infection-inflammation in dogs undergoing surgery for rupture of the cranial cruciate ligament: 902 cases (2005–2006). *J. Am. Vet. Med. Assoc.* 236 (1): 88–94.

21 Weese, J.S. (2008). A review of post-operative infections in veterinary orthopaedic surgery. *Vet. Comp. Orthop. Traumatol.* 21 (2): 99–105.

22 Munro, H.M. and Thrusfield, M.V. (2001). Battered pets': non-accidental physical injuries found in dogs and cats. *J. Small Anim. Pract.* 42 (6): 279–290.

23 Swaim, S.F., Bradley, D.M., Vaughn, D.M. et al. (1993). The greyhound dog as a model for studying pressure ulcers. *Decubitus* 6 (2): 32–35, 8–40.

24 Swaim, S.F. and Angarano, D.W. (1990). Chronic problem wounds of dog limbs. *Clin. Dermatol.* 8 (3–4): 175–186.

25 Amalsadvala, T. and Swaim, S.F. (2006). Management of hard-to-heal wounds. *Vet. Clin. North Am. Small Anim. Pract.* 36 (4): 693–711.

26 Glass, E.N., Cornetta, A.M., deLahunta, A. et al. (1998). Clinical and clinicopathologic features in 11 cats with Cuterebra larvae myiasis of the central nervous system. *J. Vet. Intern. Med.* 12 (5): 365–368.

27 Slansky, F. (2007). Feline cuterebrosis caused by a lagomorph-infesting Cuterebra spp. larva. *J. Parasitol.* 93 (4): 959–961.

28 Pelosi, A., Hauptman, J.G., Eyster, G.E. et al. (2008). Myocardial perforation by a stick foreign body in a dog. *J. Vet. Emerg. Crit. Care* 18 (2): 184–187.

29 Hartley, C., McConnell, J.F., and Doust, R. (2007). Wooden orbital foreign body in a Weimaraner. *Vet. Ophthalmol.* 10 (6): 390–393.

30 White, R.A.S. and Lane, J.G. (1988). Pharyngeal stick penetration injuries in the dog. *J. Small Anim. Pract.* 29 (1): 13–35.

31 Stein, D.J., Dodman, N.H., Borchelt, P., and Hollander, E. (1994). Behavioral disorders in veterinary practice: relevance to psychiatry. *Compr. Psychiatry* 35 (4): 275–285.

32 Scott, D.W., Miller, W.H., and Erb, H.N. (2013). Feline dermatology at Cornell University: 1407 cases (1988–2003). *J. Feline Med. Surg.* 15 (4): 307–316.

33 Aydingoz, I.E. and Mansur, A.T. (2011). Canine scabies in humans: a case report and review of the literature. *Dermatology* 223 (2): 104–106.

34 Yasukawa, K., Saito, S., Kubo, T. et al. (2010). Low-dose recombinant canine interferon-gamma for treatment of canine atopic dermatitis: an open randomized comparative trial of two doses. *Vet. Dermatol.* 21 (1): 42–49.

35 Moon-Fanelli, A.A., Dodman, N.H., and Cottam, N. (2007). Blanket and flank sucking in Doberman Pinschers. *J. Am. Vet. Med. Assoc.* 231 (6): 907–912.

36 Virga, V. (2003). Behavioral dermatology. *Vet. Clin. North Am. Small Anim. Pract.* 33 (2): 231–251, v–vi.

37 Overall, K.L. and Dunham, A.E. (2002). Clinical features and outcome in dogs and cats with obsessive-compulsive disorder: 126 cases (1989–2000). *J. Am. Vet. Med. Assoc.* 221 (10): 1445–1452.

38 Feusner, J.D., Hembacher, E., and Phillips, K.A. (2009). The mouse who couldn't stop washing: pathologic grooming in animals and humans. *CNS Spectr.* 14 (9): 503–513.

39 Famigli-Bergamini, P., Azzalini, L., Avallone, G., and Sarli, G. (2016). Pathology in practice. *J. Am. Vet. Med. Assoc.* 249 (2): 161–163.

40 De Paepe, A. and Malfait, F. (2012). The Ehlers-Danlos syndrome, a disorder with many faces. *Clin. Genet.* 82 (1): 1–11.

41 Barnett, K.C. and Cottrell, B.D. (1987). Ehlers-Danlos syndrome in a dog – ocular, cutaneous and articular abnormalities. *J. Small Anim. Pract.* 28 (10): 941–946.

42 Sequeira, J.L., Rocha, N.S., Bandarra, E.P. et al. (1999). Collagen dysplasia (cutaneous asthenia) in a cat. *Vet. Pathol.* 36 (6): 603–606.

43 Uri, M., Verin, R., Ressel, L. et al. (2015). Ehlers-Danlos syndrome associated with fatal spontaneous vascular rupture in a dog. *J. Comp. Pathol.* 152 (2–3): 211–216.

44 Barrera, R., Mane, C., Duran, E. et al. (2004). Ehlers-Danlos syndrome in a dog. *Can. Vet. J.* 45 (4): 355–356.

45 Hegreberg, G.A., Padgett, G.A., Gorham, J.R., and Henson, J.B. (1969). A connective tissue disease of dogs and mink resembling the Ehlers-Danlos syndrome of man. II. Mode of inheritance. *J. Hered.* 60 (5): 249–254.

46 Paciello, O., Lamagna, F., Lamagna, B., and Papparella, S. (2003). Ehlers-Danlos-like syndrome in 2 dogs: clinical, histologic, and ultrastructural findings. *Vet. Clin. Pathol.* 32 (1): 13–18.

47 Matthews, B.R. and Lewis, G.T. (1990). Ehlers-Danlos syndrome in a dog. *Can. Vet. J.* 31 (5): 389–390.

48 Scott, D.W., Miller, W.H., and Griffin, C.E. (1995). *Muller & Kirk's Small Animal Dermatology*, 736–805. Philadelphia: WB Saunders.

49 Furiani, N., Porcellato, I., and Brachelente, C. (2017). Reversible and cachexia-associated feline skin fragility syndrome in three cats. *Vet. Dermatol.* 28 (5): 508–e121.

50 Scott, D.W., Miller, W.H., and Griffin, C.E. (2013). *Muller and Kirk's Small Animal Dermatology*, 695–723. St Louis, MO: Elsevier Inc.

51 Rossmeisl, J.H. Jr., Scott-Moncrieff, J.C., Siems, J. et al. (2000). Hyperadrenocorticism and

hyperprogesteronemia in a cat with an adrenocortical adenocarcinoma. *J. Am. Anim. Hosp. Assoc.* 36 (6): 512–517.

52 Cross, E., Moreland, R., and Wallack, S. (2012). Feline pituitary-dependent hyperadrenocorticism and insulin resistance due to a plurihormonal adenoma. *Top. Companion Anim. Med.* 27 (1): 8–20.

53 McKiernan, B.C., Adams, W.M., and Huse, D.C. (1984). Thoracic bite wounds and associated internal injury in 11 dogs and 1 cat. *J. Am. Vet. Med. Assoc.* 184 (8): 959–964.

54 Cowell, A.K. and Penwick, R.C. (1989). Dog bite Wounds – a study of 93 cases. *Compend. Cont. Educ. Pract.* 11 (3): 313–320.

55 Trott, A. (1988). Mechanisms of surface soft tissue trauma. *Ann. Emerg. Med.* 17 (12): 1279–1283.

56 Goldstein, E.J. and Richwald, G.A. (1987). Human and animal bite wounds. *Am. Fam. Physician* 36 (1): 101–109.

57 Swaim, S.F. and Henderson, R.A. (1992). *Bite Wounds. Small Animal Wound Management*, 112–117. Philadelphia: Lippincott.

58 Swaim, S.F. (2002). Penetrating wounds. In: *The Veterinary ICU Book* (ed. W.E. Wingfield and M.R. Raffe), 967–970. Jackson Hole, WY: Teton New Media.

59 Brook, I. (2005). Management of human and animal bite wounds: an overview. *Adv. Skin Wound Care* 18 (4): 197–203.

60 Talan, D.A., Citron, D.M., Abrahamian, F.M. et al. (1999). Bacteriologic analysis of infected dog and cat bites. Emergency medicine animal bite infection study group. *N. Engl. J. Med.* 340 (2): 85–92.

61 Waldron, D.R. and Trevor, P. (1993). Management of superficial skin wounds. In: *Textbook of Small Animal Surgery* (ed. D. Slatter), 269. Philadelphia: WB Saunders.

62 Lewis, K.T. and Stiles, M. (1995). Management of cat and dog bites. *Am. Fam. Physician* 52 (2): 479–485, 89–90.

63 Pavletic, M.M. (1999). *Management of Specific Wounds. Atlas of Small Animal Reconstructive Surgery*, 66–95. Philadelphia: WB Saunders.

64 Davidson, E.B. (1998). Managing bite wounds in dogs and cats – part II. *Compend. Cont. Educ. Pract.* 20 (9): 974–991.

65 Demaria, M., Stanley, B.J., Hauptman, J.G. et al. (2011). Effects of negative pressure wound therapy on healing of open wounds in dogs. *Vet. Surg.* 40 (6): 658–669.

66 Owen, L., Hotston-Moore, A., and Holt, P. (2009). Vacuum-assisted wound closure following urine-induced skin and thigh muscle necrosis in a cat. *Vet. Comp. Orthop. Traumatol.* 22 (5): 417–421.

67 Guille, A.E., Tseng, L.W., and Orsher, R.J. (2007). Use of vacuum-assisted closure for management of a large skin wound in a cat. *J. Am. Vet. Med. Assoc.* 230 (11): 1669–1673.

68 Ben-Amotz, R., Lanz, O.I., Miller, J.M. et al. (2007). The use of vacuum-assisted closure therapy for the treatment of distal extremity wounds in 15 dogs. *Vet. Surg.* 36 (7): 684–690.

69 AVMA Model Rabies Control Ordinance: American Veterinary Medical Association. https://www.avma.org/KB/Policies/Documents/avma-model-rabies-ordinance.pdf.

70 Campbell, B.G. (2011). Managing degloving and shearing injuries. *NAVC Clinician's Brief* (October): 75–79.

71 Beardsley, S.L. and Schrader, S.C. (1995). Treatment of dogs with wounds of the limbs caused by shearing forces: 98 cases (1975–1993). *J. Am. Vet. Med. Assoc.* 207 (8): 1071–1075.

72 Benson, J.A. and Boudrieau, R.J. (2002). Severe carpal and tarsal shearing injuries treated with an immediate arthrodesis in seven dogs. *J. Am. Anim. Hosp. Assoc.* 38 (4): 370–380.

73 Diamond, D.W., Besso, J., and Boudrieau, R.J. (1999). Evaluation of joint stabilization for treatment of shearing injuries of the tarsus in 20 dogs. *J. Am. Anim. Hosp. Assoc.* 35 (2): 147–153.

74 Harasen, G.L. (2000). Tarsal shearing injuries in the dog. *Can. Vet. J.* 41 (12): 940–943.

75 Balsa, I.M. and Culp, W.T. (2015). Wound care. *Vet. Clin. North Am. Small Anim. Pract.* 45 (5): 1049–1065.

76 Campbell, B.G. (2006). Dressings, bandages, and splints for wound management in dogs and cats. *Vet. Clin. North Am. Small Anim. Pract.* 36 (4): 759–791.

77 Perez-Tamayo, R. and Ihnen, M. (1953). The effect of methionine in experimental wound healing; a morphologic study. *Am. J. Pathol.* 29 (2): 233–249.

78 Blomme, E.A., Chinn, K.S., Hardy, M.M. et al. (2003). Selective cyclooxygenase-2 inhibition does not affect the healing of cutaneous full-thickness incisional wounds in SKH-1 mice. *Br. J. Dermatol.* 148 (2): 211–223.

79 Stephens, F.O., Hunt, T.K., Jawetz, E. et al. (1971). Effect of cortisone and vitamin a on wound infection. *Am. J. Surg.* 121 (5): 569–571.

80 Laing, E.J. (1990). Problems in wound healing associated with chemotherapy and radiation therapy. *Probl. Vet. Med.* 2 (3): 433–441.

81 Amsellem, P. (2011). Complications of reconstructive surgery in companion animals. *Vet. Clin. North Am. Small Anim. Pract.* 41 (5): 995–1006, vii.

82 Tobias, K.M. and Johnston, S.A. (2012). *Veterinary Surgery: Small Animal*. St. Louis, MO: Elsevier/Saunders.

83 Davidson, J.R. (2015). Current concepts in wound management and wound healing products. *Vet. Clin. North Am. Small Anim. Pract.* 45 (3): 537–564.

84 Johnston, D.E. (1990). Care of accidental wounds. *Vet. Clin. North Am. Small Anim. Pract.* 20 (1): 27–46.

85 Sanchez, I.R., Nusbaum, K.E., Swaim, S.F. et al. (1988). Chlorhexidine diacetate and povidone-iodine cytotoxicity to canine embryonic fibroblasts and Staphylococcus aureus. *Vet. Surg.* 17 (4): 182–185.

86 Buffa, E.A., Lubbe, A.M., Verstraete, F.J., and Swaim, S.F. (1997). The effects of wound lavage solutions on canine fibroblasts: an in vitro study. *Vet. Surg.* 26 (6): 460–466.

87 Pavletic, M.M. (2010). *Atlas of Small Animal Wound Management and Reconstructive Surgery*. Ames, IA: Wiley-Blackwell.

88 Hedlund, C. (2007). Surgery of the integumentary system. In: *Small Animal Surgery* (ed. T.W. Fossum), 159–259. St. Louis, MO: Mosby Elsevier.

89 Fahie, M.A. and Shettko, D. (2007). Evidence-based wound management: a systematic review of therapeutic agents to enhance granulation and epithelialization. *Vet. Clin. North Am. Small Anim. Pract.* 37 (3): 559–577.

90 Edlich, R.F., Rodeheaver, G.T., Morgan, R.F. et al. (1988). Principles of emergency wound management. *Ann. Emerg. Med.* 17 (12): 1284–1302.

91 Stevenson, T.R., Thacker, J.G., Rodeheaver, G.T. et al. (1976). Cleansing the traumatic wound by high pressure syringe irrigation. *JACEP* 5 (1): 17–21.

92 Haury, B., Rodeheaver, G., Vensko, J. et al. (1978). Debridement: an essential component of traumatic wound care. *Am. J. Surg.* 135 (2): 238–242.

93 Hohn, D.C., MacKay, R.D., Halliday, B., and Hunt, T.K. (1976). Effect of O2 tension on microbicidal function of leukocytes in wounds and in vitro. *Surg. Forum* 27 (62): 18–20.

94 Mayet, N., Choonara, Y.E., Kumar, P. et al. (2014). A comprehensive review of advanced biopolymeric wound healing systems. *J. Pharm. Sci.* 103 (8): 2211–2230.

95 Boateng, J.S., Matthews, K.H., Stevens, H.N., and Eccleston, G.M. (2008). Wound healing dressings and drug delivery systems: a review. *J. Pharm. Sci.* 97 (8): 2892–2923.

96 Heyer, K., Augustin, M., Protz, K. et al. (2013). Effectiveness of advanced versus conventional wound dressings on healing of chronic wounds: systematic review and meta-analysis. *Dermatology* 226 (2): 172–184.

97 Alford, C.G., Caldwell, F.J., and Hanson, R. (2012). Equine distal limb wounds: new and emerging treatments. *Compend. Contin. Educ. Vet.* 34 (7): E5.

98 Armstrong, D.G., Mossel, J., Short, B. et al. (2002). Maggot debridement therapy: a primer. *J. Am. Podiatr. Med. Assoc.* 92 (7): 398–401.

99 Falch, B.M., de Weerd, L., and Sundsfjord, A. (2009). Maggot therapy in wound management. *Tidsskr. Nor. Laegeforen.* 129 (18): 1864–1867.

100 Cummings, P. (1994). Antibiotics to prevent infection in patients with dog bite wounds: a meta-analysis of randomized trials. *Ann. Emerg. Med.* 23 (3): 535–540.

101 Dire, D.J. (1992). Emergency management of dog and cat bite wounds. *Emerg. Med. Clin. North Am.* 10 (4): 719–736.

102 Krahwinkel, D.J. and Boothe, H.W. Jr. (2006). Topical and systemic medications for wounds. *Vet. Clin. North Am. Small Anim. Pract.* 36 (4): 739–757.

103 Forrest, R.D. (1982). Development of wound therapy from the dark ages to the present. *J. R. Soc. Med.* 75 (4): 268–273.

104 Mathews, K.A. and Binnington, A.G. (2002). Wound management using honey. *Compend. Cont. Educ. Pract.* 24 (1): 53–60.

105 White, J.W. (1966). Inhibine and glucose oxidase in honey: a review. *Am. Bee J.* 106: 214–216.

106 White, J.W. Jr., Subers, M.H., and Schepartz, A.I. (1963). The identification of inhibine, the antibacterial factor in honey, as hydrogen peroxide and its origin in a honey glucose-oxidase system. *Biochim. Biophys. Acta* 73: 57–70.

107 Molan, P.C. (1992). The antibacterial activity of honey .1. The nature of the antibacterial activity. *Bee World* 73 (1): 5–28.

108 Molan, P.C. (1992). The antibacterial activity of honey . 2. Variation in the potency of the antibacterial activity. *Bee World* 73 (2): 59–76.

109 Hyslop, P.A., Hinshaw, D.B., Scraufstatter, I.U. et al. (1995). Hydrogen-peroxide as a potent bacteriostatic antibiotic – implications for host-defense. *Free Radic. Biol. Med.* 19 (1): 31–37.

110 Frankel, S., Robinson, G.E., and Berenbaum, M.R. (1998). Antioxidant capacity and correlated characteristics of 14 unifloral honeys. *J. Apic. Res.* 37: 27.

111 Molan, P.C. (1999). The role of honey in the management of wounds. *J. Wound Care* 8 (8): 415–418.

112 Cooper, R.A. and Molan, P.C. (1999). Honey in wound care. *J. Wound Care* 8 (7): 340.

113 Matthews, K.A. and Binnington, A.G. (2002). Wound management using sugar. *Compend. Contin. Educ. Vet.* 24 (1): 41–52.

114 Willix, D.J., Molan, P.C., and Harfoot, C.G. (1992). A comparison of the sensitivity of wound-infecting species of bacteria to the antibacterial activity of manuka honey and other honey. *J. Appl. Bacteriol.* 73 (5): 388–394.

115 Obaseiki-Ebor, E.E. and Afonya, T.C. (1984). In-vitro evaluation of the anticandidiasis activity of honey distillate (HY-1) compared with that of some antimycotic agents. *J. Pharm. Pharmacol.* 36 (4): 283–284.

116 Dryden, M., Lockyer, G., Saeed, K., and Cooke, J. (2014). Engineered honey: in vitro antimicrobial activity of a novel topical wound care treatment. *J. Glob. Antimicrob. Resist.* 2 (3): 168–172.

117 Kaufman, T., Eichenlaub, E.H., Angel, M.F. et al. (1985). Topical acidification promotes healing of experimental deep partial thickness skin burns – a randomized double-blind preliminary-study. *Burns* 12 (2): 84–90.

118 Bergman, A., Yanai, J., Weiss, J. et al. (1983). Acceleration of wound healing by topical application of honey. An animal model. *Am. J. Surg.* 145 (3): 374–376.

119 Subrahmanyam, M. (1998). A prospective randomised clinical and histological study of superficial burn wound healing with honey and silver sulfadiazine. *Burns* 24 (2): 157–161.

120 Kamut, N. (1993). Use of sugar in infected wounds. *Trop. Dr.* 23 (4): 185–188.

121 Chirife, J., Scarmato, G., and Herszage, L. (1982). Scientific basis for use of granulated sugar in treatment of infected wounds. *Lancet* 1 (8271): 560–561.

122 Shakoor, A., Muhammad, S.A., and Kashif, M. (2011). Surgical rectification of paraphimosis associated with tumorous growth in a dog. *IJAVMS* 5 (5): 452–455.

123 Coburn, W.M. 3rd, Russell, M.A., and Hofstetter, W.L. (1997). Sucrose as an aid to manual reduction of incarcerated rectal prolapse. *Ann. Emerg. Med.* 30 (3): 347–349.

124 Hovey, M.A. and Metcalf, A.M. (1997). Incarcerated rectal prolapse – rupture and ileal evisceration after failed reduction – report of a case. *Dis. Colon Rectum* 40 (10): 1254–1257.

125 Miesner, M.D. and Anderson, D.E. (2008). Management of uterine and vaginal prolapse in the bovine. *Vet. Clin. North Am. Food Anim. Pract.* 24 (2): 409–419, ix.

126 Bohling, M.W., Henderson, R.A., Swaim, S.F. et al. (2004). Cutaneous wound healing in the cat: a macroscopic description and comparison with cutaneous wound healing in the dog. *Vet. Surg.* 33 (6): 579–587.

127 Bohling, M.W. and Henderson, R.A. (2006). Differences in cutaneous wound healing between dogs and cats. *Vet. Clin. North Am. Small Anim. Pract.* 36 (4): 687–692.

128 Taylor, G.I. and Minabe, T. (1992). The angiosomes of the mammals and other vertebrates. *Plast. Reconstr. Surg.* 89 (2): 181–215.

129 Hartmann, M., Jonsson, K., and Zederfeldt, B. (1992). Effect of tissue perfusion and oxygenation on accumulation of collagen in healing wounds. Randomized study in patients after major abdominal operations. *Eur. J. Surg.* 158 (10): 521–526.

130 Jonsson, K., Jensen, J.A., Goodson, W.H. 3rd et al. (1991). Tissue oxygenation, anemia, and perfusion in relation to wound healing in surgical patients. *Ann. Surg.* 214 (5): 605–613.

131 Grillo, H.C., Watts, G.T., and Gross, J. (1958). Studies in wound healing: I. Contraction and the wound contents. *Ann. Surg.* 148 (2): 145–160.

132 Abercrombie, M., Flint, M.H., and James, D.W. (1956). Wound contraction in relation to collagen formation in scorbutic Guinea-pigs. *J. Embryol. Exp. Morpholog.* 4 (2): 167–175.

133 Gray, M.J. (2005). Chronic axillary wound repair in a cat with omentalisation and omocervical skin flap. *J. Small Anim. Pract.* 46 (10): 499–503.

134 Lascelles, B.D., Davison, L., Dunning, M. et al. (1998). Use of omental pedicle grafts in the management of non-healing axillary wounds in 10 cats. *J. Small Anim. Pract.* 39 (10): 475–480.

135 Lascelles, B.D. and White, R.A. (2001). Combined omental pedicle grafts and thoracodorsal axial pattern flaps for the reconstruction of chronic, nonhealing axillary wounds in cats. *Vet. Surg.* 30 (4): 380–385.

136 Pavletic, M.M. (1994). Surgery of the skin and management of wounds. In: *The Cat: Diseases and Clinical Management* (ed. R.G. Sherding), 1969–1997. Edinburgh: Churchill Livingstone.

5

Hypotrichosis and Alopecia

5.1 An Introduction to Hypotrichosis and Alopecia in Companion Animal Medicine

Fur thinning and fur loss are common presentations in companion animal medicine [1–4]. *Hypotrichosis* refers to the former condition, and *alopecia* refers to the latter [2]. The lists of differential diagnoses for both conditions are quite extensive. History taking and pattern recognition by experienced clinicians facilitate diagnostic work-ups that lead to answers. Specifically, the following questions may be beneficial in narrowing down the differentials list:

- Does the patient have any other clinical signs?
- Is the fur loss regional?
- Is the fur loss symmetrical?

When affected patients present for veterinary evaluation, they may have concurrent clinical signs that provide clues as to the likely diagnosis. For example, patients that present with fur loss and pruritus are likely to have underlying inflammatory skin disease such as atopic dermatitis [2].

The location of fur thinning or fur loss is equally important. Vasculitis may result in focal alopecia at the site of vaccinations [3]. Focal alopecia may also be associated with superficial bacterial folliculitis [3]. Focal alopecia at the tail base, in combination with flea dirt, is confirmatory for flea allergy dermatitis.

Certain conditions, such as dermatophytosis and demodicosis, may cause local or generalized fur loss [1, 3–5]. When focal disease manifests, certain locations may be more likely to be affected. For example, the muzzle and feet are common sites of fur thinning or fur loss in dogs that present with juvenile-onset localized demodicosis [3, 5, 6]. By contrast, sarcoptic mange lesions in canine patients tend to concentrate on the head, pinnae, elbows, and hocks [7, 8].

The symmetry of lesions, in addition to their location, provides yet another clue. For example, the presence of bilaterally symmetrical truncal alopecia is highly suggestive of endocrine and/or metabolic disease [4]. Hypothyroidism, hyperadrenocorticism, and sex hormone imbalances must be considered in affected patients [4]. In addition, iatrogenic causes for such presentations must be ruled out [4]. Exogenous administration of glucocorticoids can induce hyperadrenocorticism [4]. Inadvertent exogenous exposure to human topical hormone replacement therapy can induce hyperestrogenism [9, 10].

The goal of this chapter is to create broad categories for causes of hypotrichosis and alopecia so that the novice clinician has a starting point for working up cases involving dermatopathy.

5.2 Species-Specific Focal Alopecia

Peri-aural hypotrichosis or alopecia is common in healthy feline patients. Sometimes these conditions are referred to as pre-auricular hypotrichosis or alopecia. Either clinical presentation is normal provided that the underlying skin is intact [11] (see Figures 5.1a–c).

The presence of skin lesions within the pre-auricular alopecic zone is suggestive of underlying disease (see Figure 5.2).

Scabs, crusts, and curvilinear excoriations may be the result of battle wounds or self-trauma. For example, cats with otitis externa or *Otodectes cynotis* infestation may exhibit pruritus, which may lead to superficial scratch wounds at the affected ear(s) (see Figures 5.3a, b).

5.3 Tardive Hypotrichosis or Alopecia

Some canine and feline patients are born with normal coats. However, as they age, they develop fur thinning or fur loss. These conditions are referred to as tardive hypotrichosis or alopecia, respectively. Fur loss may be focal, regional, or generalized. Symmetry of fur loss is common. Young adults are affected most often, although

(a)

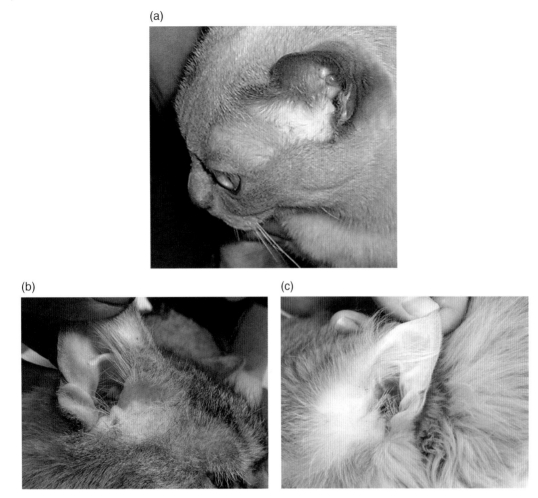

(b)   (c)

Figure 5.1 (a). Peri-aural hypotrichosis in a Tonkinese cat. (b). Peri-aural hypotrichosis in a Domestic short-haired cat. *Source:* Courtesy of Patricia Bennett, DVM. (c). Peri-aural alopecia in a Domestic Medium-haired cat. *Source:* Courtesy of Media Resources at Midwestern University.

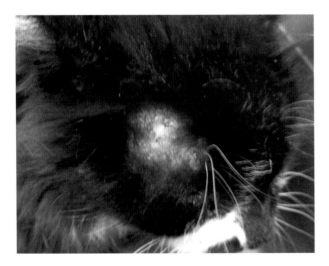

Figure 5.2 Traumatized skin in a pruritic feline patient. Note that the patient's peri-aural hypotrichosis is normal; however, the presence of scabs and crusting is not. *Source:* Courtesy of Patricia Bennett, DVM.

the condition may first become apparent when the canine patient sheds out its puppy coat [4, 12].

5.3.1 Pattern Baldness

Pattern baldness is a specific type of tardive hypotrichosis or alopecia that occurs regionally. Dogs are affected more often than cats, and certain breeds appear with frequency in the literature [4, 12].

Four types of pattern baldness have been reported in companion animal medicine [4, 12]. One type of pattern baldness is pinnal alopecia. Among dogs, this condition is specific to Dachshunds. However, cats may also be affected [4, 12]. There may be a predisposition for males [4].

Young adults experience thinning of fur along the dorsal aspect of both pinnae between six and nine months of age. Hypotrichosis progresses to alopecia over time, and exposed skin may develop hyperpigmentation. The remainder of the coat is unaffected [4, 12] (see Figures 5.4a, b).

(a)   (b)

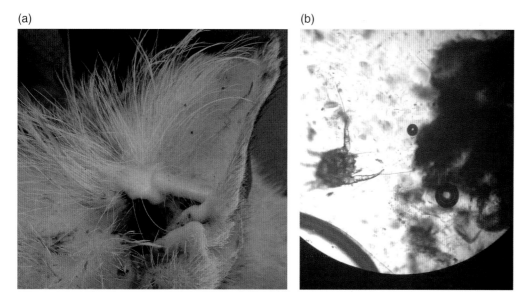

Figure 5.3 (a). Gross examination of the entrance to the external ear canal of a feline patient with otitis externa. *Source:* Courtesy of Kara Thomas, DVM, CVMA. (b). Light microscopy of an aural swab that is positive for *Otodectes cynotis*. Ear mites often induce pruritus, which may lead to curvilinear scratch marks and damage to the pre-auricular skin. *Source:* Courtesy of Kimberly Wallitsch, DVM Class of 2019, Midwestern University College of Veterinary Medicine.

(a)   (b)

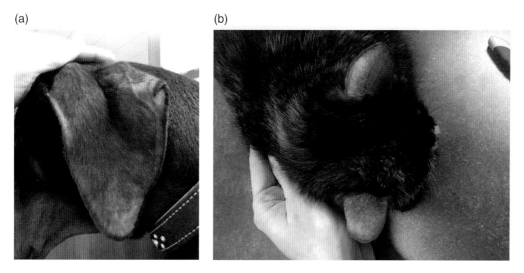

Figure 5.4 (a). Pinnal alopecia in a Dachshund. Although only the left ear is pictured here, hair loss was symmetrical in this patient. *Source:* Courtesy of Dr. Elizabeth Robbins. (b). Pinnal alopecia in a cat. *Source:* Courtesy of Sarah Bashaw, DVM.

Ventral and caudal alopecia have been reported as a second type of pattern baldness in Dachshunds, Boston Terriers, Manchester Terriers, Whippets, and Chihuahuas [4]. The age at onset and progression of the syndrome is similar to pinnal alopecia. There may be a predisposition for females [4] (see Figures 5.5a–c).

A third type of pattern baldness has been reported in Portuguese Water Dogs and American Water Spaniels [4, 12]. Alopecia can be extensive, involving not only the ventral and lateral neck, but also the trunk and thighs. Both males and females may be affected; however, the onset of estrous cycles in females may hasten or worsen alopecia [4, 12].

Greyhounds develop their own unique type of pattern baldness, bald thigh syndrome. Classically, this presents as caudal thigh hypotrichosis or alopecia; however, alopecia may extend to the ventrum [4, 12] (see Figures 5.6a, b).

Note that the skin in regions that are affected by pattern baldness is intact. The presence of lesions in these areas is suggestive of unrelated, underlying skin disease (see Figure 5.7).

(a)

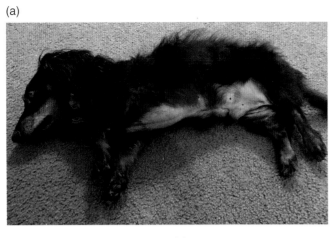

(b)

(c)

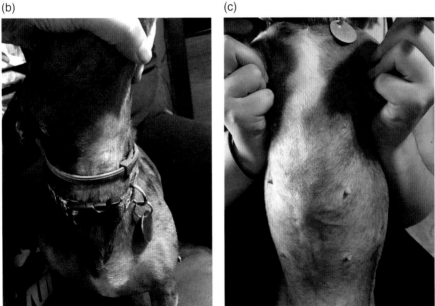

Figure 5.5 (a). Alopecia of the ventrum in a Long-haired Dachshund. *Source:* Courtesy of Hilary Lazarus, DVM. (b). Ventral neck and chest alopecia in a Dachshund. *Source:* Courtesy of Erin M. Miracle. (c). Alopecia of the ventrum in a Dachshund. *Source:* Courtesy of Erin M. Miracle.

5.3.2 Black Hair Follicular Dysplasia

Follicular dysplasia refers to abnormal growth and development of the hair follicle, leading to structurally defective hair shafts and hypotrichosis that progresses to alopecia [13]. Black hair follicular dysplasia affects black fur only, and has been reported in several breeds [12, 14, 15]. These include Dachshunds, Jack Russell Terriers, King Charles Cavalier Spaniels, Salukis, Bearded, and Border Collies, Beagles, Basset Hounds, Pointers, Gordon Setters, Doberman Pinschers, Large Münsterländer, and New Zealand Huntaway dogs [12, 14, 16–25]. An autosomal recessive mode of inheritance has been suspected [16].

Once patients become alopecic, they will not experience regrowth of the affected black fur.

Trichograms of affected hairs demonstrate clumps of melanin in the cortex and medulla in addition to other defects, including fractures of the hair cuticle [13, 17, 23, 26–28].

Patients with black hair follicular dysplasia are predisposed to follicular plugging with keratin containing melanin aggregates [19]. In addition, affected dogs may be more likely to develop secondary bacterial skin infections [19].

5.3.3 Color Dilution Alopecia

Another form of follicular dysplasia is color dilution alopecia [13, 21, 26, 29]. Any dilutely pigmented dog may be affected; however, this condition is most commonly reported in blue, red, and fawn-coated patients.

(a)

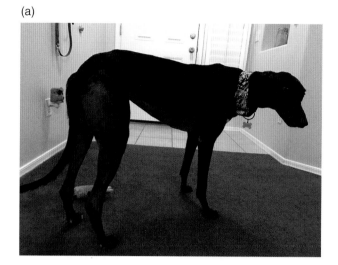

(b)

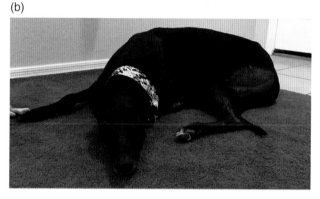

Figure 5.6 (a). Lateral view of bald thigh syndrome in a Greyhound. *Source:* Courtesy of Hilary Lazarus, DVM. (b). Alternate view of bald thigh syndrome in a Greyhound. *Source:* Courtesy of Hilary Lazarus, DVM.

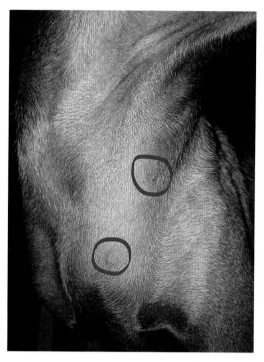

Figure 5.7 The presence of a papular rash is indicative of dermatopathy that is unrelated to ventral neck alopecia. Pyoderma was confirmed via cytological impression smears of ruptured pustules. *Source:* Courtesy of Kelly Bradley, DVM.

The most common breeds to appear in the literature include Doberman Pinschers, Miniature Pinschers, Dachshunds, Chow Chows, Standard Poodles, Great Danes, Italian Greyhounds, Whippets, Chihuahuas, Shetland Sheepdogs, Yorkshire, and Silky Terriers [12, 13, 21, 22, 29–39].

An autosomal recessive mode of inheritance has been confirmed in Wire-Haired Dachshunds, and is suspected for most other breeds [26].

A change in coat quality precedes progressive hypotrichosis. The affected fur becomes dull, dry, and brittle (see Figures 5.8a–f).

Papules and comedones may develop in alopecic regions (see Figure 5.9).

Trichogram findings are similar to those reported for black hair follicular dysplasia.

Affected patients are also predisposed to follicular plugging and secondary bacterial infections [30].

5.4 Non-Color-Linked, Cyclical Follicular Dysplasias

Follicular dysplasias are not always linked to coat color. An example is canine idiopathic recurrent flank alopecia, otherwise referred to as seasonal flank alopecia. This cyclical condition is characterized by regional alopecia regardless of coat color [13, 40–44].

Both idiopathic recurrent flank alopecia and seasonal flank alopecia are misnomers because the thorax or lumbar regions may also be affected, with or without flank involvement [40].

Both males and females, intact or neutered, may be affected [13, 42–44]. Certain breeds appear to be predisposed, including Affenpinschers, Doberman Pinschers, Boxers, English Bulldogs, Miniature Schnauzers, Miniature Poodles, Bouvier de Flandres, Airedale, and Scottish Terriers [40, 42–45].

Fur loss occurs annually and often spontaneously resolves without therapy. Affected patients have normal growth hormone activity, and intact patients have normal reproductive hormone profiles [40].

Exposed skin may become hyperpigmented (see Figure 5.10).

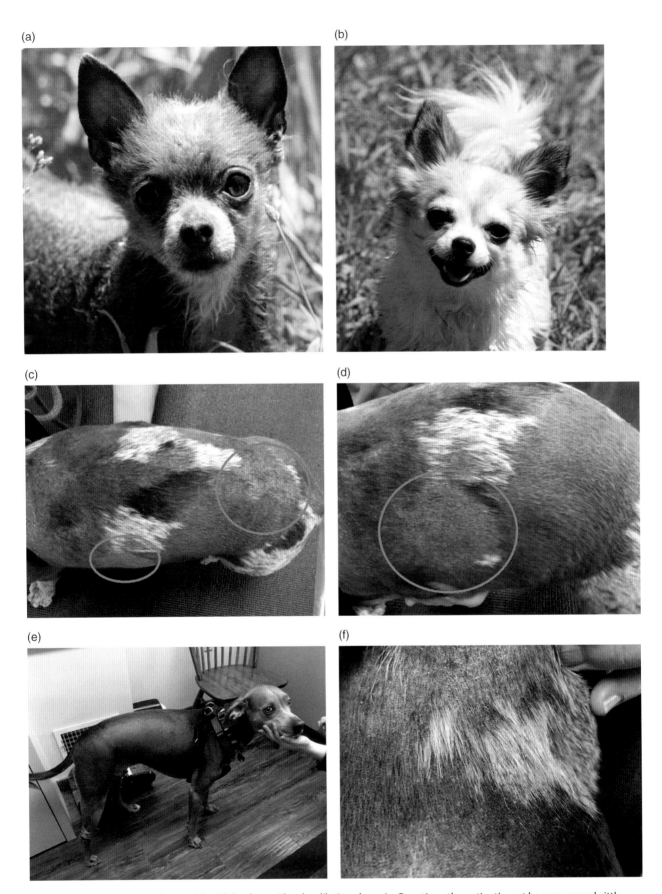

Figure 5.8 (a). Poor coat quality in a blue Chihuahua with color dilution alopecia. Over time, the patient's coat became more brittle. Progressive hypotrichosis ensued. *Source:* Courtesy of Cheri Erwin. (b). Contrast the poor coat quality in Figure 5.8a with the superior coat quality in this canine patient that lacks color dilution alopecia. *Source:* Courtesy of Cheri Erwin. (c). Color dilution alopecia in an adult Dachshund. Note the progressive loss of the blue coat color. (d). Color dilution alopecia in an adult Dachshund. Note the progressive loss of the blue coat color. (e). Color dilution alopecia in an adult dog. *Source:* Courtesy of Jackie Kucskar. (f). Color dilution alopecia in an adult dog. *Source:* Courtesy of Dr. Elizabeth Robbins.

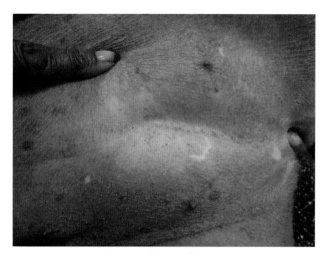

Figure 5.9 Comedones along the ventrum of a canine patient. *Source:* Courtesy of Patricia Bennett, DVM.

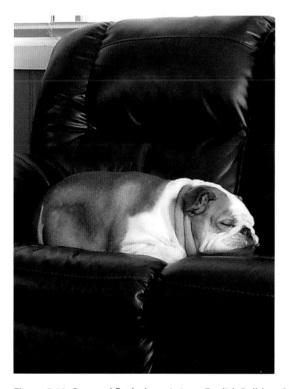

Figure 5.10 Seasonal flank alopecia in an English Bulldog. *Source:* Courtesy of Tara Beugel.

Flank alopecia may bear a striking resemblance to the bilaterally symmetrical truncal alopecia that stems from underlying endocrinopathies such as hypothyroidism, hyperadrenocorticism, hyposomatotropism, and sex-hormone-related dermatoses [42, 46–52]. Therefore, flank alopecia is a diagnosis of exclusion.

5.5 Non-Color-Linked, Non-Cyclical Follicular Dysplasias

Unlike canine idiopathic recurrent flank alopecia, follicular dysplasias such as Alopecia X are non-cyclical. Alopecia X is a condition that occurs primarily in Nordic breeds and others with plush coats [53–55]. These breeds include Pomeranians, Chow Chows, Keeshonds, Siberian Huskies, and Alaskan Malamutes [4, 53, 56, 57]. Case reports of Miniature and Toy Poodles have also appeared in the veterinary literature.

Other descriptors for this condition have included adrenal hyperplasia-like syndrome and growth hormone-responsive alopecia [4, 53–55].

Patients with Alopecia X are not systemically ill; however, they appear as if they have retained their puppy coat because of the loss of primary hairs [4]. As the condition progresses, their coats demonstrate bilaterally symmetrical truncal alopecia. Because this pattern distribution spares the head and forelimbs, it can mirror the clinical signs that are classic for hypothyroidism and hyperadrenocorticism [53]. A comprehensive diagnostic work-up is required to rule out endocrinopathy. Alopecia X is a diagnosis of exclusion.

Historically, some patients have responded to exogenous supplementation with growth hormone, much like the condition's name implies [53, 58]. Hair regrowth with treatment may be complete or partial. However, because growth hormone may increase the chance of developing diabetes mellitus, alternative therapies have been explored [53]. Anecdotally and experimentally, melatonin administration has been effective [53, 59, 60]. So, too, has mitotane and parenteral medroxyprogesterone acetate, although neither drug is without adverse effect [56, 61].

5.6 Congenital Hypotrichosis and Alopecia as Additional Causes of Non-Endocrine, Non-Inflammatory Hair Loss

Congenital hypotrichosis and alopecia may result from either a reduced number of hair follicles or structural defects in hair follicles. Most cases in companion animal medicine are due to the latter [62].

Hairless dogs are relatively uncommon. There are four primary breeds [62]:

- Mexican Hairless or Xoloitzcuintli
- Chinese Crested
- Inca Hairless
- Peruvian Inca Orchid

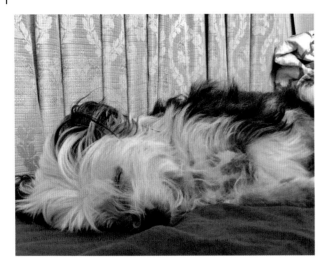

Figure 5.11 A Powderpuff Chinese Crested dog. *Source:* Courtesy of J. Chang.

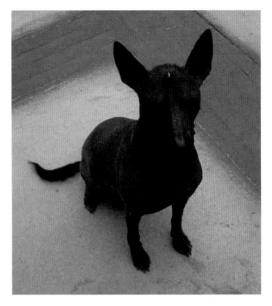

Figure 5.12 A Peruvian Inca Orchid dog. *Source:* Courtesy of Danielle Cucuzella.

The gene for hairlessness is inherited as an autosomal dominant trait [62–64]. Breedings are capable of producing both haired and hairless siblings.

Mexican Hairless dogs carry the hairless allele, Hm [62]. Patients that are homozygous dominant are almost exclusively hairless, meaning that they only have a few tufts on the dorsum of the head and at the tail tip [62]. They also often have missing or abnormally shaped teeth because both dentition and hairlessness are caused by underlying ectodermal dysplasia [62].

The hairless allele, Hr, in Chinese Crested dogs is prenatally lethal when inherited as homozygous dominant. Therefore, hairless Chinese Crested dogs are heterozygotes [62]. These patients are hairless except for the dorsum of the head, tail, and lower extremities [62]. Littermates that are fully furred are homozygous recessive for Hr, and are called "powderpuffs" [65] (see Figure 5.11).

The Peruvian Inca Orchid dog is exceptionally rare (see Figure 5.12).

There are also hairless cats. The primary breed of hairless cats in the United States is the Sphynx, whereas the Donskoy is a more popular hairless breed of cat in Russia.

Hairless crosses with haired breeds may also produce hairless offspring. Consider, for example, these lesser-known breeds:

- The Elf Cat: a hybrid of the American Curl cat and the Sphynx
- The Ukrainian Levkoy: a hybrid of the Scottish Fold cat and the Sphynx
- The Bambino: a hybrid of the Munchkin and the Sphynx

Sphynx cats lack fur except for short tufts on the ears, muzzle, tail, and feet [62] (see Figures 5.13a, b).

Comedones are prominent in both hairless dogs and cats. They represent an accumulation of keratin within plugged hair follicles [62]. In particular, comedones tend to concentrate along the topline, ventral neck, and distal extremities [66]. Sebaceous and apocrine glands may or may not be developed in hairless patients [67].

5.7 Endocrine, Non-Inflammatory Hair Loss

Endocrinopathies may result in progressive hypotrichosis to alopecia. Hormonal alopecia can be the result of [68]

- Hypothyroidism
- Hyperadrenocorticism
- Hyperestrogenism
- Exposure to human topical hormone replacement therapy.

Of the conditions listed above, hypothyroidism is the most common cause of endocrine, non-inflammatory hair loss in dogs [69]. Pathophysiology of hypothyroidism typically involves thyroid atrophy or lymphocytic thyroiditis. Either condition reduces the functional capacity of the thyroid [69].

Acquired hypothyroidism rather than congenital hypothyroidism is most typical in terms of presentation, with middle-aged to older canine patients being over-represented [69]. Commonly affected breeds include Doberman Pinschers, Golden Retrievers, Old English Sheepdogs, Irish Setters, and Great Danes [69]. Hypothyroid patients whose breeds are high risk may present with clinical signs as early as two to three years of age [69, 70].

(a)
(b)

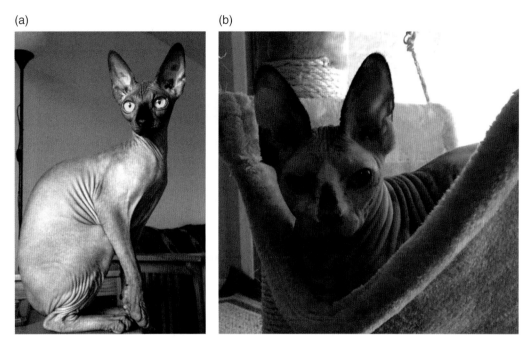

Figure 5.13 (a). A Sphynx cat. *Source:* Courtesy of Brittany Hyde, DVM. (b). A Sphynx cat. *Source:* Courtesy of Brittany Hyde, DVM.

Clients may report increased weight gain without increased daily caloric intake due to a sluggish metabolism. Their mentation may also be dull. In addition, dogs may be cold- or exercise-intolerant [69].

Multiple systems may be affected, including the following [69]:

- Central nervous system
  - Ataxia, head tilt, and seizure disorders
- Peripheral nervous system
  - Knuckling
- Cardiovascular system
  - Bradycardia
- Musculoskeletal system
  - Muscle weakness
  - Slow, stiff gait

Systems that are less likely to be involved include the following [69]:

- Gastrointestinal system
  - Constipation
- Special Senses
  - Anterior uveitis
  - Corneal lipid deposits
- Urogenital system
  - Testicular atrophy and infertility in male patients
  - Irregular cycles and infertility in female patients

Because the thyroid plays a significant role in hair growth and replacement, there are several cutaneous manifestations of disease [68, 69]. Hypothyroid patients classically present with "ring around the collar," meaning that there is an alopecic patch outlining the neck, and/or "rat tail" [69] (see Figures 5.14a, b).

Hypothyroid patients may also demonstrate the classic endocrine dermatologic abnormality, bilaterally symmetrical truncal alopecia [71].

Other common sites of alopecia include pressure points, such as over the elbows and hips [69]. Callus formation may be quite pronounced (see Figure 5.15).

Coats may also fail to regrow after clipping, or the loss of guard hairs may give the illusion that the "puppy coat" has been retained [69, 72].

Hypothyroidism in and of itself is a non-pruritic disease [69]. However, hypothyroid dogs often succumb to secondary bacterial and/or fungal infections that are likely to induce pruritus [69].

After diagnostic confirmation of hypothyroidism, treatment is initiated to supplement affected patients with thyroxine.

Canine hyperadrenocorticism, otherwise known as Cushing's syndrome, is another common cause of endocrine, non-inflammatory hair loss. Naturally occurring Cushing's syndrome results from endogenous overproduction of glucocorticoids. Exogenous sources of glucocorticoids can also cause an iatrogenic form of Cushing's syndrome. Both naturally occurring and iatrogenic Cushing's syndrome cause hair loss [69, 70].

Clients may report excessive thirst, urination, and appetite. In the medical record, this is often transcribed as "PU/PD/PP" – polyuria, polydipsia, and polyphagia. In addition, dogs may develop a pot-bellied appearance. The pendulous abdomen results from the

(a)

(b)

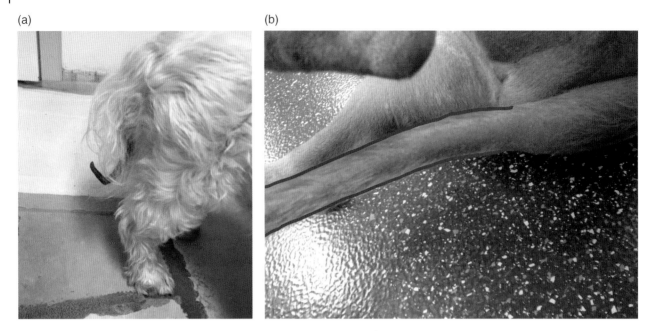

Figure 5.14 (a). "Rat Tail" in a Shih Tzu with endocrinopathy. *Source:* Courtesy of Gail Nason. (b). "Rat Tail" in a large-breed dog with hypothyroidism. *Source:* Courtesy of Patricia Bennett, DVM.

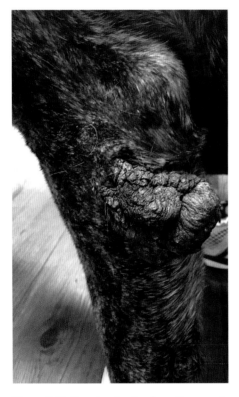

Figure 5.15 Prominent callus formation over the elbow in a hypothyroid Mastiff. *Source:* Courtesy of Sarah Bashaw, DVM.

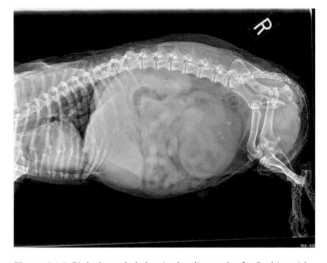

Figure 5.16 Right lateral abdominal radiograph of a Cushingoid canine patient demonstrating hepatomegaly with rounded liver margins.

glucocorticoid-induced catabolic state and fat redistribution. Hepatomegaly contributes to the pot-bellied look (see Figure 5.16).

Muscle atrophy is common in these patients, and is particularly evident around the head and face. Patients are progressively weak. They also tend to pant excessively because of glucocorticoid influence on the respiratory center, and the impact of steroids on the respiratory muscles [69, 70].

Because cortisol impacts fur growth and wound healing, there are several cutaneous manifestations of disease [69, 73]. Bilaterally symmetrical truncal hypotrichosis may or may not progress to alopecia [74]. The head and limbs are classically spared [69] (see Figures 5.17a–f).

One of the first dermatologic manifestations of Cushing's syndrome may be that the patient's coat does not shed out properly [69].

(a)

(b)

(c)

(d)

(e)

(f)

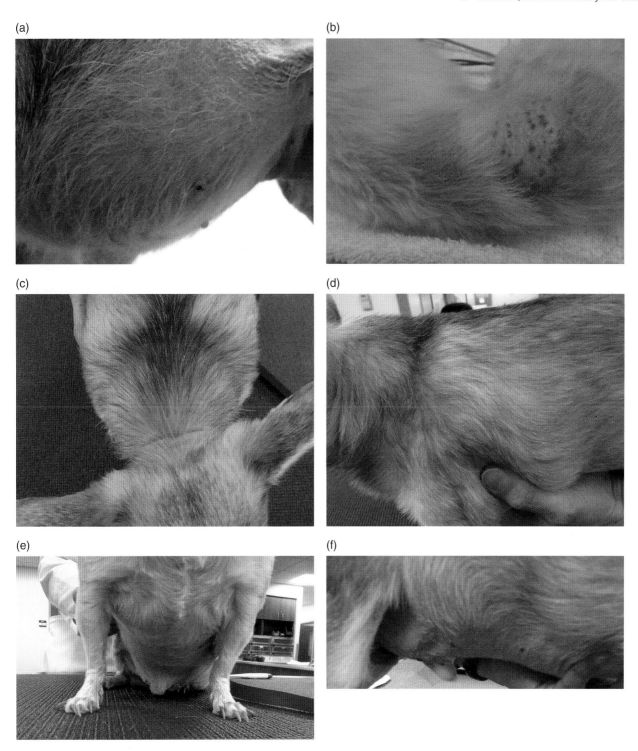

Figure 5.17 (a). Pendulous abdomen with appreciable hypotrichosis in a Cushingoid patient. *Source:* Courtesy of Patricia Bennett, DVM. (b). Truncal alopecia in a Cushingoid patient. *Source:* Courtesy of Samantha B. Thurman, DVM. (c). "Ring around the collar" classic hair loss pattern for endocrine alopecia in a canine patient with hyperadrenocorticism. *Source:* Courtesy of Patricia Bennett, DVM. (d). Truncal alopecia in a canine patient with hyperadrenocorticism. *Source:* Courtesy of Patricia Bennett, DVM. (e). Ventral alopecia in a canine patient with iatrogenic hyperadrenocorticism secondary to chronic steroid administration. *Source:* Courtesy of Patricia Bennett, DVM. (f). Alternate view of ventral alopecia in a canine patient with iatrogenic hyperadrenocorticism secondary to chronic steroid administration. *Source:* Courtesy of Patricia Bennett, DVM.

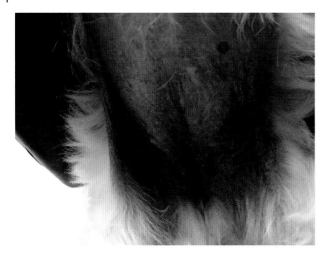

Figure 5.18 Ventral abdomen of a canine patient with chronic pyoderma. Note the extensive hyperpigmentation and lichenification of the affected skin.

(a)

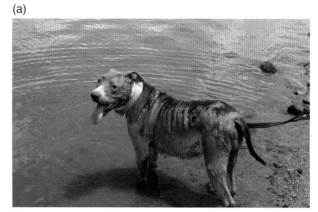

(b)

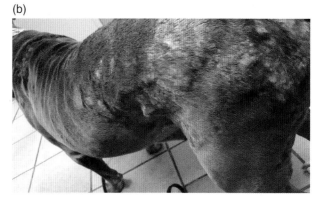

(c)

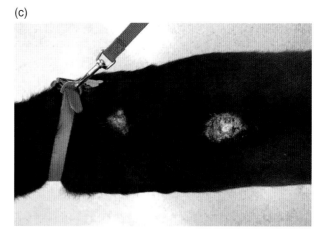

Figure 5.19 (a). Calcinosis cutis in a canine patient. *Source:* Courtesy of Danielle Cucuzella. (b). Close-up of calcinosis cutis in a canine patient. *Source:* Courtesy of Danielle Cucuzella. (c). Aerial view close-up of calcinosis cutis in a canine patient. *Source:* Courtesy of Beki Cohen Regan, DVM, DACVIM (Oncology).

As Cushing's syndrome progresses, the skin of the ventral abdominal wall becomes thinner [74]. The skin may feel paper thin [69]. It is also easily bruised due to the increased fragility of dermal vessels [69].

Secondary bacterial and fungal skin infections are common. Chronic infections may lead to hyperpigmentation of skin [74] (see Figure 5.18).

Affected patients may also develop comedones or calcinosis cutis, deposits of calcium within the dermis. These deposits may be generalized, but often increase in number over cervical, axillary, and inguinal regions [69] (see Figures 5.19a–c).

A diagnostic work-up for hyperadrenocorticism involves an investigation into the origin of the condition. If the condition is pituitary-dependent, treatment is aimed at reducing the amount of glucocorticoids that is being produced by the adrenal glands [69].

One of the more commonly used drugs is the intentionally cytotoxic drug o,p'-DDD [75]. This drug causes atrophy and necrosis of the adrenal glands, particularly the zona fasciculata and reticularis. This requires a balancing act and cautious monitoring. The clinician seeks to destroy enough of the adrenal glands to be therapeutic, without destroying so much as to induce an Addisonian crisis [69].

Alternate medications include ketoconazole and trilostane, both of which inhibit cortisol production by the adrenal glands. However, neither drug is without adverse effect.

A surgical approach to the management of pituitary-dependent hyperadrenocorticism is hypophysectomy.

Patients with adrenal-based hyperadrenocorticism may also be managed surgically, by removing the affected adrenal gland. If the tumor is non-resectable or if the risk to the patient is considered to be too great, then the patient is managed medically with o,p'-DDD; however, a larger dose is required to disable the diseased adrenal gland [69, 76, 77].

Hyperestrogenism is a much less common cause of endocrine, non-inflammatory hair loss. Endogenous estrogen is produced by the adrenal glands and gonads. Female patients may develop hyperestrogenism secondary to cystic ovaries or granulosa cell tumors, and certain types of testicular masses, such as Sertoli cell tumors, are estrogen-secreting [69, 78–80] (see Figure 5.20).

Exogenous sources of estrogen may also lead to hyperestrogenism. Consider, for example, those patients with urinary incontinence that are medically managed with estrogen. These patients are at increased risk for the development of hyperestrogenism [69, 78–80].

At high doses, estrogen inhibits hair growth in dogs [10, 81, 82]. Therefore, cutaneous manifestations of hyperestrogenism primarily involve progressive thinning of the coat and mirror those previously described for hyperadrenocorticism.

In addition, male dogs with hyperestrogenism often develop linear preputial dermatosis. This is a strip of redness and scaling between the prepuce and the scrotum along the ventral midline [69, 83].

More recently, there have been reports of canine hyperestrogenism secondary to exposure to human topical hormone replacement therapy. Wiener [10] described five such patients, male and female, intact and neutered, all of which had close contact with their

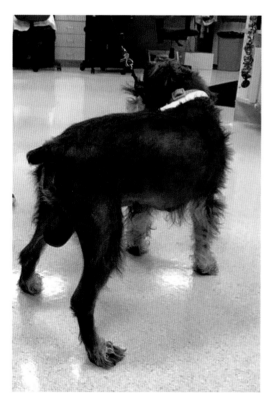

Figure 5.20 Dermatopathy in a canine patient that was subsequently diagnosed with a Sertoli cell tumor. *Source:* Courtesy of Beki Cohen.

respective owners, including that they slept in the same bed [10].

Patients varied significantly as to when skin lesions developed relative to exposure. In one patient, hypotrichosis occurred not long after the client started to use an estradiol-based cream, whereas another patient did not exhibit clinical signs until 10 months of exposure [10].

There also appears to be patient-specific predispositions to estradiol-induced fur loss in that not all patients in a multi-pet household developed clinical signs in Wiener's review, despite the same exposure to the same client [10].

When clients discontinued topical therapy or applied topical preparations in the morning as opposed to the evening, to prevent contamination of the bed and subsequent patient exposure, alopecia resolved. However, resolution was not rapid: it took months [10].

Berger et al. described six additional cases with similar findings [9]. In addition, vulvar and nipple enlargement was seen in some, but not all, of the affected patients [9].

5.8 Non-Endocrine, Inflammatory Hair Loss

All of the aforementioned causes of hypotrichosis and alopecia were non-inflammatory based upon their pathology. However, hair loss can also be the result of the following common inflammatory processes:

- Demodicosis
- Sarcoptic mange
- Dermatophytosis
- Bacterial pyoderma

Demodicosis is the condition by which the canine patient is infested with ectoparasites, *Demodex canis,* and the feline patient is infested with *Demodex cati* and/ or *Demodex gatoi* [5, 84–88].

As was described in Chapter 3, Section 3.8.1, demodicosis may result in localized or generalized disease. The former has a good prognosis, particularly in cases of juvenile onset. These cases tend to resolve spontaneously, whereas generalized demodicosis requires an investigation into the underlying disease [89].

Patients with generalized demodicosis often present with one or more of the following signs: erythema, hypotrichosis or alopecic patches with or without a papulopustular rash, folliculitis or furunculosis, scaling and follicular casts, pododermatitis, and paronychia [89–91]. The face and forelimbs are often affected first, before the disease spreads throughout the body. The patient may or may not exhibit lymphadenopathy. The patient may or may not be febrile. Refer to Chapter 3, Figures 3.12a–d for depictions of generalized disease (see Figures 5.21a–c).

Consult Chapter 3, Section 3.8.1 regarding diagnostic work-up and treatment options.

Sarcoptic mange involves infestation with the mange mite, *Sarcoptes scabiei*. *Sarcoptes scabiei* is a surface dweller that is capable of inducing zoonotic disease. Clinical signs may be mild, or, as is more often the case, patients are intensely pruritic [7].

Lesions in dogs tend to concentrate on the head, pinnae, elbows, and hocks [7, 8] (see Figure 5.22a, b).

Cats are rarely affected with this disease; however, case reports have documented feline lesions on the bridge of the nose, feet, claws, and tail [92–94].

Humans report pruritic papules along the arms and trunk [95].

Superficial skin scrapes that demonstrate the *Sarcoptes* mite are confirmatory for the disease. As was reviewed in Chapter 3, Section 3.8.1, *S. scabiei* has a very round body on cytology with long limb pedicles (refer to Chapter 3, Figure 3.15) [94].

It can be challenging to secure a positive skin scrape. It is possible that sarcoptic mange occurs with greater frequency than is diagnosed [7].

Superficial dermatophytosis, otherwise referred to as ringworm, may also cause hypotrichosis or alopecic patches. Dermatophytosis is also a zoonotic disease.

As was discussed in Chapter 3, Section 3.8.2, canine patients with ringworm tend to be infected with *Trichophyton mentagrophytes* or *Microsporum gypseum* [96–98]. *Microsporum canis* is the primary source of ringworm in cats [96–98].

(a) (b)

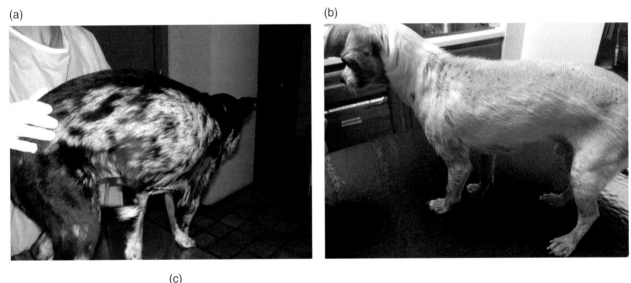

(c)

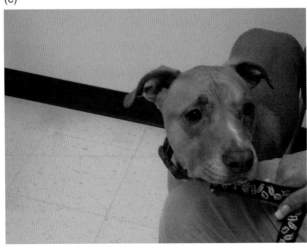

Figure 5.21 (a). Generalized demodicosis in a canine patient, demonstrating alopecic patches along the trunk. *Source:* Courtesy of Joseph Onello at Central Mesa Veterinary Hospital. (b). Generalized demodicosis in a canine patient, demonstrating facial, truncal, and limb involvement. *Source:* Courtesy of Pamela Mueller, DVM. (c). Focal demodicosis in a canine patient, demonstrating periocular involvement.

(a)

(b)

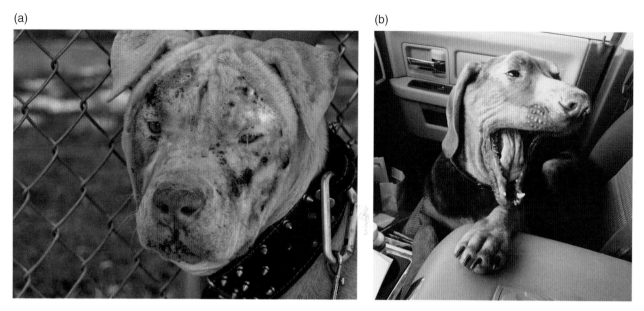

Figure 5.22 (a). Sarcoptic mange in a canine patient, demonstrating facial involvement. *Source:* Courtesy of Laura Polerecky. (b). Sarcoptic mange in a canine patient, demonstrating periocular and peri-oral hypotrichosis. *Source:* Courtesy of Lauren Bessert.

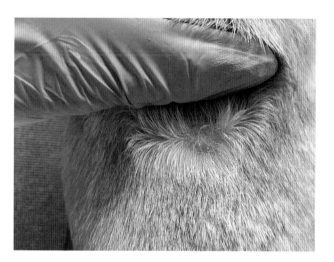

Figure 5.23 Classic circular alopecia in a canine patient with dermatophytosis. The client had dermatologic lesions as well. *Source:* Courtesy of Garrett A. Rowley, DVM.

Affected canine patients may exhibit kerion formation. Refer to Chapter 3, Figure 3.18.

Canine patients also tend to exhibit crusting or circular alopecia (see Figure 5.23).

Feline lesions from dermatophytosis tend to be more varied in presentation [97]. Partial alopecia and crusting on the face and limbs is typical (see Figures 5.24a, b).

Diagnosis of dermatophytosis is supported by positive, apple-green fluorescence of lesions with a Wood's lamp. Refer to Chapter 3, Figures 3.20a, b (see Figure 5.25).

However, only 50% of *M. canis* fluoresce, and most other species do not exhibit fluorescence. Therefore, a negative Wood's lamp does not rule out dermatophytosis.

(a)

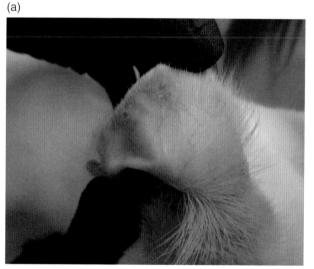

(b)

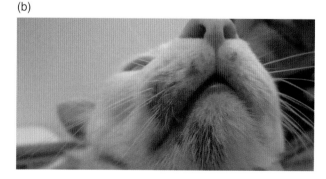

Figure 5.24 (a). Feline patient with dermatophytosis with crusting at the ventral pinna. *Source:* Courtesy of Arielle Hatcher. (b). Feline patient with dermatophytosis with crusting of the muzzle and chin. *Source:* Courtesy of Arielle Hatcher.

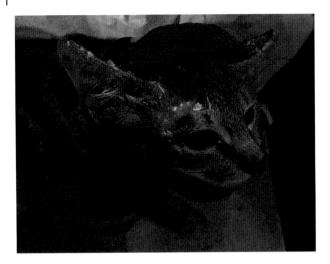

Figure 5.25 Positive fluorescence of gross lesions in a feline patient with dermatophytosis. *Source:* Courtesy of Colleen M. Cook, Midwestern University College of Veterinary Medicine, Class of 2019.

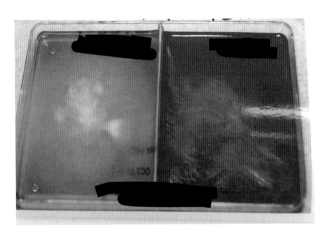

Figure 5.26 Positive fungal culture using a dual chamber culture plate. Note fungal growth on the Specialized Enhanced Sporulation Agar (ESA), far left. *Source:* Courtesy of Erin Harker, DVM.

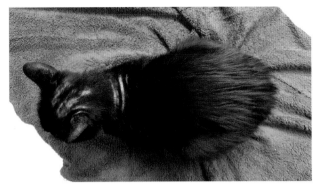

Figure 5.27 Hypotrichosis associated with flea allergy dermatitis in a cat. *Source:* Courtesy of Ballroom Dance School Manhattan.

A positive fungal culture is confirmatory for dermatophytosis (see Figure 5.26).

Another cause of inflammatory hair loss is bacterial pyoderma, in which there is bacterial infection of the skin. Pyoderma can be superficial, meaning that only the epidermis and hair follicles are affected, or pyoderma can be deep, involving the dermis.

Pyoderma may be a primary condition. More commonly, pyoderma is secondary to an underlying condition or disease. In particular, allergic skin disease is a common initiator of pyoderma. Allergic skin disease includes flea allergy dermatitis, atopic dermatitis, and food allergies.

Patients with flea allergy dermatitis develop a sensitivity reaction to flea saliva, which contains histamine-like compounds. Patients may develop immediate or delayed reactions, or both. The resulting pruritus often leads to extensive hypotrichosis and alopecia secondary to intense scratching and chewing at the coat [99] (see Figure 5.27).

Flea infestations are often visible to the naked eye (see Figures 5.28a–c).

On occasion, only flea feces are present on the patient. This so-called flea dirt is dried blood that the fleas ingested, metabolized, and expelled. To differentiate dirt from flea dirt, the clinician can gather the substance between two moistened paper towels. If a reddish-brown discoloration results from the towels being rubbed together, then the substance is likely to be flea dirt (see Figure 5.29).

Atopic dermatitis, or atopy, is an inflammatory chronic skin disease triggered by allergies [100, 101]. Age of onset of atopy is six months to three years [101–105]. Breeds that may be at increased risk of developing atopy include Boxers, Chinese Shar-Peis, Dalmatians, English Bulldogs, Labrador Retrievers, Lhasa Apsos, Miniature Schnauzers, Pugs, West Highland White Terriers, Yorkshire Terriers, Boston, and Cairn Terriers [100, 104, 106–108].

Classically, the face, ears, paws, extremities, and ventrum are involved in canine patients with atopic dermatitis [100, 102, 108] (see Figures 5.30a–f).

Clinical signs associated with atopy may be seasonal or non-seasonal [100].

Food allergies may also predispose to pyoderma and pruritus, which leads to hair loss (see Figures 5.31a, b).

Allergic skin disease requires a diagnostic investigation that may include intradermal allergy testing, otherwise known as skin testing (see Figures 5.32a, b).

As mentioned earlier, parasitic skin diseases, such as demodicosis and sarcoptic mange, may also result in pyoderma.

(a)

(b)

(c)

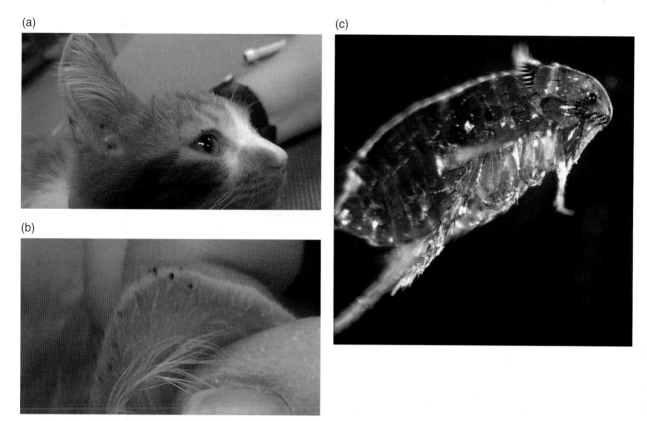

Figure 5.28 (a). Gross flea infestation in a cat. Note periocular and pinnal involvement. *Source:* Courtesy of Laura Polerecky. (b). Gross flea infestation in a cat. Note extensive pinnal involvement. *Source:* Courtesy of Laura Polerecky. (c). Microscopic image of *Ctenocephalides felis*, the cat flea. *Source:* Courtesy of Dr. Araceli Lucio-Forster, Cornell University College of Veterinary Medicine.

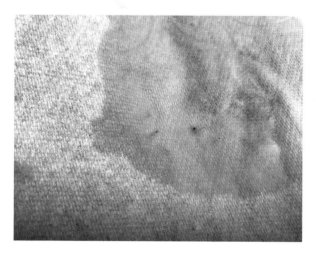

Figure 5.29 Evidence of flea dirt. *Source:* Courtesy of Jule Schweighoefer.

In addition, pyoderma may occur with greater frequency in those breeds with anatomic predispositions such as excessive skin folds (see Figures 5.33a–c).

Clinical lesions associated with pyoderma include papules, pustules, epidermal collarettes, and crusts. In breeds with short coats, papules may resemble urticaria because follicular inflammation causes the hairs to stand erect. To distinguish papules from urticaria, the clinician may attempt to epilate hairs over the questionable lesion. If the hair epilates with ease, then the lesion is likely a papule from superficial pyoderma. Hairs overlying urticaria do not epilate readily (see Figures 5.34a–f).

Mucocutaneous pyoderma is a specific type of pyoderma that affects the lips, nasal planum, nares, and peri-oral skin. Occasionally, it affects the eyelids, anus, and the external openings to the urogenital tracts [109, 110] (see Figures 5.35a, b).

Cytology of pustular contents confirms pyoderma by the presence of intracellular bacteria within neutrophils.

Pyoderma is antibiotic-responsive. The patient's pruritus must also be addressed if recovery is to be hastened.

Hair loss may also be due to inflammatory disease associated with these less common presentations [111–113]:

- Sebaceous adenitis
- Pemphigus foliaceus
- Epitheliotropic T-cell lymphoma
- Alopecia areata

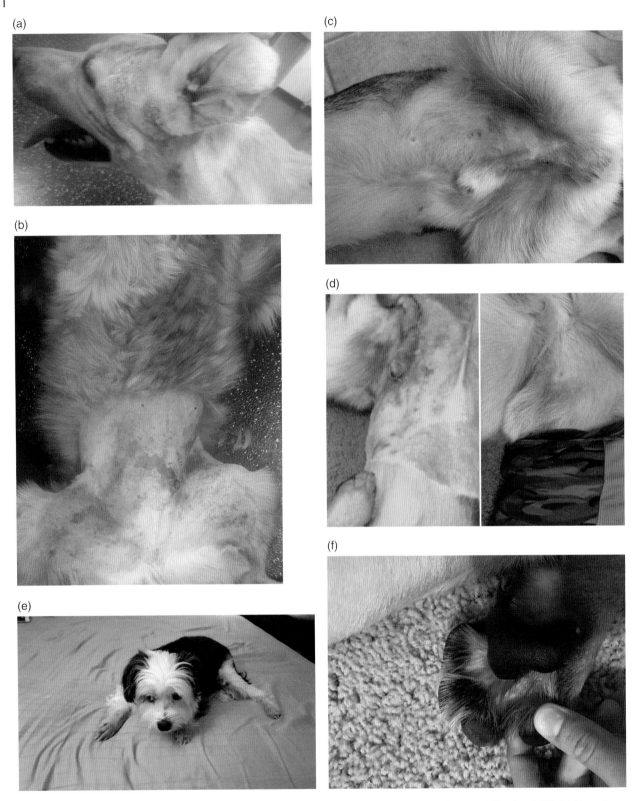

Figure 5.30 (a) Aural involvement in a canine patient with atopic dermatitis. *Source:* Courtesy of Lori A. Stillmaker, DVM. (b). Ventral involvement in a canine patient with atopic dermatitis. *Source:* Courtesy of Lori A. Stillmaker, DVM. (c). Ventral involvement in a canine patient with atopic dermatitis. *Source:* Courtesy of Jule Schweighoefer. (d). Ventral involvement in a canine patient with atopic dermatitis, pre- and post-treatment. *Source:* Courtesy of Jule Schweighoefer. (e). Distal limb involvement in a canine patient with atopic dermatitis. *Source:* Courtesy of John Chang. (f). Paw involvement in a canine patient with atopic dermatitis. *Source:* Courtesy of Jule Schweighoefer.

(a) (b)

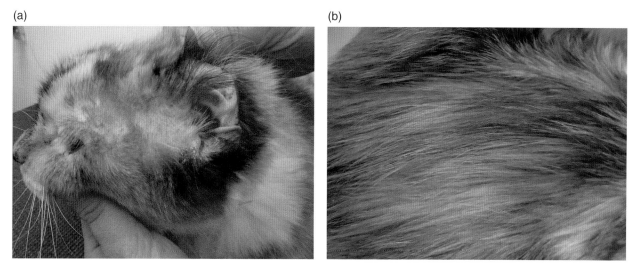

Figure 5.31 (a). Feline patient with presumptive food allergies. Note the erythema and excoriations associated with the peri-aural and pinnal regions. *Source:* Courtesy of Patricia Bennett, DVM. (b). Coat color change in a feline patient with presumptive food allergies. *Source:* Courtesy of Patricia Bennett, DVM.

(a) (b)

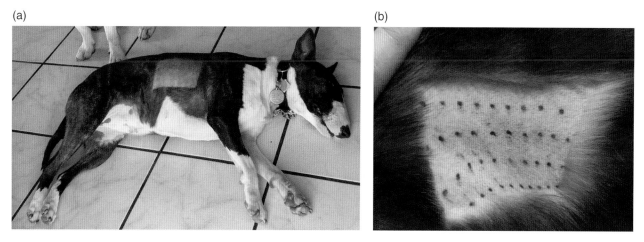

Figure 5.32 (a). Canine patient with right flank prepared for skin testing. *Source:* Courtesy of Danielle Cucuzella. (b). Feline patient undergoing intradermal allergy testing. *Source:* Courtesy of Stephanie Horwitz.

These conditions are beyond the scope of this text and require consultation of additional resources.

However, they remind the astute clinician that lesser-known conditions do occur in the companion animal population. When a diagnostic work-up has ruled out the most common presentations, it is appropriate to broaden one's list of differential diagnoses, particularly if there are concurrent clinical signs that do not fit the typical presentation. For example, hypopigmentation and ulceration of tissue, in addition to hair loss, is consistent with some presentations of canine cutaneous epitheliotropic T-cell lymphoma [112, 114] (see Figure 5.36).

Cutaneous lymphoma is not unique to dogs [111] (see Figures 5.37–c).

5.9 Hepatocutaneous Syndrome as a Cause of Hair Loss

Hepatocutaneous syndrome is a relatively uncommon disease that manifests as skin lesions [115–117]. It is a disease of many names in the medical literature, including superficial necrolytic dermatitis, necrolytic migratory erythema (NME), and metabolic epidermal necrosis (MEN) [115, 116].

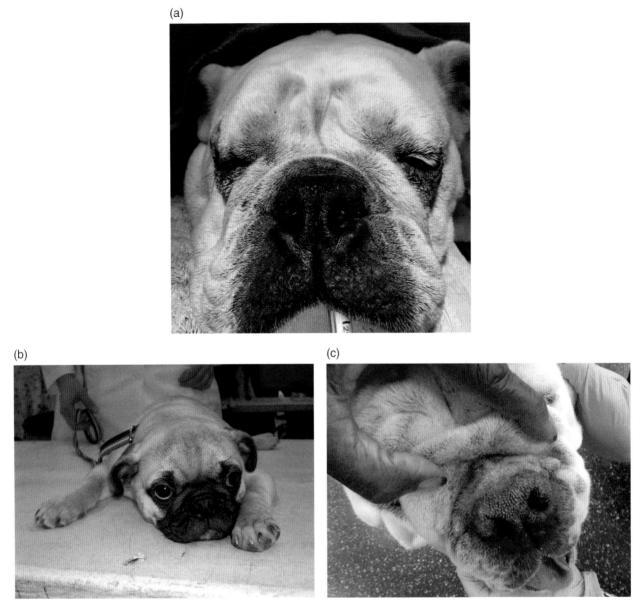

Figure 5.33 (a). English Bulldog patient demonstrating extensive nasal folds that may predispose him to pyoderma. Incidentally, this patient had recently undergone corrective surgery for entropion, hence the peri-orbital sutures. *Source:* Courtesy of Jessica Friedman, DVM. (b). Nasal folds in a Pug dog. *Source:* Courtesy of Laura Polarecky. (c). Skin fold dermatitis in an English Bulldog. *Source:* Courtesy of Patricia Bennett, DVM.

Human patients with glucagon-secreting pancreatic neoplasia present with this syndrome; however, that is not typically the case in dogs [116, 118–121]. Histopathological changes in dogs originate from the liver and are best characterized as a degenerative vacuolar hepatopathy that disrupts parenchymal architecture [117, 122]. Ultrasonography of the affected liver reveals hypoechoic nodules [117]. These cause the liver to take on a Swiss cheese or honeycomb appearance [117]. Clinicopathologic abnormalities are suggestive of hepatic dysfunction and include a non-regenerative anemia, microcytosis, and an elevated serum alkaline phosphatase [117]. Bile acids may be normal or elevated [116, 123, 124]. Affected dogs are rarely icteric [116, 123, 124].

Male dogs may be at greater risk for development of this syndrome than females, and small-to-medium breeds are over-represented [117, 123, 125]. Malteses, West Highland White Terriers, Shih Tzus, Cocker Spaniels, and Shetland Sheepdogs frequent case reports [116, 117, 123, 126].

Cats may present with either primary hepatic or pancreatic lesions [115, 116].

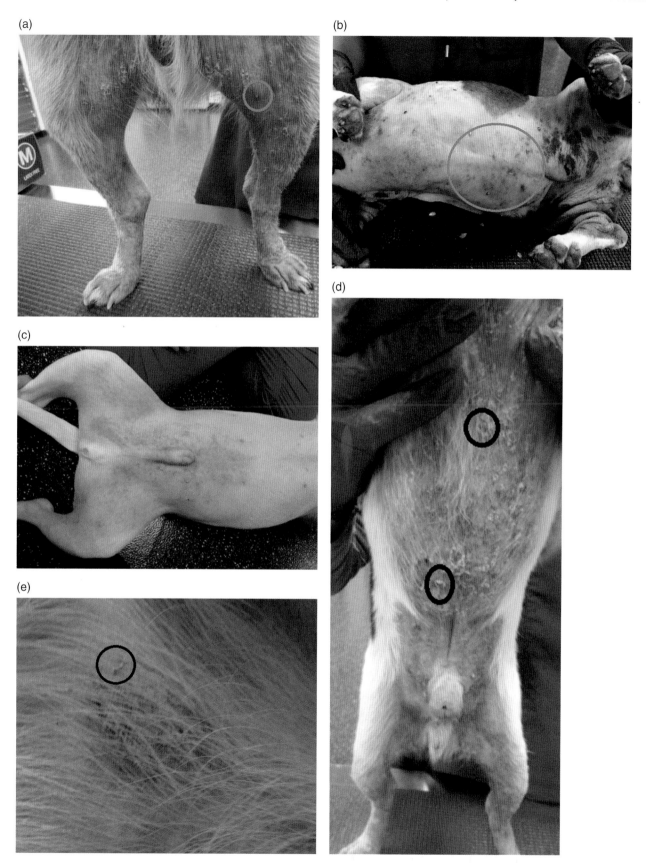

Figure 5.34 (a). Pyoderma in a canine patient. An isolated papule has been circled in blue. *Source:* Courtesy of Dr. Elizabeth Robbins. (b). Papulopustular rash along the ventrum of a canine patient with pyoderma. (c). Papulopustular rash along the ventrum of a canine patient with pyoderma. *Source:* Courtesy of Dr. Elizabeth Robbins. (d). Epidermal collarettes in a canine patient with pyoderma. *Source:* Courtesy of Dr. Elizabeth Robbins. (e). An isolated crust in a canine patient with pyoderma. *Source:* Courtesy of Patricia Bennett, DVM. (f). Papules in a short-coated canine patient. Note how these lesions could look similar to urticaria. *Source:* Courtesy of Kelly Bradley.

(f)

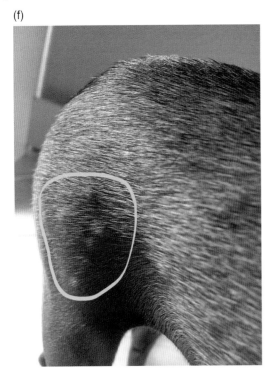

Figure 5.34 (Continued)

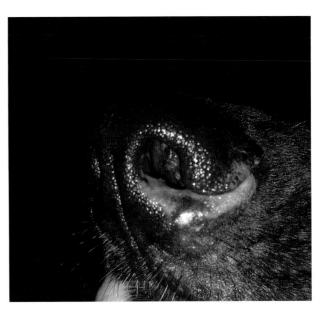

Figure 5.36 Hypopigmentation and ulceration of the tissue adjacent to the nose. This presentation resembles that which is seen in some cases of canine cutaneous epitheliotropic T-cell lymphoma. *Source:* Courtesy of Jule Schweighoefer.

(a) (b)

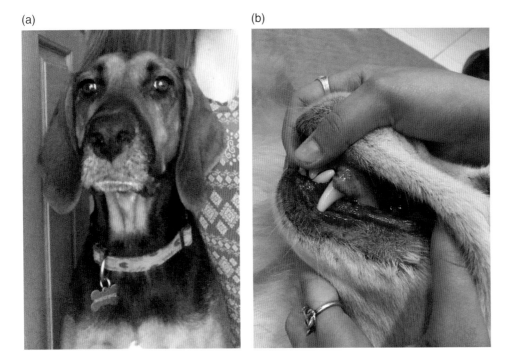

Figure 5.35 (a). Mucocutaneous pyoderma involving the muzzle of a canine patient. *Source:* Courtesy of Lauren Bessert. (b). Mucocutaneous pyoderma in a canine patient. *Source:* Courtesy of Amanda Leigh Rappaport.

Figure 5.37 (a) Confirmed case of cutaneous lymphoma in a feline patient. *Source:* Courtesy of Kelli L. Crisfulli, RVT. (b). Note the extensive involvement of the face in the same feline patient. *Source:* Courtesy of Kelli L. Crisfulli, RVT. (c). Note the involvement of the trunk in the same feline patient. *Source:* Courtesy of Kelli L. Crisfulli, RVT.

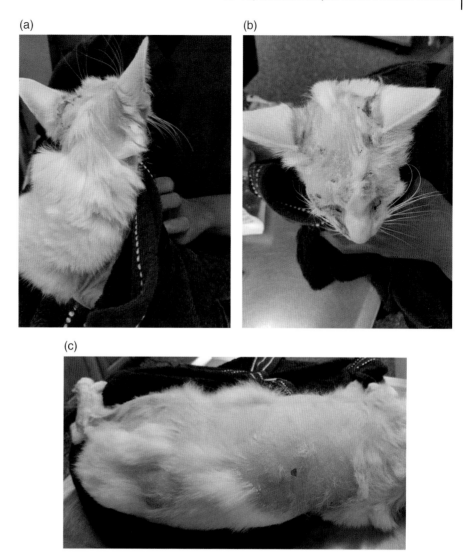

Dogs and cats typically present for chief complaints involving the skin. Ventral alopecia is the classic presentation for hepatocutaneous syndrome in the cat [115]. Dogs may also present for regional alopecia; however, the location may be more varied. One case report describes alopecia of the hip, with crusting, redness, and erosions of the muzzle, elbows, digits, and footpads [126] (see Figure 5.38).

The exposed skin may be hyper-reflective and unnaturally shiny. It is often marred by crusting, excoriations, and ulcerations.

The pathophysiology that links hepatic and cutaneous lesions is currently unknown [115, 116, 120, 122].

Although hepatocutaneous syndrome is rare, it serves as an important reminder that alopecia may be an outward reflection of underlying and potentially fatal disease. A minimum database is an important step to take in the diagnostic work-up for alopecia to rule out hepatocutaneous syndrome.

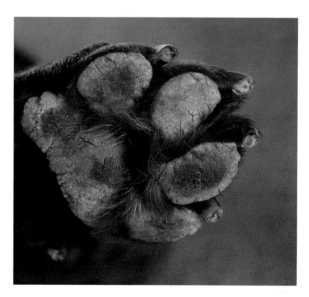

Figure 5.38 Footpad disease due to hepatocutaneous syndrome.

5.10 Chemotherapy

Approximately 65% of human patients experience chemotherapy-induced alopecia (CIA) [127, 128]. Psychologically, CIA has the potential to negatively impact self-concept and body image [129–133]. Medications that are more likely to induce CIA in humans include doxorubicin and cyclophosphamide [127]. It is not surprising that these medications induce alopecia because they target the most rapidly dividing cells in the body. Doxorubicin in particular causes hair follicle cells to undergo apoptosis [134].

Medication dose, dosing frequency, and route of administration also play a role [127].

CIA also occurs in companion animal patients, although it has been researched less extensively. Few reports track the incidence of CIA in canine and feline patients, or the psychological effect on clients that witness alopecia in their companion animals. A study by Falk et al. [127] examined the risk of injectable doxorubicin-associated alopecia in 150 dogs that had been treated at a teaching hospital from 2012 to 2014 [127]. Nineteen percent developed CIA. A greater risk was associated with curly or wire-haired coats [127]. Patients with these coats were 22 times more likely to develop alopecia [127].

An isolated case report by Cavalcanti et al. [135] also describes alopecia in a Bernese Mountain Dog that had been treated for a subcutaneous mast cell tumor (MCT) with oral toceranib phosphate, a tyrosine kinase inhibitor [135]. In addition to periocular alopecia, the patient presented with hyperkeratosis of the dorsal nasal planum and patchy depigmentation of the nasal planum and footpads [135].

Although findings from isolated reports such as this one cannot be extrapolated to the entire population of patients receiving chemotherapy, they remind us as clinicians to alert clients of the potential for hair loss with treatment. This hair loss may or may not be permanent.

5.11 Radiation Therapy

Radiation therapy is increasingly used in companion animal medicine as part of a multimodal approach to cancer treatment. It is important to prepare veterinary clients for the possibility that alopecia will develop at the radiation site(s) as an acute side effect [136–139]. Clients are often warned of the potential for damage to irradiated tissues such as the small bowel and the oropharyngeal, nasal, and urinary bladder mucosa. However, irradiated hair follicles may result in alopecia. This alopecia may resolve or it may persist indefinitely (see Figures 5.39a, b).

(a)

(b)

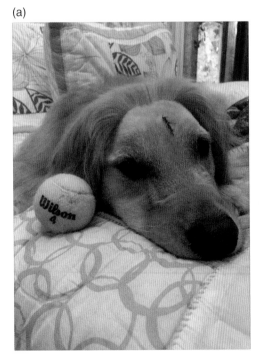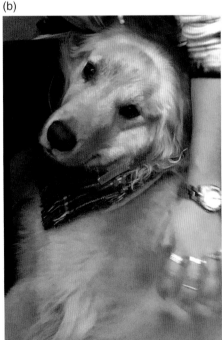

Figure 5.39 (a). Golden Retriever about to begin radiation therapy. Fur had been previously clipped for surgery. *Source:* Courtesy of Amanda Leigh Rappaport. (b). Same Golden Retriever following radiation therapy. Alopecia at the forehead persists. *Source:* Courtesy of Amanda Leigh Rappaport.

5.12 Alopecia Associated with Topical Medications

Medications that are applied topically to the skin, particularly flea and tick preventatives, may result in skin lesions, including alopecia. Although the frequency with which this occurs has not been reported in the literature, isolated case reports and compiled chemical safety studies of spot-on formulations suggest that alopecia is possible.

For example, the spot-on product, Assurity®, which contains spinetoram, caused 38% cats in a clinical trial to develop hypotrichosis or alopecia [140]. Trichogram findings were suggestive that barbering resulted in hair loss [140].

There has been increased public interest in the development of so-called "natural" flea preventatives. Public perception is often that "natural" implies *safer*. Many of these over-the-counter products contain essential oils. Peppermint oil, cinnamon oil, lemongrass oil, melaleuca oil, clove oil, and rosemary frequent the active ingredient list [141, 142].

One retrospective study found that 92% of canine and feline patients that had been exposed to essential oils developed one or more adverse effects [141]. Behavioral changes were commonly noted. In addition, adverse effects were reported for the gastrointestinal, respiratory, and central nervous systems. Many patients exhibited erythema of the skin at the site of topical application. Some patients did not live long enough to see if hair loss resulted.

The imidacloprid/flumethrin collar (Seresto®) also causes alopecia in some patients. This alopecia is transient, meaning that it resolves after the collar is permanently removed (see Figure 5.40).

Clients should be made aware that alopecia is a side effect of topical preventatives, albeit rare.

5.13 Non-Medical Causes of Hair Loss

Pressure alopecia is a phenomenon that has been reported in the human medical literature [143]. It results from ischemic changes to the skin, including the scalp, that may result from prolonged recumbence during lengthy surgical procedures. Articles of clothing, such as headbands, can also trigger the development of pressure alopecia after periods of prolonged use [143].

Although reports of a similar phenomenon are infrequent in the veterinary literature, it stands to reason that wearing articles of clothing, such as collars or harnesses, may also lead to alopecia (see Figure 5.41).

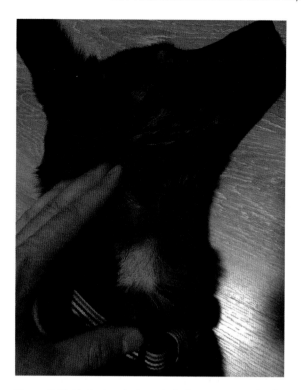

Figure 5.40 Ventral neck alopecia that was suspected to be caused by wearing a flea collar. *Source:* Courtesy of Blake and Danielle Tafoya.

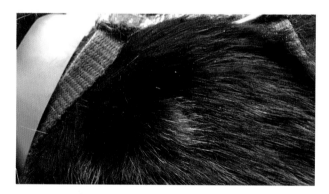

Figure 5.41 Subtle hypotrichosis in a feline patient, assumed to be due to the harness. The harness has been elevated so that the line of hypotrichosis is evident. *Source:* Courtesy of Garrett A. Rowley, DVM.

5.14 Poor Nutritional Plane as a Cause of Alopecia

Nutrition plays an important role in maintaining coat quality [144]. Poor coat quality is one of the first signs of malnutrition or malabsorptive disease [144–146]. In particular, deficiencies in zinc and/or linoleic acid can result in significant dermatoses that resolve with dietary supplementation [144, 146–149] (see Figures 5.42a, b).

5.15 Environmental Causes of Alopecia

Just as articles of clothing can cause pressure alopecia, so, too, can environmental points of contact. Consider, for example, the canine patient that spends a significant time outdoors on concrete. The frequent contact with such a hard, unyielding surface will naturally lead to

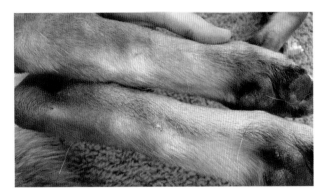

Figure 5.43 Plantar aspect of the distal hind limbs in a one-year-old German Shepherd with pressure-associated hypotrichosis due to daily bouts of running and playing on concrete. *Source:* Courtesy of Jule Schweighoefer.

hypotrichosis and potentially callus formation (see Figure 5.43).

5.16 Compulsive and/or Displacement Disorders

Over-grooming has long been recognized in a number of species, including companion animals, birds, and humans [150]. Several pathological syndromes associated with grooming have been described in cats and dogs:

- Acral lick dermatitis and flank sucking in dogs
- Psychogenic alopecia in cats or "fur mowing"

Acral lick dermatitis or acral lick granuloma is characterized as a condition by which nodules or plaques form at one or more of the distal limbs of a canine patient due to excessive licking. Over time, these lesions develop hyperpigmentation and lichenification. They also become alopecic. Secondary infections may result from repeated trauma. Deep furunculosis is not uncommon [151] (see Figure 5.44).

Acral lick lesions may be confused for bacterial or fungal granulomas. In addition, lymphoma and MCTs may present similarly [152]. Diagnostic work-ups are essential to case management so that key differentials are not missed. It is important not to assume that an acral lick lesion is an acral lick lesion until other potentially insidious possibilities have been ruled out.

(a)
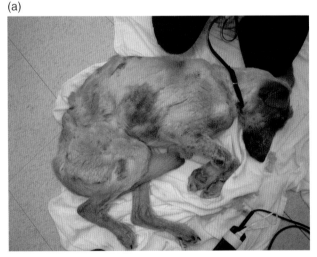

(b)
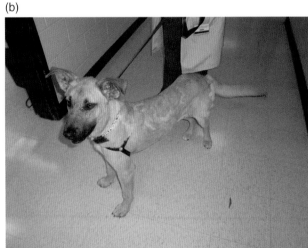

Figure 5.42 (a). Emaciated canine patient with significant nutritional deficits due to neglect. Note the poor quality of the coat and the extensive patches of alopecia. *Source:* Courtesy of Daniel Foy. (b). Same patient as in Figure 5.42a; however, the patient's nutritional plane has been increased. Note the significant improvement in coat quality. This progress took months to achieve. *Source:* Courtesy of Daniel Foy.

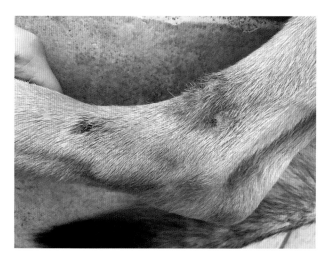

Figure 5.44 Acral lick lesions associated with the tarsus of a canine patient. *Source:* Courtesy of Jule Schweighoefer.

Flank sucking is an unusual behavior for which Doberman Pinschers appear to be predisposed [153, 154]. Patients with this syndrome mouth their flanks repeatedly, particularly at bedtime just prior to falling asleep [153, 154]. Mildly affected patients simply moisten the flank. However, in extreme cases this recurrent activity causes hypotrichosis that progresses to alopecia. When patients continue to mouth after hair loss, abrasions and open wounds may ensue [153, 155].

Psychogenic alopecia in cats involves over-grooming or so-called "fur mowing" of any one or more parts of the body (see Figures 5.45a–g).

The primary name of this syndrome, psychogenic alopecia, implies that affected patients have obsessive-compulsive tendencies that fail to cease even when they result in bodily harm. Because we as clinicians cannot ask our patients specifically what is going through their minds when they groom, it is difficult to say whether these behaviors are true compulsions.

What is known is that psychogenic alopecia is overdiagnosed, and that more often than not, these behaviors have a true underlying medical cause [150]. It would be inappropriate for a clinician to label these behaviors as psychogenic unless the diagnosis is one of exclusion, meaning that all medical and dermatological causes have been ruled out [156, 157].

Consider, for example, the cat that presents for self-induced alopecia. A case series by Waisglass et al. [156] found that only 1 in 10 cats had true psychogenic alopecia [156]. The remainder had medical causes that included adverse food reactions and atopy [156].

Review the non-endocrine causes of inflammatory hair loss that were covered in Section 5.8. All of these causes may set the stage for over-grooming.

Furthermore, diseases that cause discomfort may lead to over-grooming of the region of the body that is in pain. Cats with urinary tract disease may excessively groom their ventral abdomen. In the author's experience, cats with osteoarthritis often over-groom the joint(s) involved.

If the underlying condition is not addressed, then the patient will continue to groom excessively. The same holds true for canine patients.

Of perhaps greater concern is that sometimes patients may continue to lick even after the condition has resolved. In that case, licking may have become a habit. This is frequently the case for canine patients with acral lick dermatitis. The inciting factor has been removed, but the patient continues to traumatize the affected tissue [150, 158]. This presents case management challenges, and explains why acral lick dermatitis is one of the most frustrating skin conditions for and clinicians alike.

In addition to medical conditions that provoke over-grooming, over-grooming may also develop as a displacement behavior to cope with social environmental stressors [150, 159, 160]. These may include a change in companionship or a change in lifestyle, such as a move from outdoor to indoor living [161].

Although this misdirected behavior is more socially acceptable to the client than inappropriate elimination, spraying, or marking, collaborative efforts should be made to reduce stress to improve quality of life for the patient.

(a)

(c)

(b)

(d)

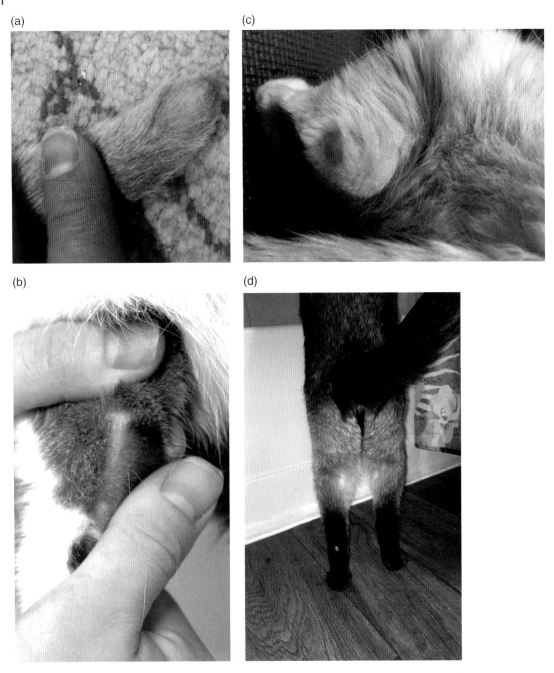

Figure 5.45 (a). Fur mowing of the tail tip of a feline patient, without any breach of skin integrity. (b). Fur mowing associated with the left hock of a feline patient. *Source:* Courtesy of the Media Resources Department at Midwestern University. (c). Fur mowing associated with the left hock of a feline patient. This lesion was bilaterally symmetrical, although symmetry is not demonstrated in this photograph. (d). Fur mowing associated with the left hock of a feline patient. This lesion was not bilaterally symmetrical, as is apparent in this photograph. *Source:* Courtesy of Natalie J. Reeser. (e). Fur mowing associated with the left medial thigh of a feline patient. This lesion was not bilaterally symmetrical. *Source:* Courtesy of Dr. Elizabeth Robbins. (f). Fur mowing with excoriations at the caudoventral abdomen of this feline patient. *Source:* Courtesy of Jeri Altizer. (g). Fur mowing of the ventral abdomen of a feline patient. *Source:* Courtesy of Meagan Alcorn.

(e)

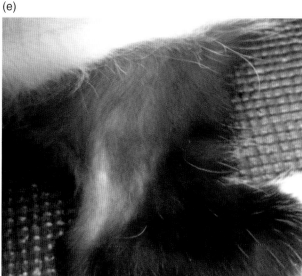

(g)

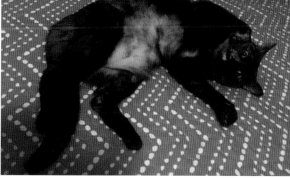

(f)

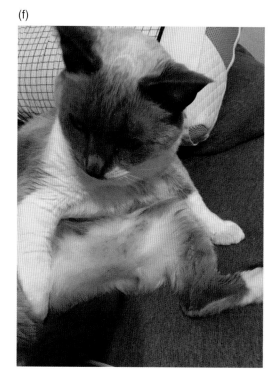

Figure 5.45 (Continued)

References

1 Moriello, K.A. (2012). Dermatology. In: *The Cat: Clinical Medicine and Management* (ed. S.E. Little), 371–424. St. Louis: Elsevier Saunders.

2 Breathnach, R.M.S. and Shipstone, M. (2006). The cat with alopecia. In: *Problem-Based Feline Medicine* (ed. J. Rand), 1052–1066. Toronto: Elsevier Saunders.

3 Kennis, R.A. (2008). Disorders causing focal Alopecia. In: *Handbook of Small Animal Practice*, 5e (ed. R.V. Morgan), 834–840. Saunders/Elsevier: St. Louis, Mo.

4 Ghubash, R.M. (2003). Disorders causing symmetrical Alopecia. In: *Handbook of Small Animal Practice*, 4e (ed. R.V. Morgan), 841–849. Philadelphia: Saunders.

5 Mueller, R.S. (2012). An update on the therapy of canine demodicosis. *Compend. Contin. Educ. Vet.* 34 (4): E1–E4.

6 Scott, D.W., Miller, W.H., and Griffin, C.E. (2001). *Canine Demodicosis. Muller & Kirk's Small Animal Dermatology*, 457–474. Philadelphia, P.A.: WB Saunders.

7 Pin, D., Bensignor, E., Carlotti, D.N., and Cadiergues, M.C. (2006). Localised sarcoptic mange in dogs: a retrospective study of 10 cases. *J. Small Anim. Pract.* 47 (10): 611–614.

8 Scott, D.W., Miller, W.H., and Griffin, C.E. (2001). *Parasitic Skin Diseases. Muller & Kirk's Small Animal Dermatology*, 476–483. Philadelphia, P.A.: W.B. Saunders.

9 Berger, D.J., Lewis, T.P., Schick, A.E. et al. (2015). Canine alopecia secondary to human topical hormone replacement therapy in six dogs. *J. Am. Anim. Hosp. Assoc.* 51 (2): 136–142.

10 Wiener, D.J., Rufenacht, S., Koch, H.J. et al. (2015). Estradiol-induced alopecia in five dogs after contact with a transdermal gel used for the treatment of postmenopausal symptoms in women. *Vet. Dermatol.* 26 (5): 393–396, e90–1.

11 Englar, R.E. (2017). *Performing the Small Animal Physical Examination*. Hoboken, N.J.: Wiley.

12 Scott, D.W., Miller, W.H., and Griffin, C.E. (2013). *Congenital and Hereditary Defects. Muller & Kirk's Small Animal Dermatology*, 573–616. St. Louis, Missouri: Elsevier, Inc.

13 Laffort-Dassot, C., Beco, L., and Carlotti, D.N. (2002). Follicular dysplasia in five Weimaraners. *Vet. Dermatol.* 13 (5): 253–260.

14 Gross, T.L., Ihrke, P.J., and Walder, E.J. (1992). *Veterinary Dermatopathology. A Macroscopic and Microscopic Evaluation of Canine and Feline Skin Disease*. St. Louis, Missouri: Mosby Year Book.

15 Selmanovitz, V.J., Markofsky, J., and Orentreich, N. (1977). Black hair follicular dysplasia in dogs. *J. Am. Vet. Med. Assoc.* 171: 1079–1081.

16 Schmutz, S.M., Moker, J.S., Clark, E.G., and Shewfelt, R. (1998). Black hair follicular dysplasia, an autosomal recessive condition in dogs. *Can. Vet. J.* 39 (10): 644–646.

17 Lewis, C.J. (1995). Black hair follicular dysplasia in UK bred salukis. *Vet. Rec.* 137 (12): 294–295.

18 Knottenbelt, C.M. and Knottenbelt, M.K. (1996). Black hair follicular dysplasia in a tricolour Jack Russell terrier. *Vet. Rec.* 138 (19): 475–476.

19 Munday, J.S., French, A.F., and McKerchar, G.R. (2009). Black-hair follicular dysplasia in a New Zealand huntaway dog. *N. Z. Vet. J.* 57 (3): 170–172.

20 von Bomhard, W., Mauldin, E.A., Schmutz, S.M. et al. (2006). Black hair follicular dysplasia in large Munsterlander dogs: clinical, histological and ultrastructural features. *Vet. Dermatol.* 17 (3): 182–188.

21 Carlotti, D.N. (1990). Canine hereditary black hair follicular dysplasia and color mutant alopecia. Clinical and histopathological aspects. In: *Advances in Veterinary Dermatology* (ed. C. Von Tscharner and H. Rew), 43–46. Philadelphia: Bailliere Tindall.

22 O'Neil, C. (1981). Hereditary disease in the dog and cat. *Compend. Contin. Educ. Vet.* 3: 791–800.

23 Hargis, A.M., Brignac, M., and Bagdadi, F. (1991). Black hair follicular dysplasia in black and white saluki dogs: differentiation from colour mutant alopecia in the Doberman pinscher by microscopic examination of hairs. *Vet. Dermatol.* 2: 69–83.

24 Dunn, K.A., Russell, M., and Boness, J.M. (1995). Black hair follicular dysplasia. *Vet. Rec.* 137 (16): 412.

25 Harper, R.C. (1978). Congenital black hair follicular dysplasia in bearded collie puppies. *Vet. Rec.* 102 (4): 87.

26 Beco, L., Fontaine, J., and Gross, T.L. (1995). Color dilution alopecia in seven dachshunds. A clinical study and the hereditary, microscopical and ultrastructural aspect of the disease. *Vet. Dermatol.* 7: 91–97.

27 Brignac, M., Foil, C.S., and Al Bagdadi, F. (1990). Microscopy of colour mutant alopecia. In: *Advances in Veterinary Dermatology* (ed. C. von Tscharner and H. Rew), 448. Philadelphia: Bailliere Tindall.

28 Prieur, D.J., Fittschen, C., and Collier, L.L. (1983). Macromelanosomes in the hair of blue Doberman pinscher dogs. *Carnivore Genetics Newsletter* 7: 242–247.

29 Austin, V.H. (1975). Blue dog disease. *Mod. Vet. Pract.* 56: 31–34.

30 Kim, J.H., Kang, K.I., Sohn, H.J. et al. (2005). Color-dilution alopecia in dogs. *J. Vet. Sci.* 6 (3): 259–261.

31 Ferrer, L., Durall, I., Closa, J., and Mascort, J. (1988). Colour mutant alopecia in Yorkshire terriers. *Vet. Rec.* 122 (15): 360–361.

32 Finnie, J.W. and Tham, V.L. (1993). Colour mutant alopecia in a kelpie x border collie dog. *Aust. Vet. J.* 70 (10): 388–389.

33 Austin, V.H. (1979). Alopecias of the dog and cat. Part II. *Mod. Vet. Pract.* 60 (2): 130–134.

34 Miller, W.J. (1990). Colour dilution alopecia in Doberman pinschers with blue or fawn coat colour: a study on the incidence and histopathology of this disorder. *Vet. Dermatol.* 1: 113–122.

35 Miller, W.H. (1990). Follicular dysplasia in adult back and red Doberman pinschers. *Vet. Dermatol.* 1: 180–187.

36 Miller, W.H. (1991). Alopecia associated with coat color dilution in 2 Yorkshire terriers, one saluki, and one mix-breed dog. *J. Am. Anim. Hosp. Assoc.* 27 (1): 39–43.

37 Briggs, O.M. and Botha, W.S. (1986). Color mutant Alopecia in a blue Italian greyhound. *J. Am. Anim. Hosp. Assoc.* 22 (5): 611–614.

38 Roperto, F., Cerundolo, R., Restucci, B. et al. (1995). Colour dilution alopecia (CDA) in ten Yorkshire terriers. *Vet. Dermatol.* 6 (4): 171–178.

39 Malik, R. and France, M.P. (1991). Hyperpigmentation and symmetrical Alopecia in 3 silky terriers. *Aust. Vet. Pract.* 21 (3): 135–138.

40 Curtis, C.F., Evans, H., and Lloyd, D.H. (1996). Investigation of the reproductive and growth hormone status of dogs affected by idiopathic recurrent flank alopecia. *J. Small Anim. Pract.* 37 (9): 417–422.

41 Muntener, T., Schuepbach-Regula, G., Frank, L. et al. (2012). Canine noninflammatory alopecia: a comprehensive evaluation of common and distinguishing histological characteristics. *Vet. Dermatol.* 23 (3): 206–e44.

42 Scott, D.W. (1990). Seasonal flank alopecia in ovariohysterectomized dogs. *Cornell Vet.* 80 (2): 187–195.

43 Miller, M.A. and Dunstan, R.W. (1993). Seasonal flank alopecia in boxers and Airedale terriers: 24 cases (1985–1992). *J. Am. Vet. Med. Assoc.* 203 (11): 1567–1572.

44 Waldman, L. (1995). Seasonal flank alopecia in affenpinschers. *J. Small Anim. Pract.* 36 (6): 271–273.

45 Schmeitzel, L.P. (1990). Sex hormone-related and growth hormone-related alopecias. *Vet. Clin. North Am. Small Anim. Pract.* 20 (6): 1579–1601.

46 Nesbitt, G.H. (1983). *Canine and Feline Dermatology: A Systematic Approach*. Philadelphia: Lea and Febiger.

47 Bagnell, B.G. (1984). Skin and associated structures. In: *Canine Medicine and Therapeutics* (ed. E.A. Chandler, J.B. Sutton and D.J. Thompson), 244–259. Oxford: Blackwell Scientific Publications.

48 Miller, W.H. (1989). Sex hormone-related dermatoses in dogs. In: *Current Veterinary Therapy*, 10e (ed. R.W. Kirk), 595–602. Philadelphia: W.B. Saunders.

49 Bush, B.M. (1984). Endocrine system. In: *Canine Medicine and Therapeutics* (ed. E.A. Chandler, J.B. Sutton and D.J. Thompson), 206–243. Oxford: Blackwell Scientific Publications.

50 Chastain, C.B. and Ganjam, V.K. (1986). *Clinical Endocrinology of Companion Animals*. Philadelphia: Lea and Febiger.

51 Shanley, K.J. and Miller, W.H. (1987). Adult-onset growth-hormone deficiency in sibling Airedale terriers. *Compend. Cont. Educ. Pract.* 9 (11): 1076–1082.

52 Medleau, L., Eigenmann, J.E., Saunders, H.M., and Goldschmidt, M.H. (1985). Congenital hypothyroidism in a dog. *J. Am. Anim. Hosp. Assoc.* 21 (3): 341–344.

53 Frank, L.A., Hnilica, K.A., and Oliver, J.W. (2004). Adrenal steroid hormone concentrations in dogs with hair cycle arrest (Alopecia X) before and during treatment with melatonin and mitotane. *Vet. Dermatol.* 15 (5): 278–284.

54 Scott, D.W., Miller, W.H., and Griffin, C.E. (eds.) (2001). Endocrine and metabolic diseases. In: *Muller and Kirk's Small Animal Dermatology*, 780–885. Philadelphia: W.B. Saunders.

55 Schmeitzel, L.P., Lothrop, C.D., and Rosenkrantz, W.S. (1995). Congenital adrenal hyperplasia-like syndrome. In: *Kirk's Current Veterinary Therapy XII* (ed. J.D. Bonagura), 600–604. Philadelphia: W.B. Saunders.

56 Frank, L.A. and Watson, J.B. (2013). Treatment of alopecia X with medroxyprogesterone acetate. *Vet. Dermatol.* 24 (6): 624–627, e153–4.

57 Brunner, M.A.T., Jagannathan, V., Waluk, D.P. et al. (2017). Novel insights into the pathways regulating the canine hair cycle and their deregulation in alopecia X. *PLoS One* 12 (10): e0186469.

58 Campbell, K.L. (1988). Growth hormone-related disorders in dogs. *Compend. Cont. Educ. Pract.* 10 (4): 477–482.

59 Paradis, M. (2000). Melatonin therapy for canine alopecia. In: *Kirk's Current Veterinary Therapy XIII* (ed. J.D. Bonagura), 546–549. Philadelphia: W.B. Saunders.

60 Paradis, M. and Alopecia, X. (2002). *Derm Dialogue* (Summer): 12–14.

61 Rosenkrantz, W.S. and Griffin, C.E. (eds.) (1992). Lysodren therapy in suspect adrenal sex hormone dermatosis. Second World Congress of Veterinary Dermatology (13–16 May). Montreal, Quebec, Canada.

62 Mecklenburg, L. (2006). An overview on congenital alopecia in domestic animals. *Vet. Dermatol.* 17 (6): 393–410.

63 Kimura, T., Ohshima, S., and Doi, K. (1992). Haematological and serum biochemical values in hairless and haired descendants of Mexican hairless dogs. *Lab. Anim.* 26 (3): 214–218.

64 Kimura, T., Ohshima, S., and Doi, K. (1993). The inheritance and breeding results of hairless descendants of Mexican hairless dogs. *Lab. Anim.* 27 (1): 55–58.

65 Robinson, R. (1985). Chinese crested dog. *J. Hered.* 76 (3): 217–218.

66 Kimura, T. and Doi, K. (1996). Spontaneous comedones on the skin of hairless descendants of Mexican hairless dogs. *Exp. Anim.* 45 (4): 377–384.

67 Kimura, T. (1996). Studies on development of hairless descendants of Mexican hairless dogs and their usefulness in dermatological science. *Exp. Anim.* 45 (1): 1–13.

68 Baker, K. (1986). Hormonal alopecia in dogs and cats. *In Pract.* 8 (2): 71–78.

69 Frank, L.A. (2006). Comparative dermatology – canine endocrine dermatoses. *Clin. Dermatol.* 24 (4): 317–325.

70 Feldman, E.C. and Nelson, R.W. (2004). *Canine and Feline Endocrinology and Reproduction*. St. Louis, Missouri: W.B. Saunders.

71 Scott-Moncrieff, J.C. (2007). Clinical signs and concurrent diseases of hypothyroidism in dogs and cats. *Vet. Clin. North Am. Small Anim. Pract.* 37 (4): 709–722, vi.

72 Credille, K.M., Slater, M.R., Moriello, K.A. et al. (2001). The effects of thyroid hormones on the skin of beagle dogs. *J. Vet. Intern. Med.* 15 (6): 539–546.

73 Stewart, L.J. (1994). The integumentary changes of hyperadrenocorticism. *Semin. Vet. Med. Surg.* 9 (3): 123–126.

74 Zur, G. and White, S.D. (2011). Hyperadrenocorticism in 10 dogs with skin lesions as the only presenting clinical signs. *J. Am. Anim. Hosp. Assoc.* 47 (6): 419–427.

75 Peterson, M.E. and Kintzer, P.P. (1997). Medical treatment of pituitary-dependent hyperadrenocorticism. Mitotane. *Vet. Clin. North Am. Small Anim. Pract.* 27 (2): 255–272.

76 Sennello, K.A., Panciera, D.L., Lanz, O.I., and Vail, D.M. (2004). Treating adrenal neoplasia in dogs and cats. *Vet. Med.* 99 (2): 172–186.

77 Anderson, C.R., Birchard, S.J., Powers, B.E. et al. (2001). Surgical treatment of adrenocortical tumors: 21 cases (1990–1996). *J. Am. Anim. Hosp. Assoc.* 37 (1): 93–97.

78 Suess, R.P. Jr., Barr, S.C., Sacre, B.J., and French, T.W. (1992). Bone marrow hypoplasia in a feminized dog with an interstitial cell tumor. *J. Am. Vet. Med. Assoc.* 200 (9): 1346–1348.

79 Barsanti, J.A., Medleau, L., and Latimer, K. (1983). Diethylstilbestrol-induced alopecia in a dog. *J. Am. Vet. Med. Assoc.* 182 (1): 63–64.

80 Peters, M.A., de Jong, F.H., Teerds, K.J. et al. (2000). Ageing, testicular tumours and the pituitary-testis axis in dogs. *J. Endocrinol.* 166 (1): 153–161.

81 Gardener, W.U. and DeVita, J. (1940). Inhibition of hair growth in dogs receiving estrogens. *Yale J. Biol. Med.* 13: 213–215.

82 Gross, T.L. and Ihrke, P.J. (2005). *Atrophic Skin Diseases of the Adnexae. Skin Diseases of the Dog and Cat*, 480–517. Oxford: Blackwell Publishing.

83 Rosychuk, R.A.W. (1998). Cutaneous manifestations of endocrine disease in dogs. *Compend. Cont. Educ. Pract.* 20 (3): 287–302.

84 Taffin, E.R., Casaert, S., Claerebout, E. et al. (2016). Morphological variability of Demodex cati in a feline immunodeficiency virus-positive cat. *J. Am. Vet. Med. Assoc.* 249 (11): 1308–1312.

85 Neel, J.A., Tarigo, J., Tater, K.C., and Grindem, C.B. (2007). Deep and superficial skin scrapings from a feline immunodeficiency virus-positive cat. *Vet. Clin. Pathol.* 36 (1): 101–104.

86 Frank, L.A., Kania, S.A., Chung, K., and Brahmbhatt, R. (2013). A molecular technique for the detection and differentiation of Demodex mites on cats. *Vet. Dermatol.* 24 (3): 367–369, e82–3.

87 Cordero, A.M., Sheinberg-Waisburd, G., Romero Nunez, C., and Heredia, R. (2017 April). Early onset canine generalized demodicosis. *Vet. Dermatol.* 29 (2): 173.

88 Bowden, D.G., Outerbridge, C.A., Kissel, M.B. et al. (2017). Canine demodicosis: a retrospective study of a veterinary hospital population in California, USA (2000–2016). *Vet. Dermatol.*.

89 Mueller, R.S., Bensignor, E., Ferrer, L. et al. (2012). Treatment of demodicosis in dogs: 2011 clinical practice guidelines. *Vet. Dermatol.* 23 (2): 86–96, e20–1.

90 Rouben, C. (2016). Claw and claw bed diseases. *Clinician's Brief* (April): 35–40.

91 Manning, T.O. (1983). Cutaneous diseases of the paw. *Clin. Dermatol.* 1 (1): 131–142.

92 Huang, H.P. and Lien, Y.H. (2013). Feline sarcoptic mange in Taiwan: a case series of five cats. *Vet. Dermatol.* 24 (4): 457–459, e104–5.

93 Malik, R., Stewart, K.M., Sousa, C.A. et al. (2006). Crusted scabies (sarcoptic mange) in four cats due to *Sarcoptes scabiei* infestation. *J. Feline Med. Surg.* 8 (5): 327–339.

94 Hawkins, J.A., McDonald, R.K., and Woody, B.J. (1987). *Sarcoptes scabiei* infestation in a cat. *J. Am. Vet. Med. Assoc.* 190 (12): 1572–1573.

95 Aydingoz, I.E. and Mansur, A.T. (2011). Canine scabies in humans: a case report and review of the literature. *Dermatology* 223 (2): 104–106.

96 Warren, S. (2013). Claw disease in dogs: part 2 – diagnosis and management of specific claw diseases. *Companion Anim.* 18 (5): 226–231.

97 Outerbridge, C.A. (2006). Mycologic disorders of the skin. *Clin. Tech. Small Anim. Pract.* 21 (3): 128–134.

98 Colombo, S., Nardoni, S., Cornegliani, L., and Mancianti, F. (2007). Prevalence of Malassezia spp. yeasts in feline nail folds: a cytological and mycological study. *Vet. Dermatol.* 18 (4): 278–283.

99 Dryden, M. (2016). Flea Allergy Dermatitis. Merck Veterinary Manual [Internet]. https://www.merckvetmanual.com/integumentary-system/fleas-and-flea-allergy-dermatitis/flea-allergy-dermatitis (accessed 16 November 2017).

100 Griffin, C.E. and DeBoer, D.J. (2001). The ACVD task force on canine atopic dermatitis (XIV): clinical manifestations of canine atopic dermatitis. *Vet. Immunol. Immunopathol.* 81 (3–4): 255–269.

101 Hillier, A. and Griffin, C.E. (2001). The ACVD task force on canine atopic dermatitis (I): incidence and prevalence. *Vet. Immunol. Immunopathol.* 81 (3–4): 147–151.

102 Nesbitt, G.H., Kedan, G.S., and Caciolo, P. (1984). Canine atopy .1. Etiology and diagnosis. *Compend. Cont. Educ. Pract.* 6 (1): 73–84.

103 Nesbitt, G.H., Kedan, G.S., and Caciolo, P. (1984). Canine atopy. 2. Management. *Compend. Cont. Educ. Pract.* 6 (3): 264–278.

104 Saridomichelakis, M.N., Koutinas, A.F., Gioulekas, D., and Leontidis, L. (1999). Canine atopic dermatitis in Greece: clinical observations and the prevalence of positive intradermal test reactions in 91 spontaneous cases. *Vet. Immunol. Immunopathol.* 69 (1): 61–73.

105 Prelaud, P., Guaguere, E., Alhaidari, Z. et al. (1998). Reevaluation of diagnostic criteria of canine atopic dermatitis. *Rev. Med. Vet.* 149 (11): 1057–1064.

106 Carlotti, D.N. and Costargent, F. (1994). Analysis of positive skin tests in 449 dogs with allergic dermatitis. *Eur. J. Comp. Anim. Pract.* 4: 42–59.

107 Halliwell, R.E. (1971). Atopic disease in the dog. *Vet. Rec.* 89 (8): 209–214.

108 Scott, D.W. (1981). Observations on canine atopy. *J. Am. Anim. Hosp. Assoc.* 17 (1): 91–100.

109 Bassett, R.J., Burton, G.G., and Robson, D.C. (2004). Antibiotic responsive ulcerative dermatoses in German shepherd dogs with mucocutaneous pyoderma. *Aust. Vet. J.* 82 (8): 485–489.

110 Gortel, K. (2013). Recognizing pyoderma more difficult than it may seem. *Vet. Clin. N. Am. Small.* 43 (1): 1–18.

111 Fontaine, J., Heimann, M., and Day, M.J. (2011). Cutaneous epitheliotropic T-cell lymphoma in the cat: a review of the literature and five new cases. *Vet. Dermatol.* 22 (5): 454–461.

112 Fontaine, J., Bovens, C., Bettenay, S., and Mueller, R.S. (2009). Canine cutaneous epitheliotropic T-cell lymphoma: a review. *Vet. Comp. Oncol.* 7 (1): 1–14.

113 Schmidt, V. (2011). Epitheliotropic T-cell cutaneous lymphoma in dogs. *Companion Anim.* 16: 49–54.

114 Gross, T.L., Ihrke, P., Walder, E.J., and Affolter, V.K. (2005). *Skin Diseases of the Dog and Cat, Clinical and Histopathological Diagnosis*. Oxford: Blackwell Science.

115 Kimmel, S.E., Christiansen, W., and Byrne, K.P. (2003). Clinicopathological, ultrasonographic, and histopathological findings of superficial necrolytic dermatitis with hepatopathy in a cat. *J. Am. Anim. Hosp. Assoc.* 39 (1): 23–27.

116 Byrne, K.P. (1999). Metabolic epidermal necrosis-hepatocutaneous syndrome. *Vet. Clin. North Am. Small Anim. Pract.* 29 (6): 1337–1355.

117 Hall-Fonte, D.L., Center, S.A., McDonough, S.P. et al. (2016). Hepatocutaneous syndrome in Shih Tzus: 31 cases (1996–2014). *J. Am. Vet. Med. Assoc.* 248 (7): 802–813.

118 Marinkovich, M.P., Botella, R., Datloff, J., and Sangueza, O.P. (1995). Necrolytic migratory erythema without glucagonoma in patients with liver disease. *J. Am. Acad. Dermatol.* 32 (4): 604–609.

119 Bond, R., McNeil, P.E., Evans, H., and Srebernik, N. (1995). Metabolic epidermal necrosis in two dogs with different underlying diseases. *Vet. Rec.* 136 (18): 466–471.

120 Miller, W.H., Scott, D.W., Buerger, R.G. et al. (1990). Necrolytic migratory erythema in dogs – a Hepatocutaneous syndrome. *J. Am. Anim. Hosp. Assoc.* 26 (6): 573–581.

121 Torres, S.M.F., Caywood, D.D., OBrien, T.D. et al. (1997). Resolution of superficial necrolytic dermatitis following excision of a glucagon-secreting pancreatic neoplasm in a dog. *J. Am. Anim. Hosp. Assoc.* 33 (4): 313–319.

122 Gross, T.L., Song, M.D., Havel, P.J., and Ihrke, P.J. (1993). Superficial necrolytic dermatitis (necrolytic migratory erythema) in dogs. *Vet. Pathol.* 30 (1): 75–81.

123 Outerbridge, C.A. (2010). Hepatocutaneous syndrome. In: *Textbook of Veterinary Internal Medicine* (ed. S.J. Ettinger and E.C. Feldman), 112–115. St. Louis, Missouri: Saunders Elsevier.

124 March, P.A., Hillier, A., Weisbrode, S.E. et al. (2004). Superficial necrolytic dermatitis in 11 dogs with a history of phenobarbital administration (1995–2002). *J. Vet. Intern. Med.* 18 (1): 65–74.

125 Outerbridge, C.A., Marks, S.L., and Rogers, Q.R. (2002). Plasma amino acid concentrations in 36 dogs with histologically confirmed superficial necrolytic dermatitis. *Vet. Dermatol.* 13 (4): 177–186.

126 Nam, A., Han, S.M., Go, D.M. et al. (2017). Long-term management with adipose tissue-derived mesenchymal stem cells and conventional treatment in a dog with Hepatocutaneous syndrome. *J. Vet. Intern. Med.* 31 (5): 1514–1519.

127 Falk, E.F., Lam, A.T., Barber, L.G., and Ferrer, L. (2017). Clinical characteristics of doxorubicin-associated alopecia in 28 dogs. *Vet. Dermatol.* 28 (2): 207–e48.

128 Trueb, R.M. (2010). Chemotherapy-induced hair loss. *Skin Therapy Lett.* 15 (7): 5–7.

129 McGarvey, E.L., Baum, L.D., Pinkerton, R.C., and Rogers, L.M. (2001). Psychological sequelae and alopecia among women with cancer. *Cancer Pract.* 9 (6): 283–289.

130 Rosman, S. (2004). Cancer and stigma: experience of patients with chemotherapy-induced alopecia. *Patient Educ. Couns.* 52 (3): 333–339.

131 Lemieux, J., Maunsell, E., and Provencher, L. (2008). Chemotherapy-induced alopecia and effects on quality of life among women with breast cancer: a literature review. *Psychooncology* 17 (4): 317–328.

132 Munstedt, K., Manthey, N., Sachsse, S., and Vahrson, H. (1997). Changes in self-concept and body image during alopecia induced cancer chemotherapy. *Support Care Cancer* 5 (2): 139–143.

133 Spiegel, D. and Giese-Davis, J. (2003). Depression and cancer: mechanisms and disease progression. *Biol. Psychiatry* 54 (3): 269–282.

134 Yun, S.J. and Kim, S.J. (2007). Hair loss pattern due to chemotherapy-induced anagen effluvium: a cross-sectional observation. *Dermatology* 215 (1): 36–40.

135 Cavalcanti, J.V.J., Hasbach, A., Barnes, K. et al. (2017). Skin depigmentation associated with toceranib phosphate in a dog. *Vet. Dermatol.* 28 (4): 400–e95.

136 McEntee, M.C. (2006). Veterinary radiation therapy: review and current state of the art. *J. Am. Anim. Hosp. Assoc.* 42 (2): 94–109.

137 Fajardo, L.F., Berthrong, M., and Anderson, R.E. (2001). *Radiation Pathology*. Oxford: Oxford University Press.

138 Harris, D., King, G.K., and Bergman, P.J. (1997). Radiation therapy toxicities. *Vet. Clin. North Am. Small Anim. Pract.* 27 (1): 37–46.

139 Gillette, E.L., LaRue, S.M., and Gillette, S.M. (1995). Normal tissue tolerance and management of radiation injury. *Semin. Vet. Med. Surg.* 10 (3): 209–213.

140 Credille, K.M., Thompson, L.A., Young, L.M. et al. (2013). Evaluation of hair loss in cats occurring after treatment with a topical flea control product. *Vet. Dermatol.* 24 (6): 602–605, e145–6.

141 Genovese, A.G., McLean, M.K., and Khan, S.A. (2012). Adverse reactions from essential oil-containing natural flea products exempted from Environmental Protection Agency regulations in dogs and cats. *J. Vet. Emerg. Crit. Care (San Antonio)* 22 (4): 470–475.

142 Villar, D., Knight, M.J., Hansen, S.R., and Buck, W.B. (1994). Toxicity of melaleuca oil and related essential oils applied topically on dogs and cats. *Vet. Hum. Toxicol.* 36 (2): 139–142.

143 Davies, K.E. and Yesudian, P. (2012). Pressure alopecia. *Int. J. Trichology* 4 (2): 64–68.

144 Marsh, K.A., Ruedisueli, F.L., Coe, S.L., and Watson, T.D.G. (2000). Effects of zinc and linoleic acid supplementation on the skin and coat quality of dogs receiving a complete and balanced diet. *Vet. Dermatol.* 11 (4): 277–284.

145 Codner, E.C. and Thatcher, C.D. (1993). Nutritional Management of Skin-Disease. *Compend. Cont. Educ. Pract.* 15 (3): 411–424.

146 Miller, W.H. Jr. (1989). Nutritional considerations in small animal dermatology. *Vet. Clin. North Am. Small Anim. Pract.* 19 (3): 497–511.

147 Campbell, K.L. (1990). Fatty-acid supplementation and skin-disease. *Vet. Clin. N. Am. Small.* 20 (6): 1475–1486.

148 Fadok, V.A. (1982). Zinc responsive dermatosis in a great-Dane – a case-report. *J. Am. Anim. Hosp. Assoc.* 18 (3): 409–414.

149 Degryse, A.D., Fransen, J., Vancutsem, J., and Ooms, L. (1987). Recurrent zinc-responsive dermatosis in a Siberian. *J. Small Anim. Pract.* 28 (8): 721–726.

150 Feusner, J.D., Hembacher, E., and Phillips, K.A. (2009). The mouse who couldn't stop washing: pathologic grooming in animals and humans. *CNS Spectr.* 14 (9): 503–513.

151 Patel, A. (2010 May). Acral lick dermatitis. *Companion Anim.* 15 (4): 43–47.

152 Denerolle, P., White, S.D., Taylor, T.S., and Vandenabeele, S.I. (2007). Organic diseases mimicking acral lick dermatitis in six dogs. *J. Am. Anim. Hosp. Assoc.* 43 (4): 215–220.

153 Moon-Fanelli, A.A., Dodman, N.H., and Cottam, N. (2007). Blanket and flank sucking in Doberman pinschers. *J. Am. Vet. Med. Assoc.* 231 (6): 907–912.

154 Houpt, K.A. (1991). Feeding and drinking behavior problems. *Vet. Clin. North Am. Small Anim. Pract.* 21 (2): 281–298.

155 Gnirs, K. and Prelaud, P. (2005). Cutaneous manifestations of neurological diseases: review of neuro-pathophysiology and diseases causing pruritus. *Vet. Dermatol.* 16 (3): 137–146.

156 Waisglass, S.E., Landsberg, G.M., Yager, J.A., and Hall, J.A. (2006). Underlying medical conditions in cats with presumptive psychogenic alopecia. *J. Am. Vet. Med. Assoc.* 228 (11): 1705–1709.

157 Virga, V. (2003). Behavioral dermatology. *Vet. Clin. North Am. Small Anim. Pract.* 33 (2): 231–251, v–vi.

158 Shumaker, A.K., Angus, J.C., Coyner, K.S. et al. (2008). Microbiological and histopathological features of canine acral lick dermatitis. *Vet. Dermatol.* 19 (5): 288–298.

159 Seksel, K. and Lindeman, M.J. (1998). Use of clomipramine in the treatment of anxiety-related and obsessive-compulsive disorders in cats. *Aust. Vet. J.* 76 (5): 317–321.

160 Sawyer, L.S., Moon-Fanelli, A.A., and Dodman, N.H. (1999). Psychogenic alopecia in cats: 11 cases (1993–1996). *J. Am. Vet. Med. Assoc.* 214 (1): 71–74.

161 Pekmezci, D., Sancak, A.A., Cakiroglu, D., and Meral, Y. (2009). Psychogenic alopecia in five cats. *Ank. Univ. Vet. Fak. Derg.* 56 (2): 145–146.

6

Infestation

6.1 An Introduction to Medical Terminology Associated with Parasitology

Parasitology is the study of organisms that exploit other organisms, so-called hosts, to support, sustain, or complete their life cycle [1]. Parasites that either live on the external surface of a host or within the skin are called ectoparasites as compared to those that live within the host, endoparasites [1]. Ectoparasites and their resultant infestations form the basis of this chapter. Whereas endoparasites *infect* their hosts, ectoparasites *infest* their host by virtue of exploiting the host's surface [1].

In addition to causing infestation, ectoparasites are frequently vectors of disease: they are capable of carrying and transmitting one or more pathogens into another organism [1]. Because ectoparasites are causative agents of disease, the perceptive clinician must consider not only which ectoparasites are present in each patient, but also which diseases they may harbor.

6.2 Lice

Lice are ectoparasites with worldwide distribution, but their abundance in large part depends upon the climate. They are more common in regions with colder climates that are less hospitable to fleas and ticks [2, 3]. They also thrive in kenneled situations because patients are in close quarters with direct contact [1, 2, 4, 5].

Within the United States, lice are relatively uncommon, in large part because many regional climates necessitate flea and tick parasiticides, most of which are effective against lice [2]. When lice infestations do occur in dogs or cats, patients tend to represent extremes of age or those that are debilitated by disease [6].

Lice are species-specific. They can, however, be transported from one host to another by inanimate objects, such as brushes or combs, or by another species acting as a fomite [7, 8].

Once they have found a host, lice have preferential regions of the body on which to reside. In dogs and cats, lice prefer the head, face, neck, ears, back, and tail [4, 9]. Long-eared dogs such as Bassett hounds and various breeds of Spaniels may be at greater risk of pediculosis, infestation with lice [4, 10, 11]. Thick and longhaired coats also provide hospitable habitats for lice to seek refuge: it may be more difficult for these dogs and cats to effectively groom out the lice [11].

There are two primary suborders of lice. The *Mallophaga* suborder of lice constitutes the chewing or biting lice. These feed on sebaceous secretions and epidermal debris, as opposed to the sucking lice, in the suborder *Anoplura*, which ingest host blood [2, 4, 8, 10, 11].

Mallophaga is a word with Greek origins: *mallos*, for hair, and *phagein*, feeding by biting [12]. Members of *Mallophaga* have large heads that are wider than the thorax to support wide mandibles adapted for chewing. Three pairs of legs attach to the thorax. These assist with clasping hair shafts to move throughout the coat [7].

There are approximately 2500 species within *Mallophaga*, many of which are hosted by birds [10]. Of importance to companion animal medicine are two species, *Trichodectes canis* and *Felicola subrostratus* [4]. The former species is dog-specific; the latter occurs only in cats [4, 5]. Nits, which are lice eggs, of both species are visible to the naked eye [2] (see Figures 6.1a–c).

Both *T. canis* and *F. subrostratus* trigger pruritus [4]. Self-inflicted scratch wounds are common. Over time, coats become dull and unkempt [4]. Scaling and crusting are often by-products of infestation [4]. Alopecic patches may occur if infestation is severe enough [4].

In addition, *T. canis* is a vector of the cestode, *Dipylidium caninum* [13]. Clinicians more often associate transmission of *D. caninum* with fleas; however, it is important to note that chewing lice also make capable vectors.

T. canis is also of increasing concern in wildlife because moderate to severe infestations have been documented in gray wolves and coyotes in Alaska [14–16].

Common Clinical Presentations in Dogs and Cats, First Edition. Ryane E. Englar.
© 2019 John Wiley & Sons, Inc. Published 2019 by John Wiley & Sons, Inc.

(a) (b) (c)

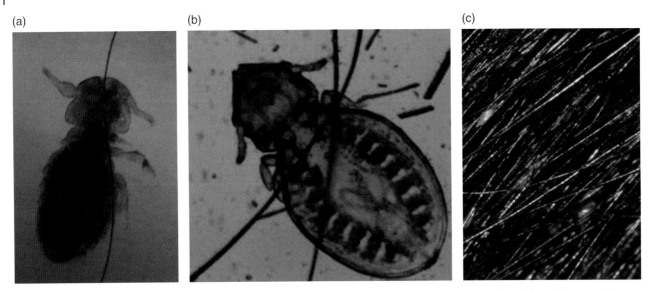

Figure 6.1 (a) *Trichodectes canis* as seen under the light microscope. This louse was collected off the coat of a debilitated puppy with a comb. *Source:* Courtesy of Kirsten Ura-Barton, DVM. (b) *Felicola subrostratus* as seen under the light microscope. This louse was collected from a debilitated geriatric cat. (c) Nits from *F. subrostratus*, on the surface of a black-coated patient.

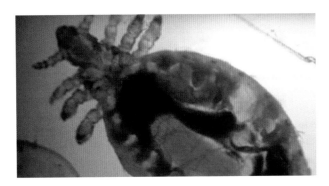

Figure 6.2 *Linognathus setosus*.

The suborder, *Anoplura*, consists of lice that are typically larger than those in *Mallophaga*, with narrower heads and more slender abdomens. Instead of possessing large mandibles for chewing, they have mouthparts that pierce the skin to feed upon capillary blood [7]. They tend to be gray in color; however, their hue becomes redder as blood meals fill their intestines. Only one species is relevant to companion animal medicine, *Linognathus setosus*. This species infests dogs only [2, 4, 7] (see Figure 6.2).

Like infestations with *Mallophaga*, *L. setosus* infestations also induce pruritus. In addition, because sucking lice consume blood meals from their hosts, they may cause significant anemia in young or debilitated patients [2, 4, 9, 12] (see Figure 6.3).

6.3 Cuterebra

Cuterebra is a genus of botflies that parasitize the dermis of rodents and rabbits. Cuterebriasis, the disease caused by such parasitism, is relevant to companion animal medicine because cats, and less commonly dogs, are atypical hosts [1, 17].

The adult botfly is approximately the size and shape of a bumblebee [18]. It lays its eggs near rodent and rabbit dens and burrows. When cats and dogs investigate these holes, they may become inadvertent, accidental hosts of hatched larvae. Larvae enter into the host via an external opening such as the nasal or oral cavity, or via a wound. Larvae then migrate beneath the skin, encyst, and develop further. Sometimes these larvae are referred to as bots or warbles [1, 17].

One or more bots may grow within a feline or canine host. The cheek and neck are common locations in the cat [18] (see Figure 6.4).

As each bot enlarges beneath the surface of the skin, a visible or palpable swelling may develop. A "breathing hole" may be evident on the skin's surface, overlying the site of bot development. This hole enlarges as the bot matures in preparation from its exit from the host [1, 17].

The third-stage larva that emerges is fully developed, dark brown-to-black in color, and covered with spines [1] (see Figure 6.5).

The warble itself may create extensive tissue damage at the site of development (see Figure 6.6).

Secondary infection of the empty cyst after the warble has exited the host may result in additional trauma.

Aberrant migration of *Cuterebra* in the cat has also been reported in the nasopharynx, oropharynx, trachea, thoracic cavity, orbit, anterior chamber of the eye, and within the central nervous system [18–33]. These complications present site-specific challenges, and may be fatal to the patient.

Improper removal of the bot through crushing may cause an anaphylactic reaction [1, 17].

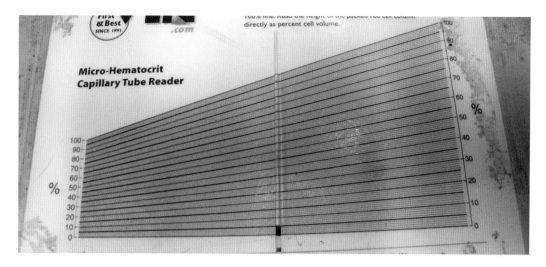

Figure 6.3 Severe anemia in a debilitated patient as evidenced by a packed cell volume of 4%. *Source:* Courtesy of Daniel Foy, MS, DVM, DACVIM, DACVECC.

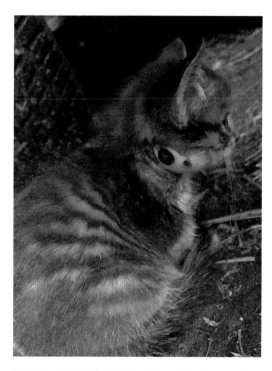

Figure 6.4 Cuterebriasis in a kitten. Note the prominent swelling caudoventral to the right mandible and extending down the neck. *Source:* Courtesy of Melanie Goble, DVM, Renewed Strength Veterinary Services; Also Megan Bell & Leroy Jenkins.

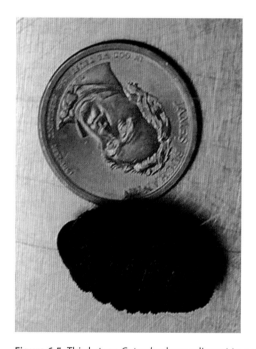

Figure 6.5 Third-stage *Cuterebra* larva adjacent to a golden dollar from the United States for size comparison. *Source:* Courtesy of Melanie Goble, DVM, Renewed Strength Veterinary Services; Also Megan Bell & Leroy Jenkins.

6.4 Fleas

Fleas are by far more common ectoparasites than lice and third-stage *Cuterebra* larvae. There are more than 2200 species and subspecies of fleas worldwide; however, only four are present in great enough numbers on cats and dogs to be a nuisance [34–36]:

- *Ctenocephalides felis felis*
- *Ctenocephalides canis*
- *Pulex simulans*
- *Echidnophaga gallinacea*

Of these four species of fleas, *C. felis felis* is most commonly seen in North America [34–37]. Although it is colloquially referred to as the cat flea, it infests both dogs and cats [34, 36].

The resulting condition of being flea-bitten is called pulicosis [37]. Unlike lice, fleas are not species-specific. Pulicosis results in high infection rates of companion animals as well as wildlife [37–44].

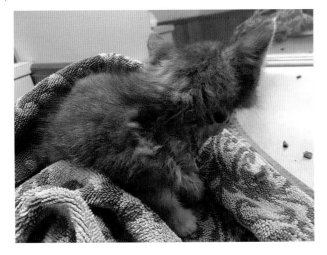

Figure 6.6 Note the significant tissue trauma sustained by this kitten with cuterebriasis. This photograph was taken after warble extraction. *Source:* Courtesy of Melanie Goble, DVM, Renewed Strength Veterinary Services; Also Megan Bell & Leroy Jenkins.

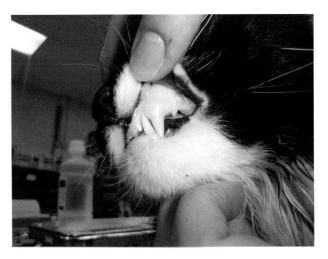

Figure 6.7 Extreme pallor associated with the mucous membranes of a debilitated cat. This cat was significantly anemic. *Source:* Courtesy of Daniel Foy, MS, DVM, DACVIM, DACVECC.

Clinicians typically identify adult fleas or flea dirt on physical examination. Adult fleas are visible to the naked eye and are grossly recognizable. Refer to Figures 5.28a–c and 5.29.

It is important to recognize that adult fleas on companion animal patients only represent approximately 5% of the total flea population [34]. Environments that house flea-infested patients rapidly become infested with eggs, larvae, and pupae [34]. In particular, larvae favor carpet fibers, where they can seek refuge from direct sunlight [34]. Heat destroys them, as does desiccation [45, 46]. Because residential environments provide microhabitats that support flea reproduction, flea control must target multiple life stages to be effective [34, 47–49]. Flea control strategies are beyond the scope of this text. However, overcoming infestations in the home represents a significant concern and challenge for the companion animal owner [34–36, 38, 47]. Maintaining an open dialogue, creating partnership with the veterinary team, and facilitating client education are invaluable to the success of a flea eradication program.

6.4.1 Fleas and Hypersensitivity Reactions

In addition to being nuisances for the patient, client, and the home environment, fleas may trigger a hypersensitive state in some patients. These individuals suffer from immediate or delayed immune reactions, or both, in response to antigenic stimulation from flea saliva. Pruritus is severe and often leads to rapid and extensive self-induced trauma to the coat [50]. Refer to Chapter 5, Section 5.8 for more information.

6.4.2 Fleas and Anemia

As was true of sucking lice, fleas can also deplete small and/or debilitated patients of their blood supply. Each female flea consumes 13.6 µl of blood per day [51]. This may not seem like a significant amount, but when a patient contains hundreds of fleas, this volume adds up. Anemia can be significant and even fatal [34–36] (see Figure 6.7).

6.4.3 Fleas as Vectors for Cestodes

Fleas can also serve as vectors for tapeworms such as *D. caninum* [34–37]. This cestode is zoonotic: humans inadvertently become infected when they unknowingly ingest whole fleas that contain it [37, 40, 52]. Consider, for example, children who may have poor handwashing hygiene.

D. caninum has worldwide distribution, but is especially prevalent in North American cats [53–62].

Adult tapeworms attach themselves to the wall of the small intestine of their feline host. As these hermaphrodites mature, eggs are produced and stored within terminal segments called proglottids. Each proglottid contains egg capsules or packets, each containing 5–30 hexacanth ova [1] (see Figure 6.8).

Once a proglottid is full of eggs, it detaches and is shed in the host's feces. Proglottids are visible to the naked eye and may resemble grains of white rice or cucumber seeds [1, 63] (see Figures 6.9a, b).

D. caninum eggs are released from terminal segments into the environment when each proglottid breaks open.

When larval stages of the cat flea, *C. felis felis,* consume these eggs, they become infected. Inside of the larval cat flea, the *D. caninum* egg matures into a larval stage, the cysticercoid. Each flea may contain dozens of cysticercoids, each of which is capable of infecting a cat when a cat ingests the flea during grooming [1].

D. caninum has a pre-patent period of two to four weeks [1, 57, 64].

In the adult cat or dog, *D. caninum* may cause perianal pruritus, but is otherwise merely an inconvenience for the patient and an eyesore for the client.

If the cestode burden is great enough, a young or debilitated patient may present for non-specific clinical signs such as an unthrifty coat and a pot-bellied appearance with abdominal distension. Diarrhea or constipation may result from heavy *D. caninum* infestation (see Figure 6.10).

Intestinal obstruction because of *D. caninum* is rare, but possible.

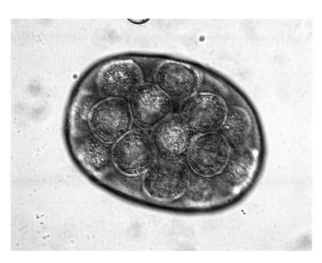

Figure 6.8 *Dipylidium caninum* egg packet. *Source:* Courtesy of Dr. Araceli Lucio-Forster, Cornell University College of Veterinary Medicine.

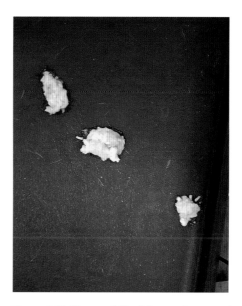

Figure 6.10 Masses of *Dipylidium caninum* proglottids from a canine patient that presented for elective sterilization surgery as part of a veterinary non-profit rural outreach program. *Source:* Courtesy of Hannah Butler.

(a)

(b)

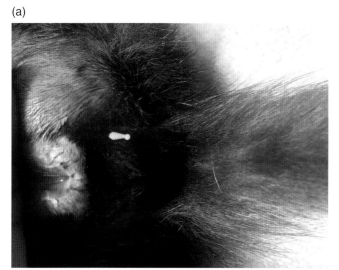

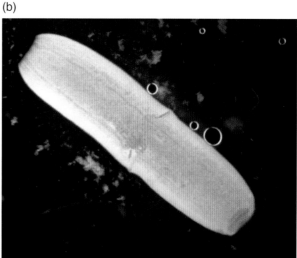

Figure 6.9 (a) *Dipylidium caninum* proglottid, grossly visible to the naked eye as it scoots across the perineal fur of this canine patient. *Source:* Courtesy of Frank Isom, DVM. (b) *D. caninum* proglottid, enlarged. *Source:* Courtesy of Dr. Araceli Lucio-Forster, Cornell University College of Veterinary Medicine.

6.4.4 Fleas as Vectors for Nematodes

In addition to transmitting cestodes, fleas also host filarial nematodes, such as *Acanthocheilonema reconditum*, synonymous with *Dipetalonema reconditum* [37, 65, 66]. Fleas ingest these nematodes as microfilariae during a blood meal. Within one to two weeks of being inside of the flea, the microfilariae mature into infective larvae. These larvae are injected into the skin of a canine host when the infected flea takes its next blood meal. As the larvae burrow into the connective tissue of the dog, they mature into adults that then reproduce to continue the life cycle.

Infected dogs are typically asymptomatic. Adult *D. reconditum* may be discovered as an incidental finding on necropsy. In addition to subcutaneous tissues, these nematodes invade body cavities and kidneys. *D. reconditum* microfilariae may also be identified on a blood smear. The inexperienced veterinary student may confuse *D. reconditum* with the canine heartworm, *Dirofilaria immitis*; however, these can be readily differentiated based upon size and shape. *Dirofilaria immitis* is much larger than *D. reconditum*. In addition, *Dirofilaria immitis* classically has a straight tail and tapered head as compared to *D. reconditum*, which has a button-hook tail and a blunted head.

Although *D. reconditum* is not of particular concern to canine patients, it can also affect humans bitten by infected fleas. Although humans represent dead-end hosts, *D. reconditum* larvae can create pathology in connective tissue as well as in other organs, including the human eye [66–69].

6.4.5 Fleas as Vectors for Other Pathogens

In addition to filarial nematodes, fleas are capable of transmitting the following pathogens [34, 70–73]:

- *Rickettsia typhi*
- *Rickettsia felis*
- *Bartonella henselae*
- *Mycoplasma haemofelis*
- *Yersinia pestis*

R. typhi is the causative agent of murine fever in humans. *R. felis* causes cat-flea typhus, otherwise known as flea-borne spotted fever. Both represent global threats to human health and are beyond the scope of this text [74–84]. However, it is the responsibility of veterinarians to be aware that these conditions do exist and have been linked to fleas collected from cats [75, 76]. Continued partnership with the human medical profession should improve understanding of the spread of these diseases and the need for widespread flea control to reduce the risk that either disease will be contracted.

B. henselae is the vector-transmitted causative agent of bartonellosis, otherwise referred to as cat scratch fever [85]. It is zoonotic. Humans are thought to be infected when wounds caused by cat scratches are inoculated with flea feces [85, 86]. It is also possible that flea feces could contaminate feline saliva, which in turn would contaminate bite wounds in humans [85].

Cat scratch fever is of concern to humans because it can induce local or systemic disease. Locally, it manifests as self-limiting lymphadenopathy that resolves within two to four months [87]. Up to 10% of patients may develop atypical presentations, for example, oculoglandular syndrome [87, 88]. Oculoglandular syndrome is characterized by progressive lymphadenopathy that involves pre-auricular rather than submandibular regions. Oculoglandular syndrome is also associated with non-suppurative, painless conjunctivitis [88]. Other patients may complain of neurological symptoms such as headaches. Cranial or peripheral nerve complaints, with and without mental status changes and encephalopathy, seizures, and neuroretinitis have also been reported [85, 88–92].

Domestic cats are considered the primary mammalian reservoir host for *B. henselae*. Wild cats in the United States and abroad are also exposed to this gram-negative bacteria [85]. Antibodies to *B. henselae* have been identified in 17% of African lions, 18% of Floridian panthers, 28% of Texan mountain lions, 31% of African cheetahs, and 30–53% of Californian wild felids, captive and free [85, 93–95].

B. henselae are a diverse collection of genetically distinct bacteria, meaning that two 16S ribosomal ribonucleic acid (rRNA) types exist, with two subgroups of each [85, 96]. There are regional differences in infection rates because the prevalence of different types and subtypes varies depending upon geography [97–101]. Co-infection with different types and subtypes is also possible [97, 102, 103].

Cats that are infected with *B. henselae*, either via natural or experimental means, tend to be asymptomatic [95, 97]. When cats succumb to experimental infection, clinical signs tend to be mild [103–105]. Infections among naturally infected cats are rarely reported; however, isolated cases of uveitis and endocarditis have been reported [106–109].

Chronic, recurrent bacteremia is common in cats with *B. henselae* although it is difficult to rule out the possibility that these cats have been re-exposed and/or re-infected [103, 110–112]. Diagnosis and treatment are beyond the scope of this text. However, it is important to note that because of the potential for relapses, treatment presents a challenge. It is difficult to establish when the patient is truly free and clear of *B. henselae* [85].

M. haemofelis, formerly known as *Haemobartonella felis*, are bacteria that attach to the external surface of host erythrocytes and cause hemolytic anemia [113, 114]. Fleas and other arthropod vectors, such as ticks and mosquitoes, transmit this pathogen through blood meals [113]. Transfusions also serve as a mode of transmission for *M. haemofelis* [115].

Infection with *M. haemofelis* is worldwide; however, prevalence rates vary by region of the globe [116–121]. Among anemic feline patients in the United States, the prevalence of *M. haemofelis* is 25% [122].

Outdoor male cats appear to be at increased risk of infection [114, 120, 123].

Infections tend to be subclinical in cats unless there is concurrent immunosuppression [113]. According to some, but not all studies, clinical signs are more likely to develop in cats that are infected with feline immunodeficiency virus (FIV) or feline leukemia virus (FeLV) [114, 120, 124–126]. Infected cats may also alternate between clinical and subclinical periods of disease, in which there are cyclical phases of anemia [123, 127].

When clinical infection is present, it tends to be severe. Anemia results from increased fragility of infected erythrocytes and extravascular hemolysis [114, 128–132]. Under experimental conditions, infected erythrocytes are rapidly removed from circulation: within three hours, infected red blood cells may decline from 90% to less than 1% of the circulating population [126, 133, 134].

Clinically ill patients present with non-specific signs resulting from anemia including lethargy, depression, weakness, and inappetence [114]. Patient pallor, tachypnea, and tachycardia are supportive of presumptive anemia, which is confirmed via hemogram [114]. Refer to Figure 6.7 for visual depiction of pallor that was associated with significant anemia in a feline patient.

Blood smears from infected cats may demonstrate autoagglutination (see Figure 6.11).

There is low sensitivity for cytological detection of *M. haemofelis,* which appear as epierythrocytic bacteria [114] (see Figure 6.12).

False positives may result when basophilic stain precipitates are mistaken for bacteria [114] (see Figure 6.13).

Y. pestis is the causative agent of plague, known during Medieval times as "the Black Death" [135]. As a reportable disease, plague is of particular concern because it is zoonotic and often fatal [135]. Fleas act as vectors. Fleabite transmission is most common; however, infected rodents or lagomorphs may transmit disease if they are ingested [135, 136]. Infection may be localized. The bubonic form results in abscesses and draining tracts. In cats, necrotic stomatitis may develop secondary to ingesting infected tissue, and local lymph nodes, such as the mandibular and sublingual, may become swollen. Cats may also present with primary pulmonary disease or septicemia [135–139].

It is important to note that *C. felis felis* is not an efficient transmitter of plague, and is therefore not responsible for the majority of cases involving disease transmission. More typically, plague is spread by the tropical or Oriental rat flea, *Xenopsylla cheopis.*

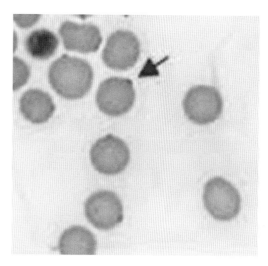

Figure 6.12 *Mycoplasma haemofelis* on a feline blood smear. The red arrow is pointing to an infected erythrocyte. Note the location of the epierythrocytic bacteria.

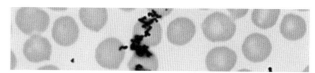

Figure 6.13 Stain precipitate as an artifact of slide preparation for blood smear analysis. Note how stain precipitate could be mistaken for *Mycoplasma haemofelis* if it overlaid an erythrocyte in such a way as to give the illusion of epierythrocytic bacteria.

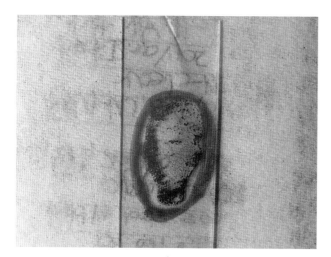

Figure 6.11 Autoagglutination on a blood smear. *Source:* Courtesy of Dr. Lisa Keenan.

6.5 Ticks

Fleas are not the only ectoparasite of concern as a prominent vector of disease. Ticks represent a veterinary and human health threat by virtue of the pathogens they harbor.

Unlike fleas, ticks have extensive life cycles that may take up to three years to complete as each undergoes four distinct life stages:

- Egg
- Six-legged larva
- Eight-legged nymph
- Adult

Most ticks rely upon different host animals to support each stage of their life cycle. An exception is the brown dog tick, *Rhipicephalus sanguineus*, which is capable of being a one-host tick, exploiting the dog at all stages of its life cycle [140].

Many ticks never complete their full life cycle because they do not find an appropriate host to provide their next blood meal.

Blood meals cause ticks to swell enormously. When fed, female ticks may grow to a size that is 100 times her body weight [34, 141, 142].

Fed, swollen ticks are said to be engorged with blood (see Figures 6.14a, b).

6.5.1 Tick Family Classification

For classification purposes, ticks can be divided into two primary families [34]:

- Soft-bodied ticks, Argasidae
- Hard-bodied ticks, Ixodidae

Hard-bodied, or so-called hard ticks, are characterized by their scutums, a protective shield that covers their dorsum [34]. The color or pattern of the scutum may assist with species identification [34]. In addition, certain species may be recognized by their posterior indentations or festoons [34]. Hard ticks also have the head or capitum positioned in front of the scutum.

Within the United States, hard-bodied ticks are prevalent and are of greatest concern as vectors of disease. Common ticks include the [34]:

- Lone Star tick, *Amblyomma americanum*
- Gulf Coast tick, *Amblyomma maculatum*
- Black-legged or deer tick, *Ixodes scapularis*
- Western black-legged tick, *Ixodes pacificus*
- Rocky Mountain wood tick, *Dermacentor andersoni*
- Pacific Coast tick, *Dermacentor occidentalis*
- American dog tick, *Dermacentor variabilis*
- Brown dog tick, *R. sanguineus* (see Figures 6.15–6.18.)

The spinose ear tick, *Otobius megnini*, is the only soft-bodied tick of concern as a parasite of North

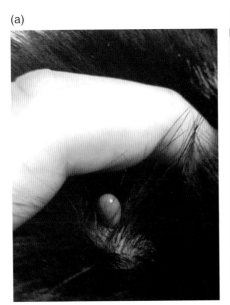
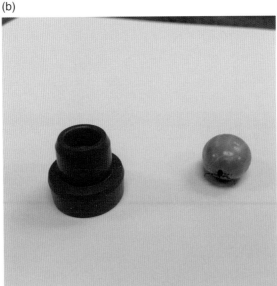

Figure 6.14 (a) Engorged tick attached to the forehead of a canine patient. *Source:* Courtesy of Kimberly Wallitsch. (b) Engorged tick, detached from its canine host. Rubber top from a red top blood tube has been placed in the photograph as a size comparison. *Source:* Courtesy of Daniel Foy, MS, DVM, DACVIM, DACVECC.

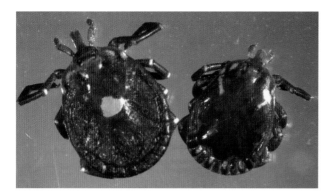

Figure 6.15 Male and female adult Lone Star ticks, *Amblyomma americanum*. The female is on the left. Note the presence of a single white dot against the brown scutum that distinguishes the female from the male. *Source:* Courtesy of Dr. Araceli Lucio-Forster, Cornell University College of Veterinary Medicine.

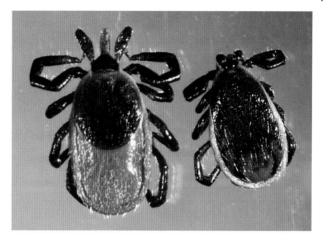

Figure 6.16 Male and female adult black-legged ticks, *Ixodes scapularis*. The female is on the left. Note the characteristic orange-red body surrounding the black scutum. *Source:* Courtesy of Dr. Araceli Lucio-Forster, Cornell University College of Veterinary Medicine.

(a)

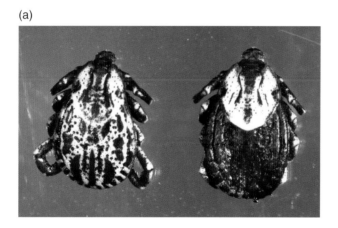

(b)   (c)

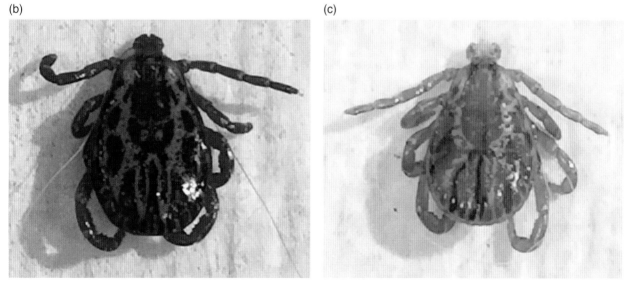

Figure 6.17 (a) Male and female adult American dog ticks, *Dermacentor variabilis*. The female is on the right. *Source:* Courtesy of Dr. Araceli Lucio-Forster, Cornell University College of Veterinary Medicine. (b) Adult male American dog tick, *D. variabilis*, representing color variation. *Source:* Courtesy of J.W. Allen. (c) Adult male American dog tick, *D. variabilis*, representing color variation. *Source:* Courtesy of J.W. Allen.

(a)

(b)

(c)

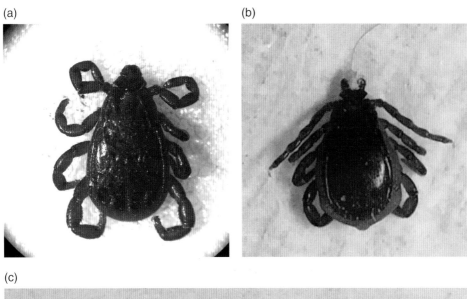

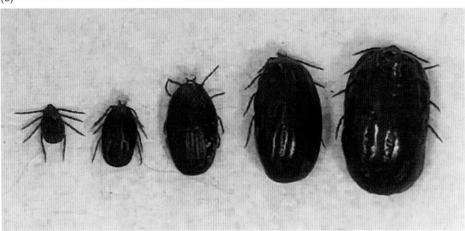

Figure 6.18 (a) Adult male brown dog tick, *Rhipicephalus sanguineus. Source:* Courtesy of Dr. Araceli Lucio-Forster, Cornell University College of Veterinary Medicine. (b) Adult male brown dog tick, *R. sanguineus. Source:* Courtesy of J.W. Allen. (c) Adult female brown dog ticks, *R. sanguineus,* representing varying stages of engorgement. *Source:* Courtesy of J.W. Allen.

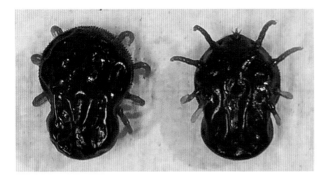

Figure 6.19 Adult spinose ear ticks, *Otobius megnini.* The tick on the left demonstrates a dorsal-ventral (DV) view; the tick on the right demonstrates a ventral-dorsal (VD) view. *Source:* Courtesy of J.W. Allen.

American mammals [34]. Soft-bodied ticks lack scutums. In addition, the capitum sits under the body [34] (see Figure 6.19).

6.5.2 Tick Identification on Physical Examination

Ticks may feed on any part of their host, and therefore can be found throughout the coat (see Figure 6.20).

Some ticks appear have site-specific preferences. For example, *R. sanguineus* prefers the ears or interdigital spaces [34] (see Figure 6.21).

Note that careful examination during a comprehensive physical examination is critical to accuracy with

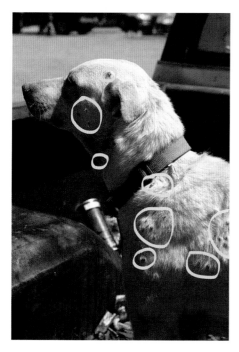

Figure 6.20 Adult dog with a coat that is infested with ticks encircled in yellow. *Source:* Courtesy of Laura Polerecky.

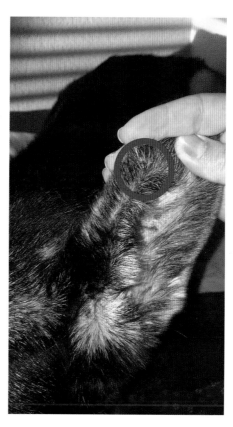

Figure 6.22 Integumentary growth on the pinna of a canine patient. Note how it resembles a tick and could easily be mistaken for one if the clinician was cursory with the physical examination. *Source:* Courtesy of Samantha Gans.

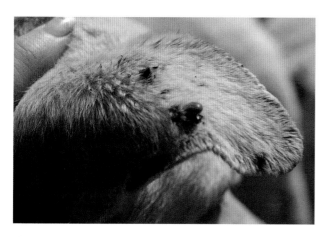

Figure 6.21 Tick attachment to the pinna of an adult dog. *Source:* Courtesy of Laura Polerecky.

diagnosis making. It may sound obvious; however, cutaneous nodules may bear striking resemblance to ticks (see Figure 6.22).

Clinicians should therefore take care to be thorough.

Tick infestations on canine and feline patients can be extraordinary (see Figure 6.23).

Ticks may also cause pruritus at attachment sites. This may lead to intense scratching, chewing, or biting that can result in thinning or the hair coat or self-trauma (see Figure 6.24).

Alternatively, the patient's coat may bear no evidence of ticks other than skin erythema, crusting, and scabbing at the site of prior tick attachment (see Figure 6.25).

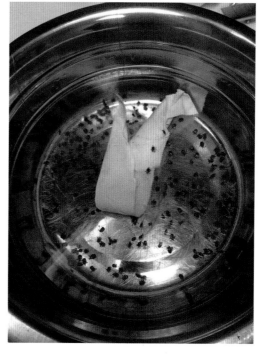

Figure 6.23 The result of tick removal from an infested coat of a canine patient. *Source:* Courtesy of Kimberly Wallitsch.

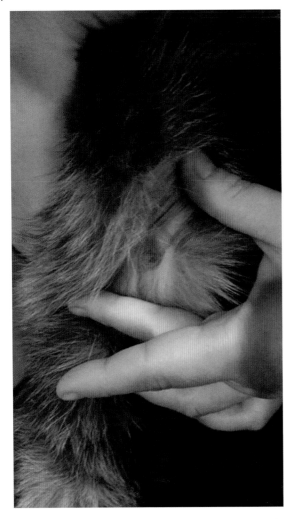

Figure 6.24 Alopecic patch and superficial wound secondary to over-grooming at site of tick attachment. *Source:* Courtesy of Kelli L. Crisfulli, RVT.

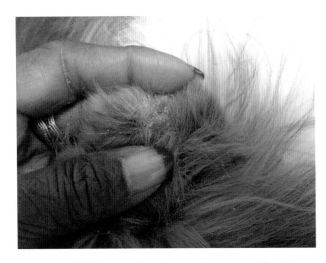

Figure 6.25 Erythema and crusting as cutaneous reactions to prior tick attachment in a canine patient. *Source:* Courtesy of Patricia Bennett, CVM.

6.5.3 Introduction to Ticks as Vectors of Disease

Despite their potential for inciting skin disease, ticks are of greater concern because they harbor and transmit blood-borne diseases, including the following:

- Anaplasmosis [34, 143, 144]
  - Causative agents: *Anaplasma phagocytophilum, Anaplasma platys*
  - Vectors: *I. scapularis, I. pacificus*
- Ehrlichiosis [34, 144, 145]
  - Causative agents: *Ehrlichia ewingii, Ehrlichia canis, Ehrlichia chaffeensis*
  - Vector: *Amblyomma* spp., *R. sanguineus, D. variabilis*
- Borreliosis or Lyme disease [34, 143, 146–148]
  - Causative agent: *Borrelia burgdorferi*
  - Vector: *I. scapularis, I. pacificus, Ixodes dammini*
- Babesiosis [143, 149, 150]
  - Causative agent: *Babesia canis, Babesia gibsoni*
  - Vector: *R. sanguineus*
- Cytauxzoonosis [34, 151–153]
  - Causative agent: *Cytauxzoon felis*
  - Vectors: *Amblyomma* spp., *D. variabilis*
- Rocky Mountain Spotted Fever [34, 143, 154, 155]
  - Causative agent: *Rickettsia rickettsii*
  - Vectors: *D. variabilis, D. andersoni, R. sanguineus*
- Tick paralysis [34]
  - Vectors: *D. variabilis, D. andersoni*
- American canine hepatozoonosis [34, 153, 156]
  - Causative agent: *Hepatozoon americanum*
  - Vectors: *A. maculatum, R. sanguineus*
  - Unique details of transmission: ingestion of the tick is required for dogs to become infected [156]
- Tularemia [34, 157]
  - Causative agent: *Francisella tularensis*
  - Vectors: *Amblyomma* spp., *D. variabilis, D. andersoni*
- Q Fever [34, 155, 158, 159]
  - Causative agent: *Coxiella burnetii*
  - Vectors: *O. megnini, R. sanguineus*

This list is not intended to be comprehensive, just as this chapter is not intended to be a comprehensive review of parasitology. Rather, the goal is to introduce these pathogens as considerations for tick-borne disease as well as to emphasize those presentations that are more likely to be seen in clinical practice:

- Anaplasmosis
- Ehrlichiosis
- Borreliosis

6.5.4 Anaplasmosis

Anaplasmosis in dogs may be caused by *A. phagocytophilum, A. platys,* or co-infection with both [144]. When patients present with concurrent ehrlichiosis,

(a)
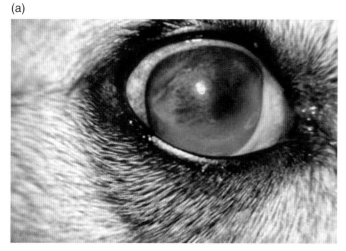

(b)
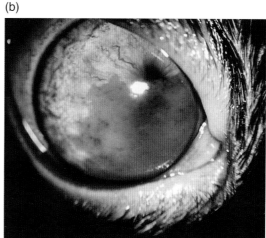

Figure 6.26 (a) Uveitis in a canine patient. (b) Uveitis in a feline patient.

clinical disease is much more severe; disease with *Anaplasma* spp. alone is classically mild [144, 160–164].

A. phagocytophilum causes non-specific clinical signs such as lethargy, depression, fever, and anorexia [144]. Lameness associated with polyarthritis may occur [165–168]. Patients may also present with gastrointestinal upset or evidence of abnormal bleeding, such as epistaxis [165–168].

A. platys tends to be associated with cyclical, recurrent thrombocytopenia [144]. Most dogs remain asymptomatic despite very low platelet counts [144, 169]. However, there have been reports of clinical disease in canine patients that presented for bleeding and anterior uveitis [161, 169–171] (see Figures 6.26a, b).

Although cats are not a reservoir host, they, too, can be infected from being fed upon by *Anaplasma*(+) ticks. Recent studies have demonstrated antibodies against *Anaplasma* spp. in 4.3% of cats in the United States and 30% of cats in endemic regions [172, 173].

Because clinical signs of anaplasmosis in cats are similar to dogs in that they are non-specific, it can be challenging to establish if the patient's malaise is in fact due to infection with *Anaplasma* spp. or if there is other underlying disease. Exposure to *Anaplasma* spp. and antibody production in response are not guarantees of disease or active infection.

6.5.5 Ehrlichiosis

Ehrlichiosis in North American dogs is primarily due to infection with *E. canis*; however, *E. ewingii* and *E. chaffeensis* may also cause disease, particularly in heavy tick regions such as south-central United States [144, 174, 175]. Some regions may have as high as 59% of dogs testing positive for antibodies to *Ehrlichia* spp. [175].

Much as was the case for anaplasmosis, many dogs are subclinical for ehrlichiosis [144]. Other patients demonstrate the same non-specific signs of disease as those infected with *Anaplasma* spp. [144]. Clinical disease may be acute or chronic. Lameness secondary to polyarthritis is common [144].

In addition to myalgia, patients may present with lymphadenopathy and/or splenomegaly [176, 177]. Overt bleeding is possible, including petechiations, ecchymoses, hyphema, retinal hemorrhage, and hematuria [144] (see Figures 6.27a–g).

Neuropathies are rarely reported; however, patients may present with ataxia, head tilt, nystagmus, or seizures [144, 178, 179]. Patients may be thrombocytopenic [144, 177, 178].

Cats may also succumb to ehrlichiosis [144, 180]. Clinical presentations of infected cats mirror those in dogs. In addition, cats may develop concurrent anemia and pancytopenia [70, 144, 180–183].

6.5.6 Borreliosis

Borreliosis, otherwise known as Lyme disease, is a zoonosis. The causative agent, *Borrelia burgdorferi*, is a spirochete that lives in the midgut of infected ticks. Ticks feed on their hosts for multiple days. For the first 12–24 hours of a bite, ticks feed, but do not transmit *B. burgdorferi*. During this time, spirochetes migrate from the tick midgut to the salivary glands. As they undergo this migration, they also remodel their outer surface proteins so that they are less likely to be recognized by the next host's immune defenses. OspA-presenting bacteria switch to their outer proteins to OspC [148, 184–187].

Immune evasion by *B. burgdorferi* persists once bacteria are injected into the new host via the tick's saliva [148]. Lyme disease may be subclinical. However,

(a)

(b)

(c)

(d)

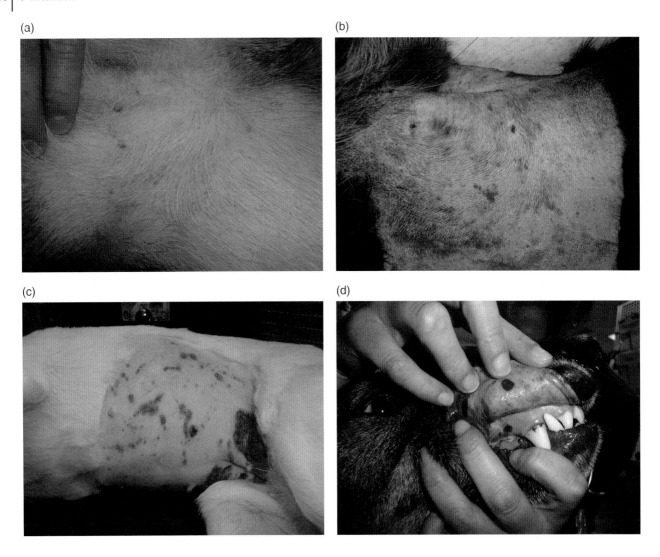

Figure 6.27 (a) Petechiations along the ventrum of a canine patient. *Source:* Courtesy of Daniel Foy, MS, DVM, DACVIM, DACVECC. (b) Petechiations along the ventrum of a canine patient. *Source:* Courtesy of Daniel Foy, MS, DVM, DACVIM, DACVECC. (c) Ecchymoses associated with the ventrum and inguinal region of a canine patient. *Source:* Courtesy of Daniel Foy, MS, DVM, DACVIM, DACVECC. (d) Petechiations and ecchymoses associated with the oral mucous membranes of a canine patient. *Source:* Courtesy of Daniel Foy, MS, DVM, DACVIM, DACVECC. (e) Petechiations associated with the penile shaft of a canine patient. *Source:* Courtesy of Daniel Foy, MS, DVM, DACVIM, DACVECC. (f) Scleral hemorrhage in a canine patient. *Source:* Courtesy of Daniel Foy, MS, DVM, DACVIM, DACVECC. (g) Hyphema in a canine patient. *Source:* Courtesy of Shirley Yang, DVM.

more commonly, Lyme disease presents as acutely debilitating disease that may or may not be cyclical. Because hosts often have difficulty eliminating *B. burgdorferi* from the body, Lyme disease may become chronic [148].

Dogs and cats do not experience Borreliosis in three distinct stages as do humans [148]. They also do not develop erythema migrans, the classic bull's-eye rash with which infected human patients present [148].

Tick bites frequently go unnoticed, and Lyme disease is diagnosed well after the fact. Days to weeks after the

initial infection, dogs may develop non-specific signs of malaise: fever, lethargy, and lymphadenopathy. These tend to be short-lived [148].

When disease is experimentally induced, infected dogs present with lameness two to six months after infection [188, 189]. Lameness starts at the limb nearest the site of the tick bite, and then appears to spread [188, 189]. Lameness may be intermittent or progressive. It may also appear to jump from limb to limb [188, 189].

Certain breeds such as Golden Retrievers, Labrador Retrievers, and Bernese Mountain Dogs also appear

(e)

(f)

(g)

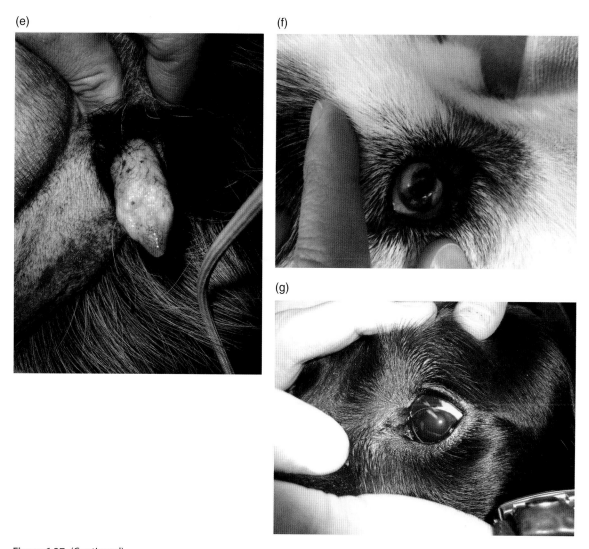

Figure 6.27 (Continued)

predisposed to the development of so-called Lyme nephritis, a glomerulopathy in which there is dramatic, progressive protein loss. Patients present with azotemia, uremia, proteinuria, and peripheral edema. The disease is often fatal [148, 190, 191].

Cats are also exposed to Borreliosis through tick bites. Little is known about the clinical features of Borreliosis in cats because of limited case reports; however, lameness, fever, fatigue, and anorexia appear to be presenting complaints [146].

6.5.7 Introduction to Diagnostics

Diagnosis and treatment options are beyond the scope of this text, but it is important to note that blood smears can be diagnostic for anaplasmosis or ehrlichiosis by identifying characteristic morulae within infected cells, such as monocytes and neutrophils [144]. However, the yield of morulae is low in many infected animals [144] (see Figure 6.28a).

Antibody detection is often used to supplement or confirm a diagnosis as through the use of point-of-care assays such as the 3Dx/4Dx SNAP tests manufactured by IDEXX Laboratories. These test for *E. canis* and *A. phagocytophilum*; however, the analytes may also react with antibodies generated against *E. chaffeensis* and *A. platys*, respectively [144, 192, 193]. Note that although these tableside tests were developed for dogs, they are not species-specific. They can also be used as diagnostic assays in cats [194] (see Figures 6.28b–e).

Note that positive results for these tableside assays demonstrate exposure, but not necessarily active infection.

(a) (b)

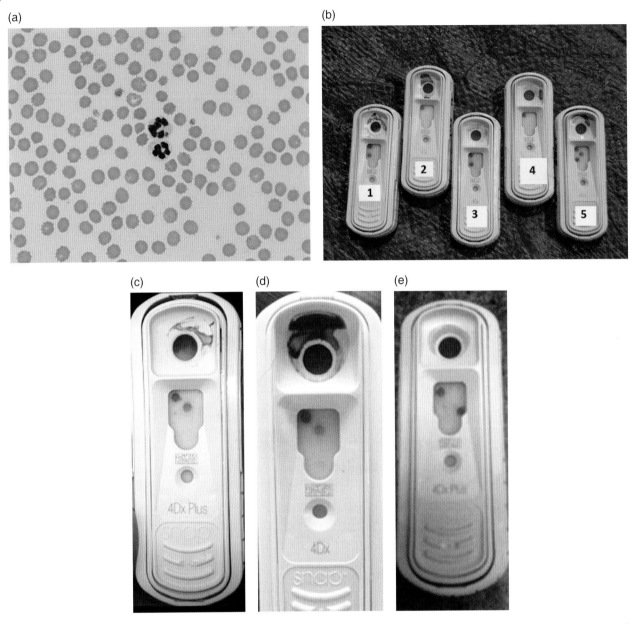

(c)　　　　(d)　　　　(e)

Figure 6.28 (a) *Anaplasma phagocytophilum* morulae within a canine neutrophil at 100×. *Source:* Courtesy of Nora Springer. (b) Point-of-care 4DX IDEXX SNAP tests for *Ehrlichia canis, A. phagocytophilum, Borrelia burgdorferi,* and *Dirofilaria immitis.* Tests #1 and #3 are positive for *E. canis.* Tests #2 and #4 are negative. Test #5 is positive for both *E. canis and A. phagocytophilum. Source:* Courtesy of Laura Polerecky. (c) Point-of-care 4DX IDEXX SNAP test that is positive for *A. phagocytophilum.* (d) Point-of-care 4DX IDEXX SNAP test that is positive for both *A. phagocytophilum* and *B. burgdorferi.* Note that the positive for *B. burgdorferi* is faint. (e) Point-of-care 4DX IDEXX SNAP test that is positive for *Dirofilaria immitis.*

6.5.8 Cytauxzoonosis

Cytauxzoonosis is yet another tick-borne disease [34, 151–153]. Although it occurs with far less frequency than the aforementioned diseases, it does warrant investigation as infection with *C. felis* is often fatal [195–198].

C. felis is a protozoon that typically infects the bobcat, *Lynx rufus,* as the reservoir host [195, 199]. Bobcats recover quickly from infection; however, they become

persistent carriers of infection [152, 200]. Ticks acquire *C. felis* when they feed upon infected bobcats. If they then feed upon domestic cats, cats become subsequently infected and succumb to severe illness within two weeks of the tick bite [199, 201].

Young, outdoor cats, particularly those in rural areas, where contact with ticks is common, are most at risk [195, 202].

(a) (b)

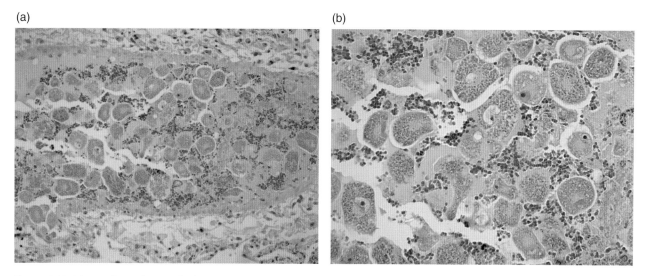

Figure 6.29 (a) Vascular occlusion of a feline pulmonary vessel secondary to infection with *Cytauxzoon felis*. Low magnification. *Source:* Courtesy of Dr. Araceli Lucio-Forster, Cornell University College of Veterinary Medicine, and Dwight D. Bowman, PhD. (b) Same cytology as in Figure 6.29a, only at 20× magnification. *Source:* Courtesy of Dr. Araceli Lucio-Forster, Cornell University College of Veterinary Medicine, and Dwight D. Bowman, PhD.

Illness results from a combination of pathology. Ticks inoculate sporozoites of *C. felis* into the new host. These sporozoites multiply within feline mononuclear cells. As they multiply, they distend the infected cells with schizonts. These cells disseminate throughout the body, where at any point they can obstruct the vasculature much like thrombi, causing local or systemic organ failure [195, 203–206]. Hepatic and pulmonary obstruction are common [204] (see Figures 6.29a. b).

The resultant clinical signs pertain to the specific type of organ dysfunction. For example, cats with pulmonary obstruction commonly present with tachypnea, dyspnea, and open-mouth breathing.

Other clinical signs may include depression, anorexia, and icterus. The patient may be febrile unless moribund, in which case hypothermia is more typical [195, 196].

Lymphadenopathy and splenomegaly are common findings on physical examination. Abdominal palpation may be painful. There may be evidence of internal bleeding such as petechiations or ecchymoses [195, 196, 205–210]. Patients decline rapidly.

C. felis schizonts create further damage to host tissues by dividing into merozoites that then rupture out of infected mononuclear cells. These merozoites are phagocytosed by erythrocytes, and may be observed as piroplasms on a blood smear. These are characteristic signet-ring-shaped, intraerythrocytic structures that stain deeply purple with Wright-Giemsa prep [195]. Less characteristic shapes include bipolar oval or round structures, and tetrad bodies [195].

Hemolysis may occur during early phases of infection. Erythroparasitemia also allows *C. felis* to be transmitted to other hosts when the next tick attaches for a blood meal [195, 211–214].

6.6 Mites

Mites are also ectoparasites.

Mites are similar to ticks in that both organisms belong to the arachnid class of ectoparasites. Adult arachnids have two body segments: a fused head and thorax, and an abdomen.

Unlike ticks, which are visible to the naked eye, mites cannot be visualized without microscopy.

There are many species of mites. For the purposes of this text, the reader should consider the six most common species in companion animal medicine:

- *Demodex* spp.
- *Sarcoptes scabiei*
- *Notoedres cati*
- *Cheyletiella* spp.
- *Otodectes cynotis*
- *Trombicula* spp.

Review Chapter 3, Section 3.8.1 and Chapter 5, Section 5.8 on demodicosis. Recall that demodicosis refers to canine infestation with *Demodex canis* and feline infestation with *Demodex cati* or *Demodex gatoi* [215–220].

Demodicosis may result in localized or generalized disease. Cases involving juvenile onset of localized disease typically have a good prognosis in that they tend to resolve spontaneously, whereas adult onset of generalized demodicosis results from underlying disease [221].

Infestation with *Demodex* spp. causes erythema, hypotrichosis or alopecic patches with or without a papulopustular rash, folliculitis or furunculosis, scaling and follicular casts, pododermatitis, and/or paronychia [221–223]. The face and forelimbs are often involved. Recall Chapter 3, Figures 3.12a–d and Chapter 5, Figures 5.21a–c.

Deep skin scrapings are required to unearth the cigar-shaped *D. canis* from deep within the hair follicle, whereas *D. gatoi* is a surface dweller. Superficial scrapings for *D. gatoi* will suffice. Yield of scrapings is typically high, and a diagnosis can be easily made.

Refer to Chapter 3, Figures 3.13 and 3.14 to differentiate *D. canis* from *D. gatoi*.

Review Chapter 5, Section 5.8 on sarcoptic mange. Recall that sarcoptic mange involves infestation with surface dweller *S. scabiei*, a zoonotic mite. Canine lesions concentrate on the head, pinnae, elbows, and hocks [224, 225]. Recall Chapter 5, Figures 5.22a, b.

Cats are rarely infested with *S. scabiei*. When they are, lesions typically involve the bridge of the nose, feet, claws, and tail [226–228].

Because this mite is zoonotic, humans can also be infested. Infested humans develop severe pruritus and a papular rash along the arms and trunk [229].

Superficial skin scrapes confirm the diagnosis of sarcoptic mange. However, the yield of mites is low, and false negatives are common [224, 228].

Refer to Chapter 3, Figure 3.15 for classic cytology of *S. scabiei*.

N. cati is infrequently seen in cats; however, it occurs with greater frequency than *S. scabiei*. Recall from Chapter 3, Section 3.8.1 that *N. cati* causes crusting and scaling of the face and pinnae as well as paronychia [4, 230]. Chronically affected skin may become hyperpigmented and/or thickened [4].

Superficial skin scrapings confirm the diagnosis (see Figure 6.30).

Like *Sarcoptes* spp., *N. cati* is also zoonotic [230]. In addition, dogs may be transiently affected [4].

Cheyletiella spp. are also mange mites. Two species are of particular importance to companion animal medicine: *Cheyletiella yasguri* infests dogs whereas *Cheyletiella blakei* infests cats [4].

Unlike *D. canis*, *Cheyletiella* spp. do not burrow within hair follicles. Instead, they are surface dwellers that feed on lymph after piercing the skin with chelicerae [4]. In particular, they prefer the head and topline of cats [4].

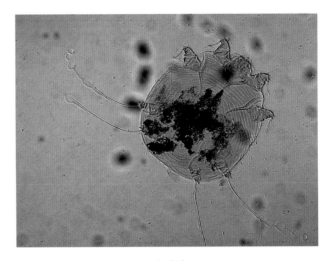

Figure 6.30 *Notoedres cati* under light microscopy, 100× magnification. *Source:* Courtesy of Dr. Araceli Lucio-Forster, Cornell University College of Veterinary Medicine.

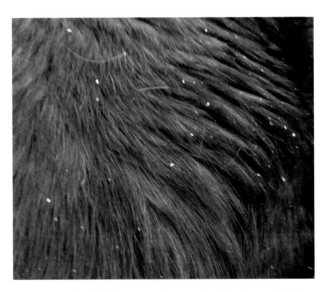

Figure 6.31 *Cheyletiella* spp. can be mistaken for dandruff in this feline patient.

As they move up and down the trunk of the body, they create the appearance of "walking dandruff" [4] (see Figure 6.31).

Exfoliative skin lesions are common. Scale may be extensive and may pile up in such a way that it looks like bran in the coat.

Alopecic patches are rare, but may occur secondary to pruritus. Patients may also exhibit hyperesthesia along planes inhabited by the mites.

Diagnosis is via skin scrapings and/or examination of combings and Scotch tape preps. Adult mites are large in size and have characteristic mouth parts with curved or hooked palpi that are visible under light microscopy (see Figures 6.32a, b).

(a) (b)

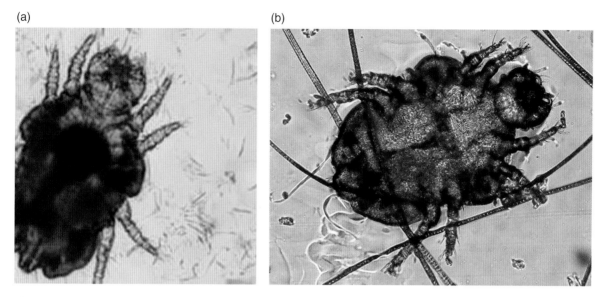

Figure 6.32 (a) *Cheyletiella* as seen through light microscopy. It is difficult to appreciate the curved palpi in this image. (b) *Cheyletiella* as seen through light microscopy. It is easy to appreciate the curved palpi in this image.

(a) (b)

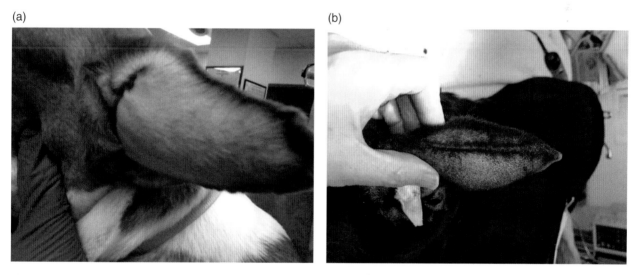

Figure 6.33 (a) Aural hematoma in a canine patient. Only the left ear is affected. *Source:* Courtesy of Patricia Bennett. (b) Alternate view of aural hematoma in a canine patient. *Source:* Courtesy of Samantha B. Thurman, DVM.

Like *Sarcoptes* spp. and *Notoedres* spp., *Cheyletiella* spp. are also zoonotic [231]. Infested humans complain of a pruritic, papular rash [231].

O. cynotis are more commonly seen in cats and dogs than *Sarcoptes, Notoedres,* and *Cheyletiella* spp. They prefer to inhabit the external ear canal, where they cause local irritation and inflammation [4]. As infestation progresses, affected patients accumulate a classic "coffee ground" debris within the ear canal [4]. This debris is dark brown cerumen laced with dried blood and mite feces [4].

Aural pruritus may be intense. Self-trauma is common and may include excoriations from scratching [4]. Refer to Chapter 5, Figure 5.2.

In addition, aural hematomas may result from violent headshaking (see Figures 6.33a, b).

O. cynotis infestations can be confirmed through magnified otoscopy or via light microscopy using a mineral oil slide prep. Refer to Chapter 5, Figure 5.3b (also see Figure 6.34).

Trombiculidae mite larvae or "chiggers" can also infest cats and dogs. Nymphs and adults do not require a host; however, the larvae do. They are abundant in the environment during the late summer and early autumn months, and hence their colloquial name, "harvest mites." These six-legged larvae tend to be orange-red in color, and they prefer to inhabit areas that are not thickly furred, such as the ears, around the eyes, between the toes, bridge of the nose, and abdomen [4, 232]. They pierce the skin with chelicerae, inject digestive enzymes into the skin, and feed on the liquefied tissues that result. Pruritus is the most common result of infestation [4, 232].

Diagnosis is via direct observation on the patient and examination under light microscopy (see Figure 6.35).

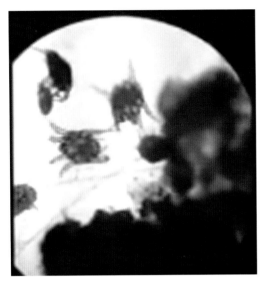

Figure 6.34 *Otodectes cynotis* mites as seen through light microscopy. *Source:* Courtesy of Tiffany N. Hall, DVM.

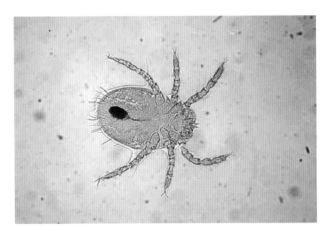

Figure 6.35 *Trombiculidae* mite larva as seen through light microscopy.

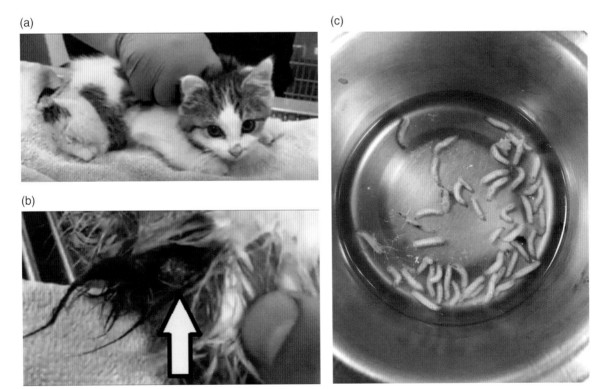

Figure 6.36 (a) Stray kitten that presented for perineal myiasis. *Source:* Courtesy of Dr. Andrew Queler, OSU'99. (b) Close-up of perineal myiasis. *Source:* Courtesy of Dr. Andrew Queler, OSU'99. (c) Close-up of maggots in a stainless steel dish. These had previously been extracted from a patient. *Source:* Courtesy of Nicole K. Spooner, DVM.

6.7 Myiasis

Infestation of host tissue with fly larvae, maggots, is called myiasis [233]. Larvae may infest openings to body cavities, such as the mouth, nose, ears, and entrances to digestive and urinary tracts. However, in companion animal medicine, myiasis is most typically associated with wounds and open draining tracts [233] (see Figures 6.36a–c).

Wounds offer prime locations for larval colonization because they offer diseased tissue upon which the larvae can snack. For this reason, necrotic tumors may also harbor maggots [233].

Resolution of the wound, as through debridement and surgical closure, will eliminate myiasis. However, secondary infections may require initiation of treatment with systemic antibiotics.

References

1 Bowman, D.D. and Georgi, J.R. (2009). *Georgis' Parasitology for Veterinarians*, 9e, ix, 451 p. St. Louis, MO: Saunders/Elsevier.

2 Kohler-Aanesen, H., Saari, S., Armstrong, R. et al. (2017). Efficacy of fluralaner (Bravecto chewable tablets) for the treatment of naturally acquired *Linognathus setosus* infestations on dogs. *Parasit. Vectors* 10 (1): 426.

3 Hanssen, I., Mencke, N., Asskildt, H. et al. (1999). Field study on the insecticidal efficacy of advantage against natural infestations of dogs with lice. *Parasitol. Res.* 85 (4): 347–348.

4 Arther, R.G. (2009). Mites and lice: biology and control. *Vet. Clin. North Am. Small Anim. Pract.* 39 (6): 1159–1171, vii.

5 Shanks, D.J., Gautier, P., McTier, T.L. et al. (2003). Efficacy of selamectin against biting lice on dogs and cats. *Vet. Rec.* 152 (8): 234–237.

6 Stanneck, D., Kruedewagen, E.M., Fourie, J.J. et al. (2012). Efficacy of an imidacloprid/flumethrin collar against fleas, ticks, mites and lice on dogs. *Parasit. Vectors* 5: 102.

7 Hendrix, C.M. and Robinson, E. (2017). *Diagnostic Parasitology for Veterinary Technicians*, 5e, xliv, 384 p. St. Louis, Missouri: Elsevier Inc.

8 Wall, R. and Shearer, D. (1997). Lice (Phthiraptera). In: *Veterinary Entomology: Arthropod Ectoparasites of Veterinary Importance* (ed. R. Wall and D. Shearer), 284–312. Dordrecht: Springer Netherlands.

9 Gunnarsson, L., Zakrisson, G., Christensson, D., and Uggla, A. (2004). Efficacy of selamectin in the treatment of nasal mite (*Pneumonyssoides caninum*) infection in dogs. *J. Am. Anim. Hosp. Assoc.* 40 (5): 400–404.

10 Benelli, G., Caselli, A., Di Giuseppe, G., and Canale, A. (2018). Control of biting lice, Mallophaga – a review. *Acta Trop.* 177: 211–219.

11 Urquhart, G.M., Armour, J., Duncan, J.L. et al. (1987). *Veterinary Parasitology*. U.K.: Longman Scientific and Technical.

12 Mehlhorn, H., Walldorf, V., Abdel-Ghaffar, F. et al. (2012). Biting and bloodsucking lice of dogs – treatment by means of a neem seed extract (MiteStop(R), Wash Away Dog). *Parasitol. Res.* 110 (2): 769–773.

13 Kuzner, J., Turk, S., Grace, S. et al. (2013). Confirmation of the efficacy of a novel fipronil spot-on for the treatment and control of fleas, ticks and chewing lice on dogs. *Vet. Parasitol.* 193 (1–3): 245–251.

14 Durden, L.A. (2001). Lice (Phtiraptera). In: *Parasitic Diseases of Wild Mammals* (ed. W.M. Samuel, M.J. Pybus and A.A. Kocan), 3–17. Ames, Iowa: Iowa State University Press.

15 Schwartz, C.C., Stephenson, R., and Wilson, N. (1983). *Trichodectes canis* on the gray wolf and coyote on Kenai Peninsula, Alaska. *J. Wildl. Dis.* 19 (4): 372–373.

16 Woldstad, T.M., Dullen, K.N., Hundertmark, K.J., and Beckmen, K.B. (2014). Restricted evaluation of *Trichodectes canis* (Phthiraptera: Trichodectidae) detection methods in Alaska gray wolves. *Int. J. Parasitol. Parasites Wildl.* 3 (3): 239–241.

17 Wall, R. and Shearer, D. (2001). *Veterinary Ectoparasites: Biology, Pathology, and Control*. Oxford: Blackwell Science, Ltd.

18 Fischer, K. (1983). Cuterebra larvae in domestic cats. *Vet. Med. Small Anim. Clin.* 78 (8): 1231–1233.

19 Hendrix, C.M., Cox, N.R., Clemonschevis, C.L. et al. (1989). Aberrant intracranial myiasis caused by larval Cuterebra infection. *Compend. Contin. Educ. Pract.* 11 (5): 550–562.

20 Kazacos, K.R., Bright, R.M., Johnson, K.E. et al. (1980). Cuterebra sp as a cause of pharyngeal myiasis in cats. *J. Am. Anim. Hosp. Assoc.* 16 (5): 773–776.

21 Thirloway, L. (1982). Aberrant migration of a Cuterebra larva in a cat. *Vet. Med. Small Anim. Clin.* 77 (4): 619–620.

22 Wolf, A.M. (1979). Cuterebra larva in the nasal passage of a kitten. *Feline Pract.* 9 (1): 25–26.

23 Johnson, B.W., Helper, L.C., and Szajerski, M.E. (1988). Intraocular Cuterebra in a cat. *J. Am. Vet. Med. Assoc.* 193 (7): 829–830.

24 Slansky, F. (2007). Feline cuterebrosis caused by a lagomorph-infesting *Cuterebra* spp. larva. *J. Parasitol.* 93 (4): 959–961.

25 Cook, J.R., Levesque, D.C., and Nuehring, L.P. (1985). Intracranial cuterebral myiasis causing acute lateralizing meningoencephalitis in 2 cats. *J. Am. Anim. Hosp. Assoc.* 21 (2): 279–284.

26 Dvorak, L.D., Bay, J.D., Crouch, D.T., and Corwin, R.M. (2000). Successful treatment of intratracheal cuterebrosis in two cats. *J. Am. Anim. Hosp. Assoc.* 36 (4): 304–308.

27 Fitzgerald, S.D., Johnson, C.A., and Peck, E.J. (1996). A fatal case of intrathoracic cuterebriasis in a cat. *J. Am. Anim. Hosp. Assoc.* 32 (4): 353–357.

28 Glass, E.N., Cornetta, A.M., de Lahunta, A. et al. (1998). Clinical and clinicopathologic features in 11 cats with Cuterebra larvae myiasis of the central nervous system. *J. Vet. Intern. Med.* 12 (5): 365–368.

29 Harris, B.P., Miller, P.E., Bloss, J.R., and Pellitteri, P.J. (2000). Ophthalmomyiasis interna anterior associated with Cuterebra spp in a cat. *J. Am. Vet. Med. Assoc.* 216 (3): 352–355, 45.

30 Hatziolos, B.C. (1966). Cuterebra larva in the brain of a cat. *J. Am. Vet. Med. Assoc.* 148 (7): 787–793.

31 King, J.M. (2000). Cuterebra species infection in a cat. *Vet. Med.* 95 (4): 291.

32 Stiles, J. and Rankin, A. (2006). Ophthalmomyiasis interna anterior in a cat: surgical resolution. *Vet. Ophthalmol.* 9 (3): 165–168.

33 Wyman, M., Starkey, R., Weisbrode, S. et al. (2005). Ophthalmomyiasis (interna posterior) of the posterior segment and central nervous system myiasis: Cuterebra spp. in a cat. *Vet. Ophthalmol.* 8 (2): 77–80.

34 Blagburn, B.L. and Dryden, M.W. (2009). Biology, treatment, and control of flea and tick infestations. *Vet. Clin. North Am. Small Anim. Pract.* 39 (6): 1173–1200.

35 Dryden, M.W. and Rust, M.K. (1994). The cat flea – biology, ecology and control. *Vet. Parasitol.* 52 (1–2): 1–19.

36 Rust, M.K. and Dryden, M.W. (1997). The biology, ecology, and management of the cat flea. *Annu. Rev. Entomol.* 42: 451–473.

37 Traversa, D. (2013). Fleas infesting pets in the era of emerging extra-intestinal nematodes. *Parasit. Vectors* 6: 59.

38 Rust, M.K. (2005). Advances in the control of *Ctenocephalides felis* (cat flea) on cats and dogs. *Trends Parasitol.* 21 (5): 232–236.

39 Durden, L.A. and Hinckle, N.C. (2009). Fleas (Siphonaptera). In: *Medical and Veterinary Entology* (ed. G.R. Mullen and L.A. Durden), 115–136. San Diego: Academic Press.

40 Dobler, G. and Pfeffer, M. (2011). Fleas as parasites of the family Canidae. *Parasit. Vectors* 4: 139.

41 Beck, W., Boch, K., Mackensen, H. et al. (2006). Qualitative and quantitative observations on the flea population dynamics of dogs and cats in several areas of Germany. *Vet. Parasitol.* 137 (1–2): 130–136.

42 Bond, R., Riddle, A., Mottram, L. et al. (2007). Survey of flea infestation in dogs and cats in the United Kingdom during 2005. *Vet. Rec.* 160 (15): 503–506.

43 Capelli, G., Montarsi, F., Porcellato, E. et al. (2009). Occurrence of *Rickettsia felis* in dog and cat fleas (*Ctenocephalides felis*) from Italy. *Parasit. Vectors* 2 (Suppl 1): S8.

44 Farkas, R., Gyurkovszky, M., Solymosi, N., and Beugnet, F. (2009). Prevalence of flea infestation in dogs and cats in Hungary combined with a survey of owner awareness. *Med. Vet. Entomol.* 23 (3): 187–194.

45 Silverman, J., Rust, M.K., and Reierson, D.A. (1981). Influence of temperature and humidity on survival and development of the cat flea, *Ctenocephalides felis* (Siphonaptera: Pulicidae). *J. Med. Entomol.* 18 (1): 78–83.

46 Thiemann, T., Fielden, L.J., and Kelrick, M.I. (2003). Water uptake in the cat flea *Ctenocephalides felis* (Pulicidae: Siphonaptera). *J. Insect Physiol.* 49 (12): 1085–1092.

47 Blagburn, B.L. (2002). Changing trends in ectoparasite control. In: *Advances in Veterinary Dermatology* (ed. K. Thoday, C. Foil and R. Bond), 69–68. Oxford: Blackwell Publishing.

48 Perrins, N. and Hendricks, A. (2007). Recent advances in flea control. *In Pract.* 29 (4): 202–207.

49 Marsella, R. (1999). Advances in flea control. *Vet. Clin. North Am. Small* 29 (6): 1407–1424.

50 Dryden M. (2016). Flea Allergy Dermatitis. Merck Veterinary Manual [Internet]. https://www.merckvetmanual.com/integumentary-system/fleas-and-flea-allergy-dermatitis/flea-allergy-dermatitis (accessed 16 November 2017).

51 Dryden, M.W. and Gaafar, S.M. (1991). Blood consumption by the cat flea, *Ctenocephalides felis* (Siphonaptera: Pulicidae). *J. Med. Entomol.* 28 (3): 394–400.

52 Kramer, F. and Mencke, N. (2001). *Flea Biology and Control*. Berlin, Germany: Springer-Verlag Berlin and Heidelberg GmbH & Co.

53 Flick, S.C. (1973). Endoparasites in cats: current practice and opinions. *Feline Pract.* 4: 21–34.

54 Hitchcock, D.J. (1953). Incidence of gastro-intestinal parasites in some Michigan kittens. *North Am. Vet.* 34: 428–429.

55 Arundel, J.H. (1970). Control of helminth parasites of dogs and cats. *Aust. Vet. J.* 46 (4): 164–168.

56 Baker, M.K., Lange, L., Verster, A., and van der Plaat, S. (1989). A survey of helminths in domestic cats in the Pretoria area of Transvaal, Republic of South Africa. Part 1: the prevalence and comparison of burdens of helminths in adult and juvenile cats. *J. S. Afr. Vet. Assoc.* 60 (3): 139–142.

57 Boreham, R.E. and Boreham, P.F.L. (1990). *Dipylidium-Caninum* – life-cycle, epizootiology, and control. *Compend. Contin. Educ. Pract.* 12 (5): 667–675.

58 Collins, G.H. (1973). A limited survey of gastro-intestinal helminths of dogs and cats. *N. Z. Vet. J.* 21 (8): 175–176.

59 Coman, B.J. (1972). A survey of the gastro-intestinal parasites of the feral cat in Victoria. *Aust. Vet. J.* 48 (4): 133–136.

60 Coman, B.J. (1972). Helminth parasites of the dingo and feral dog in Victoria with some notes on the diet of the host. *Aust. Vet. J.* 48 (8): 456–461.

61 Coman, B.J., Jones, E.H., and Driesen, M.A. (1981). Helminth parasites and arthropods of feral cats. *Aust. Vet. J.* 57 (7): 324–327.

62 Engbaek, K., Madsen, H., and Larsen, S.O. (1984). A survey of helminths in stray cats from Copenhagen with ecological aspects. *Z. Parasitenkd.* 70 (1): 87–94.

63 Griffiths, H.J. (1978). *Handbook of Veterinary Parasitology*. Minnesota: University of Minnesota.

64 Fourie, J.J., Crafford, D., Horak, I.G., and Stanneck, D. (2012). Prophylactic treatment of flea-infested cats with an imidacloprid/flumethrin collar to forestall infection with *Dipylidium caninum*. *Parasit. Vectors* 5: 151.

65 Brianti, E., Gaglio, G., Napoli, E. et al. (2012). New insights into the ecology and biology of *Acanthocheilonema reconditum* (Grassi, 1889) causing canine subcutaneous filariosis. *Parasitology* 139 (4): 530–536.

66 Huynh, T., Thean, J., and Maini, R. (2001). *Dipetalonema reconditum* in the human eye. *Br. J. Ophthalmol.* 85 (11): 1391–1392.

67 Curi, A.L. and Marback, E. (2012). Orbital parasitosis. *Ocul. Immunol. Inflamm.* 20 (4): 239–243.

68 John, M., Mathew, S.M., Sebastian, V. et al. (2012). Multiple live subconjunctival dipetalonema: report of a case. *Indian J. Ophthalmol.* 60 (3): 228–229.

69 Tarello, W. (2004). Identification and treatment of Dipetalonema grassii microfilariae in a cat from Central Italy. *Vet. Rec.* 155 (18): 565–566.

70 Breitschwerdt, E.B. (2008). Feline bartonellosis and cat scratch disease. *Vet. Immunol. Immunopathol.* 123 (1–2): 167–171.

71 Kamrani, A., Parreira, V.R., Greenwood, J., and Prescott, J.F. (2008). The prevalence of Bartonella, hemoplasma, and *Rickettsia felis* infections in domestic cats and in cat fleas in Ontario. *Can. J. Vet. Res.* 72 (5): 411–419.

72 Woods, J.E., Brewer, M.M., Hawley, J.R. et al. (2005). Evaluation of experimental transmission of Candidatus Mycoplasma haemominutum and *Mycoplasma haemofelis* by Ctenocephalides felis to cats. *Am. J. Vet. Res.* 66 (6): 1008–1012.

73 Eisen, R.J., Borchert, J.N., Holmes, J.L. et al. (2008). Early-phase transmission of *Yersinia pestis* by cat fleas (*Ctenocephalides felis*) and their potential role as vectors in a plague-endemic region of Uganda. *Am. J. Trop. Med. Hyg.* 78 (6): 949–956.

74 Williams, M., Izzard, L., Graves, S.R. et al. (2011). First probable Australian cases of human infection with *Rickettsia felis* (cat-flea typhus). *Med. J. Aust.* 194 (1): 41–43.

75 Maina, A.N., Fogarty, C., Krueger, L. et al. (2016). Rickettsial infections among *Ctenocephalides felis* and host animals during a flea-borne rickettsioses outbreak in Orange County, California. *PLoS One* 11 (8): e0160604.

76 Billeter, S.A., Diniz, P.P., Jett, L.A. et al. (2016). Detection of Rickettsia species in fleas collected from cats in regions endemic and nonendemic for flea-borne rickettsioses in California. *Vector Borne Zoonotic Dis.* 16 (3): 151–156.

77 Reif, K.E. and Macaluso, K.R. (2009). Ecology of *Rickettsia felis*: a review. *J. Med. Entomol.* 46 (4): 723–736.

78 Parola, P. (2011). *Rickettsia felis*: from a rare disease in the USA to a common cause of fever in sub-Saharan Africa. *Clin. Microbiol. Infect.* 17 (7): 996–1000.

79 Angelakis, E., Mediannikov, O., Parola, P., and Raoult, D. (2016). *Rickettsia felis*: the complex journey of an emergent human pathogen. *Trends Parasitol.* 32 (7): 554–564.

80 Perez-Osorio, C.E., Zavala-Velazquez, J.E., Leon, J.J.A., and Zavala-Castro, J.E. (2008). *Rickettsia felis* as emergent global threat for humans. *Emerg. Infect. Dis.* 14 (7): 1019–1023.

81 Zavala-Castro, J.E., Dzul-Rosado, K.R., Leon, J.J.A. et al. (2008). An increase in human cases of spotted fever rickettsiosis in Yucatan, Mexico, involving children. *Am. J. Trop. Med. Hyg.* 79 (6): 907–910.

82 Wiggers, R.J., Martin, M.C., and Bouyer, D. (2005). *Rickettsia felis* infection rates in an east Texas population. *Tex. Med.* 101 (2): 56–58.

83 Civen, R. and Ngo, V. (2008). Murine typhus: an unrecognized suburban vectorborne disease. *Clin. Infect. Dis.* 46 (6): 913–918.

84 Liddell, P.W. and Sparks, M.J. (2012). Murine typhus: endemic Rickettsia in Southwest Texas. *Clin. Lab. Sci.* 25 (2): 81–87.

85 Guptill, L. (2010). Feline bartonellosis. *Vet. Clin. North Am. Small Anim. Pract.* 40 (6): 1073–1090.

86 Foil, L., Andress, E., Freeland, R.L. et al. (1998). Experimental infection of domestic cats with *Bartonella henselae* by inoculation of *Ctenocephalides felis* (Siphonaptera: Pulicidae) feces. *J. Med. Entomol.* 35 (5): 625–628.

87 Moriarty, R.A. and Margileth, A.M. (1987). Cat scratch disease. *Infect. Dis. Clin. North Am.* 1 (3): 575–590.

88 English, R. (2006). Cat-scratch disease. *Pediatr. Rev.* 27 (4): 123–128; quiz 8.

89 Slater, L.N., Welch, D.F., Hensel, D., and Coody, D.W. (1990). A newly recognized fastidious gram-negative pathogen as a cause of fever and bacteremia. *N. Engl. J. Med.* 323 (23): 1587–1593.

90 Wong, M.T., Dolan, M.J., Lattuada, C.P. Jr. et al. (1995). Neuroretinitis, aseptic meningitis, and lymphadenitis associated with Bartonella (Rochalimaea) henselae infection in immunocompetent patients and patients infected with human immunodeficiency virus type 1. *Clin. Infect. Dis.* 21 (2): 352–360.

91 De La Rosa, G.R., Barnett, B.J., Ericsson, C.D., and Turk, J.B. (2001). Native valve endocarditis due to *Bartonella henselae* in a middle-aged human immunodeficiency virus-negative woman. *J. Clin. Microbiol.* 39 (9): 3417–3419.

92 Fournier, P.E., Lelievre, H., Eykyn, S.J. et al. (2001). Epidemiologic and clinical characteristics of Bartonella quintana and *Bartonella henselae* endocarditis: a study of 48 patients. *Medicine (Baltimore)* 80 (4): 245–251.

93 Rotstein, D.S., Taylor, S.K., Bradley, J., and Brieitschwerdt, E.B. (2000). Prevalence of *Bartonella henselae* antibody in Florida panthers. *J. Wildl. Dis.* 36 (1): 157–160.

94 Yamamoto, K., Chomel, B.B., Lowenstine, L.J. et al. (1998). *Bartonella henselae* antibody prevalence in free-ranging and captive wild felids from California. *J. Wildl. Dis.* 34 (1): 56–63.

95 Molia, S., Chomel, B.B., Kasten, R.W. et al. (2004). Prevalence of Bartonella infection in wild African lions (Panthera leo) and cheetahs (Acinonyx jubatus). *Vet. Microbiol.* 100 (1–2): 31–41.

96 Zeaiter, Z., Fournier, P.E., and Raoult, D. (2002). Genomic variation of *Bartonella henselae* strains detected in lymph nodes of patients with cat scratch disease. *J. Clin. Microbiol.* 40 (3): 1023–1030.

97 Guptill, L., Wu, C.C., HogenEsch, H. et al. (2004). Prevalence, risk factors, and genetic diversity of *Bartonella henselae* infections in pet cats in four regions of the United States. *J. Clin. Microbiol.* 42 (2): 652–659.

98 Maruyama, S., Kasten, R.W., Boulouis, H.J. et al. (2001). Genomic diversity of *Bartonella henselae* isolates from domestic cats from Japan, the USA and France by pulsed-field gel electrophoresis. *Vet. Microbiol.* 79 (4): 337–349.

99 Bergmans, A.M., de Jong, C.M., van Amerongen, G. et al. (1997). Prevalence of Bartonella species in domestic cats in The Netherlands. *J. Clin. Microbiol.* 35 (9): 2256–2261.

100 Heller, R., Artois, M., Xemar, V. et al. (1997). Prevalence of *Bartonella henselae* and Bartonella clarridgeiae in stray cats. *J. Clin. Microbiol.* 35 (6): 1327–1331.

101 Gurfield, A.N., Boulouis, H.J., Chomel, B.B. et al. (2001). Epidemiology of Bartonella infection in domestic cats in France. *Vet. Microbiol.* 80 (2): 185–198.

102 Gurfield, A.N., Boulouis, H.J., Chomel, B.B. et al. (1997). Coinfection with Bartonella clarridgeiae and *Bartonella henselae* and with different *Bartonella henselae* strains in domestic cats. *J. Clin. Microbiol.* 35 (8): 2120–2123.

103 Kordick, D.L., Brown, T.T., Shin, K., and Breitschwerdt, E.B. (1999). Clinical and pathologic evaluation of chronic *Bartonella henselae* or Bartonella clarridgeiae infection in cats. *J. Clin. Microbiol.* 37 (5): 1536–1547.

104 Guptill, L., Slater, L., Wu, C.C. et al. (1997). Experimental infection of young specific pathogen-free cats with *Bartonella henselae*. *J. Infect. Dis.* 176 (1): 206–216.

105 O'Reilly, K.L., Bauer, R.W., Freeland, R.L. et al. (1999). Acute clinical disease in cats following infection with a pathogenic strain of *Bartonella henselae* (LSU16). *Infect. Immun.* 67 (6): 3066–3072.

106 Lappin, M.R. and Black, J.C. (1999). Bartonella spp infection as a possible cause of uveitis in a cat. *J. Am. Vet. Med. Assoc.* 214 (8): 1205–1207.

107 Lappin, M.R., Kordick, D.L., and Breitschwerdt, E.B. (2000). Bartonella spp antibodies and DNA in aqueous humour of cats. *J. Feline Med. Surg.* 2 (1): 61–68.

108 Chomel, B.B., Kasten, R.W., Williams, C. et al. (2009). Bartonella endocarditis: a pathology shared by animal reservoirsand patients. *Ann. N. Y. Acad. Sci.* 1166: 120–126.

109 Perez, C., Hummel, J.B., Keene, B.W. et al. (2010). Successful treatment of *Bartonella henselae* endocarditis in a cat. *J. Feline Med. Surg.* 12 (6): 483–486.

110 Arvand, M., Viezens, J., and Berghoff, J. (2008). Prolonged *Bartonella henselae* bacteremia caused by reinfection in cats. *Emerg. Infect. Dis.* 14 (1): 152–154.

111 Guptill, L., Slater, L., Wu, C.C. et al. (1999). Immune response of neonatal specific pathogen-free cats to experimental infection with *Bartonella henselae*. *Vet. Immunol. Immunopathol.* 71 (3–4): 233–243.

112 Kordick, D.L., Wilson, K.H., Sexton, D.J. et al. (1995). Prolonged Bartonella bacteremia in cats associated with cat-scratch disease patients. *J. Clin. Microbiol.* 33 (12): 3245–3251.

113 Bergmann, M., Englert, T., Stuetzer, B. et al. (2017). Risk factors of different hemoplasma species infections in cats. *BMC Vet. Res.* 13: 1–6.

114 Sykes, J.E. (2010). Feline hemotropic mycoplasmas. *Vet. Clin. North Am. Small Anim. Pract.* 40 (6): 1157–1170.

115 Museux, K., Boretti, F.S., Willi, B. et al. (2009). In vivo transmission studies of 'Candidatus Mycoplasma turicensis' in the domestic cat. *Vet. Res.* 40 (5): 1–14.

116 Just, F. and Pfister, K. (2007). Detection frequency of haemoplasma infections of the domestic cat in Germany. *Berl. Munch. Tierarztl. Wochenschr.* 120 (5–6): 197–201.

117 Laberke, S., Just, F., Pfister, K., and Hartmann, K. (2010). Prevalence of feline haemoplasma infection in cats in Southern Bavaria, Germany, and infection risk factor analysis. *Berl. Munch. Tierarztl. Wochenschr.* 123 (1–2): 42–48.

118 Lobetti, R.G. and Tasker, S. (2004). Diagnosis of feline haemoplasma infection using a real-time PCR assay. *J. S. Afr. Vet. Assoc.* 75 (2): 94–99.

119 Reynolds, C.A. and Lappin, M.R. (2007). "Candidatus Mycoplasma haemominutum" infections in 21 client-owned cats. *J. Am. Anim. Hosp. Assoc.* 43 (5): 249–257.

120 Willi, B., Boretti, F.S., Baumgartner, C. et al. (2006). Prevalence, risk factor analysis, and follow-up of infections caused by three feline hemoplasma species in cats in Switzerland. *J. Clin. Microbiol.* 44 (3): 961–969.

121 Willi, B., Tasker, S., Boretti, F.S. et al. (2006). Phylogenetic analysis of "Candidatus Mycoplasma turicensis" isolates from pet cats in the United Kingdom, Australia, and South Africa, with analysis of risk factors for infection. *J. Clin. Microbiol.* 44 (12): 4430–4435.

122 Messick, J.B. (2003). New perspectives about Hemotrophic mycoplasma (formerly, Haemobartonella and Eperythrozoon species) infections in dogs and cats. *Vet. Clin. North Am. Small Anim. Pract.* 33 (6): 1453–1465.

123 Foley, J.E., Harrus, S., Poland, A. et al. (1998). Molecular, clinical, and pathologic comparison of two distinct strains of *Haemobartonella felis* in domestic cats. *Am. J. Vet. Res.* 59 (12): 1581–1588.

124 Gentilini, F., Novacco, M., Turba, M.E. et al. (2009). Use of combined conventional and real-time PCR to determine the epidemiology of feline haemoplasma infections in northern Italy. *J. Feline Med. Surg.* 11 (4): 277–285.

125 George, J.W., Rideout, B.A., Griffey, S.M., and Pedersen, N.C. (2002). Effect of preexisting FeLV infection or FeLV and feline immunodeficiency virus coinfection on pathogenicity of the small variant of *Haemobartonella felis* in cats. *Am. J. Vet. Res.* 63 (8): 1172–1178.

126 Sykes, J.E., Terry, J.C., Lindsay, L.L., and Owens, S.D. (2008). Prevalences of various hemoplasma species among cats in the United States with possible hemoplasmosis. *J. Am. Vet. Med. Assoc.* 232 (3): 372–379.

127 Weingart, C., Tasker, S., and Kohn, B. (2016). Infection with haemoplasma species in 22 cats with anaemia. *J. Feline Med. Surg.* 18 (2): 129–136.

128 Willi, B., Boretti, F.S., Cattori, V. et al. (2005). Identification, molecular characterization, and experimental transmission of a new hemoplasma isolate from a cat with hemolytic anemia in Switzerland. *J. Clin. Microbiol.* 43 (6): 2581–2585.

129 Zulty, J.C. and Kociba, G.J. (1990). Cold agglutinins in cats with haemobartonellosis. *J. Am. Vet. Med. Assoc.* 196 (6): 907–910.

130 Maede, Y. and Hata, R. (1975). Studies on feline haemobartonellosis. II. The mechanism of anemia produced by infection with *Haemobartonella felis*. *Nippon Juigaku Zasshi* 37 (1): 49–54.

131 Maede, Y. (1975). Studies on feline haemobartonellosis. IV. Lifespan of erythrocytes of cats infected with *Haemobartonella felis*. *Nippon Juigaku Zasshi* 37 (5): 269–272.

132 Groebel, K., Hoelzle, K., Wittenbrink, M.M. et al. (2009). Mycoplasma suis invades porcine erythrocytes. *Infect. Immun.* 77 (2): 576–584.

133 Harvey, J.W. and Gaskin, J.M. (1977). Experimental feline hemobartonellosis. *J. Am. Anim. Hosp. Assoc.* 13 (1): 28–38.

134 Alleman, A.R., Pate, M.G., Harvey, J.W. et al. (1999). Western immunoblot analysis of the antigens of *Haemobartonella felis* with sera from experimentally infected cats. *J. Clin. Microbiol.* 37 (5): 1474–1479.

135 Pennisi, M.G., Egberink, H., Hartmann, K. et al. (2013). *Yersinia pestis* infection in cats: ABCD guidelines on prevention and management. *J. Feline Med. Surg.* 15 (7): 582–584.

136 Eidson, M., Thilsted, J.P., and Rollag, O.J. (1991). Clinical, clinicopathologic, and pathologic features of plague in cats: 119 cases (1977–1988). *J. Am. Vet. Med. Assoc.* 199 (9): 1191–1197.

137 Carlson, M.E. (1996). *Yersinia pestis* infection in cats. *Feline Pract.* 24 (6): 22–24.

138 Gasper, P.W., Barnes, A.M., Quan, T.J. et al. (1993). Plague (*Yersinia pestis*) in cats: description of experimentally induced disease. *J. Med. Entomol.* 30 (1): 20–26.

139 Chomel, B. (2012). Plague. In: *Infectious Diseases of the Dog and Cat* (ed. C.E. Greene), 469–476. Philadelphia: WB Saunders.

140 Dryden, M.W. (2009). Flea and tick control in the 21st century: challenges and opportunities. *Vet. Dermatol.* 20 (5–6): 435–440.

141 Kaufman, W.R. (1989). Tick-host interaction: a synthesis of current concepts. *Parasitol. Today* 5 (2): 47–56.

142 Sonenshine, D.E. (1991). The midgut. In: *Biology of Ticks*, vol. 1 (ed. D.E. Sonenshine), 159–176. New York: Oxford University Press.

143 Sonenshine, D.E., Lane, R.S., and Nicholson, W.L. (2002). Ticks (Ixodida). In: *Medical and Veterinary Entomology* (ed. G.R. Mullen and L.A. Durden), 517–558. Amsterdam: Academic Press Elsevier Science.

144 Little, S.E. (2010). Ehrlichiosis and anaplasmosis in dogs and cats. *Vet. Clin. North Am. Small Anim. Pract.* 40 (6): 1121–1140.

145 Childs, J.E. and Paddock, C.D. (2003). The ascendancy of *Amblyomma americanum* as a vector of pathogens affecting humans in the United States. *Annu. Rev. Entomol.* 48: 307–337.

146 Magnarelli, L.A., Anderson, J.F., Levine, H.R., and Levy, S.A. (1990). Tick parasitism and antibodies to *Borrelia burgdorferi* in cats. *J. Am. Vet. Med. Assoc.* 197 (1): 63–66.

147 Little, S.E., Heise, S.R., Blagburn, B.L. et al. (2010). Lyme borreliosis in dogs and humans in the USA. *Trends Parasitol.* 26 (4): 213–218.

148 Krupka, I. and Straubinger, R.K. (2010). Lyme borreliosis in dogs and cats: background, diagnosis, treatment and prevention of infections with *Borrelia burgdorferi* sensu stricto. *Vet. Clin. North Am. Small Anim. Pract.* 40 (6): 1103–1119.

149 Sanogo, Y.O., Davoust, B., Inokuma, H. et al. (2003). First evidence of *Anaplasma platys* in *Rhipicephalus sanguineus* (Acari: Ixodida) collected from dogs in Africa. *Onderstepoort J. Vet. Res.* 70 (3): 205–212.

150 Higuchi, S., Kuroda, H., Hoshi, H. et al. (1999). Development of *Babesia gibsoni* in the midgut of the nymphal stage of the tick, *Rhipicephalus sanguineus*. *J. Vet. Med. Sci.* 61 (6): 697–699.

151 Reichard, M.V., Meinkoth, J.H., Edwards, A.C. et al. (2009). Transmission of *Cytauxzoon felis* to a domestic cat by *Amblyomma americanum*. *Vet. Parasitol.* 161 (1–2): 110–115.

152 Blouin, E.F., Kocan, A.A., Kocan, K.M., and Hair, J. (1987). Evidence of a limited schizogonous cycle for *Cytauxzoon felis* in bobcats following exposure to infected ticks. *J. Wildl. Dis.* 23 (3): 499–501.

153 Hoskins, J.D. (1991). Canine haemobartonellosis, canine hepatozoonosis, and feline cytauxzoonosis. *Vet. Clin. North Am. Small Anim. Pract.* 21 (1): 129–140.

154 Demma, L.J., Eremeeva, M., Nicholson, W.L. et al. (2006). An outbreak of Rocky Mountain spotted fever associated with a novel tick vector, *Rhipicephalus sanguineus*, in Arizona, 2004: preliminary report. *Ann. N. Y. Acad. Sci.* 1078: 342–343.

155 Dantas-Torres, F. (2008). The brown dog tick, *Rhipicephalus sanguineus* (Latreille, 1806) (Acari: Ixodidae): from taxonomy to control. *Vet. Parasitol.* 152 (3–4): 173–185.

156 Ewing, S.A. and Panciera, R.J. (2003). American canine hepatozoonosis. *Clin. Microbiol. Rev.* 16 (4): 688–697.

157 Sonenshine, D.E. (1993). Tick-borne diseases. In: *Biology of Ticks*, vol. 2 (ed. D.E. Sonenshine), 255–319. New York: Oxford University Press.

158 Eklund, C.M., Kohls, G.M., and Jellison, W.L. (1958). Isolation of Colorado tick fever virus from rodents in Colorado. *Science* 128 (3321): 413.

159 Jellison, W.L., Bell, E.J., and Huebner, R.J. (1958). Q fever studies in Southern California. IV. Occurrence of *Coxiella burnetii* in the spinose ear tick, *Otobius megnini*. *Public Health Rep.* 63: 1483–1489.

160 Kordick, S.K., Breitschwerdt, E.B., Hegarty, B.C. et al. (1999). Coinfection with multiple tick-borne pathogens in a Walker Hound kennel in North Carolina. *J. Clin. Microbiol.* 37 (8): 2631–2638.

161 Harvey, J.W. (2006). Thrombocytotropic anaplasmosis (A. platys infection). In: *Infectious Diseases of the Dog and Cat* (ed. C.E. Greene), 229–231. St. Louis, MO: Saunders Elsevier.

162 Gaunt, S., Beall, M., Stillman, B. et al. (2010). Experimental infection and co-infection of dogs with *Anaplasma platys* and *Ehrlichia canis*: hematologic, serologic and molecular findings. *Parasit. Vectors* 3 (1): 33.

163 Hua, P., Yuhai, M., Shide, T. et al. (2000). Canine ehrlichiosis caused simultaneously by *Ehrlichia canis* and Ehrlichia platys. *Microbiol. Immunol.* 44 (9): 737–739.

164 Suksawat, J., Pitulle, C., Arraga-Alvarado, C. et al. (2001). Coinfection with three Ehrlichia species in dogs from Thailand and Venezuela with emphasis on consideration of 16S ribosomal DNA secondary structure. *J. Clin. Microbiol.* 39 (1): 90–93.

165 Egenvall, A.E., Hedhammar, A.A., and Bjoersdorff, A.I. (1997). Clinical features and serology of 14 dogs affected by granulocytic ehrlichiosis in Sweden. *Vet. Rec.* 140 (9): 222–226.

166 Kohn, B., Galke, D., Beelitz, P., and Pfister, K. (2008). Clinical features of canine granulocytic anaplasmosis in 18 naturally infected dogs. *J. Vet. Intern. Med.* 22 (6): 1289–1295.

167 Poitout, F.M., Shinozaki, J.K., Stockwell, P.J. et al. (2005). Genetic variants of *Anaplasma phagocytophilum* infecting dogs in Western Washington State. *J. Clin. Microbiol.* 43 (2): 796–801.

168 Greig, B., Asanovich, K.M., Armstrong, P.J., and Dumler, J.S. (1996). Geographic, clinical, serologic, and molecular evidence of granulocytic ehrlichiosis, a likely zoonotic disease, in Minnesota and Wisconsin dogs. *J. Clin. Microbiol.* 34 (1): 44–48.

169 Harvey, J.W., Simpson, C.F., and Gaskin, J.M. (1978). Cyclic thrombocytopenia induced by a Rickettsia-like agent in dogs. *J. Infect. Dis.* 137 (2): 182–188.

170 Abarca, K., Lopez, J., Perret, C. et al. (2007). *Anaplasma platys* in dogs, Chile. *Emerg. Infect. Dis.* 13 (9): 1392–1395.

171 Glaze, M.B. and Gaunt, S.D. (1986). Uveitis associated with Ehrlichia platys infection in a dog. *J. Am. Vet. Med. Assoc.* 189 (8): 916–917.

172 Billeter, S.A., Spencer, J.A., Griffin, B. et al. (2007). Prevalence of *Anaplasma phagocytophilum* in domestic felines in the United States. *Vet. Parasitol.* 147 (1–2): 194–198.

173 Magnarelli, L.A., Bushmich, S.L., IJdo, J.W., and Fikrig, E. (2005). Seroprevalence of antibodies against *Borrelia burgdorferi* and *Anaplasma phagocytophilum* in cats. *Am. J. Vet. Res.* 66 (11): 1895–1899.

174 Liddell, A.M., Stockham, S.L., Scott, M.A. et al. (2003). Predominance of *Ehrlichia ewingii* in Missouri dogs. *J. Clin. Microbiol.* 41 (10): 4617–4622.

175 Little, S.E., O'Connor, T.P., Hempstead, J. et al. (2010). *Ehrlichia ewingii* infection and exposure rates in dogs from the southcentral United States. *Vet. Parasitol.* 172 (3–4): 355–360.

176 Harrus, S. and Waner, T. (2011). Diagnosis of canine monocytotropic ehrlichiosis (*Ehrlichia canis*): an overview. *Vet. J.* 187 (3): 292–296.

177 Stich, R.W., Schaefer, J.J., Bremer, W.G. et al. (2008). Host surveys, ixodid tick biology and transmission scenarios as related to the tick-borne pathogen, *Ehrlichia canis. Vet. Parasitol.* 158 (4): 256–273.

178 Neer, T.M. and Harrus, S. (2006). Canine monocytotropic ehrlichiosis and neorickettsiosis (E. Canis, E. Chaffeensis, E. ruminantium, N. sennetsu, and N. risticii infections). In: *Infectious Diseases of the Dog and Cat* (ed. C.E. Greene), 203–216. St. Louis, MO: Saunders Elsevier.

179 Goodman, R.A., Hawkins, E.C., Olby, N.J. et al. (2003). Molecular identification of *Ehrlichia ewingii* infection in dogs: 15 cases (1997–2001). *J. Am. Vet. Med. Assoc.* 222 (8): 1102–1107.

180 Stubbs, C.J., Holland, C.J., Relf, J.S. et al. (2000). Feline ehrlichiosis. *Compend. Contin. Educ. Pract.* 22 (4): 307–318.

181 Tarello, W. (2005). Microscopic and clinical evidence for Anaplasma (Ehrlichia) phagocytophilum infection in Italian cats. *Vet. Rec.* 156 (24): 772–774.

182 Bjoersdorff, A., Svendenius, L., Owens, J.H., and Massung, R.F. (1999). Feline granulocytic ehrlichiosis – a report of a new clinical entity and characterisation of the infectious agent. *J. Small Anim. Pract.* 40 (1): 20–24.

183 Lappin, M.R., Breitschwerdt, E.B., Jensen, W.A. et al. (2004). Molecular and serologic evidence of *Anaplasma phagocytophilum* infection in cats in North America. *J. Am. Vet. Med. Assoc.* 225 (6): 893–896, 79.

184 Grimm, D., Tilly, K., Byram, R. et al. (2004). Outer-surface protein C of the Lyme disease spirochete: a protein induced in ticks for infection of mammals. *Proc. Natl. Acad. Sci. U. S. A.* 101 (9): 3142–3147.

185 Ribeiro, J.M., Mather, T.N., Piesman, J., and Spielman, A. (1987). Dissemination and salivary delivery of Lyme disease spirochetes in vector ticks (Acari: Ixodidae). *J. Med. Entomol.* 24 (2): 201–205.

186 Schwan, T.G., Piesman, J., Golde, W.T. et al. (1995). Induction of an outer surface protein on *Borrelia burgdorferi* during tick feeding. *Proc. Natl. Acad. Sci. U. S. A.* 92 (7): 2909–2913.

187 deSilva, A.M., Telford, S.R., Brunet, L.R. et al. (1996). *Borrelia burgdorferi* OspA is an arthropod-specific transmission-blocking Lyme disease vaccine. *J. Exp. Med.* 183 (1): 271–275.

188 Straubinger, R.K., Summers, B.A., Chang, Y.F., and Appel, M.J. (1997). Persistence of *Borrelia burgdorferi* in experimentally infected dogs after antibiotic treatment. *J. Clin. Microbiol.* 35 (1): 111–116.

189 Straubinger, R.K., Straubinger, A.F., Harter, L. et al. (1997). *Borrelia burgdorferi* migrates into joint capsules and causes an up-regulation of interleukin-8 in synovial membranes of dogs experimentally infected with ticks. *Infect. Immun.* 65 (4): 1273–1285.

190 Grauer, G.F., Burgess, E.C., Cooley, A.J., and Hagee, J.H. (1988). Renal lesions associated with Borrelia-burgdorferi infection in a dog. *J. Am. Vet. Med. Assoc.* 193 (2): 237–239.

191 Dambach, D.M., Smith, C.A., Lewis, R.M., and VanWinkle, T.J. (1997). Morphologic, immunohistochemical, and ultrastructural characterization of a distinctive renal lesion in dogs putatively associated with *Borrelia burgdorferi* infection: 49 cases (1987–1992). *Vet. Pathol.* 34 (2): 85–96.

192 O'Connor, T.P., Hanscom, J.L., Hegarty, B.C. et al. (2006). Comparison of an indirect immunofluorescence assay, western blot analysis, and a commercially available ELISA for detection of *Ehrlichia canis* antibodies in canine sera. *Am. J. Vet. Res.* 67 (2): 206–210.

193 Diniz, P.P., Beall, M.J., Omark, K. et al. (2010). High prevalence of tick-borne pathogens in dogs from an Indian reservation in northeastern Arizona. *Vector Borne Zoonotic Dis.* 10 (2): 117–123.

194 Levy, S.A., O'Connor, T.P., Hanscom, J.L., and Shields, P. (2003). Evaluation of a canine C6 ELISA Lyme disease test for the determination of the infection status of cats naturally exposed to *Borrelia burgdorferi*. *Vet. Ther.* 4 (2): 172–177.

195 Sherrill, M.K. and Cohn, L.A. (2015). Cytauxzoonosis: diagnosis and treatment of an emerging disease. *J. Feline Med. Surg.* 17 (11): 940–948.

196 Birkenheuer, A.J., Cohn, L.A., Levy, M.G. et al. (2008). Atovaquone and azithromycin for the treatment of *Cytauxzoon felis*. *J. Vet. Intern. Med.* 22 (3): 703–704.

197 Meinkoth, J.H. and Kocan, A.A. (2005). Feline cytauxzoonosis. *Vet. Clin. North Am. Small Anim. Pract.* 35 (1): 89–101, vi.

198 Wang, J.L., Li, T.T., Liu, G.H. et al. (2017). Two Tales of *Cytauxzoon felis* infections in domestic cats. *Clin. Microbiol. Rev.* 30 (4): 861–885.

199 Blouin, E.F., Kocan, A.A., Glenn, B.L. et al. (1984). Transmission of *Cytauxzoon felis* Kier, 1979 from bobcats, Felis rufus (Schreber), to domestic cats by *Dermacentor variabilis* (Say). *J. Wildl. Dis.* 20 (3): 241–242.

200 Cowell, R.L., Fox, J.C., Panciera, R.J., and Tyler, R.D. (1988). Detection of Anticytauxzoon antibodies in cats infected with a Cytauxzoon organism from bobcats. *Vet. Parasitol.* 28 (1–2): 43–52.

201 Wagner, J.E. (1976). A fatal cytauxzoonosis-like disease in cats. *J. Am. Vet. Med. Assoc.* 168 (7): 585–588.

202 Reichard, M.V., Baum, K.A., Cadenhead, S.C., and Snider, T.A. (2008). Temporal occurrence and environmental risk factors associated with cytauxzoonosis in domestic cats. *Vet. Parasitol.* 152 (3–4): 314–320.

203 Kocan, A.A., Kocan, K.M., Blouin, E.F., and Mukolwe, S.W. (1992). A redescription of schizogony of *Cytauxzoon felis* in the domestic cat. *Ann. N. Y. Acad. Sci.* 653: 161–167.

204 Simpson, C.F., Harvey, J.W., Lawman, M.J. et al. (1985). Ultrastructure of schizonts in the liver of cats with experimentally induced cytauxzoonosis. *Am. J. Vet. Res.* 46 (2): 384–390.

205 Birkenheuer, A.J., Le, J.A., Valenzisi, A.M. et al. (2006). *Cytauxzoon felis* infection in cats in the mid-Atlantic states: 34 cases (1998–2004). *J. Am. Vet. Med. Assoc.* 228 (4): 568–571.

206 Jackson, C.B. and Fisher, T. (2006). Fatal cytauxzoonosis in a Kentucky cat (Felis domesticus). *Vet. Parasitol.* 139 (1–3): 192–195.

207 Hoover, J.P., Walker, D.B., and Hedges, J.D. (1994). Cytauxzoonosis in cats: eight cases (1985–1992). *J. Am. Vet. Med. Assoc.* 205 (3): 455–460.

208 Meier, H.T. and Moore, L.E. (2000). Feline cytauxzoonosis: a case report and literature review. *J. Am. Anim. Hosp. Assoc.* 36 (6): 493–496.

209 Bondy, P.J., Cohn, L.A., and Kerl, M.E. (2005). Feline cytauxzoonosis. *Compend. Contin. Educ. Pract.* 27 (1): 69–75.

210 Cohn, L.A. and Birkenheuer, A.J. (2011). Cytauxzoonosis. In: *Infectious Diseases of the Dog and Cat* (ed. C.E. Greene), 764–770. St. Louis, MO: Saunders Elsevier.

211 Haber, M.D., Tucker, M.D., Marr, H.S. et al. (2007). The detection of *Cytauxzoon felis* in apparently healthy free-roaming cats in the USA. *Vet. Parasitol.* 146 (3–4): 316–320.

212 Meinkoth, J., Kocan, A.A., Whitworth, L. et al. (2000). Cats surviving natural infection with *Cytauxzoon felis*: 18 cases (1997–1998). *J. Vet. Intern. Med.* 14 (5): 521–525.

213 Brown, H.M., Latimer, K.S., Erikson, L.E. et al. (2008). Detection of persistent *Cytauxzoon felis* infection by polymerase chain reaction in three asymptomatic domestic cats. *J. Vet. Diagn. Investig.* 20 (4): 485–488.

214 Brown, H.M., Lockhart, J.M., Latimer, K.S., and Peterson, D.S. (2010). Identification and genetic characterization of *Cytauxzoon felis* in asymptomatic domestic cats and bobcats. *Vet. Parasitol.* 172 (3–4): 311–316.

215 Taffin, E.R., Casaert, S., Claerebout, E. et al. (2016). Morphological variability of *Demodex cati* in a feline immunodeficiency virus-positive cat. *J. Am. Vet. Med. Assoc.* 249 (11): 1308–1312.

216 Neel, J.A., Tarigo, J., Tater, K.C., and Grindem, C.B. (2007). Deep and superficial skin scrapings from a feline immunodeficiency virus-positive cat. *Vet. Clin. Pathol.* 36 (1): 101–104.

217 Frank, L.A., Kania, S.A., Chung, K., and Brahmbhatt, R. (2013). A molecular technique for the detection and differentiation of Demodex mites on cats. *Vet. Dermatol.* 24 (3): 367–369, e82–3.

218 Cordero, A.M., Sheinberg-Waisburd, G., Romero Nunez, C., and Heredia, R. (2018). Early onset canine generalized demodicosis. *Vet. Dermatol.* 29 (2): 173.

219 Bowden, D.G., Outerbridge, C.A., Kissel, M.B. et al. (2018). Canine demodicosis: a retrospective study of a veterinary hospital population in California, USA (2000-2016). *Vet. Dermatol.* 29 (1): 19–e10.

220 Mueller, R.S. (2012). An update on the therapy of canine demodicosis. *Compend. Contin. Educ. Vet.* 34 (4): E1–E4.

221 Mueller, R.S., Bensignor, E., Ferrer, L. et al. (2012). Treatment of demodicosis in dogs: 2011 clinical practice guidelines. *Vet. Dermatol.* 23 (2): 86–96, e20–1.

222 Rouben, C. (2016). Claw and claw bed diseases. *Clinician's Brief* (April): 35–40.

223 Manning, T.O. (1983). Cutaneous diseases of the paw. *Clin. Dermatol.* 1 (1): 131–142.

224 Pin, D., Bensignor, E., Carlotti, D.N., and Cadiergues, M.C. (2006). Localised sarcoptic mange in dogs: a retrospective study of 10 cases. *J. Small Anim. Pract.* 47 (10): 611–614.

225 Scott, D.W., Miller, W.H., and Griffin, C.E. (2001). *Parasitic Skin Diseases. Muller & Kirk's Small Animal Dermatology*, 476–483. Philadelphia, PA: W.B. Saunders.

226 Huang, H.P. and Lien, Y.H. (2013). Feline sarcoptic mange in Taiwan: a case series of five cats. *Vet. Dermatol.* 24 (4): 457–459, e104–5.

227 Malik, R., Stewart, K.M., Sousa, C.A. et al. (2006). Crusted scabies (sarcoptic mange) in four cats due to *Sarcoptes scabiei* infestation. *J. Feline Med. Surg.* 8 (5): 327–339.

228 Hawkins, J.A., McDonald, R.K., and Woody, B.J. (1987). *Sarcoptes scabiei* infestation in a cat. *J. Am. Vet. Med. Assoc.* 190 (12): 1572–1573.

229 Aydingoz, I.E. and Mansur, A.T. (2011). Canine scabies in humans: a case report and review of the literature. *Dermatology* 223 (2): 104–106.

230 Sivajothi, S., Sudhakara Reddy, B., Rayulu, V.C., and Sreedevi, C. (2015). *Notoedres cati* in cats and its management. *J. Parasit. Dis.* 39 (2): 303–305.

231 Wall, R. and Shearer, D. (1997). *Veterinary Ectoparasites: Biology, Pathology & Control*. Oxford: Blackwell Science.

232 Schneider, T. (2006). *Veterinary Parasitology, Special Excerpt*. Stuttgart: Parey.

233 Mathison, B.A. and Pritt, B.S. (2014). Laboratory identification of arthropod ectoparasites. *Clin. Microbiol. Rev.* 27 (1): 48–67.

7

Skin Fragility

7.1 Introduction to Skin Fragility Syndromes in Companion Animal Medicine

Skin fragility refers to one or more dermatological syndromes that result in thinning of the skin and spontaneous tearing. These syndromes rarely appear as case presentations in clinical practice because the frequency with which they arise in canine and feline patients is quite low. When complications from these syndromes present themselves as wounds, they may be initially mistaken for traumatic injuries. It is often not until wounds recur repeatedly in the absence of trauma that a thorough diagnostic investigation is launched into the underlying cause.

Skin fragility syndromes of companion animals may be congenital, inherited, or acquired [1]. Congenital syndromes are often present at birth or shortly thereafter and result from a developmental abnormality as opposed to inherited defects. Acquired skin fragility syndromes occur secondary to underlying diseases processes, such as endocrinopathy, infectious disease, or neoplasia.

In canine and feline practice, skin fragility syndromes are most often acquired [1]. Treatment involves management of the underlying condition as well as any wounds present. However, surgical closure of wounds presents additional challenges because wound healing tends to be compromised in these patients.

7.2 Inherited Skin Fragility Syndromes

Three skin fragility syndromes are thought to be inherited in dogs and cats:

- Ehlers–Danlos syndrome
- Cutaneous Asthenia syndrome
- Epidermolysis bullosa

In the medical literature, some authors consider cutaneous asthenia syndrome to be synonymous with Ehlers–Danlos syndrome [1, 2]. However, cutaneous asthenia syndrome only impacts the skin, causing skin tears, whereas true Ehlers–Danlos syndrome impacts all connective tissue by virtue of defective collagen synthesis or assembly [2, 3]. The resultant connective tissue is weak. This interferes with the structure, function, and integrity of the skin joints, muscles, ligaments, vasculature, and ocular tissues [3–5].

Ehlers–Danlos syndrome was first introduced in Chapter 4, Section 4.1. It is more likely to occur in cats than dogs, and patients tend to present at a young age [6].

Note that Ehlers–Danlos syndrome is not unique to dogs and cats. The syndrome has also been reported in mink, rabbits, horses, sheep, cattle, and humans [2, 3, 7–19].

Ehlers–Danlos syndrome is inherited as autosomal dominant [2, 4, 20–22].

Patients with this syndrome have abnormal collagen. This is apparent on histopathologic examination of full thickness skin biopsies [2]. There are fewer collagen fibers in patients with Ehlers–Danlos syndrome [2]. Fibers that are present tend to be shortened and/or fragmented [1]. These form the basis of abnormal clusters of collagen bundles [22].

In addition, the epidermis and dermis of patients are atypically thin, and the skin as a whole has poor tensile strength [2, 22]. This results in inferior puncture resistance and skin tearing tendencies [1, 17, 23]. A primary function of the integument is to act as a mechanical barrier [24]. The patient with Ehlers–Danlos syndrome has an abnormal response to stretch and strain that compromises the integrity of the skin, making it more likely to tear.

Patients often present with gaping "fish-mouth" wounds that require primary closure [11, 25, 26]. Wound dehiscence is common. When wounds do heal, scars often appear sunken because of inadequate collagen deposition [11, 27]. Sometimes these scars are referred to as cigarette paper scars in the literature because of their shiny and depigmented appearance, covered by an insufficiently thin layer of epidermis [2, 5, 11, 25, 28].

Because the skin is not the only tissue composed of collagen, other tissues may also be compromised. For example, the walls of vasculature may be equally compromised [27]. Patients with Ehlers–Danlos syndrome that experience minor trauma often bleed excessively [27]. Hematoma formation and extensive bruising are common sequelae for injuries that would be trivial in those without this syndrome [27].

Patients with Ehlers–Danlos syndrome may also develop joint laxity [2, 5, 11]. This may manifest as bouts of lameness for which there is no obvious cause. An isolated case report appears in the veterinary literature, describing right hind limb lameness and medial patellar luxation in an intact male Spaniel cross with Ehlers–Danlos syndrome at 11 months of age [2].

Ocular abnormalities, if present, may include lens opacifications, lens subluxations, corneal dystrophy, or any combinations thereof [2, 22, 29]. Corneal edema is possible, and pupillary light reflexes may be sluggish [2, 4].

Patients with Ehlers–Danlos syndrome may have concurrent ocular, orthopedic, and cutaneous defects. However, more often they present with a constellation of signs in one or two systems, rather than all three [2]. Cutaneous abnormalities are most common [2]. Of these, skin fragility is a typical presentation.

In addition to skin fragility, patients with Ehlers–Danlos syndrome may also demonstrate skin hyperextensibility [2, 4]. Skin hyperextensibility can be thought of as skin stretchiness. Normal skin has a certain "give" or "pull" that is to be expected. Consider, for example, the skin at the nape of the neck that is used for scruffing

a cat. There is a certain amount of skin stretch and resilience that the clinician has grown to expect. Skin hyperextensibility is when the skin exceeds the expected amount of stretch. Skin stretch is overexaggerated (see Figures 7.1a, b).

As demonstrated in Figures 7.1a, and b, when skin hyperextensibility is extreme, it is unmistakable.

However, mild cases may be less easy to detect, and subjectivity may play a role as the clinician assesses whether or not the skin overstretches.

To eliminate the guesswork, the ability of the skin to stretch can be quantified using the extensibility index [2]. Traction is applied manually to the dorsolumbar skin. The vertical height of this stretch is recorded. This height is then divided by the patient's body length, as represented by the distance from the occipital crest to the base of the tail [2].

Normal patients have ratios that range from 0.08 to 0.15. Therefore, their extensibility index is said to fall between 8 and 15% [21]. Patients with Ehlers–Danlos syndrome have nearly twice that, ranging from 17 to 25% [21].

Note that some patients with Ehlers–Danlos syndrome only have hyperextensibility. Others only have fragility. Some have both [2, 4].

Patients that experience skin fragility may have up to a 40-fold reduction in tensile strength [25]. Such skin lacks the ability to serve as an effective mechanical barrier and is prone to tears. These tears are termed dermatosparaxis, which translates to "torn skin" [3] (see Figure 7.2).

The severity of skin fragility depends upon the individual patient. Skin fragility may be mild or life-threatening, or somewhere in between [27].

(a)

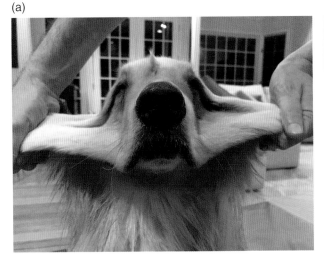

(b)

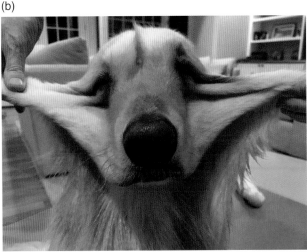

Figure 7.1 (a) Canine patient with appreciable skin hyperextensibility as a result of Ehlers–Danlos syndrome. Erika Sox Burns, DVM, DACVIM-SAIM. (b) Alternate view of a canine patient with extreme skin hyperextensibility. *Source:* Courtesy of Erika Sox Burns, DVM, DACVIM-SAIM.

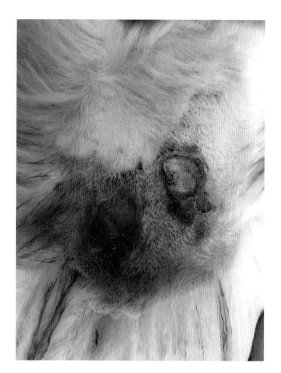

Figure 7.2 Ventral neck wounds in a canine patient with Ehlers–Danlos syndrome. *Source:* Courtesy of Erika Sox Burns, DVM, DACVIM-SAIM.

Wounds are frustrating sequelae of Ehlers–Danlos syndrome for veterinary clients because they arise without obvious trauma. A case report by Famigli-Bergamini describes three wounds that were sustained within a time frame of six months in a four-year-old intact female Dachshund dog [25]. The thorax was involved twice and the shoulder once. These lesions can be quite large: the third wound in this Dachshund measured four by seven centimeters [25]. A year later, the patient re-presented for wounds along the ventral thorax, ventral abdomen, and left flank [25].

The cost of care that is required to manage the patient appropriately may lead to a discussion of euthanasia, particularly in patients that present repeatedly for extensive and/or recurrent wounds [25].

Vascular involvement also carries a guarded to poor prognosis because there is a risk that vessels or hollow organs will rupture [10, 27]. This may result in sudden death from exsanguination.

On the other hand, mild cases of Ehlers–Danlos syndrome carry a favorable prognosis provided that owners can manage wound care and reduce the risk of self-injury by being cautious about the environment in which the patient is housed [11].

Cutaneous asthenia syndrome is another hereditary skin fragility disorder, the name of which translates to "weak skin." It is similar to Ehlers–Danlos syndrome, but affects only the skin [3]. There may be several subtypes of cutaneous asthenia syndrome, given that both autosomal dominant and autosomal recessive patterns of inheritance have been documented [2, 3, 11–18, 30, 31].

Certain breeds of cats are overrepresented in the medical literature, including Himalayans and Burmese [16, 30, 31]. Domestic shorthaired cats may also be at increased risk [17, 18].

In all species except Burmese cats, cutaneous asthenia syndrome is characterized by skin tears secondary to skin fragility [3]. Burmese cats appear to be unique in that they do not always present with skin wounds [3]. Instead, they may simply develop atrophic alopecia and necrotic eschars that are suggestive of vascular injury [3].

A diagnosis of cutaneous asthenia syndrome can be made based upon history and an abnormally elevated extensibility index. However, just as is the case for Ehlers–Danlos syndrome, histopathologic examination of full thickness skin biopsies is required for the diagnosis to be definitive [3]. Unfortunately, light microscopy may result in false negatives because cutaneous changes may be very subtle [15, 23, 32–34]. Electron microscopy may be necessary to identify these subtleties and provide the clinician with a more accurate diagnosis [17, 23, 32, 35].

Epidermolysis bullosa is a third inherited skin fragility syndrome in dogs and cats. Whereas Ehlers–Danlos and cutaneous asthenia syndromes involve defective collagen, epidermolysis bullosa involves mutations of proteins that form the cytoskeleton of keratinocytes and the basement membrane zone [36–38].

In affected humans, the following genes have been identified as having mutations: PRP1, DSP, KRT5, KRT14, PLEC1, ITGA6, ITGB4, LAMA3, LAMB3, LAMC2, COL17A1, and COL7A1. These genes code for various keratins, integrins, laminins, and collagens [39, 40]. The resultant proteins lack the cystoskeletal arrangement that is required to provide a solid foundation. As a result, affected patients experience dermoepidermal separation [1].

Clinical signs involve fragile skin and mucous membranes [39]. Those regions of the body that are exposed to frictional stress are particularly susceptible to damage, specifically, the oral cavity and the skin that covers the limbs [41, 42].

Ulcers develop along the gums, hard and soft palates, tongue, cheek, and lip mucosa [39]. Blisters also form on the skin of affected humans; however, they are far less commonly seen in veterinary patients [39]. When sloughing of the skin occurs, it tends to be limited to the footpads of cats [43]. Claws are considered extensions of the skin. These, too, are susceptible to sloughing [43].

All congenital and inherited skin fragility syndromes are rare. Of the three that have been described here, epidermolysis bullosa is the most rare [43, 44]. These syndromes are discussed in brief here not because they will be diagnosed every day in clinical practice, but rather so that the savvy clinician is aware of their existence if and when that one clinical case presents itself. Young patients that present for wounds without a history of known trauma, especially when they do so repeatedly, should be considered in light of these three syndromes.

7.3 Acquired Skin Fragility Syndromes

Acquired skin fragility syndromes occur in dogs and cats with greater frequency than congenital or inherited ones [1]. The challenge is in recognizing that an underlying condition is present that will require medical management. Without addressing the underlying condition, the patient will succumb to additional complications of disease rather than just skin fragility.

7.3.1 Infectious Disease

7.3.1.1 Feline Infectious Peritonitis
Acquired skin fragility syndromes may also result from underlying infectious disease, although such instances are recorded less often in the medical literature.

The first report of skin fragility syndrome due to feline infectious peritonitis (FIP) was published in 2007 [45]. The patient was a six-year-old female spayed domestic shorthaired cat that presented on emergency for abnormal behavior, anorexia, and weight loss. On presentation, the patient was depressed, dehydrated, and cachectic. There was abdominal distension. A fluid wave was palpable. A 3 cm tear over the left flank was an incidental finding [45].

Following admission to the hospital for diagnostic work-up, the patient sustained skin tearing during gentle restraint over the neck. This restraint resulted in a second wound that measured 7-by-15 cm. The patient was humanely euthanized [45].

Pre- and postmortem findings were consistent with FIP. The diagnosis of FIP was confirmed via indirect immunohistochemistry to detect FIP protein in formalin-fixed tissues [45].

Histopathologic examination of the skin identified changes that were consistent with skin fragility syndrome: epidermal atrophy and dermal thinning [45].

7.3.1.2 Histoplasmosis
The first report of skin fragility syndrome due to disseminated histoplasmosis was published in 2011 [1]. The patient was a four-year-old female spayed domestic shorthaired cat that presented for depression, weight loss, anorexia, and diarrhea. The patient was febrile on presentation and had a 5-by-5 cm patch of skin on the dorsal neck in which the epidermis had entirely separated from the dermis. According to the client, this patch of skin was sustained during transport to the veterinary clinic. This history is suggestive of a wound sustained due to skin fragility. The patient was subsequently diagnosed with histoplasmosis [1].

Histoplasmosis is a fungal disease caused by the soilborne *Histoplasma capsulatum* [46]. Within the United States, *H. capsulatum* concentrates around the Ohio, Missouri, and Mississippi rivers [1, 46]. Infection in companion animals is thought to occur when patients inadvertently inhale microconidia [1, 46]. The yeast subsequently reaches the lower respiratory tract, where it replicates [46]. Locally, disease impacts the pulmonary system. However, infection may spread through blood or lymph [46]. Systemic disease is most common in infected cats that are clinical for histoplasmosis.

Patients less than four years of age are most susceptible as are those with weakened immunity [1, 46].

The pathophysiology that links histoplasmosis and skin fragility is unknown. However, skin fragility was confirmed at necropsy following humane euthanasia of the patient that was described in the 2011 case report. Additional areas of skin sloughing were identified along the dorsum and forelimbs. Histopathology confirmed epidermal atrophy and dermal edema. The latter would have resulted in skin sloughing [1].

7.3.2 Hyperadrenocorticism

Hyperadrenocorticism was first introduced in Chapter 5. In particular, Section 5.7 covered hyperadrenocorticism as a leading cause of endocrine, non-inflammatory alopecia. The classic pattern of alopecia that is seen in Cushingoid patients is bilaterally symmetrical and truncal, sparing the head and limbs [47, 48].

Recall that hyperadrenocorticism is also known as Cushing's syndrome. This syndrome results from an excess of circulating glucocorticoids.

Spontaneous Cushing's syndrome occurs when glucocorticoids are endogenously overproduced [49–53]. This overproduction may stem from inappropriate, unchecked secretion of cortisol by the adrenal glands themselves, as from adrenocortical neoplasia. Alternatively, the pituitary gland may oversecrete adrenocorticotropic hormone, ACTH. ACTH in turn stimulates the adrenal glands to produce more cortisol than the body needs [49–53].

Pituitary-dependent hyperadrenocorticism is more common than adrenal, and accounts for 80–85% of diagnosed cases [49–53]. Pituitary adenomas occur with greater frequency than adenocarcinomas [49–55].

Most are microadenomas, meaning that the diameter of the tumor is less than 10 mm. Only one in 10 dogs presents with macroadenomas at the time of diagnosis [55, 56]. As tumors grow, they compress the pituitary gland. They may also extend into the hypothalamus. Their progression may induce neurological signs; however, because tumor growth rate is quite slow, neuropathy is infrequent [49].

Adrenal-dependent hyperadrenocorticism is typically unilateral, and accounts for 10–15% of Cushingoid patients [49–53, 57]. Canine cases are equally split between naturally occurring adrenal adenomas and carcinomas [49–53, 58]. Both types, adenomas and carcinomas, also occur in cats [58, 59].

Carcinomas carry a worse prognosis because they tend to be invasive [49–53]. When there is right-sided involvement, there is significant concern for invasion of the caudal vena cava and metastasis to the liver, lung, and kidney [51].

Cushing's syndrome may also be triggered by prolonged administration or excessive dosing of exogenous glucocorticoids, such as prednisone [49–53].

Both naturally occurring and iatrogenic Cushing's syndrome cause hair loss [48, 60]. In addition to alopecia, common presenting complaints include "PU/PD/PP," polyuria, polydipsia, and polyphagia. In addition, patients may become pot-bellied due to fat redistribution, and they tend to pant excessively [48, 60].

Middle-aged to older dogs are more commonly affected [49–53]. Pituitary-dependent hyperadrenocorticism may occur with greater frequency in breeds such as Poodles, Dachshunds, and Terriers [49]. Large breeds and female dogs may have greater risk of developing adrenal tumors [52, 61].

Skin lesions may be the only clinical sign of hyperadrenocorticism [47].

Thin skin may be apparent on the physical exam [47, 49, 62–64]. Skin may develop translucency, allowing for greater visualization of superficial blood vessels, or it may take on an aged, wrinkled appearance [62] (see Figure 7.3).

The skin's texture may also change. It may feel like paper [65].

Hyperadrenocorticism is associated with skin fragility. It has been estimated that one in every three cats with Cushing's syndrome has fragile skin [65]. This subset of patients is at increased risk of skin tearing [64–66]. Tears may result from routine handling or grooming [65]. Sheets of skin may also tear off with minor trauma [45].

7.3.3 Additional Paraneoplastic Syndromes

Paraneoplastic syndrome refers to a constellation of clinical signs in one region or body system that results from the presence of cancer elsewhere in the body [67]. Instead

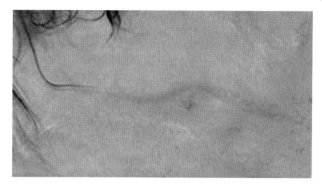

Figure 7.3 Prominent subcutaneous vessels in a Cushingoid patient.

of these clinical signs being triggered by local disease such as a mass effect, they are induced by humoral factors [67]. For example, neoplastic cells may secrete hormones or cytokines, which then act remotely on other regions of the body. Alternatively, the tumor itself may trigger an immune response that sets off a cascade of events with far-reaching impact.

Patients may present with paraneoplastic syndrome before cancer has been diagnosed [67]. Recognizing certain patterns of clinical signs should prompt an investigation that leads to diagnosis and expedites case management.

Hyperadrenocorticism is one of the most common diseases in companion animal medicine that results in paraneoplastic syndrome [67]. Note how overproduction of endogenous cortisol from either a pituitary or adrenal tumor exerts distant effects on the body [67, 68].

A second example of paraneoplastic syndrome is hypercalcemia of malignancy. For example, thyroid carcinoma is just one type of neoplasia that results in markedly increased serum calcium and ionized calcium levels [69–74]. Lymphomas, lymphosarcomas, anal sac adenocarcinoma, and multiple myeloma have also been associated with hypercalcemia [70, 75–77]. Hypercalcemia may cause changes in appetite, alterations in gut motility, causing either diarrhea or constipation, nausea and/or vomiting, and PU/PD.

Lymphoma has also been linked to skin fragility syndrome in a 2013 case report by Crosaz et al. [78]. The patient was an 11-year-old female spayed domestic short-haired cat that presented for evaluation of a 2-by-7 cm wound on the right flank. No known trauma had been sustained by the cat, and the cat's lifestyle was indoor only. Relevant physical examination findings included a paper-like texture to the skin, with several star-shaped lesions. During gentle restraint, the ventral abdominal skin overlying these lesions tore [78]. During the diagnostic work-up, the patient arrested. Postmortem examination included histopathologic analysis of the skin. This analysis revealed epidermal and dermal atrophy, both of which are consistent with skin fragility syndrome.

Lesser known paraneoplastic syndromes may also impact the skin, causing skin fragility syndrome. Consider, for example, hepatocutaneous syndrome, which was first introduced in Chapter 5, Section 5.9 as a cause of alopecia. Hepatocutaneous syndrome is an uncommon paraneoplastic disease that has also been called superficial necrolytic dermatitis, necrolytic migratory erythema (NME), and metabolic epidermal necrosis (MEN) [79, 80].

Although the pathophysiology remains to be determined, glucagon-secreting pancreatic neoplasia, pancreatic adenocarcinoma, extrapancreatic glucagonoma, and degenerative vacuolar hepatopathies result in thin, fragile skin [67, 79–83].

7.3.4 Other Causes of Skin Fragility

Non-neoplastic hepatopathies such as cholangiohepatitis and hepatic lipidosis may also result in skin fragility syndrome [45, 84]. A 2010 case report by Daniel et al. of a nine-year-old female spayed domestic shorthaired cat describes accidental skin tearing between the shoulder blades while being held and petted by the client. The

patient had a six-week history of vomiting and weight loss, and was icteric on presentation. The diagnostic work-up subsequently confirmed hepatic disease [84].

There have also been isolated reports in the medical literature that demonstrate an apparent link between cachexia and skin fragility syndrome [85]. It is thought that cachexia inhibits collagen production in predisposed patients, resulting in thin and easily damaged skin [85]. In cachexic patients, skin fragility appears to be reversible [85].

7.3.5 Concluding Thoughts about Skin Fragility

Skin fragility syndromes are unusual and rarely seen in clinical practice. However, histories of atraumatic or recurrent wounds warrant investigation. Such wounds may be indicative of underlying, more insidious disease or a condition such as Ehlers–Danlos syndrome that is likely to result in repeat episodes. In either case, client and staff education is critical so that all members of the veterinary team understand the need to tread lightly, and that even gentle restraint may have serious consequences.

References

1 Tamulevicus, A.M., Harkin, K., Janardhan, K., and Debey, B.M. (2011). Disseminated histoplasmosis accompanied by cutaneous fragility in a cat. *J. Am. Anim. Hosp. Assoc.* 47 (3): e36–e41.

2 Matthews, B.R. and Lewis, G.T. (1990). Ehlers-Danlos syndrome in a dog. *Can. Vet. J.* 31 (5): 389–390.

3 Hansen, N., Foster, S.F., Burrows, A.K. et al. (2015). Cutaneous asthenia (Ehlers-Danlos-like syndrome) of Burmese cats. *J. Feline Med. Surg.* 17 (11): 954–963.

4 Barnett, K.C. and Cottrell, B.D. (1987). Ehlers-Danlos syndrome in a dog – ocular, cutaneous and articular abnormalities. *J. Small Anim. Pract.* 28 (10): 941–946.

5 Paciello, O., Lamagna, F., Lamagna, B., and Papparella, S. (2003). Ehlers-Danlos-like syndrome in 2 dogs: clinical, histologic, and ultrastructural findings. *Vet. Clin. Pathol.* 32 (1): 13–18.

6 Paterson, S. (2008). Congenital and hereditary skin diseases. In: *Manual of Skin Diseases of the Dog and Cat*, 251–252. Oxford: Wiley Blackwell.

7 Smith, L.T., Wertelecki, W., Milstone, L.M. et al. (1992). Human dermatosparaxis: a form of Ehlers-Danlos syndrome that results from failure to remove the amino-terminal propeptide of type I procollagen. *Am. J. Hum. Genet.* 51 (2): 235–244.

8 Beighton, P., De Paepe, A., Steinmann, B. et al. (1998). Ehlers-Danlos syndromes: revised nosology,

Villefranche, 1997. Ehlers-Danlos National Foundation (USA) and Ehlers-Danlos Support Group (UK). *Am. J. Med. Genet.* 77 (1): 31–37.

9 Mao, J.R. and Bristow, J. (2001). The Ehlers-Danlos syndrome: on beyond collagens. *J. Clin. Invest.* 107 (9): 1063–1069.

10 Malfait, F. and De Paepe, A. (2014). The Ehlers-Danlos syndrome. *Adv. Exp. Med. Biol.* 802: 129–143.

11 Barrera, R., Mane, C., Duran, E. et al. (2004). Ehlers-Danlos syndrome in a dog. *Can. Vet. J.* 45 (4): 355–356.

12 Marshall, V.L., Secombe, C., and Nicholls, P.K. (2011). Cutaneous asthenia in a Warmblood foal. *Aust. Vet. J.* 89 (3): 77–81.

13 White, S.D., Affolter, V.K., Bannasch, D.L. et al. (2004). Hereditary equine regional dermal asthenia ("hyperelastosis cutis") in 50 horses: clinical, histological, immunohistological and ultrastructural findings. *Vet. Dermatol.* 15 (4): 207–217.

14 White, S.D., Affolter, V.K., Schultheiss, P.C. et al. (2007). Clinical and pathological findings in a HERDA-affected foal for 1.5 years of life. *Vet. Dermatol.* 18 (1): 36–40.

15 Sinke, J.D., van Dijk, J.E., and Willemse, T. (1997). A case of Ehlers-Danlos-like syndrome in a rabbit with a review of the disease in other species. *Vet. Q.* 19 (4): 182–185.

16 Holbrook, K.A., Byers, P.H., Counts, D.F., and Hegreberg, G.A. (1980). Dermatosparaxis in a Himalayan cat: II. Ultrastructural studies of dermal collagen. *J. Invest. Dermatol.* 74 (2): 100–104.

17 Sequeira, J.L., Rocha, N.S., Bandarra, E.P. et al. (1999). Collagen dysplasia (cutaneous asthenia) in a cat. *Vet. Pathol.* 36 (6): 603–606.

18 Szczepanik, M., Golynski, M., Wilkolek, P. et al. (2006). Ehlers-Danlos syndrome (cutaneous asthenia) – a report of three cases in cats. *B. Vet. Inst. Pulawy.* 50 (4): 609–612.

19 Counts, D.F., Byers, P.H., Holbrook, K.A., and Hegreberg, G.A. (1980). Dermatosparaxis in a Himalayan cat: I. Biochemical studies of dermal collagen. *J. Invest. Dermatol.* 74 (2): 96–99.

20 Muller, G.H., Kirk, R.W., and Scott, D.W. (1983). *Small Animal Dermatology*, 561–565. Toronto: W.B. Saunders.

21 Minor, R.R., Lein, D.H., Patterson, D.F. et al. (1983). Defects in collagen fibrillogenesis causing hyperextensible, fragile skin in dogs. *J. Am. Vet. Med. Assoc.* 182 (2): 142–148.

22 Hegreberg, G.A., Padgett, G.A., and Page, R.C. (eds.) (1970). *The Ehlers-Danlos syndrome of dogs and mink. Symp Proc III, Animal Models for Biological Research*. Washington: Natl Acad Sci.

23 Benitah, N., Matousek, J.L., Barnes, R.F. et al. (2004). Diaphragmatic and perineal hernias associated with cutaneous asthenia in a cat. *J. Am. Vet. Med. Assoc.* 224 (5): 706–709, 698.

24 Yang, W., Sherman, V.R., Gludovatz, B. et al. (2015). On the tear resistance of skin. *Nat. Commun.* 6: 6649.

25 Famigli-Bergamini, P., Azzalini, L., Avallone, G., and Sarli, G. (2016). Pathology in practice. *J. Am. Vet. Med. Assoc.* 249 (2): 161–163.

26 Scott, D.W., Miller, W.H., and Griffin, C.E. (1995). *Muller & Kirk's Small Animal Dermatology*, 736–805. Philadelphia: W.B. Saunders.

27 Uri, M., Verin, R., Ressel, L. et al. (2015). Ehlers-Danlos syndrome associated with fatal spontaneous vascular rupture in a dog. *J. Comp. Pathol.* 152 (2–3): 211–216.

28 De Paepe, A. and Malfait, F. (2012). The Ehlers-Danlos syndrome, a disorder with many faces. *Clin. Genet.* 82 (1): 1–11.

29 Anderson, J.H. and Brown, R.E. (1978). Cutaneous asthenia in a dog. *J. Am. Vet. Med. Assoc.* 173 (6): 742–743.

30 Dokuzeylul, B., Altun, E.D., Ozdogan, T.H. et al. (2013). Cutaneous asthenia (Ehlers-Danlos syndrome) in a cat. *Turk. J. Vet. Anim. Sci.* 37 (2): 245–249.

31 Burton, G., Stenzel, D., and Mason, K.V. (2000). Cutaneous asthenia in Burmese cats: a vasculopathy? *Vet. Dermatol.* 11 (Suppl): 31.

32 Patterson, D.F. and Minor, R.R. (1977). Hereditary fragility and hyperextensibility of the skin of cats. A defect in collagen fibrillogenesis. *Lab. Investig.* 37 (2): 170–179.

33 Fernandez, C.J., Scott, D.W., Erb, H.N., and Minor, R.R. (1998). Staining abnormalities of dermal collagen in cats with cutaneous asthenia or acquired skin fragility as demonstrated with Masson's trichrome stain. *Vet. Dermatol.* 9 (1): 49–54.

34 Brounts, S.H., Rashmir-Raven, A.M., and Black, S.S. (2001). Zonal dermal separation: a distinctive histopathological lesion associated with hyperelastosis cutis in a Quarter Horse. *Vet. Dermatol.* 12 (4): 219–224.

35 Hegreberg, G.A. (1982). Animal models of collagen disease. *Prog. Clin. Biol. Res.* 94: 229–244.

36 Solovan, C., Ciolan, M., and Olariu, L. (2005). The biomolecular and ultrastructural basis of epidermolysis bullosa. *Acta Dermatovenerol. Alp. Pannonica Adriat.* 14 (4): 127–135.

37 Masunaga, T. (2006). Epidermal basement membrane: its molecular organization and blistering disorders. *Connect. Tissue Res.* 47 (2): 55–66.

38 Castiglia, D. and Zambruno, G. (2010). Molecular testing in epidermolysis bullosa. *Dermatol. Clin.* 28 (2): 223–229, vii–viii.

39 Medeiros, G.X. and Riet-Correa, F. (2015). Epidermolysis bullosa in animals: a review. *Vet. Dermatol.* 26 (1): 3–13, e1–2.

40 Fine, J.D., Eady, R.A., Bauer, E.A. et al. (2008). The classification of inherited epidermolysis bullosa (EB): report of the third international consensus meeting on diagnosis and classification of EB. *J. Am. Acad. Dermatol.* 58 (6): 931–950.

41 Bruckner-Tuderman, L., McGrath, J.A., Robinson, E.C., and Uitto, J. (2010). Animal models of epidermolysis bullosa: update 2010. *J. Invest. Dermatol.* 130 (6): 1485–1488.

42 Sawamura, D., Nakano, H., and Matsuzaki, Y. (2010). Overview of epidermolysis bullosa. *J. Dermatol.* 37 (3): 214–219.

43 Olivry, T., Dunston, S.M., and Marinkovich, M.P. (1999). Reduced anchoring fibril formation and collagen VII immunoreactivity in feline dystrophic epidermolysis bullosa. *Vet. Pathol.* 36 (6): 616–618.

44 White, S.D., Dunstan, R.W., Olivry, T. et al. (1993). Dystrophic (dermolytic) epidermolysis bullosa in a cat. *Vet. Dermatol.* 4: 91–95.

45 Trotman, T.K., Mauldin, E., Hoffmann, V. et al. (2007). Skin fragility syndrome in a cat with feline infectious peritonitis and hepatic lipidosis. *Vet. Dermatol.* 18 (5): 365–369.

46 Greene, C.E. (2006). Histoplasmosis. In: *Infectious Diseases of the Dog and Cat* (ed. C.E. Green), 577–584. St. Louis, M.O.: W.B. Saunders.

47 Zur, G. and White, S.D. (2011). Hyperadrenocorticism in 10 dogs with skin lesions as the only presenting clinical signs. *J. Am. Anim. Hosp. Assoc.* 47 (6): 419–427.

48 Frank, L.A. (2006). Comparative dermatology — canine endocrine dermatoses. *Clin. Dermatol.* 24 (4): 317–325.

49 Peterson, M.E. (2007). Diagnosis of hyperadrenocorticism in dogs. *Clin. Tech. Small Anim. Pract.* 22 (1): 2–11.

50 Peterson, M.E. (1984). Hyperadrenocorticism. *Vet. Clin. North Am. Small Anim. Pract.* 14 (4): 731–749.

51 Herrtage, M.E. (2004). Canine hyperadrenocorticism. In: *Manual of Endocrinology*, 3e (ed. C.T. Mooney and M.E. Peterson), 50–171. Quedgeley, Gloucester: British Small Animal Veterinary Association.

52 Feldman, E.C. and Nelson, R.W. (2004). Canine hyperadrenocorticism (Cushing's syndrome). In: *Canine and Feline Endocrinology and Reproduction*, 252–357. Philadelphia, P.A: W.B. Saunders.

53 Kintzer, P.P. and Peterson, M.E. (2006). Diseases of the adrenal gland. In: *Manual of Small Animal Practice*, 3e (ed. S.J. Birchard and R.G. Sherding), 357–375. Philadelphia, P.A: Saunders Elsevier.

54 Capen, C.C., Martin, S.L., and Koestner, A. (1967). Neoplasms in adenohypophysis of dogs — a clinical and pathologic study. *Pathol. Vet.* 4 (4): 301–325.

55 Peterson, M.E., Krieger, D.T., Drucker, W.D., and Halmi, N.S. (1982). Immuno-cytochemical study of the hypophysis in 2k dogs with pituitary-dependent hyperadrenocorticism. *Acta Endocrinol.* 101 (1): 15–24.

56 Duesberg, C.A., Feldman, E.C., Nelson, R.W. et al. (1995). Magnetic resonance imaging for diagnosis of pituitary macrotumors in dogs. *J. Am. Vet. Med Assoc.* 206 (5): 657–662.

57 Ford, S.L., Feldman, E.C., and Nelson, R.W. (1993). Hyperadrenocorticism caused by bilateral adrenocortical neoplasia in dogs: four cases (1983–1988). *J. Am. Vet. Med. Assoc.* 202 (5): 789–792.

58 DeClue, A.E., Breshears, L.A., Pardo, I.D. et al. (2005). Hyperaldosteronism and hyperprogesteronism in a cat with an adrenal cortical carcinoma. *J. Vet. Intern. Med.* 19 (3): 355–358.

59 Rossmeisl, J.H. Jr., Scott-Moncrieff, J.C., Siems, J. et al. (2000). Hyperadrenocorticism and hyperprogesteronemia in a cat with an adrenocortical adenocarcinoma. *J. Am. Anim. Hosp. Assoc.* 36 (6): 512–517.

60 Feldman, E.C. and Nelson, R.W. (2004). *Canine and Feline Endocrinology and Reproduction*. St. Louis, Missouri: W.B. Saunders.

61 Reusch, C.E. and Feldman, E.C. (1991). Canine hyperadrenocorticism due to adrenocortical neoplasia. Pretreatment evaluation of 41 dogs. *J. Vet. Intern. Med.* 5 (1): 3–10.

62 Nelson, R.W., Feldman, E.C., and Smith, M.C. (1988). Hyperadrenocorticism in cats: seven cases (1978–1987). *J. Am. Vet. Med. Assoc.* 193 (2): 245–250.

63 Lien, Y.H., Huang, H.P., and Chang, P.H. (2006). Iatrogenic hyperadrenocorticism in 12 cats. *J. Am. Anim. Hosp. Assoc.* 42 (6): 414–423.

64 Watson, P.J. and Herrtage, M.E. (1998). Hyperadrenocorticism in six cats. *J. Small. Anim. Pract.* 39 (4): 175–184.

65 Boland, L.A. and Barrs, V.R. (2017). Peculiarities of feline hyperadrenocorticism: update on diagnosis and treatment. *J. Feline Med. Surg.* 19 (9): 933–947.

66 Valentin, S.Y., Cortright, C.C., Nelson, R.W. et al. (2014). Clinical findings, diagnostic test results, and treatment outcome in cats with spontaneous hyperadrenocorticism: 30 cases. *J. Vet. Intern. Med.* 28 (2): 481–487.

67 Turek, M.M. (2003). Cutaneous paraneoplastic syndromes in dogs and cats: a review of the literature. *Vet. Dermatol.* 14 (6): 279–296.

68 Fox, L.E. (1995). The paraneoplastic disorders. In: *Kirk's Current Veterinary Therapy II: Small Animal Practice* (ed. J.D. Bonagura and R.W. Kirk), 530–542. Philadelphia, P.A: W.B. Saunders.

69 Lane, A.E. and Wyatt, K.M. (2012). Paraneoplastic hypercalcemia in a dog with thyroid carcinoma. *Can. Vet. J.* 53 (10): 1101–1104.

70 Elliott, J., Dobson, J.M., Dunn, J.K. et al. (1991). Hypercalcemia in the dog – a study of 40 cases. *J. Small Anim. Pract.* 32 (11): 564–571.

71 Messinger, J.S., Windham, W.R., and Ward, C.R. (2009). Ionized hypercalcemia in dogs: a retrospective study of 109 cases (1998–2003). *J. Vet. Intern. Med.* 23 (3): 514–519.

72 Withrow, S.J. and Vail, D.M. (2007). *Withrow and MacEwen's Small Animal Clinical Oncology*. St. Louis, M.O.: Saunders Elsevier.

73 Ettinger, S.J. (2005). *Textbook of Veterinary Internal Medicine*. Philadelphia, P.A.: Elsevier Saunders.

74 Feldman, E.C. and Nelson, R.W. (1996). *Canine and Feline Endocrinology and Reproduction*. Philadelphia, P.A.: W.B. Saunders.

75 Hammer, A.S. and Couto, C.G. (1994). Complications of multiple-myeloma. *J. Am. Anim. Hosp. Assoc.* 30 (1): 9–14.

76 Meuten, D.J., Kociba, G.J., Capen, C.C. et al. (1983). Hypercalcemia in dogs with lymphosarcoma. Biochemical, ultrastructural, and histomorphometric investigations. *Lab. Investig.* 49 (5): 553–562.

77 Meuten, D.J., Segre, G.V., Capen, C.C. et al. (1983). Hypercalcemia in dogs with adenocarcinoma derived from apocrine glands of the anal sac. Biochemical and histomorphometric investigations. *Lab. Investig.* 48 (4): 428–435.

78 Crosaz, O., Vilaplana-Grosso, F., Alleaume, C. et al. (2013). Skin fragility syndrome in a cat with multicentric follicular lymphoma. *J. Feline Med. Surg.* 15 (10): 953–958.

79 Kimmel, S.E., Christiansen, W., and Byrne, K.P. (2003). Clinicopathological, ultrasonographic, and histopathological findings of superficial necrolytic dermatitis with hepatopathy in a cat. *J. Am. Anim. Hosp. Assoc.* 39 (1): 23–27.

80 Byrne, K.P. (1999). Metabolic epidermal necrosis-hepatocutaneous syndrome. *Vet. Clin. North Am. Small Anim. Pract.* 29 (6): 1337–1355.

81 Miller, W.H., Scott, D.W., Buerger, R.G. et al. (1990). Necrolytic migratory erythema in dogs – a hepatocutaneous syndrome. *J. Am. Anim. Hosp. Assoc.* 26 (6): 573–581.

82 Gross, T.L., Song, M.D., Havel, P.J., and Ihrke, P.J. (1993). Superficial necrolytic dermatitis (necrolytic migratory erythema) in dogs. *Vet. Pathol.* 30 (1): 75–81.

83 Mizuno, T., Hiraoka, H., Yoshioka, C. et al. (2009). Superficial necrolytic dermatitis associated with extrapancreatic glucagonoma in a dog. *Vet. Dermatol.* 20 (1): 72–79.

84 Daniel, A.G., Lucas, S.R., Junior, A.R. et al. (2010). Skin fragility syndrome in a cat with cholangiohepatitis and hepatic lipidosis. *J. Feline Med. Surg.* 12 (2): 151–155.

85 Furiani, N., Porcellato, I., and Brachelente, C. (2017). Reversible and cachexia-associated feline skin fragility syndrome in three cats. *Vet. Dermatol.* 28 (5): 508–e121.

8

Changes in Coat Color

8.1 Introduction to the Value of Coat Color

Coat color is an important aesthetic feature for some companion animal owners. Coat color may be characteristic of a certain breed of dog or cat, or coat color may be a preference that owners seek when looking to adopt or purchase a new companion. Anecdotally, it has been suggested that coat color discrimination influences adoptability. The popular press has historically reported that black dogs and cats experience lower adoption rates, longer average length of availability for adoption (LOA), and higher euthanasia rates at animal shelters [1].

Although more recent reports in the medical literature suggest otherwise, it is important to recognize that human perceptions and stereotypes about coat color exist [1–6]. A 2012 study by Delgado et al. evaluated public perceptions online via an anonymous survey questionnaire. Results suggested that orange cats were seen as friendlier than others; white cats were considered to be more reserved; and tri-color cats were labeled as intolerant or aloof [7].

Within the veterinary field, stereotypes perpetuate this idea that calico cats have "cattitude" and tortoiseshell cats have "tortitude." These beliefs suggest that black, orange, and white-patched cats are more likely to possess aggressive tendencies than other colored coats.

These biases may or may not be accurate [7–9]. Coat coloration in cats and dogs is complex, and although personality may play a role, the extent to which it does remains to be determined.

Even so, coat color matters to a select population of companion animal owners. Coat color may be of particular importance to breeders given that buyer preferences dictate that which is marketable and at what cost.

Coat color is also a very visible phenotypic characteristic. Clients are readily able to detect changes in coat color and may present patients to clinical practice for evaluation.

Coat color changes are generally benign and may even represent normal development of the breed. However, it is prudent to review the most common causes of coat color changes, if for no other reason than to advance client education if or when these changes present themselves.

8.2 Point Coloration: An Expected Coat Color Change over Time

Certain breeds of cats are known for their color-point coat patterns. These include the Siamese, Burmese, Tonkinese, Balinese, Birman, Singapura, and Himalayan cats [10–12].

Color-point coat patterns are those in which distinct areas of the body are highlighted with color. In the breeds listed above, faces and extremities (ears, paws, and tails) may be darker than other areas of the body. These highlighted body parts are said to be "pointed."

Points develop in cats due to acromelanism [12–16]. This is a condition in which temperature dictates where pigmentation develops on the coat.

Thermal influence over coat color stems from a mutation of the albino gene that results in temperature-dependent tyrosinase [14]. Tyrosinase is an enzyme that, at the level of the hair bulb, assists with melanin formation [10, 14, 16–19].

In color-point cats, tyrosinase is active only at cooler temperatures. Areas of the body that register at core body temperature, such as the torso, remain under-pigmented compared to areas of the body that are cooler, such as extremities [10, 17–19].

Colors of points have breed-specific names. For example, Siamese cats are typically referred to as seal points (brown), flame points (red-orange), blue points (gray), and lilac (lavender) points (see Figures 8.1a–d)

Tonkinese cats have similar color points; however, the Siamese color-point lingo does not exist among

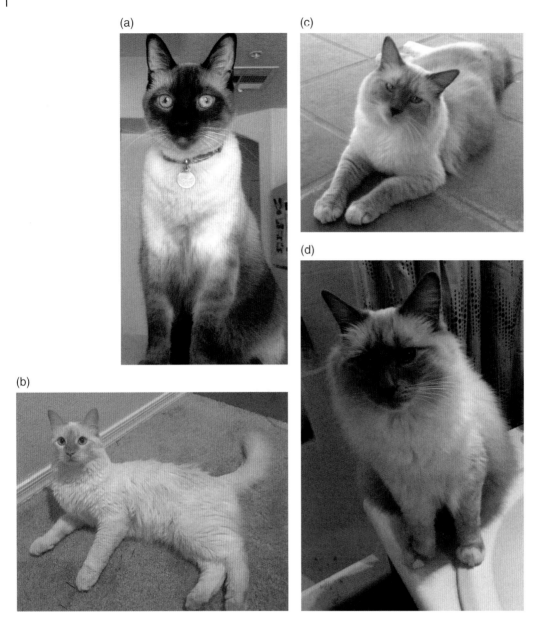

Figure 8.1 (a) An example of a seal point Siamese. *Source:* Courtesy of Kyley Olson. (b) An example of a flame point Siamese. *Source:* Courtesy of Amanda D. Schellinger. (c) An example of a blue point Siamese. *Source:* Courtesy of Lydia McDaniel, DVM. (d) An example of a lilac point Siamese. *Source:* Courtesy of Lydia McDaniel, DVM.

Tonkinese breeders. For example, a "seal point" Tonkinese would be referred to as having the base coat color, champagne. Likewise, a "lilac point" Tonkinese would be considered platinum (see Figures 8.2a, b).

Color-point cats are born without points. Kittens are white at birth because tyrosinase is inactivated by the homogenously warm environment of the queen's uterus.

Points develop as kittens age, as different regions of the body are exposed to different temperatures. Cooler regions of the body (the face, muzzle, extremities, and tail) darken relative to the torso, which remains lighter.

Color points become obvious by four weeks of age, particularly in seal point Siamese or champagne Tonkinese (see Figures 8.3a–e).

Color points may be less obvious in lilac Siamese or platinum Tonkinese because the frosty gray points are less apparent than the chocolate brown. The same could be same for flame-point Siamese. The points are much softer. However, with age, these subtler points do become more striking (see Figures 8.4a–i).

Because tyrosinase in cats with acromelanism is temperature sensitive, geography plays an additional role in

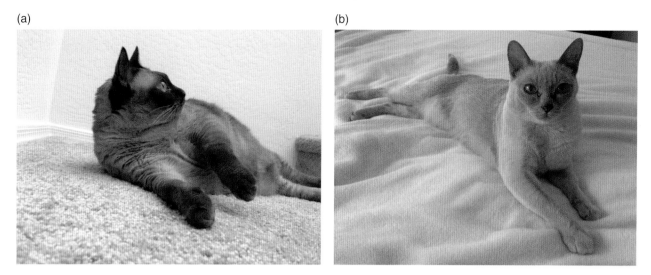

Figure 8.2 (a) An example of a champagne mink Tonkinese. (b) An example of a platinum solid Tonkinese.

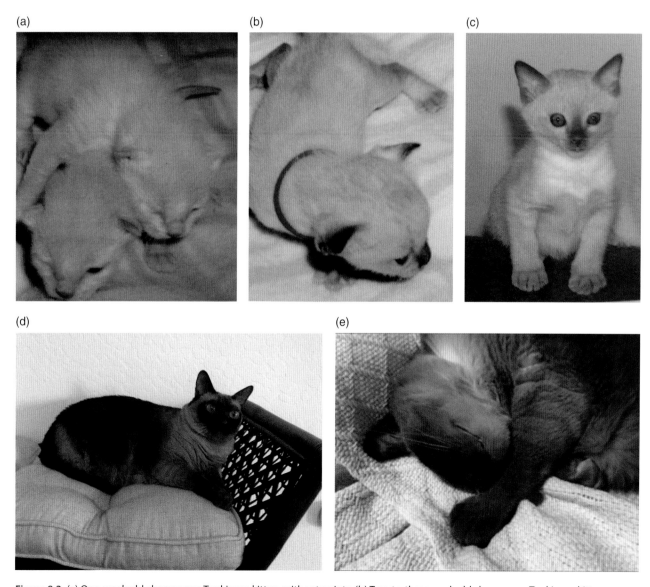

Figure 8.3 (a) One-week old champagne Tonkinese kitten, without points. (b) Two-to-three week old champagne Tonkinese kitten, developing points. (c) Two-month old champagne Tonkinese kitten, developing points. (d) Ten-year old champagne Tonkinese cat with established points. (e) Thirteen-year-old champagne Tonkinese cat with established points.

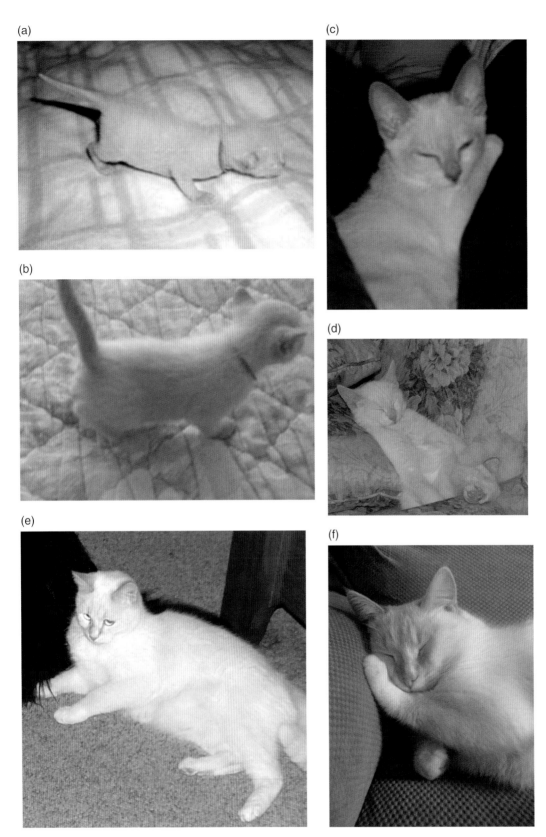

Figure 8.4 (a) One-week old Tonkinese platinum kitten, without points. (b) Two-to-three-week-old platinum Tonkinese kitten, developing points. (c) Two-month-old platinum Tonkinese kitten, developing points. (d) Six-month-old flame-point Siamese cat. *Source:* Courtesy of Kathy and Kenneth Knowles. (e) One-year-old flame-point Siamese cat. *Source:* Courtesy of Kathy and Kenneth Knowles. (f) Two-year-old flame-point Siamese cat. *Source:* Courtesy of Kathy and Kenneth Knowles. (g) Three-year-old flame-point Siamese cat. *Source:* Courtesy of Kathy and Kenneth Knowles. (h) Ten-year-old platinum Tonkinese cat with established points. (i) Thirteen-year old platinum and champagne Tonkinese cats side-by-side for comparison.

(g)

(h)

(i)

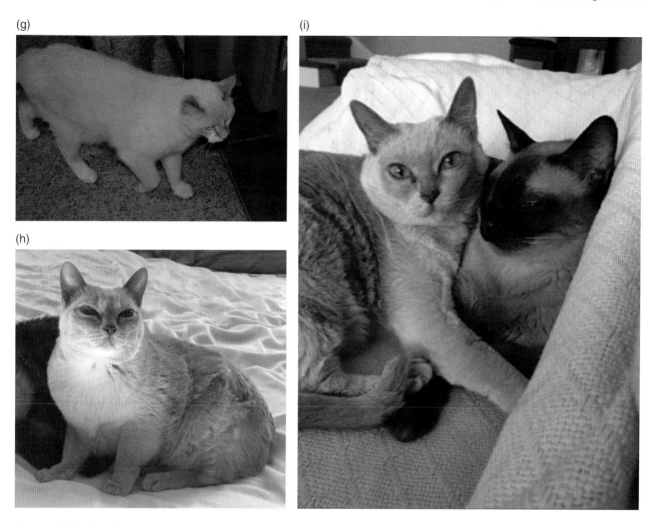

Figure 8.4 (Continued)

determining how dark points will become. Color-point cats that live in cooler climates tend to have darker, more distinct points than those cats that live in warmer regions of the world. If the climate is sufficiently cold, color-point cats may also develop bilateral truncal darkening [12, 13, 15]. Exclusively outdoor color-point cats in a cold climate may experience a coat color change in which the whole body darkens [15]. They in essence lose their points.

Additionally, consider how coat clipping may impact coat color. Shaving the ventral abdomen in preparation for ovariohysterectomy, for example, creates a temporary region of chilled skin. As fur regrows, pigment production may be enhanced given that tyrosinase has now been activated. This will result in a darkened ventral abdomen, more so than would have been seen had the region not been shaved. Note that this color change is temporary; however, it will not resolve until the next hair cycle [12, 13].

Inflammation is another factor that affects heat production. Consider, for example, a febrile kitten with an upper respiratory infection. If there is sufficient inflammation of the nasal passageways and sinus cavities, local temperature at the face may inactivate tyrosinase. New fur growth will be unpigmented, affecting the depth and richness of the expected facial mask [15].

Finally, consider obesity. Obese patients have an excess of fat as an insulator. The skin is in effect further from the core body temperature, making it cooler than expected, much like the extremities. Obese color-point cats are therefore more likely to have darkening along the trunk because tyrosinase is activated in this now cooler region. Like inflammation, obesity may be fleeting. If obese patients slim down, in effect removing that excess layer of insulation, the temperature of the trunk warms. Tyrosinase subsequently inactivates. Fur that grows during the next cycle will not appear as pigmented [15].

8.3 Whitening of the Fur

Certain conditions may impair or destroy pigment-producing cells, melanocytes [12, 20, 21]. This results in depigmentation of the hair shaft such that the fur appears to whiten. The appropriate medical terminology for whitening of the fur is leukotrichia [12, 20, 21].

Several conditions may result in graying of the fur and eventual leukotrichia. These include the following [20–29]:

- Natural aging*
- Stress*
- Pregnancy*
- Nutrition*
- Trauma*
- Dietary deficiency
- Systemic illness
- Vitiligo*
- Radiation therapy*
- Drug reactions*
- Post-inflammatory folliculitis
- Breed-specific tyrosinase deficiency in Chow Chow dogs
- Alopecia areata
- Oculocutaneous syndromes such as Vogt-Koyanagi-Harada (VKH)
- Epitheliotropic lymphoma

The starred conditions above will be touched upon in this chapter.

Leukotrichia may also be idiopathic, meaning that the cause is unknown. This was most recently documented by White et al. in 1990, in which seven of nine pups in a litter of Labrador Retrievers developed progressive leukotrichia [25]. Initially, leukotrichia involved facial fur, including fur around the eyes. By 10 weeks of age, leukotrichia had extended to the neck, dorsum, and feet. At 14 weeks of age, leukotrichia began to spontaneously resolve. An underlying cause was never identified [25].

8.3.1 Natural Aging

Natural aging causes leukotrichia in companion animals just as in humans. As dogs and cats age, melanocytes die. When hair follicles contain fewer melanocytes, fur contains less melanin. Over time, the affected fur takes on a more transparent color such as silvery gray. As the population of melanocytes continues to deplete, gray fur becomes whiter. In dogs, the facial hairs tend to lose pigment first. The muzzle is often affected. Dogs also often become whiter at the fur around the eyes (see Figures 8.5a–e).

8.3.2 Premature Aging

Companion animal patients may also develop premature graying (see Figures 8.6a–c).

Premature graying has been studied more thoroughly in humans than in companion animals. Genetics is thought to play a role in humans and presumably influences graying in dogs and cats, too [30].

In addition to genetics, anxiety may be a contributing factor for companion animal patients [30]. Indeed, stressful events in humans have been linked to premature graying [30–34]. This includes stress at the cellular level as well as emotionally driven stress such as can be found in the workplace [33].

Stress may also be physiological, for example, the stress associated with the physiologic state of pregnancy. There are isolated case reports of pregnant Siamese cats that developed so-called "goggle eyes." The term, "goggle eyes", refers to peri-ocular leukotrichia that coincides with pregnancy [29].

Leukotrichia secondary to stress may or may not resolve after the stressful event.

Note that neither age-related nor premature leukotrichia is of any medical consequence. It is purely cosmetic.

8.3.3 Nutrition

Certain nutritional deficiencies can result in progressive graying of the coat. Specifically, a deficiency in copper, zinc, or both grays the coat, which will be especially noticeable in a previously black-coated dog or cat [35]. To prevent this, commercial diets exceed the minimum requirements for both elements. However, dogs and cats that receive home-prepared diets may become deficient [36].

8.3.4 Trauma

Leukotrichia may also result from traumatic events that damage melanocytes (see Figure 8.7).

Pigment does not typically return to these damaged regions, which remain white for the lifetime of the patient.

8.3.5 Vitiligo

The pigmentary abnormalities that were outlined in Sections 8.3.1, 8.3.2, and 8.3.3 were acquired. However, depigmentation of the coat can also be hereditary or familial. Vitiligo is a familial disease in Siamese cats and in certain breeds of dog, such as the Rottweiler. Vitiligo has also been described in humans, horses, cattle, mice, and rabbits [21, 37–41].

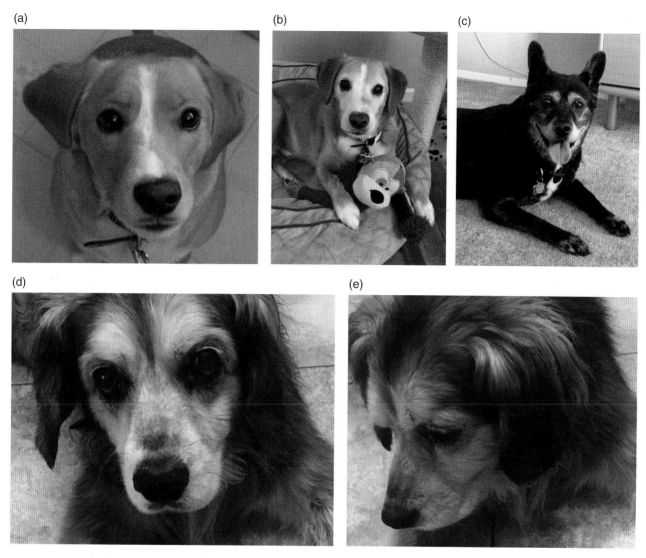

Figure 8.5 (a) Bicolored canine patient prior to age-related graying. *Source:* Courtesy of Gina Olmsted, DVM, DACVIM (Oncology). (b) Same bicolored canine patient pictured in Figure 8.5a, demonstrating age-related leukotrichia. *Source:* Courtesy of Gina Olmsted, DVM, DACVIM (Oncology). (c) Aged canine patient, demonstrating natural onset of leukotrichia. *Source:* Courtesy of the Burches. (d) Head-on view of aged canine patient, demonstrating leukotrichia. *Source:* Courtesy of Jennifer Sodetz, DVM. (e) Side view of aged canine patient, demonstrating leukotrichia. *Source:* Courtesy of Jennifer Sodetz, DVM.

As young adults, affected patients undergo depigmentation of the coat that may or may not involve the claws. Depigmentation is typically symmetrical in terms of distribution. Lesions may be global or focal, involving, for instance, only the face or around the eyes. Other regions that are commonly affected include the nose, lips, footpads, scrotum, and perineum. The oral mucosa may also be involved [21, 37, 38, 42–44].

Although clinical signs may wax and wane, complete remission is unlikely.

Note that clinical presentation and history may be suggestive of vitiligo, but are not pathognomonic. An extensive work-up is indicated to rule out contact allergy, nutritional deficiency, epitheliotropic lymphoma, systemic lupus erythematosus (SLE), discoid lupus erythematosus, panleukopenia, feline leukemia, and endocrinopathies [21].

8.3.6 Radiation Therapy

Radiation therapy is one arm of case management for companion animal patients with primary bone tumors, such as osteosarcoma and fibrosarcoma, lymphomas, carcinomas, such as apocrine gland anal sac carcinoma, and lymph node metastasis [45–53].

Radiation therapy uses high-energy x-rays, gamma rays, and other charged particles as part of curative or

(a)

(b)

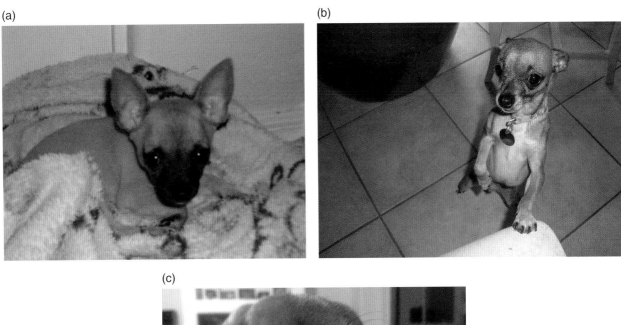

(c)

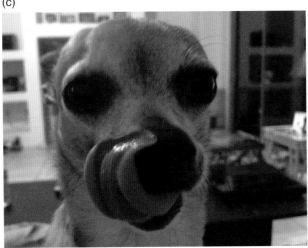

Figure 8.6 (a) Chihuahua puppy prior to the onset of premature graying. *Source:* Courtesy of Amanda Talbott, MWU veterinary student. (b) Same canine patient pictured in Figure 8.6a, demonstrating premature graying at three years of age. *Source:* Courtesy of Amanda Talbott, MWU veterinary student. (c) Same canine patient pictured in Figure 8.6a, demonstrating leukotrichia at eight years of age. *Source:* Courtesy of Amanda Talbott, MWU veterinary student.

palliative therapy to reduce tumor size and clean up surgical margins. In addition to targeting cancer, radiation therapy may have unintended consequences, particularly when it contacts normal, healthy tissue [45–53].

These consequences may be acute or delayed. Localized alopecia is a common acute effect.

When hair regrows, its color may have changed dramatically. Leukotrichia is a frequent late effect of radiation therapy (see Figure 8.8).

Late effects may develop months to years after treatment. They may or may not be reversible. The extent to which they occur often depends upon the dose of radiation per fraction. The larger the dose, the more likely there are to be adverse effects [45–53].

8.3.7 Drug Reactions

Tyrosine kinase inhibitors are known to induce reversible skin depigmentation in humans and, rarely, dogs. Depigmentation may begin as early as the first week of treatment. Once the treatment is discontinued, pigment is restored [54].

Cavalcanti et al. [54] describes the first published case in the veterinary literature. An 11-year-old intact male Bernese mountain dog with a low-grade mast cell tumor developed cutaneous lesions during treatment with oral toceranib phosphate. Three weeks into treatment, the patient developed periorbital leukotrichia and depigmentation. In addition, the dog's nasal planum

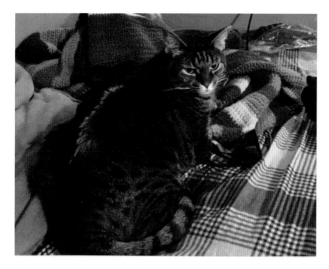

Figure 8.7 Feline patient with a white stripe of fur along dorsal midline, where full thickness skin trauma had been sustained previously. *Source:* Courtesy of Ophelia ("Ophie") Nedrow and her humans Annette Sugden and Michael Nedrow.

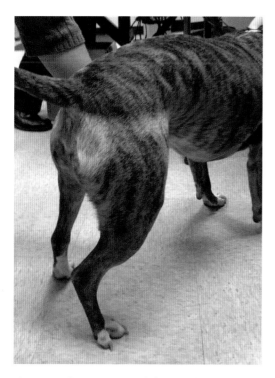

Figure 8.8 Canine patient exhibiting right-sided perineal leukotrichia secondary to radiation therapy to manage an apocrine gland anal sac carcinoma. *Source:* Courtesy of Beki Cohen Regan, DVM, DACVIM (Oncology).

was hyperkeratotic and became crusted over. There was an overall loss of the normal cobblestone architecture. Human patients who have been prescribed pharmaceutical agents in the same class also report

cutaneous lesions, including dry skin, pruritus, and desquamation [55–59].

8.4 "Red Hair Syndrome"

"Red Hair Syndrome" refers to the progressive change in coat color from black to red or rust-brown. "Red Hair Syndrome" results from one or more dietary deficiencies.

Diets that are deficient in protein will transform the coat to red-brown, particularly at the flanks, ventral abdomen, and paws [60]. The same may be seen in patients that suffer from malnutrition and/or malabsorptive gastrointestinal disease [60].

Additional nutrients of interest are phenylalanine and tyrosine. The former is an essential amino acid; the latter is a precursor of melanin [61, 62]. These amino acids are important constituents of proteins that influence coat color. When levels of tyrosine are low in the diet, reddish-brown pheomelanin synthesis is preferred over black-colored eumelanin [63, 64]. The result is the development of a progressively rust-brown to reddish coat in black-coated dogs and cats [63].

When dietary deficiencies are corrected, black coats are restored [35, 61]. "Red Hair Syndrome" is therefore reversible.

The amount of phenylalanine and tyrosine that cats require for growth is insufficient to maintain a black hair coat [35, 61, 65–67]. Therefore, diets must exceed growth requirements such that the sum of both amino acids in kibble should be 1.5% or higher [35].

Commercial dog food should also contain sufficient phenylalanine and tyrosine to exceed growth requirements in order to maintain an optimal black color coat [63].

8.5 Allergies and Tear Staining

Dogs and cats with allergic skin disease may experience coat-color changes from black to red for reasons yet to be determined (see Figures 8.9a–b).

Additionally, skin irritation that results in excessive licking or grooming may also discolor any fur red or rust-brown. The same is true of excessive tearing, so-called epiphora. This is particularly prominent in light-coated dogs, of which the Maltese, Miniature poodle, and Toy poodle are overrepresented [68] (see Figures 8.10a–c).

The red or rust-brown color stems from the composition of tears and saliva [68–71]. Both body fluids contain

(a)

(b)

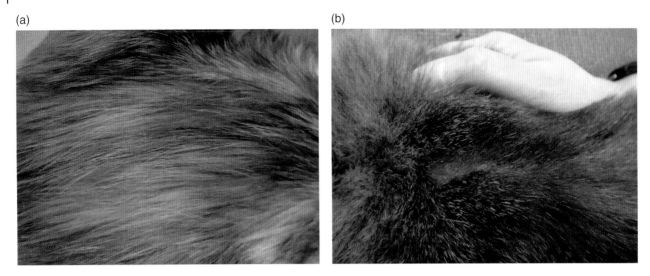

Figure 8.9 (a) Feline patient with allergic skin disease. Note the coat color change from black to rust-orange. *Source:* Courtesy of Patricia Bennett, DVM. (b) Canine patient with allergic skin disease. Note the coat color change from black to rust-orange. *Source:* Courtesy of Patricia Bennett, DVM.

(a)

(b)

(c)

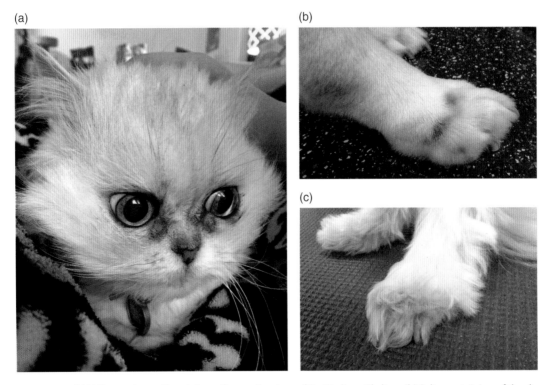

Figure 8.10 (a) Feline patient with epiphora. *Source:* Courtesy of Dr. Madison Skelton. (b) Salivary staining of the dorsal aspect of the right forepaw in a canine patient with atopy. *Source:* Courtesy of Patricia Bennett, DVM. (c) Salivary staining of the left forepaw in a canine patient with *Malassezia* overgrowth. *Source:* Courtesy of Patricia Bennett, DVM.

porphyrins [35, 72]. These are natural stains. The stains themselves are a cosmetic concern only. However, the savvy clinician should look for an underlying cause that may be addressed.

Some causes are more readily treated than others. For example, underlying skin allergies are medically manageable, whereas tear overflow from abnormal conformation is more likely to be a persistent problem [73].

References

1 Svoboda, H.J. and Hoffman, C.L. (2015). Investigating the role of coat colour, age, sex, and breed on outcomes for dogs at two animal shelters in the United States. *Anim. Welf.* 24 (4): 497–506.

2 Woodward, L., Milliken, J., and Humy, S. (2012). Give a dog a bad name and hang him: evaluating big, black dog syndrome. *Soc. Anim.* 20 (3): 236–253.

3 Protopopova, A., Gilmour, A.J., Weiss, R.H. et al. (2012). The effects of social training and other factors on adoption success of shelter dogs. *Appl. Anim. Behav. Sci.* 142 (1–2): 61–68.

4 Diesel, G., Smith, H., and Pfeiffer, D.U. (2007). Factors affecting time to adoption of dogs re-homed by a charity in the UK. *Anim. Welf.* 16 (3): 353–360.

5 Brown, W.P., Davidson, J.P., and Zuefle, M.E. (2013). Effects of phenotypic characteristics on the length of stay of dogs at two no kill animal shelters. *J. Appl. Anim. Welf. Sci.* 16 (1): 2–18.

6 Brown, W.P. and Morgan, K.T. (2015). Age, breed designation, coat color, and coat pattern influenced the length of stay of cats at a no-kill shelter. *J. Appl. Anim. Welf. Sci.* 18 (2): 169–180.

7 Delgado, M.M., Munera, J.D., and Reevy, G.M. (2012). Human perceptions of coat color as an indicator of domestic cat personality. *Anthrozoös* 25 (4): 427–440.

8 Ledger, R. and O'Farrell, V. (eds.) (1996). *Factors influencing the reactions of cats to humans and novel objects*. Proceedings of the 30th International Congress of the ISAE. Guelph: Co. K. L. Campbell Centre for the Study of Animal Welfare.

9 Munera, J. (2010). *Domestic cats: Coat color and personality*. Florida: New College of Florida.

10 Stokking, L.B. and Campbell, K.C. (2004). Disorders of pigmentation. In: *Small Animal Dermatology Secrets* (ed. K.C. Campbell), 352–355. Philadelphia: Hanley & Belfus.

11 Gebhardt, R.H., Pond, G., and Raleigh, I. (1979). *A Standard Guide to Cat Breeds*, 319. New York: McGraw-Hill.

12 Miller, W.H., Griffin, C.E., Campbell, K.L. et al. (2013). *Muller & Kirk's Small Animal Dermatology*, 7e, ix, 938 p. St. Louis, Mo.: Elsevier.

13 Maxie, M.G. (2016). *Jubb, Kennedy, and Palmer's Pathology of Domestic Animals*, 6e, 3 volumes. St. Louis, Missouri: Elsevier.

14 van Grouw, H. (2012). What colour is that sparrow? A case study: colour aberrations in the house sparrow passer domesticus. *Intern. Stud. Sparrows* 36: 30–55.

15 McCannon-Collier, M. and Davis, K.L. (1992). *Siamese Cats: Everything about Acquisition, Care, Nutrition, Behavior, Health Care, and Breeding*. Hauppauge, N.Y.: Barron's Educational Series, Inc.

16 Kaas, J.H. (2005). Serendipity and the Siamese cat: the discovery that genes for coat and eye pigment affect the brain. *ILAR J.* 46 (4): 357–363.

17 Association CF. Cat Colors FAQ: Cat Color Genetics. http://www.fanciers.com/other-faqs/color-genetics.html (accessed 3 April 2019).

18 Lyons, L.A., Imes, D.L., Rah, H.C., and Grahn, R.A. (2005). Tyrosinase mutations associated with Siamese and Burmese patterns in the domestic cat (Felis catus). *Anim. Genet.* 36 (2): 119–126.

19 Ye, X.C., Pegado, V., Patel, M.S., and Wasserman, W.W. (2014). Strabismus genetics across a spectrum of eye misalignment disorders. *Clin. Genet.* 86 (2): 103–111.

20 Classen, J., Bettenay, S.V., and Mueller, R.S. (2017). Seasonal leukotrichia in a German shepherd dog. A case report. *Tierarztl Prax Ausg K Kleintiere Heimtiere* 45 (1): 46–51.

21 Lopez, R., Ginel, P.J., Molleda, J.M. et al. (1994). A clinical, pathological and immunopathological study of vitiligo in a Siamese cat. *Vet. Dermatol.* 5 (1): 27–32.

22 Lee, D.Y., Kim, C.R., Park, J.H., and Lee, J.H. (2011). The incidence of leukotrichia in segmental vitiligo: implication of poor response to medical treatment. *Int. J. Dermatol.* 50 (8): 925–927.

23 Rosenkrantz, W.S. and Gross, T.L. (eds.) (2001). *Epitheliotropic lymphocytic adnexal infiltration with leukotrichia in a boxer*. Norfolk: NAVDF.

24 Tobin, D.J., Gardner, S.H., Luther, P.B. et al. (2003). A natural canine homologue of alopecia areata in humans. *Br. J. Dermatol.* 149 (5): 938–950.

25 White, S.D. and Batch, S. (1990). Leukotrichia in a litter of Labrador retrievers. *J. Am. Anim. Hosp. Assoc.* 26 (3): 319–321.

26 Engstrom, D. (1966). Tyrosinase deficiency in the chow chow. In: *Current Veterinary Therapy* (ed. R.W. Kirk), 352. Philadelphia: W.B. Saunders.

27 Kern, T.J., Walton, D.K., Riis, R.C. et al. (1985). Uveitis associated with poliosis and vitiligo in six dogs. *J. Am. Vet. Med. Assoc.* 187 (4): 408–414.

28 Campbell, K.L., Mclaughlin, S.A., and Reynolds, H.A. (1986). Generalized leukoderma and Poliosis following uveitis in a dog. *J. Am. Anim. Hosp. Assoc.* 22 (1): 121–124.

29 Little, S. (2012). *The Cat: Clinical Medicine and Management*. St. Louis, Missouri: Saunders.

30 King, C., Smith, T.J., Grandin, T., and Borchelt, P. (2016). Anxiety and impulsivity: factors associated with premature graying in young dogs. *Appl. Anim. Behav. Sci.* 185: 78–85.

31 Kauser, S., Westgate, G.E., Green, M.R., and Tobin, D.J. (2011). Human hair follicle and epidermal melanocytes exhibit striking differences in their aging profile which involves catalase. *J. Invest. Dermatol.* 131 (4): 979–982.

32 Kocaman, S.A., Cetin, M., Durakoglugil, M.E. et al. (2012). The degree of premature hair graying as an independent risk marker for coronary artery disease: a predictor of biological age rather than chronological age. *Anadolu Kardiyol Derg* 12 (6): 457–463.

33 Tenibiaje, D.J. (2013). Work-related stress. *Eur. J. Bus. Soc. Sci.* 1: 73–80.

34 Tobin, D.J. and Paus, R. (2001). Graying: gerontobiology of the hair follicle pigmentary unit. *Exp. Gerontol.* 36 (1): 29–54.

35 Beynen, A.C. (2017). Diet and hair color in cats and dogs. *Creature Companion* (June): 34–35.

36 Dillitzer, N., Becker, N., and Kienzle, E. (2011). Intake of minerals, trace elements and vitamins in bone and raw food rations in adult dogs. *Br. J. Nutr.* 106: S53 S56.

37 Boissy, R.E., Moellmann, G.E., and Lerner, A.B. (1987). Morphology of melanocytes in hair bulbs and eyes of vitiligo mice. *Am. J. Pathol.* 127: 380–388.

38 Naughton, G.K., Mahaffey, M., and Bystryn, J.C. (eds.) (1986). Antibodies to surface antigens of pigmented cells in animals with vitiligo. Proceedings for the Society for Experimental Biology and Medicine.

39 Naughton, G.K., Eisinger, M., and Bystryn, J.C. (1983). Antibodies to normal human melanocytes in vitiligo. *J. Exp. Med.* 158 (1): 246–251.

40 Mozos, E., Novales, M., Millan, J., and Sierra, M. (1991). Focal hypopigmentation in horses resembling Arabian fading syndrome. *Equine Vet. Educ.* 3: 122–125.

41 Hayashi, T., Tsuruno, M., Ohtake, O. et al. (1989). *Studies on vitiligo vulgaris in Japanese black cattle. Bulletin of the Faculty of Agriculture*, vol. 42, 199–204. Tottori University.

42 Scott, D.W. and Randolph, J.F. (1989). Vitiligo in 2 old-English sheepdog littermates and in a dachshund with juvenile-onset diabetes-mellitus. *Companion Anim. Pract.* 19 (3): 18–22.

43 Sherding, R.G. (1994.). Diseases of the skin. In: *The Cat: Diseases and Clinical Management*, 2e (ed. R.G. Sherding), 1994–2046. Philadelphia, PA, New York, NY: W.B. Saunders.

44 Muller, G.H., Kirk, R.W., and Scott, D.W. (1989). Pigmentary abnormalities. In: *Small Animal Dermatology*, 705–714. Philadelphia: W.B. Saunders.

45 McDonald, C., Looper, J., and Greene, S. (2012). Response rate and duration associated with a 4Gy 5 fraction palliative radiation protocol. *Vet. Radiol. Ultrasound* 53 (3): 358–364.

46 Lawrence, J., Forrest, L., Adams, W. et al. (2008). Four-fraction radiation therapy for macroscopic soft tissue sarcomas in 16 dogs. *J. Am. Anim. Hosp. Assoc.* 44 (3): 100–108.

47 Hillers, K.R., Lana, S.E., Fuller, C.R., and LaRue, S.M. (2007). Effects of palliative radiation therapy on nonsplenic hemangiosarcoma in dogs. *J. Am. Anim. Hosp. Assoc.* 43 (4): 187–192.

48 Liptak, J.M., Dernell, W.S., Ehrhart, E.J. et al. (2004). Retroperitoneal sarcomas in dogs: 14 cases (1992–2002). *J. Am. Vet. Med. Assoc.* 224 (9): 1471–1477.

49 Plavec, T., Kessler, M., Kandel, B. et al. (2006). Palliative radiotherapy as treatment for non-resectable soft tissue sarcomas in the dog – a report of 15 cases. *Vet. Comp. Oncol.* 4 (2): 98–103.

50 Poirier, V.J., Bley, C.R., Roos, M., and Kaser-Hotz, B. (2006). Efficacy of radiation therapy for the treatment of macroscopic canine oral soft tissue sarcoma. *In Vivo* 20 (3): 415–419.

51 Pfeiffer, I. (2016). Canine thyroid carcinoma in 4-year-old American bulldog: Radiation oncology perspective. DVM360.

52 Lurie, D.M., Kent, M.S., Fry, M.M., and Theon, A.P. (2008). A toxicity study of low-dose rate half-body irradiation and chemotherapy in dogs with lymphoma. *Vet. Comp. Oncol.* 6 (4): 257–267.

53 Ramirez, O. 3rd, Dodge, R.K., Page, R.L. et al. (1999). Palliative radiotherapy of appendicular osteosarcoma in 95 dogs. *Vet. Radiol. Ultrasound* 40 (5): 517–522.

54 Cavalcanti, J.V.J., Hasbach, A., Barnes, K. et al. (2017). Skin depigmentation associated with toceranib phosphate in a dog. *Vet. Dermatol.* 28 (4): 400–e95.

55 Autier, J., Escudier, B., Wechsler, J. et al. (2008). Prospective study of the cutaneous adverse effects of sorafenib, a novel multikinase inhibitor. *Arch. Dermatol.* 144 (7): 886–892.

56 Al Enazi, M.M., Kadry, R., and Mitwali, H. (2009). Skin depigmentation induced by sunitinib treatment of renal cell carcinoma. *J. Am. Acad. Dermatol.* 61 (5): 905–906.

57 Sternberg, C.N., Davis, I.D., Mardiak, J. et al. (2010). Pazopanib in locally advanced or metastatic renal cell carcinoma: results of a randomized phase III trial. *J. Clin. Oncol.* 28 (6): 1061–1068.

58 Lacouture, M.E., Reilly, L.M., Gerami, P., and Guitart, J. (2008). Hand foot skin reaction in cancer patients treated with the multikinase inhibitors sorafenib and sunitinib. *Ann. Oncol.* 19 (11): 1955–1961.

59 Giacchero, D., Ramacciotti, C., Arnault, J.P. et al. (2012). A new spectrum of skin toxic effects associated with the multikinase inhibitor vandetanib. *Arch. Dermatol.* 148 (12): 1418–1420.

60 Hadlow, W.J. (1997). Dubbing animal diseases with color. *Vet. Pathol.* 34 (1): 74–78.

61 Morris, J.G., Yu, S.G., and Rogers, Q.R. (2002). Red hair in black cats is reversed by addition of tyrosine to the diet. *J. Nutr.* 132 (6): 1646s–1648s.

62 Rogers, Q.R. and Morris, J.G. (1979). Essentiality of amino acids for the growing kitten. *J. Nutr.* 109 (4): 718–723.

63 Watson, A., Servet, E., Hervera, M., and Biourge, V.C. (2015). Tyrosine supplementation and hair coat pigmentation in puppies with black coats – a pilot study. *J. Appl. Anim. Nutr.* 3: e10.

64 Slominski, A. (1989). L-tyrosine induces synthesis of melanogenesis related proteins. *Life Sci.* 45 (19): 1799–1803.

65 Anderson, P.J.B., Rogers, Q.R., and Morris, J.G. (2002). Cats require more dietary phenylalanine or tyrosine for melanin deposition in hair than for maximal growth. *J. Nutr.* 132 (7): 2037–2042.

66 Williams, J.M., Morris, J.G., and Rogers, Q.R. (1987). Phenylalanine requirement of kittens and the sparing effect of tyrosine. *J. Nutr.* 117 (6): 1102–1107.

67 Yu, S., Rogers, Q.R., and Morris, J.G. (2001). Effect of low levels of dietary tyrosine on the hair colour of cats. *J. Small Anim. Pract.* 42 (4): 176–180.

68 Maggs, D.J., Miller, P.E., Ofri, R., and Slatter, D.H. (2013). *Slatter's Fundamentals of Veterinary Ophthalmology*, 5e, x, 506 p. St. Louis, MO: Elsevier.

69 Carwardine, P.C. (1976). Metronidazole in the treatment of tear staining in dogs. *Vet. Rec.* 98 (3): 59.

70 Yi, N.Y., Park, S.A., Jeong, M.B. et al. (2006). Medial canthoplasty for epiphora in dogs: a retrospective study of 23 cases. *J. Am. Anim. Hosp. Assoc.* 42 (6): 435–439.

71 Roberts, S.R. (1962). Dog tear secretion and tear proteins. *J. Small Anim. Pract.* 3 (1): 1–5.

72 Natalija, M.M., Popovic, N., Lazarevic, M., and Ljiljana, M. (2010). The role of ambrosia Artemisiifolia allergen in canine atopic dermatitis. *Acta Vet. (Beogr)* 60 (2–3): 183–196.

73 Farnworth, M.J., Chen, R., Packer, R.M. et al. (2016). Flat feline faces: is Brachycephaly associated with respiratory abnormalities in the domestic cat (Felis catus)? *PLoS One* 11 (8): e0161777.

9

Changes in Pigmentation

9.1 Introduction to Coat and Skin Pigmentation

Melanin is a natural pigment produced within melanocytes following biochemical reactions involving the amino acid, tyrosine [1]. Melanin is a primary determinant of skin and coat color [2]. In mammals, the agouti gene determines the distribution of melanin within each individual [3, 4]. Which types of melanin are present and in which ratios further modify coat color [3, 4]. There are two primary types of melanin [1, 3–9]:

- Eumelanin
- Pheomelanin

Black is the default color for eumelanin. Unaltered eumelanin confers a black coat or skin. However, the presence of one or more genes may modify eumelanin such that the black shade is muted.

Black may be softened into liver (brown), blue (gray), or isabella (light brown) variations. In essence, these genes are dilutors: they reduce eumelanin from its full strength to create partial colors. Blue and isabella are considered dilutions [5, 6] (see Figures 9.1a–g).

In addition to conferring color to the skin and coat, eumelanin contributes color to the nose and irises. Brown-eyed dogs are so because of eumelanin. When eumelanin is diluted, iridal pigment lightens to an amber or gold. This color is akin to what we might consider hazel in humans [5, 6].

Unlike eumelanin, pheomelanin contributes to coat color only. The default color for pheomelanin is red. Like eumelanin, genes may modify pheomelanin to create softer shades of red. These include oranges, creams, golds, yellows, and tans [5, 6]. Pheomelanin can also be darkened to create the rich mahogany color that is appreciated in certain Golden Retrievers and Irish Setters (see Figures 9.2a–e).

Melanism refers to having pigment in the skin or coat. Its natural opposite is albinism, the lack of pigmentation. Patients that are albino are white-coated due to lack of

pigment. Albino patients may also possess red eyes. In these clinical cases, the irises appear red not because of red pigment, but because of the visibility of blood vessels showing through the uncolored iris.

The aforementioned examples pertain to the influence of melanin on coat color. Refer to Chapter 8, Section 8.2 for a discussion about how temperature can affect melanin in patients with point coloration, such as Siamese cats.

This chapter will focus on the influence of melanin on the skin and changes in pigmentation over time. Because pheomelanin affects only the coat, this chapter will exclusively concentrate on eumelanin.

Note that variations in skin color are normal in dogs and cats. There is not a "one-size-fits-all." It is common for our companion animal patients to display patches of skin of various shades, including pink, tan, brown, and black.

These darker splotches, so-called tar spots, age spots, or pigment spots, represent concentrations of eumelanin. Such patches are most noticeable in shorthaired dogs along the ventral abdomen and medial limbs, where fur coverage is least (see Figures 9.3a, b).

9.2 Hereditary Hyperpigmentation of the Skin

Hyperpigmentation results from increased deposition of melanin within the skin [10]. There are various reasons for hyperpigmentation to develop in a companion animal patient. Hereditary hyperpigmentation is particularly common in solid orange or orange-faced cats and is referred to as lentigo simplex [10, 11]. Lentigo simplex has also been reported in cream, red, and tricolor cats [12]. There is one isolated report in the medical literature that confirms lentigines in a silver-coated cat [13].

Cats with lentigo simplex develop flattened areas of pigment that range in size from 1–10 mm [11, 14]. These lesions often develop when patients are less than one year old. Lesions typically enlarge with age, increase in number, and/or coalesce [10, 11].

Common Clinical Presentations in Dogs and Cats, First Edition. Ryane E. Englar.
© 2019 John Wiley & Sons, Inc. Published 2019 by John Wiley & Sons, Inc.

(a)

(b)

(c)

(d)

(f)

(e)

(g)

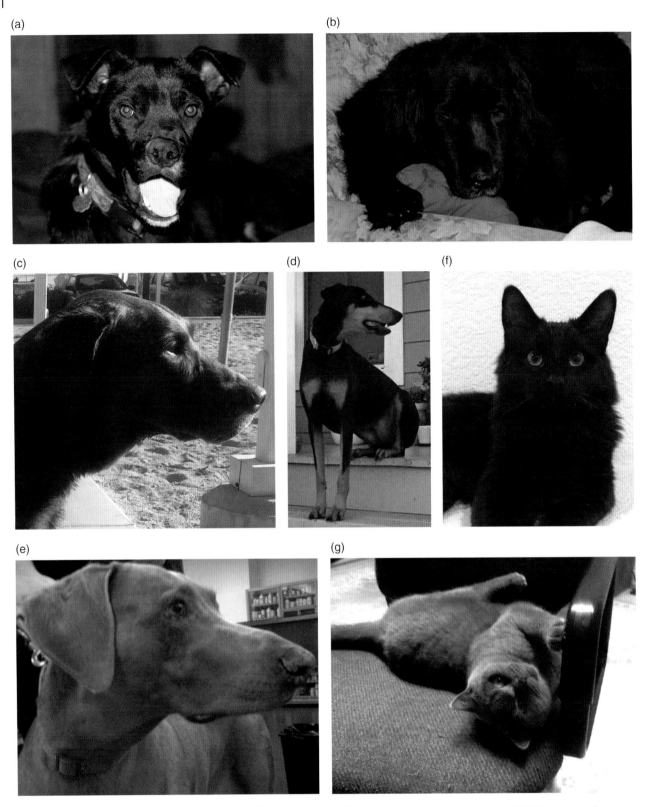

Figure 9.1 (a) An example of an all-black, shorthaired mixed breed dog. *Source:* Courtesy of Laura Polerecky, LVT. (b) Example of a longhaired, black Newfoundland dog. *Source:* Courtesy of Kathryn Knowles. (c) An example of a solid brown dog. *Source:* Courtesy of Jess Darmofal, DVM. (d) An example of a Doberman dog. The black regions of the coat are due to eumelanin. *Source:* Courtesy of Michael and Naomi Englar. (e) An example of a solid blue coat in a Weimaraner dog. *Source:* Courtesy of Dr. Elizabeth Robbins. (f) An example of a solid black cat. *Source:* Courtesy of Amanda Coleman, DVM. (g) An example of a solid blue coat in a British Shorthair cat. *Source:* Courtesy of Richard and Jill Englar, Bliss and Gwen.

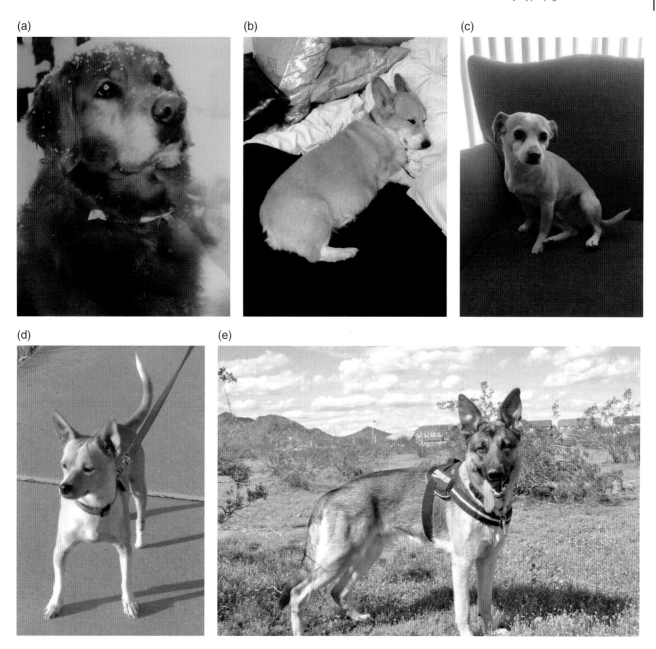

Figure 9.2 (a) Example of a mahogany coat in a Golden retriever dog. *Source:* Courtesy of the Adler Family. (b) Example of an orange-gold coat in a dog. *Source:* Courtesy of Rayeann Solano, DVM. (c) Example of a tan coat color in a mixed breed dog. *Source:* Courtesy of Kimberly Vu. (d) An example of a light tan-cream colored dog. *Source:* Courtesy of Ann Marie Wronkowski. (e) Example of a sable coat of a German shepherd dog. A mix of eumelanin and pheomelanin causes the sable. *Source:* Courtesy of Jule Schweighoefer.

These black-brown macules or patches can appear anywhere on the skin; however, they are particularly concentrated at the nose, lips, eyelids, oral mucosa, hard palate, and pinnae [11, 14, 15] (see Figures 9.4a–e).

Lentigo simplex rarely occurs in dogs [16, 17]. The presentation is similar to cats. Black macules develop as early as five months old [13]. These lesions may increase in number or size as the patient ages [17]. Occasionally, they fade in terms of color, without changing size or shape [17]. One lesion is called a lentigo; multiple lesions are called lentigines [14].

All lesions remain flat and do not induce an inflammatory response [11]. Their presence is purely cosmetic. However, they are grossly difficult to distinguish from melanoma [11, 14]. Lesions that become raised or develop traits that are otherwise uncharacteristic of lentigines should be removed via excisional biopsy and submitted for histopathology.

(a)   (b)

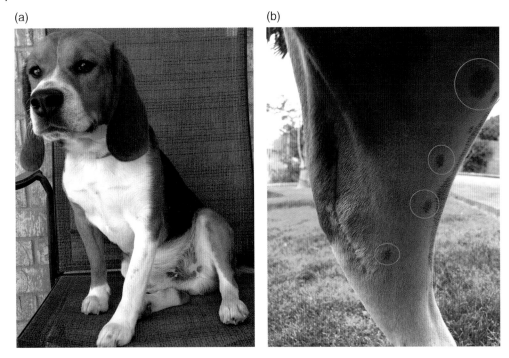

Figure 9.3 (a) Normal variation of skin pigmentation in a canine patient, most noticeable at the groin. Note the mottled appearance. *Source:* Courtesy of Jordanne M. Diaz. (b) Normal variation of skin pigmentation in a canine patient, most noticeable at the medial hind limb. Note the mottled appearance. The circled regions demonstrate areas of increased eumelanin concentration. *Source:* Courtesy of Kiefer Hazard, DVM.

9.3 Non-Inherited, Acquired Hyperpigmentation of the Skin

In addition to hereditary hyperpigmentation, melanin deposition can increase in response to inflammation and/or underlying disease. In other words, hyperpigmentation can be acquired. The following outlines the most common causes of acquired hyperpigmentation in companion animal patients:

- Mite infestation
- Endocrinopathy
- *Malassezia* dermatitis
- Bacterial dermatitis
- Contact sensitivity
- Neoplasia

This list is not intended to be exhaustive. It is a starting point for the preclinical veterinary student who is building a list of plausible differential diagnoses for the presenting complaint, hyperpigmentation.

9.3.1 Demodicosis and Skin Hyperpigmentation

Mite infestations result in appreciable inflammation of the skin. In particular, infestation with *Demodex*

spp. may be associated with the development of skin hyperpigmentation.

Review Chapter 3, Section 3.8.1, Chapter 5, Section 5.8, and Chapter 6, Section 6.6 on demodicosis. Recall that demodicosis involves canine infestation with *Demodex canis* and feline infestation with *Demodex cati* or *Demodex gatoi* [18–23]. Such infestations result in localized or generalized inflammatory skin disease.

Affected patients classically present with erythema, hypotrichosis, or alopecic patches with or without a papulopustular rash, folliculitis, or furunculosis, scaling and follicular casts, pododermatitis, and/or paronychia [24–26].

In a small percentage of cases, hyperpigmentation may also result from demodicosis in dogs and cats [27] (see Figures 9.5a–c).

This change in skin pigmentation is an incidental finding [27, 28]. In other words, it is supportive of, but not pathognomonic for demodicosis. Skin scrapings are required for a definitive diagnosis. Recall that deep skin scrapings are required to unearth the cigar-shaped *D. canis* from the hair follicle, whereas *D. gatoi* is a surface dweller. Superficial scrapings for *D. gatoi* will suffice.

Note that hyperpigmentation secondary to demodicosis is highly variable among individuals within the same species. It also appears to be a species-dependent

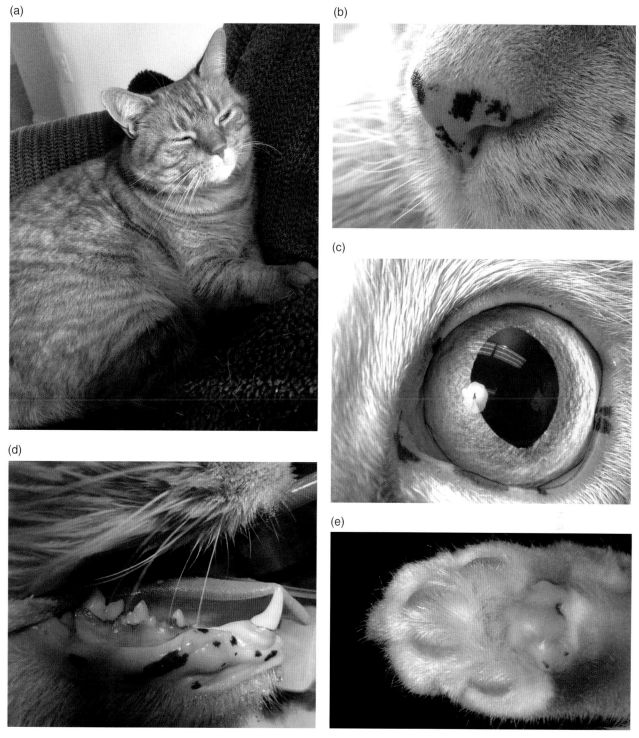

Figure 9.4 (a) An example of an orange or so-called ginger cat. Lentigo simplex is frequently inherited in cats with this coat color. *Source:* Courtesy of Richard and Jill Englar, and Boo Radley. (b) Examples of lesions from lentigo simplex on the nose of a feline patient. (c) Examples of lesions from lentigo simplex on the eyelids of a feline patient. *Source:* Courtesy of Media Resources at Midwestern University. (d) Examples of lesions from lentigo simplex on the oral mucosa of a feline patient. *Source:* Courtesy of Genevieve LaFerriere, DVM. (e) Examples of lesions from lentigo simplex on the metatarsal pad.

(a)

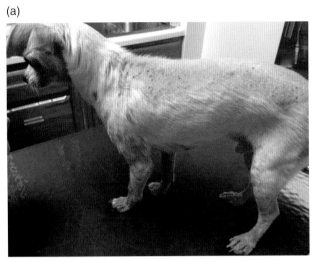

(b)   (c)

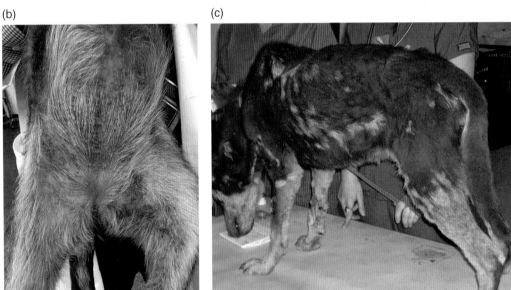

Figure 9.5 (a) Generalized demodicosis in a canine patient. Note that the patient has very subtle hyperpigmentation along the dorsolateral trunk. *Source:* Courtesy of Pamela Mueller, DVM. (b) Generalized demodicosis in a canine patient. Note that there are regions of subtle hyperpigmentation along the ventral abdomen, along with a severe, concurrent papulopustular rash. (c) Generalized demodicosis in a canine patient. Note the regions of hyperpigmentation, particularly on the distal limbs. The affected skin appears grayer than is normal for this patient. *Source:* Courtesy of Laura Polerecky, LVT.

response [27]. For example, hamsters and humans may also develop hyperpigmentation secondary to demodicosis, whereas pigs, cattle, and horses do not [27, 29–33].

In humans, hyperpigmentation is attributed to the fact that healing skin exhibits increased melanocyte activity [34].

It is unclear what triggers hyperpigmentation in dogs and cats with mite infestations. It has been speculated that the underlying inflammation causes increased vascularity within the dermis [27]. This may in turn stimulate melanocytes to increase their activity [27]. The expected result would be increased production and deposition of melanin.

9.3.2 Endocrinopathy and Skin Hyperpigmentation

Hormonal imbalances may also lead to acquired or secondary skin hyperpigmentation [27].

Consider, for example, the fact that the pituitary gland produces melanocyte-stimulating hormone, MSH [34]. The pituitary gland receives feedback from the adrenal cortex with regard to production and secretion of MSH [34]. Pathology at the level of the adrenal cortex may contribute to abnormal feedback to the pituitary gland concerning the body's need for MSH [27]. If MSH levels increase, then hyperpigmentation will result [27]. This pathway has been explored in human medicine [34]. It has been theorized that companion animal patients may react via the same mechanisms.

Other endocrinopathies do not directly impact the adrenal axis, yet still may result in hyperpigmentation of the skin. Hypothyroidism is perhaps the best example because it occurs commonly in dogs, and hypothyroid dogs often develop hyperpigmentation [35, 36]. In a 1999 study by Dixon et al., as many as one in five dogs with hypothyroidism developed hyperpigmentation [37].

Recall from Chapter 5, Section 5.7 that hypothyroidism is the most common cause of endocrine, non-inflammatory hair loss [35, 38]. Hypothyroid patients classically present with bilaterally symmetrical truncal alopecia, "ring around the collar," and/or "rat tail" [35, 39] (see Figures 5.14a, b).

When hyperpigmentation occurs, it is most evident at alopecic sites as an incidental finding. Because hyperpigmentation is supportive of, but not pathognomonic for hypothyroidism, follow-up bloodwork is indicated to achieve a definitive diagnosis. Typically, this consists of a complete blood count (CBC), serum biochemistry, and a full thyroid panel including thyroxine (T4), free T4 (fT4), and thyroid-stimulating hormone (TSH). Dogs with classic textbook hypothyroidism demonstrate low values for both T4 and fT4 in spite of an elevated TSH.

Treatment for canine hypothyroidism typically involves lifelong oral supplementation of synthetic T4.

9.3.3 *Malassezia* Overgrowth and Skin Hyperpigmentation

Recall from Chapter 3, Section 3.8.2 that *Malassezia pachydermatis* is a commensal fungal organism that is found on the surface of the skin in normal dogs and cats [40, 41]. *Malassezia* has also been isolated from the ear canals and anal sacs of healthy dogs, and within the nail folds of healthy cats [41, 42].

Malassezia dermatitis results from yeast overgrowth. This often manifests as progressive accumulation of dark brown, greasy exudate at the nail base, nail staining, or the development of brittle, excessively flaky nails (see Figures 9.6a, b).

Patients with *Malassezia* dermatitis are often pruritic and exacerbate the inflammatory component of disease through self-trauma. Constant licking at and scratching of the skin leads to pronounced thickening of the skin, lichenification.

Chronically affected skin also tends to darken in pigment. This hyperpigmentation resolves with medical treatment.

Depending upon the distribution and the severity of the lesions, medical management may involve topical and/or oral administration of antifungal drugs, with or without antihistamines. Occasionally, oral or injectable steroids are administered to reduce the itch if pruritus is resulting in self-injury.

Note that resolution is a slow process, and full recovery may take months (see Figures 9.7a, b).

9.3.4 Pyoderma and Skin Hyperpigmentation

Recall from Chapter 5, Section 5.8 that pyoderma refers to bacterial infection of the skin. This infection may be superficial or deep, focal or generalized. Most often, pyoderma is secondary to an underlying condition or disease, such as allergic skin disease. This catchall phrase

(a)

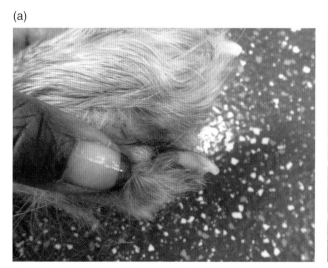

(b)

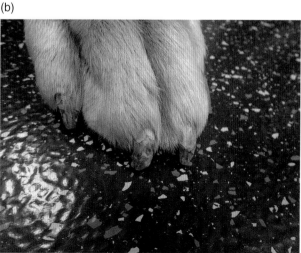

Figure 9.6 (a) Evidence of nail staining secondary to *Malassezia* dermatitis. *Source:* Courtesy of Patricia Bennett, DVM. (b) Onychomycosis in a canine patient. *Source:* Courtesy of Patricia Bennett, DVM.

(a)

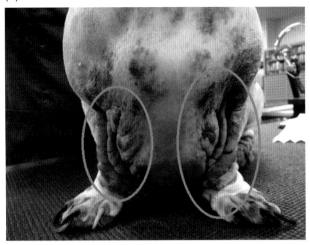

(b)

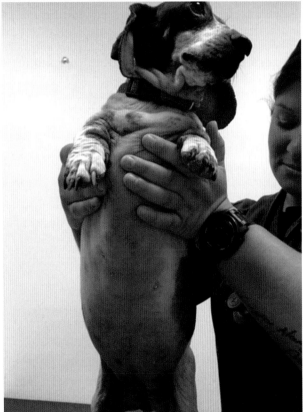

Figure 9.7 (a) Severe *Malassezia* dermatitis in a canine patient. Note the extensive lichenification and hyperpigmentation of the ventral abdomen. *Source:* Courtesy of Dr. Elizabeth Robbins. (b) Same patient as depicted in Figure 9.7a, following two months of medical treatment. Note the improvement in the skin: the lichenification has resolved, and the skin has resumed its normal shade of pink. *Source:* Courtesy of Dr. Elizabeth Robbins.

includes flea allergy dermatitis, atopic dermatitis, and food allergies [43, 44].

Hallmark signs of pyoderma include primary and secondary skin lesions, including the following (see Figures 9.8a–f):

- Papules
- Pustules
- Papulopustular rash
- Collarettes
- Crusts
- Scale

When pyoderma is chronic, either because it has yet to be treated or it is refractory to treatment, the skin may darken in pigment [45, 46] (see Figure 9.9).

As is true of the other conditions outlined in Section 9.2, hyperpigmentation is supportive of, but not pathognomonic for pyoderma.

Cytology is confirmatory for bacterial dermatitis. Impression smears of sterilely ruptured pustules should yield intracellular bacteria. Cocci are supportive of a presumptive diagnosis of Staphylococcal pyoderma.

9.3.5 Contact Sensitivity and Skin Hyperpigmentation

Allergic contact hypersensitivity more commonly occurs in humans than in dogs or cats in large part because the coat of most companion animal patients functions as a protective barrier [47]. When allergic contact reactions occur, they tend to limit themselves to those regions of the body that are naturally less haired, such as the ventral abdomen, medial thighs, and the interdigital skin or between footpads [47].

Hairless breeds present additional concerns because their lack of fur coverage puts them at increased risk for skin exposure to and contact with environmental irritants. A 2007 study by Kimura demonstrated sensitivities specific to a colony of Mexican Hairless Dogs housed in stainless steel cages [47]. Although these dogs required 8–12 months of sensitization to develop spontaneously occurring contact dermatitis, they did ultimately present with macroscopic lesions that included macules and papules [47].

As exposure to the inciting agent persisted, inflammatory dermatitis developed and progressed [47]. Chronic lesions included lichenification and hyperpigmentation [47]. In addition, the skin became dry and scaly. Some patients also developed skin fissures [47].

Patients clinically improved when they were relocated from stainless steel housing to concrete flooring with concrete and wooden resting areas [47].

Follow-up patch testing of affected patients with metal salts confirmed underlying sensitivity to the constituents of stainless steel cages, including chromium [47]. Chromium has been reported in the human medical literature as a cause of occupational dermatitis [48–58]. Human males appear to be predisposed [47]. Likewise, male hairless dogs appear more likely to develop allergic contact hypersensitivity [47].

The implications of these findings are that the housing of hairless breeds must be considered in light of their

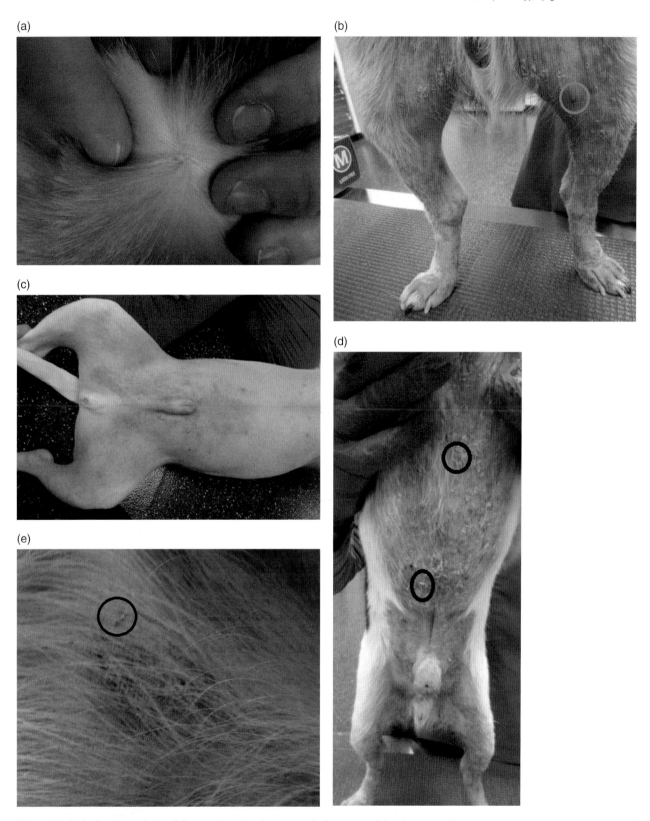

Figure 9.8 (a) Isolated papule in a feline patient. Papules are small elevations of the skin, typically measuring <1.0 cm. *Source:* Courtesy of Patricia Bennett, DVM. (b) Canine patient with pyoderma. Note the isolated pustule that has been encircled in blue. A pustule is a pus-filled papule. *Source:* Courtesy of Dr. Elizabeth Robbins. (c) Canine patient with papulopustular rash secondary to pyoderma. *Source:* Courtesy of Dr. Elizabeth Robbins. (d) Epidermal collarettes in a canine patient with pyoderma. Collarettes refer to the damaged rings of skin that are left behind after pustules rupture. *Source:* Courtesy of Dr. Elizabeth Robbins. (e) Isolated crust in a canine patient with pyoderma. A crust is dried exudate and keratin. *Source:* Courtesy of Patricia Bennett, DVM. (f) Scale in a canine patient with pyoderma. Scale refers to loose flakes of skin, otherwise known as dandruff. *Source:* Courtesy of Patricia Bennett, DVM.

(f)

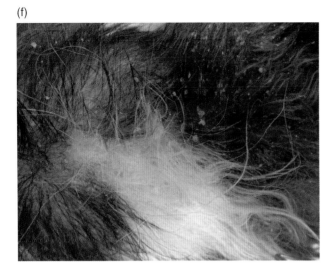

Figure 9.8 (Continued)

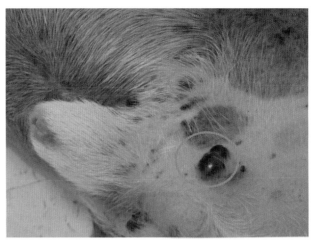

Figure 9.10 Melanocytic nodules in a canine patient. *Source:* Courtesy of Patricia Bennett.

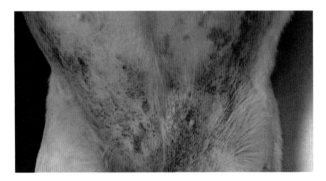

Figure 9.9 Hyperpigmentation in a canine patient with pyoderma. *Source:* Courtesy of Beki Cohen Regan, DVM, DACVIM (Oncology).

potential to cause underlying dermatopathy. If a hairless breed presents with hyperpigmentation, among other skin lesions, then careful history taking should elicit information about the patient's residence, including where, if at all, it is kenneled. A patient that is housed within stainless steel for long periods may be prone to the development of contact hypersensitivity. In that situation, removal of the source of the allergen should constitute effective treatment.

9.3.6 Neoplastic Disease and Skin Hyperpigmentation

Melanocytic tumors are relatively rare in companion animal patients [59]. They account for less than 4% of all skin tumors in dogs and less than 1% of all skin tumors in cats [60] (see Figure 9.10).

In dogs, the eyelids and forelimbs are preferred locations for cutaneous melanomas, that is, melanocytic tumors without known or proven metastatic potential [60]. Certain breeds, including the Miniature and Standard Schnauzer, Doberman Pinscher, Irish Setter, and Golden Retriever are predisposed [60].

Abdominal, perineal, and scrotal skin are preferred sites for cutaneous malignant melanomas in dogs [60]. Both the Miniature and Standard schnauzer are predisposed to malignancy, along with the Scottish terrier [60].

Cats tend to develop malignant melanoma at the ears and eyelids [60]. This is of concern because both sites are prime locations for lentigines.

The only way to differentiate these lesions from malignancies is histologic examination [60]. Excision of presumptive lesions is advisable if there is a significant change in the nature of one or more lentigines [10, 60].

The presence of lentigines, however, in and of itself does not make the patient more likely to develop melanoma [12].

9.3.7 Other Causes of Skin Hyperpigmentation

Hyperpigmentation is a clinical sign rather than a diagnosis. It is also a common presentation for dermatopathies. When it appears, it is a sign to investigate further.

The common causes of acquired hyperpigmentation have been outlined here. There are many other causes that have not been noted. If and when hyperpigmentation is present in a patient that does not fit the aforementioned scenarios, it would be wise for the reader to seek additional resources and the expert assistance of a veterinary dermatologist.

9.4 Cosmetic Depigmentation of the Nasal Planum

Not all dermatopathies result in hyperpigmentation of the skin. Some result in loss of pigmentation. This depigmentation may be generalized or focal, cosmetic or pathologic.

There are two primary focal cosmetic changes that may occur to the nasal planum of the canine patient:

- Dudley nose
- Snow nose

Dudley nose is more commonly seen in Doberman Pinschers, Afghan Hounds, Irish Setters, Pointers, Poodles, Samoyeds, Labrador Retrievers, and white German Shepherd Dogs [61, 62].

The nasal planum of a patient with Dudley nose is darkly pigmented at birth. Then, for unknown reasons, the color fades over time to a flesh-colored pale brown or pink [61–63] (see Figures 9.11a, b).

Dudley nose is primarily an aesthetic concern for breeders, who may consider it a fault. However, these patients may be at increased risk of nasal solar dermatitis. This results from prolonged exposure to ultraviolet (UV) light. The application of topical sunscreen may help to protect these depigmented areas from becoming overexposed to sunlight.

Snow nose carries the same appearance as Dudley nose. However, it represents seasonal rather than age-related depigmentation of the nasal planum. During winter months, the nasal planum undergoes depigmentation. The nasal planum subsequently regains pigment over the spring and summer months [61–63] (see Figures 9.12a–c).

The mechanism by which this occurs is also unknown. Labrador Retrievers, Golden Retrievers, Bernese Mountain Dogs, and Huskies appear to be predisposed [61, 62].

As is advised for Dudley nose, topical sunscreen may help to protect those with snow nose from sunburn due to overexposure of the depigmented regions to UV light.

9.5 Pathologic Depigmentation of the Nasal Planum

Not all depigmentation is a reflection of age or seasonal change. Fungal and immune-mediated pathology can also result in nasal depigmentation.

Deep mycoses, such as blastomycosis and aspergillosis, have been implicated in cases that present with depigmentation of the nasal planum [63–69].

9.5.1 Blastomycosis and the Nasal Planum

Blastomycosis is a systemic fungal infection that infects patients primarily through inhalation of *Blastomyces dermatitidis* spores [65]. The inhaled spores subsequently establish colonies within the respiratory tract [65]. Because the organism spreads through lymphatics as well as the bloodstream, distant sites may be colonized.

B. dermatitidis is endemic to North American soil [65, 66]. Those who reside near the Mississippi, Missouri, and Ohio River valleys are most at risk for contracting disease [65]. Although cats may develop blastomycosis, dogs and humans are more likely to succumb than other species [65, 70, 71].

Young adult, large-breed dogs, such as Golden Retrievers and Doberman Pinschers, are overrepresented [65, 66, 72, 73]. Some studies demonstrate an apparent predisposition for disease in male dogs [65, 73, 74]. This mirrors what is seen in human medicine [75].

Clinical signs of blastomycosis in dogs vary widely depending upon how well the organism disseminates throughout the patient's body [65]. Patients with disseminated disease often present with a multitude of clinical signs that affect several organ systems [65].

Initially, vague signs may predominate [65]. Affected dogs may present for anorexia and generalized malaise. Weight loss may persist over an extended period of weeks to months [65].

Pulmonary infection results in tachypnea, dyspnea, and/or cyanosis in 65–85% of canine patients [65]. Thirty to fifty percent of dogs present with concurrent lymphadenopathy [65]. The same percentage of dogs develop cutaneous signs, including nodules, papules, plaques, and depigmentation lesions of the nasal planum [65] (see Figure 9.13).

Twenty to fifty percent of dogs develop glaucoma secondary to ocular involvement. Others may develop anterior uveitis, chorioretinitis, and/or retinal detachment.

Figure 9.11 (a) Dudley nose in a yellow Labrador Retriever dog. The nose of this patient used to be jet black. The shade has since faded to a pale brown. (b) Dudley nose in a yellow Labrador Retriever dog. The nose of this patient used to be jet black. The shade has since faded to a light pink.

(a)

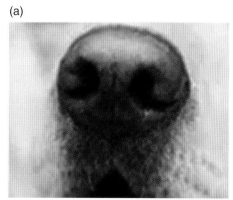

(b)

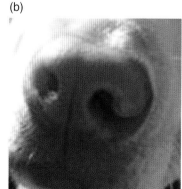

(a)

(b)

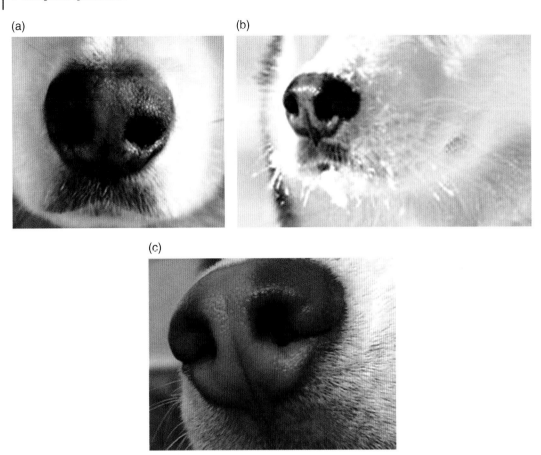

(c)

Figure 9.12 (a) Snow nose in a Husky dog. Note the subtlety of this lesion, which is just beginning to appear in the winter months. (b) Progressive snow nose in a Husky dog. Note how this lesion has expanded as compared to what is pictured in Figure 9.12a. (c) Extreme representation of snow nose in a mixed breed dog. Note how the entire nasal planum has transformed into a shade of pale-brown pink.

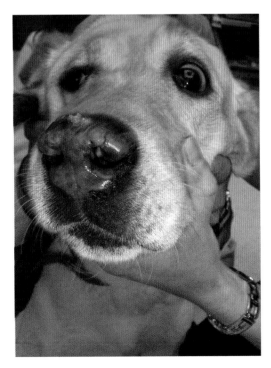

Figure 9.13 Nasal depigmentation in a canine patient that was ultimately diagnosed with blastomycosis. *Source:* Courtesy of Daniel Foy, MS, DVM, DACVIM, DACVECC.

Ten to fifteen percent of dogs develop bone involvement, particularly in those regions distal to the elbow and stifle [65].

Infrequently, blastomycosis causes claw and claw bed disease, including paronychia [40, 41, 65].

Cats with blastomycosis are less likely to present as described above [65]. Instead, their clinical signs more typically reflect central nervous system or dermal involvement, as through the development of abscesses [65, 71, 76, 77].

The diagnostic work-up for blastomycosis is beyond the scope of this text; however, identification of organisms from aspirates or biopsies yields a definitive diagnosis [65]. Organisms typically appear on cytology as broad-based, budding yeast (see Figures 9.14a–d).

Members of the veterinary team who handle specimens must exhibit great caution, because blastomycosis has the potential to be zoonotic [65, 78, 79].

Treatment for blastomycosis is beyond the scope of this text, but requires long-term systemic administration of antifungal agents such as ketoconazole, itraconazole, fluconazole, and/or amphotericin B [63]. Concurrent use of prescription non-steroidal anti-inflammatory drugs (NSAIDS) does not appear to improve survival for dogs with pulmonary blastomycosis [80].

(a)

(b)

(c)

(d)

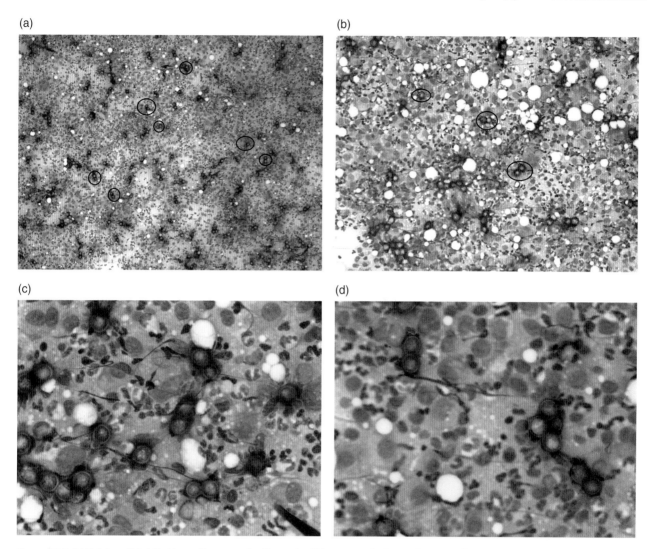

Figure 9.14 (a) Cytology (10×) that is confirmatory of a diagnosis of blastomycosis. *Source:* Courtesy of Daniel Foy, MS, DVM, DACVIM, DACVECC. (b) Cytology (20×) that is confirmatory of a diagnosis of blastomycosis. *Source:* Courtesy of Daniel Foy, MS, DVM, DACVIM, DACVECC. (c) Cytology (40×) that is confirmatory of a diagnosis of blastomycosis. *Source:* Courtesy of Daniel Foy, MS, DVM, DACVIM, DACVECC. (d) Cytology (50×) that is confirmatory of a diagnosis of blastomycosis. *Source:* Courtesy of Daniel Foy, MS, DVM, DACVIM, DACVECC.

9.5.2 Aspergillosis and the Nasal Planum

Aspergillosis is a fungal infection that is caused by *Aspergillus fumigatus* [67]. The infection may be systemic or focal. Sinonasal aspergillosis is relatively common in dogs.

As many as one in three dogs that present for chronic sinorhinitis have sinonasal aspergillosis [68, 81]. Long-snouted dogs, such as German Shepherd Dogs and Rottweilers, are overrepresented [67]. Most dogs are also less than seven years of age at the time of diagnosis [81].

A. fumigatus is ubiquitous in the environment [82]. Its spores are present in soil, decaying organic material, water, and dust [82]. Inhalation is most typically the route by which infection is established [83–88].

Healthy patients evade infection because of anatomic and physiologic protective mechanisms. These include nasal sinuses and mucus, both of which trap debris. In addition, the ciliary lining of respiratory passages functions to sweeps debris out of the airways.

A. fumigatus is opportunistic as a pathogen because it induces primary infection in patients that are immuno-compromised [82]. These patients develop sneezing and nasal discharge that is mucoid to mucopurulent. Occasionally, epistaxis results [82, 89, 90].

Sinonasal *A. fumigatus* may also develop secondary to nasal trauma, including the presence of a nasal foreign body or other space-occupying lesion, such as neoplasia [67].

The nares of a patient with sinonasal aspergillosis may become ulcerated. More commonly, there is partial to complete depigmentation of the nasal planum and/or the epithelium of the alar fold [82, 89, 90] (see Figures 9.15a–c).

As sinonasal disease progresses, nasal turbinates are destroyed [82, 91]. The cribriform plate, nasal bones, and orbit may also become damaged [82, 92, 93].

(a)

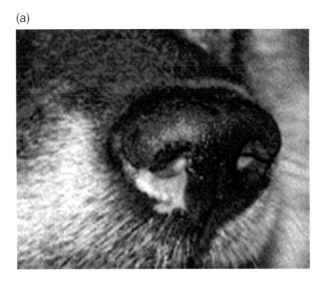

(b)   (c)

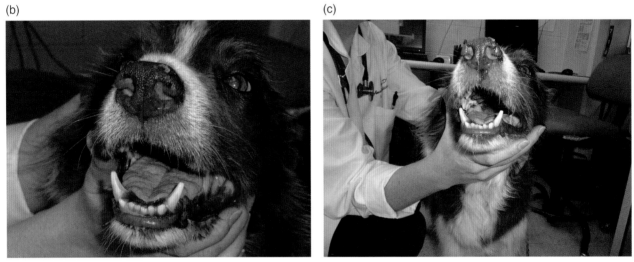

Figure 9.15 (a) Depigmentation of the right nare in a canine patient that was subsequently diagnosed with sinonasal aspergillosis. *Source:* Courtesy of Daniel Foy, MS, DVM, DACVIM, DACVECC. (b) Depigmentation of the entire nasal planum in a canine patient that was subsequently diagnosed with sinonasal aspergillosis. *Source:* Courtesy of Daniel Foy, MS, DVM, DACVIM, DACVECC. (c) Same patient as depicted in Figure 9.15b. Note the presence of blood-tinged, mucoid nasal discharge. *Source:* Courtesy of Daniel Foy, MS, DVM, DACVIM, DACVECC.

The diagnostic work-up for sinonasal aspergillosis is beyond the scope of this text. However, the pathway to diagnosis typically includes advanced imaging, such as computed tomography, to identify the extent of turbinate destruction, and/or rhinoscopy. Rhinoscopy allows for direct visualization of the nasal passageways, which may reveal the presence of one or more foreign bodies, such as grass awns, or fungal plaques [67].

Fungal plaques as seen via rhinoscopy appear to line the mucosa as various shades of white, yellow, or light green.

Plaques may also coalesce into a neoplastic growth, so-called fungal granulomas. These may be dislodged through flushing of the nasal cavity with saline, and can be quite extensive (see Figure 9.16).

Histopathologic analysis of these samples and biopsies of adjacent tissue are essential. The diagnosis is confirmed via microscopic visualization of hyphae invading nasal tissue [67] (see Figures 9.17a, b).

Treatment for sinonasal aspergillosis is beyond the scope of this text, but may involve sinus trephination with lavage and administration of antifungal agents [67]. If the cribriform plate is intact, local therapy can be used to manage disease more effectively than systemic administration of antifungal agents [67]. Historically, enilconazole emulsions were delivered to the nasal chambers and frontal sinuses via surgically implanted tubes [94]. Clotrimazole infusions under general anesthesia are equally efficacious [95].

Note that cats can also succumb to sinonasal aspergillosis. However, cats are by far more likely to develop sino-orbital aspergillosis [69, 96–109]. Accordingly, cats most often present with exophthalmos rather than with pigmentary changes of the nasal planum [69, 96–109].

9.5.3 Immune-Mediated Disease and the Nasal Planum

In addition to deep mycoses, immune-mediated pathology such as discoid lupus erythematosus (DLE) can also result in nasal depigmentation (see Figures 9.18a, b).

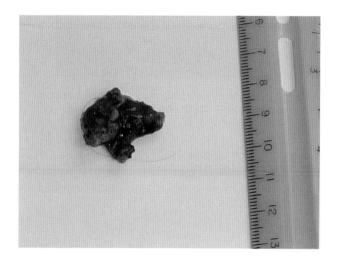

Figure 9.16 Fungal granuloma in a canine patient with sinonasal aspergillosis. *Source:* Courtesy of Daniel Foy, MS, DVM, DACVIM, DACVECC.

In addition to depigmentation of the nasal planum, DLE is often characterized by erythema, erosions, crusting, and scaling.

Note that DLE lesions are not limited to the nasal planum. They may also extend to the muzzle, peri-oral and peri-ocular skin, the pinnae, oral cavity, and the nictitans [63].

Grossly, DLE is impossible to distinguish from cutaneous lymphoma, which also causes depigmentation of the nasal planum, with and without ulcerative lesions [63].

Diagnosis of DLE is via histopathology [63].

Patients with a diagnosis of DLE are medically managed using systemic immunosuppressive agents [63]. A recent case report by Rossi et al. demonstrated remission with oral tetracycline and oral niacinamide [110].

9.6 Idiopathic Depigmentation of the Skin

Recall that vitiligo was introduced in Chapter 8, Section 8.3.5 as a familial disease in Siamese cats and in certain breeds of dog. The Rottweiler and Doberman Pinscher are overrepresented [63, 111].

Affected patients typically undergo symmetrical depigmentation of the coat. Lesions may affect the whole body, or they may be localized to the face or around the eyes [112–117].

In addition to depigmentation of the coat, patients with vitiligo also experience reduced to absent skin pigment. This progressive depigmentation may or may not include the nasal planum.

(a)

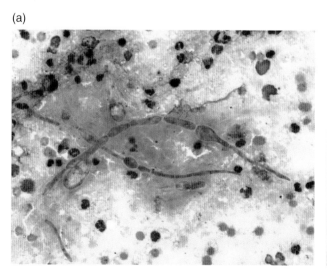

(b)

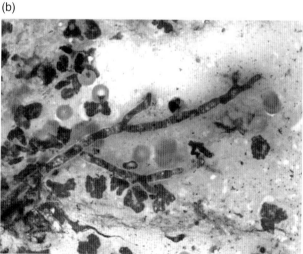

Figure 9.17 (a) Cytology (50x) that is confirmatory of a diagnosis of aspergillosis. Note the characteristic fungal hyphae. *Source:* Courtesy of Daniel Foy, MS, DVM, DACVIM, DACVECC. (b) Cytology (100×) that is confirmatory of a diagnosis of aspergillosis. Note the characteristic fungal hyphae. *Source:* Courtesy of Daniel Foy, MS, DVM, DACVIM, DACVECC.

(a)　　　　　　　　　　　(b)

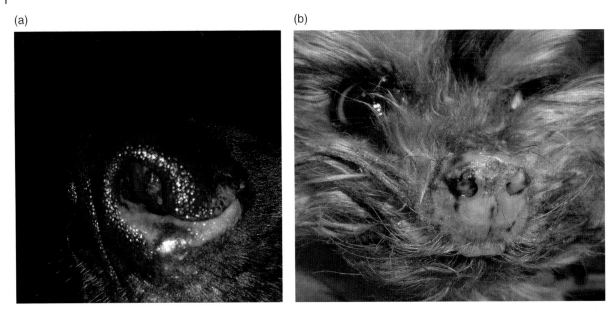

Figure 9.18 (a) Depigmentation of the left nare in a canine patient that was subsequently diagnosed with discoid lupus erythematosus (DLE). (b) Depigmentation and crusting of the nasal planum in a canine patient for which discoid lupus erythematosus (DLE) was a top differential diagnosis. *Source:* Courtesy of Daniel Foy, MS, DVM, DACVIM, DACVECC.

Histopathology is required for definitive diagnosis of vitiligo. Grossly, lesions are difficult to distinguish from other pathology, including DLE [112].

Treatment for vitiligo is not warranted. However, as was the case for Dudley nose and snow nose, sunscreen on hairless regions such as the nasal planum may reduce the risk of sunburn.

References

1 Lin, J.Y. and Fisher, D.E. (2007). Melanocyte biology and skin pigmentation. *Nature* 445 (7130): 843–850.

2 Jimbow, K., Quevedo, W.C. Jr., Fitzpatrick, T.B., and Szabo, G. (1976). Some aspects of melanin biology: 1950–1975. *J. Invest. Dermatol.* 67 (1): 72–89.

3 Meneely, P.M. and Meneely, P.M. (2014). *Genetic Analysis: Genes, Genomes, and Networks in Eukaryotes*, 6e, xxvi, 552 p. Oxford: Oxford University Press.

4 Griffiths, A.J.F., Miller, J.H., Suzuki, D.T. et al. (2000). Gene interaction in coat color of mammals. In: *An Introduction to Genetic Analysis*, 7e (ed. A.J.F. Griffiths, J.H. Miller and D.T. Suzuki). New York: W.H. Freeman.

5 Buzhardt, L. (2018). Genetics Basics - Coat Color Genetics in Dogs. https://vcahospitals.com/know-your-pet/genetics-basics-coat-color-genetics-in-dogs (accessed 22 April 2019).

6 Chapell, J. (2017). Two Different Kinds of Pigment. www.doggenetics.co.uk/pigment.html.

7 Bowling, S.A. (2016). Canine Color Genetics. http://bowlingsite.mcf.com/Genetics/ColorGen.html.

8 Schmutz, S.M. (2016). Genetics of Coat Color and Type in Dogs. http://homepage.usask.ca/~schmutz/dogcolors.html.

9 Newton, J.M., Wilkie, A.L., He, L. et al. (2000). Melanocortin 1 receptor variation in the domestic dog. *Mamm. Genome* 11 (1): 24–30.

10 Patel, A. and Forsythe, P.J. (2008). *Saunders Solutions in Veterinary Practice: Small Animal Dermatology*, 1e. China: Saunders, Ltd.

11 Little, S. (2012). *The Cat: Clinical Medicine and Management*, 1e. St. Louis, Missouri: Saunders Elsevier.

12 Scott, D.W. (1987). Lentigo simplex in orange cats. *Companion Anim. Pract.* 1 (2): 23–25.

13 Nash, S. and Paulsen, D. (1990). Generalized lentigines in a silver cat. *J. Am. Vet. Med. Assoc.* 196 (9): 1500–1501.

14 Hnilica, K. and Patterson, A.P. (2017). *Small Animal Dermatology: A Color Atlas and Therapeutic Guide*. St. Louis, Missouri: Elsevier, Inc.

15 Friberg, C. (2006). Feline facial dermatoses. *Vet. Clin. North Am. Small Anim. Pract.* 36 (1): 115–140, vi–vii.

16 Vanrensburg, I.B.J. and Briggs, O.M. (1986). Pathology of canine lentiginosis profusa. *J. S. Afr. Vet. Assoc.* 57 (3): 159–161.

17 Muller, G.H., Kirk, R.W., and Scott, D.W. (1983). Pigmentary abnormalities. In: *Small Animal Dermatology*, 594. Philadelphia: W.B. Saunders, Co.

18 Taffin, E.R., Casaert, S., Claerebout, E. et al. (2016). Morphological variability of Demodex cati in a feline immunodeficiency virus-positive cat. *J. Am. Vet. Med. Assoc.* 249 (11): 1308–1312.

19 Neel, J.A., Tarigo, J., Tater, K.C., and Grindem, C.B. (2007). Deep and superficial skin scrapings from a feline immunodeficiency virus-positive cat. *Vet. Clin. Pathol.* 36 (1): 101–104.

20 Frank, L.A., Kania, S.A., Chung, K., and Brahmbhatt, R. (2013). A molecular technique for the detection and differentiation of Demodex mites on cats. *Vet. Dermatol.* 24 (3): 367–369, e82–3.

21 Cordero, A.M., Sheinberg-Waisburd, G., Romero Nunez, C., and Heredia, R. (2017). Early onset canine generalized demodicosis. *Vet. Dermatol.* 29 (2): 173.

22 Bowden, D.G., Outerbridge, C.A., Kissel, M.B. et al. (2017). Canine demodicosis: a retrospective study of a veterinary hospital population in California, USA (2000–2016). *Vet. Dermatol.* 29 (1): 19-e10.

23 Mueller, R.S. (2012). An update on the therapy of canine demodicosis. *Compend. Contin. Educ. Vet.* 34 (4): E1–E4.

24 Mueller, R.S., Bensignor, E., Ferrer, L. et al. (2012). Treatment of demodicosis in dogs: 2011 clinical practice guidelines. *Vet. Dermatol.* 23 (2): 86–96, e20–1.

25 Rouben, C. (2016). Claw and claw bed diseases. *Clinician's Brief* (April): 35–40.

26 Manning, T.O. (1983). Cutaneous diseases of the paw. *Clin. Dermatol.* 1 (1): 131–142.

27 Baker, K.P. (1975). Hyperpigmentation of the skin in canine demodicosis. *Vet. Parasitol.* 1: 193–197.

28 Ackerman, L. (1984). Demodicosis in cats. *Mod. Vet. Pract.* 65 (10): 751–752.

29 Bennison, J.C. (1943). Demodicosis of horses with particular reference to equine members of the genus Demodex. *JR Army Vet. Corps.* 14: 34–39.

30 Bwangamoi, O. (1970). The pathogenesis of demodicosis in cattle in East Africa. *Br. Vet. J.* 127: 30–33.

31 Nemestri, L. and Szeky, A. (1966). Demodicosis of swine. *Acta Vet. Acad. Sci. Hung.* 16: 251–261.

32 Nutting, W.B. and Rauch, H. (1963). Distribution of Demodex Aurati in host (Mesocricetus auratus) skin complex. *J. Parasitol.* 49 (2): 323–329.

33 Oppong, E.N.W. (1970). *Aspects of Bovine Demodicosis, Streptothricosis, and Besnoitiosis in the Accra Plains of Ghana*. Ireland: Universtiy of Dublin.

34 Snell, R.S. (1963). A study of the melanocytes and melanin in a healing deep wound. *J. Anat.* 97: 243–253.

35 Frank, L.A. (2006). Comparative dermatology–canine endocrine dermatoses. *Clin. Dermatol.* 24 (4): 317–325.

36 Nesbitt, G.H., Izzo, J., Peterson, L., and Wilkins, R.J. (1980). Canine hypothyroidism: a retrospective study of 108 cases. *J. Am. Vet. Med. Assoc.* 177 (11): 1117–1122.

37 Dixon, R.M., Reid, S.W., and Mooney, C.T. (1999). Epidemiological, clinical, haematological and biochemical characteristics of canine hypothyroidism. *Vet. Rec.* 145 (17): 481–487.

38 Baker, K. (1986). Hormonal alopecia in dogs and cats. *In Pract.* 8 (2): 71–78.

39 Scott-Moncrieff, J.C. (2007). Clinical signs and concurrent diseases of hypothyroidism in dogs and cats. *Vet. Clin. North Am. Small Anim. Pract.* 37 (4): 709–722, vi.

40 Warren, S. (2013). Claw disease in dogs: part 2 – diagnosis and management of specific claw diseases. *Companion Anim.* 18 (5): 226–231.

41 Outerbridge, C.A. (2006). Mycologic disorders of the skin. *Clin. Tech. Small Anim. Pract.* 21 (3): 128–134.

42 Colombo, S., Nardoni, S., Cornegliani, L., and Mancianti, F. (2007). Prevalence of Malassezia spp. yeasts in feline nail folds: a cytological and mycological study. *Vet. Dermatol.* 18 (4): 278–283.

43 Griffin, C.E. and DeBoer, D.J. (2001). The ACVD task force on canine atopic dermatitis (XIV): clinical manifestations of canine atopic dermatitis. *Vet. Immunol. Immunopathol.* 81 (3–4): 255–269.

44 Maina, E., Galzerano, M., and Noli, C. (2014). Perianal pruritus in dogs with skin disease. *Vet. Dermatol.* 25 (3): 204–209, e51–2.

45 Maynard, L., Reme, C.A., and Viaud, S. (2011). Comparison of two shampoos for the treatment of canine Malassezia dermatitis: a randomised controlled trial. *J. Small Anim. Pract.* 52 (11): 566–572.

46 Pin, D., Carlotti, D.N., Jasmin, P. et al. (2006). Prospective study of bacterial overgrowth syndrome in eight dogs. *Vet. Rec.* 158 (13): 437–441.

47 Kimura, T. (2007). Contact hypersensitivity to stainless steel cages (chromium metal) in hairless descendants of Mexican hairless dogs. *Environ. Toxicol.* 22 (2): 176–184.

48 Bock, M., Schmidt, A., Bruckner, T., and Diepgen, T.L. (2003). Occupational skin disease in the construction industry. *Br. J. Dermatol.* 149 (6): 1165–1171.

49 Bruynzeel, D.P., Hennipman, G., and van Ketel, W.G. (1988). Irritant contact dermatitis and chrome-passivated metal. *Contact Dermatitis* 19 (3): 175–179.

50 Burden, D.J. and Eedy, D.J. (1991). Orthodontic headgear related to allergic contact dermatitis: a case report. *Br. Dent. J.* 170 (12): 447–448.

51 Gad, S.C. (1989). Acute and chronic systemic chromium toxicity. *Sci. Total Environ.* 86 (1–2): 149–157.

52 Hansen, K.S. (1983). Occupational dermatoses in hospital cleaning women. *Contact Dermatitis* 9 (5): 343–351.

53 Hansen, M.B., Rydin, S., Menne, T., and Duus, J.J. (2002). Quantitative aspects of contact allergy to chromium and exposure to chrome-tanned leather. *Contact Dermatitis* 47 (3): 127–134.

54 Kim, M.H., Choi, Y.W., Choi, H.Y., and Myung, K.B. (2001). Prurigo pigmentosa from contact allergy to chrome in detergent. *Contact Dermatitis* 44 (5): 289–292.

55 Lee, H.S. and Goh, C.L. (1988). Occupational dermatosis among chrome platers. *Contact Dermatitis* 18 (2): 89–93.

56 Nygren, O. and Wahlberg, J.E. (1998). Speciation of chromium in tanned leather gloves and relapse of chromium allergy from tanned leather samples. *Analyst* 123 (5): 935–937.

57 Papa, G., Romano, A., Quaratino, D. et al. (2000). Contact dermatoses in metal workers. *Int. J. Immunopathol. Pharmacol.* 13 (1): 43–47.

58 Williams, N. (1996). A survey of respiratory and dermatological disease in the chrome plating industry in the West Midlands, UK. *Occup. Med. (Lond.)* 46 (6): 432–434.

59 Day, M.J. and Lucke, V.M. (1995). Melanocytic neoplasia in the cat. *J. Small Anim. Pract.* 36 (5): 207–213.

60 Goldschmidt, M.H. (1994). Pigmented lesions of the skin. *Clin. Dermatol.* 12 (4): 507–514.

61 AKC. (2015). Loss of Pigmentation in Dogs. https://www.akc.org/expert-advice/health/loss-of-pigmentation-in-dogs.

62 Isenhart, P. (2013). The Dog's Nose: How it works and skin conditions. https://petmassage.com/the-dogs-nose-how-it-works-and-skin-conditions.

63 White, S.D. (1994). Diseases of the nasal planum. *Vet. Clin. North Am. Small Anim. Pract.* 24 (5): 887–895.

64 Cohn, L.A. (2014). Canine nasal disease. *Vet. Clin. North Am. Small Anim. Pract.* 44 (1): 75–89.

65 Kerl, M.E. (2003). Update on canine and feline fungal diseases. *Vet. Clin. North Am. Small Anim. Pract.* 33 (4): 721–747.

66 Werner, A. and Norton, F. (2011). Blastomycosis. *Compend. Contin. Educ. Vet.* 33 (8): E1–E4; quiz E5.

67 Benitah, N. (2006). Canine nasal aspergillosis. *Clin. Tech. Small Anim. Pract.* 21 (2): 82–88.

68 Epstein, S. and Hardy, R. (2011). Clinical resolution of nasal aspergillosis following therapy with a homeopathic remedy in a dog. *J. Am. Anim. Hosp. Assoc.* 47 (6): e110–e115.

69 Barrs, V.R. and Talbot, J.J. (2014). Feline aspergillosis. *Vet. Clin. North Am. Small Anim. Pract.* 44 (1): 51–73.

70 Legendre, A. (1998). Blastomycosis. In: *Infectious Diseases of the Dog and Cat*, 2e (ed. C. Greene), 371–377. Philadelphia: W.B. Saunders.

71 Miller, P.E., Miller, L.M., and Schoster, J.V. (1990). Feline Blastomycosis – a report of 3 cases and literature-review (1961 to 1988). *J. Am. Anim. Hosp. Assoc.* 26 (4): 417–424.

72 Baumgardner, D.J., Buggy, B.P., Mattson, B.J. et al. (1992). Epidemiology of blastomycosis in a region of high endemicity in north central Wisconsin. *Clin. Infect. Dis.* 15 (4): 629–635.

73 Arceneaux, K.A., Taboada, J., and Hosgood, G. (1998). Blastomycosis in dogs: 115 cases (1980–1995). *J. Am. Vet. Med. Assoc.* 213 (5): 658–664.

74 Rudmann, D.G., Coolman, B.R., Perez, C.M., and Glickman, L.T. (1992). Evaluation of risk factors for blastomycosis in dogs: 857 cases (1980–1990). *J. Am. Vet. Med. Assoc.* 201 (11): 1754–1759.

75 Pappas, P.G. (2004). Blastomycosis. *Semin. Respir. Crit. Care Med.* 25 (2): 113–121.

76 Taboda, J. (2000). Systemic mycoses. In: *Textbook of Veterinary Internal Medicine. 1*, 5e (ed. S.J. Ettinger and E.C. Feldman), 453–476. Philadelphia: W.B. Saunders.

77 Gionfriddo, J.R. (2000). Feline systemic fungal infections. *Vet. Clin. North Am. Small Anim. Pract.* 30 (5): 1029–1050.

78 Cote, E., Barr, S.C., and Allen, C. (1997). Possible transmission of blastomycosis dermatitidis via culture specimen. *J. Am. Vet. Med. Assoc.* 210 (4): 479–480.

79 Ramsey, D.T. (1994). Blastomycosis in a veterinarian. *J. Am. Vet. Med. Assoc.* 205 (7): 968.

80 Walton, R.A.L., Wey, A., and Hall, K.E. (2017). A retrospective study of anti-inflammatory use in dogs with pulmonary blastomycosis: 139 cases (2002–2012). *J. Vet. Emerg. Crit. Care (San Antonio)* 27 (4): 439–443.

81 Sharp, N.J. (1998). Canine nasal aspergillosis-penicilliosis. In: *Infectious Diseases of the Dog and Cat*, 2e (ed. C. Greene), 404–409. Philadelphia: W.B. Saunders, Co.

82 Magro, M., Sykes, J., Vishkautsan, P., and Martinez-Lopez, B. (2017). Spatial patterns and impacts of environmental and climatic factors on canine sinonasal aspergillosis in Northern California. *Front. Vet. Sci.* 4: 104.

83 Mullins, J., Harvey, R., and Seaton, A. (1976). Sources and incidence of airborne Aspergillus fumigatus (Fres). *Clin. Allergy* 6 (3): 209–217.

84 Warris, A., Klaassen, C.H., Meis, J.F. et al. (2003). Molecular epidemiology of Aspergillus fumigatus isolates recovered from water, air, and patients shows two clusters of genetically distinct strains. *J. Clin. Microbiol.* 41 (9): 4101–4106.

85 Curtis, L., Cali, S., Conroy, L. et al. (2005). Aspergillus surveillance project at a large tertiary-care hospital. *J. Hosp. Infect.* 59 (3): 188–196.

86 Haines, J. (1995). Aspergillus in compost – straw man or fatal flaw. *Biocycle* 36 (4): 32–35.

87 Streifel, A.J., Lauer, J.L., Vesley, D. et al. (1983). Aspergillus-Fumigatus and other Thermotolerant fungi generated by hospital building demolition. *Appl. Environ. Microbiol.* 46 (2): 375–378.

88 Ren, P., Jankun, T.M., Belanger, K. et al. (2001). The relation between fungal propagules in indoor air and home characteristics. *Allergy* 56 (5): 419–424.

89 Day, M.J. (2009). Canine sino-nasal aspergillosis: parallels with human disease. *Med. Mycol.* 47 (Suppl 1): S315–S323.

90 Sharp, N.J. and Harvey, C.E. (1991). Aspergillosis: report on diagnosis and treatment. *Tijdschr. Diergeneeskd.* 116 (Suppl 1): 35S–37S.

91 Zonderland, J.L., Stork, C.K., Saunders, J.H. et al. (2002). Intranasal infusion of enilconazole for treatment of sinonasal aspergillosis in dogs. *J. Am. Vet. Med. Assoc.* 221 (10): 1421–1425.

92 Sharp, N.J.H., Harvey, C.E., and Obrien, J.A. (1991). Treatment of canine nasal aspergillosis penicilliosis with fluconazole (Uk-49,858). *J. Small Anim. Pract.* 32 (10): 513–516.

93 Saunders, J.H., Zonderland, J.L., Clercx, C. et al. (2002). Computed tomographic findings in 35 dogs with nasal aspergillosis. *Vet. Radiol. Ultrasound* 43 (1): 5–9.

94 Sharp, N.J., Sullivan, M., Harvey, C.E., and Webb, T. (1993). Treatment of canine nasal aspergillosis with enilconazole. *J. Vet. Intern. Med.* 7 (1): 40–43.

95 Mathews, K.G., Davidson, A.P., Koblik, P.D. et al. (1998). Comparison of topical administration of clotrimazole through surgically placed versus nonsurgically placed catheters for treatment of nasal aspergillosis in dogs: 60 cases (1990–1996). *J. Am. Vet. Med. Assoc.* 213 (4): 501–506.

96 Wilkinson, G.T., Sutton, R.H., and Grono, L.R. (1982). Aspergillus Spp infection associated with orbital cellulitis and sinusitis in a cat. *J. Small Anim. Pract.* 23 (3): 127–131.

97 Goodall, S.A., Lane, J.G., and Warnock, D.W. (1984). The diagnosis and treatment of a case of nasal aspergillosis in a cat. *J. Small Anim. Pract.* 25 (10): 627–633.

98 Davies, C. and Troy, G.C. (1996). Deep mycotic infections in cats. *J. Am. Anim. Hosp. Assoc.* 32 (5): 380–391.

99 Hamilton, H.L., Whitley, R.D., and McLaughlin, S.A. (2000). Exophthalmos secondary to aspergillosis in a cat. *J. Am. Anim. Hosp. Assoc.* 36 (4): 343–347.

100 Tomsa, K., Glaus, T.A., Zimmer, C., and Greene, C.E. (2003). Fungal rhinitis and sinusitis in three cats. *J. Am. Vet. Med. Assoc.* 222 (10): 1380–1384.

101 Barrs, V.R., Halliday, C., Martin, P. et al. (2012). Sinonasal and sino-orbital aspergillosis in 23 cats: aetiology, clinicopathological features and treatment outcomes. *Vet. J.* 191 (1): 58–64.

102 Declercq, J., Declercq, L., and Fincioen, S. (2012). Unilateral sino-orbital and subcutaneous aspergillosis in a cat. *Vlaams. Diergen. Tijds.* 81 (6): 357–362.

103 Kano, R., Shibahashi, A., Fujino, Y. et al. (2013). Two cases of feline orbital aspergillosis due to Aspergillus udagawae and A-viridinutans. *J. Vet. Med. Sci.* 75 (1): 7–10.

104 Malik, R., Vogelnest, L., O'Brien, C.R. et al. (2004). Infections and some other conditions affecting the skin and subcutis of the naso-ocular region of cats – clinical experience 1987–2003. *J. Feline Med. Surg.* 6 (6): 383–390.

105 Karnik, K., Reichle, J.K., Fischetti, A.J., and Goggin, J.M. (2009). Computed tomographic findings of fungal rhinitis and sinusitis in cats. *Vet. Radiol. Ultrasound* 50 (1): 65–68.

106 Furrow, E. and Groman, R.P. (2009). Intranasal infusion of clotrimazole for the treatment of nasal aspergillosis in two cats. *J. Am. Vet. Med. Assoc.* 235 (10): 1188–1193.

107 Barachetti, L., Mortellaro, C.M., Di Giancamillo, M. et al. (2009). Bilateral orbital and nasal aspergillosis in a cat. *Vet. Ophthalmol.* 12 (3): 176–182.

108 Giordano, C., Gianella, P., Bo, S. et al. (2010). Invasive mould infections of the naso-orbital region of cats: a case involving Aspergillus fumigatus and an aetiological review. *J. Feline Med. Surg.* 12 (9): 714–723.

109 Smith, L.N. and Hoffman, S.B. (2010). A case series of unilateral orbital aspergillosis in three cats and treatment with voriconazole. *Vet. Ophthalmol.* 13 (3): 190–203.

110 Rossi, M.A., Messenger, L.M., Linder, K.E., and Olivry, T. (2015). Generalized canine discoid lupus erythematosus responsive to tetracycline and niacinamide therapy. *J. Am. Anim. Hosp. Assoc.* 51 (3): 171–175.

111 Gaugere, E. and Alhaidari, Z. (1989). Disorders of melanin pigmentation in the skin of dogs and cats. In: *Current Veterinary Therapy X* (ed. R.W. Kirk), 628–632. Philadelphia: W.B. Saunders.

112 Lopez, R., Ginel, P.J., Molleda, J.M. et al. (1994). A clinical, pathological and immunopathological study of vitiligo in a Siamese cat. *Vet. Dermatol.* 5 (1): 27–32.

113 Boissy, R.E., Moellmann, G.E., and Lerner, A.B. (1987). Morphology of melanocytes in hair bulbs and eyes of vitiligo mice. *Am. J. Pathol.* 127: 380–388.

114 Naughton, G.K., Mahaffey, M., and Bystryn, J.C. (eds.) (1986). Antibodies to surface antigens of pigmented cells in animals with vitiligo. *Proc. Soc. Exp. Biol. Med.* 181 (3): 423–426.

115 Scott, D.W. and Randolph, J.F. (1989). Vitiligo in 2 old-English sheepdog littermates and in a dachshund with juvenile-onset diabetes-mellitus. *Companion Anim. Pract.* 19 (3): 18–22.

116 Sherding, R.G. (1994). Diseases of the skin. In: *The Cat: Diseases and Clinical Management*, 2e (ed. R.G. Sherding), 1994–2046. Philadelphia, PA; New York, NY: W.B. Saunders.

117 Muller, G.H., Kirk, R.W., and Scott, D.W. (1989). Pigmentary abnormalities. In: *Small Animal Dermatology*, 705–714. Philadelphia: W.B. Saunders.

10

Nasal and Footpad Hyperkeratosis

10.1 Introduction to Hyperkeratosis

The stratum corneum is the outermost layer of the epidermis [1–3]. When this layer thickens, as from an overproduction of keratin, the result is grossly visible, hyperplastic skin. This appearance is termed hyperkeratosis [1].

Hyperkeratosis often develops in regions of the body that are exposed to persistent pressure or irritation [1]. It can be thought of as the skin's attempt to protect itself. This provides a simplistic explanation for the development of calluses and corns in people with improperly fitted shoes.

Companion animal patients may also develop calluses. One of the most common examples that comes to mind is the elbow callus. This occurs most often in large to giant breed dogs in response to chronic pressure applied to a poorly cushioned pressure point, the elbow. Elbow calluses also develop in recumbent patients of any size for similar reasons [4] (see Figure 10.1).

Nasal and footpad hyperkeratosis are frequently encountered in clinical practice. These may occur in isolation of one another or they may occur concurrently [1]. Clients may present the patient for evaluation of either, or hyperkeratosis may be an incidental finding on physical examination.

Consider how hyperkeratosis transforms the appearance of the patient. Although its color may vary, the surface of the nasal planum is typically shiny, with a smooth-to-cobblestone texture [5, 6]. The healthy nasal planum may also appear moistened due to serous nasal secretions (see Figures 10.2a–d).

When the nasal planum develops hyperkeratosis, it is overtaken by dryness. Frond-like projections may develop at the nasal planum's surface [1]. These fronds are proliferations of keratin. In addition, the once pliable nasal planum becomes firm [5, 6] (see Figures 10.3a–c).

If the nasal planum is sufficiently dry, it may crack and fissure. This results in pain and bleeding [5, 6]. Secondary infection may also develop.

Consider also the appearance of a normal footpad in a companion animal patient. Footpads may vary in color and extent of wear. The cat or dog that spends most of its life standing on a concrete surface will have more calloused footpads than the patient that spends all of its life indoors (see Figures 10.4a–d).

Much like the nasal planum, footpads with hyperkeratosis develop frond-like projections of keratin [7, 8]. Hyperkeratotic footpads may also accumulate excessive crusts, with or without fissures developing between them [8] (see Figures 10.5a–c).

When fissures develop, they may result in lameness secondary to pain [8]. Secondary infection is also possible [8].

Nasal and footpad hyperkeratosis are not pathognomonic for one specific disease [5]. When one or both appear, they may be purely age-related and/or cosmetic [5, 9]. However, they could also be a reflection of underlying infectious, inflammatory, or neoplastic disease [5]. The following is a list of the most reported causes of nasal and footpad hyperkeratosis [1, 5, 9–11]:

- Familial hyperkeratosis
- Zinc-responsive dermatosis
- Disease-induced hyperkeratosis

Infectious causes of nasal and footpad hyperkeratosis include the following [1, 5, 9, 10, 12]:

- Canine Distemper Virus (CDV)
- *Dirofilaria repens*
- Leishmaniasis

Immune-mediated diseases that result in nasal and footpad hyperkeratosis include the following [1, 5, 9, 10, 13, 14]:

- Pemphigus foliaceus
- Systemic lupus erythematosus (SLE)

Neoplastic diseases such as cutaneous lymphoma, hepatocutaneous syndrome, and glucagonoma may cause nasal and footpad hyperkeratosis. However, these conditions are quite rare in companion animal patients [1, 5].

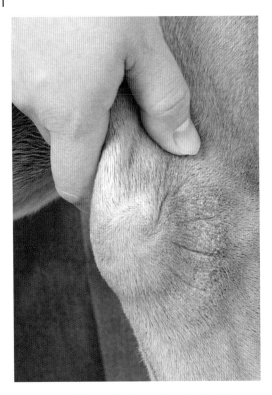

Figure 10.1 Elbow callus in an otherwise healthy young adult Great Dane. This patient had bilateral elbow calluses. Only the right side is pictured here. *Source:* Courtesy of the Media Resources Department at Midwestern University.

History taking and a comprehensive physical examination are important first steps to establish if the presenting patient is otherwise healthy or if additional complaints point toward more systemic disease.

Not every cause as outlined above will be covered here. The goal of this chapter is to introduce the reader to the primary causes of hyperkeratosis within the companion animal population.

10.2 Idiopathic Hyperkeratosis

Note that diagnostic investigation of hyperkeratosis may be inconclusive. Cases of nasal and footpad hyperkeratosis in otherwise asymptomatic canine patients may be idiopathic. These cases most often develop in aged [1, 9, 10, 15]. These dogs may or may not respond to therapeutic attempts to soften the excessive keratin with petroleum jelly, propylene glycol, salicylic acid, and/or tretinoin gel [1, 5, 16].

10.3 Hereditary Hyperkeratosis

Hereditary nasal parakeratosis (HNP) was first described in Labrador retriever and Labrador retriever crosses in two separate studies by Page et al. and Peters et al. in 2003 [9, 16]. Parakeratosis refers to the principle histologic feature that these patients share, parakeratotic hyperkeratosis [9, 16]. This specific type of hyperkeratosis defines the condition by which cells of the stratum corneum proliferate extensively and retain their nuclei [9, 16]. The presence of these nucleated squames may reflect incomplete differentiation or an underlying inflammatory process [16]. In humans, parakeratotic hyperkeratosis is a response to inflammation, as is seen in psoriasis [16]. Whether or not inflammation is an inciting factor in dogs with HNP remains to be determined.

Patients with HNP develop nasal hyperkeratosis as young adults, typically between 6 and 12 months of age [9, 16]. Of the 18 cases that were described by Page, the majority did not have concurrent footpad disease [9].

Dogs with HNP have gray-to-brown accumulations of keratin [9]. Concurrent depigmentation of the nasal planum is rare, but possible (see Figures 10.6a, b).

These hyperkeratotic lesions do not appear to worsen with sunlight. Some owners report that they improve after the dog's nose is moistened by rain or snow [9].

Dogs with HNP are otherwise healthy [9, 16].

HNP does not appear to be sex-linked in terms of its inheritance: males and females are affected equally. HNP does not also appear to favor certain coat colors [16]. Page et al. proposed an autosomal recessive inheritance, but this has yet to be confirmed [9].

Treatment is not necessary. However, some dogs may response to the use of topical propylene glycol or other emollients, such as petroleum jelly [9, 16]. In these patients, treatment is not curative. Treatment reduces lesions, but must be continued indefinitely to retain beneficial effects [16].

A second inherited condition that involves a thickened stratum corneum is digital hyperkeratosis (DH), otherwise referred to as hereditary footpad hyperkeratosis (HFH). HFH is inherited among Irish Terriers as an autosomal recessive trait [17]. This condition was first described by Binder et al. in 2000 [18]. It has also been described in Kerry Blue Terriers and Dogues de Bordeaux [18–21].

Patients with HFH develop appreciable calluses on the palmar and plantar surfaces of all four feet. As these lesions progress, they are prone to cracking. The resultant pain causes lameness [18].

Much like HNP, HFH lesions arise as early as 18 weeks of age [18]. By the time the patient is six months old, paw pads are encrusted with keratin [18]. Keratin accumulation can be quite extreme, resulting in deposits up to 5 mm deep.

Histopathologic lesions classically reflect orthokeratotic hyperkeratosis. This means that cells are anucleate as compared to those in HNP [17, 18, 22].

In addition, the claws of affected Irish Setters may be unnaturally rounded [18].

(a)

(c)

(b)

(d)

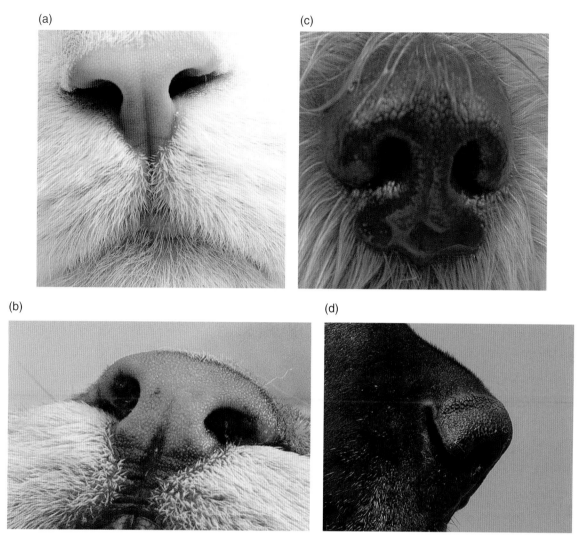

Figure 10.2 (a) Head-on view of a normal, pink nasal planum in a feline patient. *Source:* Courtesy of the Media Resources Department at Midwestern University. (b) Three-quarter view of a normal, rust-brown nasal planum in a feline patient. *Source:* Courtesy of the Media Resources Department at Midwestern University. (c) Head-on view of a normal, black nasal planum in a canine patient. Note the smooth, moist surface. (d) Side-view of a normal, black nasal planum in a canine patient. Note that the surface texture is cobblestone.

Treatment is palliative. Its aim is to soften the keratinaceous debris [18]. In addition, pads may need to be filed [18].

10.4 Zinc-Responsive Dermatosis

The body is dependent upon zinc to maintain function [23]. As a constituent of more than 70 metalloenzymes, zinc participates in carbohydrate, protein, lipid, and nucleic acid metabolism [23, 24]. Zinc also modulates the immune response and regulates wound healing [23–27].

Within the body, zinc is stored primarily in muscle, bone, teeth, and skin [23, 28, 29]. Concerning the skin, the epidermis contains by far more zinc than the dermis [28, 29]. The highest concentrations of epidermal zinc are in the nasal planum and footpads [30].

Because the body's reserves of zinc are limited, patients rely upon dietary zinc to maintain function [23, 31]. As expected, certain physiologic states require more zinc than others [23]. Zinc requirements are greater for those young patients that are still growing and in adults that are reproductively active [31, 32]. Pregnancy, lactation, and illness may raise requirements for zinc by two to three times [32].

Certain ingredients in the diet may also raise zinc requirements [23]. For example, diets that are high in plant proteins such as soy decrease the body's ability to absorb zinc [23, 33–35]. Vegetarian-based diets may therefore require supplemental zinc to compensate for this reduction in zinc utilization. Additionally, excess intake of calcium, iron, and copper may also reduce zinc absorption by the intestines [23, 33–35].

One-fifth of the body's zinc is stored in skin [23, 28, 29]. Therefore, zinc deficiencies often result in dermatosis.

(a)

(b)

(c)

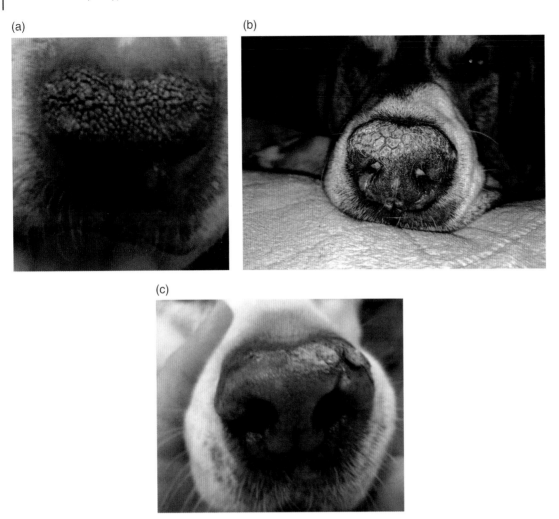

Figure 10.3 (a) Frond-like projections on the nasal planum due to nasal hyperkeratosis. (b) Nasal hyperkeratosis in an adult dog. *Source:* Courtesy of Gregory J. Costanzo, DVM. (c) Cracking and crusting of the nasal planum, associated with nasal hyperkeratosis.

This is true of dogs and cats, but also cattle, sheep, goats, pigs, and humans [31, 36–41]. Among companion animal patients, zinc-responsive dermatosis is more likely to occur in the dog.

There are two syndromes related to zinc-responsive dermatosis in the dog [23]. Syndrome 1 is the result of an inherited defect that reduces the body's ability to absorb zinc through the intestines [42, 43]. Siberian Huskies and Alaskan Malamutes are overrepresented [42, 43]. Age of onset is typically young: 41% develop lesions prior to two years old [23, 44].

Footpad hyperkeratosis is common in affected dogs. In addition, these patients typically present with focal alopecia and crusting, most notably around the eyes, ears, nose, and mouth [23] (see Figures 10.7a, b).

Syndrome 2 occurs when patients consume zinc-deficient diets and diets high in soy or calcium. Any breed has the potential to be affected. Patients tend to exhibit clinical signs as puppies during periods of rapid growth.

In additional to nasal and footpad hyperkeratosis, these dogs may also demonstrate vague signs of malaise, such as depression, poor growth, and anorexia [23].

Signalment, particularly age and breed, as well as familial and dietary history are instrumental in making a presumptive diagnosis [23]. Because it is difficult to accurately quantify zinc levels in serum, plasma, and hair in dogs, zinc supplementation is a more appropriate diagnostic test [23]. If patients that are supplemented with zinc demonstrate a positive response, then the diagnosis of zinc-associated dermatosis is said to be confirmed [23].

Dogs with Syndrome 1 should respond to zinc supplementation [23]. Over 88% of patients experience complete remission. Note, however, that the time for this to occur is highly variable. A study by Colombini et al. [44] demonstrated full recovery within 3 to 210 days of initiating therapy [44]. If therapy is discontinued, then lesions recur. Lesions may also recur if the dosage schedule is

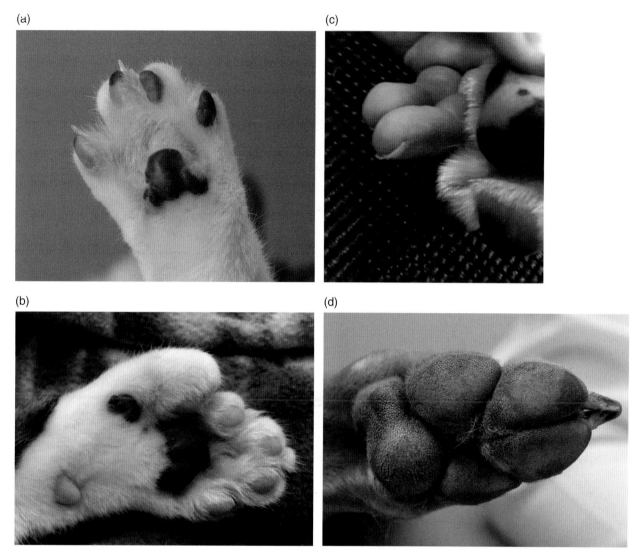

Figure 10.4 (a) Normal footpads in a feline patient. *Source:* Courtesy of the Media Resources Department at Midwestern University. (b) Normal footpads in a feline patient with polydactyly. *Source:* Courtesy of Karen Burks, DVM. (c) Normal footpads in a canine patient. (d) Normal footpads in a Great Dane dog.

altered [11, 23, 44, 45]. Zinc supplementation is therefore required for life [23].

Dogs with Syndrome 2 need only an adjustment in diet to experience resolution of signs within one-and-a-half months [23, 46]. It is thought that remission takes weeks to attain because previously depleted zinc reserves must be rebuilt. For reasons that are not entirely understood, some puppies require supplementation throughout the physiologic state of growth [10, 46]. For these patients, it is not until they reach maturity that supplementation can cease.

Daily supplementation is typically via the oral route of administration [23]. If the patient fails to respond or if the patient develops emesis secondary to oral supplementation, then once-weekly injectable therapy may be indicated [42].

10.5 CDV and "Hard Pad Disease"

CDV is an enveloped, single-stranded RNA virus within the genus *Morbillivirus* and family Paramyxoviridae [47, 48]. Although this discussion will focus on the disease as it has been characterized in the dog, it is important to recognize that CDV also impacts wild canids as well as species within the families Mustelidae, Procyonidae, Ursidae, and Viverridae [47]. In addition, wild felids and those in captivity are susceptible to CDV [49, 50].

In dogs, CDV results in systemic disease that most notably impacts the respiratory, gastrointestinal, and neurological systems [47]. The modified-live vaccine for CDV in the 1950s has significantly reduced the incidence of this disease [47, 51, 52]. However, CDV continues to

(a)

(b)

(c)

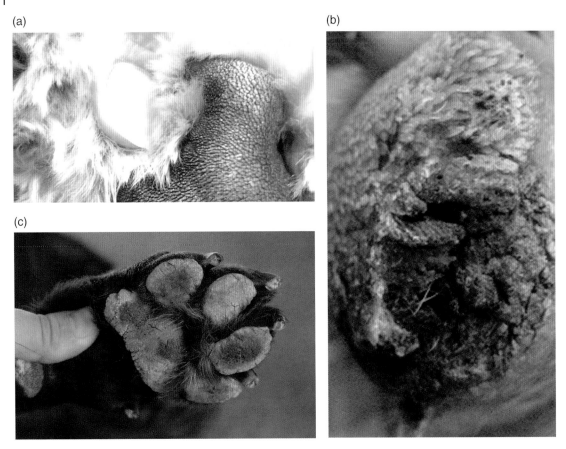

Figure 10.5 (a) Mild frond-like projections in a canine patient with footpad hyperkeratosis. (b) More pronounced frond-like projections in a canine patient with footpad hyperkeratosis. (c) Marked crusting of the footpads in a canine patient. *Source:* Courtesy of Jackie Kucskar, DVM.

(a)

(b)

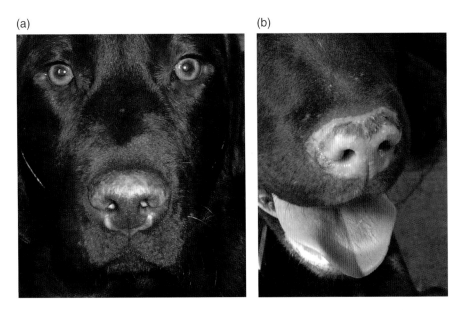

Figure 10.6 (a) Early depigmentation of the nose, attributed to hereditary nasal parakeratosis (HNP) of Labrador retrievers. *Source:* Courtesy of Jackie Kucskar, DVM. (b) Progressive nasal depigmentation with the accumulation of frond-like projections on dorsal rim of the nasal planum, attributed to hereditary nasal parakeratosis (HNP) of Labrador retrievers. *Source:* Courtesy of Jackie Kucskar, DVM.

(a) (b)

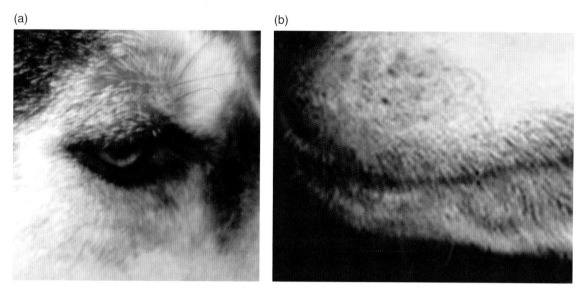

Figure 10.7 (a) Peri-orbital alopecia in a Northern Breed dog with zinc-responsive dermatosis. (b) Alopecic crusting around the mouth in a Northern Breed dog with zinc-responsive dermatosis.

be diagnosed globally, with isolated reports of CDV even among vaccinated animals [53, 54].

Young patients are more susceptible than the aged, particularly as maternally derived immunity wanes in three-to-six-month-old pups [47]. The prevalence of CDV also appears to increase during the colder months [47].

Disease transmission is via aerosol or direct contact with an infected animal [47]. Body fluids contain high levels of virus [55].

Infected patients experience a significant drop in CD4+ lymphocytes [47, 56, 57]. The result is that they become severely immunosuppressed [47]. Initially, patients may develop a transient fever three to six days after infection [47]. Clients may report generalized malaise, including lethargy, depression, and anorexia [47]. Ocular and nasal discharge may develop [47].

CDV spreads to the epithelium within six to nine days post-infection [47, 58–60]. Nasal and footpad hyperkeratosis are commonly reported findings in dogs with CDV [47, 60, 61] (see Figure 10.8).

Because of the frequency with which hyperkeratosis arises, CDV is sometimes referred to as "hard pad disease" [15, 60, 62–66]. It is important to note, however, that CDV is not the only condition that results in hard pads and that grossly these clinical signs are indistinguishable from zinc-related dermatosis and other aforementioned causes of hyperkeratosis [15, 60, 67, 68].

Other classic signs of CDV that do not involve the integumentary system include enamel hypoplasia (see Figure 10.9).

Neurological signs that result from CDV are late onset, and typically do not arise until 20 or more days after infection [47]. These are beyond the scope of this chapter.

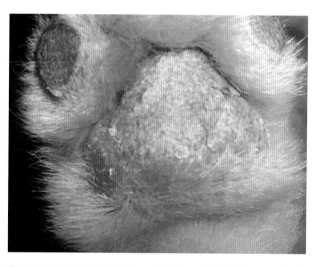

Figure 10.8 Footpad hyperkeratosis in a patient that succumbed to Canine Distemper Virus (CDV).

However, textbook cases of neurological CDV frequently describe rhythmic, involuntary jerking of one or more muscle groups [69]. This state is referred to as myoclonus. When such tics involve the head and jaw, the patient may appear as if chewing gum [47].

10.6 Hepatocutaneous Syndrome and Glucagonoma

Refer to Chapter 5, Section 5.9 and Chapter 7, Section 7.3.3 as an introduction to hepatocutaneous syndrome as a cause of alopecia and skin fragility. Recall that hepatocutaneous syndrome is relatively uncommon in

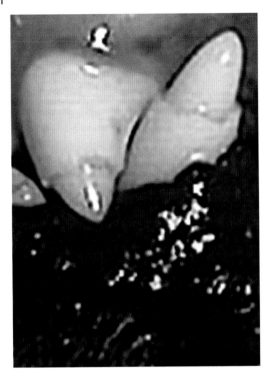

Figure 10.9 Enamel hypoplasia in a patient that was infected with Canine Distemper Virus (CDV).

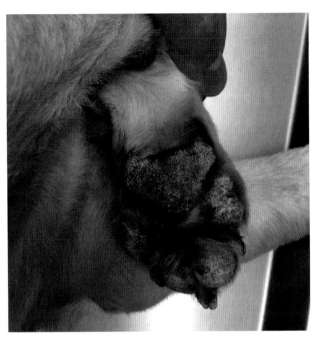

Figure 10.10 Footpad hyperkeratosis secondary to glucagonoma in a canine patient. *Source:* Courtesy of Rodolfo Oliveira Leal, DVM (Portugal), PhD, Dipl. ECVIM-CA (Internal Medicine).

companion animal patients as a paraneoplastic disease and has several pseudonyms, including superficial necrolytic dermatitis and necrolytic migratory erythema (NME) [70, 71].

Hepatocutaneous syndrome may result from hepatic or pancreatic disease. Glucagon-secreting pancreatic masses are more common in humans than in dogs or cats. However, when they develop, glucagonomas have the potential to induce footpad hyperkeratosis [71–76] (see Figure 10.10).

Patients with this condition are not limited to lesions of the footpad. They often present with crusting over pressure points, and erosions on the muzzle and around the eyes [8]. Affected patients also tend to be systemically ill [8]. Serum biochemistry findings for these patients typically yields elevations in liver enzymes, bile acids, and glucose. Serum albumin is often depressed [8]. These changes support the need to pursue diagnostic imaging [8]. The liver takes on a classic honeycomb appearance on ultrasound [77].

References

1 Miller, W.H., Griffin, C.E., Campbell, K.L. et al. (2013). *Muller & Kirk's Small Animal Dermatology*, 7e, ix, 938 p. St. Louis, MO: Elsevier.

2 Moriello, K.A. and Mason, I.S. (1995). *Handbook of Small Animal Dermatology*, 1e, xv, 334 p., 8 p. of plates p. Oxford England; Tarrytown, N.Y., U.S.A.: Pergamon.

3 Medleau, L. and Hnilica, K.A. (2006). *Small Animal Dermatology: A Color Atlas and Therapeutic Guide*, 2e, xvii, 526 p. St. Louis, MO: Saunders Elsevier.

4 Fossum, T.W., Duprey, L.P., and O'Connor, D. (2007). Surgery of the integumentary system. In: *Small Animal Surgery*, 3e (ed. T.W. Fossum, L.P. Duprey and D. O'Connor), 159–259. Boston, MA: Elsevier.

5 Catarino, M., Combarros-Garcia, D., Mimouni, P. et al. (2017). Control of canine idiopathic nasal hyperkeratosis with a natural skin restorative balm: a randomized double-blind placebo-controlled study. *Vet. Dermatol.*

6 Gross, T.L., Ihrke, P.J., and Walder, E.J. (2005). *Skin Diseases of the Dog and Cat: Clinical and Histopathologic Diagnosis*, 2e. Oxford, U.K.: Blackwell Science Ltd.

7 Medleau, L. and Hnilica, K.A. (2006). Idiopathic nasodigital hyperkeratosis. In: *Small Animal Dermatology: A Color Atlas and Therapeutic Guide*, 2e (ed. L. Medleau and K.A. Hnilica), 316–318. St. Louis, MO: Saunders Elsevier.

8 Werner, A. (2016). *Top 5 Causes of Crusted Paw in Dogs Clinician's Brief* (June).

9 Page, N., Paradis, M., Lapointe, J.M., and Dunstan, R.W. (2003). Hereditary nasal parakeratosis in Labrador retrievers. *Vet. Dermatol.* 14 (2): 103–110.

10 Kwochka, K.W. (1993). Primary keratinization disorders of dogs. In: *Current Veterinary Dermatology, the Science and Art of Therapy* (ed. C.E. Griffin, K.W. Kwochka and J.M. Macdonald), 176–190. St. Louis, MO: Mosby Year Book.

11 Kunkle, G.A. (1980). Zinc-responsive dermatoses in dogs. In: *Current Veterinary Therapy VII* (ed. R.W. Kirk), 472–476. Philadelphia: W.B. Saunders Co.

12 Ciaramella, P., Oliva, G., Luna, R.D. et al. (1997). A retrospective clinical study of canine leishmaniasis in 150 dogs naturally infected by Leishmania infantum. *Vet. Rec.* 141 (21): 539–543.

13 Ihrke, P.J., Stannard, A.A., Ardans, A.A. et al. (1985). Pemphigus foliaceus of the footpads in three dogs. *J. Am. Vet. Med. Assoc.* 186 (1): 67–69.

14 August, J.R. and Chickering, W.R. (1985). Pemphigus foliaceus causing lameness in 4 dogs. *Compend. Contin. Educ. Pract.* 7 (11): 894–902.

15 Yager, J.A. and Wilcock, B.P. (1994). *Color Atlas and Text of Surgical Pathology of the Dog and Cat, Dermatopathology and Skin Tumors*. London: Wolfe Publishing.

16 Peters, J., Scott, D.W., Erb, H.N., and Miller, W.H. (2003). Hereditary nasal parakeratosis in Labrador retrievers: 11 new cases and a retrospective study on the presence of accumulations of serum ('serum lakes') in the epidermis of parakeratotic dermatoses and inflamed nasal plana of dogs. *Vet. Dermatol.* 14 (4): 197–203.

17 Drogemuller, M., Jagannathan, V., Becker, D. et al. (2014). A mutation in the FAM83G gene in dogs with hereditary footpad hyperkeratosis (HFH). *PLoS Genet.* 10 (5): e1004370.

18 Binder, H., Arnold, S., Schelling, C. et al. (2000). Palmoplantar hyperkeratosis in Irish terriers: evidence of autosomal recessive inheritance. *J. Small Anim. Pract.* 41 (2): 52–55.

19 Paradis, M. (1992). Footpad hyperkeratosis in a family of Dogues de Bordeaux. *Vet. Dermatol.* 3: 75–78.

20 Kral, F. and Schwartzman, R.M. (1964). *Veterinary and Comparative Dermatology*. Philadelphia: J.B. Lippincott.

21 Scott, D.W., Miller, W.H., and Griffin, C.E. (1995). Congenital and hereditary defects. In: *Muller and Kirk's Smal Animal Dermatology*, 5e, 754–755. Philadelphia: W.B. Saunders.

22 Schleifer, S.G., Versteeg, S.A., van Oost, B., and Willemse, T. (2003). Familial footpad hyperkeratosis and inheritance of keratin 2, keratin 9, and desmoglein 1 in two pedigrees of Irish terriers. *Am. J. Vet. Res.* 64 (6): 715–720.

23 Colombini, S. (1999). Canine zinc-responsive dermatosis. *Vet. Clin. North Am. Small Anim. Pract.* 29 (6): 1373–1383.

24 Chvapil, M. (1976). Effect of zinc on cells and biomembranes. *Med. Clin. North Am.* 60 (4): 799–812.

25 Riordan, J.F. (1976). Biochemistry of zinc. *Med. Clin. North Am.* 60 (4): 661–674.

26 Pekarek, R.S., Sandstead, H.H., Jacob, R.A., and Barcome, D.F. (1979). Abnormal cellular immune responses during acquired zinc deficiency. *Am. J. Clin. Nutr.* 32 (7): 1466–1471.

27 Norris, D. (1985). Zinc and cutaneous inflammation. *Arch. Dermatol.* 121 (8): 985–989.

28 Molokhia, M.M. and Portnoy, B. (1969). Neutron activation analysis of trace elements in skin. 3. Zinc in normal skin. *Br. J. Dermatol.* 81 (10): 759–762.

29 Neldner, K.H. (1980). The zinc compound test. *Arch. Dermatol.* 116 (1): 39–40.

30 Lansdown, A.B. and Sampson, B. (1997). Trace metals in keratinising epithelia in beagle dogs. *Vet. Rec.* 141 (22): 571–572.

31 Hurley, L.S. and Swenerton, H. (1971). Lack of mobilization of bone and liver zinc under teratogenic conditions of zinc deficiency in rats. *J. Nutr.* 101 (5): 597–603.

32 Council, N.R. (1985). *Nutrient Requirements of Dogs*. Washington, D.C.: National Academy Press.

33 Underwood, E.J. (1977). *Trace Elements in Human and Animal Nutrition*, 4e. New York: Academic Press.

34 Hunt, J.R., Johnson, P.E., and Swan, P.B. (1987). Dietary conditions influencing relative zinc availability from foods to the rat and correlations with Invitro measurements. *J. Nutr.* 117 (11): 1913–1923.

35 Becker, W.M. and Hoekstra, W.G. (1971). The intestinal absorption of zinc. In: *Intestinal Absorption of Metal Ions, Trace Elements, and Radionuclides* (ed. S.C. Skoryna and D. Waldron-Edward), 229–256. Oxford: Pergamon Press.

36 Fadok, V.A. (1982). Zinc responsive dermatosis in a great-Dane – a case-report. *J. Am. Anim. Hosp. Assoc.* 18 (3): 409–414.

37 Kane, E., Morris, J.G., Rogers, Q.R. et al. (1981). Zinc-deficiency in the cat. *J. Nutr.* 111 (3): 488–495.

38 Lewis, P.K., Hoekstra, W.G., Grummer, R.H., and Phillips, P.H. (1956). The effect of certain nutritional factors including calcium, phosphorus and zinc on parakeratosis in swine. *J. Anim. Sci.* 15 (3): 741–751.

39 Miller, J.K. and Miller, W.J. (1962). Experimental zinc deficiency and recovery of calves. *J. Nutr.* 76 (4): 467–474.

40 Nelson, D.R., Wolff, W.A., Blodgett, D.J. et al. (1984). Zinc-deficiency in sheep and goats – 3 field cases. *J. Am. Vet. Med. Assoc.* 184 (12): 1480–1485.

41 Wells, B.T. and Winkelmann, R.K. (1961). Acrodermatitis Enteropathica – report of 6 cases. *Arch. Dermatol.* 84 (1): 40–52.

42 Willemse, T. (1992). Zinc-related cutaneous disorders of dogs. In: *Kirk's Current Veterinary Therapy XI* (ed. R.W. Kirk and J.D. Bonagura), 532–534. Philadelphia: W.B. Saunders.

43 Brown, R.G., Hoag, G.N., Smart, M.E., and Mitchell, L.H. (1978). Alaskan malamute chondrodysplasia. V. Decreased gut zinc absorption. *Growth* 42 (1): 1–6.

44 Colombini, S. and Dunstan, R.W. (1997). Zinc-responsive dermatosis in northern-breed dogs: 17 cases (1990–1996). *J. Am. Vet. Med. Assoc.* 211 (4): 451–453.

45 Degryse, A.D., Fransen, J., Vancutsem, J., and Ooms, L. (1987). Recurrent zinc-responsive dermatosis in a Siberian. *J. Small Anim. Pract.* 28 (8): 721–726.

46 Scott, D.W., Miller, W.H., and Griffen, C.E. (1995). Nutritional skin diseases. In: *Muller and Kirk's Small Animal Dermatology*, 5e, 897. Philadelphia: W.B. Saunders.

47 Martella, V., Elia, G., and Buonavoglia, C. (2008). Canine distemper virus. *Vet. Clin. North Am. Small Anim. Pract.* 38 (4): 787–797, vii–viii.

48 van Regenmortel, H.V.M., Fauquet, C.M., and Bishop, D.H.L. (2000). *Virus Taxonomy. Seventh Report of the International Committee on Taxonomy of Viruses.* New York: Academic Press.

49 Harder, T.C., Kenter, M., Vos, H. et al. (1996). Canine distemper virus from diseased large felids: biological properties and phylogenetic relationships. *J. Gen. Virol.* 77 (Pt 3): 397–405.

50 Roelke-Parker, M.E., Munson, L., Packer, C. et al. (1996). A canine distemper virus epidemic in Serengeti lions (Panthera leo). *Nature* 379 (6564): 441–445.

51 Appel, M.J. (1987). Canine distemper virus. In: *Virus Infection of Carnivores* (ed. M.J. Appel), 133–159. Amsterdam: Elsevier.

52 Appel, M.J. and Summers, B.A. (1995). Pathogenicity of morbilliviruses for terrestrial carnivores. *Vet. Microbiol.* 44 (2–4): 187–191.

53 Blixenkrone-Moller, M., Svansson, V., Appel, M. et al. (1992). Antigenic relationships between field isolates of morbilliviruses from different carnivores. *Arch. Virol.* 123 (3–4): 279–294.

54 Decaro, N., Camero, M., Greco, G. et al. (2004). Canine distemper and related diseases: report of a severe outbreak in a kennel. *New Microbiol.* 27 (2): 177–181.

55 Elia, G., Decaro, N., Martella, V. et al. (2006). Detection of canine distemper virus in dogs by real-time RT-PCR. *J. Virol. Methods* 136 (1–2): 171–176.

56 Appel, M.J. (1969). Pathogenesis of canine distemper. *Am. J. Vet. Res.* 30 (7): 1167–1182.

57 Iwatsuki, K., Okita, M., Ochikubo, F. et al. (1995). Immunohistochemical analysis of the lymphoid organs of dogs naturally infected with canine distemper virus. *J. Comp. Pathol.* 113 (2): 185–190.

58 Appel, M.J., Shek, W.R., and Summers, B.A. (1982). Lymphocyte-mediated immune cytotoxicity in dogs infected with virulent canine distemper virus. *Infect. Immun.* 37 (2): 592–600.

59 Winters, K.A., Mathes, L.E., Krakowka, S., and Olsen, R.G. (1983). Immunoglobulin class response to canine-distemper virus in Gnotobiotic dogs. *Vet. Immunol. Immunopathol.* 5 (2): 209–215.

60 Engelhardt, P., Wyder, M., Zurbriggen, A., and Grone, A. (2005). Canine distemper virus associated proliferation of canine footpad keratinocytes in vitro. *Vet. Microbiol.* 107 (1–2): 1–12.

61 Greene, E.C. and Appel, M.J. (1990). Canine distemper virus. In: *Infectious Diseases of the Dog and Cat* (ed. E.C. Greene), 226–241. Philadelphia: W.B. Saunders.

62 Grone, A., Doherr, M.G., and Zurbriggen, A. (2004). Canine distemper virus infection of canine footpad epidermis. *Vet. Dermatol.* 15 (3): 159–167.

63 Grone, A., Doherr, M.G., and Zurbriggen, A. (2004). Up-regulation of cytokeratin expression in canine distemper virus-infected canine footpad epidermis. *Vet. Dermatol.* 15 (3): 168–174.

64 Mac, I.A., Trevan, D.J., and Montgomerie, R.F. (1948). Observations on canine encephalitis. *Vet. Rec.* 60 (49): 635–644.

65 Koutinas, A.F., Baumgartner, W., Tontis, D. et al. (2004). Histopathology and immunohistochemistry of canine distemper virus-induced footpad hyperkeratosis (hard pad disease) in dogs with natural canine distemper. *Vet. Pathol.* 41 (1): 2–9.

66 Grone, A., Groeters, S., Koutinas, A. et al. (2003). Non-cytocidal infection of keratinocytes by canine distemper virus in the so-called hard pad disease of canine distemper. *Vet. Microbiol.* 96 (2): 157–163.

67 Scott, W.D., Miller, W.H., and Griffin, C.E. (2001). *Small Animal Dermatology.* Philadelphia: W.B. Saunders.

68 Friess, M., Engelhardt, P., Dobbelaere, D. et al. (2005). Reduced nuclear translocation of nuclear factor (NF)-kappaB p65 in the footpad epidermis of dogs infected with distemper virus. *J. Comp. Pathol.* 132 (1): 82–89.

69 Tipold, A., Vandevelde, M., and Jaggy, A. (1992). Neurological manifestations of canine-distemper virus-infection. *J. Small Anim. Pract.* 33 (10): 466–470.

70 Kimmel, S.E., Christiansen, W., and Byrne, K.P. (2003). Clinicopathological, ultrasonographic, and histopathological findings of superficial necrolytic dermatitis with hepatopathy in a cat. *J. Am. Anim. Hosp. Assoc.* 39 (1): 23–27.

71 Byrne, K.P. (1999). Metabolic epidermal necrosis-hepatocutaneous syndrome. *Vet. Clin. North Am. Small Anim. Pract.* 29 (6): 1337–1355.

72 Marinkovich, M.P., Botella, R., Datloff, J., and Sangueza, O.P. (1995). Necrolytic migratory erythema without glucagonoma in patients with liver disease. *J. Am. Acad. Dermatol.* 32 (4): 604–609.

73 Bond, R., McNeil, P.E., Evans, H., and Srebernik, N. (1995). Metabolic epidermal necrosis in two dogs with different underlying diseases. *Vet. Rec.* 136 (18): 466–471.

74 Miller, W.H., Scott, D.W., Buerger, R.G. et al. (1990). Necrolytic migratory erythema in dogs – a

Hepatocutaneous syndrome. *J. Am. Anim. Hosp. Assoc.* 26 (6): 573–581.

75 Torres, S.M.F., Caywood, D.D., OBrien, T.D. et al. (1997). Resolution of superficial necrolytic dermatitis following excision of a glucagon-secreting pancreatic neoplasm in a dog. *J. Am. Anim. Hosp. Assoc.* 33 (4): 313–319.

76 Oberkirchner, U., Linder, K.E., Zadrozny, L., and Olivry, T. (2010). Successful treatment of canine necrolytic migratory erythema (superficial necrolytic dermatitis) due to metastatic glucagonoma with octreotide. *Vet. Dermatol.* 21 (5): 510–516.

77 Gross, T.L., Song, M.D., Havel, P.J., and Ihrke, P.J. (1993). Superficial necrolytic dermatitis (necrolytic migratory erythema) in dogs. *Vet. Pathol.* 30 (1): 75–81.

11

Erythematous Wheals and Angioedema

11.1 Introduction to Terminology

Veterinary dermatologists recognize a wide variety of skin lesions. Such lesions may be primary or secondary. Primary lesions are the direct result of underlying dermatopathy. For example, consider bacterial pyoderma, which was introduced in Chapter 9, Section 9.3.4. Primary lesions for pyoderma include papules and pustules [1, 2].

11.1.1 Wheals

Allergic skin disease may also be described in terms of its primary lesion, the wheal. Sometimes referred to as a hive or a welt, a wheal is a spontaneous, focal, erythematous elevation of the skin that is caused by dermal edema [3, 4]. Wheals may be rounded or flat-topped depending upon how much fluid accumulates in the layer of skin just below the surface. Most wheals are pruritic [1, 2].

Wheals are not unique to companion animal patients. Wheals are also characteristic of allergic skin disease in humans (see Figures 11.1a–c).

Because humans lack fur, wheals are easier to identify in human patients. For the same reason, wheals are easier to see in canine and feline patients in the regions that are sparsely haired, such as the ventral abdomen and the medial thighs (see Figure 11.2).

In dogs and cats, wheals may be mistaken for those primary skin lesions that occur in bacterial folliculitis (see Figure 11.3).

Parting the overlaying fur facilitates identification of one or more wheals. When more than one wheal is present, the patient is said to have hives or urticaria [3, 5–7].

11.1.2 Angioedema

Wheals may occur with or without angioedema [3, 5–7]. Angioedema refers to significant swelling of the deeper layers of the skin, the dermis and subcutis [8]. This most often occurs at the distal extremities and head [8] (see Figures 11.4a–d).

11.1.3 Anaphylaxis

Urticaria and angioedema suggest that the patient is having an anaphylactic reaction [3]. Anaphylaxis is a severe hypersensitivity reaction that can cause fatality [3, 9–16].

Anaphylaxis may be mediated through immunoglobulin E (IgE) or alternate pathways, including IgG, immunoglobulin M (IgM), and complement system activation [13, 15, 16]. There are also non-immunologic causes of anaphylaxis, such as thermal extremes [13, 15, 16].

This chapter will focus on IgE-mediated anaphylaxis. This type of anaphylaxis relies upon histamine as a primary mediator [13]. Histamine is stored within certain cells of the body, mast cells. Mast cells are one of many components of normal connective tissue [17]. In the dog, mast cells are found in greatest numbers in the skin, lung, gut, and liver [18, 19].

Mast cells participate in inflammatory, immune, and neuroimmune responses [13]. When mast cells are activated during an anaphylactic reaction, they rapidly release mediators, including histamine. The release of histamine from mast cells increases vascular permeability [13]. This leakiness of capillaries contributes to edema, a cardinal sign of inflammation [13].

In addition to histamine, mast cell granules also contain heparin, proteases, and proteoglycans [13]. These mediators potentiate the body's inflammatory response [13].

The subsequent activation of phospholipase A magnifies inflammation through the creation of prostaglandin D2 and leukotrienes (LTB4, LTC4, LTD4, and LTE4) [13, 20–26]. Furthermore, the release of cytokines IL-4, IL-5, IL-6, IL-8, IL-9, IL-13, and IL-33, and tumor necrosis factor (TNF-α) contribute to shock [13, 27, 28].

Eighty percent of human patients who experience anaphylaxis demonstrate cutaneous signs such as urticaria [3, 9, 11, 29]. According to a 2017 study by Rostaher et al., 67% of dogs with anaphylaxis develop wheals; 70.8% develop angioedema; and 37.5% develop both [3].

In addition, because the liver is the major shock organ for dogs, many canine patients develop vomiting and diarrhea [3, 30–36].

(a)

(b)

(c)

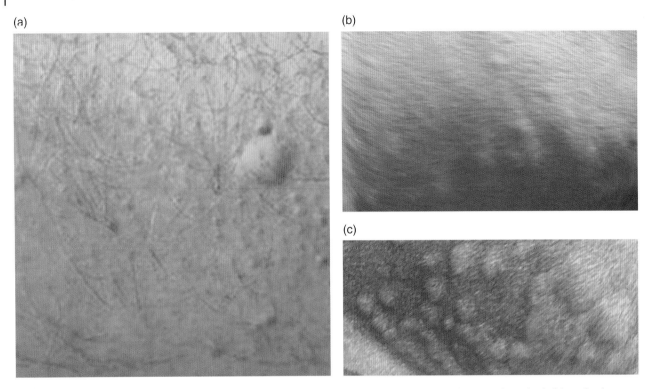

Figure 11.1 (a) Wheal in a human patient with allergic skin disease. (b) Wheals in a white-coated dog. Note how the hidden wheals appear to raise the fur. (c) Wheals in a brown-coated dog.

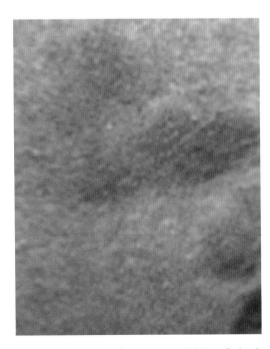

Figure 11.2 Consider the improved visibility of wheals along the ventral abdominal skin of this dog.

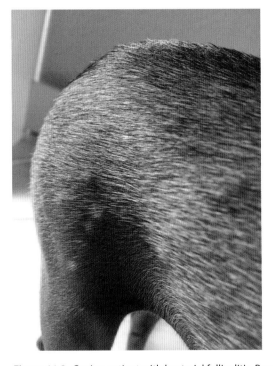

Figure 11.3 Canine patient with bacterial folliculitis. Because the primary skin lesions (papules and pustules) are hidden beneath the fur, the fur has the appearance of being elevated or raised. This gives the illusion that this patient has hives along the craniolateral right thigh. *Source:* Courtesy of Kelly Bradley, DVM.

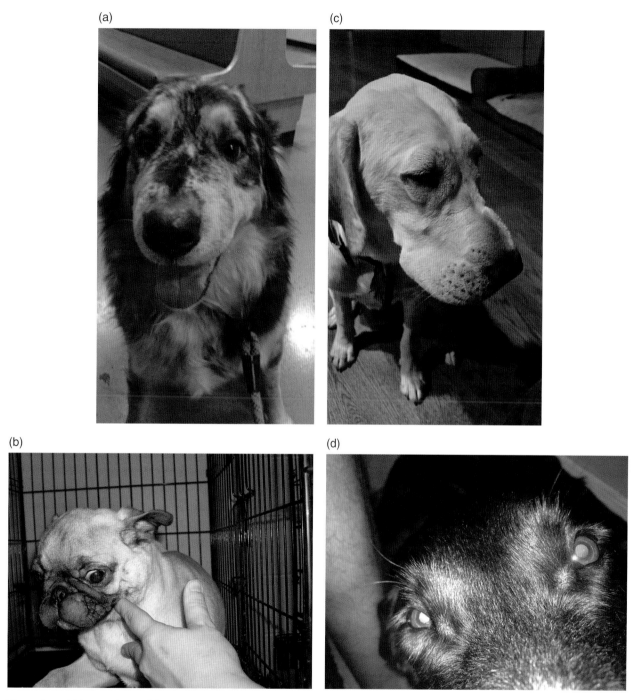

Figure 11.4 (a) Angioedema of the muzzle of a canine patient, secondary to a bee sting. *Source:* Courtesy of Lauren Bessert. (b) Facial angioedema in a Pug dog secondary to an adverse reaction to an injectable vaccination. *Source:* Courtesy of Laura Polerecky, LVT. (c) Canine angioedema without a known cause. *Source:* Courtesy of Amber May. (d) Angioedema concentrated around the right eye, resulting from an adjacent bee sting. *Source:* Courtesy of Ben Turner.

Cats, on the other hand, tend to develop respiratory distress because the lung is their primary shock organ [13, 30, 33–35, 37–40].

Additional sequelae for both dogs and cats may include hypersalivation, incoordination, and hypovolemic shock [13, 33, 41–43].

Treatment for anaphylaxis is beyond the scope of this text; however, the patient's need for care is urgent. The extent of treatment that is required depends upon each individual presentation. However, medical management is typically aimed at countering hypovolemic shock to restore blood pressure via fluid therapy and vasopressors, such as epinephrine [13]. Additionally, oxygen, antihistamines, glucocorticoids, and bronchodilators may be of immediate assistance [3, 4, 13, 33, 44, 45].

11.2 Triggers for Urticaria and Anaphylaxis

Ideally, the cause of urticaria and anaphylaxis is established to reduce the risk of recurrence secondary to re-exposure [3]. Known causes of both in companion animal patients include the following [3, 5, 21, 33, 46–55]:

- Vaccines
- Transfusions
- Envenomation
- Drugs, including anesthetic agents and radiocontrast media

Anecdotal case reports appear in the veterinary literature that suggest food may also trigger anaphylaxis in dogs [3]. Peanut ingestion by a nine-year-old Schnauzer dog and walnut ingestion by a five-year-old Vizsla dog resulted in erythematous wheals and gastrointestinal signs [56, 57].

Reports of additional triggers, such as stress, appear in the human literature [3]. Whether or not stress is a trigger for veterinary patients remains to be determined.

Because so many factors may contribute to an anaphylactic reaction, thorough history taking is essential [3]. Careful review of past pertinent medical records by the attending clinician is also critical to pinpoint any potential triggers, such as prescription drug therapy.

Additionally, when planning medical management that is known to trigger anaphylaxis, it is critical that the veterinary team anticipate potential problems and communicate these to the client before problems arise. Troubleshooting problems early is more likely to result in favorable patient outcomes.

When no overt cause of anaphylaxis has been identified through history taking or review of the patient's medical record, a diagnostic investigation is launched. This may involve intradermal testing, IgE serology, or the submission of surgical biopsies for histopathologic analysis (see Figure 11.5).

11.2.1 Vaccines as a Trigger for Urticaria and Anaphylaxis

The goal of administering immunizations is to prevent disease, both in the individual and within the population [42, 58]. Although we do not tend to think of companion animal medicine from the perspective of "herd health," that is precisely what vaccinations aim to do.

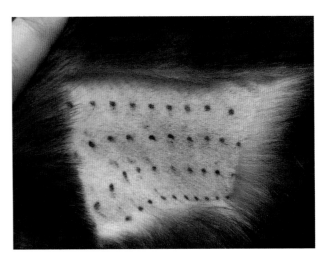

Figure 11.5 Feline intradermal skin testing. *Source:* Courtesy of Stephanie Horwitz.

No vaccine is without risk. Despite being vetted by the United States Department of Agriculture (USDA) for efficacy, potency, purity, and safety, vaccines may still cause unexpected responses or so-called adverse events [58]. The majority of these responses do not require medical management [58]. For example, vaccines often induce one to two days of general malaise, with or without fever [59]. These symptoms tend to be self-limiting [58].

However, type 1 hypersensitivity reactions may result [42, 58, 60]. When these do, they typically occur shortly after vaccination, on the order of minutes to hours [58]. Pruritus and urticaria are anticipated sequelae of type 1 hypersensitivity reactions. Gastrointestinal signs, angioedema, respiratory, and circulatory collapse are possible [58, 59]. Anaphylaxis represents a serious reaction to vaccination.

Few studies explore the frequency with which vaccine reactions, severe or otherwise, occur.

The most comprehensive study to date was conducted by Moore et al. in 2005 [61]. Electronic records from 1,226,159 dogs at 360 veterinary hospitals were examined between January 1, 2002 and December 31, 2003 for evidence of nonspecific vaccine reactions, allergic reactions, urticaria, shock, or anaphylaxis [61]. During that two-year period, there were 4,678 adverse events associated with administering 3,439,576 vaccine doses [61]. There were, in other words, 38.2 adverse events for every 10,000 dogs [61].

Additional analysis was performed on a random sample of 400 affected dogs [61]. Of these dogs, 30.8% presented with facial swelling and 20.8% presented with urticaria [61]. Fifteen percent exhibited generalized pruritus [61]. One in ten affected dogs presented with vomiting, and 8% of dogs developed vaccinated site swelling or soreness [61].

According to Moore et al., risk of vaccine reaction was proportional to the number of vaccinations that were administered on the same visit. Patients that received more than one vaccine were at greater risk of developing an adverse reaction. In dogs that weighed less than 10 kg (22 pounds), each additional vaccine that was administered increased the risk of an adverse event by 27% [61]. In dogs that weighed greater than 10 kg, each vaccination increased the risk by 12% [61].

According to Moore et al., risk of vaccine reaction was also greater in young adults. Dogs that were between one and three years of age had a 35–64% greater risk of developing a vaccine reaction as compared to those between the ages of two and nine months [61].

Certain breeds appear to be predisposed to vaccine-associated hypersensitivity reactions [42, 61]. Among small breeds of dogs, Chihuahuas, Dachshunds, Pugs, Boston terriers, and Miniature Pinschers seem more likely to experience an adverse reaction [42, 61]. Boxers are overrepresented among large breeds [42, 61].

Moore et al. also conducted a comprehensive study in 2007 to explore the frequency with which adverse responses to vaccines occur in cats [43]. Electronic records from 496,189 cats at 329 veterinary hospitals were examined between January 1, 2002 and December 31, 2004 [43]. During that three-year period, adverse events occurred in 51.6 out of every 10,000 cats [43].

Additional analysis was performed on a random sample of 1699 affected cats [43]. Of these cats, 54.2% had localized swelling or soreness at the site of vaccination [43]. Vomiting occurred in one in four cats [43]. Less than 6% of cats presented for facial swelling, and 1.9% presented for pruritus [43].

One-year-old cats appeared to be most at risk of developing an adverse reaction [43]. However, unlike canine patients, certain breeds of cats did not seem to be predisposed [43]. There was no statistically significant difference between the frequency of adverse reactions in purebreds (Siamese, Himalayan, Persian, and Maine Coon) and the frequency in Domestic short-, medium-, and long-haired cats [43].

The development of urticaria and anaphylaxis are important reasons for the veterinary profession to maintain an open dialogue with clients. Transparency in communication is essential so that patients that do react adversely to vaccinations receive the medical care that they require urgently.

The potential severity of vaccine reactions is another reason why veterinarians should re-examine vaccination protocols. The public is increasingly concerned about the possibility of over-vaccinating. It is the role of the veterinary profession to determine the validity of this concern and to continue to push for the safety and efficacy of those vaccinations that continue to be listed as core vaccinations.

However, the development of urticaria and anaphylaxis are not the only reason for vaccination protocols to be reviewed. Links have been established between the development of canine autoimmune disease and vaccination [60]. Consider, for example, such diseases as immune-mediated hemolytic anemia (IMHA), immune-mediated thrombocytopenia (IMTP), and polyarthritis [62–64]. Concerns have also been raised that implicate vaccinations in feline injection-site sarcomas [65–72].

Veterinarians are therefore responsible for conducting risk assessment in each patient. Vaccination recommendations should be tailored to the individual based upon the likelihood of exposure to disease depending upon lifestyle, among other risk factors [73].

11.2.2 Insects as a Trigger for Urticaria and Anaphylaxis

Anaphylaxis due to insect stings rarely appears in the veterinary literature. However, isolated case reports demonstrate that dogs and presumably cats are susceptible to stings from insects within the order Hymenoptera [30, 52, 74–79].

Two families of stinging insects within Hymenoptera will be considered briefly here [80]:

- The family *Apoidea*
- The family *Vespoidea*

Apoidea members include the honeybees and bumblebees, as compared to wasps, hornets, and yellow jackets, which are members of *Vespoidea*. Both deliver a sting to their target [80] (see Figures 11.6a, b).

Members of *Apoidea* deliver a single sting, after which they die. This is a function of the fact that the stinger is barbed and embeds in the target. Following the sting, the stinger is ripped out of the insect's abdomen [80].

Members of *Vespoidea*, on the other hand, lack barbs. The stinger does not remain attached to the target. This allows the stinging insect to sting the victim repeatedly, without dying [80, 81].

Neither *Apoidea* nor *Vespoidea* are capable of titrating the potency of their sting. Each sting delivers a standard amount of venom [80].

Companion animal patients may succumb to anaphylaxis after a single sting [80]. The dose that the target receives is less important than the individual's underlying sensitivity to the venom.

All patients that are stung develop localized pain and swelling. However, not all develop anaphylactic reactions; those that do present for urticaria and angioedema. The respiratory and gastrointestinal tracts may or may not be involved. Hypotension and sudden death are also potential sequelae [80].

(a)

(b)

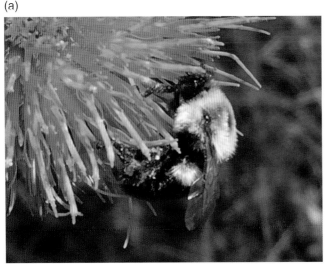

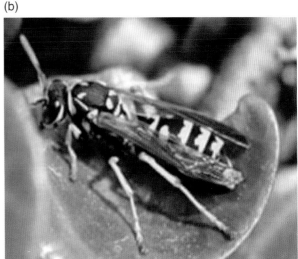

Figure 11.6 (a) Member of the family *Apoidea*. (b) Member of the family *Vespoidea*.

Rarely, patients may develop delayed hypersensitivity reactions that consist of a rash days to weeks after envenomation [80].

One case report describes acute kidney injury in a dog with pre-existing renal compromise following bee envenomation [74]. This mirrors pathology that has been reported in human victims of insect stings [82].

11.2.3 Snake Envenomation as a Trigger for Anaphylaxis

Anaphylaxis is not a typical presentation for victims of snakebite envenomation [83]. However, it is possible. Because venom is a mixture of proteins, it is capable of sensitizing the body to its constituents [83].

Patients who have previously experienced envenomation have circulating antibodies against venom proteins [83–85]. If they were to again become victims of envenomation, their bodies would be primed to react [83]. There are isolated case reports in the human medical literature of type 1 hypersensitivity reactions that are thought to be the result of circulating IgE or IgG [83].

It is reasonable to assume that the same potential exists in companion animal patients. For that reason, a brief overview of snake envenomation will be covered here.

There are two families of venomous snakes in North America [86]:

- The family *Crotalidae*
- The family *Elapidae*

Crotalids include rattlesnakes, cottonmouths, and copperheads [86]. Crotalids are colloquially referred to as pit vipers because they have a so-called pit, a heat-seeking

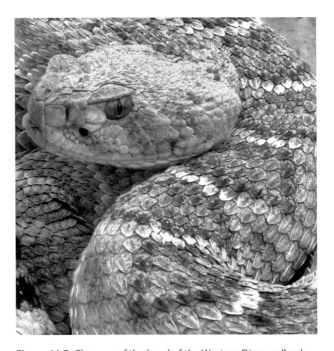

Figure 11.7 Close-up of the head of the Western Diamondback Rattlesnake, *Crotalus atrox*.

organ, between their eye and their nose [86]. In addition to this pit, other distinguishing features include diamond-shaped heads, elliptical eyes, and retractable fangs [86, 87] (see Figure 11.7).

Unlike stinging insects, crotalids can control the amount of venom that they release [86]. They may choose to empty all contents of their venom gland, for instance, when they are intending to kill their prey; or they may choose to deliver a warning dose as a defense mechanism [87]. They also have the capacity to "dry

(a)

(c)

(b)

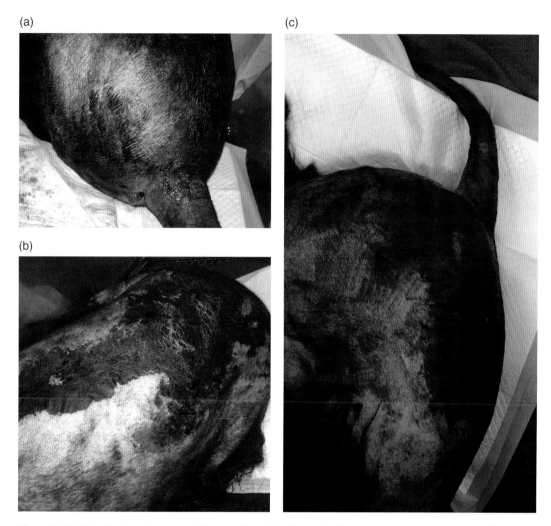

Figure 11.8 (a) Marked erythema and inflammation of the hind end of a canine patient that experienced envenomation by a pit viper. *Source:* Courtesy of Sarah McN. S. Kendig. (b) Extensive necrosis along the dorsum of a canine patient that experienced envenomation by a pit viper. *Source:* Courtesy of Sarah McN. S. Kendig. (c) Extensive necrosis along the perineum and tail of a canine patient that experienced envenomation by a pit viper. *Source:* Courtesy of Sarah McN. S. Kendig.

bite," meaning that no venom is released [86]. As many as one in four bites are "dry" [88].

Because the purpose of crotalid venom is to pre-digest prey, its contents are rich in metalloproteinases, hyaluronidases, and collagenases [86]. These collectively break apart connective tissue, driving the venom into deeper tissues. Extensive skin damage, myonecrosis, hemorrhage, and systemic inflammation result [86, 89].

Urticaria is not typically seen in cases of snake envenomation. Instead, cellulitis predominates [86].

Swelling at the bite site is pronounced. Dogs are typically bitten on the head, whereas cats tend to be bitten on the front legs [86].

Fang marks may or may not be visible. If they are, they often ooze blood or serum. Snakebites are exceedingly painful, and victims develop severe coagulopathies. Petechiations and ecchymoses are frequently identified on physical examination [86].

Tissue damage is extensive. Skin becomes necrotic rapidly [86] (see Figures 11.8a–c).

Clinical signs are more extensive in dogs than in cats. Cats may be more resistant to crotalid venom [86, 87].

Compared to crotalid envenomation, elapsid envenomation is less often associated with extreme inflammation, angioedema, and anaphylaxis. Instead, neurological presentations are more typical of coral snake envenomations. The victim tends to present with generalized muscle weakness that progresses to paralysis. Ultimately, respiratory paralysis results in death if the patient does not receive immediate medical attention [86, 90].

11.2.4 Mast Cell Tumor Degranulation as a Trigger for Urticaria and Anaphylaxis

Recall from Section 11.1.3 that mast cells are an expected population of cells in all patients. These cells play an important role in inflammatory and immune responses as a direct result of the mediators that they contain within granules.

When mast cells are called into action, they undergo degranulation; that is, they release the contents of their cytoplasmic granules into the surrounding tissues.

The granules of mast cells contain proteoglycans. This is important because certain cytological stains and dyes are capable of binding these proteoglycans, thus making it possible to identify mast cells easily in tissue, even under light microscopy [91, 92]. Mast cells appear under the microscope to be round cells that contain a variable number of purple-red cytoplasmic granules [91, 93–96] (see Figures 11.9a, b).

Degranulation serves a purpose in the normal patient. The release of cytokines by mast cells recruits other cells to the area of injury. In this way, mast cells mediate the body's response to inflammation [17].

However, mast cell tumors (MCTs) can also develop in which this cell type is overrepresented. MCTs can form anywhere, including the liver and the spleen; however, the skin is a common location for dogs [17, 97].

Some clinicians call cutaneous MCTs the "great pretender" because they have no distinct pathognomonic appearance. They truly can look like any other tumor type (see Figures 11.10a–d).

Cutaneous MCTs that are low grade and well differentiated often, but not always, appear as solitary, slow-growing nodules [96, 98]. Undifferentiated cutaneous MCTs tend to grow more rapidly and ulcerate [96, 98].

Sometimes lesions are poorly defined, particularly when they are located on distal extremities [91]. Here, they may be mistaken for acral lick dermatitis based upon gross appearance [91].

Because cutaneous MCTs do not have a classic appearance, the differential diagnosis list for any cutaneous mass should always include MCT [91, 99]. Fine-needle aspiration is an important diagnostic tool because it allows for cytological examination, which is diagnostic [91].

Any dog can develop a MCT. However, certain breeds appear to have a predisposition for their development. These breeds include Boxers, Boston terriers, English Bulldogs, Bull terriers, Staffordshire terriers, Cocker spaniels, Labrador retrievers, Golden Retrievers, and Schnauzers [17, 91, 94, 96, 100–105].

There does not appear to be predisposition for MCTs based upon gender [91, 98, 100, 104–107].

Most dogs are between 7.5 and 9 years of age at the time of diagnosis [91, 93, 94, 98, 99, 104–111]. However, MCTs have been diagnosed in canine patients less than six months of age [108, 112, 113]. Boxers also appear more likely to develop MCTs at younger ages than other breeds [105, 109].

Patients with cutaneous MCTs often present for evaluation of a newly discovered growth rather than for the local or systemic effects that result from mast cell degranulation [19, 91, 94, 114]. The trunk and extremities are the most common anatomic locations for cutaneous MCTs to appear in dogs [94, 102, 106, 115, 116]. The scrotum and perineum are less frequently involved [103]. Cutaneous MCTs in cats tend to concentrate on the head, neck, and trunk [117, 118].

A significant concern associated with MCT is that they can degranulate spontaneously, for example, during palpation or even during surgical manipulation of a

(a)

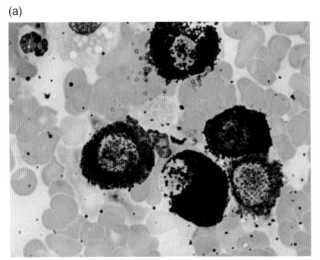

(b)

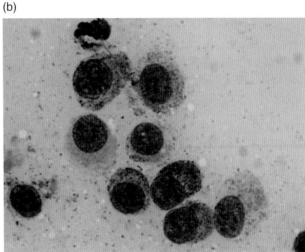

Figure 11.9 (a) Cytological appearance of mast cells degranulating. Note the deep purple staining granules. *Source:* Courtesy of Erin M. Harker, DVM. (b) Additional example demonstrating the classic cytological appearance of mast cells.

cutaneous mass [17, 18, 94, 98, 99]. This may result in systemic effects due to histamine release. If severe enough, the release of histamine into the circulation may cause gastric and duodenal ulceration [17, 119, 120].

Histamine release may also induce anaphylaxis [17, 121]. Surgical manipulation of MCTs therefore presents great risk to the patient if the patient is not pre-medicated with prophylactic gastroprotectants and antihistamines to combat anticipated degranulation.

11.2.5 Prescription Drugs as a Trigger for Urticaria and Anaphylaxis

All medications have the potential to cause harm. When medications are prescribed or administered to the patient, the clinician must take care to weigh the anticipated benefits against the potential for adverse outcomes.

A handful of drugs have been reported to cause anaphylactic reactions. Although the incidence is low and case

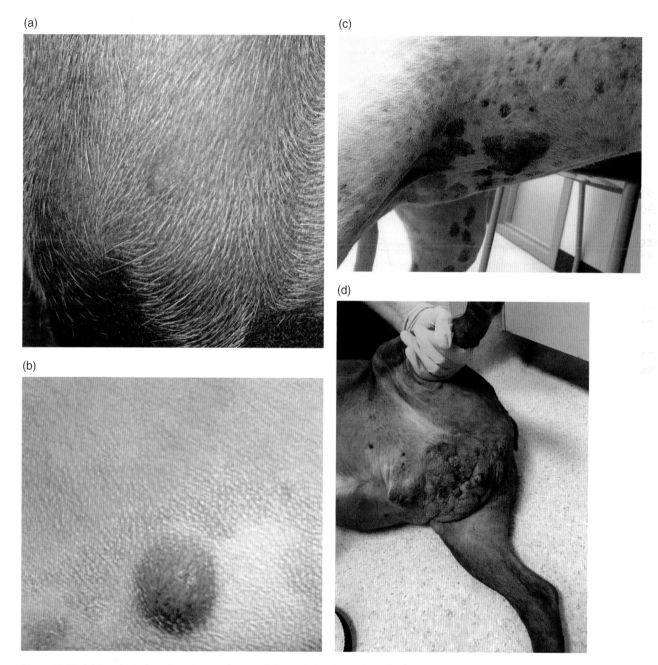

Figure 11.10 (a) Papular lesion along the cranioventral chest of a canine patient. This lesion was subsequently diagnosed as a mast cell tumor (MCT) via fine-needle aspirate cytology. (b) Raised cutaneous MCT along the ventrum of a canine patient. (c) Ulcerated MCT along the ventral abdomen of a canine patient. (d) Extensive inguinal MCT in a canine patient. *Source:* Courtesy of Beki Cohen Regan, DVM, DACVIM (Oncology).

reports are sporadic, medication-induced anaphylaxis is a real phenomenon. For patient safety, it is therefore imperative that clinicians be cognizant of what they are administering and what ill effects these agents may potentially cause.

Propofol is one such drug that has been known to cause anaphylactic reactions in humans and dogs alike [122]. Propofol is an injectable agent that is administered to induce anesthesia. During brief, invasive procedures, it may also be used to maintain anesthesia. Given that it is injected, propofol is produced in liquid form as a drug suspended in an emulsion of egg yolk lecithin and soybean oil [122]. Both eggs and soy have been implicated in food allergies in dogs [123].

Humans who have underlying allergies to eggs and/or soy are at risk for developing propofol-induced anaphylaxis [122, 124, 125]. Although the risk that muscle relaxants, latex, antibiotics, colloids, and sedatives will lead to an anaphylactic reaction is much greater, anesthesiologists are reluctant to administer propofol to humans with known egg or soy allergies [122, 126, 127].

Propofol is routinely used in anesthetic plans for canine patients [122]. A 2017 study by Onuma et al. was the first of its kind to evaluate the risk of using propofol in egg- or soy-allergic canine patients [122]. Although the number of patients that were enrolled in the study was low [21], dogs that tested with high levels of IgE against egg/chicken or soy were more likely to react adversely, with anaphylactic reactions, than those without [122]. For the purposes of this study, anaphylactic reactions included flushing of the skin; hypotension; significant respiratory depression, more so than would be expected secondary to propofol administration; and respiratory arrest [122].

Caution must therefore be taken when administering propofol to veterinary patients, most of whom will not have been previously tested for food allergies. If anaphylaxis is going to result, it is most likely to occur within two to three minutes following propofol administration [122, 125, 128]. Being prepared to respond appropriately to an anaphylactic reaction is an important step toward managing patient safety. Patients with known prior reactions to propofol should receive alternate induction and/or maintenance agents.

Isolated anecdotal reports also suggest that certain agents in topical ophthalmic preparations may induce anaphylaxis in feline patients [41, 129]. Topical antimicrobial agents are routinely prescribed in clinical practice to manage such presenting complaints as conjunctivitis, keratitis, and corneal ulceration [41]. Commonly prescribed preparations include bacitracin, neomycin, and polymyxin B (BNP), with or without a corticosteroid. These agents may also be used in combination with a

lubricant to moisten the ocular surface when it is compromised, as from keratoconjunctivitis sicca [41].

Historically, neomycin has been blamed for anaphylactoid reactions in cats. However, a 2011 study by Hume-Smith et al. determined that polymyxin B, not neomycin, was present in ophthalmic preps that had been given to 61 cats that experienced anaphylaxis within 4 hours of topical administration [41]. Roughly half of the cats experienced anaphylaxis much more quickly, within 10 minutes of receiving the drug [41].

Unfortunately, extraneous variables make it impossible at this time to make a definitive link between polymyxin B and anaphylaxis. For example, the case report by Plunkett in 2000 describes a cat that developed anaphylaxis following administration of both proparacaine and neomycin-polymyxin-corticosteroid [129]. Proparacaine could have caused the anaphylactic reaction as opposed to polymyxin. Alternatively, the patient could have been sensitive to neomycin or the corticosteroid.

The take-away message from these anecdotes is that all medications, not just injectable ones, have the potential for adverse effects. Topical medications are often considered benign. However, these medications may also result in fatalities [41]. Clinicians should therefore strive to be cautious in their approach to the treatment of ocular maladies. For example, when treating conjunctivitis, clinicians should avoid the tendency to prescribe ophthalmic antimicrobial agents unless the causative agent of the conjunctivitis has been confirmed [41].

It may be particularly prudent to avoid the use of preparations that include polymyxin B in cats whenever possible because neurotoxicity, including neuromuscular blockade, has also been reported as a potential and severe adverse effect [41, 130–132].

11.3 Differential Diagnoses for Facial Swelling

Recall that angioedema is suggestive that a patient is having an anaphylactic reaction. However, it is important to note that anaphylaxis is not the only cause of facial swelling. There are other causes of facial swelling that can mirror angioedema.

Consider, for example, canine juvenile cellulitis. This condition, also known as puppy strangles, typically targets canine patients less than four months old [133]. These patients present with progressive cutaneous lesions including pustules, crusts, and alopecic patches at the muzzle and peri-ocular skin [133]. Facial lesions frequently spread. Pinnal, ventral abdominal, genital, and perineal involvement is common [133].

Mandibular lymphadenopathy develops [133]. As lymph nodes in this region enlarge, they create the illusion of a puffy face and neck.

The seasoned clinician will not mistake canine juvenile cellulitis for angioedema secondary to anaphylaxis [133]. The appearance of the former, paired with the history, is sufficient for a presumptive diagnosis. However, as veterinary students make their way onto the clinic floor, many are experiencing most of clinical practice for the very first time. Were a patient with puppy strangles to present on emergency, it is easy to see how they might consider anaphylaxis as a differential diagnosis.

Congenital or fetal anasarca is another condition that is characterized by extensive swelling. Colloquially, congenital anasarca is referred to as the "water baby" or "walrus baby" defect [134, 135]. More commonly seen in brachycephalic breeds, affected patients retain excessive amounts of water in utero [134, 135]. Because these newborns are so edematous, they frequently block the entrance to the birth canal. This obstruction causes dystocia [134, 135].

When delivered via cesarean section, the condition of these pups is unmistakable: they look like miniature water balloons (see Figure 11.11).

The case presentation for anasarca is difficult to mistake for any other condition if the clinician is experienced and/or if s/he has been provided with the history and patient signalment, specifically the age.

However, to the novice, the patient depicted in Figure 11.11 may bear a striking resemblance to one suffering from angioedema.

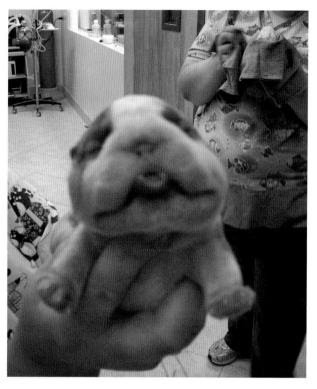

Figure 11.11 The classic appearance of congenital anasarca in an English bulldog puppy that was delivered via cesarean section.

Therefore, it is important for any clinician-in-training to consider all possibilities and to recall the importance of both taking a comprehensive case history and performing a thorough physical examination.

References

1 Rijnberk, A. and van Sluijs, F.J. (2009). *Medical History and Physical Examination in Companion Animals*, 2e, viii, 333 p. Edinburgh; New York: Saunders/Elsevier.

2 Miller, W.H., Griffin, C.E., Campbell, K.L. et al. (2013). *Muller & Kirk's Small Animal Dermatology*, 7e, ix, 938 p. St. Louis, Mo.: Elsevier.

3 Rostaher, A., Hofer-Inteeworn, N., Kummerle-Fraune, C. et al. (2017). Triggers, risk factors and clinico-pathological features of urticaria in dogs – a prospective observational study of 24 cases. *Vet. Dermatol.* 28 (1): 38–e9.

4 Nast, A., Griffiths, C.E., Hay, R. et al. (2016). The 2016 international league of dermatological societies' revised glossary for the description of cutaneous lesions. *Br. J. Dermatol.* 174 (6): 1351–1358.

5 Hill, P. (2014). Canine urticaria and angioedema. In: *Veterinary Allergy* (ed. C. Noli, A.P. Foster and W. Rosenkrantz), 195–200. Somerset, N.J.: Wiley.

6 Prelaud, P. (2008). Urticaria and angio-edema. In: *A Practical Guide to Canine Dermatology* (ed. E. Guaguere and P. Prelaud), 265–269. Paris: Merial.

7 Miller, W.H., Griffin, C.E., and Campbell, K.L. (2013). Hypersensitivity disorders. In: *Muller and Kirk's Small Animal Dermatology*, 363–432. St. Louis, M.O.: Elsevier Mosby.

8 Moellman, J.J., Bernstein, J.A., Lindsell, C. et al. (2014). A consensus parameter for the evaluation and management of angioedema in the emergency department. *Acad. Emerg. Med.* 21 (4): 469–484.

9 Brown, S.G. (2004). Clinical features and severity grading of anaphylaxis. *J. Allergy Clin. Immunol.* 114 (2): 371–376.

10 Dhami, S., Panesar, S.S., Roberts, G. et al. (2014). Management of anaphylaxis: a systematic review. *Allergy* 69 (2): 168–175.

11 Sampson, H.A., Munoz-Furlong, A., Campbell, R.L. et al. (2006). Second symposium on the definition and management of anaphylaxis: summary report--second National Institute of allergy and infectious disease/food allergy and anaphylaxis network symposium. *Ann. Emerg. Med.* 47 (4): 373–380.

12 Muraro, A., Roberts, G., Worm, M. et al. (2014). Anaphylaxis: guidelines from the European academy of allergy and clinical immunology. *Allergy* 69 (8): 1026–1045.

13 Shmuel, D.L. and Cortes, Y. (2013). Anaphylaxis in dogs and cats. *J. Vet. Emerg. Crit. Care (San Antonio)* 23 (4): 377–394.

14 Lucke, W.C. and Thomas, H. Jr. (1983). Anaphylaxis: pathophysiology, clinical presentations and treatment. *J. Emerg. Med.* 1 (1): 83–95.

15 Simons, F.E. (2008). 9. Anaphylaxis. *J. Allergy Clin. Immunol.* 121 (2 Suppl): S402–S407; quiz S20.

16 Simons, F.E., Ardusso, L.R., Bilo, M.B. et al. (2011). World Allergy Organization anaphylaxis guidelines: summary. *J. Allergy Clin. Immunol.* 127 (3): 587–593; e1–22.

17 Misdorp, W. (2004). Mast cells and canine mast cell tumours. A review. *Vet. Q.* 26 (4): 156–169.

18 Dean, P.W. (1988). Mast-cell tumors in dogs – diagnosis, treatment, and prognosis. *Vet. Med.* 83 (2): 185–188.

19 O'Keefe, D.A. (1990). Canine mast cell tumors. *Vet. Clin. North Am. Small Anim. Pract.* 20 (4): 1105–1115.

20 Johnson, R.F. and Peebles, R.S. (2004). Anaphylactic shock: pathophysiology, recognition, and treatment. *Semin. Respir. Crit. Care Med.* 25 (6): 695–703.

21 Schaer, M., Ginn, P.E., and Hanel, R.M. (2005). A case of fatal anaphylaxis in a dog associated with a dexamethasone suppression test. *J. Vet. Emerg. Crit. Care* 15 (3): 213–216.

22 Khan, B.Q. and Kemp, S.F. (2011). Pathophysiology of anaphylaxis. *Curr. Opin. Allergy Clin. Immunol.* 11 (4): 319–325.

23 Strait, R.T., Morris, S.C., and Finkelman, F.D. (2006). IgG-blocking antibodies inhibit IgE-mediated anaphylaxis in vivo through both antigen interception and Fc gamma RIIb cross-linking. *J. Clin. Invest.* 116 (3): 833–841.

24 Jonsson, F., Mancardi, D.A., Kita, Y. et al. (2011). Mouse and human neutrophils induce anaphylaxis. *J. Clin. Investig.* 121 (4): 1484–1496.

25 Lieberman, P. (2003). Anaphylaxis and anaphylactoid reactions. In: *Middleton's Allergy: Principles and Practice*, 6e (ed. N.F. Adkinson, J.W. Yunginger and W.W. Busse), 1497–1522. St. Louis, MO: Mosby-Year Book.

26 Tran, P.T. and Muelleman, R.L. (2006). Allergy, hypersensitivity and anaphylaxis. In: *Rosen's Emergency Medicine: Concepts and Clinical Practice* (ed. J.A. Marx, R.S. Hockberger and R.M. Walls), 1818–1838. Philadelphia: Mosby Elsevier.

27 Pushparaj, P.N., Tay, H.K., H'Ng, S.C. et al. (2009). The cytokine interleukin-33 mediates anaphylactic shock. *Proc. Natl. Acad. Sci. U. S. A.* 106 (24): 9773–9778.

28 Simons, F.E. (2009). Anaphylaxis: recent advances in assessment and treatment. *J. Allergy Clin. Immunol.* 124 (4): 625–636; quiz 37–8.

29 Ditto, A.M., Harris, K.E., Krasnick, J. et al. (1996). Idiopathic anaphylaxis: a series of 335 cases. *Ann. Allergy Asthma Immunol.* 77 (4): 285–291.

30 Wadell, L. (2010). Systemic anaphylaxis. In: *Textbook of Veterinary Internal Medicine Expert Consult*, 7e (ed. S. Ettinger and E.C. Feldman), 531–534. Paris: Saunders.

31 Akcasu, A. and West, G.B. (1960). Anaphylaxis in the dog. *Int. Arch. Allergy Appl. Immunol.* 16: 326–335.

32 Dean, H.R. and Webb, R.A. (1924). The morbid anatomy and histology of anaphylaxis in the dog. *J. Pathol. Bacteriol.* 27: 51–64.

33 Dowling, P.M. (2015). Anaphylaxis. In: *Small Animal Critical Care Medicine* (ed. D.C.S. Hopper), 807–811. St. Louis, M.O.: W.B. Saunders.

34 Quantz, J.E., Miles, M.S., Reed, A.L., and White, G.A. (2009). Elevation of alanine transaminase and gallbladder wall abnormalities as biomarkers of anaphylaxis in canine hypersensitivity patients. *J. Vet. Emerg. Crit. Care (San Antonio)* 19 (6): 536–544.

35 Cohen, R.D. (1995). Systemic anaphylaxis. In: *Kirk's Current Veterinary Therapy XII: Small Animal Practice* (ed. J.D. Bonagura and R.W. Kirk), 458–460. Philadelphia: W.B. Saunders.

36 Boothe, D.M. (2002). Adverse reactions to therapeutic drugs in the CCU patient. In: *The Veterinary ICU Book* (ed. W.E. Wingfield and M.R. Raffe), 1049–1056. Jackson Hole, WY: Teton New Media.

37 Litster, A. and Atwell, R. (2006). Physiological and haematological findings and clinical observations in a model of acute systemic anaphylaxis in Dirofilaria immitis-sensitised cats. *Aust. Vet. J.* 84 (5): 151–157.

38 Aitken, I.D. and McCusker, H.B. (1969). Feline anaphylaxis: some observations. *Vet. Rec.* 84 (3): 58–61.

39 McCusker, H.B. and Aitken, I.D. (1966). Anaphylaxis in the cat. *J. Pathol. Bacteriol.* 91 (1): 282–285.

40 Greenberger, P.A., Rotskoff, B.D., and Lifschultz, B. (2007). Fatal anaphylaxis: postmortem findings and associated comorbid diseases. *Ann. Allergy Asthma Immunol.* 98 (3): 252–257.

41 Hume-Smith, K.M., Groth, A.D., Rishniw, M. et al. (2011). Anaphylactic events observed within 4 h of ocular application of an antibiotic-containing ophthalmic preparation: 61 cats (1993–2010). *J. Feline Med. Surg.* 13 (10): 744–751.

42 Moore, G.E. and HogenEsch, H. (2010). Adverse vaccinal events in dogs and cats. *Vet. Clin. North Am. Small Anim. Pract.* 40 (3): 393–407.

43 Moore, G.E., DeSantis-Kerr, A.C., Guptill, L.F. et al. (2007). Adverse events after vaccine administration in cats: 2,560 cases (2002–2005). *J. Am. Vet. Med. Assoc.* 231 (1): 94–100.

44 Simons, F.E., Ardusso, L.R., Bilo, M.B. et al. (2014). International consensus on (ICON) anaphylaxis. *World Allergy Organ. J.* 7 (1): 9.

45 Worm, M., Eckermann, O., Dolle, S. et al. (2014). Triggers and treatment of anaphylaxis an analysis of 4000 cases from Germany, Austria and Switzerland. *Dtsch. Arztebl. Int.* 111 (21): 367–375.

46 Ohmori, K., Masuda, K., Sakaguchi, M. et al. (2002). A retrospective study on adverse reactions to canine vaccines in Japan. *J. Vet. Med. Sci.* 64 (9): 851–853.

47 Johnson, R.A., Simmons, K.T., Fast, J.P. et al. (2011). Histamine release associated with intravenous delivery of a fluorocarbon-based sevoflurane emulsion in canines. *J. Pharm. Sci.* 100 (7): 2685–2692.

48 Armitage-Chan, E. (2010). Anaphylaxis and anaesthesia. *Vet. Anaesth. Analg.* 37 (4): 306–310.

49 Day, M.J. (2005). The canine model of dietary hypersensitivity. *Proc. Nutr. Soc.* 64 (4): 458–464.

50 Teuber, S.S., Del Val, G., Morigasaki, S. et al. (2002). The atopic dog as a model of peanut and tree nut food allergy. *J. Allergy Clin. Immunol.* 110 (6): 921–927.

51 Boord, M. (2014). Venomous insect hypersensitivity. In: *Veterinary Allergy* (ed. C. Noli, A.P. Foster and W. Rosenkrantz), 191–194. Somerset, NJ: Wiley.

52 Cowell, A.K., Cowell, R.L., Tyler, R.D., and Nieves, M.A. (1991). Severe systemic reactions to hymenoptera stings in three dogs. *J. Am. Vet. Med. Assoc.* 198 (6): 1014–1016.

53 Tocci, L.J. (2010). Transfusion medicine in small animal practice. *Vet. Clin. North Am. Small Anim. Pract.* 40 (3): 485–494.

54 Rosenberg, M., Patterson, R., Kelly, J.F., and Harris, K.E. (1977). Acute urticaria and bronchospasm following radiographic contrast-media in a dog. *J. Allergy Clin. Immunol.* 59 (4): 339–340.

55 Edom, G. (2002). The uncertainty of the toxic effect of stings from the urtica nettle on hunting dogs. *Vet. Hum. Toxicol.* 44 (1): 42–44.

56 Kang, M.H. and Park, H.M. (2012). Putative peanut allergy-induced urticaria in a dog. *Can. Vet. J.* 53 (11): 1203–1206.

57 Rostaher, A., Fischer, N.M., Kummerle-Fraune, C. et al. (2017). Probable walnut-induced anaphylactic reaction in a dog. *Vet. Dermatol.* 28 (2): 251–e66.

58 Davis-Wurzler, G.M. (2006). Current vaccination strategies in puppies and kittens. *Vet. Clin. North Am. Small Anim. Pract.* 36 (3): 607–640, vii.

59 Tizard, I. (2004). The use of vaccines. In: *Veterinary Immunology: An Introduction*, 259–271. Philadelphia: Saunders Elsevier.

60 Day, M.J. (2006). Vaccine side effects: fact and fiction. *Vet. Microbiol.* 117 (1): 51–58.

61 Moore, G.E., Guptill, L.F., Ward, M.P. et al. (2005). Adverse events diagnosed within three days of vaccine administration in dogs. *J. Am. Vet. Med. Assoc.* 227 (7): 1102–1108.

62 McAnulty, J.F. and Rudd, R.G. (1985). Thrombocytopenia associated with vaccination of a dog with a modified-live paramyxovirus vaccine. *J. Am. Vet. Med. Assoc.* 186 (11): 1217–1219.

63 Duval, D. and Giger, U. (1996). Vaccine-associated immune-mediated hemolytic anemia in the dog. *J. Vet. Intern. Med.* 10 (5): 290–295.

64 Kohn, B., Garner, M., Lubke, S. et al. (2003). Polyarthritis following vaccination in four dogs. *Vet. Comp. Orthopaed.* 16 (1): 6–10.

65 Meyer, E.K. (2001). Vaccine-associated adverse events. *Vet. Clin. North Am. Small Anim. Pract.* 31 (3): 493–514, vi.

66 Lester, S., Clemett, T., and Burt, A. (1996). Vaccine site-associated sarcomas in cats: clinical experience and a laboratory review (1982–1993). *J. Am. Anim. Hosp. Assoc.* 32 (2): 91–95.

67 Kass, P.H., Barnes, W.G. Jr., Spangler, W.L. et al. (1993). Epidemiologic evidence for a causal relation between vaccination and fibrosarcoma tumorigenesis in cats. *J. Am. Vet. Med. Assoc.* 203 (3): 396–405.

68 Hendrick, M.J. (1999). Feline vaccine-associated sarcomas. *Cancer Investig.* 17 (4): 273–277.

69 Hendrick, M.J. and Brooks, J.J. (1994). Postvaccinal sarcomas in the cat: histology and immunohistochemistry. *Vet. Pathol.* 31 (1): 126–129.

70 Hendrick, M.J. and Goldschmidt, M.H. (1991). Do injection site reactions induce fibrosarcomas in cats? *J. Am. Vet. Med. Assoc.* 199 (8): 968.

71 Hendrick, M.J., Kass, P.H., McGill, L.D., and Tizard, I.R. (1994). Postvaccinal sarcomas in cats. *J. Natl. Cancer Inst.* 86 (5): 341–343.

72 Hendrick, M.J., Shofer, F.S., Goldschmidt, M.H. et al. (1994). Comparison of fibrosarcomas that developed at vaccination sites and at nonvaccination sites in cats: 239 cases (1991–1992). *J. Am. Vet. Med. Assoc.* 205 (10): 1425–1429.

73 Glickman, L.T. (1999). Weighing the risks and benefits of vaccination. *Adv. Vet. Med.* 41: 701–713.

74 Buckley, G.J., Corrie, C., Bandt, C., and Schaer, M. (2017). Kidney injury in a dog following bee sting-associated anaphylaxis. *Can. Vet. J.* 58 (3): 265–269.

75 Thomas, E., Mandell, D.C., and Waddell, L.S. (2013). Survival after anaphylaxis induced by a bumblebee

sting in a dog. *J. Am. Anim. Hosp. Assoc.* 49 (3): 210–215.

76 Waddell, L.S. and Drobatz, K.J. (1999). Massive envenomation by Vespula spp in two dogs. *J. Vet. Emerg. Crit. Care* 9 (2): 67–71.

77 Noble, S.J. and Armstrong, P.J. (1999). Bee sting envenomation resulting in secondary immune-mediated hemolytic anemia in two dogs. *J. Am. Vet. Med. Assoc.* 214 (7): 1026–1027, 1.

78 Walker, T., Tidwell, A.S., Rozanski, E.A. et al. (2005). Imaging diagnosis: acute lung injury following massive bee envenomation in a dog. *Vet. Radiol. Ultrasound* 46 (4): 300–303.

79 Wysoke, J.M., Bland van-den Berg, P., and Marshall, C. (1990). Bee sting-induced haemolysis, spherocytosis and neural dysfunction in three dogs. *J. S. Afr. Vet. Assoc.* 61 (1): 29–32.

80 Fitzgerald, K.T. and Flood, A.A. (2006). Hymenoptera stings. *Clin. Tech. Small Anim. Pract.* 21 (4): 194–204.

81 Goddard, J. (2000). *Physician's Guide to Arthropods of Medical Importance*. Philadelphia: W.B. Saunders.

82 Bresolin, N.L., Carvalho, L.C., Goes, E.C. et al. (2002). Acute renal failure following massive attack by Africanized bee stings. *Pediatr. Nephrol.* 17 (8): 625–627.

83 Ryan, K.C. and Caravati, E.M. (1994). Life-threatening anaphylaxis following envenomation by 2 different species of Crotalidae. *J. Wilderness Med.* 5 (3): 263–268.

84 Kopp, P., Dahinden, C.A., and Mullner, G. (1993). Allergic reaction to snake-venom after repeated bites of vipera-aspis. *Clin. Exp. Allergy* 23 (3): 231–232.

85 Wadee, A.A. and Rabson, A.R. (1987). Development of specific IgE antibodies after repeated exposure to snake-venom. *J. Allergy Clin. Immunol.* 80 (5): 695–698.

86 Gilliam, L.L. and Brunker, J. (2011). North American snake envenomation in the dog and cat. *Vet. Clin. North Am. Small Anim. Pract.* 41 (6): 1239–1259.

87 Peterson, M.E. (2006). Snake bite: pit vipers. *Clin. Tech. Small Anim. Pract.* 21 (4): 174–182.

88 Gold, B.S. and Wingert, W.A. (1994). Snake venom poisoning in the United States: a review of therapeutic practice. *South. Med. J.* 87 (6): 579–589.

89 Holstege, C.P., Miller, M.B., Wermuth, M. et al. (1997). Crotalid snake envenomation. *Crit. Care Clin.* 13 (4): 889–921.

90 Marks, S.L., Mannella, C., and Schaer, M. (1990). Coral Snake envenomation in the dog – report of 4 cases and review of the literature. *J. Am. Anim. Hosp. Assoc.* 26 (6): 629–634.

91 Welle, M.M., Bley, C.R., Howard, J., and Rufenacht, S. (2008). Canine mast cell tumours: a review of the pathogenesis, clinical features, pathology and treatment. *Vet. Dermatol.* 19 (6): 321–339.

92 Huntley, J.F. (1992). Mast cells and basophils: a review of their heterogeneity and function. *J. Comp. Pathol.* 107 (4): 349–372.

93 Govier, S.M. (2003). Principles of treatment for mast cell tumors. *Clin. Tech. Small Anim. Pract.* 18 (2): 103–106.

94 Rabanal, R. and Ferrer, L. (eds.) (2002). *Mast Cell Tumors: From the Molecular Biology to the Clinic*. Nice: ISVD.

95 Tams, T.R. and Macy, D.W. (1981). Canine mast cell tumors. *Compend. Contin. Educ. Pract.* 17: 869–878.

96 Bostock, D.E. (1986). Neoplasms of the skin and subcutaneous tissues in dogs and cats. *Br. Vet. J.* 142 (1): 1–19.

97 London, C.A. and Seguin, B. (2003). Mast cell tumors in the dog. *Vet. Clin. North Am. Small Anim. Pract.* 33 (3): 473–489, v.

98 Thamm, D.H. and Vail, D.M. (2007). Mast cell tumors. In: *Withrow & MacEwen's Small Animal Clinical Oncology*, 4e (ed. S.J. Withrow and D.M. Vail), 402–424. St. Louis, M.O.: Saunders Elsevier.

99 Scott, D.W., Miller, W.H., and Griffin, C.G. (2001). Mast cell tumor. In: *Small Animal Dermatology*, 6e (ed. D.W. Scott, W.H. Miller and C.G. Griffin), 1320–1330. St. Louis, MO: W.B. Saunders.

100 Peters, J.A. (1969). Canine mastocytoma: excess risk as related to ancestry. *J. Natl. Cancer Inst.* 42 (3): 435–443.

101 Priester, W.A. and McKay, F.W. (1980). The occurrence of tumors in domestic animals. *Natl. Cancer Inst. Monogr.* (54): 1–210.

102 Rothwell, T.L., Howlett, C.R., Middleton, D.J. et al. (1987). Skin neoplasms of dogs in Sydney. *Aust. Vet. J.* 64 (6): 161–164.

103 Goldschmidt, M.H. and Shofer, F.S. (1992). Mast cell tumors. In: *Skin Tumors of the Dog and Cat* (ed. A.T.B. Edney), 231–251. New York: Pergamon Press.

104 Patnaik, A.K., Ehler, W.J., and MacEwen, E.G. (1984). Canine cutaneous mast cell tumor: morphologic grading and survival time in 83 dogs. *Vet. Pathol.* 21 (5): 469–474.

105 Baker-Gabb, M., Hunt, G.B., and France, M.P. (2003). Soft tissue sarcomas and mast cell tumours in dogs; clinical behaviour and response to surgery. *Aust. Vet. J.* 81 (12): 732–738.

106 Brodey, R.S. (1970). Canine and feline neoplasia. *Adv. Vet. Sci. Comp. Med.* 14: 309–354.

107 Howard, E.B., Sawa, T.R., Nielsen, S.W., and Kenyon, A.J. (1969). Mastocytoma and gastroduodenal ulceration. Gastric and duodenal ulcers in dogs with mastocytoma. *Pathol. Vet.* 6 (2): 146–158.

108 Conroy, J.D. (1983). Canine skin tumors. *J. Am. Anim. Hosp. Assoc.* 19 (1): 91–114.

109 Bensignor, E., Delisle, F., and Devauchelle, P. (1996). A retrospective study of 84 cases of mast cell tumours in dogs. In: *Advances in Veterinary Dermatology* (ed. K.W. Kwochka, T. Willemse and G. Von Tscharner), 560–561. Oxford, U.K.: Butterworth-Heinemann.

110 Bensignor, E., Fontaine, J.J., Delisle, F., and Devauchelle, P. (1996). Mast cell tumors in dogs: an anotomoclinical and therapeutical study of 85 cases. *Recl. Med. Vet.* 172 (7–8): 351–358.

111 Dobson, J.M. and Scase, T.J. (2007). Advances in the diagnosis and management of cutaneous mast cell tumours in dogs. *J. Small Anim. Pract.* 48 (8): 424–431.

112 Davis, B.J., Page, R., Sannes, P.L., and Meuten, D.J. (1992). Cutaneous mastocytosis in a dog. *Vet. Pathol.* 29 (4): 363–365.

113 Mukaratirwa, S., Chipunza, J., Chitanga, S. et al. (2005). Canine cutaneous neoplasms: prevalence and influence of age, sex and site on the presence and potential malignancy of cutaneous neoplasms in dogs from Zimbabwe. *J. S. Afr. Vet. Assoc.* 76 (2): 59–62.

114 Lemarie, R.J., Lemarie, S.L., and Hedlund, C.S. (1995). Mast-cell tumors – clinical management. *Compend. Contin. Educ. Pract.* 17 (9): 1085–1101.

115 Bostock, D.E. (1973). The prognosis following surgical removal of mastocytomas in dogs. *J. Small Anim. Pract.* 14 (1): 27–41.

116 Sfiligoi, G., Rassnick, K.M., Scarlett, J.M. et al. (2005). Outcome of dogs with mast cell tumors in the inguinal or perineal region versus other cutaneous locations: 124 cases (1990–2001). *J. Am. Vet. Med. Assoc.* 226 (8): 1368–1374.

117 Garcia JL. (2013). Journal Scan: Feline mast cell tumors: An overview with a view to a cure. DVM360 [Internet]. http://veterinarymedicine.dvm360.com/journal-scan-feline-mast-cell-tumors-overview-with-view-cure.

118 Henry, C. and Herrera, C. (2013). Mast cell tumors in cats: clinical update and possible new treatment avenues. *J. Feline Med. Surg.* 15 (1): 41–47.

119 Byers, J.C. and Fleischman, R.W. (1981). Peptic-ulcers associated with a mast-cell tumor in a dog. *Canine Pract.* 8 (3): 42–44.

120 Fox, L.E., Rosenthal, R.C., Twedt, D.C. et al. (1990). Plasma histamine and gastrin-concentrations in 17 dogs with mast-cell tumors. *J. Vet. Intern. Med.* 4 (5): 242–246.

121 Rogers, K.S. (1996). Mast cell tumors: dilemmas of diagnosis and treatment. *Vet. Clin. North Am. Small Anim. Pract.* 26 (1): 87–102.

122 Onuma, M., Terada, M., Ono, S. et al. (2017). Incidence of anaphylactic reactions after propofol administration in dogs. *J. Vet. Med. Sci.* 79 (8): 1446–1452.

123 Jeffers, J.G., Meyer, E.K., and Sosis, E.J. (1996). Responses of dogs with food allergies to single-ingredient dietary provocation. *J. Am. Vet. Med. Assoc.* 209 (3): 608–611.

124 Cochico, S.G. (2012). Propofol allergy: assessing for patient risks. *AORN J.* 96 (4): 398–405; quiz 6–8.

125 Tashkandi, J. (2010). My patient is allergic to eggs, can i use propofol? A case report and review. *Saudi J Anaesth* 4 (3): 207–208.

126 Mertes, P.M., Alla, F., Trechot, P. et al. (2011). Groupe d'Etudes des reactions Anaphylactoides P. anaphylaxis during anesthesia in France: an 8-year national survey. *J. Allergy Clin. Immunol.* 128 (2): 366–373.

127 Masuda, K. (2014). Urticaria and anaphylaxis during anesthesia. *Arerugi* 63 (5): 682–685.

128 Laxenaire, M.C., Mata-Bermejo, E., Moneret-Vautrin, D.A., and Gueant, J.L. (1992). Life-threatening anaphylactoid reactions to propofol (Diprivan). *Anesthesiology* 77 (2): 275–280.

129 Plunkett, S.J. (2000). Anaphylaxis to ophthalmic medication in a cat. *J. Vet. Emerg. Crit. Care* 10 (3): 169–171.

130 Lee, C., Ricker, S., and Katz, R.L. (1979). Autonomic block, cardiovascular depression and histamine release produced by polymyxin B in the cat. *Can. Anaesth. Soc. J.* 26 (3): 196–200.

131 Falagas, M.E. and Kasiakou, S.K. (2006). Toxicity of polymyxins: a systematic review of the evidence from old and recent studies. *Crit. Care* 10 (1): R27.

132 Singh, Y.N., Marshall, I.G., and Harvey, A.L. (1982). Pre- and postjunctional blocking effects of aminoglycoside, polymyxin, tetracycline and lincosamide antibiotics. *Br. J. Anaesth.* 54 (12): 1295–1306.

133 Davidson, A.P. (2006). Juvenile Cellulitis. *NAVC Clinician's Brief* (March): 21–22.

134 Cunto, M., Zambelli, D., Castagnetti, C. et al. (2015). Diagnosis and treatment of Foetal anasarca in two English bulldog puppies. *Pak. Vet. J.* 35 (2): 251–253.

135 Hopper, B.J., Richardson, J.L., and Lester, N.V. (2004). Spontaneous antenatal resolution of canine hydrops fetalis diagnosed by ultrasound. *J. Small Anim. Pract.* 45 (1): 2–8.

12

Papules and Pustules

12.1 Introduction to Papules and Pustules as Primary Skin Lesions

Primary skin lesions are the result of underlying skin pathology. Recall that wheals were introduced as primary skin lesions for allergic skin disease in Chapter 11. Wheals are not the only type of primary skin lesion. Although there are several, the two most commonly identified primary skin lesions on physical examination of dogs and cats are papules and pustules.

Papules are small, solid elevations of the skin, typically measuring less than 1 cm [1] (see Figures 12.1a, b).

Papules may appear as isolated lesions, as depicted in Figures 12.1a, b, or papules may coalesce, creating a plaque (see Figures 12.2a, b).

Papules may or may not involve hair follicles [1]. Many are the result of inflammation, and appear pink or red in color [1].

Pustules are pus-filled papules [1]. The accumulated purulent material may make the lesion appear yellowish-gold (see Figure 12.3).

When pustules rupture, they leave behind a temporary "footprint" as evidence that they were once there. This "footprint" is called an epidermal collarette. An epidermal collarette is a circular rim that outlines where the pustule used to be. It consists of peeling skin that will eventually flake off (see Figures 12.4a, b).

Epidermal collarettes are secondary lesions [1].

Crusts can also be secondary lesions [1]. Crusts represent a mixture of pus, serum, and dried exudate [1]. When a pustule ruptures, its contents may be incorporated into a crust. Crusts may adhere to the fur, which makes them more likely to be seen in haired regions of the body as opposed to those regions where fur is sparse [1] (see Figures 12.5a–c).

12.2 Causes of Papules and Pustules as Primary Skin Lesions

There are many causes for the development of papules and pustules. These causes can be lumped into two main categories, infectious and noninfectious. Of these two categories, infectious causes of papules and pustules are most likely.

Papules and pustules may represent primary skin disease, as in cases of bacterial pyoderma [2, 3].

Alternatively, papules and pustules may develop secondary to an underlying condition, such as the following [1–4]:

- Demodicosis
- Dermatophytosis
- Endocrinopathies
- Ectoparasite infestation
- Hypersensitivity reactions
- Immunodeficiency syndromes
- Primary or secondary seborrhea

Papules and pustules may also result from the use of immunosuppressive drugs or the prolonged use of corticosteroids [4].

12.3 Infectious Causes of Papules and Pustules as Primary Skin Lesions

12.3.1 Canine Pyoderma

Pyoderma is a common diagnosis among canine patients that present for skin disease [5–12]. Pyoderma is the condition by which skin becomes infected [5].

When pyoderma is limited to the hair follicles and epidermis, it is considered superficial. Sometimes, this

(a) (b)

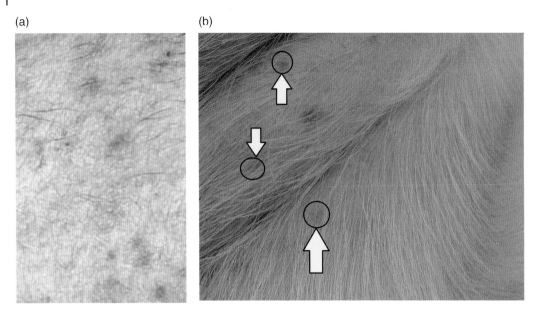

Figure 12.1 (a) Isolated papules along the ventrum of a canine patient. (b) Isolated papules along the ventral abdomen of a canine patient.

(a)

(b)

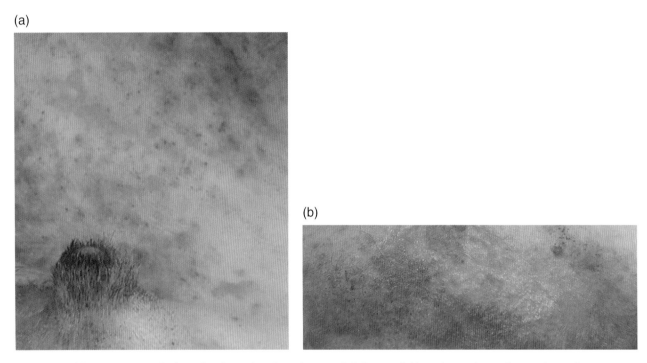

Figure 12.2 (a) Numerous papules have fused together along the ventral abdomen of this canine patient to form a plaque. *Source: Courtesy of Lori A. Stillmaker, DVM.* (b) Extensive plaque formation along the ventrum of a canine patient. *Source: Courtesy of Lori A. Stillmaker, DVM.*

condition is referred to as superficial bacterial folliculitis to indicate follicular involvement [2, 13].

Deep pyoderma involves the dermis. This condition may or may not be associated with furunculosis, deep-seated infection of tissue adjacent to the hair follicle, resulting in abscess formation [13].

In canine patients, superficial pyoderma predominates [2, 12, 14]. Most often, it is caused by commensal bacteria that constitute the normal skin flora in a healthy patient [2]. Historically, *Staphylococcus intermedius* predominated among isolates from clinical cases [3, 15, 16]. However, retrospective analysis has demonstrated that such organisms were in fact *Staphylococcus pseudintermedius* [17].

S. pseudintermedius still causes the majority of cases of superficial pyoderma in dogs that present to clinical practice today [3, 17, 18]. *S. pseudintermedius* is an opportunistic pathogen [2, 19, 20]. It quietly colonizes the skin and mucosa of healthy patients, including oral, nasal, anal, and genital sites [21].

Certain conditions and factors prime *S. pseudintermedius* to become pathogenic [22, 23]. These so-called "host factors" increase the susceptibility of certain patients to disease [3]. For example, patients with one or more endocrinopathies, underlying flea allergy dermatitis, or abnormal cornification of the skin may be predisposed to pyoderma [3]. Their skin constitutes a compromised barrier.

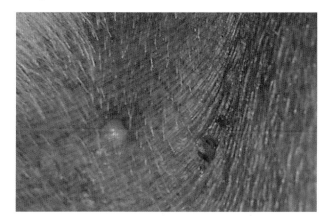

Figure 12.3 Isolated pustule along the ventral abdomen of a canine patient.

Dogs also more readily succumb to pyoderma as compared to other mammals [2, 3, 21]. This may be due to the fact that, compared to other species, dogs have a thinner stratum corneum, less intercellular lipids, and an elevated pH [13, 21].

In addition to *S. pseudintermedius*, dogs may be colonized or infected by other *Staphylococcus* sp. For example, *Staphylococcus aureus* and *Staphylococcus schleiferi* have been implicated as etiologic agents of canine superficial pyoderma [12, 24, 25].

Certain dog breeds appear to be at greater risk for development of pyoderma. These include Labrador retrievers, Golden retrievers, German Shepherds, Cocker spaniels, and West Highland White terriers, among other terrier breeds [5].

Affected dogs with pyoderma may or may not be pruritic. Pruritus, when present, may or may not be severe [3].

Papules and pustules are the classic textbook lesions for pyoderma. In the past, many clinicians instituted topical and/or systemic antibiotic therapy based upon gross appearance alone [2]. However, it is important to recognize that papules and pustules are not pathognomonic for pyoderma. Pustules may in fact be sterile [1]. Furthermore, the development of antibiotic resistant strains of *Staphylococcus*, such as methicillin-resistant *Staphylococcus pseudintermedius* (MRSP), makes it imperative that clinicians pursue definitive diagnosis, culture, and sensitivity testing [2]. Finally, not all dogs present with these classic lesions. Many shorthaired dogs with pyoderma present with moth-eaten coats in the absence of papules and pustules, and Cocker spaniels

(a)

(b)

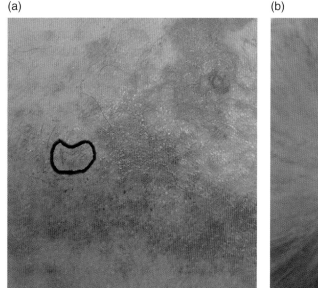
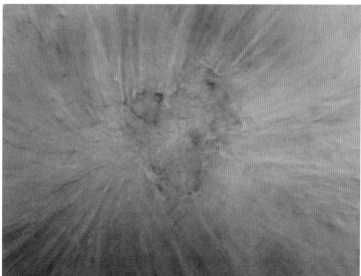

Figure 12.4 (a) Epidermal collarette along the ventrum of a canine patient. The lesion has been outlined in black. *Source:* Courtesy of Lori A. Stillmaker, DVM. (b) Epidermal collarette along the dorsum of a canine patient. *Source:* Courtesy of Crystal Melton.

(a)

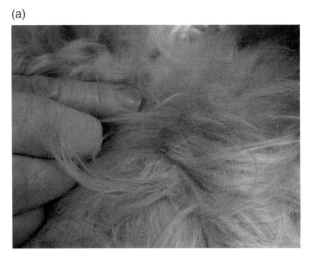

(b)   (c)

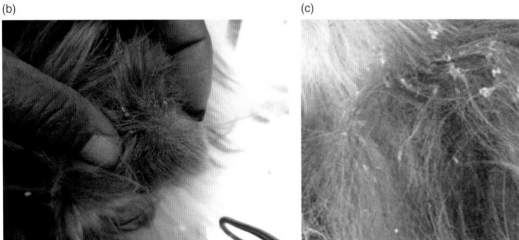

Figure 12.5 (a) Isolated crust in a canine patient. *Source:* Courtesy of Patricia Bennett, DVM. (b) Isolated crusts in a feline patient. *Source:* Courtesy of Patricia Bennett, DVM. (c) Many crusts adhered to the fur coat of a canine patient. *Source:* Courtesy of Crystal Melton.

often present with vegetative plaques that might grossly be suggestive of seborrhea [3] (see Figures 12.6a–c).

If the clinician were only looking for papules or pustules as a screening test for pyoderma, these atypical cases would escape diagnosis. The takeaway message is that dogs presenting with skin disease require dermatological work-ups [3, 12].

Skin cytology is a valuable tool that can provide rapid insight with minimal investment of time and cost [2, 3, 21]. There are a variety of methods of sample collection, depending upon the lesion type.

When patients present with one or more pustules, at least one representative lesion should be sampled. This requires the pustule to first be ruptured with a sterile needle or the edge of a microscope slide [21]. This allows for its liquid contents to be transferred onto a microscope slide by touching the slide gently to the surface of the skin that includes the lesion [21]. The exudate may be heat-fixed to the slide or allowed to

air dry. There are differences in opinion as to which method is preferred.

The dried slide is subsequently stained [21]. A common stain that is used in veterinary practice is the modified Wright's stain [21]. Commercially, this is marketed as the product, Diff-Quik.

The stained slide is then examined via light microscopy, initially under low magnification to find a region of interest. Once this region, a thin layer of material, has been identified, the magnification is raised. The oil immersion lens (1000× magnification) and bright illumination allow for the identification of bacteria [21].

Note that the modified Wright's stain cannot differentiate Gram-positive from Gram-negative bacteria. Both stain deep blue [21].

Bacteria may be extracellular or intracellular. Cytological confirmation of pyoderma involves the demonstration of bacteria within neutrophils [2, 3, 12]. Because *S. pseudintermedius* is the most common cause

(a)

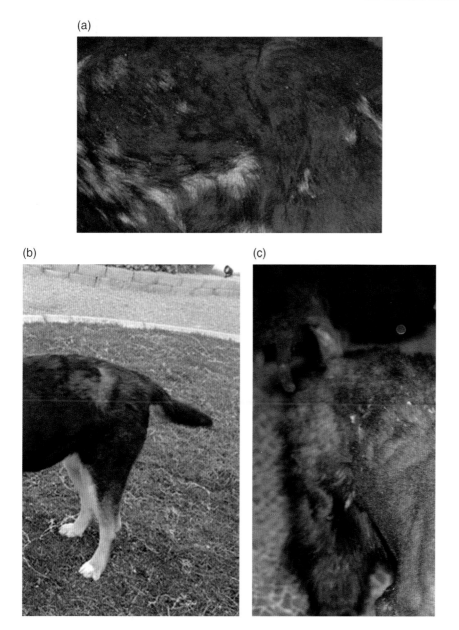

(b)

(c)

Figure 12.6 (a) The left lateral thorax and abdomen of this patient with skin disease has a moth-eaten appearance. *Source:* Courtesy of Laura Polerecky, LVT. (b) The dorsolateral left flank of this canine patient with pyoderma has a moth-eaten appearance. *Source:* Courtesy of Danielle Nicole. (c) The trunk and proximal tail of this canine patient has a moth-eaten appearance secondary to pyoderma. *Source:* Courtesy of Laura Polerecky, LVT.

of pyoderma, intracellular bacteria are typically cocci [21]. Cocci may be paired. Sometimes they form groupings or clusters [21]. The presence of intracellular bacilli is suggestive of pyoderma [21, 26]. Sometimes cytology demonstrates a mixed bacterial population. If the sample had been taken from an open wound, this can make it difficult to determine if bacteria are a byproduct of contamination or if they are in fact the primary etiologic agent [21] (see Figures 12.7a–c).

When bacteria are present, their numbers are typically estimated and lumped into a subjective rating scale [21].

For example, some clinics make use zero, +1, +2, +3, and +4 in an attempt to quantify bacterial counts. This facilitates tracking of the patient's response to treatment, once medications have been prescribed.

Note that bacteria are not the only organisms that can be identified via light microscopy. In addition, lesions may demonstrate an overgrowth of yeast, such as *Malassezia* sp. [3, 12, 21] (see Figure 12.8).

Yeast overgrowth may be secondary to pyoderma, or *Malassezia* dermatitis may have compromised the skin such that a secondary bacterial infection resulted.

(a)

(b)

(c)

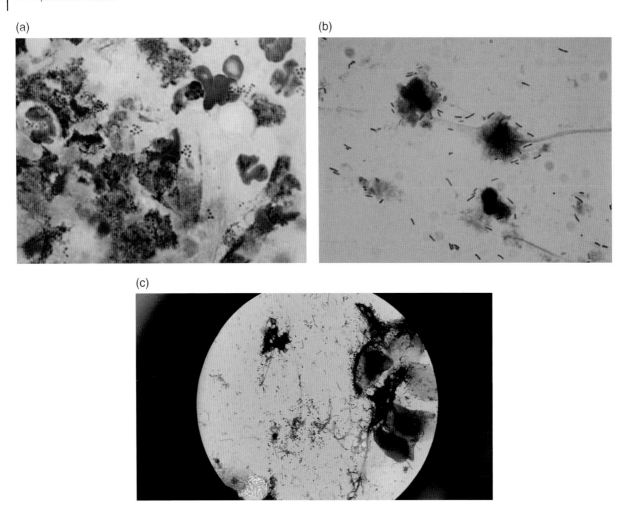

Figure 12.7 (a) Intracellular and extracellular cocci from a skin lesion. This is confirmatory for pyoderma. (b) Extracellular rod-shaped bacteria from a skin lesion. (c) Mixed bacterial population (rods and cocci) from an aural swab of a canine patient with severe otitis externa. *Source:* Courtesy of Kelli L. Crisfulli, RVT.

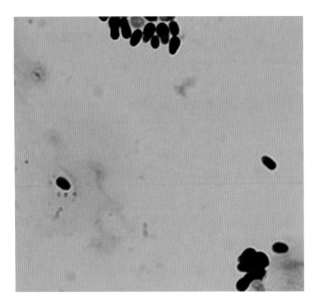

Figure 12.8 Cytological confirmation of yeast from a skin impression smear. Yeast are larger than bacteria and, if budding, demonstrate the classic shoe-print or peanut shape.

In either case, both conditions must be addressed in order for the patient to experience resolution of clinical signs.

Fungal hyphae are much less commonly seen; however, these are readily differentiated from yeast and bacteria based upon appearance alone (see Figures 12.9a, b).

In addition to evaluating cytology for bacteria, yeast, and other organisms, it is important to consider the morphology of white blood cells as these represent the body's response to an underlying infection [3]. In particular, neutrophils should be examined.

In cases of pyoderma, patients typically demonstrate neutrophilic inflammation [3, 21]. The affected neutrophils are frequently referred to as degenerate. Degenerate neutrophils have morphologic abnormalities such as swollen nuclei. This may cause the nucleus of each to appear lighter in color than is expected and smudged [21, 27].

Neutrophils may also become hypersegmented, meaning that the nucleus develops more lobes or segments than is typical [27] (see Figures 12.10a, b).

(a)

(b)

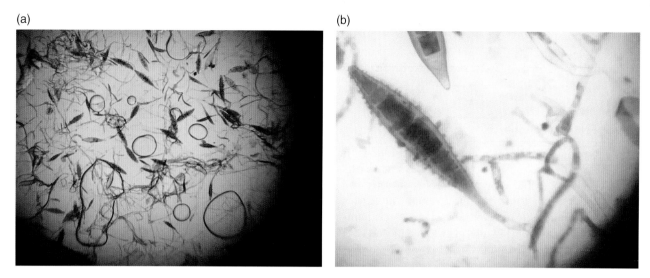

Figure 12.9 (a) Fungal hyphae of *Microsporum* sp. *Source:* Courtesy of Jennifer Lang. (b) Close-up of fungal hyphae of *Microsporum* sp. *Source:* Courtesy of Jennifer Lang.

(a)   (b)

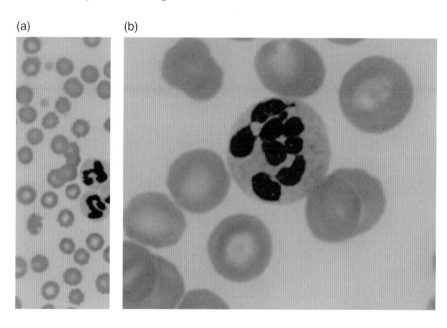

Figure 12.10 (a) Example of two normal neutrophils. Although this image is taken from a blood smear rather than skin cytology, it demonstrates the appearance of normal neutrophils. Contrast the morphology of these with the neutrophil in Figure 12.10b. (b) Example of hypersegmented neutrophil. Although this image is taken from a blood smear rather than from skin cytology, it demonstrates the increased number of lobes that is characteristic of a hypersegmented neutrophil. *Source:* Courtesy of Nora Springer, DVM, DACVP.

Infection may also cause neutrophils to rupture. These contents are evident on cytology as streaks of nuclear material [21].

Historically, antibiotic therapy for pyoderma has been initiated based upon history, physical examination findings, and cytological identification of intracellular bacteria [2, 12]. In fact, pyoderma represents one of the greatest reasons that veterinarians reach for antimicrobials in clinical practice [12, 14, 28, 29]. However, the development of antibiotic resistance, particularly among *Staphylococcus* sp., raises significant concerns about treating pyoderma without a bacterial culture and susceptibility panel [2]. In particular, methicillin resistance is a growing concern [3, 12]. When organisms are methicillin-resistant, they will not respond to treatment with any member of the beta-lactam family of antibiotics [3].

In addition, multi-drug resistance (MDR) is increasing among microbial populations. A study in 2009 by Bemis et al. demonstrated that over 90% of methicillin-resistant *S. pseudintermedius* were also multi-drug resistant [30].

To more appropriately manage the use of antibiotics for pyoderma, guidelines were recently developed and published by the Antimicrobial Guidelines Working Group of the International Society for Companion Animal Infectious Diseases [12]. These guidelines identify clinical scenarios in which bacterial culture is indicated. Bacterial culture is particularly important in cases of chronic disease or in those patients with recurrent pyoderma [2, 3, 12].

Samples for culture are ideally collected from pustules [12]. Note that a culture may be taken at any time from a pustule, even if the patient is currently receiving systemic antibiotics [2, 31].

In the event that a pustule is not available for culture, culturing an epidermal collarette or crust is also an effective strategy [3, 32, 33].

12.3.2 Feline Pyoderma

Although pyoderma is a common diagnosis in dogs, it is important to recognize that it can also occur in cats [34–37]. A 2012 publication by Scott et al. reviewed 1,407 feline cases that presented to Cornell University's Teaching Hospital and received one or more dermatological diagnoses [9]. One in ten cats was diagnosed with bacterial folliculitis [9]. Unlike dogs, cats do not appear to have breed predilections [34].

Cats with bacterial infections of the skin often have concurrent disease such as allergic skin disease, secondary to food or fleas [34, 38–40]. Mange mite infestations, including *Demodex* sp. and *Notoedres cati,* may also contribute to secondary infection [34].

When pyoderma occurs in cats, the condition may mirror the clinical appearance that is seen in dogs. More commonly, however, feline pyoderma presents as superficial crusts and erosions. This presentation is often referred to as miliary dermatitis in the veterinary literature [34, 40] (see Figure 12.11).

Other lesions, such as "rodent ulcers" and eosinophilic plaques, are often seen concurrently with feline pyoderma [34, 41, 42] (see Figures 12.12a, b).

Diagnosis of pyoderma in the cat is the same as in the dog: a supportive history, compatible physical examination findings, and cytological demonstration of inflammatory changes in neutrophils and intracellular bacteria [41].

The challenge associated with feline pyoderma is in recognizing that the classic appearance of it as is seen in dogs does not always present in cats. Cats may have atypical lesions or lesions that are less characteristic. This reiterates the need for a diagnostic work-up, rather than basing treatment decisions on gross appearance alone.

(a)

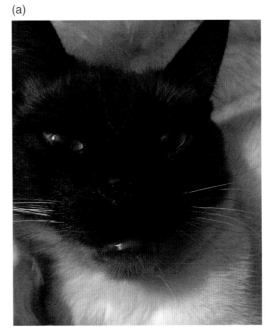

(b)

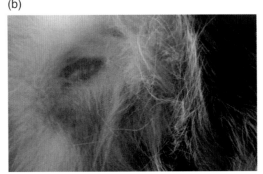

Figure 12.12 (a) Eosinophilic granuloma, or so-called "rodent ulcer," at the lower lip of a feline patient. (b) Eosinophilic plaque along the ventrum of a feline patient. *Source:* Courtesy of Dr. Elizabeth Robbins.

Figure 12.11 Classic appearance of miliary dermatitis along the dorsum of a feline patient. Note that the eroded papules form crusts at the skin's surface.

12.3.3 The Importance of Identifying the Primary Underlying Cause

Pyoderma may be a primary condition. However, it is often secondary to an assortment of underlying medical maladies [1–3]. If these maladies are not unearthed, then the patient is at risk of relapse or recurrence of pyoderma because the primary, predisposing issue has not been addressed or resolved [2].

Consider, for example, pyoderma in feline patients with underlying food allergy. Prior to diagnosis, these patients typically present for non-seasonal, recurrent flares of facial, cervical, truncal, or ventral abdominal pruritus [39, 43]. On physical examination, these patients tend to have multiple lesions of the skin, including alopecia and crusting [39]. Miliary dermatitis is also possible [39]. In patients with facial involvement, lesions tend to concentrate in the pre-auricular region [39].

Secondary pyoderma is common [39]. A 2013 study by Vogelnest et al. demonstrated that 47% of cats who were subsequently diagnosed with adverse food reactions had concurrent pyoderma [39].

If these patients were only treated for pyoderma and no further diagnostic work-up was attempted, they would likely demonstrate a positive response initially, only to relapse or experience recurrence after discontinuing treatment.

When treatment recurs, it is important to investigate further.

Coming back to the example of cats with suspected food allergies, elimination diets are indicated [39]. This may include home-prepared diets, commercial diets with a novel source of protein and/or carbohydrate, and commercial hydrolyzed diets [39]. Confirmed cases demonstrate marked improvement during the dietary phase, only to relapse when the initial diet is reintroduced [39].

Dermatologic investigations are often extensive because so many dermatologic conditions share so many of the same features in terms of lesions. Patients may benefit from an assortment of diagnostic tests to rule out various dermatopathies.

For example, evaluation of the coat via Wood's lamp or individual hairs via trichogram, as well as fungal culture, are important diagnostic tests to rule in or rule out dermatophytosis [12]. Refer to Chapter 3, Section 3.8.2 and Chapter 5, Section 5.8 for more information on managing this condition.

In addition, superficial and deep skin scrapes play an important role in diagnosing concurrent mange mite infestations [12]. Refer to the above-mentioned for more information on mange.

Impression smears and acetate tape preps may confirm the presence of *Malassezia* dermatitis. Refer to Chapter 3, Section 3.8.2 for more information on yeast overgrowth, particularly that which is associated with the nails.

Although these diagnostic tools may not be used in every clinical case of pyoderma that presents as a first-time offense, their use is critical when cases are refractory to treatment [12].

12.3.4 The Importance of Unearthing Other Causes for Persistence or Recurrence of Pyoderma

It is important to remember that patients may also experience relapses and recurrences of pyoderma without concurrent medical conditions. In these patients, pyoderma may be complicated by extraneous factors such as

- Poor client compliance
- Inappropriate treatment
- Inappropriate duration of treatment.

Client compliance is an important factor for the success of any treatment regime. The patient is only capable of responding to treatment if the treatment is administered as prescribed. Veterinarians are responsible for ensuring that prescribing instructions are clear and understood by the client. When prescribing at-home therapy, veterinarians should also take care to elicit the client's perspective as to which course of action will be easiest for the client. For example, are liquid medications more easily administered to the patient in question than tablets?

The veterinary team is also responsible for follow-up during treatment to determine if the patient is indeed receiving the prescribed medication on schedule. If the patient is not responding to treatment, it could be because doses were inadvertently missed or intentionally skipped due to patient intolerance of being pilled. In these situations, it is critical to arm the client with strategies to improve the administration of medication or devise an alternate approach, such as hospital boarding, to allow the patient to receive medication on schedule.

History-taking during recheck appointments is critical to identifying compliance issues. Establishing a plan and opening doors of communication at the initial visit are key to troubleshooting potential problem areas before they arise.

In addition to client compliance, the treatment plan itself may have been inappropriate. Consider, for example, the prescribed drug and the duration of therapy. A 2014 publication by Summers et al. examined the prescribing practices of primary care veterinarians that were managing cases of canine pyoderma. Of the 683 dogs that were included in the study, 97% were prescribed a systemic antibiotic [5].

The most common prescriptions for pyoderma include amoxicillin-clavulanic acid, cephalexin, and clindamycin [5]. Although these medications are appropriate on paper for the management of canine pyoderma, they may be increasingly less effective *in vivo* because of developing antimicrobial resistance [3, 5, 12, 44, 45].

Bacterial culture and susceptibility panels demonstrate which antibiotics demonstrate efficacy against the etiologic agent(s); however, this diagnostic tool was employed in only 2% of all cases in Summers's study [5].

Furthermore, one in four dogs in Summers's study were underdosed; that is, they were prescribed doses that are insufficient to achieve therapeutic levels [5].

Finally, treatment duration was insufficient in 40% of cases: antibiotics were prescribed for less than 14 days [5]. Although patients that respond well to therapy are expected to have fewer lesions and less discomfort within the first two weeks of treatment, a minimum of 21 days of antibiotic treatment is indicated for superficial pyoderma [2]. Other recommendations in the current veterinary literature include treating the patient for one to two weeks beyond clinical resolution of signs as determined by physical examination [2, 13]. In either case, a 10-day course of antibiotics is insufficient.

This study serves as an important reminder that decisions we make as clinicians impact patient outcomes. Sometimes, disease persists because microbes develop resistances to therapy. However, there are other occasions when patient care factors hinder or even prevent disease resolution. It is important to consider these factors every time there is a perceived drug failure so that if there is an underlying issue surrounding patient care, it is addressed.

For example, performing a bacterial culture and susceptibility panel may indicate the need to prescribe less commonly used antibiotics, such as amikacin and chloramphenicol, in order to target bacterial populations that have developed resistance against beta-lactams [3].

12.4 Noninfectious Causes of Papules and Pustules as Primary Skin Lesions

Historically, pustules were considered the result of infectious disease until proved otherwise. However, as our understanding of clinical medicine has expanded, and as our reliance upon cytology as a diagnostic tool has grown, it has become apparent that pustules may also represent sterile disease processes [1]. Immune-mediated conditions, such as pemphigus foliaceus, come to mind [1].

Recall from Chapter 3, Section 3.8.3 that pemphigus foliaceus is one type of immune-mediated disease that targets the skin and mucous membranes [46–48]. As disease progresses, keratinocytes separate from one another [49], causing crusting and erosive lesions. Because the nails are an extension of the integumentary system, the nail beds are frequently involved. Paronychia may occur in as many as one-third of feline patients with pemphigus foliaceus [49, 50].

In these cases, cytology plays an important role in establishing pemphigus as a presumptive diagnosis. Rather than assuming that one or more pustules is evidence of pyoderma, a representative lesion is sampled. When the contents of a pustule from a patient with pemphigus are sampled, the sample will be devoid of bacteria. Neutrophils may or may not be present. Unlike that which is seen in cases of pyoderma, those neutrophils that are present are not degenerate [51].

Furthermore, any keratinocytes that are evident on cytology are considered acantholytic [51]. This means that there are free-floating rafts of cells that have lost their anchor to the epidermis.

Acantholytic keratinocytes are not pathognomonic for pemphigus foliaceus. A definitive diagnosis of pemphigus must come from a biopsy [51]. The best lesion to sample for biopsy includes one or more pustules. A second-best lesion to sample is a crust. Crusts may keep micropustules hidden from view [51].

Identification of acantholytic keratinocytes on histopathologic examination is confirmatory for pemphigus foliaceus [51].

Pemphigus foliaceus may predispose the patient to secondary bacterial infections that then require antimicrobial therapy. However, the crux of medical management of uncomplicated cases is the long-term administration of immunosuppressive agents.

Although the incidence of pemphigus foliaceus in companion animals is low compared to pyoderma, the existence of immune-mediated conditions serve as an important reminder that misdiagnosis is possible if treatment is based upon gross lesions alone. Pustules are often, but not always, the result of infectious disease.

References

1 Craig, M. (2009). Lesion morphology in veterinary dermatology. *UK Vet.* 14 (3): 1–4.
2 Bajwa, J. (2016). Canine superficial pyoderma and therapeutic considerations. *Can. Vet. J.* 57 (2): 204–206.
3 Bloom, P. (2014). Canine superficial bacterial folliculitis: current understanding of its etiology, diagnosis and treatment. *Vet. J.* 199 (2): 217–222.
4 DeBoer, D.J. (1990). Strategies for management of recurrent pyoderma in dogs. *Vet. Clin. North Am. Small Anim. Pract.* 20 (6): 1509–1524.
5 Summers, J.F., Hendricks, A., and Brodbelt, D.C. (2014). Prescribing practices of primary-care veterinary practitioners in dogs diagnosed with bacterial pyoderma. *BMC Vet. Res.* 10: 240.

6 Hill, P.B., Lo, A., Eden, C.A. et al. (2006). Survey of the prevalence, diagnosis and treatment of dermatological conditions in small animals in general practice. *Vet. Rec.* 158 (16): 533–539.

7 Lund, E.M., Armstrong, P.J., Kirk, C.A. et al. (1999). Health status and population characteristics of dogs and cats examined at private veterinary practices in the United States. *J. Am. Vet. Med. Assoc.* 214 (9): 1336–1341.

8 Sischo, W.M., Ihrke, P.J., and Franti, C.E. (1989). Regional distribution of ten common skin diseases in dogs. *J. Am. Vet. Med. Assoc.* 195 (6): 752–756.

9 Scott, D.W. and Paradis, M. (1990). A survey of canine and feline skin disorders seen in a university practice: Small Animal Clinic, University of Montreal, Saint-Hyacinthe, Quebec (1987–1988). *Can. Vet. J.* 31 (12): 830–835.

10 Wells, D.L. and Hepper, P.G. (1999). Prevalence of disease in dogs purchased from an animal rescue shelter. *Vet. Rec.* 144 (2): 35–38.

11 Freeman, L.M., Abood, S.K., Fascetti, A.J. et al. (2006). Disease prevalence among dogs and cats in the United States and Australia and proportions of dogs and cats that receive therapeutic diets or dietary supplements. *J. Am. Vet. Med. Assoc.* 229 (4): 531–534.

12 Hillier, A., Lloyd, D.H., Weese, J.S. et al. (2014). Guidelines for the diagnosis and antimicrobial therapy of canine superficial bacterial folliculitis (Antimicrobial Guidelines Working Group of the International Society for Companion Animal Infectious Diseases). *Vet. Dermatol.* 25 (3): 163–175, e42-3.

13 Miller, W.H., Griffin, C.E., and Campbell, K.L. (2013). *Muller and Kirk's Small Animal Dermatology*. St. Louis, MO: Elsevier.

14 Guardabassi, L., Houser, G.A., Frank, L.A., and Papich, M.G. (2008). Guidelines for antimicrobial use in dogs and cats. In: (ed. L. Guardabassi, L.B. Jensen and H. Kruse), *Guide to antimicrobial use in animals*, (pp. 183–206). Oxford, UK: Wiley-Blackwell.

15 Cox, H.U., Newman, S.S., Roy, A.F., and Hoskins, J.D. (1984). Species of Staphylococcus isolated from animal infections. *Cornell Vet.* 74 (2): 124–135.

16 Medleau, L., Long, R.E., Brown, J., and Miller, W.H. (1986). Frequency and antimicrobial susceptibility of Staphylococcus species isolated from canine pyodermas. *Am. J. Vet. Res.* 47 (2): 229–231.

17 Devriese, L.A., Vancanneyt, M., Baele, M. et al. (2005). Staphylococcus pseudintermedius sp. nov., a coagulase-positive species from animals. *Int. J. Syst. Evol. Microbiol.* 55 (Pt 4): 1569–1573.

18 Sasaki, T., Kikuchi, K., Tanaka, Y. et al. (2007). Reclassification of phenotypically identified Staphylococcus intermedius strains. *J. Clin. Microbiol.* 45 (9): 2770–2778.

19 Paul, N.C., Damborg, P., and Guardabassi, L. (2015). Dam-to-offspring transmission and persistence of Staphylococcus pseudintermedius clones within dog families. *Vet. Dermatol.* 25 (3): e2.

20 Bannoehr, J. and Guardabassi, L. (2012). Staphylococcus pseudintermedius in the dog: taxonomy, diagnostics, ecology, epidemiology and pathogenicity. *Vet. Dermatol.* 23 (4): 253–266, e51-2.

21 Gortel, K. (2013). Recognizing pyoderma: more difficult than it may seem. *Vet. Clin. North Am. Small Anim. Pract.* 43 (1): 1–18.

22 Gortel, K., Campbell, K.L., Kakoma, I. et al. (1999). Methicillin resistance among staphylococci isolated from dogs. *Am. J. Vet. Res.* 60 (12): 1526–1530.

23 Jones, R.D., Kania, S.A., Rohrbach, B.W. et al. (2007). Prevalence of oxacillin- and multidrug-resistant staphylococci in clinical samples from dogs: 1,772 samples (2001–2005). *J. Am. Vet. Med. Assoc.* 230 (2): 221–227.

24 Cain, C.L., Morris, D.O., O'Shea, K., and Rankin, S.C. (2011). Genotypic relatedness and phenotypic characterization of Staphylococcus schleiferi subspecies in clinical samples from dogs. *Am. J. Vet. Res.* 72 (1): 96–102.

25 Frank, L.A., Kania, S.A., Hnilica, K.A. et al. (2003). Isolation of Staphylococcus schleiferi from dogs with pyoderma. *J. Am. Vet. Med. Assoc.* 222 (4): 451–454.

26 Morris DO, editor. (2011). Unusual Pyoderma. 25th Annual Congress of the ESVD-ECVD 2011 (7–10 September); Brussels (Belgium).

27 Tornquist, S.J. (ed.) (2009). *Cytology of inflammation and infectious diseases*. San Diego: CVC.

28 Baker, S.A., Van-Balen, J., Lu, B. et al. (2012). Antimicrobial drug use in dogs prior to admission to a veterinary teaching hospital. *J. Am. Vet. Med. Assoc.* 241 (2): 210–217.

29 Rantala, M., Holso, K., Lillas, A. et al. (2004). Survey of condition-based prescribing of antimicrobial drugs for dogs at a veterinary teaching hospital. *Vet. Rec.* 155 (9): 259–262.

30 Bemis, D.A., Jones, R.D., Frank, L.A., and Kania, S.A. (2009). Evaluation of susceptibility test breakpoints used to predict mecA-mediated resistance in Staphylococcus pseudintermedius isolated from dogs. *J. Vet. Diagn. Investig.* 21 (1): 53–58.

31 Barber, M. (1961). Methicillin-resistant staphylococci. *J. Clin. Pathol.* 14: 385–393.

32 White, S.D., Brown, A.E., Chapman, P.L. et al. (2005). Evaluation of aerobic bacteriologic culture of epidermal collarette specimens in dogs with superficial pyoderma. *J. Am. Vet. Med. Assoc.* 226 (6): 904–908.

33 Vaughan DF, Lemarie SL, editors. (2008). Comparison of culture and susceptibility results of superficial versus biopsy specimens in dogs with superficial pyoderma. North American Veterinary Dermatology Forum in Denver, Colorado (9–12 April 2008).

34 Wildermuth, B.E., Griffin, C.E., and Rosenkrantz, W.S. (2006). Feline pyoderma therapy. *Clin. Tech. Small Anim. Pract.* 21 (3): 150–156.

35 White, S.D. (1991). Pyoderma in five cats. *J. Am. Vet. Med. Assoc.* 27: 141–146.

36 Icen, H. and Yesilmen, S. (2008). Staphylococcal pyoderma in a cat: a case report. *J. Anim. Vet. Adv.* 7 (10): 1332–1334.

37 Medleau, L., Rakich, P.M., Latimer, K.S., and Grant, J.B. (1991). Superficial pyoderma in the cat – diagnosing an uncommon skin disorder. *Vet. Med.* 86 (8): 807–811.

38 Ravens, P.A., Xu, B.J., and Vogelnest, L.J. (2014). Feline atopic dermatitis: a retrospective study of 45 cases (2001–2012). *Vet. Dermatol.* 25 (2): 95–102, e27-8.

39 Vogelnest, L.J. and Cheng, K.Y. (2013). Cutaneous adverse food reactions in cats: retrospective evaluation of 17 cases in a dermatology referral population (2001–2011). *Aust. Vet. J.* 91 (11): 443–451.

40 Favrot, C. (2013). Feline non-flea induced hypersensitivity dermatitis: clinical features, diagnosis and treatment. *J. Feline Med. Surg.* 15 (9): 778–784.

41 Yu, H.W. and Vogelnest, L.J. (2012). Feline superficial pyoderma: a retrospective study of 52 cases (2001–2011). *Vet. Dermatol.* 23 (5): 448–e86.

42 Mueller, R.S. (1999). Bacterial dermatoses. In: *A Practical Guide to Feline Dermatology* (ed. E. Guagere and P. Prelaud), 6.1–6.11. Paris: Merial.

43 Bryan, J. and Frank, L.A. (2010). Food allergy in the cat: a diagnosis by elimination. *J. Feline Med. Surg.* 12 (11): 861–866.

44 Beco, L., Guaguere, E., Lorente Mendez, C. et al. (2013). Suggested guidelines for using systemic antimicrobials in bacterial skin infections (1): diagnosis based on clinical presentation, cytology and culture. *Vet. Rec.* 172 (3): 72–78.

45 Summers, J.F., Brodbelt, D.C., Forsythe, P.J. et al. (2012). The effectiveness of systemic antimicrobial treatment in canine superficial and deep pyoderma: a systematic review. *Vet. Dermatol.* 23 (4): 305–329, e61.

46 Côté, E. (2015). *Clinical Veterinary Advisor. Dogs and Cats*, 3e, xxxvii, 1642 p. St. Louis, Missouri: Elsevier Mosby.

47 Preziosi, D.E., Goldschmidt, M.H., Greek, J.S. et al. (2003). Feline pemphigus foliaceus: a retrospective analysis of 57 cases. *Vet. Dermatol.* 14 (6): 313–321.

48 Simpson, D.L. and Burton, G.G. (2013). Use of prednisolone as monotherapy in the treatment of feline pemphigus foliaceus: a retrospective study of 37 cats. *Vet. Dermatol.* 24 (6): 598–601, e143-4.

49 Rouben, C. (2016). Claw and Claw Bed Diseases. *Clinician's Brief* (April): 35–40.

50 Miller, W.H., Griffin, C.E., and Campbell, K.L. (2012). *Diseases of Eyelids, Claws, Anal Sacs, and Ears. Muller and Kirk's Small Animal Dermatology*, 7e, 731–739. Philadelphia, P.A: WB Saunders.

51 Tater KC, Olivry T. (2010). Canine and feline pemphigus foliaceus: Improving your chances of a successful outcome. DVM 360 [Internet]. http://veterinarymedicine.dvm360.com/canine-and-feline-pemphigus-foliaceus-improving-your-chances-successful-outcome?id=&sk=&date=&%0A%09%09%09&pageID=4.

13

Scale and Crusts

13.1 Introduction to Scale as a Clinical Sign

The integumentary system serves many purposes, not the least of which is to form a protective barrier or shield for the organism that it is intended to envelop [1]. Although commensals reside on the skin, they are prevented from breaching the skin's surface as long as it is intact [1]. Skin surface lipids and the appropriate production of sebum by the sebaceous glands play a critical role in maintaining skin surface pH and integrity [2–5]. They also guard against excessive water loss [1].

In order to maintain a functional epidermal barrier, epithelial cells must continually regenerate [6, 7]. Regeneration allows those cells that have sloughed to be replaced. This process is referred to as desquamation [8].

Healthy skin undergoes desquamation. Basal epidermal cells replicate via mitosis constantly in order to produce replacement keratinocytes [7]. Thousands of these replacement cells are produced daily so that at all times the stratum corneum has a contiguous layer of anucleate, flat, keratinized cells [7]. On average, the maturation process for a keratinocyte takes 21–22 days [7, 9].

Unlike snakes, which shed their skin entirely in one piece, companion animals such as dogs and cats shed individual cells over time. These individual cells tend not to be noticed on the patient or in the environment.

Scale occurs when desquamated cells accumulate and are now visible to the naked eye [8]. Visualization of scale is enhanced in dark-coated patients because it stands out readily against a dark brown or black backdrop. Sometimes clients refer to this scale as "dandruff" (see Figures 13.1a, b).

Scale may consist of isolated specks, larger flakes, or adherent sheets [8] (see Figure 13.2).

Recall from Chapter 6, Section 6.6 that specks of scale can be mistaken for *Cheyletiella* sp., hence the name for the condition that is caused by this mange mite, "walking dandruff" [10].

The amount of scale that a patient has may be affected by environmental factors. Consider, for example, how low-humidity environments impact the skin. These increase the rate of desquamation because the skin surface is drier than normal [2, 11].

Other environmental contributing factors include chronic exposure to forced-air heat, blow drying of the coat, and over-shampooing [7].

Patient factors also contribute to the amount of scale. For example, patients with pemphigus foliaceus have poor cohesion between keratinocytes [11, 12]. Classically, this results in inappropriate separation between layers of the skin. Vesicle and bullae formation are typical lesions for pemphigus. However, decreased cohesion may also result in increased scale.

Some patients do not have pemphigus or extenuating environmental pressures, yet they still present with excessive scale. Veterinary clients and clinicians alike often report that these patients have *seborrhea*. It is important to keep in mind that seborrhea is a clinical descriptor as opposed to a diagnosis [1, 2].

Historically, seborrhea was subdivided into *Seborrhea sicca* and *Seborrhea oleosa* [1, 13]. The former refers to excessively dry skin, whereas the latter refers to skin that feels progressively greasy. The wetness associated with *S. oleosa* is frequently associated with secondary bacterial and/or fungal infections with associated pruritus, with or without hyperkeratosis [2] (see Figures 13.3a–e).

In reality, patients may fluctuate between both extremes. In other words, there is often overlap between seborrhea sicca and seborrhea oleosa, and neither term facilitates identification of the underlying disease [1].

Seborrheic skin lesions vary tremendously between patients [2]. In addition to scale, patients with seborrhea may also present with accumulations of waxy material that adhere to hair shafts [6]. Patients with seborrhea may develop secondary folliculitis, crusting, and alopecia [6]. If accumulations of scale, wax, or crusts become irritating, then erythema of affected skin may develop [2, 14].

Patients with seborrhea may also develop digital hyperkeratosis [1, 7]. In these cases, keratin accumulates in regions of the pads that are not weight bearing [7].

(a) (b)

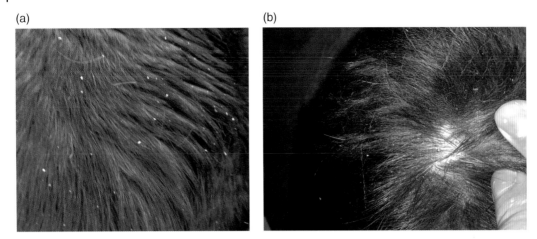

Figure 13.1 (a) Isolated scale in a Tonkinese cat. (b) Isolated scale in a canine patient. *Source:* Courtesy of Blake and Danielle Tafoya.

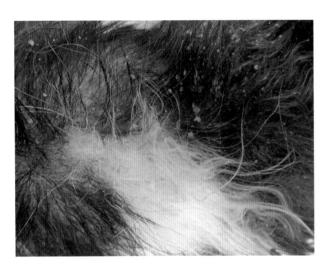

Figure 13.2 Flakes of scale in a canine patient. *Source:* Courtesy of Patricia Bennett, DVM.

For this reason, the carpal pads are most frequently affected [7]. Because these pads represent non-contact areas, the accumulated keratin is not worn off [7]. In and of themselves, hardened paw pads are not painful. However, they may become painful if cracks and fissures develop, exposing deeper tissue [7]. Refer to Chapter 10 to recall additional causes of hyperkeratosis that must be considered if a patient presents with so-called "hard pad disease."

Patients with seborrhea may also develop hyperplastic sebaceous glands at the tail base or the proximal third of the tail [7]. These patients develop what appears to be a swollen tail base, with or without hyperpigmented skin and comedones [7]. A primary rule out for this condition is testicular neoplasia [7, 15].

Seborrhea is the byproduct of abnormal keratinization [1, 2, 6, 11, 13, 14, 16, 17]. In the majority of cases, this abnormal keratinization results from an overproliferation of the epidermis [2, 17].

Epidermal hyperproliferation may result from an intrinsic defect [1]. Consider, for example, an inherited

disorder of cornification. This condition constitutes primary seborrhea [1].

Epidermal hyperproliferation may also be secondary to any condition that increases the rate at which basal epidermal cells undergo mitosis [1, 2]. For example, dermatitis speeds up epidermal turnover time [2].

Other factors that stimulate epidermal basal cell mitosis include prostaglandins, estrogens, and radiation therapy [2]. Deficiencies in vitamin A and the hormone, thyroxine, also increase the rate of epidermal turnover [2].

13.1.1 Primary Seborrhea

Primary seborrhea is most often reported in American cocker spaniels and Irish setters [2, 6, 9, 18]. Other breeds that are predisposed include English springer spaniels, West Highland white terriers, Dachshunds, Bassett hounds, Labrador retrievers, Golden retrievers, and German shepherd dogs [2, 6, 7, 9, 14, 18–22].

Affected dogs are typically young adults at time of onset. Patients typically present before their second birthday with clinical signs that progress as they age [7].

Any part of the body may be affected by seborrhea; however, the topline is commonly involved [7]. In addition, seborrheic areas tend to be those in which skin overlaps [7]. Consider, for example, the axillary, inguinal, ventral neck, and interdigital regions. These are common locations for seborrhea because they are intertriginous [7]. For similar reasons, dogs with skin folds may be at increased risk for developing seborrheic skin (see Figure 13.4).

Patients with seborrhea may present with concurrent otitis externa [13]. When present, otitis externa may affect one or both ears. There is no classic presentation for seborrhea-associated otitis (see Figures 13.5a–d).

All presentations of otitis externa should undergo otoscopic examination and cytology, to establish whether antibacterial and/or antifungal therapy is indicated. Aural cultures may be advised, particularly in cases involving mixed bacterial populations.

(a)　(b)

(c)　(d)　(e)

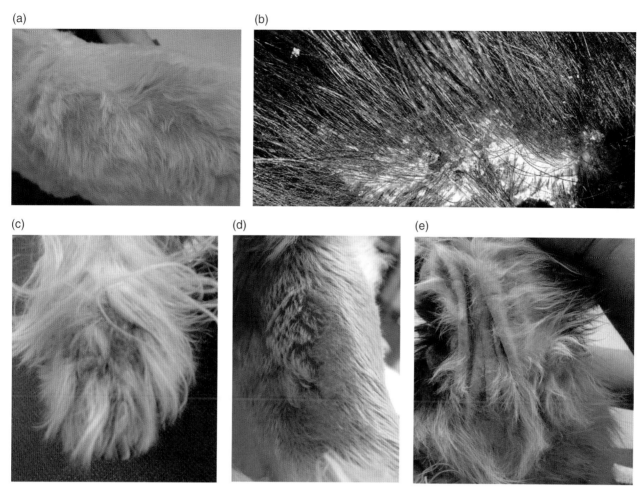

Figure 13.3 (a) Seborrhea sicca in a white-coated canine patient. Scale is difficult to appreciate due to the light coat color. If you were to palpate the skin, its surface would not feel oily. (b) Seborrhea sicca in a black-coated canine patient. Note how it is easier to appreciate the scale against a black coat. The skin's surface of this patient is dry to the touch. (c) Dorsum of a canine patient's paw. This patient has seborrhea oleosa. If you were to palpate the skin, its surface would feel characteristically greasy. It would also likely be malodorous. (d) Seborrhea oleosa associated with the forearm of this canine patient. You can appreciate from the photograph how moist the region of the body is, and how the skin's surface is also quite inflamed as a result of concurrent pyoderma. *Source:* Courtesy of Patricia Bennett, DVM. (e) Seborrhea oleosa associated with the ventral neck of a canine patient. You can appreciate the greasy feel of this skin's surface. *Source:* Courtesy of Patricia Bennett, DVM.

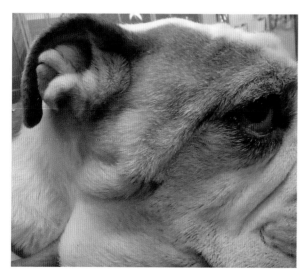

Figure 13.4 This canine patient presented for seborrhea. Note that the facial and nasal folds are contributing factors because seborrhea tends to target intertriginous areas.

Patients with primary seborrhea experience accelerated epidermal turnover time [2, 6, 9]. Maturation of keratinocytes is reduced from the expected three weeks to eight days [2, 7, 9]. This promotes the accumulation of scale.

In addition, these patients experience a shift in the types of skin surface lipids that are produced by their sebaceous glands. In the normal patient, the health, integrity, and permeability of the skin barrier is maintained primarily by sterol and wax esters [2, 3, 5]. Cholesterol is scant. So, too, are triglycerides and free fatty acids [2, 3, 5].

By contrast, seborrheic skin is often deficient in linoleic acid [23]. This impairs the skin's ability to serve as a semipermeable barrier to the outside world.

In addition, seborrheic skin is characterized as having less diester waxes and more free fatty acids [5]. Free fatty acids are irritating to the skin. When overabundant, they have the potential to incite inflammation [5].

(a)

(b)

(c)

(d)

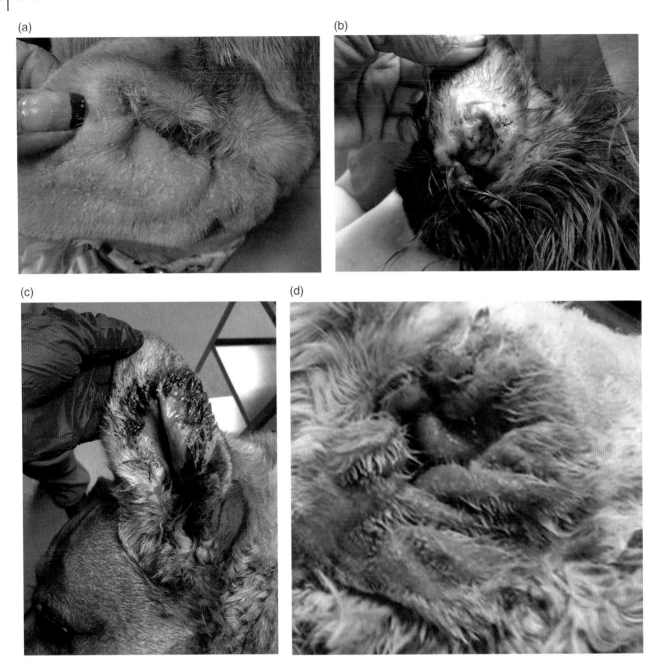

Figure 13.5 (a) Fungal otitis externa in a canine patient. Although only one pinna is shown here, this condition was characterized by bilateral otitis, with moderate pinnal inflammation and copious flaky aural debris. (b) Fungal otitis externa in a canine patient. Note that the aural debris is significantly less dry than that which is pictured in Figure 13.5a. *Source:* Courtesy of Patricia Bennett, DVM. (c) This canine patient developed severe bacterial otitis externa with copious amounts of putrid, purulent aural debris. (d) This canine patient developed recurrent mixed fungal and bacterial otitis externa with marked inflammation. Appreciate that the entrance to the external ear canal is stenotic. *Source:* Courtesy of Dr. Stephanie Harris.

Free fatty acids also tend to create strong, unpleasant odors that are displeasing to the veterinary client [24]. Such odors are often described as being rancid [2, 25].

The shift in lipid composition in seborrheic skin also reduces surface bacteriostatic properties, thus encouraging bacterial and fungal growth [24]. Normal skin houses a multitude of commensal and opportunistic organisms

[26–28]. It has been estimated that every square centimeter of healthy skin contains 100–200 aerobic organisms [13].

However, when the lipid profile of the skin shifts in cases of seborrhea, secondary infection with *Staphylococcus* and *Streptococcus* sp. is common [3, 29–31]. A study by Ihrke et al. reported that the mean aerobic flora count was 50 times greater in seborrheic dogs than in those within the control group [32]. These opportunistic invaders perpetuate dermatitis and contribute to malodor [24]. Refer to Chapter 12, Section 12.3.1 for descriptions of bacterial pyoderma. Pruritus is frequently associated with pyoderma.

Overgrowth with *Malassezia* sp. is also common in seborrheic skin [3, 26, 29–31, 33]. In particular, seborrheic skin hosts increased populations of *Malassezia pachydermatis* [26]. From the perspective of diagnostic medicine, these populations are most often isolated from the groin, neck, interdigital spaces, and ear canals [26].

Seborrheic skin also supports overgrowth of *Candida* sp. [26]. *Candida parapsilosis* preferentially resides within the perianal region [26].

When primary seborrhea occurs, its distribution within the patient is typically generalized. However, primary seborrhea may also be focal. One example is canine ear margin seborrhea [7, 34]. Dachshunds and Beagles appear to be predisposed to this condition [2]. In affected patients, scale targets the ear margins. Over time, patients develop follicular plugs or keratin mats along the perimeter of the pinnae [7, 34] (see Figure 13.6).

In severe cases of canine ear margin seborrhea, the edges of the pinnae may crack and fissure. This may aggravate the underlying skin and cause bleeding [7, 34]. Pinnal edges may also develop patchy alopecia [7, 34] (see Figure 13.7).

The appearance of canine ear margin seborrhea resembles that of canine sarcoptic mange. However, patients with sarcoptic mange are extraordinarily pruritic, as compared to patients with canine ear margin seborrhea, which are not [34].

A second example of focal seborrhea is Schnauzer Comedone Syndrome [2, 8]. Comedones are colloquially referred to as blackheads. These are specific types of papules that are formed when sebaceous ducts and hair follicles are plugged by debris. Patients that develop this syndrome tend to be Miniature Schnauzers. These

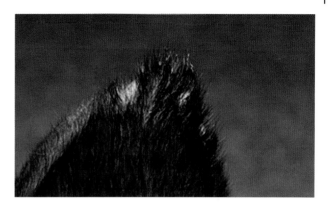

Figure 13.7 Patchy alopecia along the ear margin in a canine patient with focal seborrhea.

patients present as young adults with comedones concentrated along their toplines [2].

It is important to relay to the veterinary client that primary seborrhea cannot be cured [1]. Affected patients require lifelong medical management to reduce scale, greasiness, secondary infection, and odor [2, 11, 13, 16, 18].

In particular, hydrating shampoos, rinses, creams, and gels are of value in restoring moisture to those patients with exceptionally dry skin [2, 11, 13, 16, 18]. Emollients and humectants are common ingredients in moisturizing preparations [24]. Examples of the former include coconut, cottonseed, and olive oils [24]. These reduce loss of water through the skin [24]. So, too, do certain hydrocarbons and fats, including lanolin [24].

Humectants attract water from the environment to increase the water content at the skin's surface [24]. These include propylene glycol, sodium lactate, and glycerin [24].

Combination products often incorporate additional ingredients into these moisturizing preparations, including diphenhydramine and pramoxine, to reduce itch; colloidal oatmeal, to help the skin retain its moisture; and chlorhexidine, to flush the hair follicles [24].

Antiseborrheic formulations also play a role in medical management because they effectively remove scale and other debris [2, 11, 13, 16, 18]. Popular active ingredients in canine products that achieve this function include sulfur, salicylic acid, selenium sulfide, coal tar, and benzoyl peroxide [2, 24, 29]. Some products often serve more than one function. For example, salicylic acid is both keratinolytic and hydrating [2]. The latter property is achieved when salicylic acid reduces canine skin pH. This facilitates hydration of the keratin [2].

In-depth therapeutic plans are beyond the scope of this chapter. Because seborrheic skin is so variable, there is no one "right" plan of attack. Treatment plans must be tailored to the patient and modified based upon the patient's response to therapy.

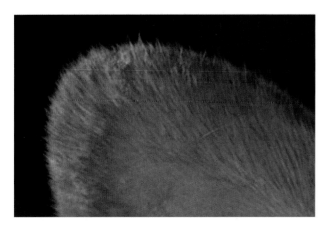

Figure 13.6 Scaling associated with the ear margin.

13.1.2 Secondary Seborrhea

By far, clinical cases of secondary seborrhea that present to the general practitioner outnumber those of primary seborrhea [7]. Patients with secondary seborrhea present similarly as those with primary seborrhea. However, rather than having an inherent defect in cornification, they have one or more triggers that caused seborrhea. In order to establish the underlying cause(s) of disease, patients with secondary seborrhea require an extensive diagnostic work-up [7]. Without exploring the trigger(s) for seborrhea, the clinical sign of scale will persist and/or recur.

There are innumerable causes of secondary seborrhea, the most common of which include [7, 8, 13, 14]:

- Allergies
  - Atopy
  - Contact allergy
  - Flea bite hypersensitivity
  - Food allergy
- Autoimmune conditions
  - Pemphigus foliaceus
  - Systemic lupus erythematosus (SLE)
- Dermatophytosis
- Ectoparasite infestation
  - Demodicosis
  - Pediculosis
  - *Otodectes cynotis*
  - Scabies
- Endocrinopathies
  - Hypothyroidism
  - Hyperadrenocorticism
- Neoplasia
  - Cutaneous T-cell Lymphoma
- Nutritional deficiencies
  - Vitamin A
  - Zinc

Refer to Chapter 5 for a review of atopy and dermatophytosis; Chapter 6 for ectoparasites; Chapter 9 for endocrinopathies and immune-mediated disease; and Chapter 10 for zinc deficiency syndromes.

Because this list of differential diagnoses is extensive, yet not exhaustive, a clinician cannot identify scale on physical examination and automatically establish a cause.

As with many dermatopathies, the importance of a comprehensive history cannot be overstated [7]. Age and breed may provide important clues. For example, consider the Siberian husky or Alaskan malamute. These cold-weather breeds are overrepresented for zinc-responsive dermatosis [1, 8, 35–38]. On the other hand, West Highland white terriers are the poster children for skin allergies [1]. Cocker spaniels more often present with primary than secondary seborrhea; however, they may also have concurrent deficiencies in vitamin A [1, 8].

History taking also may reveal important details that assist with the prioritization of differential diagnoses. For example, patients that are not pruritic are less likely to have allergic or parasitic skin disease [7]. Patients that present at middle to older age for polydipsia (PD) and polyuria (PU) are more likely to have an underlying endocrinopathy [7]. If the patient has underlying hypothyroidism, it may be heat-seeking and gain weight despite no changes in caloric intake [8]. If the PU/PD patient exhibits excessive panting and apparent muscle weakness, it may have underlying hyperadrenocorticism [8].

The physical examination provides clues about the likelihood of certain disease pathways. For example, that same middle-aged patient with PU/PD may also have bilaterally symmetrical truncal alopecia. This distribution pattern is supportive of an underlying endocrine imbalance [7].

The presence of papules and pustules are suggestive of concurrent pyoderma. Pyoderma frequently occurs in patients with seborrheic skin [7]. However, erythema is more commonly seen, along with easier-than-anticipated epilation [7].

The aggressiveness of the clinician's diagnostic approach depends in large part upon the client's level of frustration and the severity of the lesions [7]. Some clients may elect to do a step-by-step work-up; others may elect to pursue multiple diagnostic tests at once.

When patients present with seborrhea, most require one or more of the following tests to provide confirmation of one or more underlying diseases [1, 7]:

- Wood's Lamp, trichogram, and dermatophyte cultures to rule out dermatophytosis
- Superficial and deep skin scrapes to rule out mange mites
- Fine-needle aspirates (FNAs) and impression smears of primary lesions, such as pustules, to rule out pyoderma, with or without bacterial culture
- Ear cytology, with or without bacterial culture
- Baseline bloodwork, including complete blood count, chemistry panel, and hormonal assays
- Fecal analysis
- Skin biopsy
- Food trials
- Intradermal allergy testing
- Response to ectoparasite preventative

Allergies are a common cause of seborrhea, whereas pyoderma is often secondary to seborrheic disease [7]. In particular, flea allergy dermatitis causes a classic distribution pattern of lesions at the tail base and dorsal lumbosacral area [7]. The caudal thighs may also be involved [7]. Contrast that distribution with those regions that are more typically seen in atopic patients: the face, ears, feet, axillae, and ventral abdomen [7].

Sarcoptic mange also has preferred sites to target on the body: ear margins, lateral elbows, and hocks [7]. Patients infested with *Sarcoptes* may also exhibit a positive pinnal-pedal reflex [7, 39].

Endocrinopathies are also a common cause of seborrheic skin [7]. Recall that thyroxine deficiency, as occurs in hypothyroid patients, increases the rate of epidermal turnover [2]. This results in an accumulation of scale.

The bottom line is that seborrheic skin requires a diagnostic investigation to treat the root(s) of the issue. Without taking measures to address, if not resolve, the underlying issue, the clinician is tossing darts in the dark.

Spot treatments to address seborrheic skin may provide short-term comfort; however, they do not prevent the disease from persisting, progressing, or recurring [8].

Systemic antibiotics are frequently employed due to the high rate of concurrent pyoderma; topical and/or systemic anti-fungals are added as needed to manage cases of *Malassezia* overgrowth [14].

Zinc supplementation will facilitate the healing of seborrheic skin in dogs with inherited or acquired deficiencies, and oral synthetic retinoids may be of some benefit, particularly to the subset of vitamin A-deficient Cocker spaniels [14, 40].

Coat clipping may help the veterinary client to stay on top of lesions as they emerge [14].

13.1.3 Other Causes of Scale

The most common causes of scale have been outlined here as disorders of cornification. However, ichthyosis should also be mentioned as a rare defect that impairs the way in which the stratum corneum forms [8, 41]. There are several different subtypes of ichthyosis.

The one that is most familiar to veterinary practitioners is associated with young Golden retrievers [41]. These patients are typically diagnosed when they are under one-year old [41]. Affected dogs have recently demonstrated a shared mutation in the PNPLA 1 gene [41, 42]. These patients present with thick sheets of white-to-gray, adherent scale [1, 41]. Scale can be peeled off like tissue paper [1]. It comes off in very large flakes that can easily be the size of dimes [1]. Affected Golden retrievers are non-pruritic in the absence of concurrent pyoderma.

Jack Russell terriers also develop a type of ichthyosis as a result of a mutation in the gene TGMI. Because TGMI plays an important role in forming the exterior of the corneocyte, the mutation leads to abnormal connections between cells. Secondary infection, particularly yeast overgrowth syndromes, are common [41, 43].

More recently, a similar disorder has been identified in American bulldogs. Disease is accelerated in this breed and develops before weaning [41, 44, 45]. Affected patients

developed a wrinkled appearance to the abdominal skin because of the way in which scale adheres to the glabrous skin [1, 41]. The mutation involves the gene ICHTHYN, and impairs lipid metabolism [41, 42, 45, 46].

Diagnostic tests have been established to identify and remove carriers within the breeding pool.

13.2 Introduction to Crusts as a Clinical Sign

Crusts were first introduced in Chapter 12, Section 12.1 as a type of secondary skin lesion that is essentially a concretion of pus, serum, and dried exudate [47]. Crusts often adhere to the coat. However, they eventually break free from the skin's surface like scale. Refer to Chapter 12, Figures 12.5a–c.

As was discussed in Section 12.3.2, crusts are commonly seen in cats with miliary dermatitis, as from pyoderma [48, 49]. Pyoderma is the most common cause of crusting. However, there are three other causes that warrant further investigation here [50]:

- Fly bite dermatitis
- Feline mosquito bite hypersensitivity
- Squamous cell carcinoma (SCC)

Although these causes occur with less frequency in clinical practice, their presentations are important for the novice clinician to recognize as potential differentials for crusts.

Fly bite dermatitis is typically caused by [50]

- The stable fly, *Stomoxys calcitrans*, a member of the family, Muscidae
- The black fly or buffalo gnat, a member of the family *Simuliidae*.

Other biting insects of interest include the sand fly and the mosquito.

Fly bite dermatitis occurs most often during the warmer months of the year, spring and summer. Stable flies typically target the ear margins of cats and dogs with erect ears, and the ear folds of those in which the ears are floppy [50]. Short-coated, outdoor patients are most often affected because the coat is thin and offers less protection than a dense coat [50].

Affected ears become erythematous and/or alopecic at the sites of bites [50]. Bite wounds, however small, exude serum and blood. Although the amount of ooze is scant, it dries to form crusts that irritate the ear margins [50] (see Figures 13.8a, b).

If flies are exceptionally populous, they may attack the upper limbs and trunk.

Lesions tend to be pruritic, but self-limiting. Lesions spontaneously resolve if the patient transitions to an

(a)

(b)

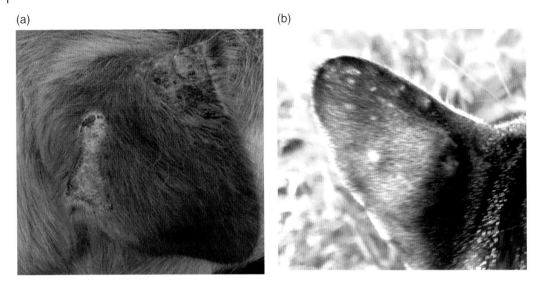

Figure 13.8 (a) Fly bite lesions in a canine patient. (b) Fly bite lesions in a feline patient.

indoor lifestyle and/or when seasons change such that flies are no longer pests.

Black fly bites have a much more recognizable appearance. These rings of erythema predominate on the ventral abdomen, where fur is sparse [50] (see Figure 13.9).

Clients may mistake these for the classic "bull's-eye" lesion that is associated with Lyme disease in human patients.

Black fly bites may be more irritating than stable fly bites, and may require topical therapy to squelch the associated itch.

Feline mosquito bite hypersensitivity is unique to cats [14, 34, 50, 51]. Lesions are seasonal: they develop in predominantly outdoor cats over summer and regress during the fall months [34]. Dark-coated cats appear to be more at risk than light-coated cats [34].

Lesions develop in response to a Type 1 hypersensitivity reaction to mosquito saliva [50, 52]. Facial eruptions are most common, particularly at the bridge of the nose [14, 34, 50, 51]. The nasal planum in entirety may also be affected [14].

Papules and crusts are the predominant lesions [14, 34, 50, 51]. Secondary alopecia is common as surface lesions become erosive and exudative [14, 34, 50, 51] (see Figures 13.10a, b).

It is important to inform veterinary clients that most products that are marketed as insect repellants for humans are unsafe for cats [52]. Consider, for example, products that contain N,N-Diethyl-meta-toluamide (also called DEET or diethyltoluamide) or a permethrin base [52].

Lesions resolve spontaneously as the mosquito season ends or if patients are transitioned into an exclusively indoor lifestyle [14, 34, 50, 51]. Lesions will recur during

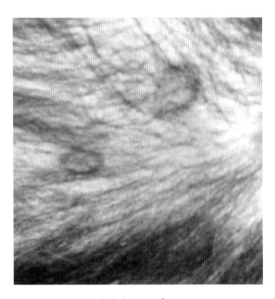

Figure 13.9 Ventral abdomen of a canine patient. Note the classic pattern of erythema that is associated with black fly bites.

subsequent mosquito seasons if patients are re-exposed. Annual re-exposure is thought to worsen the severity of lesions [34]. In the severest of cases, the muzzle, pinnae, periorbital skin, and flexor surfaces of the carpi may also be involved [34]. Biopsies of affected skin demonstrate significant dermal eosinophilic inflammation [34].

Few other diseases cause lesions that are similar in appearance. Feline herpesvirus ulcerative dermatitis and feline calicivirus-associated virulent systemic disease may both cause ulcerative facial dermatitis [53]. In addition, the cat with feline calicivirus-associated virulent systemic disease also tends to present with severe limb edema [53].

(b)

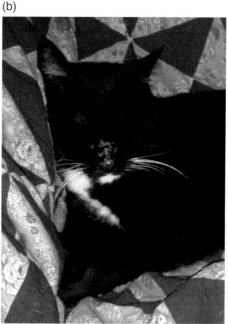

(a)

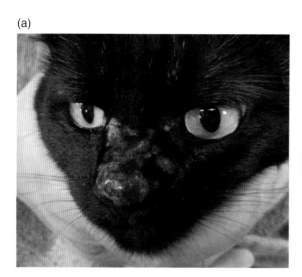

Figure 13.10 (a) Erosive, ulcerative lesions of the nasal planum in a feline patient afflicted with mosquito bite hypersensitivity. *Source:* Courtesy of Dr. Elizabeth Robbins. (b) Feline patient that is recovering from mosquito bite hypersensitivity. Note that the skin is no longer erosive or ulcerative. It is scabbed over and in the process of healing. *Source:* Courtesy of Juliane Daggett, MBS, DVM.

In both situations, the affected cat presents as being systemically ill [53]. This is in stark contrast to the cat that presents for mosquito bite hypersensitivity. Other than being painful and potentially pruritic, the mosquito-bitten cat is systemically healthy [54].

SCC may also present with crusting of the nasal planum [55]. SCC at this site occurs with greater frequency in the cat than dog, particularly if the cat is white-coated [55]. White-coated cats are 13 times more at risk than cats with other coat colors [56].

Cats with SCC of the nasal planum present with erosive lesions that proliferate over time [55]. Clients may initially present the patient for what appears to be a non-healing cat scratch on the nasal planum only to find that it never goes away [57]. These lesions are slow-growing. They invade local tissue for months to years before they metastasize [55].

Because SCC of the nasal planum is persistent, it does not fit with the classic presentation of mosquito bite hypersensitivity, in which the lesions resolve at the conclusion of mosquito season.

SCC also tends to present simultaneously in other regions of the body, such as the eyelids or pinnae [57].

Diagnosis of SCC is via biopsy [57].

References

1 Moriello K. (2015). Stopping the Scales, Greasiness and Odor of Seborrhea in Shelter and Foster Home Dogs. Maddie's Institute [Internet]: https://www.maddiesfund.org/assets/documents/Institute/Stopping%20 Seborrhea%20-%20Transcript.pdf.

2 Campbell, K.L. (1994). Seborrheic skin disorders and their treatment in dogs. *Clin. Dermatol.* 12 (4): 551–558.

3 Sharaf, D.M., Clark, S.J., and Downing, D.T. (1977). Skin surface lipids of the dog. *Lipids* 12 (10): 786.

4 Ziboh, V.A. and Chapkin, R.S. (1987). Biologic significance of polyunsaturated fatty acids in the skin. *Arch. Dermatol.* 123 (12): 1686a–1690a.

5 Horowitz, L.N. and Ihrke, P.J. (1977). Canine seborrhea. In: *Current Veterinary Therapy VI* (ed. R.W. Kirk), 519–524. Philadephia, PA: W.B. Saunders.

6 Baker, B.B. and Maibach, H.I. (1987). Epidermal cell renewal in seborrheic skin of dogs. *Am. J. Vet. Res.* 48 (4): 726–728.

7 Shanley, K.J. (1990). The seborrheic disease complex. An approach to underlying causes and therapies. *Vet. Clin. North Am. Small Anim. Pract.* 20 (6): 1557–1577.

8 Bloom, P. (2007). Canine scaling disorders. *NAVC Clinician's Brief* (July): 9–13.

9 Kwochka, K.W. and Rademakers, A.M. (1989). Cell proliferation of epidermis, hair follicles, and sebaceous glands of beagles and cocker spaniels with healthy skin. *Am. J. Vet. Res.* 50 (4): 587–591.

10 Arther, R.G. (2009). Mites and lice: biology and control. *Vet. Clin. North Am. Small Anim. Pract.* 39 (6): 1159–1171, vii.

11 Campbell, K.L. (1985). Seborrhea. *Dermatol. Rep.* 4 (3): 1–8.

12 Spindler, V., Eming, R., Schmidt, E. et al. (2018). Mechanisms causing loss of keratinocyte cohesion in pemphigus. *J. Invest. Dermatol.* 138 (1): 32–37.

13 Ihrke, P.J. (1979). Canine seborrheic disease complex. *Vet. Clin. N. Am.* 9 (1): 93–106.

14 Schaer, M. and Gaschen, F. (2016). *Clinical Medicine of the Dog and Cat*. Boca Raton, FL: Taylor & Francis Group, LLC.

15 Miller, W.H. (1989). Sex hormone-related dermatoses in dogs. In: *Current Veterinary Therapy X* (ed. R.W. Kirk), 595–602. Philadelphia, PA: Saunders.

16 Halliwell, R.E. (1979). Seborrhea in the dog. *Compend. Contin. Educ. Pract. Vet.* 1: 227–236.

17 Kwochka, K.W. (1993). Overview of normal keratinization and cutaneous scaling disorders of dogs. In: *Current Veterinary Dermatology* (ed. C.E. Griffin, K.W. Kwochka and J.M. MacDonald), 167–175. St Louis: Mosby Year Book.

18 Muller, G.H., Kirk, R.W., and Scott, D.W. (1983). *Small Animal Dermatology*. Philadelphia, PA: W.B. Saunders Co.

19 Scott, D.W. and Miller, W.H. (1996). Primary seborrhoea in English springer spaniels: a retrospective study of 14 cases. *J. Small Anim. Pract.* 37 (4): 173–178.

20 Kwochka, K.W. (1993). Cutaneous scaling disorders in the dog. In: *Manual of Small Animal Dermatology* (ed. P.H. Locke, R.G. Harvey and I.S. Mason), 52–59. Cheltenham: British Small Animal Veterinary Association.

21 Kwochka, K.W. and Smeak, D.D. (1990). The cellular defect in idiopathic seborrhea of cocker spaniels. In: *Advances in Veterinary Dermatology* (ed. R.E. Halliwell and C. von Tscharner), 265–277. Philadelphia, PA: Bailliere Tindall.

22 Yager, J.A. and Wilcock, B.P. (1994). *Color Atlas and Text of Surgical Pathology of the Dog and Cat. Dermatopathology and Skin Tumors*. London: Mosby Year Book.

23 Campbell, K.L. and Davis, C.A. (1990). Effects of thyroid hormones on serum and cutaneous fatty acid concentrations in dogs. *Am. J. Vet. Res.* 51 (5): 752–756.

24 Nesbitt GH, editor. (2008). Management of canine keratinization (seborrheic) disorders. CVC, Washington, D.C.: DVM 360.

25 Raczkowski, J.J. (1984). *Pathogenic Studies of Canine Seborrheic Skin Disease in the West Highland White Terrier Breed*. Manhattan, KS: Kansas State University.

26 Yurayart, C., Chindamporn, A., Suradhat, S. et al. (2011). Comparative analysis of the frequency, distribution and population sizes of yeasts associated with canine seborrheic dermatitis and healthy skin. *Vet. Microbiol.* 148 (2–4): 356–362.

27 Kennis, R.A., Rosser, E.J. Jr., Olivier, N.B., and Walker, R.W. (1996). Quantity and distribution of Malassezia organisms on the skin of clinically normal dogs. *J. Am. Vet. Med. Assoc.* 208 (7): 1048–1051.

28 Uchida, Y., Mizutani, M., Kubo, T. et al. (1992). Otitis externa induced with Malassezia pachydermatis in dogs and the efficacy of pimaricin. *J. Vet. Med. Sci.* 54 (4): 611–614.

29 Anderson, W.N. (1974). Treatment regimen for seborrhea of dogs. *J. Am. Vet. Med. Assoc.* 164 (11): 1111–1113.

30 Plant, J.D., Rosenkrantz, W.S., and Griffin, C.E. (1992). Factors associated with and prevalence of high Malassezia pachydermatis numbers on dog skin. *J. Am. Vet. Med. Assoc.* 201 (6): 879–882.

31 Sparber, F. and LeibundGut-Landmann, S. (2017). Host responses to Malassezia spp. in the mammalian skin. *Front. Immunol.* 8: 1614.

32 Ihrke, P.J., Schwartzman, R.M., Mcginley, K. et al. (1978). Microbiology of normal and seborrheic canine skin. *Am. J. Vet. Res.* 39 (9): 1487–1489.

33 Yurayart, C., Nuchnoul, N., Moolkum, P. et al. (2013). Antifungal agent susceptibilities and interpretation of Malassezia pachydermatis and Candida parapsilosis isolated from dogs with and without seborrheic dermatitis skin. *Med. Mycol.* 51 (7): 721–730.

34 Gross, T.L., Ihrke, P.J., Walder, E.J., and Affolter, V.K. (2005). *Skin Diseases of the Dog and Cat*, 2e. Ames, Iowa: Blackwell Publishing.

35 Willemse, T. (1992). Zinc-related cutaneous disorders of dogs. In: *Kirk's Current Veterinary Therapy XI* (ed. R.W. Kirk and J.D. Bonagura), 532–534. Philadelphia: W.B. Saunders.

36 Brown, R.G., Hoag, G.N., Smart, M.E., and Mitchell, L.H. (1978). Alaskan Malamute chondrodysplasia. V. Decreased gut zinc absorption. *Growth* 42 (1): 1–6.

37 Colombini, S. (1999). Canine zinc-responsive dermatosis. *Vet. Clin. North Am. Small Anim. Pract.* 29 (6): 1373–1383.

38 Colombini, S. and Dunstan, R.W. (1997). Zinc-responsive dermatosis in northern-breed dogs: 17 cases (1990–1996). *J. Am. Vet. Med. Assoc.* 211 (4): 451–453.

39 Shanley, K.J. (1990). Interpreting dermatologic lesions, Part II, Diagnostic techniques. *Vet. Tech.* 11: 149–156.

40 Werner, A.H. and Power, H.T. (1994). Retinoids in veterinary dermatology. *Clin. Dermatol.* 12 (4): 579–586.

41 Mauldin, E.A. (2013). Canine ichthyosis and related disorders of cornification. *Vet. Clin. North Am. Small Anim. Pract.* 43 (1): 89–97.

42 Grall, A., Guaguere, E., Planchais, S. et al. (2012). PNPLA1 mutations cause autosomal recessive congenital ichthyosis in golden retriever dogs and humans. *Nat. Genet.* 44 (2): 140–147.

43 Credille, K.M., Minor, J.S., Barnhart, K.F. et al. (2009). Transglutaminase 1-deficient recessive lamellar ichthyosis associated with a LINE-1 insertion in Jack Russell terrier dogs. *Br. J. Dermatol.* 161 (2): 265–272.

44 Mauldin EA, Casal ML, editors. (2008). Autosomal recessive ichthyosis in the American bulldog. North American Veterinary Forum Proceedings; Denver, CO.

45 Mauldin EA, Casal ML, editors. (2010). The molecular characterization of American bulldog ichthyosis. International Society of Veterinary Dermatopathology; Portland, Oregon.

46 Dahlqvist, J., Klar, J., Hausser, I. et al. (2007). Congenital ichthyosis: mutations in ichthyin are associated with specific structural abnormalities in the granular layer of epidermis. *J. Med. Genet.* 44 (10): 615–620.

47 Craig, M. (2009). Lesion morphology in veterinary dermatology. *UK Vet.* 14 (3): 1–4.

48 Wildermuth, B.E., Griffin, C.E., and Rosenkrantz, W.S. (2006). Feline pyoderma therapy. *Clin. Tech. Small Anim. Pract.* 21 (3): 150–156.

49 Favrot, C. (2013). Feline non-flea induced hypersensitivity dermatitis: clinical features, diagnosis and treatment. *J. Feline Med. Surg.* 15 (9): 778–784.

50 Nuttall, T., Harvey, R.G., and McKeever, P.J. (2009). *Skin Diseases of the Dog and Cat.* Boca Raton, FL: Taylor & Francis Group.

51 August, J.R. (2010). *Consultations in Feline Internal Medicine.* St. Louis, MO: Saunders.

52 Diesel, A. (2017). Cutaneous hypersensitivity dermatoses in the feline patient: a review of allergic skin disease in cats. *Vet. Sci.* 4 (2): E25.

53 Nagata, M. (2013). Applied dermatology: the cutaneous viral dermatoses in dogs and cats. *Compend. Contin. Educ. Vet.* 35 (7): E1.

54 Kunkle, G.A. (2006). Feline facial dermatoses challenge. *NAVC Clinician's Brief* (March): 16–19.

55 Thomson, M. (2007). Squamous cell carcinoma of the nasal planum in cats and dogs. *Clin. Tech. Small Anim. Pract.* 22 (2): 42–45.

56 Dorn, C.R., Taylor, D.O., and Schneider, R. (1971). Sunlight exposure and risk of developing cutaneous and oral squamous cell carcinomas in white cats. *J. Natl. Cancer Inst.* 46 (5): 1073–1078.

57 Murphy, S. (2013). Cutaneous squamous cell carcinoma in the cat: current understanding and treatment approaches. *J. Feline Med. Surg.* 15 (5): 401–407.

14

Skin Nodules and Tumors

14.1 Introduction to Terminology

Skin lesions can be classified as primary and secondary. Recall from Chapter 12 that primary lesions are the direct result of an underlying skin condition. They are, in a sense, the first responders.

Papules were introduced in Chapter 12 as one type of primary lesion. These are small, solid elevations of the skin that typically measure less than 1 cm in width [1]. A nodule is essentially a large papule, measuring 1 cm or more in diameter [1]. In addition to being larger, a nodule tends to invade the skin more deeply than a papule [1]. Rather than just involving the epidermis, a nodule typically invades the dermis, if not the subcutaneous tissues [1]. A tumor is a large nodule [1]. A tumor may involve one or more skin layers [1]. It is important to note that while most papules and nodules look and feel alike, there is no such classic appearance for tumors. Tumors come in a variety of sizes, shapes, consistencies, and textures (see Figures 14.1a–m).

14.2 Tracking Characteristics of Tumors over Time

As is evident from Figures 14.1a–m, no two tumors look or feel alike. Patients may also have more than one tumor, and tumors may either remain static or grow over time. Growth rates of tumors vary, in large part depending upon tumor type and location. Some are slow-growing and may be monitored over time by the veterinary client and clinician; others experience rapid growth that necessitates speedy intervention. Tumors may also change over time. The surface of a smooth tumor may become erosive or ulcerative, or what used to be a freely moveable tumor may become anchored to underlying tissue.

Because of the potential for tumor characteristics to change, it is critical that the veterinarian identify lesions in the medical record and describe to them in such a way that allows tumors to be tracked over time.

When one or more tumors are identified on physical exam, the veterinarian should document the following characteristics in the medical record:

- How many tumors?
- What size(s) are the tumors?
- Where are the tumors located?
- How long have they been present?
- How are the tumors configured?
- What is their surface texture? Are they smooth or erosive?
- What is their consistency? Are they homogenously soft or firm, or are they heterogeneous?
- How deep on palpation do the tumors appear to extend?
- Do any important neighboring anatomical structures appear to be involved?
- Are the tumors freely moveable or are they fixed in space?
- How have the tumors progressed or changed, based upon the client's reported history?
- How have the tumors progressed or changed, based upon the clinician's past assessment?
- Are the tumors painful on palpation?

In addition to documenting tumors in the text of the medical record, many veterinarians also make use of a "skin map," that is, an outline of the patient from the left, right, dorsal, and ventral views. This is particularly useful for veterinarians to keep track of a patient that has multiple lesions. The "skin map" provides a visual representation of the size and location of tumors, and notes how tumors appear to be progressing or regressing.

Photo documentation of tumors may also be helpful, particularly in electronic medical records where they can be uploaded directly into the patient's file.

The veterinarian may estimate tumor size. However, because tumor size factors into decision making when it comes to assessing how much the tumor has grown over time and whether or not it requires incisional or excisional biopsy, accuracy of measurements is critical. Measurement of tumor size should ultimately be done using calipers rather than guestimates. Calipers are a

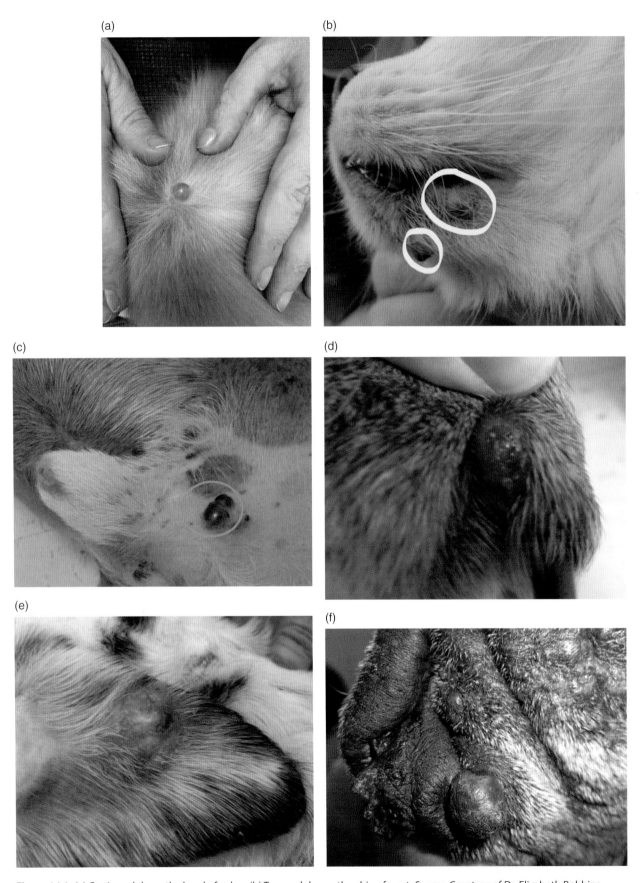

Figure 14.1 (a) Cystic nodule on the head of a dog. (b) Two nodules on the chin of a cat. *Source:* Courtesy of Dr. Elizabeth Robbins. (c) Melanotic nodules at the groin of a dog. (d) Ulcerative interdigital nodule in a dog. *Source:* Courtesy of Patricia Bennett, DVM. (e) Tumor associated with the ventral aspect of a canine pinna. *Source:* Courtesy of Patricia Bennett, DVM. (f) Tumor associated with the lower lip fold in a dog. *Source:* Courtesy of Dr. Elizabeth Robbins.

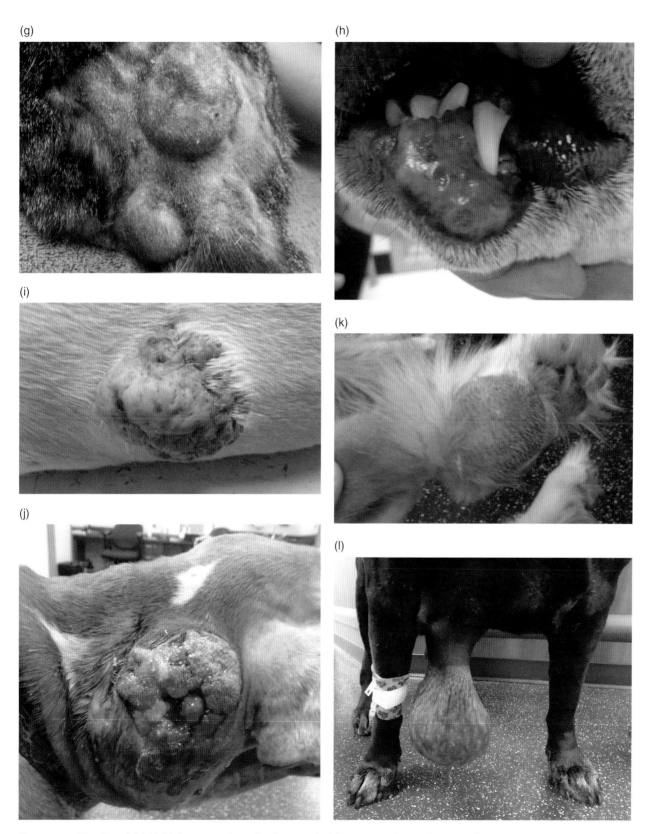

Figure 14.1 (Continued) (g) Multiple tumors along the dorsum of a feline patient. *Source:* Courtesy of Samantha B. Thurman, DVM. (h) Erosive tumor associated with the lower left lip of a canine patient. *Source:* Courtesy of Patricia Bennett, DVM. (i) Cauliflower-like tumor along the dorsum of a dog. (j) Extensive, ulcerative tumor caudal to the right pinna of a dog. (k) Tumor associated with the plantar aspect of a dog's right hind paw. *Source:* Courtesy of Patricia Bennett, DVM. (l). Pendulous tumor arising from the right axillary region of a canine patient. (m). Extensive, firm, anchored tumor arising from the right inguinal and flank regions of a canine patient. *Source:* Courtesy of Pamela Mueller, DVM.

(m)

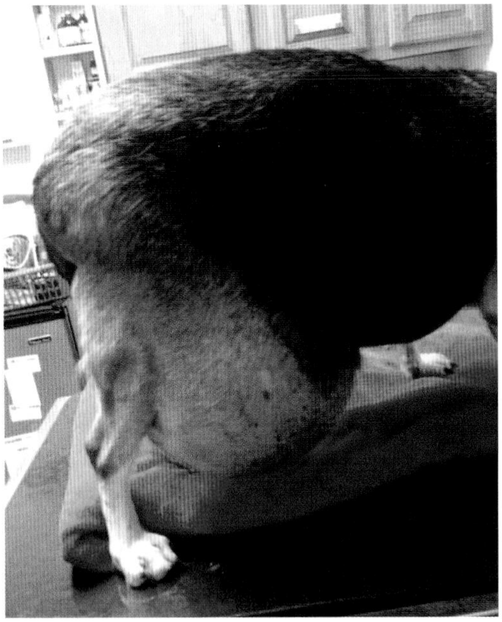

Figure 14.1 (Continued)

handy instrument to measure dimensions. Their use in human medicine is advised to improve accuracy at the time of diagnosis and to more accurately chart the patient's response to treatment [2] (see Figures 14.2a, b).

14.3 Important Diagnostic Tools for Evaluation of Tumors

Because most tumor types do not have a characteristic appearance, veterinarians require additional tools beyond the physical examination to assist with diagnosis and treatment options.

One inexpensive, minimally invasive diagnostic tool is fine-needle aspiration and cytologic examination [3, 4]. Fine-needle aspiration is a rapid diagnostic test in the sense that it can be performed in the clinic, at the time of the appointment, and the results can be read before the patient is discharged to the client. The patient does not require general anesthesia, and risks for bleeding and infection are low [3].

Although fine-needle aspiration does not provide the same quality of sample as does a biopsy, it is an important starting point for medical or surgical planning [3]. For example, consider mast cell tumors (MCTs). These are easily diagnosed via fine-needle aspiration and cytologic examination [3, 5]. Refer to Chapter 11, Figures 11.9a, b to recall the appearance of mast cells under light microscopy.

The advantage of knowing that the patient has a MCT prior to surgery is invaluable. Recall from Chapter 11 that mast cells degranulate spontaneously, releasing histamine and other inflammatory mediators into the circulation [6–10]. Degranulation is probable during surgical manipulation of the tumor. If this release is severe, the patient may go into a state of anaphylactic shock or experience gastrointestinal ulceration [6, 11, 12]. Knowing that a tumor consists of mast cells prepares the surgeon for these possible sequelae [6, 13]. Surgical candidates for MCT excision or resection are typically prophylactically prescribed gastroprotectants and antihistamines to combat the potential risk for degranulation.

Fine-needle aspiration also provides a presumptive diagnosis for such tumor types as lipomas, sebaceous cysts, other round cell tumors, and inflammatory processes, including abscesses [3].

Any structure that can be palpated on physical examination can be aspirated [4]. The use of ultrasonography is helpful for the aspiration of internal structures that either cannot be felt on examination or are adjacent to vital structures [4].

Different techniques for fine-needle aspiration have been published [3, 4]. The needle-off technique is when the needle, sans syringe, is inserted, manipulated, and redirected into the tissue of interest to obtain a sufficient sample. The needle is withdrawn. A syringe containing four to six milliliters of air is then attached to the needle to expel the sample onto a slide [4]. Be sure that the bevel of the needle is pointing down toward the slide so that the sample is directed onto the slide rather than into the surrounding air [4].

The needle-off technique is advantageous for working in and around small regions of the body, where having a syringe attached to the needle would get in the way [4]. Consider, for example, feline lymph nodes. These would present a challenge if the needle had to redirected with an attached syringe. There is just not sufficient space to accommodate the equipment needed [4].

The needle-on technique provides true aspiration. A six-cubic-centiliter (cc) syringe is attached to a 20 or 22 gauge needle. The seal to the syringe is broken, but all air is subsequently removed so that the syringe is empty. As soon as the beveled aspect of the needle has been inserted into the mass, the clinician draws back on the plunger. Aspiration results in negative pressure. When the clinician releases the plunger, the plunger returns to its default position. The clinician repeats this process three to five times. Suction is released on the syringe before the needle is withdrawn from the tissue [4]. The needle is removed from the syringe. Air is then drawn into the syringe. The needle is reattached to the syringe so that the sample can be expelled onto the slide [4].

(a)

(b)

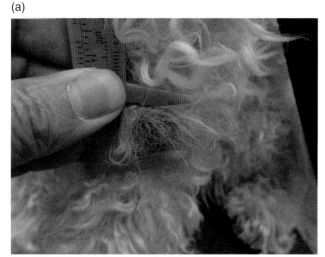
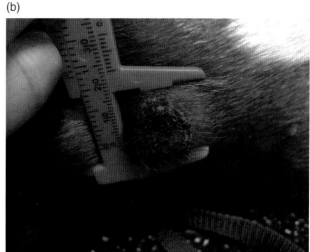

Figure 14.2 (a) Using calipers to quantify tumor size in a white dog. *Source:* Courtesy of Patricia Bennett, DVM. (b) Using calipers to quantify tumor size in a black dog. *Source:* Courtesy of Samantha B. Thurman, DVM.

The needle-on technique may be more successful at releasing cells from a firm mass because of the negative pressure that is generated in the process of true aspiration [4]. It may also be less painful for the patient than to have the needle redirected again and again, as occurs with the needle-off technique [4].

Regardless of technique, the result should be a sample that can be spread out among four to six slides [3, 4].

An advantage of creating multiple slides from a single sample is that the content of each slide will be thinner. Slides cannot be read if samples are allowed to dry as thick beads of material [4].

Creating smears also helps to distribute the material evenly [4].

Consult a cytology text for pointers on how to create even slides with minimal disruption to the cellular content of each sample.

Slides must be dry and stained before being read by the veterinarian [3, 4]. The stained slide is then examined via light microscopy, initially under low magnification to find a region of interest. Once this region has been identified, the magnification is raised.

A common stain that is used in veterinary practice is the modified Wright's stain [14]. Commercially, this is marketed as the product Diff-Quik.

Slides may also be submitted for cytologic examination by a clinical pathologist. A primary advantage of this consultation is the experience that the clinical pathologist brings to the table. In addition, the pathologist may be able to provide additional details, such as the tumor's tissue of origin, by means of special stains [3].

Cytology from fine-needle aspiration is imperfect in the sense that it may or may not obtain a representative population of cells for diagnosis. A biopsy has the potential to provide more information because its sample size is larger.

However, cytology is an important starting point to guide patient planning [3].

When the results of cytology suggest that surgical excision of the tumor is in the best interest of the patient, or when the cytologic examination is inconclusive, a biopsy may be necessary.

There are three main types of biopsies [15]:

- Punch biopsy
- Incisional biopsy
- Excisional biopsy

Punch biopsies are single-use tools to sample tissue [15]. The lesion is centered under the punch. The punch is pressed firmly against the skin and rotated in one direction. When the punch reaches the subcutis, the sampler feels a significant decrease in resistance. At this point, the punch is removed, and the tissue section is grasped with tissue forceps. If necessary, the attachment of the sample to adjacent tissue is snipped using iris scissors. The defect is closed using one cruciate suture or several simple interrupted sutures, depending upon the size of the punch [15].

For most lesions, a six-millimeter (mm) punch is used. However, lesions on the nasal planum or footpads may require a smaller tool, such as a four-mm punch [15].

Punch biopsy tools dull readily when reused on the same patient. This can lead to artifact from tissue compression. Replace punches as necessary when sampling more than one lesion on a given patient [15].

Punch biopsies are more effective when used to sample small lesions such as papules or crusts. Incisional or excisional biopsies are more often employed for nodules and tumors [15]. These techniques offer the ability to sample deeper, including muscle planes that may be bridged by the tumor [15].

An incisional biopsy samples a fraction of the tumor; an excisional biopsy removes the tumor in its entirety. An incisional biopsy may be preferred as the initial approach to a tumor in order to secure the diagnosis and then determine the extent of surgical margins that are required for a complete excision. An excisional biopsy may also not be possible without radical reconstruction.

Keep in mind that no one diagnostic tool is perfect. Biopsy results may be inconclusive. Biopsy results may not provide a definitive answer; however, they may effectively rule out one or more differential diagnoses. They may also narrow the scope of possibilities to one group of diseases, for example, allergic skin disease. In these circumstances, the clinician must take on the role of detective. S/he must combine information that was obtained from the biopsy and piece that together with the patient's history, presenting complaint, and physical examination findings to determine what is most likely for the patient and where to go from here [15].

14.4 Common Skin Tumors of Dogs and Cats

The takeaway message from this chapter is that skin tumors require more investment by the clinician than just history taking and gross observational skills. Skin tumors require a diagnostic investigation to determine how best to approach these lesions. In particular, veterinary clients want answers to the following questions:

- Is the tumor painful?
- Is the tumor cancerous?
- Will the tumor continue to grow?
- Does the tumor need to be surgically excised?

Most of these questions cannot be answered without additional information, as from a diagnostic work-up.

That being said, certain tumor types and certain tumor locations predominate. It behooves the novice clinician to become familiar with and be able to recognize what some of these are so that s/he has a baseline of knowledge in terms of how to proceed.

In the dog, the majority of skin tumors are benign [16, 17]. By contrast, in the cat, the majority of skin tumors are malignant [16–19].

A handful of studies in the veterinary medical literature explore the incidence of skin tumor types in dogs and cats [18–24].

Sebaceous adenomas and perianal adenomas are common in dogs [16]. Intact male dogs are overrepresented when it comes to the latter [25].

MCTs are common in the dog and represent 11–27% of skin malignancies [16, 26–28]. Digital squamous cell carcinoma (SCC) and melanoma are also common in the dog [16, 29, 30].

Young dogs are at greater risk for cutaneous histiocytoma and viral papillomas [24, 31, 32].

One of the largest, most recent studies to be published on cutaneous tumors in cats was conducted by Ho et al. in 2017. This study examined more than 9000 skin tumors in cats throughout the United Kingdom during a seven-year period [18]. The top five skin tumors in this population of cats were the following [18]:

- Basal cell tumor
- Fibrosarcoma
- SCC
- MCT
- Lipoma

These results are consistent with other studies involving feline cutaneous tumors [18, 20, 21, 33, 34].

According to Ho's study, certain breeds, including the Himalayan and Snowshoe, appear to have an increased risk for cutaneous tumor development [18]. Other breeds, such as the Siamese, Burmese, and Birman, appear to have reduced risk [18].

When only malignant skin tumors are considered, no purebred is at increased risk. However, the Siamese, Burmese, and Birman continue to experience risk reduction [18]. So, too, do the Persian, Ragdoll, British Blue, and Norwegian Forest Cat breeds [18].

The goal of this chapter is not to cover every cutaneous tumor type in dogs and cats; whole texts are devoted to canine and feline oncology.

Instead, the goal of this chapter is to highlight certain skin tumors that veterinarians may see in clinical practice. Additional resources can then be consulted for a comprehensive discussion on medical and/or surgical management.

14.4.1 Papillomas

Papillomas are also known as warts. They more commonly occur in dogs than cats and are most often associated with papillomavirus, a double-stranded, non-enveloped DNA virus [35].

More than one syndrome of papillomatosis exists in dogs [35, 36]. Of these, canine oral papillomatosis manifests most often in clinical practice.

Canine oral papillomatosis is contagious dog-to-dog [35]. Direct contact allows for viral transmission between patients. In addition, virus may be spread by fomites when abraded skin is involved [36].

Dogs are typically young adults, less than two years of age, at the time of presentation [35]. Unlike most tumors,

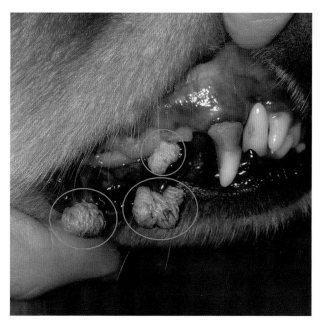

Figure 14.3 Canine oral papillomatosis. *Source:* Courtesy of Paola Bazan Steyling.

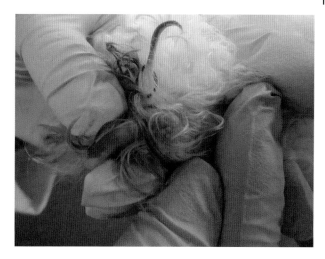

Figure 14.4 Cutaneous papilloma associated with the digit of a canine patient. *Source:* Courtesy of Patricia Bennett, DVM.

lesions have a classic appearance with frond-like projections. These lesions preferentially target the oral cavity, eyelids, and skin [36, 37] (see Figure 14.3).

Histologically, the fronds that are visible to the naked eye are composed of thickened layers of squamous epithelium [38].

Most lesions spontaneously regress within one to three months of developing and therefore require no treatment [35, 39]. Historically, benign neglect has been the typical approach for this tumor type unless lesions interfere with daily activities such as eating, due to chronic irritation and inflammation that may be associated with secondary infection.

It is important to note that in rare cases, progression to SCC is possible [35, 36, 39, 40]. Therefore, lesions that persist may need to be addressed surgically or at least monitored for changes in tumor characteristics that may suggest a progression toward insidious disease.

In addition to oral papillomas, papillomas may be cutaneous. Cutaneous papillomas tend to occur in older dogs, particularly Cocker spaniels and Kerry blue terriers [36]. These carry the same classic appearance as oral papillomas; however, these concentrate around the head, eyelids, and feet [36] (see Figure 14.4).

Wart-like lesions include fibropapillomas, or skin tags. These also represent proliferations of squamous epithelium, but they lack the classic frond-like appearance of viral-induced papillomas. They also tend to be solitary and slow-growing (see Figures 14.5a–d).

Skin tags are most often benign. Surgery is typically pursued for cosmetic reasons or if the lesion's presence causes irritation. For example, skin tags associated with the eyelid may contact the cornea, causing corneal irritation and triggering epiphora [41].

14.4.2 Cutaneous Histiocytomas

Cutaneous histiocytomas are common, benign, localized tumors [42, 43]. They result from an over-proliferation of histiocytes, immune cells that are engaged in phagocytosis and antigen presentation during the inflammatory process [42, 44]. In other words, what constitutes a normal response to inflammation by the immune system goes into overdrive [42]. Cutaneous histiocytomas therefore constitute an inappropriate immune response [42].

Cutaneous histiocytomas are characterized by nodules that concentrate on the head, neck, limbs, perineum, and scrotum [42, 44–49]. Lesions tend to be fast-growing and dome-shaped [42, 45, 46] (see Figure 14.6).

Young dogs under the age of three years old are most often affected [46]. Solitary lesions are most typical; however, Shar Pei dogs appear to be predisposed to developing one or more cutaneous histiocytomas [45, 46].

Fine-needle aspiration and cytologic examination confirm the presence of a round cell tumor. Unlike MCTs, which contain cytoplasmic purple-staining granules, cutaneous histiocytomas contain abundant light basophilic cytoplasm without vacuoles or granular material. Nuclei are round to oval in shape and may be eccentrically placed [42] (see Figure 14.7).

Most cutaneous histiocytomas spontaneously regress, although the process may take weeks to months [36]. Regression appears to be faster, on the order of six weeks, when lesions are solitary, whereas regression may take upwards of 10 months for multiple lesions [42, 45, 46].

Note that cutaneous histiocytoma is distinct from systemic histiocytosis (SH), which more commonly

(a)

(b)

(c)

(d)

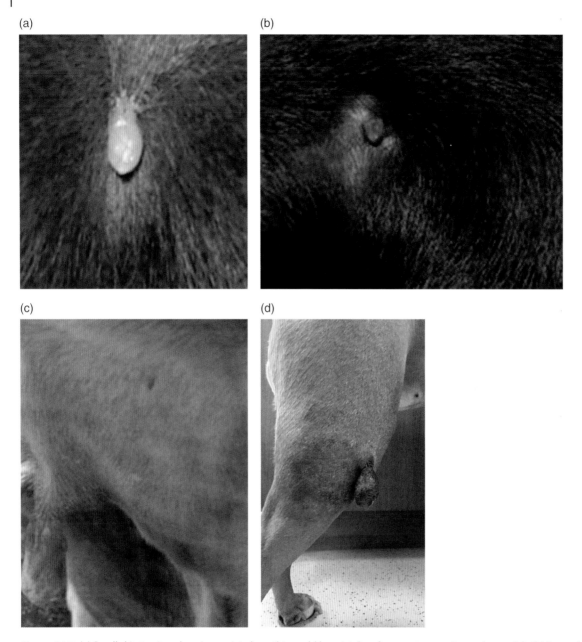

Figure 14.5 (a) Small skin tag in a dog. Appreciate how this could be mistaken for an ectoparasite, such as a tick. (b) Second example of a small skin tag in a dog. (c) Large, pendulous skin tag on the chest of a dog. Note how it attaches to the body via a stalk. (d) Pendulous skin tag at the lateral aspect of the right stifle of a dog.

presents in Bernese mountain dogs [42, 44–49]. Patients with SH have multiple organ involvement in addition to cutaneous lesions and therefore present as systematically ill [42, 44, 45, 50, 51].

14.4.3 Mast Cell Tumors

MCTs occur more commonly in dogs than in cats, and may occur in both cutaneous and visceral forms [16]. Canine cutaneous MCTs tend to prefer the trunk, perineal region, and the extremities [52]. By contrast, feline cutaneous MCTs tend to prefer the head and neck [22].

Refer to Chapter 11, Section 11.2.4 for a description of MCT cytology, degranulation, and associated sequelae.

It is important to recognize that MCTs can be readily identified on cytologic examination; however, histologic grading of the tumor and staging of the disease is critical to obtain an accurate prognosis. Depending upon tumor grade, surgery may be reattempted to create wider margins. Radiotherapy, chemotherapy, or immunotherapy may also be prescribed [36].

All MCTs have malignancy potential, and may metastasize to regional lymph nodes, the spleen, liver, or bone marrow [36]. Examination of these sites via other

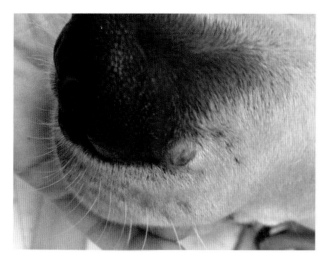

Figure 14.6 Cutaneous histiocytoma associated with the nose in a canine patient.

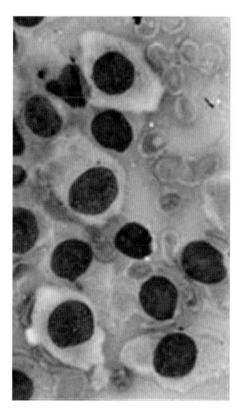

Figure 14.7 Cytology of a cutaneous histiocytoma in a canine patient.

diagnostic modalities, such as thoracic radiography and abdominal ultrasound, is important for patient planning.

14.4.4 Sebaceous Adenomas

Sebaceous adenomas are common benign tumors that arise from the sebaceous or sweat glands. These tumors tend to be age-related, meaning that they become more

common findings on physical examination of older patients [53–58]. It is especially common for aged patients to develop more than one.

Cocker spaniels, huskies, Alaskan malamutes, and Samoyeds may be predisposed to developing sebaceous adenomas [54, 56].

These raised lesions may occur anywhere on the body. However, the preferred locations appear to be the head and trunk [53, 57]. In particular, sebaceous adenomas favor the eyelids [54, 56, 59].

Rarely, sebaceous adenomas develop in association with the mammary or salivary glands [53, 60–62].

It is common for sebaceous adenomas to be mistaken for papillomas [36]. They tend to arise from a narrow stalk and may appear to be multilobulated. The tumors themselves are alopecic (see Figures 14.8a–c).

Unlike papillomas, sebaceous adenomas do not spontaneously resolve. Surgical excision may be performed for cosmetic purposes or to remove a growth that is irritating to the patient. For example, eyelid masses may inhibit the patient from opening the eye or may trigger excessive tear production by contacting the cornea. Epiphora may also result in crusty eyelids from an accumulation of dried tear discharge. This discharge may be irritating to the patient as well as aesthetically displeasing to the client.

Clients need to be forewarned that recurrence is frequent, particularly after incomplete surgical removal [53, 54, 56].

14.4.5 Lipomas

Lipomas are subcutaneous, benign fatty tumors that occur more commonly in dogs than cats [63]. In September 2017, they were considered to be the number one health condition in pedigree dogs [64].

Lipomas can develop anywhere on the body. They can remain small or can grow to become quite large (see Figures 14.9a–d).

Classically, lipomas palpate as soft, squishy lumps beneath the skin's surface. They tend to have some mobility on palpation; however, as they grow larger, they may become anchored or pinned between tissues. They also may run out of space to grow, for example, if they develop on distal limbs or the ventral chest.

Most dogs with one lipoma will develop more as they age.

Historically, lipomas have been "diagnosed" by feel alone. However, this is misleading and poses a threat to the health of the patient. Lipomas cannot be distinguished grossly from infiltrative lipomas, which invade local tissues, including muscle and fascia. They also cannot be distinguished from liposarcomas by appearance alone. These exhibit malignancy and have metastatic potential.

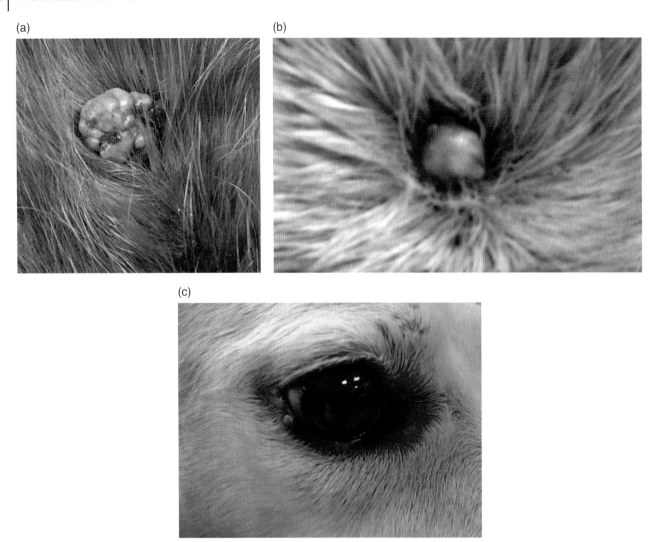

Figure 14.8 (a) Mottled pink and gray, fleshy sebaceous adenoma on the lateral surface of the thigh of a canine patient. (b) Pink, fleshy sebaceous adenoma on the dorsum of a canine patient. (c) Sebaceous adenoma associated with the lower eyelid of this canine patient. *Source:* Courtesy of Patricia Bennett, DVM.

All growths should therefore be subject to fine-needle aspiration and cytologic examination. Simple lipomas consist of lipocytes and cytologically are difficult to differentiate from adipose tissue [63]. However, identification of spindle cells from an aspirated sample should raise the veterinarian's index of suspicion that a more insidious disease process may be underway [65].

It is also important to consider that lipomas can invade body cavities. Although 98% of lipomas occur at subcutaneous sites alone, they may extend into or arise from intrathoracic, intra-abdominal, and intra-pelvic sites [63, 65–74]. In these unusual cases, clinical signs result from compression or entrapment of other organs, such as intestinal strangulation by lipoma [63].

14.4.6 Mammary Tumors

Canine and feline mammary tumors are relatively common. In female cats, mammary neoplasia is the third most common tumor type [75–77].

As in humans, there is appreciable hormonal risk associated with mammary cancer in dogs and cats. Although estrogens and progesterones are important for normal development of the mammary glands in both species, chronic exposure has been linked to tumor formation [78].

When dogs are spayed before their first estrus, the risk of developing mammary neoplasia is 0.5%. When ovariohysterectomy is delayed to just before the second estrus, risk rises to 8%. Spaying a dog any time after the second estrus results in an increased risk of 26% [77, 78].

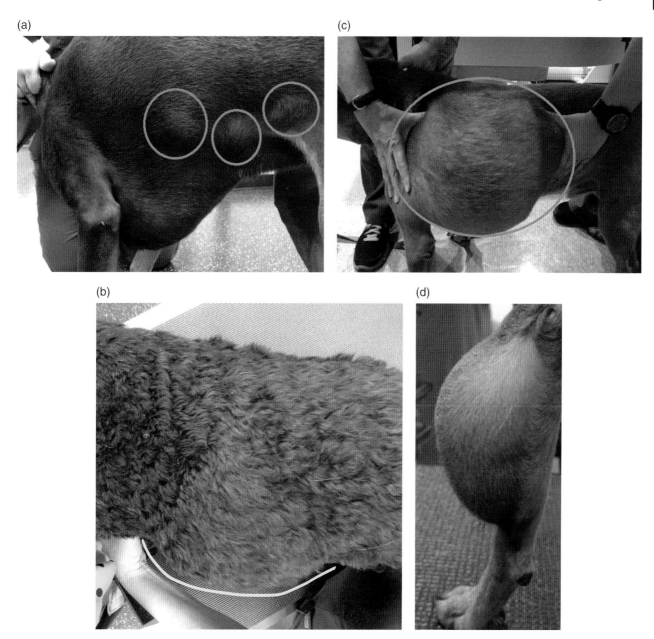

Figure 14.9 (a) Canine patient with three visible and palpable lipomas. (b) Large lipoma associated with the left lateral body wall of this canine patient. (c) Extensive lipoma overtaking the left lateral body wall of this canine patient. *Source:* Courtesy of Samantha B. Thurman, DVM. (d) Lipoma overtaking the limb of this canine patient. *Source:* Courtesy of Patricia Bennett, DVM.

Other risk factors include obesity at a young age and ingestion of a diet high in red meat [79].

Certain canine breeds appear to be predisposed to mammary neoplasia, including Toy and Miniature Poodles, English Springer Spaniels, Brittany Spaniels, Cocker Spaniels, English Setters, Pointers, German Shepherds, Maltese Yorkshire Terriers, and Dachshunds [78, 80, 81].

Roughly 50% of canine mammary tumors are malignant [78, 82, 83]. Of those malignant tumor types, tubular carcinoma or adenocarcinoma is most common in dogs [78]. This tumor tends to metastasize to the regional lymph nodes and the lungs via the lymphatic system [78].

Affected dogs tend to present to the veterinarian healthy at initial diagnosis [78]. The veterinary client may have palpated one or more masses in the mammary chain, or the veterinarian may have discovered these as incidental findings on a routine physical examination [78].

Affected patients tend to be older. They are usually either sexually intact, or they have a history of being spayed at a later age [78].

Dogs have five pairs of mammary glands. More typically, mammary neoplasia in the dog involves the caudal fourth and/or fifth pairs [78] (see Figures 14.10a–c).

Fine-needle aspiration and cytologic examination are inferior to biopsies for the diagnosis of mammary neoplasia. It is often difficult to differentiate between malignant and benign types [78]. Therefore, biopsy is the preferred tool for the initial diagnostic work-up [78].

Mammary neoplasia in the dog tends to be mixed, meaning that more than one type of neoplasia can be present in a given tumor. Additionally, different tumors may represent different cytologic types. It is therefore critical that all tumors be biopsied [78, 84, 85].

Because of the potential for metastasis to the lungs, three-view thoracic radiographs are an important step in the diagnostic approach [78].

In the feline patient, mammary neoplasia is much more frequently associated with malignancy [75, 76]. Eighty to ninety percent of mammary tumors are malignant in cats [76, 86, 87].

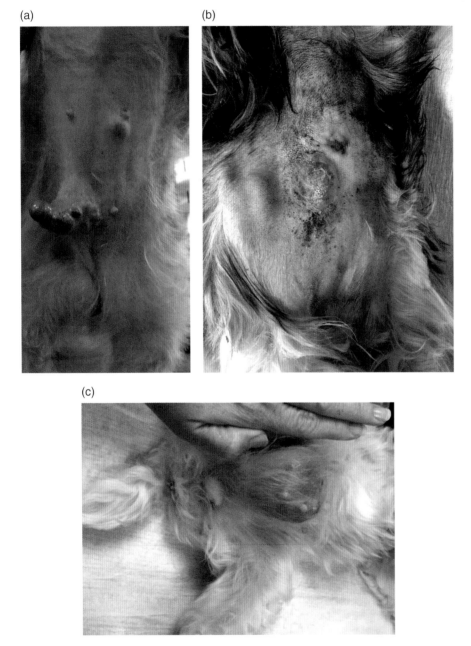

Figure 14.10 (a) Mammary neoplasia in a canine patient. *Source:* Courtesy of Kara Thomas, DVM, CVMA. (b) Erosive mammary neoplasia in a canine patient. *Source:* Courtesy of Dr. Stephanie Harris. (c) Mammary neoplasia in a canine patient. *Source:* Courtesy of Samantha B. Thurman, DVM.

Much like dogs, aged, intact cats also experience an increased risk for development of mammary cancer. The risk is seven times greater in intact cats than those that are altered [88]. In addition, the use of progestins to curb behavioral aggression or prevent pregnancy increases the risk, in both males and females [89, 90].

Siamese and other Oriental breeds may be at increased risk [75].

Cats have four pairs of mammary glands. Like dogs, the caudal glands of cats appear to develop mammary neoplasia more frequently than the cranial ones [91, 92].

A mammary mass may be solitary; however, multiple masses, with multiple gland involvement, are common in cats [75]. Lesions may be discrete and unattached to surrounding tissue, or they may be anchored [75]. Surface erosion or ulceration is possible [75]. Most mammary tumors in cats are adenocarcinomas [75].

Significant swelling and pain tend to be associated with inflammatory carcinomas [93]. Even so, looks can be deceiving. Fibroadenomatous hyperplasia in younger cats may be mistaken for malignant disease [76]. Confirmation of mammary neoplasia is critical for patient planning. Because malignancies occur so much more frequently in cats than dogs, fine-needle aspiration is an acceptable place to begin in terms of one's diagnostic approach [75].

Complete staging is indicated for those in which mammary neoplasia is present to determine the extent of disease [75]. Aspiration of drainage lymph nodes and three-view chest radiographs are essential diagnostic tools.

Surgical resection of one or both chains is considered the mainstay of treatment. Bilateral chain mastectomy can be performed at once or it can be staged [75].

It is important to recognize that mammary malignancies are more likely in cats than dogs and that prognosis is guarded. Local recurrence or metastasis hastens death.

14.4.7 Anal Gland Tumors

Perianal tumors occur more often in dogs than cats. These include perianal adenomas and anal sac adenocarcinomas. Perineal swelling or discomfort may be the first sign of disease [94] (see Figures 14.11a, b).

When perianal or anal sac masses are of significant size, they often cause compression of the anal canal. Affected patients may present with a history of dyschezia. For this reason, this tumor type will be discussed in Part Six of the textbook, within chapters that emphasize the digestive system.

14.5 Less Common Skin Tumors of Dogs and Cats

Not all tumors commonly occur in dogs and cats, and not all tumor types can be touched upon in this text. However, one tumor type in particular will be covered here that constitutes an important contagious tumor of dogs [95]. That tumor type is canine transmissible venereal tumor (TVT).

Although TVT is relatively uncommon in North America and North and Central Europe, it is enzootic throughout most of the world [95]. In particular, it is concentrated in tropical and subtropical regions, including Puerto Rico, Papua New Guinea, and Central and South America [95, 96]. TVT is the most common tumor

(a)

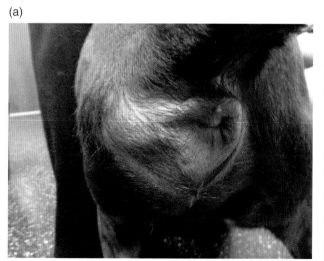

(b)

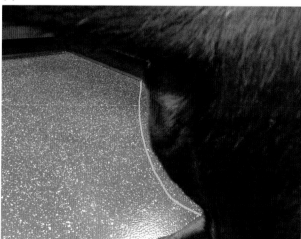

Figure 14.11 (a) Appreciable swelling of the canine perineum due to anal sac tumor, as viewed head-on. *Source:* Courtesy of Patricia Bennett, DVM. (b) Side view of perineal swelling due to anal sac tumor. *Source:* Courtesy of Patricia Bennett, DVM.

(a) (b)

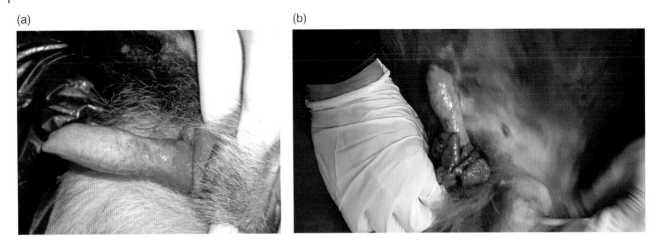

Figure 14.12 (a) Transmissible venereal tumor (TVT) at the base of a canine penis. *Source:* Courtesy of Laura Polerecky, LVT. (b) TVT at the base and along the shaft of a canine penis. *Source:* Courtesy of Hannah Butler.

type in dogs in the Bahamas, Japan, and India [97–99]. In addition, TVT extends into the canine populations of south-western France, Ireland, China, the Far East, the Middle East, and parts of Africa [95–97].

As veterinarians and veterinary students engage in outreach to other nations and communities, including those outlined above, they are likely to experience this tumor.

Although TVT is found predominantly on the external genitalia, it has been known to invade the skin, which is why it is being discussed here [97, 100–104]. Isolated case reports of TVT in the soft palate, oral, nasal, and conjunctival mucosa have also appeared in the veterinary literature [95, 100, 105–108].

TVT is spread when tumor cells are deposited on damaged epithelial surfaces [95, 100]. The act of mating is abrasive to genital surfaces. Additionally, those behaviors that occur in canine populations, such as licking, biting, and scratching at genitalia, perpetuate transmission between mucous membranes.

Young, sexually mature, and sexually active dogs are most at risk for development of TVT [95, 100]. There have also been isolated cases that support transmission from the dam to her pups [109].

Lesions in both males and females vary in shape and size. TVT may take on a cauliflower appearance by developing fronds, much like a papilloma, or it may be multilobulated [95]. The smallest lesions are on the order of micrometers; contrast that to large masses upwards of 15 cm [95]. The surface integrity of the tumor is likely to be compromised. Ulcerations, hemorrhage, and secondary infections are common [95].

In males, lesions most often concentrate at the bulbus glandis. Less frequently, they appear on the shaft or the glans penis [95] (see Figures 14.12a, b).

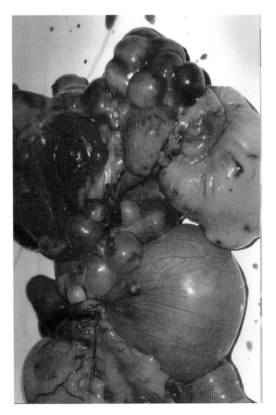

Figure 14.13 Transmissible venereal tumor (TVT) associated with canine ovaries. *Source:* Courtesy of Laura Polerecky, LVT.

In females, lesions more frequently occur at the vestibule. Less frequently, they are visible within the vagina or at the vulvar lips [95].

During surgical exploration, as during an ovariohysterectomy, lesions have also been found in the ovaries [100] (see Figure 14.13).

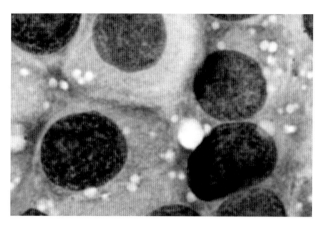

Figure 14.14 Round cell tumor appearance of transmissible venereal tumor (TVT). Note the large nucleus, eccentrically placed nucleolus, and basophilic, vacuolated cytoplasm.

Diagnosis is via history taking, physical examination findings, cytologic examination, and histology [95]. On cytology, TVT is a round cell tumor. Associated cells are large, with large nuclei, and an eccentrically placed nucleolus [100]. Because the nucleus is large, each cell has only a thin rim of basophilic cytoplasm that may or may not contain vacuoles (see Figure 14.14).

Excisional surgery, chemotherapy, immunotherapy, and radiotherapy have been attempted as a means to eliminate this tumor [95]. However, tumors regress in healthy, immunocompetent dogs [95]. Only those dogs with immunosuppression, ocular, or central nervous system involvement carry a guarded prognosis [95].

References

1 Craig, M. (2009). Lesion morphology in veterinary dermatology. *UK Vet.* 14 (3): 1–4.

2 Wasson, J., Amonoo-Kuofi, K., Scrivens, J., and Pfleiderer, A. (2012). Caliper measurement to improve clinical assessment of palpable neck lumps. *Ann. R. Coll. Surg. Engl.* 94 (4): 256–260.

3 Impellizeri JA. (2012). Skills laboratory: how to make a high-quality slide from a fine-needle aspirate. Vet. Med. DVM360. (May). http://veterinarymedicine.dvm360.com/skills-laboratory-how-make-high-quality-slide-fine-needle-aspirate.

4 Garrett, L. (2010). Fine-needle aspiration. *NAVC Clinician's Brief* (June): 61–66.

5 Welle, M.M., Bley, C.R., Howard, J., and Rufenacht, S. (2008). Canine mast cell tumours: a review of the pathogenesis, clinical features, pathology and treatment. *Vet. Dermatol.* 19 (6): 321–339.

6 Misdorp, W. (2004). Mast cells and canine mast cell tumours. A review. *Vet. Q.* 26 (4): 156–169.

7 Dean, P.W. (1988). Mast-cell tumors in dogs – diagnosis, treatment, and prognosis. *Vet. Med.* 83 (2): 185–188, 190–92.

8 Thamm, D.H. and Vail, D.M. (2007). Mast cell tumors. In: *Withrow & MacEwen's Small Animal Clinical Oncology*, 4e (ed. S.J. Withrow and D.M. Vail), 402–424. St. Louis, MO: Saunders Elsevier.

9 Rabanal, R. and Ferrer, L. (eds.) (2002). *Mast Cell Tumors: From the Molecular Biology to the Clinic.* ISVD; Nice.

10 Scott, D.W., Miller, W.H., and Griffin, C.G. (2001). Mast cell tumor. In: *Small Animal Dermatology*, 6e (ed. D.W. Scott, W.H. Miller and C.G. Griffin), 1320–1330. St. Louis, MO: W.B. Saunders.

11 Byers, J.C. and Fleischman, R.W. (1981). Peptic-ulcers associated with a mast-cell tumor in a dog. *Canine Pract.* 8 (3): 42–44.

12 Fox, L.E., Rosenthal, R.C., Twedt, D.C. et al. (1990). Plasma histamine and gastrin-concentrations in 17 dogs with mast-cell tumors. *J. Vet. Intern. Med.* 4 (5): 242–246.

13 Rogers, K.S. (1996). Mast cell tumors: dilemmas of diagnosis and treatment. *Vet. Clin. North Am. Small Anim. Pract.* 26 (1): 87–102.

14 Gortel, K. (2013). Recognizing pyoderma: more difficult than it may seem. *Vet. Clin. North Am. Small Anim. Pract.* 43 (1): 1–18.

15 Bartlett, S. (2017). Dermatology diagnostics: cutaneous biopsy. *Today's Veterinary Practice* 7 (4). https://todaysveterinarypractice.com/dermatology-details-dermatology-diagnostics-cutaneous-biopsy/ (accessed 3 May 2019).

16 Meleo, K.A. (1997). Tumors of the skin and associated structures. *Vet. Clin. North Am. Small Anim. Pract.* 27 (1): 73–94.

17 Ogilvie, G.K. and Moore, A.S. (1995). *Manging the Veterinary Cancer Patient.* Trenton: Veterinary Learning Systems.

18 Ho, N.T., Smith, K.C., and Dobromylskyj, M.J. (2017). Retrospective study of more than 9000 feline cutaneous tumours in the United Kingdom: 2006–2013. *J. Feline Med. Surg.* 20 (2): 128–134. 1098612X17699477.

19 Schmidt, J.M., North, S.M., Freeman, K.P., and Ramiro-Ibanez, F. (2010). Feline paediatric oncology: retrospective assessment of 233 tumours from cats up to one year (1993 to 2008). *J. Small Anim. Pract.* 51 (6): 306–311.

20 Graf, R., Gruntzig, K., Boo, G. et al. (2016). Swiss feline cancer registry 1965–2008: the influence of sex, breed and age on tumour types and tumour locations. *J. Comp. Pathol.* 154 (2–3): 195–210.

21 Miller, M.A., Nelson, S.L., Turk, J.R. et al. (1991). Cutaneous neoplasia in 340 cats. *Vet. Pathol.* 28 (5): 389–395.

22 Buerger, R.G. and Scott, D.W. (1987). Cutaneous mast cell neoplasia in cats: 14 cases (1975–1985). *J. Am. Vet. Med. Assoc.* 190 (11): 1440–1444.

23 Fox, L.E. (1995). Feline cutaneous and subcutaneous neoplasms. *Vet. Clin. North Am. Small Anim. Pract.* 25 (4): 961–979.

24 Schmidt, J.M., North, S.M., Freeman, K.P., and Ramiro-Ibanez, F. (2010). Canine paediatric oncology: retrospective assessment of 9522 tumours in dogs up to 12 months (1993–2008). *Vet. Comp. Oncol.* 8 (4): 283–292.

25 Susaneck, S.J. and Withrow, S.J. (1989). Tumors of the skin and subcutaneous tissues. In: *Clinical Veterinary Oncology* (ed. S.J. Withrow and E.G. MacEwen), 139. Philadelphia, PA: JB Lippincott.

26 Cohen, D., Reif, J.S., Brodey, R.S., and Keiser, H. (1974). Epidemiological analysis of the most prevalent sites and types of canine neoplasia observed in a veterinary hospital. *Cancer Res.* 34 (11): 2859–2868.

27 Dorn, C.R., Taylor, D.O., Schneider, R. et al. (1968). Survey of animal neoplasms in alameda and contra costa counties, California. II. Cancer morbidity in dogs and cats from Alameda County. *J. Natl. Cancer Inst.* 40 (2): 307–318.

28 Priester, W.A. (1973). Skin tumors in domestic animals. Data from 12 United States and Canadian colleges of veterinary medicine. *J. Natl. Cancer Inst.* 50 (2): 457–466.

29 Marino, D.J., Matthiesen, D.T., Stefanacci, J.D., and Moroff, S.D. (1995). Evaluation of dogs with digit masses: 117 cases (1981–1991). *J. Am. Vet. Med. Assoc.* 207 (6): 726–728.

30 Obrien, M.G., Berg, J., and Engler, S.J. (1992). Treatment by digital amputation of subungual squamous-cell carcinoma in dogs – 21 cases (1987–1988). *J. Am. Vet. Med. Assoc.* 201 (5): 759–761.

31 Moore, P.F. and Affolter, V.K. (2009). Histiocytic disease complex. In: *Kirk's Current Veterinary Therapy XIV: Small Animal Practice* (ed. T. Bonagura), 348–351. St. Louis, MO: Elsevier Science.

32 Teifke, J.P., Lohr, C.V., and Shirasawa, H. (1998). Detection of canine oral papillomavirus-DNA in canine oral squamous cell carcinomas and p53 overexpressing skin papillomas of the dog using the polymerase chain reaction and non-radioactive in situ hybridization. *Vet. Microbiol.* 60 (2–4): 119–130.

33 Bostock, D.E. (1986). Neoplasms of the skin and subcutaneous tissues in dogs and cats. *Br. Vet. J.* 142 (1): 1–19.

34 Jorger, K. (1988). Skin tumors in cats. Occurrence and frequency in the research material (biopsies from 1984–1987) of the Institute for Veterinary Pathology, Zurich. *Schweiz. Arch. Tierheilkd.* 130 (10): 559–569.

35 Bianchi, M.V., Casagrande, R.A., Watanabe, T.T.N. et al. (2012). Canine papillomatosis: a retrospective study of 24 cases (2001–2011) and immunohistochemical characterization. *Pesqui. Vet. Bras.* 32 (7): 653–657.

36 Lewis, D. (2011). Dermatologic disorders. In: *Clinical Medicine of the Dog and Cat*, 2e (ed. M. Schaer), 9–48. London: Manson Publishing.

37 Goldschmidt, M.H. and Hendrick, M.J. (2002). Tumors of the skin and soft tissues. In: *Tumors in Domestic Animals*, 4e (ed. D.J. Meuten), 45–118. Ames, Iowa: Iowa State Press.

38 Gross, T.L., Ihrke, P.J., Walder, E.J., and Affolter, V.K. (2005). *Skin Diseases of the Dog and Cat: Clinical and Histopathologic Diagnosis*. Oxford: Blackwell.

39 Munday, J.S., Thomson, N.A., and Luff, J.A. (2017). Papillomaviruses in dogs and cats. *Vet. J.* 225: 23–31.

40 Nicholls, P.K. and Stanley, M.A. (1999). Canine papillomavirus – a centenary review. *J. Comp. Pathol.* 120 (3): 219–233.

41 Villalobos, A.E. (2018). *The Merck Veterinary Manual*. Kenilworth, NJ, USA: Merck Sharp & Dohme Corp., a subsidiary of Merck & Co., Inc.

42 Coomer, A. and Liptak, J.M. (2008). Canine histiocytic diseases. *Compendium* 30 (4): 202–217.

43 Ramsey, I.K., McKay, J.S., Rudorf, H., and Dobson, J.M. (1996). Malignant histiocytosis in three Bernese mountain dogs. *Vet. Rec.* 138 (18): 440–444.

44 Affolter, V.K. and Moore, P.F. (2000). Canine cutaneous and systemic histiocytosis: reactive histiocytosis of dermal dendritic cells. *Am. J. Dermatopathol.* 22 (1): 40–48.

45 Affolter, V.K. and Moore, P.F. (eds.) (1999). *Canine Histiocytic Proliferative Disease*. AAVD.

46 Moore, P.F. and Affolter, V.K. (2005). Canine and feline histiocytic diseases. In: *Textbook of Veterinary Internal Medicine* (ed. S.J. Ettinger and E.C. Feldman), 779–782. St. Louis: Elsevier Saunders.

47 Paterson, S., Boydell, P., and Pike, R. (1995). Systemic histiocytosis in the Bernese mountain dog. *J. Small Anim. Pract.* 36 (5): 233–236.

48 Moore, P.F. (1984). Systemic histiocytosis of Bernese mountain dogs. *Vet. Pathol.* 21 (6): 554–563.

49 Mays, M.B. and Bergeron, J.A. (1986). Cutaneous histiocytosis in dogs. *J. Am. Vet. Med. Assoc.* 188 (4): 377–381.

50 Affolter, V.K. and Moore, P.F. (2002). Localized and disseminated histiocytic sarcoma of dendritic cell origin in dogs. *Vet. Pathol.* 39 (1): 74–83.

51 Austin, B.R. and Henderson, R.A. (2003). What is your diagnosis. *J. Am. Vet. Med. Assoc.* 223 (11): 1569–1570.

52 Macy, D.W. and MacEwen, E.G. (1989). Mast cell tumors. In: *Clinical Veterinary Oncology* (ed. S.J.

Wlthrow and E.G. MacEwen), 156. Philadelphia, PA: WB Saunders.

53 Strafuss, A.C. (1976). Sebaceous gland adenomas in dogs. *J. Am. Vet. Med. Assoc.* 169 (6): 640–642.

54 Pullet, L.T. and Stannard, A.A. (1990). Tumor of the skin of soft tissues. In: *Tumors in Domestic Animals*, 3e (ed. J.E. Moulton), 23–87. California: University of California Press.

55 Roberts, S.M., Severin, G.A., and Lavach, J.D. (1986). Prevalence and treatment of palpebral neoplasms in the dog: 200 cases (1975–1983). *J. Am. Vet. Med. Assoc.* 189 (10): 1355–1359.

56 Vail, M.D. and Withrow, S.J. (1996). Tumors of the skin and subcutaneous tissue. In: *Small Animal Clinical Oncology* (ed. S.J. Withrow and E.G. MacEwen), 167–191. Pennsylvania: W.B. Saunders Company.

57 Halouzka, R. and Nevole, M. (1976). Sebaceous gland tumors in dogs. *Vet. Med. (Praha).* 21 (9): 565–572.

58 Muller, G.H., Kirk, R.W., and Scott, D.W. (1989). Neoplastic diseases. In: *Small Animal Dermatology* (ed. J. Dyson), 844–958. Philadelphia: W.B. Saunders Company.

59 Krehbiel, J.D. and Langham, R.F. (1975). Eyelid neoplasms of dogs. *Am. J. Vet. Res.* 36 (1): 115–119.

60 Yasuno, K., Takagi, Y., Kobayashi, R. et al. (2011). Mammary adenoma with sebaceous differentiation in a dog. *J. Vet. Diagn. Investig.* 23 (4): 832–835.

61 Smrkovski, O.A., LeBlanc, A.K., Smith, S.H. et al. (2006). Carcinoma ex pleomorphic adenoma with sebaceous differentiation in the mandibular salivary gland of a dog. *Vet. Pathol.* 43 (3): 374–377.

62 Go, D.M., Lee, S.H., Woo, S.H., and Kim, D.Y. (2017). Intra-oral sebaceous gland tumours in two dogs. *J. Comp. Pathol.* 157 (4): 296–298.

63 Mayhew, P.D. and Brockman, D.J. (2002). Body cavity lipomas in six dogs. *J. Small Anim. Pract.* 43 (4): 177–181.

64 British Veterinary Association. (2017). Lipomas found to be number one disorder among Kennel Club dogs. https://veterinaryrecord.bmj.com/content/vetrec/181/12/306.full.pdf (accessed 14 January 2018).

65 Avallone, G., Pellegrino, V., Muscatello, L.V. et al. (2017). Spindle cell lipoma in dogs. *Vet. Pathol.* 54 (5): 792–794.

66 Teunissen, G.H. (1977). Intrathoracic lipoma in a dog. *Tijdschr Diergeneeskd.* 102 (2): 113–116.

67 McLaughlin, R. Jr. and Kuzma, A.B. (1991). Intestinal strangulation caused by intra-abdominal lipomas in a dog. *J. Am. Vet. Med. Assoc.* 199 (11): 1610–1611.

68 Mullins, R.A., Bergamino, C., and Kirby, B.M. (2017). What is your diagnosis? *J. Am. Vet. Med. Assoc.* 250 (6): 615–617.

69 Bergman, P.J., Withrow, S.J., Straw, R.C., and Powers, B.E. (1994). Infiltrative lipoma in dogs: 16 cases (1981–1992). *J. Am. Vet. Med. Assoc.* 205 (2): 322–324.

70 Miles, J. and Clarke, D. (2001). Intrathoracic lipoma in a Labrador retriever. *J. Small Anim. Pract.* 42 (1): 26–28.

71 Regan, R.C., Northrup, N.C., Sharma, A., and Ellis, A.E. (2015). What is your diagnosis? *J. Am. Vet. Med. Assoc.* 247 (12): 1365–1367.

72 Ben-Amotz, R., Ellison, G.W., Thompson, M.S. et al. (2007). Pericardial lipoma in a geriatric dog with an incidentally discovered thoracic mass. *J. Small Anim. Pract.* 48 (10): 596–599.

73 Klosterman, E.S., Heng, H.G., Freeman, L.J., and Childress, M.O. (2012). Transdiaphragmatic extension of a retroperitoneal lipoma into the intrathoracic extrapleural space via the lumbocostal trigone in a dog. *J. Am. Vet. Med. Assoc.* 240 (8): 978–982.

74 Simpson, D.J., Hunt, G.B., Church, D.B., and Beck, J.A. (1999). Benign masses in the pericardium of two dogs. *Aust. Vet. J.* 77 (4): 225–229.

75 Morris, J. (2013). Mammary tumours in the cat: size matters, so early intervention saves lives. *J. Feline Med. Surg.* 15 (5): 391–400.

76 Gimenez, F., Hecht, S., Craig, L.E., and Legendre, A.M. (2010). Early detection, aggressive therapy: optimizing the management of feline mammary masses. *J. Feline Med. Surg.* 12 (3): 214–224.

77 Schneider, R., Dorn, C.R., and Taylor, D.O. (1969). Factors influencing canine mammary cancer development and postsurgical survival. *J. Natl. Cancer Inst.* 43 (6): 1249–1261.

78 Sorenmo, K. (2003). Canine mammary gland tumors. *Vet. Clin. North Am. Small Anim. Pract.* 33 (3): 573–596.

79 Perez Alenza, D., Rutteman, G.R., Pena, L. et al. (1998). Relation between habitual diet and canine mammary tumors in a case-control study. *J. Vet. Intern. Med.* 12 (3): 132–139.

80 Kurzman, I.D. and Gilbertson, S.R. (1986). Prognostic factors in canine mammary tumors. *Semin. Vet. Med. Surg.* 1 (1): 25–32.

81 Yamagami, T., Kobayashi, T., Takahashi, K., and Sugiyama, M. (1996). Prognosis for canine malignant mammary tumors based on TNM and histologic classification. *J. Vet. Med. Sci.* 58 (11): 1079–1083.

82 Misdorp, W., Cotchin, E., Hampe, J.F. et al. (1973). Canine malignant mammary-tumors .3. Special types of carcinomas malignant mixed tumors. *Vet. Pathol.* 10 (3): 241–256.

83 Priester, W.A. and Mantel, N. (1971). Occurrence of tumors in domestic animals – data from 12 United-States and Canadian Colleges of Veterinary Medicine. *J. Natl. Cancer Inst.* 47 (6): 1333–1334.

84 Fowler, E.H., Wilson, G.P., and Koestner, A. (1974). Biologic behavior of canine mammary neoplasms based on a histogenetic classification. *Vet. Pathol.* 11 (3): 212–229.

85 Benjamin, S.A., Lee, A.C., and Saunders, W.J. (1999). Classification and behavior of canine mammary epithelial neoplasms based on life-span observations in beagles. *Vet. Pathol.* 36 (5): 423–436.

86 Carpenter, J. (1987). Tumor and tumor-like lesions. In: *Diseases of the Cat: Medicine and Surgery* (ed. J. Holzworth), 406–596. Philadelphia: W.B. Saunders.

87 Allen, H.L. (1973). Feline mammary hypertrophy. *Vet. Pathol.* 10 (6): 501–508.

88 Misdorp, W., Romijn, A., and Hart, A.A. (1991). Feline mammary tumors: a case-control study of hormonal factors. *Anticancer Res.* 11 (5): 1793–1797.

89 Jacobs, T.M., Hoppe, B.R., Poehlmann, C.E. et al. (2010). Mammary adenocarcinomas in three male cats exposed to medroxyprogesterone acetate (1990–2006). *J. Feline Med. Surg.* 12 (2): 169–174.

90 Keskin, A., Yilmazbas, G., Yilmaz, R. et al. (2009). Pathological abnormalities after long-term administration of medroxyprogesterone acetate in a queen. *J. Feline Med. Surg.* 11 (6): 518–521.

91 Zappulli, V., De Zan, G., Cardazzo, B. et al. (2005). Feline mammary tumours in comparative oncology. *J. Dairy Res.* 72: 98–106.

92 Moore, A.S. and Ogilvie, G.K. (2001). Mammary tumors. In: *Feline Oncology: A Comprehensive Guide to Compassionate Care* (ed. G.K. Ogilvie and A.S. Moore), 355–367. Trenton, N.J: Veterinary Learning Systems.

93 Hahn, K.A. and Adams, W.H. (1997). Feline mammary neoplasia: biological behavior, diagnosis, and treatment alternatives. *Feline Pract.* 25 (2): 5–11.

94 Burgess KE, Barber LG, Gauthier M. (2009). Identifying and treating anal sac adenocarcinoma in dogs. http://veterinarymedicine.dvm360.com/identifying-and-treating-anal-sac-adenocarcinoma-dogs.

95 Ganguly, B., Das, U., and Das, A.K. (2016). Canine transmissible venereal tumour: a review. *Vet. Comp. Oncol.* 14 (1): 1–12.

96 Rust, J.H. (1949). Transmissible lymphosarcoma in the dog. *J. Am. Vet. Med. Assoc.* 114 (862): 10–14.

97 Higgins, D.A. (1966). Observations on the canine transmissible venereal tumour as seen in the Bahamas. *Vet. Rec.* 79 (3): 67–71.

98 Tateyama, S., Nazaka, H., Ashizawa, H. et al. (1986). Neoplasm in animals studied at Miyazaki University in 1970–1979. *J. Jpn. Vet. Med. Assoc.* 39: 242–247.

99 Singh, P., Singh, K., Sharma, D.K. et al. (1991). A survey of tumors in domestic-animals. *Indian Vet. J.* 68 (8): 721–725.

100 Vermooten, M.I. (1987). Canine transmissible venereal tumor (TVT): a review. *J. S. Afr. Vet. Assoc.* 58 (3): 147–150.

101 Weir, E.C., Pond, M.J., Duncan, J.R., and Polzin, D.J. (1978). Extra-genital occurrence of transmissible venereal tumor in dog – literature-review and case-reports. *J. Am. Anim. Hosp. Assoc.* 14 (4): 532–536.

102 van Rensburg, I.B. and Petrick, S.W. (1980). Extragenital malignant transmissible venereal tumour in a bitch. *J. S. Afr. Vet. Assoc.* 51 (3): 199–201.

103 Holmes, J.M. (1981). A 125IUdR technique for measuring the cell loss from subcutaneously growing canine transmissible venereal tumours. *Res. Vet. Sci.* 31 (3): 306–311.

104 Duncan, J.R. and Prasse, K.W. (1979). Cytology of canine cutaneous round cell tumors. Mast cell tumor, histiocytoma, lymphosarcoma and transmissible venereal tumor. *Vet. Pathol.* 16 (6): 673–679.

105 Bright, R.M., Gorman, N.T., Probst, C.W., and Goring, R.L. (1983). Transmissible venereal tumor of the soft palate in a dog. *J. Am. Vet. Med. Assoc.* 183 (8): 893–895.

106 Milo, J. and Snead, E. (2014). A case of ocular canine transmissible venereal tumor. *Can. Vet. J.* 55 (1): 1245–1249.

107 Komnenou, A.T., Thomas, A.L., Kyriazis, A.P. et al. (2015). Ocular manifestations of canine transmissible venereal tumour: a retrospective study of 25 cases in Greece. *Vet. Rec.* 176 (20): 523.

108 Papazoglou, L.G., Koutinas, A.F., Plevraki, A.G., and Tontis, D. (2001). Primary intranasal transmissible venereal tumour in the dog: a retrospective study of six spontaneous cases. *J. Vet. Med. A Physiol. Pathol. Clin. Med.* 48 (7): 391–400.

109 Marcos, R., Santos, M., Marrinhas, C., and Rocha, E. (2006). Cutaneous transmissible venereal tumor without genital involvement in a prepubertal female dog. *Vet. Clin. Pathol.* 35 (1): 106–109.

Part Three

Eyes and Ears

15

Acute Blindness

15.1 Description of Clinical Sign

When it occurs, acute blindness is typically bilateral [1]. Although some owners are able to identify unilateral blindness, most patients are able to compensate sufficiently so that unilateral blindness goes undetected [1].

The acutely blind patient typically presents for sudden disorientation. This may include bumping into familiar objects within the home environment. Alternatively, the patient may be reluctant to use the stairs or jump on or off the furniture [1].

The client may also have noticed persistent mydriasis of both eyes, regardless of ambient lighting (see Figures 15.1a–c).

Mydriasis is particularly noticeable to owners of feline patients because the normal pupil shape of a cat is a vertical slit when lighting is adequate [2] (see Figure 15.2).

When the feline pupil shape becomes rounded like a dog's even in direct sunlight, the change is strikingly apparent and atypical.

It is important to note that pupils also dilate when the sympathetic nervous system is activated. This response is particularly strong in cats that are undergoing the "fight or flight" response. Keep in mind that a cat with saucer-like pupils in a well-lit room may be fearful or defensively aggressive rather than acutely blind [2].

15.2 Additional Physical Examination Features Suggestive of Vision Loss

Patients that are bilaterally avisual lack menace responses in both eyes. The menace response tests the optic (II) and facial (VII) cranial nerves [2, 3].

The menace response is a test in which the clinician makes a sudden movement toward each eye with his hand. Each eye is tested separately [2, 3].

If the patient is visual, it will observe the threat. Assuming that both cranial nerves II and VII are intact, and their pathways to the brain and brainstem are functional, the patient will blink as a protective function [2, 3].

If the patient is avisual, the patient will not observe the threat and will not blink in response to the menacing gesture [2, 3].

Note that when performing the menace response, it is important not to create excessive air currents or touch the eyelids inadvertently in the process. Doing so may result in the anticipated outcome (blinking). However, the blink will be due to touch as a stimulus rather than vision [4, 5].

Other tests that may be employed to evaluate vision include "tracking" and maze tests [6].

"Tracking" tests involve dropping a small, innocuous object, such as a cotton ball, directly in front of the patient, and to both the patient's right and left sides. This allows for testing of each visual field. The object is typically dropped from a height of 20–30 cm. Visual patients follow the course of the falling object with their eye. This test may need to be repeated more than once in order to capture the patient's attention. A patient that consistently does not track the cotton ball may have reduced or absent vision [6].

Laser pointers are another handy tool to test tracking, particularly in feline examinations [6].

Maze tests involve the placement of stationary objects around the room. This effectively creates an obstacle course through which the patient is expected to navigate. Objects need not be fancy. Basic clinic essentials such as chairs and buckets are efficient and effective tools. The patient is placed on one side of the maze and is called to, by either the client or a member of the veterinary team who is stationed on the opposite side of the maze. A patient that is avisual is likely to bump or stumble into objects [6].

The maze test should be performed both in the light and in the dark to test photopic and scotopic vision, respectively [6]. Obstacle set-up should be altered between the photopic and scotopic tests to prevent the patient from memorizing the appropriate navigational course [6].

Common Clinical Presentations in Dogs and Cats, First Edition. Ryane E. Englar.
© 2019 John Wiley & Sons, Inc. Published 2019 by John Wiley & Sons, Inc.

(a)

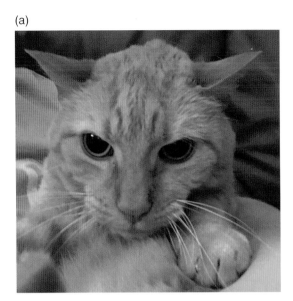

(b)   (c)

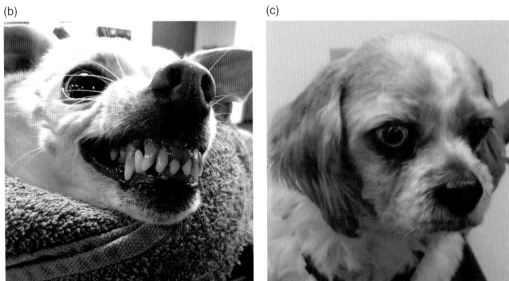

Figure 15.1 (a) Bilateral mydriasis in a feline patient. Note that this patient is not acutely blind; he is agitated as is evident by his ear carriage. However, mydriasis would have the same appearance in an acutely blind patient. *Source:* Courtesy of Rachel A. Karner. (b) Mydriasis in a canine patient. Although this photograph only depicts the right eye, both pupils were sufficiently dilated to the point that it was challenging to discern a rim of iris. Like the patient in Figure 15.1a, this dog is not acutely blind; he is reacting aggressively. However, mydriasis would have the same appearance in an acutely blind patient. *Source:* Courtesy of Media Resources at Midwestern University. (c) Mydriasis in a canine patient. This patient is blind. Mydriasis is readily apparent in this patient because the patient's right eye has a light blue iris, the rim of which stands out against the round, dilated, black pupil.

One challenge associated with maze tests is that patients may not always cooperate. A patient may refuse to navigate through the maze. In this case, it is difficult to assess if there is a true visual deficit or if the patient's reluctance is purely behavioral [6].

Cats, in particular, are notorious for refusing to complete the maze test. They have a tendency to freeze, making the test inconclusive [6].

15.3 Relevant Physical Examination Features that Assist with Disease Localization

Vision is complicated because its pathway involves far more than just the eyes. Vision requires the eyes to take in information and transmit that information to the brain via the optic nerve [1, 7].

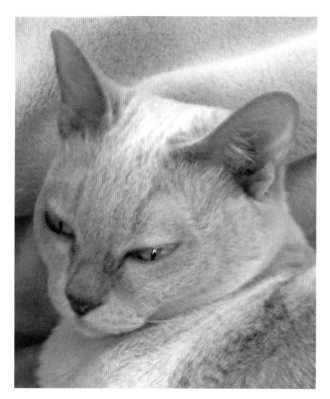

Figure 15.2 Normal pupil shape in a feline patient that is exposed to appropriate ambient lighting. Appreciate the vertical slit appearance.

In the dog, approximately 75% of optic nerve fibers from the right eye and 75% from the left eye cross at the base of the brain, at the optic chiasm. From here, these fibers course through the optic tracts into the brain [1, 7].

The complexity of this pathway is worth noting because in order for the patient to be visual, the patient must not only have functional eyes, but also functional optic nerves, optic tracts, and visual cortex [1, 7]. We often assume that avisual patients are blind because of ocular disease when in fact avisual patients may have functionally normal eyes and an abnormal brain [1, 7].

Visual deficits can therefore result from lesions anywhere in the eye–brain pathway [1, 7]. The three most common sites for lesions along the pathway that result in blindness include [1, 7]

- Retina
- Optic nerve(s)
- Visual cortex.

15.3.1 The Pupillary Light Reflex

To facilitate lesion location, the clinician can test direct and consensual pupillary light reflexes (PLRs) [1].

Intact PLRs confirm that the optic (II) and oculomotor (III) cranial nerves are functioning [4, 5].

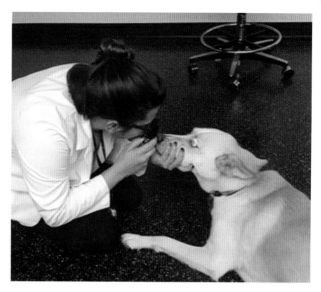

Figure 15.3 Using a direct ophthalmoscope in a canine patient. *Source:* Courtesy of Sarah Ciamello.

To test for intact PLRs, a bright light is directed at each eye. This light may come from a pen light or a direct ophthalmoscope (see Figure 15.3).

The eye at which the light is directed should constrict its pupil rapidly and remain small as long as the light source is persistent. This test assesses the direct PLR. A positive, direct PLR test is one in which the pupil into which light is directed becomes miotic. This is considered normal [4, 5].

The indirect or consensual PLR evaluates the contralateral eye. For instance, if a bright light is directed at the left eye, the right eye should also exhibit miosis. A positive, indirect PLR test is one in which the pupil of the contralateral eye becomes miotic. This is considered normal [4, 5].

Positive direct and indirect PLRs do not guarantee that the patient is visual. However, their presence or absence can facilitate lesion localization [1, 4, 5]. This is because the PLR and vision share the same neuroanatomical pathway until they reach the lateral geniculate nucleus [1].

When lesions occur at or rostral to the lateral geniculate nucleus, meaning that they occur at one or both optic tracts, the optic chiasm, optic nerve, or retina, the patient will lack both menace responses and PLRs [1].

However, when lesions that cause blindness occur beyond the lateral geniculate nucleus, PLRs will still be intact despite absent menace responses [1]. This is important to remember because PLRs will be present in a patient who is cortically blind [4, 5].

Testing for PLRs is therefore a critical test to use early on in the diagnostic approach to a patient that presents with acute blindness [1].

15.3.2 An Introduction to Fundoscopy

Fundoscopy is just as important as testing for PLRs in an acutely blind patient [1]. Fundoscopy allows the clinician to evaluate the deepest layers of the globe, including the retina, the choroid, and the optic disc [2].

In the healthy patient, the retina is transparent, and the pigmented portion of the choroid shines through [2]. In addition to visualizing the choroid, it is also possible to see the optic disc, a pink-white, triangular-to-round region where the nerve fibers of the retina pool together [2].

Dorsal to the optic disc, there is a hemi-spherical zone called the tapetum lucidum. The tapetum lucidum increases the light that is available to photoreceptors. This creates "eyeshine" when light is directed at the patient [4, 8, 9] (see Figure 15.4).

The normal canine and feline fundus varies in color from blue-green to orange-yellow [4, 8, 9] (see Figures 15.5a, b).

Colors vary between individuals [4, 8, 9].

Some patients have a reduced-to-absent tapetal region, and the non-tapetal fundus lacks pigment. The result is a subalbinotic fundus [10] (see Figure 15.6).

Dogs with merle coats; dogs or cats with blue irises; and dogs or cats with heterochromic irises are more likely to have a subalbinotic fundus [10]. This is considered normal variation [10].

Being able to recognize what constitutes a normal fundus is important so that the clinician is able to differentiate this appearance from the abnormal.

Learning how to perform a proper fundic exam is beyond the scope of this text. Consult the reference, *Performing the Small Animal Physical Examination*, for tips on techniques.

This chapter emphasizes the detection of abnormalities when they arise.

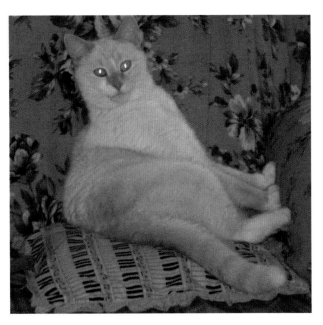

Figure 15.4 Note the "eyeshine" that is caused by a normal structure, the tapetum lucidum, in this feline patient. *Source:* Courtesy of Kathryn Knowles.

(a)   (b)

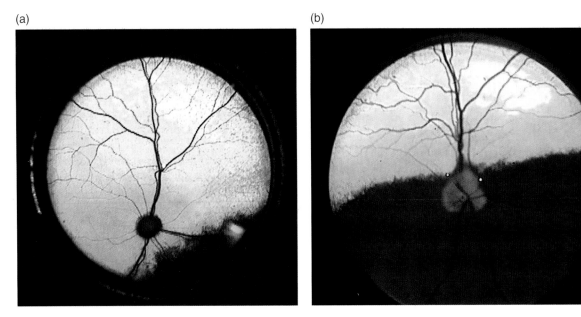

Figure 15.5 (a) The normal feline fundus. *Source:* Courtesy of D.J. Haeussler, Jr., MS, DVM, DACVO. (b) Example of the normal canine fundus. *Source:* Courtesy of D.J. Haeussler, Jr., MS, DVM, DACVO.

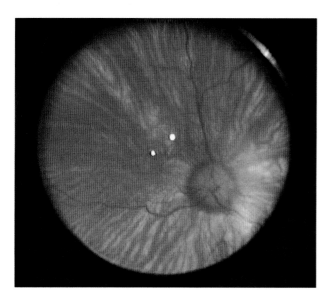

Figure 15.6 The subalbinotic fundus in a canine patient. *Source:* Courtesy of D.J. Haeussler, Jr., MS, DVM, DACVO.

15.4 Diseases of the Retina that May Result in Acute Blindness

Several retinal diseases may result in acute blindness. Those that the clinician is most likely to encounter in clinical practice include the following [1]:

- Retinal dysplasia
- Retinal detachment
- Sudden acquired retinal degeneration syndrome (SARDS)
- Fluoroquinolone retinopathy
- Retinal degeneration secondary to ketamine and methylnitrosurea

15.4.1 Retinal Dysplasia

Retinal dysplasia is a condition in which the retina does not develop or differentiate as expected [1, 11].

The retina should be a flat anatomical structure. When dysplasia occurs focally, the retina develops one or more folds that may impair vision [1, 11].

Acute blindness is more often the result of complete retinal dysplasia [1, 11]. These cases involve either nonattachment of the retina at birth due to extreme developmental anomaly or acute onset of retinal detachment. The details of retinal detachment will be covered in Section 15.4.2.

The following canine breeds are predisposed to developing retinal disease in its severest form: Bedlington terriers, Springer spaniels, Labrador retrievers, and Samoyeds [1, 11–15]. Other affected breeds that have appeared in the veterinary literature include Cocker spaniels, Yorkshire terriers, Beagles, and Rottweilers [11].

A hereditary basis has been identified in most of these breeds [1, 11]. However, retinal dysplasia does not have to be genetic. Retinal dysplasia may result from other patient and environmental factors, including exposure to canine herpesvirus and radiation [16, 17].

Cats are less likely to develop retinal dysplasia than dogs. The disease appears to be inherited in certain lines of Abyssinian and Somali cats [18].

Canine and feline patients with inherited retinal dysplasia present at an early age [1]. Initially, affected pups may be mistaken for being clumsy when in fact they have visual deficits [19].

Early screening of pups via fundoscopy will identify those with characteristics of retinal dysplasia [20]. Affected pups should not be bred [1].

15.4.2 Retinal Detachment

Retinal detachments refer to the separation of retinal layers from the retinal pigment epithelium (RPE). The RPE nourishes the neurosensory retina, absorbs scattered light, and forms the blood-retinal barrier [1]. When the RPE and neurosensory retina are no longer in close contact, vision is acutely disrupted.

Human patients who experience retinal detachment often complain of photopsia, that is, flashes of light within their peripheral vision. They may also report a gradual darkening of their peripheral vision. This may be described as a shadow or a curtain that is pulled over their field of vision.

We cannot ask veterinary patients what it is that they experience during a retinal detachment; however, their retinas detach for many of the same reasons that human retinas do [1]:

- Rhegmatogenous retinal detachment
- Exudative retinal detachment
- Tractional retinal detachment
- Traumatic retinal detachment

15.4.2.1 Rhegmatogenous Retinal Detachments

Rhegmatogenous retinal detachments occur when the retina is perforated by one or more tears. These tears allow the vitreous body in the posterior chamber of the eye to leak behind the retina, causing it to bulge and ultimately peel away from the RPE [1].

In health, the vitreous body is a jellylike material that sits as a spacer between the cranial lens and the caudal retina. Its purpose is to cushion both the lens and the retina. To serve that purpose, it is firmly attached to both [1].

Over time, the gel like consistency of the vitreous body may liquefy because of age or disease [1].

Additionally, certain breeds, such as the Papillon, Shih Tzu, Havanese, Brussels Griffon, Chihuahua, Italian

Greyhound, and Whippet, are predisposed to degeneration of the vitreous [1].

As the vitreous body liquefies, it no longer supports the retina, and in fact, its increased mobility can jar the retina. Tears in the retina may form because of the tension caused by the tugging of the liquefied vitreous against its retinal attachment points [1].

More commonly, rhegmatogenous retinal detachments occur secondary to diseases of the lens or lens instability [21, 22]. Cataracts, for example, as well as their surgical correction via phacoemulsification, increase the chance of retinal detachment [23–26]. So, too, does surgical extraction of an unstable lens [22].

15.4.2.2 Exudative Retinal Detachments

Exudative retinal detachments occur when contents from the choroidal vasculature leak into and accumulate within the space between the neurosensory retina and the RPE. These contents include the by-products of chorioretinitis, which may be triggered by bacteria, fungi, viruses, parasites, or protozoa [1, 27–37].

In the cat, toxoplasmosis can result in chorioretinitis [38]. In addition, the most common viral causes of chorioretinitis include feline immunodeficiency virus (FIV), feline leukemia virus (FeLV), and feline infectious peritonitis (FIP) [38, 39].

Fungal diseases such as cryptococcosis, blastomycosis, histoplasmosis, candidiasis, and coccidioidomycosis have also been implicated, in both dogs and cats [38, 40–42].

In the dog, chorioretinitis is less common and more often related to rare diseases or rare presentations of more common disease. For example, *Toxocara canis* is a common canine roundworm that is frequently implicated in gastrointestinal disease; however, isolated case reports demonstrate that it can result in chorioretinitis [43]. Canine brucellosis and prototheosis can also both result in chorioretinitis [44–46]; so, too, can *Sarcocystis neurona* [47].

More commonly, exudative retinal detachments result from underlying systemic hypertension [48].

In cats, hypertension is characterized as having persistently elevated, indirect systolic blood pressure at greater than 160–170 mmHg and/or elevated diastolic pressures greater than 100 mmHg [48–53].

In dogs, hypertension is characterized as having persistency elevated, indirect systolic pressures of 180–200 mmHg and/or elevated diastolic pressures greater than 100 mmHg [50, 54, 55].

This sustained elevation in systolic blood pressure impacts the arterial system and by extension, the eyes, kidneys, heart, and brain [49]. These so-called target organs are critically impacted by hypertension prior to other tissues in the body because they depend upon a rich arterial supply [49].

In companion animal medicine, systemic hypertension is common [38, 50, 51, 56–60]. It may be primary or secondary to underlying disease [49–51, 56, 61, 62]. Primary systemic hypertension is more common in dogs than cats, although it may be more common in cats than was once believed [50, 59, 63–66].

Secondary systemic hypertension results most typically from renal disease [49–53, 58, 61, 67–69]. In addition, systemic hypertension has been associated with hyperthyroidism, acromegaly, diabetes mellitus, chronic anemia, erythropoietin treatment, and high salt diets in cats [50–52, 58, 62, 70, 71].

Patients with hyperadrenocorticism, pheochromocytomas, and primary hyperaldosteronism may also develop systemic hypertension with target organ damage [49, 50, 62, 72, 73].

Hypothyroidism in dogs may cause hypertension; however, this is reserved for those cases that are complicated by severe hypercholesterolemia and atherosclerosis [50, 74]. These patients have reduced vascular compliance that may over time lead to increased blood pressure as a compensatory mechanism [74].

Retinopathy, with associated blindness, is one of the most common sequelae of systemic hypertension [51, 52, 57]. In the early stages of disease, hypertensive retinopathy may be characterized by retinal edema [49]. As hypertension persists, retinal hemorrhages may be observed during fundoscopy [49, 51, 52, 59, 62, 69] (see Figures 15.7a, b).

Retinal hemorrhages may be focal, discrete, and small, as in pinpoint dots, or they may be geographic and extensive [75].

Retinal detachment represents the most significant ocular change that is associated with hypertensive retinopathy. Retinal detachment occurs when disease is advanced and/or hypertension is extreme (see Figures 15.8a, b).

Early lesions in hypertensive retinopathy are not easy to detect. If systolic blood pressure is not routinely measured on physical examination, the presenting complaint of blindness secondary to retinal detachment is often the first sign that the veterinary patient is hypertensive [49].

An additional concern in veterinary medicine is "white-coat syndrome" or so-called "white-coat hypertension." "White-coat hypertension" is the condition by which stress in a clinical setting activates the sympathetic nervous system in some, but not all patients. This results in situational hypertension. Although transient, this hypertension may still damage target organs [76–79].

White-coat syndrome has been reported in dogs as well as cats [80, 81].

In cats with pre-existing target organ disease, such as renal insufficiency, the magnitude of white-coat-induced hypertension is greater and prolonged [81]. This may potentiate hypertensive retinopathy and hasten retinal detachment.

(a)   (b)

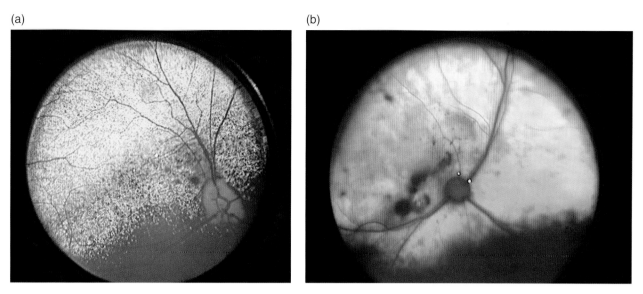

Figure 15.7 (a) Subretinal hemorrhage associated with canine systemic hypertension. *Source:* Courtesy of D.J. Haeussler, Jr., MS, DVM, DACVO. (b) Subretinal hemorrhage associated with feline systemic hypertension. *Source:* Courtesy of D.J. Haeussler, Jr., MS, DVM, DACVO.

(a)   (b)

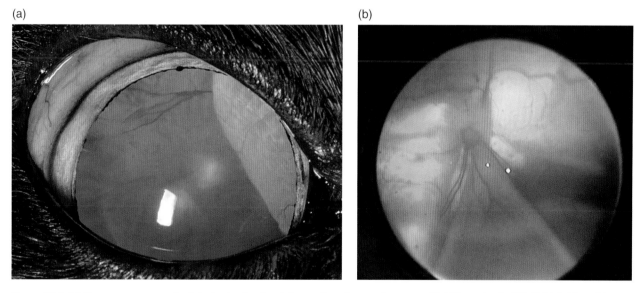

Figure 15.8 (a) Gross appearance of a detached retina in a feline patient. *Source:* Courtesy of D.J. Haeussler, Jr., MS, DVM, DACVO. (b) Fundic appearance of a detached retina in a feline patient. *Source:* Courtesy of D.J. Haeussler, Jr., MS, DVM, DACVO.

15.4.2.3 Tractional Retinal Detachments

Tractional retinal detachments occur when the retina proliferates and/or undergoes extensive neovascularization. Retinal dysplasia and diabetes mellitus are examples of conditions that involve this type of retinopathy. In both cases, the retina mechanically peels away from the underlying RPE [1].

15.4.2.4 Traumatic Retinal Detachments

Traumatic retinal detachments have been documented in the human medical literature. In humans, retinal detachments have occurred after high-force, high-speed blows to the globe [82, 83]. Consider, for example, being hit in the eye with a baseball, or suffering a punch or kick to the face [82]. The time window for detachment varies tremendously [82]. Detachment does not have to be sudden. It may occur weeks to years after the initial insult [82]. It is reasonable to assume that traumatic retinal detachments could also develop in companion animals.

There is one isolated case report in which non-ocular trauma in a canine patient resulted in bacteremia [84]. The infectious organism, oxacillin-resistant *Staphylococcus aureus*, caused the patient's right eye to develop endogenous endophthalmitis [84]. This led to unilateral retinal detachment [84].

15.4.2.5 Drug-Induced Retinal Detachments

There are isolated case reports of dogs that developed unilateral or bilateral retinal detachments after ingesting an overdose of phenylpropanolamine (PPA) [85, 86]. PPA is a synthetic, sympathomimetic drug that is prescribed to manage urinary incontinence in dogs by improving urinary sphincter control [85, 87–90]. At concentrations that are higher than prescribed, PPA potentiates the activity of catecholamines such as epinephrine by preventing them from being metabolized [85, 91, 92]. This may result in severe tachycardia and systemic hypertension that can induce target organ damage [85].

15.4.3 Sudden Acquired Retinal Degeneration Syndrome

SARDS is a condition of unknown etiology that targets middle-aged to older dogs [1, 93, 94]. SARDS has been suspected, but not yet proven in cats [39].

The disease is fast progressing, and blindness develops over the course of days to weeks [94]. Not all, but some patients present with concurrent clinical signs that are suggestive of hyperadrenocorticism [1, 94]. This subset of affected dogs exhibits polyuria (PU), polydipsia (PD), polyphagia (PP), and weight gain [1, 94].

In the early stages of disease, there are no apparent abnormalities on fundoscopy [1, 94]. Patients are diagnosed via electroretinogram (ERG) [1, 94]. The ERG measures the electrical activity of the retina in response to a light stimulus. Patients with SARDS exhibit zero electrical activity [1, 94, 95].

Until an effective treatment exists, the prognosis for the vision of these patients in terms of a return to function is poor [1, 94].

15.4.4 Fluoroquinolone Retinopathy

Enrofloxacin is a type of fluoroquinolone antibiotic. When prescribed to dogs and cats at a conservative oral dosage of 2.5 mg/kg, every 12 h, enrofloxacin did not induce retinopathy [96].

However, when the drug label was expanded to include a dosing range of 5 to 20 mg/kg per day, either administered as a split or a single dose, adverse effects in cats began to appear in the veterinary literature [96]. A small percentage of cats developed blindness [96, 97]. Blindness was partial or complete, and tended to occur within 2–14 days after treatment with enrofloxacin [96]. In most cases, blindness was permanent [96]. Today, the incidence is estimated to be 1 out of 122,414 cats [96].

Affected cats have increased tapetal reflectivity on fundoscopic examination [96]. In addition, the retinal vessels are attenuated [96]. These changes are suggestive of retinal degeneration [96].

Affected patients also have negative responses to the ERG [96].

Dose and patient age appear to influence which cats are sensitive to enrofloxacin [96, 97]. A 2001 study by Gelatt et al. demonstrated that 16 out of 17 cats that developed blindness secondary to enrofloxacin treatment had a daily dose that exceeded 5 mg/kg [97]. The only patient that developed blindness following a lower dosage of enrofloxacin (4.6 mg/kg) was 15 years old [97]. It is suspected that underlying renal or hepatic insufficiency, both of which are more likely in elderly patients, elevates the risk for retinal toxicity [96].

It is suspected that other fluoroquinolones, such as marbofloxacin and orbifloxacin, may induce retinal degeneration in cats [96]. Cats should therefore be treated with caution when prescribing this type of antibiotic.

15.4.5 Taurine-Deficient Retinopathy

Taurine is an essential amino acid in the cat, meaning that it is a required constituent of the feline diet. Taurine is responsible for maintaining the function of the photoreceptor cells [98–102].

When cats are either not fed taurine or are fed taurine-deficient diets, they develop retinal degeneration [98–102]. Retinal degeneration will occur as soon as taurine levels drop below 50% of that which is considered normal [100].

Lesions are variable between patients; however, as disease worsens, a band-shaped hyperreflective lesion is identifiable on ophthalmoscopy. This band extends from the nasal to temporal quadrants [98].

At-risk cats include those who are fed commercial dog food instead of cat food [98].

Dogs are able to synthesize taurine from methionine [103]. Because taurine is not an essential amino acid in the dog, dog food is not required to supplement taurine at the level that is required for cats. Commercial dog food is therefore an inappropriate dietary choice for cats.

Cats are also at risk for taurine-deficient retinopathy if they ingest a homemade vegetarian diet that is not supplemented for taurine. Because taurine is found in animal-based proteins, cereal grain-based diets do not provide adequate levels of taurine for functional vision [98, 103].

Incidentally, taurine deficiency does not only compromise ocular health. It also causes dilated cardiomyopathy (DCM) in cats [104–108].

Cats with taurine-deficient retinopathy benefit from an extensive cardiovascular work-up, including an echocardiogram, to determine if concurrent cardiomyopathy is present.

15.4.6 Retinal Degeneration Secondary to Ketamine and Methylnitrosurea

Ketamine is frequently used as an induction agent for feline patients. When ketamine was combined with methylnitrosurea in an isolated research study, patients developed acute blindness within five days of drug administration [109]. Histopathologic evaluation confirmed retinal degeneration. This was an unexpected adverse outcome for the project. Which drug led to blindness in cats was unclear. However, ketamine is also used as a dissociative anesthetic in humans, and transient blindness has been reported in human patients as an adverse effect [110]. This suggests that ketamine may indeed be linked to central blindness through mechanisms that are not yet understood.

15.5 Diseases of the Optic Nerve that May Result in Acute Blindness

The retina is not the only tissue in the eye–brain pathway that is responsible for visual deficits [1, 7]. Lesions may also involve the optic nerve [1, 7].

There are two main types of optic nerve pathology:

- Optic neuritis
- Optic nerve trauma

Optic neuritis is inflammation of the optic nerve, which is essentially an extension of the retina [1]. Although cats may develop optic neuritis, the condition is more likely to occur in dogs [1].

There are many causes of optic neuritis, including the following [1]:

- Infectious disease
- Immune-mediated disease
- Neoplastic disease
- Inflammatory disease
- Idiopathic disease

Infectious agents include canine distemper virus (CDV), cryptococcosis, blastomycosis, histoplasmosis, toxoplasmosis, protothecosis, and monocytic ehrlichiosis, which is caused by *Ehrlichia canis* [1, 34, 37, 94, 111–119].

The most common immune-mediated disease that has been implicated in cases involving optic neuritis is granulomatous meningoencephalomyelitis (GME) [1, 94, 111, 120, 121].

Meningiomas and lymphomas are the most common neoplastic causes of optic neuritis [94].

Cellulitis and orbital abscesses can also contribute to or induce optic neuritis [94].

All of these factors can result in acute onset of blindness.

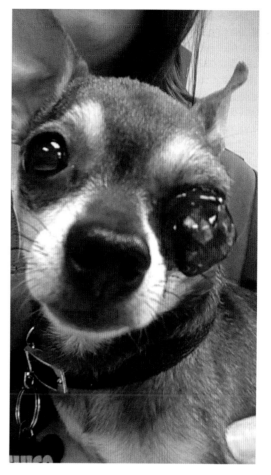

Figure 15.9 Unilateral proptosis in a canine patient. *Source:* Courtesy of Frank Isom, DVM.

Optic nerve trauma can also lead to blindness. Consider, for example, the patient that experiences proptosis. Proptosis occurs when the globe is displaced rostrally (see Figure 15.9).

In companion animal medicine, proptosis is commonly the result of being hit by a car or attacked by another animal [122]. Proptosis is more easily achieved in brachycephalic breeds on account of their shallow orbits [122]. Proptosis may also occur inadvertently in brachycephalic breeds due to heavy-handed restraint around the head and neck [122].

When proptosis occurs, the eyelids become trapped in an unnatural position caudal to the globe [122]. The resulting venous congestion creates inflammation, which puts pressure on the retrobulbar contents [122]. The result is acute blindness [122].

Although proptosed globes can be replaced within the eye socket, prognosis remains guarded [122]. Vision may or may not return, depending upon the degree to which the optic nerve was stretched.

Factors that improve prognosis include skull shape. Brachycephalic breeds tend to have a more favorable prognosis following proptosis [123]. In addition, patients that had direct or consensual PLRs at initial presentation for proptosis are more likely to regain vision [123].

Note that it is difficult to prognosticate immediately following surgical replacement whether or not vision will be regained. It may remain unclear until one to two weeks following recovery whether the patient will be visual again and, if so, to what degree [122].

Because vision may not be regained, many owners elect to enucleate the proptosed globe rather than replace it [123].

15.6 Diseases of the Visual Cortex that Result in Acute Blindness

Acute blindness may also result from transient or permanent damage to the visual cortex [1, 7]. Conditions that most often impact the visual cortex include the following [124, 125]:

- Seizures and the post-ictal phase
- Ischemic encephalopathies
  - Anesthetic complications
  - Hypoglycemia
  - Heavy metal toxicosis
  - Use of mouth gags in cats
- Neoplasia

15.6.1 Seizures and Transient Blindness

Seizures occur when the brain exhibits abnormal electrical activity that results in involuntary muscular activity and/or altered consciousness [126]. There are many types of seizures; however, the generalized tonic–clonic seizure is most often recognized by the veterinary client due to whole body involvement, particularly the limbs and jaw [126]. The postictal phase follows each seizure and may involve a change in awareness that is recognized by the owner as being abnormal for the patient [126]. The duration of this postictal phase is variable; however, the average is four hours, during which time the patient may be restless, pacing, or centrally blind [124–126]. This blindness is transient; however, it is important to inform owners of epileptic dogs and cats that it can occur [124, 125].

Any underlying condition that precipitates a seizure can therefore also be linked to transient blindness. Consider, for example, hypoglycemia of toy puppies, hypoglycemia secondary to insulinoma, hepatic encephalopathy, and uremia secondary to renal dysfunction [126].

15.6.2 Ischemic Encephalopathies and Acute Blindness

Primary anesthetic complications in veterinary medicine include intra-operative hypotension [127–129], opioid-induced dysphoria [130–132], cardiac dysrhythmias [129], post-operative regurgitation and vomiting [133], aspiration pneumonia [134], cerebellar dysfunction [135], blindness or deafness in cats [136–138], and death [139]. Of these, hypotension is cited most frequently [137]. A study by Gaynor et al. documented that hypotension occurred in 7% of cases involving anesthetized dogs and 8% of cases involving anesthetized cats at a university teaching hospital [129].

Cerebral blood flow depends upon adequate perfusion to the brain. Cerebral perfusion in turn is the result of systemic arterial pressure minus intracranial pressure [137]. When hypotension is mild, autoregulatory mechanisms within the body compensate for reduced systemic arterial pressure in order to maintain constant cerebral perfusion [137]. However, when hypotension is severe and systemic arterial pressure drops below 50 mmHg, compensation is no longer adequate [137]. Cerebral perfusion experiences a significant drop [140]. Ischemia impacts the entire brain; however, certain regions appear to be more sensitive to hypoxia [137]. These regions include the occipital lobe, which houses the visual processing center of the brain [137]. Transient or permanent blindness may result [137].

Cats appear to be particularly sensitive to hypoxia, so much so that a condition has been named to reflect the damage that ischemia does to their brains: feline ischemic encephalopathy (FIE) [137]. FIE results from hypotension secondary to anesthetic complications. FIE also results from hypoglycemia and heavy metal toxicosis, such as lead [137]. At necropsy, these patients demonstrate significant cerebral lesions, in particular, acute cortical neuronal necrosis [137, 141, 142].

Cats also have unique blood flow to the brain that predisposes them to complications following certain procedures. Specifically, consider that the internal carotid artery in cats is not the primary source of cerebral perfusion [143]. Instead, the maxillary artery is responsible for supplying the majority of blood to the brain [143–146].

Although this unique feline anatomy has been known for decades, it was only recently discovered to have significant implications for dental procedures [143, 147–149]. If maxillary arterial flow is compromised, then so too is cerebral brain flow.

The path of the maxillary artery in the cat involves the caudal mandible. When the mouth is opened maximally, as when a spring-loaded mouth gag is in place during a dental or endoscopic procedure, the maxillary artery may be partially or fully occluded [143, 147–149].

A retrospective study of 20 cats with post-anesthetic cortical blindness was conducted by Stiles et al. in 2012 [148]. Sixteen of twenty cats underwent procedures that involved the use of mouth gags [148]. This led to investigations into maxillary artery blood flow. These investigations confirmed that blood occlusion was associated with maximal opening of the mouth as caused by the use of spring-loaded mouth gags, and that such occlusion was responsible for central blindness [143, 147].

This is a wake-up call to the veterinary profession that maximal opening of the mouth in cats may lead to transient, if not permanent, damage and therefore should be avoided when at all possible [149]. Trading out spring-loaded mouth gags for a one-inch (42 mm) plastic needle cap is not sufficient. This, too, can occlude maxillary artery flow [147]. Instead, shorter plastic gags that measure 20–30 mm are advised [149].

15.6.3 Neoplasia and Acute Blindness

Of all brain tumors, meningiomas occur most frequently in dogs and cats [1, 150–152]. Although blindness may occur, it is relatively infrequent. Only about 1 in 10 cats with intracranial neoplasia present as blind [152].

15.7 Other Conditions that May Result in Acute Blindness

Keep in mind that there are many other conditions that may result in acute blindness. This chapter attempted to cover the most common of these.

Two conditions in particular have not been mentioned here that may lead to acute blindness: cataracts and glaucoma. Because these conditions are more readily recognized by other characteristic features, such as lens opacities for cataracts and buphthalmos for glaucoma, these conditions will be reserved for subsequent chapters.

References

1 Meekins, J.M. (2015). Acute blindness. *Top Companion Anim. Med.* 30 (3): 118–125.

2 Englar, R.E. (2017). *Performing the Small Animal Physical Examination*. Hoboken, NJ: Wiley.

3 Chrisman CL. (2006). The Neurologic Examination; (January):[11–6 pp.]. https://www.cliniciansbrief.com/sites/default/files/sites/cliniciansbrief.com/files/7.pdf.

4 Rijnberk, A. and van Sluijs, F.S. (2009). *Medical History and Physical Examination in Companion Animals*, 333 p. The Netherlands: Elsevier Limited.

5 DeLahunta, A., Glass, E., and Kent, M. (2015). *Veterinary Neuroanatomy and Clinical Neurology*, 4e, 409–454. St. Louis, MO: Elsevier/Saunders.

6 Maggs, D.J., Miller, P.E., and Ofri, R. (2013). *Slatter's Fundamentals of Veterinary Ophthalmology*. St. Louis, MO: Saunders.

7 Cook C. (2009). What Do They See & How Do We Know? Clean Run [Internet]:[61–6 pp.]. http://veterinaryvision.com/wp-content/uploads/2012/06/VisionInDogsPart1.pdf.

8 Maggs, D.J., Miller, P.E., Ofri, R., and Slatter, D.H. (2013). *Slatter's Fundamentals of Veterinary Ophthalmology*, 5e, x, 506 p. St. Louis, MO: Elsevier.

9 Ketring, K.L. and Glaze, M.B. (2012). *Atlas of Feline Ophthalmology*, 2e, xviii, 172 p. Chichester, West Sussex, UK; Ames, Iowa: Wiley-Blackwell.

10 Esson, D.W. (2015). Chapter 5: The normal subalbinotic fundus. In: *Clinical Atlas of Canine and Feline Ophthalmic Disease* (ed. D.W. Esson), 10–15. Wiley.

11 Dietz, H.H. (1985). Retinal dysplasia in dogs–a review. *Nord. Vet. Med.* 37 (1): 1–9.

12 Aroch, I., Ofri, R., and Aizenberg, I. (1996). Haematological, ocular and skeletal abnormalities in a Samoyed family. *J. Small Anim. Pract.* 37 (7): 333–339.

13 Ashton, N., Barnett, K.C., and Sachs, D.D. (1968). Retinal dysplasia in the Sealyham terrier. *J. Pathol. Bacteriol.* 96 (2): 269–272.

14 Barnett, K.C., Bjorck, G.R., and Kock, E. (1970). Hereditary retinal dysplasia in Labrador Retriever in England and Sweden. *J. Small Anim. Pract.* 10 (12): 755–759.

15 O'Toole, D., Young, S., Severin, G.A., and Neumann, S. (1983). Retinal dysplasia of English springer spaniel dogs: light microscopy of the postnatal lesions. *Vet. Pathol.* 20 (3): 298–311.

16 Albert, D.M., Lahav, M., Carmichael, L.E., and Percy, D.H. (1976). Canine herpes-induced retinal dysplasia and associated ocular anomalies. *Investig. Ophthalmol.* 15 (4): 267–278.

17 Shively, J.N., Phemister, R.D., Epling, G.P., and Jensen, R. (1970). Pathogenesis of radiation-induced retinal dysplasia. *Investig. Ophthalmol.* 9 (11): 888–900.

18 Tilley, L.P. and Smith, F.W.K. (2007). *Blackwell's Five-Minute Veterinary Consult: Canine and Feline.* Ames, Iowa: Blackwell.

19 Aguirre, G. (1973). Hereditary retinal diseases in small animals. *Vet. Clin. North Am.* 3 (3): 515–528.

20 Holle, D.M., Stankovics, M.E., Sarna, C.S., and Aguirre, G.D. (1999). The geographic form of retinal dysplasia in

dogs is not always a congenital abnormality. *Vet. Ophthalmol.* 2 (1): 61–66.

21 Nasisse, M.P. and Glover, T.L. (1997). Clinical signs, concurrent diseases, and risk factors associated with retinal detachment in dogs. *Prog. Vet. Comp. Ophthalmol.* 3: 87–91.

22 Glover, T.L., Davidson, M.G., Nasisse, M.P., and Olivero, D.K. (1995). The intracapsular extraction of displaced lenses in dogs: a retrospective study of 57 cases (1984–1990). *J. Am. Anim. Hosp. Assoc.* 31 (1): 77–81.

23 Sigle, K.J. and Nasisse, M.P. (2006). Long-term complications after phacoemulsification for cataract removal in dogs: 172 cases (1995–2002). *J. Am. Vet. Med. Assoc.* 228 (1): 74–79.

24 Davidson, M.G., Nasisse, M.P., Jamieson, V.E. et al. (1991). Phacoemulsification and intraocular lens implantatioon: a study of surgical results in 182 dogs. *Prog. Vet. Comp. Ophthalmol.* 1: 233–238.

25 Klein, H.E., Krohne, S.G., Moore, G.E., and Stiles, J. (2011). Postoperative complications and visual outcomes of phacoemulsification in 103 dogs (179 eyes): 2006–2008. *Vet. Ophthalmol.* 14 (2): 114–120.

26 Miller, T.R., Whitley, R.D., Meek, L.A. et al. (1987). Phacofragmentation and aspiration for cataract extraction in dogs: 56 cases (1980–1984). *J. Am. Vet. Med. Assoc.* 190 (12): 1577–1580.

27 Stiles, J. (2000). Canine rickettsial infections. *Vet. Clin. North Am. Small Anim. Pract.* 30 (5): 1135–1149.

28 Townsend, W.M., Stiles, J., and Krohne, S.G. (2006). Leptospirosis and panuveitis in a dog. *Vet. Ophthalmol.* 9 (3): 169–173.

29 Wilkinson, G.T. (1979). Feline cryptococcosis – review and 7 case-reports. *J. Small Anim. Pract.* 20 (12): 749–768.

30 Rodenbiker, H.T. and Ganley, J.P. (1980). Ocular coccidioidomycosis. *Surv. Ophthalmol.* 24 (5): 263–290.

31 Nasisse, M.P., Vanee, R.T., and Wright, B. (1985). Ocular changes in a Cat with disseminated blastomycosis. *J. Am. Vet. Med. Assoc.* 187 (6): 629–631.

32 Krohne, S.G. (2000). Canine systemic fungal infections. *Vet. Clin. N. Am. Small* 30 (5): 1063–1090.

33 Greene, R.T. and Troy, G.C. (1995(March/April)). Coccidioidomycosis in 48 Cats – a retrospective study (1984–1993). *J. Vet. Intern. Med.* 9 (2): 86–91.

34 Gwin, R.M., Makley, T.A., Wyman, M., and Werling, K. (1980). Multifocal ocular histoplasmosis in a dog and cat. *J. Am. Vet. Med. Assoc.* 176 (7): 638–642.

35 Gionfriddo, J.R. (2000). Feline systemic fungal infections. *Vet. Clin. N. Am. Small* 30 (5): 1029–1050.

36 Davidson, M.G. (2000). Toxoplasmosis. *Vet. Clin. N. Am. Small* 30 (5): 1051–1062.

37 Bloom, J.D., Hamor, R.E., and Gerding, P.A. Jr. (1996). Ocular blastomycosis in dogs: 73 cases, 108 eyes (1985–1993). *J. Am. Vet. Med. Assoc.* 209 (7): 1271–1274.

38 Stiles, J. (1999). Ocular manifestations of systemic disease. Part 2: the cat. In: *Veterinary Ophthalmology* (ed. K.N. Gelatt), 1448–1473. Philadelphia: Lippincott/ Williams & Wilkins.

39 Glaze, M.B. and Gelatt, K.N. (1999). Feline ophthalmology. In: *Veterinary Ophthalmology* (ed. K. N. Gelatt), 997–1052. Philadelphia: Lippincott/ Williams & Wilkins.

40 Graves, T.K., Barger, A.M., Adams, B., and Krockenberger, M.B. (2005). Diagnosis of systemic cryptococcosis by fecal cytology in a dog. *Vet. Clin. Pathol.* 34 (4): 409–412.

41 Angell, J.A., Merideth, R.E., Shively, J.N., and Sigler, R.L. (1987). Ocular lesions associated with coccidioidomycosis in dogs: 35 cases (1980–1985). *J. Am. Vet. Med. Assoc.* 190 (10): 1319–1322.

42 Shively, J.N. and Whiteman, C.E. (1970). Ocular lesions in disseminated coccidioidomycosis in 2 dogs. *Pathol. Vet.* 7 (1): 1–6.

43 Macarie, S., Calugaru, M., Kaucsar, E., and Bintintan, R. (2005). Toxocara canis central chorioretinitis. *Oftalmologia* 49 (3): 22–24.

44 Hollingsworth, S.R. (2000). Canine prototothecosis. *Vet. Clin. North Am. Small Anim. Pract.* 30 (5): 1091–1101.

45 Shank, A.M., Dubielzig, R.D., and Teixeira, L.B. (2015). Canine ocular prototothecosis: a review of 14 cases. *Vet. Ophthalmol.* 18 (5): 437–442.

46 Ledbetter, E.C., Landry, M.P., Stokol, T. et al. (2009). Brucella canis endophthalmitis in 3 dogs: clinical features, diagnosis, and treatment. *Vet. Ophthalmol.* 12 (3): 183–191.

47 Dubey, J.P., Black, S.S., Verma, S.K. et al. (2014). *Sarcocystis neurona* schizonts-associated encephalitis, chorioretinitis, and myositis in a two-month-old dog simulating toxoplasmosis, and presence of mature sarcocysts in muscles. *Vet. Parasitol.* 202 (3–4): 194–200.

48 Samsom, J., Rogers, K., and Wood, J.L. (2004). Blood pressure assessment in healthy cats and cats with hypertensive retinopathy. *Am. J. Vet. Res.* 65 (2): 245–252.

49 Maggio, F., DeFrancesco, T.C., Atkins, C.E. et al. (2000). Ocular lesions associated with systemic hypertension in cats: 69 cases (1985–1998). *J. Am. Vet. Med. Assoc.* 217 (5): 695–702.

50 Henik, R.A. (1997). Systemic hypertension and its management. *Vet. Clin. North Am. Small Anim. Pract.* 27 (6): 1355–1372.

51 Littman, M.P. (1994). Spontaneous systemic hypertension in 24 cats. *J. Vet. Intern. Med.* 8 (2): 79–86.

52 Morgan, R.V. (1986). Systemic hypertension in four cats: ocular and medical findings. *J. Am. Anim. Hosp. Assoc.* 22: 615–621.

53 Stiles, J., Polzin, D.J., and Bistner, S.I. (1994). The prevalence of retinopathy in Cats with systemic hypertension and chronic-renal-failure or hyperthyroidism. *J. Am. Anim. Hosp. Assoc.* 30 (6): 564–572.

54 Remillard, R.L., Ross, J.N., and Eddy, J.B. (1991). Variance of indirect blood pressure measurements and prevalence of hypertension in clinically normal dogs. *Am. J. Vet. Res.* 52 (4): 561–565.

55 Ritchie, C.M., Sheridan, B., Fraser, R. et al. (1990). Studies on the pathogenesis of hypertension in Cushing's disease and acromegaly. *Q. J. Med.* 76 (280): 855–867.

56 Komaromy, A.M., Andrew, S.E., Denis, H.M. et al. (2004). Hypertensive retinopathy and choroidopathy in a cat. *Vet. Ophthalmol.* 7 (1): 3–9.

57 Littman, M.P. (2000). Hypertension. In: *Textbook of Veterinary Internal Medicine*, 5e (ed. S.J. Ettinger), 179–182. Philadelphia: W.B. Saunders.

58 Kobayashi, D.L., Peterson, M.E., Graves, T.K. et al. (1990). Hypertension in cats with chronic renal failure or hyperthyroidism. *J. Vet. Intern. Med.* 4 (2): 58–62.

59 Sansom, J., Barnett, K.C., Dunn, K.A. et al. (1994). Ocular-disease associated with hypertension in 16 Cats. *J. Small Anim. Pract.* 35 (12): 604–611.

60 Elliott, J., Barber, P.J., Syme, H.M. et al. (2001). Feline hypertension: clinical findings and response to antihypertensive treatment in 30 cases. *J. Small Anim. Pract.* 42 (3): 122–129.

61 Henik, R.A., Snyder, P.S., and Volk, L.M. (1997). Treatment of systemic hypertension in cats with amlodipine besylate. *J. Am. Anim. Hosp. Assoc.* 33 (3): 226–234.

62 Turner, J.L., Brogdon, J.D., Lees, G.E., and Greco, D.S. (1990). Idiopathic Hypertension in a Cat with Secondary Hypertensive Retinopathy Associated with a High-Salt Diet. *J. Am. Anim. Hosp. Assoc.* 26 (6): 647–651.

63 Brown, S.A. and Henik, R.A. (1998). Diagnosis and treatment of systemic hypertension. *Vet. Clin. North Am. Small Anim. Pract.* 28 (6): 1481–1494. ix.

64 Bovee, K.C., Littman, M.P., Saleh, F. et al. (1986). Essential hereditary hypertension in dogs: a new animal model. *J. Hypertens. Suppl.* 4 (5): S172–S171.

65 Tippett, F.E., Padgett, G.A., Eyster, G. et al. (1987). Primary hypertension in a colony of dogs. *Hypertension* 9 (1): 49–58.

66 Littman, M.P., Robertson, J.L., and Bovee, K.C. (1988). Spontaneous systemic hypertension in dogs: five cases (1981–1983). *J. Am. Vet. Med. Assoc.* 193 (4): 486–494.

67 Ross, L.A. (1992). Hypertension and chronic renal failure. *Semin. Vet. Med. Surg.* 7 (3): 221–226.

68 Jensen, J., Henik, R.A., Brownfield, M., and Armstrong, J. (1997). Plasma renin activity and angiotensin I and aldosterone concentrations in cats with hypertension associated with chronic renal disease. *Am. J. Vet. Res.* 58 (5): 535–540.

69 Snyder, P.S. (1998). Amlodipine: a randomized, blinded clinical trial in 9 cats with systemic hypertension. *J. Vet. Intern. Med.* 12 (3): 157–162.

70 Peterson, M.E., Taylor, R.S., Greco, D.S. et al. (1990). Acromegaly in 14 cats. *J. Vet. Intern. Med.* 4 (4): 192–201.

71 Cowgill, L.D., James, K.M., Levy, J.K. et al. (1998). Use of recombinant human erythropoietin for management of anemia in dogs and cats with renal failure. *J. Am. Vet. Med. Assoc.* 212 (4): 521–528.

72 Chun, R., Jakovljevic, S., Morrison, W.B. et al. (1997). Apocrine gland adenocarcinoma and pheochromocytoma in a cat. *J. Am. Anim. Hosp. Assoc.* 33 (1): 33–36.

73 Flood, S.M., Randolph, J.F., Gelzer, A.R., and Refsal, K. (1999). Primary hyperaldosteronism in two cats. *J. Am. Anim. Hosp. Assoc.* 35 (5): 411–416.

74 Gwin, R.M., Gelatt, K.N., Terrell, T.G., and Hood, C.I. (1978). Hypertensive retinopathy associated with hypo-thyroidism, hypercholesterolemia, and renal-failure in a dog. *J. Am. Anim. Hosp. Assoc.* 14 (2): 200–209.

75 Crispin, S.M. and Mould, J.R. (2001). Systemic hypertensive disease and the feline fundus. *Vet. Ophthalmol.* 4 (2): 131–140.

76 Verdecchia, P., Schillaci, G., Borgioni, C. et al. (1995). White coat hypertension and white coat effect – similarities and differences. *Am. J. Hypertens.* 8 (8): 790–798.

77 Ogedegbe, G. (2008). White-coat effect: unraveling its mechanisms. *Am. J. Hypertens.* 21 (2): 135.

78 Cardillo, C., Defelice, F., Campia, U., and Folli, G. (1993). Psychophysiological reactivity and cardiac end-organ changes in white coat hypertension. *Hypertension* 21 (6): 836–844.

79 Palmer, B.F. (2001). Impaired renal autoregulation: Implications for the genesis of hypertension and hypertension-induced renal injury. *Am. J. Med. Sci.* 321 (6): 388–400.

80 Marino, C.L., Cober, R.E., Iazbik, M.C., and Couto, C.G. (2011). White-coat effect on systemic blood pressure in retired racing greyhounds. *J. Vet. Intern. Med.* 25 (4): 861–865.

81 Belew, A.M., Barlett, T., and Brown, S.A. (1999). Evaluation of the white-coat effect in cats. *J. Vet. Intern. Med.* 13 (2): 134–142.

82 Ruiz, R.S. (1969). Traumatic retinal detachments. *Br. J. Ophthalmol.* 53 (1): 59–61.

83 Johnston, P.B. (1991). Traumatic retinal detachment. *Br. J. Ophthalmol.* 75 (1): 18–21.

84 Alasil, T., Eljammal, S., Scartozzi, R., and Eliott, D. (2008). Rhegmatogenous retinal detachment after a lower extremity dog bite: a case report. *Cases J.* 1 (1): 218.

85 Ginn, J.A., Bentley, E., and Stepien, R.L. (2013). Systemic hypertension and hypertensive retinopathy following PPA overdose in a dog. *J. Am. Anim. Hosp. Assoc.* 49 (1): 46–53.

86 Crandell, J.M. and Ware, W.A. (2005). Cardiac toxicity from phenylpropanolamine overdose in a dog. *J. Am. Anim. Hosp. Assoc.* 41 (6): 413–420.

87 Bacon, N.J., Oni, O., and White, R.A. (2002). Treatment of urethral sphincter mechanism incompetence in 11 bitches with a sustained-release formulation of phenylpropanolamine hydrochloride. *Vet. Rec.* 151 (13): 373–376.

88 Byron, J.K., March, P.A., Chew, D.J., and DiBartola, S.P. (2007). Effect of phenylpropanolamine and pseudoephedrine on the urethral pressure profile and continence scores of incontinent female dogs. *J. Vet. Intern. Med.* 21 (1): 47–53.

89 Hamaide, A.J., Grand, J.G., Farnir, F. et al. (2006). Urodynamic and morphologic changes in the lower portion of the urogenital tract after administration of estriol alone and in combination with phenylpropanolamine in sexually intact and spayed female dogs. *Am. J. Vet. Res.* 67 (5): 901–908.

90 Scott, L., Leddy, M., Bernay, F., and Davot, J.L. (2002). Evaluation of phenylpropanolamine in the treatment of urethral sphincter mechanism incompetence in the bitch. *J. Small Anim. Pract.* 43 (11): 493–496.

91 Kanfer, I., Dowse, R., and Vuma, V. (1993). Pharmacokinetics of oral decongestants. *Pharmacotherapy* 13 (6 Pt 2): 116S–128S.

92 Yu, P.H. (1986). Inhibition of monoamine oxidase activity by phenylpropanolamine, an anorectic agent. *Res. Commun. Chem. Pathol. Pharmacol.* 51 (2): 163–171.

93 Vainisi, S.J., Schmidt, G.M., and West, C.S. (1983). Metabolic toxic retinopathy preliminary report. *Trans. Am. Coll. Vet. Ophthalmol.* 14: 76–81.

94 Montgomery, K.W., van der Woerdt, A., and Cottrill, N.B. (2008). Acute blindness in dogs: sudden acquired retinal degeneration syndrome versus neurological disease (140 cases, 2000–2006). *Vet. Ophthalmol.* 11 (5): 314–320.

95 van der Woerdt, A., Nasisse, M.P., and Davidson, M.G. (1991). Sudden acquired retinal degeneration in the dog: clinical and laboratory findings in 36 cases. *Prog. Vet. Comp. Ophthalmol.* 1: 11–18.

96 Wiebe, V. and Hamilton, P. (2002). Fluoroquinolone-induced retinal degeneration in cats. *J. Am. Vet. Med. Assoc.* 221 (11): 1568–1571.

97 Gelatt, K.N., van der Woerdt, A., Ketring, K.L. et al. (2001). Enrofloxacin-associated retinal degeneration in cats. *Vet. Ophthalmol.* 4 (2): 99–106.

98 Aguirre, G.D. (1978). Retinal degeneration associated with the feeding of dog foods to cats. *J. Am. Vet. Med. Assoc.* 172 (7): 791–796.

99 Schmidt, S.Y., Berson, E.L., and Hayes, K.C. (1976). Retinal degeneration in cats fed casein. I. Taurine deficiency. *Investig. Ophthalmol.* 15 (1): 47–52.

100 Schmidt, S.Y., Berson, E.L., Watson, G., and Huang, C. (1977). Retinal degeneration in cats fed casein. III. Taurine deficiency and ERG amplitudes. *Invest. Ophthalmol. Vis. Sci.* 16 (7): 673–678.

101 Berson, E.L., Hayes, K.C., Rabin, A.R. et al. (1976). Retinal degeneration in cats fed casein. II. Supplementation with methionine, cysteine, or taurine. *Investig. Ophthalmol.* 15 (1): 52–58.

102 Hayes, K.C. (1976). A review on the biological function of taurine. *Nutr. Rev.* 34 (6): 161–165.

103 Hayes, K.C. (1982). Nutritional problems in cats: taurine deficiency and vitamin A excess. *Can. Vet. J.* 23 (1): 2–5.

104 Novotny, M.J., Hogan, P.M., and Flannigan, G. (1994). Echocardiographic evidence for myocardial failure induced by taurine deficiency in domestic cats. *Can. J. Vet. Res.* 58 (1): 6–12.

105 Sisson, D.D., Knight, D.H., Helinski, C. et al. (1991). Plasma taurine concentrations and M-mode echocardiographic measures in healthy cats and in cats with dilated cardiomyopathy. *J. Vet. Intern. Med.* 5 (4): 232–238.

106 Pion, P.D., Kittleson, M.D., Rogers, Q.R., and Morris, J.G. (1987). Myocardial failure in cats associated with low plasma taurine: a reversible cardiomyopathy. *Science* 237 (4816): 764–768.

107 Pion, P.D., Kittleson, M.D., Rogers, Q.R., and Morris, J.G. (1990). Taurine deficiency myocardial failure in the domestic cat. *Prog. Clin. Biol. Res.* 351: 423–430.

108 Pion, P.D., Kittleson, M.D., Thomas, W.P. et al. (1992). Clinical findings in cats with dilated cardiomyopathy and relationship of findings to taurine deficiency. *J. Am. Vet. Med. Assoc.* 201 (2): 267–274.

109 Schaller, J.P., Wyman, M., Weisbrode, S.E., and Olsen, R.G. (1981). Induction of retinal degeneration in cats by methylnitrosourea and ketamine hydrochloride. *Vet. Pathol.* 18 (2): 239–247.

110 Fine, J., Weissman, J., and Finestone, S.C. (1974). Side effects after ketamine anesthesia: transient blindness. *Anesth. Analg.* 53 (1): 72–74.

111 Nafe, L.A. and Carter, J.D. (1981). Canine optic neuritis. *Compend. Contin. Educ. Pract. Vet.* 3: 68–79.

112 Fischer, C.A. (1971). Retinal and retinochoroidal lesions in early neuropathic canine distemper. *J. Am. Vet. Med. Assoc.* 158 (6): 740–752.

113 Fischer, C.A. and Jones, G.T. (1972). Optic neuritis in dogs. *J. Am. Vet. Med. Assoc.* 160 (1): 68–79.

114 Jergens, A.E., Wheeler, C.A., and Collier, L.L. (1986). Cryptococcosis involving the eye and central nervous system of a dog. *J. Am. Vet. Med. Assoc.* 189 (3): 302–304.

115 Gelatt, K.N., McGill, L.D., and Perman, V. (1973). Ocular and systemic cryptococcosis in a dog. *J. Am. Vet. Med. Assoc.* 162 (5): 370–375.

116 Wilson, R.W., Van Dreumel, A.A., and JNR, H. (1973). Urogenital and ocular lesions in canine blastomycosis. *Vet. Pathol.* 10 (1): 1–11.

117 Buyukmihci, N. (1982). Ocular lesions of blastomycosis in the dog. *J. Am. Vet. Med. Assoc.* 180 (4): 426–431.

118 Schultze, A.E., Ring, R.D., and Morgan, R.V. (1998). Clinical, cytologic and histopathologic manifestations of prototheosis in two dogs. *Vet. Ophthalmol.* 1: 239–243.

119 Leiva, M., Naranjo, C., and Pena, M.T. (2005). Ocular signs of canine monocytic ehrlichiosis: a retrospective study in dogs from Barcelona. *Spain. Vet. Ophthalmol.* 8 (6): 387–393.

120 Smith, R.I.E. (1995). A case of ocular granulomatous meningoencephalitis in a German-shepherd dog presenting as bilateral uveitis. *Aust. Vet. Pract.* 25 (2): 73–78.

121 Munana, K.R. and Luttgen, P.J. (1998). Prognostic factors for dogs with granulomatous meningoencephalomyelitis: 42 cases (1982–1996). *J. Am. Vet. Med. Assoc.* 212 (12): 1902–1906.

122 Kennard G. Ocular emergencies: Presenting signs, initial exam and treatment (Proceedings)2009. Available from: http://veterinarycalendar.dvm360.com/ocular-emergencies-presenting-signs-initial-exam-and-treatment-proceedings.

123 Gilger, B.C., Hamilton, H.L., Wilkie, D.A. et al. (1995). Traumatic ocular proptoses in dogs and cats: 84 cases (1980–1993). *J. Am. Vet. Med. Assoc.* 206 (8): 1186–1190.

124 Jutkowitz LA. (2008). Emergency management of seizures (Proceedings). DVM360 [Internet]. http://veterinarycalendar.dvm360.com/emergency-management-seizures-proceedings.

125 Pakozdy, A., Leschnik, M., Sarchahi, A.A. et al. (2010). Clinical comparison of primary versus secondary epilepsy in 125 cats. *J. Feline Med. Surg.* 12 (12): 910–916.

126 Rusbridge, C. (2014). Canine idiopathic epilepsy. *In Pract.* 36: 17–23.

127 Iizuka, T., Kamata, M., Yanagawa, M., and Nishimura, R. (2013). Incidence of intraoperative hypotension during isoflurane-fentanyl and propofol-fentanyl anaesthesia in dogs. *Vet. J.* 198 (1): 289–291.

128 Mazzaferro, E. and Wagner, A.E. (2001). Hypotension during anesthesia in dogs and cats: recognition, causes, and treatment. *Compend. Contin. Educ. Pract. Vet.* 23: 728–737.

129 Gaynor, J.S., Dunlop, C.I., Wagner, A.E. et al. (1999). Complications and mortality associated with anesthesia in dogs and cats. *J. Am. Anim. Hosp. Assoc.* 35 (1): 13–17.

130 Becker, W.M., Mama, K.R., Rao, S. et al. (2013). Prevalence of dysphoria after fentanyl in dogs undergoing stifle surgery. *Vet. Surg.* 42 (3): 302–307.

131 Vaisanen, M., Oksanen, H., and Vainio, O. (2004). Postoperative signs in 96 dogs undergoing soft tissue surgery. *Vet. Rec.* 155 (23): 729–733.

132 Light, G.S., Hardie, E.M., and Young, M.S. (1993). Pain and anxiety behaviors of dogs during intravenous catherization after premidication with placebo, acepromazine or oxymorphone. *Appl. Anim. Behav. Sci.* 37: 331–343.

133 Davies, J.A., Fransson, B.A., Davis, A.M. et al. (2015). Incidence of and risk factors for postoperative regurgitation and vomiting in dogs: 244 cases (2000–2012). *J. Am. Vet. Med. Assoc.* 246 (3): 327–335.

134 Ovbey, D.H., Wilson, D.V., Bednarski, R.M. et al. (2014). Prevalence and risk factors for canine post-anesthetic aspiration pneumonia (1999–2009): a multicenter study. *Vet. Anaesth. Analg.* 41 (2): 127–136.

135 Shamir, M., Goelman, G., and Chai, O. (2004). Postanesthetic cerebellar dysfunction in cats. Journal of veterinary internal medicine/American College of Veterinary. *Intern. Med.* 18 (3): 368–369.

136 Barton-Lamb, A.L., Martin-Flores, M., Scrivani, P.V. et al. (2013). Evaluation of maxillary arterial blood flow in anesthetized cats with the mouth closed and open. *Vet. J.* 196 (3): 325–331.

137 Jurk, I.R., Thibodeau, M.S., Whitney, K. et al. (2001). Acute vision loss after general anesthesia in a cat. *Vet. Ophthalmol.* 4 (2): 155–158.

138 Son, W.-G., Seo, K.-M., Lee, I. et al. (2009). Acute temporary visual loss after general anesthesia in a cat. *J. Vet. Clin.* 26: 480–482.

139 KW, C. and LW, H. (1990). A survey of anaesthesia in small animal practice: AVA/BSAVA report. *J. Vet. Anaesth.* 17: 4–10.

140 Adams, J.H. (1989). Cerebral infarction – its pathogenesis and interpretation. *J. Pathol.* 157 (4): 281–282.

141 Auer, R.N. and Siesjo, B.K. (1988). Biological differences between ischemia, hypoglycemia, and epilepsy. *Ann. Neurol.* 24 (6): 699–707.

142 Garcia, J.H. (1983). Ischemic injuries of the brain. Morphologic evolution. *Arch. Pathol. Lab. Med.* 107 (4): 157–161.

143 Barton-Lamb, A.L., Martin-Flores, M., Scrivani, P.V. et al. (2013). Evaluation of maxillary arterial blood flow in anesthetized cats with the mouth closed and open. *Vet. J.* 196 (3): 325–331.

144 Gillilan, L.A. (1976). Extra-cranial and intracranial blood-supply to brains of dog and cat. *Am. J. Anat.* 146 (3): 237–253.

145 Kumar, A.J., Hochwald, G.M., and Kricheff, I. (1976). Angiographic study of carotid arterial and jugular venous systems in cat. *Am. J. Anat.* 145 (3): 357–369.

146 Davies, D.D. and Story, H.E. (1943). *The Carotid Circulation in the Domestic Cat*, Zoological Series, vol. 28, 5–47. Field Museum of Natural History.

147 Martin-Flores, M., Scrivani, P.V., Loew, E. et al. (2014). Maximal and submaximal mouth opening with mouth gags in cats: implications for maxillary artery blood flow. *Vet. J.* 200 (1): 60–64.

148 Stiles, J., Weil, A.B., Packer, R.A., and Lantz, G.C. (2012). Post-anesthetic cortical blindness in cats: twenty cases. *Vet. J.* 193 (2): 367–373.

149 Reiter, A.M. (2014). Open wide: blindness in cats after the use of mouth gags. *Vet. J.* 201 (1): 5–6.

150 Heidner, G.L., Kornegay, J.N., Page, R.L. et al. (1991). Analysis of survival in a retrospective study of 86 dogs with brain tumors. *J. Vet. Intern. Med.* 5 (4): 219–226.

151 Bagley, R.S., Gavin, P.R., Moore, M.P. et al. (1999). Clinical signs associated with brain tumors in dogs: 97 cases (1992–1997). *J. Am. Vet. Med. Assoc.* 215 (6): 818–819.

152 Troxel, M.T., Vite, C.H., Van Winkle, T.J. et al. (2003). Feline intracranial neoplasia: retrospective review of 160 cases (1985–2001). *J. Vet. Intern. Med.* 17 (6): 850–859.

16

Hyphema

16.1 Description of Hyphema

A disruption in the blood–ocular barrier may result in blood pooling within the anterior chamber of the eye [1–3]. This clinical sign is referred to as hyphema [2–6].

Complete hyphema occurs when blood fills the entire anterior chamber, making it difficult to examine intraocular structures [7] (see Figures 16.1a, b).

If aqueous circulation is compromised or if blood is present in the anterior chamber for five to seven days, it may undergo a color change from red to blue-black [7]. This color change reflects decreased oxygenation [7]. Because of its blue-black appearance, this clinical presentation has historically been referred to as "eight-ball hyphema" [8].

Hyphema can also be incomplete. This tends to occur in cases in which hemorrhage is not ongoing. As a result, blood does not fill the entire anterior chamber. What blood is present settles out along the ventral anterior chamber, and a line of demarcation is visible [7] (see Figure 16.2).

Blood within the anterior chamber may or may not be clotted [4].

16.2 Primary Causes of Hyphema

Innumerable diseases affect the blood–ocular barrier [5]. Of these, the top causes of hyphema in clinical practice include the following [5]:

- Trauma
- Bleeding disorders
  - Inherited
  - Secondary to toxicosis
- Infectious disease
- Immune-mediated disease
- Systemic hypertension
- Anterior uveitis
- Neoplasia

16.2.1 Trauma

Proptosis was first introduced in Chapter 15, Section 15.5 in association with blunt force head trauma and excessively forceful restraint in brachycephalic breeds [9]. Hyphema frequently results from proptosis and is a poor prognostic indicator for the globe's return to function [5, 10].

Other traumatic causes of canine and feline hyphema include automobile accidents, facial bite wounds, horse kicks to the head, and cat scratches to the eye [5, 11]. Falls from great heights may also cause hyphema [5].

Because hyphema obscures intraocular structures, fundoscopy may not be possible. Given that blunt force head trauma may also result in retinal detachments, it is critical that patients be monitored closely and evaluated via other modalities. Ocular ultrasonography may facilitate the diagnosis of retinal detachment when anterior chamber opacity is too murky to appreciate the fundus through routine ophthalmoscopy [12, 13].

Beyond ocular investigation, patients that have sustained traumatic injury require a whole-body, comprehensive assessment involving bloodwork and diagnostic imaging. It is critical to rule out the possibility that, in these patients, other tissues and organs were injured [5].

16.2.2 Bleeding Disorders

Bleeding disorders may result from thrombocytopenia, hemolytic and non-hemolytic anemia, and other coagulopathies [5, 14–18]. Although it is possible to inherit one or more of these conditions, acquired coagulopathies occur more commonly in veterinary medicine [5].

Blood may pool within any compartment of the body, including the anterior chamber. Other compartments to investigate in a patient with hyphema include the thoracic and abdominal cavities [5].

Ingestion of anticoagulant rodenticides is a common clinical emergency that results in pooling of blood within one or more compartments [5]. These products prevent

(a)

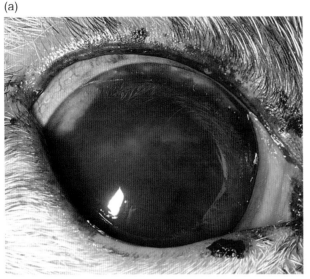

(b)

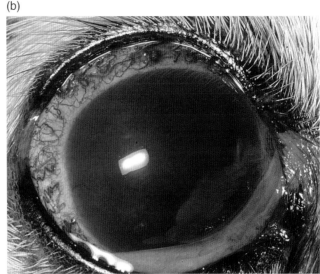

Figure 16.1 (a) Gross appearance of complete hyphema in the feline patient. *Source:* Courtesy of D.J. Haeussler, Jr., MS, DVM, DACVO. (b) Gross appearance of complete hyphema in the canine patient. *Source:* Courtesy of D.J. Haeussler, Jr., MS, DVM, DACVO.

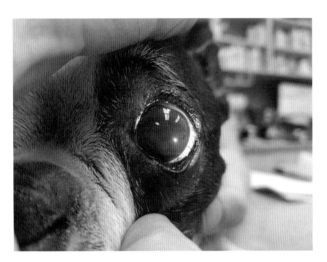

Figure 16.2 Incomplete hyphema in the canine patient. Note the line of demarcation, otherwise referred to as the "gravity line." *Source:* Courtesy of Andrew Tornell, DVM.

the recycling of vitamin K-dependent coagulation factors II, VII, IX, and X. Without the ability to regenerate these factors, the victim is ill-equipped to deal with micro-bleeds over time [5]. Unless treatment is initiated rapidly, this condition will result in exsanguination and death.

A prolonged prothrombin time (PT) is suggestive of anticoagulant rodenticide toxicity [19].

In addition to coagulation factors, platelets are also necessary to form an effective clot. Thrombocytopenia is the condition by which a patient has fewer than normal platelets [3, 5]. To the trained eye, a platelet count is easy to estimate on a blood smear [19].

When platelets are insufficient in number, the result is easy-to-detect hemorrhage throughout the skin, sclera, and mucous membranes. These tissues may exhibit pinpoint bleeds called petechiae, or larger patches of hemorrhage, ecchymoses [5] (see Figures 16.3a–f).

Thrombocytopenia may be immune-mediated, in which case platelets are destroyed by the body failing to recognize them as "self," or thrombocytopenia may be the result of infectious agents [14, 15, 20–22]. Some of the more common infectious agents that result in thrombocytopenia include the following [3, 19]:

- Bacteria
  - *Leptospira* spp., the causative agents of leptospirosis
  - *Borrelia burgdorferi*, the causative agent of Lyme disease
  - *Ehrlichia canis*, the infectious agent of canine monocytic ehrlichiosis
  - *Rickettsia rickettsia*, the infectious agent of Rocky Mountain Spotted Fever
  - *Anaplasma phagocytophilum* or *Anaplasma platys*, the causative agents of anaplasmosis
- Viruses
  - Canine and feline herpesvirus
  - Canine distemper virus (CDV)
  - Canine adenovirus (CAV)
  - Canine parvovirus (CPV)
  - Feline panleukopenia virus
  - Feline leukemia virus (FeLV)
  - Feline immunodeficiency virus (FIV)
- Fungi
  - Candidiasis
  - Histoplasmosis

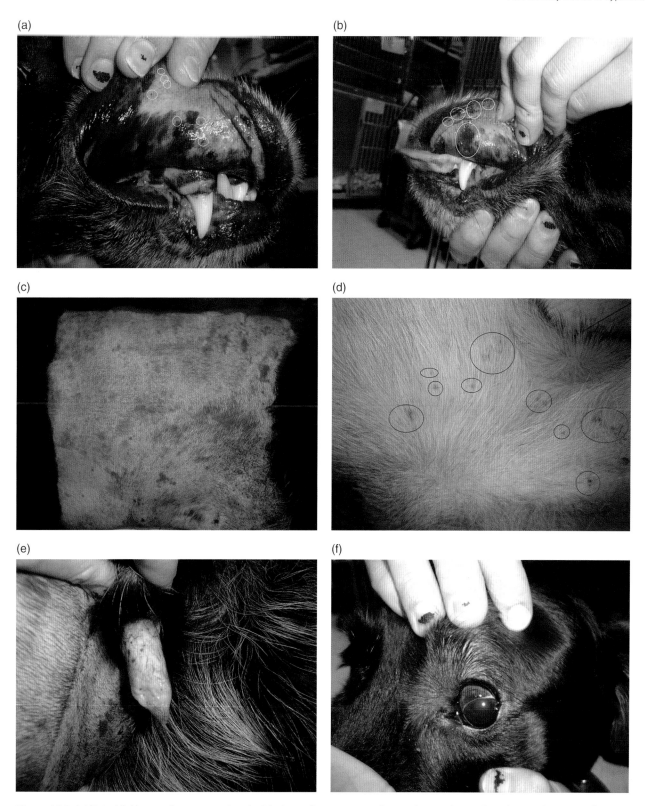

Figure 16.3 (a) Petechial hemorrhages associated with the oral mucous membranes in a canine patient. *Source:* Courtesy of Daniel Foy, MS, DVM, DACVIM, DACVECC. (b) Petechial hemorrhages and ecchymoses associated with the oral mucous membranes in a canine patient. *Source:* Courtesy of Daniel Foy, MS, DVM, DACVIM, DACVECC. (c) Petechiae associated with the flank of a shaved canine patient. *Source:* Courtesy of Daniel Foy, MS, DVM, DACVIM, DACVECC. (d) Petechiae associated with the caudoventral abdomen of a canine patient. *Source:* Courtesy of Daniel Foy, MS, DVM, DACVIM, DACVECC. (e) Petechial hemorrhages on the penile mucosa of a canine patient. *Source:* Courtesy of Daniel Foy, MS, DVM, DACVIM, DACVECC. (f) Scleral hemorrhage in a canine patient with hyphema. *Source:* Courtesy of Daniel Foy, MS, DVM, DACVIM, DACVECC.

- Protozoa
  - Leishmaniasis
  - *Cytauxzoon felis,* the causative agent of cytauxzoonosis
- Other Parasites
  - *Dirofilaria immitis*, the causative agent of canine and feline heartworm disease (HWD)

Thrombocytopenia may also be the result of myeloproliferative disorders, including lymphoma [3].

Excessive irradiation or production of estrogen by the body can further suppress platelet production in the bone marrow, leading to shortages [3]. Consider, for example, male dogs with Sertoli cell tumors [3].

Thrombocytopenia may also be drug-induced, as from antibiotics such as cephalosporins, penicillins, and trimethoprim-sulfamethoxazole [19]. In addition, H2-receptor antagonists and furosemide have also been linked to isolated cases of thrombocytopenia [19].

On the contrary, platelets may be normal in terms of number, but abnormal in terms of function [3]. Consider, for example, defects in platelet adhesion or aggregation [3]. One example of an inherited thrombocytopathy is von Willebrand disease (VWD) [3]. Although VWD can occur in any dog and, more rarely, cats, it is most frequently associated with Doberman Pinscher dogs [23].

Acquired thrombocytopathy can also result in hyphema. This may be drug-induced, as through the administration of non-steroidal anti-inflammatory drugs (NSAIDs) or corticosteroids [3].

Hyphema may also result from immune-mediated hemolytic anemia (IMHA) [3]. Certain breeds of dogs are predisposed to IMHA, including Cocker Spaniels, English Springer Spaniels, Irish Setters, Collies, and Poodles. Among dogs, middle-aged females are most at risk [19, 24, 25].

IMHA may be idiopathic in origin, or it may be triggered by a drug, vaccine, or infectious, inflammatory, or neoplastic process [26].

Cats do not appear to have a breed predisposition for IMHA, and most typically IMHA is triggered by an underlying disease [27].

Canine and feline patients with IMHA typically present as being lethargic and weak. Owners of historically active dogs may report that they have become unusually exercise-intolerant. Mucous membranes are pale [26].

To compensate for reduced oxygenation secondary to low erythrocyte counts, patients become tachycardic, with bounding pulses. They may or may not develop a hemic murmur [26].

If hemolysis is severe, mucous membranes may become icteric [26].

When blood samples are taken from patients with IMHA, they may exhibit spontaneous agglutination. This occurs when levels of antibodies against

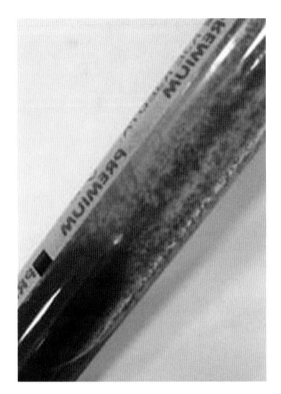

Figure 16.4 Spontaneous agglutination in a blood collection tube in a patient with IMHA.

erythrocytes become so high as to cause them to attach to more than one cell [26]. This is visible to the naked eye as specks against the wall of a blood collection tube (see Figure 16.4).

Patients with IMHA may also test positive on the slide agglutination test. EDTA-anticoagulated blood is mixed with saline on a microscope slide, and evaluated for evidence of macroagglutination [26].

Macroagglutination is abnormal and is suggestive of IMHA [26] (see Figure 16.5).

Microagglutination can be confirmed microscopically. Erythrocytes will bunch together like a grape cluster [26].

Patients with intravascular hemolysis may also develop discolored urine secondary to hemoglobinuria. The urine is said to take on a "port wine" appearance [26] (see Figure 16.6).

Non-hemolytic anemia may also cause hyphema when it is severe and acute. Consider, for example, significant ectoparasite infestation in a kitten or puppy. If hemoglobin reduces to less than 5 mg/dl, then global hemorrhage may result [3]. Patients with this degree of anemia are critically ill and at grave risk of death [3].

16.2.3 Systemic Hypertension

Systemic hypertension was introduced in Chapter 15, Section 15.4.2 with regard to its potential to cause hypertensive retinopathy. Recall that in cats, hypertension is

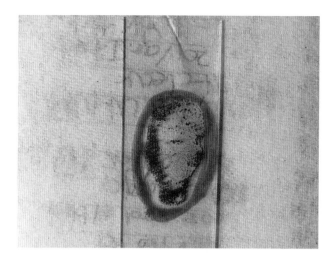

Figure 16.5 Positive slide agglutination test in a canine patient with IMHA. *Source:* Courtesy of Dr. Lisa Keenan.

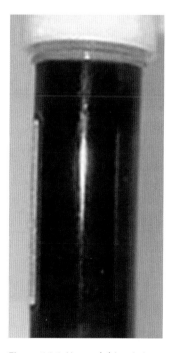

Figure 16.6 Hemoglobinuria in a canine patient with IMHA.

characterized as having persistently elevated, indirect systolic blood pressure at greater than 160–170 mmHg and/or elevated diastolic pressures greater than 100 mmHg [28–33]. By contrast, hypertension in dogs is characterized as having persistently elevated, indirect systolic pressures of 180–200 mmHg and/or elevated diastolic pressures greater than 100 mmHg [30, 34, 35].

When systemic hypertension persists, retinal detachment is the most common clinical sign [5]. However, systemic hypertension may also result in hyphema [5]. Hyphema results when arterial endothelial cells become so damaged by hypertension that they develop increased

vascular permeability [5, 36]. This causes the vasculature to be leaky. When vasculature is leaky at the level of the blood–ocular barrier, hyphema may result.

16.2.4 Anterior Uveitis

The uvea of the eye sits immediately beneath the sclera, and includes the iris, ciliary body, and the choroid [37]. It is considered to be the middle layer of the eye [37].

Any portion of the uvea can become inflamed. Anterior uveitis refers to inflammation of the iris and ciliary body [37].

One complication of anterior uveitis is that the underlying inflammation undermines the blood–ocular barrier. This causes leakage of protein and erythrocytes into the anterior chamber [37].

Patients typically present with "red eye," due to episcleral injection, photophobia, and ocular pain, as evident by blepharospasm [37, 38] (see Figures 16.7a, b).

As material continues to leak across the blood–ocular barrier, the anterior chamber may take on a cloudy or hazy appearance. This fogginess is called aqueous flare (see Figure 16.8).

Aqueous flare is most visible when a slit beam is used to cast light through the aqueous humor [38].

When uveitis is severe, hyphema may develop.

If uveitis is suspected, intraocular pressure (IOP) can be assessed as a confirmatory tool. When IOP is low, for example, less than 10 mmHg, uveitis is probable [38–40].

Patients that are suspected to have uveitis benefit from a thorough diagnostic investigation that includes a complete blood count, serum biochemistry profile, urinalysis, titers for tick-borne diseases, and thoracic and abdominal imaging [38]. Ocular ultrasonography may also be of benefit in assessing the health of the posterior uvea, particularly if aqueous flare and/or hyphema prevent a thorough fundic examination [38].

A comprehensive work-up for uveitis is essential because there are so many possible causes. These will be discussed in Chapter 17.

16.2.5 Neoplasia

Primary intraocular tumors, such as iris melanoma, may cause hyphema. These typically only affect one globe [5]. It may be difficult to diagnose an intraocular tumor when complete hyphema is present because it will obscure intraocular detail [41].

Other examples of primary intraocular tumors that result in hyphema include ciliary body hemangiosarcoma [3].

Primarily intraocular lymphoma is more common in cats than dogs [5]. When dogs develop hyphema because of lymphoma, it is typically due to multicentric disease [5].

(a)   (b)

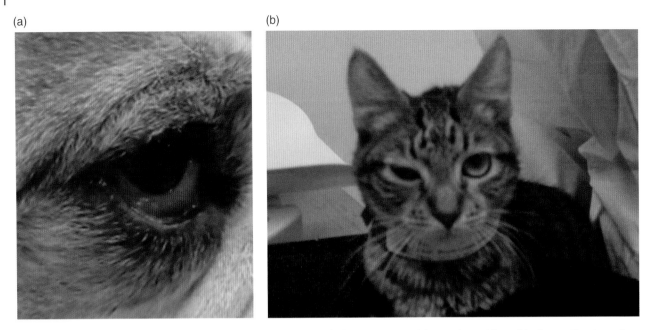

Figure 16.7 (a) Episcleral injection in a canine patient. (b) Unilateral blepharospasm in a feline patient with uveitis. *Source:* Courtesy of Patricia Bennett, DVM.

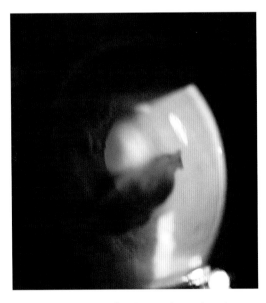

Figure 16.8 Aqueous flare in a canine patient. In a normal, healthy eye, the aqueous humor should appear clear when the light of a slit beam passes through it. Note how in this patient, the aqueous humor appears blurry and cloudy. *Source:* Courtesy of D.J. Haeussler, Jr., MS, DVM, DACVO.

16.3 Sequelae to Hyphema

Historically, poor visual outcomes have been reported for patients with hyphema [1, 42]. However, the prognosis for the patient's restoration of vision is dependent upon the underlying cause of the hyphema.

For example, hyphema secondary to retinal detachment is linked to a reduced chance that vision will be restored in the affected eye(s) [4].

In addition to visual deficits, hyphema may result in the development of cataracts, secondary glaucoma, and posterior synechiae [6]. Posterior synechiae are adhesions that pathologically attach the iris to the lens.

16.4 Important Considerations for History Taking

Hyphema is more likely to be the result of systemic than primary ocular disease [43]. Because so many etiologies can explain hyphema, it is critical that the clinician obtain a complete history. Asking certain questions may make certain rule-outs more or less likely. Important questions include the following [7]:

- Serologic status: FeLV, FIV, and HWD have been linked to the development of hyphema.
- Lifestyle, including travel history: Certain geographic regions experience increased rates of ehrlichiosis and Rocky Mountain Spotted Fever.
- Exposure to anticoagulant rodenticides: Hyphema may develop within five to seven days of ingestion.
- Prior illness: Recent illness may have compromised the immune status of the patient, making them more susceptible to diseases that induce hyphema.
- Vaccination history: Vaccinations are one potential trigger for IMHA, which may result in hyphema.

- Recently prescribed medications: These may be another potential trigger for IMHA.
- History of ocular signs prior to the development of hyphema: These may be suggestive that there is underlying uveitis or an alternate ocular concern that needs to be addressed to resolve the problem.

Comprehensive history taking and a thorough physical examination provide the clinician with important baseline data. Diagnostic tests must be tailored to the patient on the basis of these findings. For example, infectious disease testing should be performed if it is indicated based upon the patient's travel history or geographic location [7].

References

1 Jinks, M.R., Olea-Popelka, F., and Freeman, K.S. (2018). Causes and outcomes of dogs presenting with hyphema to a referral hospital in Colorado: a retrospective analysis of 99 cases. *Vet. Ophthalmol.* 21 (2): 160–166.

2 Hendrix, D.V.H. (2013). Diseases and surgery of the canine anterior uvea. In: *Veterinary Ophthalmology* (ed. K.N. Gelatt, B.C. Gilger and T.J. Kern), 1146–1198. Oxford: Wiley-Blackwell.

3 Komaromy, A.M., Ramsey, D.T., Brooks, D.E. et al. (1999). Hyphema. Part I. Pathophysiologic considerations. *Comp. Cont. Educ. Pract.* 21 (11): 1064.

4 Nelms, S.R., Nasisse, M.P., Davidson, M.G., and Kirschner, S.E. (1993). Hyphema associated with retinal disease in dogs: 17 cases (1986–1991). *J. Am. Vet. Med. Assoc.* 202 (8): 1289–1292.

5 Telle, M.R. and Betbeze, C. (2015). Hyphema: considerations in the small animal patient. *Top. Companion Anim. Med.* 30 (3): 97–106.

6 Nelson, R.W. and Couto, C.G. (2009). Disorders of hemostasis. In: *Small Animal Internal Medicine* (ed. R.W. Nelson and C.G. Couto), 1242–1259. Missouri: Mosby Elsevier.

7 Komaromy, A.M., Ramsey, D.T., Brooks, D.E. et al. (2000). Hyphema. Part II. Diagnosis and treatment. *Comp. Cont. Educ. Pract.* 22 (1): 74–79.

8 Collins, B.K. and Moore, C.P. (1999). Diseases and surgery of the canine anterior uvea. In: *Veterinary Ophthalmology* (ed. K.N. Gelatt), 755–795. Baltimore: Lippincott Williams & Wilkins.

9 Kennard G. (2009). Ocular emergencies: Presenting signs, initial exam and treatment (Proceedings). DVM360 [Internet]. http://veterinarycalendar. dvm360.com/ocular-emergencies-presenting-signs-initial-exam-and-treatment-proceedings.

10 Book, B.P., van der Woerdt, A., and Wilkie, D.A. (2008). Ultrasonographic abnormalities in eyes with traumatic hyphema obscuring intraocular structures: 33 cases (1991–2002). *J. Vet. Emerg. Crit. Car.* 18 (4): 383–387.

11 Winston, S.M. (1981). Ocular emergencies. *Vet. Clin. North Am. Small Anim. Pract.* 11 (1): 59–76.

12 Plummer, G. (2016). Retinal detachment. *Clinician's Brief.*

13 Labruyere, J.J., Hartley, C., and Holloway, A. (2011). Contrast-enhanced ultrasonography in the differentiation of retinal detachment and vitreous membrane in dogs and cats. *J. Small Anim. Pract.* 52 (10): 522–530.

14 Boudreaux, M.K. (1996). Platelets and coagulation – An update. *Vet. Clin. North Am. Small Anim. Pract.* 26 (5): 1065–1087.

15 Peterson, J.L., Couto, C.G., and Wellman, M.L. (1995). Hemostatic disorders in cats – a retrospective study and review of the literature. *J. Vet. Intern. Med.* 9 (5): 298–303.

16 Fogh, J.M. and Fogh, I.T. (1988). Inherited coagulation disorders. *Vet. Clin. North Am. Small Anim. Pract.* 18 (1): 231–243.

17 Hart, S.W. and Nolte, I. (1994). Hemostatic disorders in feline immunodeficiency virus-seropositive cats. *J. Vet. Intern. Med.* 8 (5): 355–362.

18 Lisciandro, S.C., Hohenhaus, A., and Brooks, M. (1998). Coagulation abnormalities in 22 cats with naturally occurring liver disease. *J. Vet. Intern. Med.* 12 (2): 71–75.

19 Fulks, M. and Sinnott, V. (2013). Canine and feline coagulopathy. *Clinician's Brief* (November): 77–82.

20 Mackin, A. (1995). Canine Immune-Mediated Thrombocytopenia 3. *Comp. Cont. Educ. Pract.* 17 (4): 515–535.

21 Jordan, H.L., Grindem, C.B., and Breitschwerdt, E.B. (1993). Thrombocytopenia in cats – a retrospective study of 41 cases. *J. Vet. Intern. Med.* 7 (5): 261–265.

22 Shelton, G.H. and Linenberger, M.L. (1995). Hematologic abnormalities associated with retroviral infections in the cat. *Semin. Vet. Med. Surg.* 10 (4): 220–233.

23 Johnstone, I.B. (1986). Canine Von Willebrand's disease: a common inherited bleeding disorder in Doberman pinscher dogs. *Can. Vet. J.* 27 (9): 315–318.

24 Balch, A. and Mackin, A. (2007). Canine immune-mediated hemolytic anemia: treatment and prognosis. *Compend. Contin. Educ. Vet.* 29 (4): 230–238; quiz 9.

25 Carr, A.P., Panciera, D.L., and Kidd, L. (2002). Prognostic factors for mortality and thromboembolism in canine immune-mediated hemolytic anemia: a retrospective study of 72 dogs. *J. Vet. Intern. Med.* 16 (5): 504–509.

26 Archer T. (2013). Diagnosis of Immune Mediated Hemolytic Anemia. Today's Veterinary Practice [Internet]. 3(4): http://todaysveterinarypractice.navc. com/diagnosis-of-immune-mediated-hemolytic-anemia.

27 August, J. (2006). Immune-mediated hemolytic anemia. In: *Consultations in Feline Internal Medicine*, vol. 6 (ed. J. August), 617–627. St. Louis: Saunders.

28 Maggio, F., DeFrancesco, T.C., Atkins, C.E. et al. (2000). Ocular lesions associated with systemic hypertension in cats: 69 cases (1985–1998). *J. Am. Vet. Med. Assoc.* 217 (5): 695–702.

29 Samsom, J., Rogers, K., and Wood, J.L. (2004). Blood pressure assessment in healthy cats and cats with hypertensive retinopathy. *Am. J. Vet. Res.* 65 (2): 245–252.

30 Henik, R.A. (1997). Systemic hypertension and its management. *Vet. Clin. North Am. Small Anim. Pract.* 27 (6): 1355–1372.

31 Littman, M.P. (1994). Spontaneous systemic hypertension in 24 cats. *J. Vet. Intern. Med.* 8 (2): 79–86.

32 Morgan, R.V. (1986). Systemic hypertension in four cats: ocular and medical findings. *J. Am. Anim. Hosp. Assoc.* 22: 615–621.

33 Stiles, J., Polzin, D.J., and Bistner, S.I. (1994). The prevalence of retinopathy in cats with systemic hypertension and chronic-renal-failure or hyperthyroidism. *J. Am. Anim. Hosp. Assoc.* 30 (6): 564–572.

34 Remillard, R.L., Ross, J.N., and Eddy, J.B. (1991). Variance of indirect blood pressure measurements and prevalence of hypertension in clinically normal dogs. *Am. J. Vet. Res.* 52 (4): 561–565.

35 Ritchie, C.M., Sheridan, B., Fraser, R. et al. (1990). Studies on the pathogenesis of hypertension in Cushing's disease and acromegaly. *Q. J. Med.* 76 (280): 855–867.

36 Ware, W.A. (2009). Systemic arterial hypertension. In: *Small Animal Internal Medicine* (ed. R.W. Nelson and C.G. Couto), 184–191. Missouri: Mosby Elsevier.

37 Wasik, B. and Adkins, E. (2010). Canine anterior uveitis. *Compend. Contin. Educ. Vet* 32 (11): E1.

38 Laminack, E.B., Myrna, K., and Moore, P.A. (2013). Clinical approach to the canine red eye. *Today's Veterinary Practice* (May/June).

39 Ollivier, F.J. and Plummer, C.E. (2007). The eye examination and diagnostic procedures. In: *Veterinary Opthalmology* (ed. K.N. Gelatt), 438–483. Ames, Iowa: Blackwell.

40 Moore, P.A. (2001). Examination techniques and interpretation of ophthalmic findings. *Clin. Tech. Small Anim. Pract.* 16 (1): 1–12.

41 Wilcock, B.P. and Peiffer, R.L. Jr. (1986). Morphology and behavior of primary ocular melanomas in 91 dogs. *Vet. Pathol.* 23 (4): 418–424.

42 Bliss CD, Sila GH, Morreale RJ, editors. (2009). A survey of concurrent findings in canine and feline patients presenting for hyphema at a private referral clinic in Michigan from 2004 to 2008. 40th Annual Meeting of the American College of Veterinary Ophthalmologists; Chicago, IL: Veterinary Ophthalmology.

43 Martins, T.B. and Barros, C.S.L. (2015). Red eyes in the necropsy floor: twenty cases of hyphema in dogs and cats. *Pesqui Vet. Brasil.* 35 (1): 55–61.

17

Hypopyon

17.1 Description of Hypopyon

As is true of hyphema, patients that present with hypopyon also accumulate abnormal material within the anterior chamber of the eye. However, as opposed to blood, hypopyon refers to the accumulation of purulent material, that is, white blood cells [1–3]. Pus may overtake the entire chamber [1, 3]. Alternatively, small quantities may settle out to the ventral aspect of the anterior chamber, creating a line of demarcation between normal and abnormal contents (see Figures 17.1a–e).

Hypopyon may appear milky white to yellow in appearance [1, 3].

In mild cases, it may be difficult to appreciate, particularly if the patient's third eyelid is elevated [1]. Using a strong light to highlight the anterior chamber as well as ventroflexing the patient's head to artificially depress the third eyelid may facilitate visualization of hypopyon [1].

Hypopyon may be mistaken for a fibrin clot in the anterior chamber. However, unlike hypopyon, a fibrin clot does not settle out into a line of demarcation [3].

17.2 Primary Causes of Hypopyon

Hypopyon occurs when the blood–ocular barrier breaks down, allowing for cellular entry into the anterior chamber [1, 3].

The most common cause of hypopyon is anterior uveitis [1, 3]. Less commonly, hypopyon is associated with intraocular lymphoma [1, 3].

17.3 Anterior Uveitis as the Primary Cause of Hypopyon

Recall from Chapter 16, Section 16.2.4 that anterior uveitis is inflammation of the iris and ciliary body [4].

Classic signs of anterior uveitis include "red eye." This is the result of episcleral injection [4, 5]. In addition, patients with anterior uveitis tend to be light-sensitive and exhibit ocular pain through blepharospasm [4, 5].

As anterior uveitis progresses, the anterior chamber tends to take on a hazy appearance [4, 5]. This is referred to as having aqueous flare. Refer to Chapter 16, Figure 16.8.

Aqueous flare may be overt or subtle. When there is any question as to its presence, the use of a slit beam can provide visual confirmation. In a normal, healthy eye, the aqueous humor should appear clear when the light of the slit beam passes through it. In a patient with uveitis, the aqueous humor is foggy. This "fog" changes the way that light is refracted and is thus apparent when the light of the slit beam passes through [5].

Patients with uveitis also tend to have low intraocular pressure (IOP) [5–7].

Uveitis has many rule-outs [4, 8–12].

17.3.1 Noninfectious Causes of Uveitis

Most instances of uveitis in companion animal patients are noninfectious [4, 8]. These include cases of traumatic uveitis, uveitis secondary to corneal ulceration, and lens-induced uveitis (LIU) [4, 8–12]. LIU is often associated with cataracts [4]. When cataracts resorb, lens-associated protein may leak out through the capsule [4]. This can cause a mild uveitis to develop [4]. This uveitis is typically responsive to anti-inflammatory therapy [4].

In addition, intraocular neoplasia can cause uveitis. Certain breeds appear to be overrepresented in the veterinary literature, including Rottweilers, Golden Retrievers, Labrador Retrievers, and German Shepherds [4]. Melanomas and epithelial ciliary body tumors represent the most common primary intraocular tumors, whereas lymphomas and hemangiosarcomas cause secondary intraocular neoplasia [4, 8–12].

Of primary intraocular tumors, iris and uveal melanomas are most common [4, 9, 13]. Neither tumor type has a high rate of metastasis [9, 13–15].

Of secondary intraocular tumors, lymphoma is most likely [13, 16].

Common Clinical Presentations in Dogs and Cats, First Edition. Ryane E. Englar.

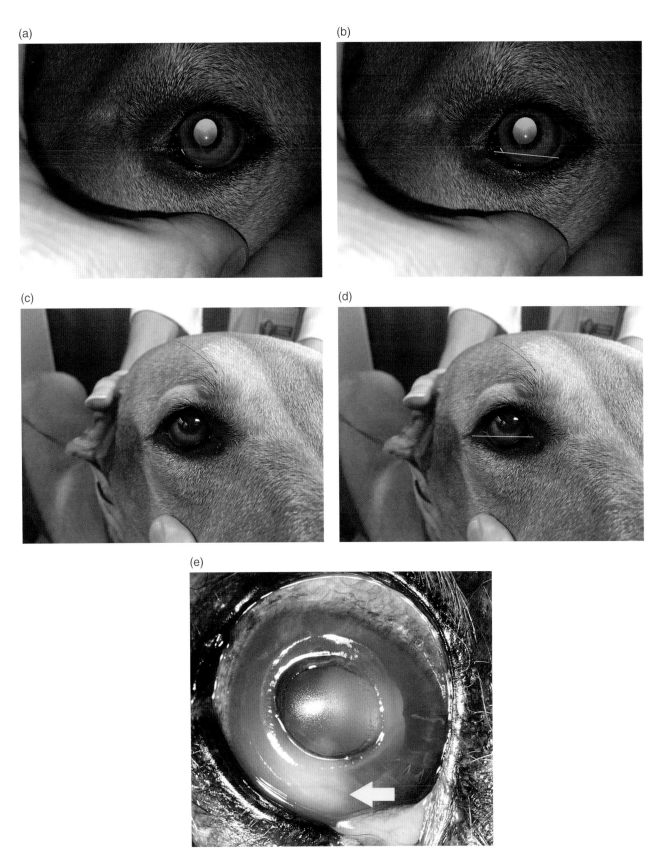

Figure 17.1 (a) Canine patient with hypopyon of the left eye. You can appreciate that a line of demarcation is evident where an accumulation of white blood cells has settled out along the floor of the anterior chamber. *Source:* Courtesy of Daniel Foy, MS, DVM, DACVIM, DACVECC. (b) Same patient as in Figure 17.1a, with the line of demarcation outlined in yellow. *Source:* Courtesy of Daniel Foy, MS, DVM, DACVIM, DACVECC. (c) Canine patient with hypopyon of the right eye. You can appreciate that a line of demarcation is evident where an accumulation of white blood cells has settled out along the floor of the anterior chamber. *Source:* Courtesy of Daniel Foy, MS, DVM, DACVIM, DACVECC. (d) Same patient as in Figure 17.1c, with the line of demarcation outlined in yellow. *Source:* Courtesy of Daniel Foy, MS, DVM, DACVIM, DACVECC. (e) Canine patient with a descemetocele, a severe condition in which the cornea is thinned to the point that only the Descemet membrane remains. Beneath the cornea, you can appreciate the presence of hypopyon, as noted by the solid yellow arrow. *Source:* Courtesy of D.J. Haeussler, Jr., MS, DVM, DACVO.

Uveitis may also be caused by breed-specific conditions. Consider, for example, pigmentary uveitis of Golden Retriever dogs [17–19]. Patients are often middle-aged at onset, and may present with concurrent uveal cysts. Disease is bilateral and progressive [19]. Although topical and systemic therapy may slow disease progression, it frequently leads to serious sequelae [19]. Over time, the by-products of inflammation may obstruct the drainage of the aqueous humor [4, 19]. In these patients, secondary glaucoma is likely [19]. As secondary glaucoma develops, the IOP rises [4].

Pigmentary uveitis of Golden Retriever dogs is inherited; however, the mode of inheritance is unknown [19].

Another breed-specific cause of noninfectious uveitis is uveodermatologic syndrome [4, 20–24]. Breeds that are most at risk include Siberian Huskies, Alaskan Malamutes, Akitas, and Samoyeds [4, 20–24]. This condition is similar to Vogt-Koyanagi-Harada syndrome in humans; however, dogs only seem to develop skin and ocular changes [25, 26].

Affected dogs are thought to experience immune-mediated destruction of melanocytes. This results in progressive depigmentation of the skin. In particular, the nose, eyelids, lips, footpads, perineum, and scrotum are impacted. Skin issues are cosmetic; however, concurrent ocular changes are severe. Uveitis is painful and may over time lead to blindness [4, 20–24].

Noninfectious etiologies of uveitis are often easily identified through a combination of history taking and physical examination. Breed, signalment, and examination findings are often enough to establish a working diagnosis [4].

Infectious etiologies are not as easily discovered, because they lack distinguishing features based on history taking and physical examination alone [4]. There are also so many potential causes of infectious uveitis that the prospect of launching a diagnostic investigation for each is daunting. The list of rule-outs seems endless.

17.3.2 Infectious Causes of Uveitis

The most common infectious causes of uveitis include the following [4, 10, 12, 27–42]:

- Algal
  - Protothecosis
- Bacterial
  - Borreliosis
  - Brucellosis
  - Feline bartonellosis
  - Leptospirosis
- Feline Viral
  - Feline immunodeficiency virus (FIV)
  - Feline infectious peritonitis (FIP)

- Feline leukemia virus (FeLV)
- Feline rhinotracheitis
- Fungal
  - Blastomycosis
  - Candidiasis
  - Canine disseminated aspergillosis
  - Coccidioidomycosis
- Protozoa
  - Leishmaniasis
  - *Neospora caninum*
  - Toxoplasmosis
  - *Trypanosoma evansi*
- Tick-borne
  - *Ehrlichia canis*, the causative agent of canine monocytic ehrlichiosis
  - *Rickettsia rickettsia*, the causative agent of Rocky Mountain Spotted Fever

Few clients are able to pursue a work-up for each potential rule-out, so prioritization is important. Consider, for example, how geographical location influences fungal disease. Patients that live in or have traveled to Arizona and other desert regions of the southwestern United States are at greater risk for coccidioidomycosis; patients within the Mississippi and Ohio River valleys are at greater risk for blastomycosis; and patients along the southeastern coast are at greater risk for protothecosis [4, 42].

An extensive discussion on each etiologic agent of disease is beyond the scope of this text. An internal medicine or infectious disease reference should be consulted for more information about each agent of interest or the pathogenesis of disease.

17.3.3 Idiopathic Uveitis

Despite the clinician's best efforts to identify the source of uveitis in a given patient, nearly two-thirds of cases in dogs are idiopathic [4, 16]. These patients tend to be middle-aged and present for unilateral uveitis [4, 16].

17.4 Diagnostic Tools to Evaluate Hypopyon

Patients with infectious uveitis tend to present with systemic signs of illness rather than just uveitis [4]. For example, these patients may have a fever or generalized lymphadenopathy [4].

Because of the potential for concurrent hematologic or organ dysfunction, baseline diagnostic tests are important for any patient that is suspected to have an underlying infection [4]. These include a complete blood count (CBC), serum biochemistry profile, and urinalysis [4].

Depending upon the causative agent, some patients may be anemic, thrombocytopenic, or pancytopenic [4]. These diagnostic clues help to narrow down the list of rule-outs. Additionally, blood smears may facilitate identification of the causative agent [4].

Anterior chamber centesis can also be performed in the anesthetized patient to obtain a sample of the aqueous humor [1, 3]. Patients are typically referred to board-certified veterinary ophthalmologists to undergo this type of procedure. The potential for causing iatrogenic damage is great if the clinician has not received training in the proper technique.

In clinical cases that warrant enucleation of the eye, the globe should be submitted for sample culture and histopathologic examination [4]. This may facilitate a diagnosis of neoplasia.

References

1 Côté, E. (2015). Clinical veterinary advisor. In: *Dogs and Cats*, 3e, xxxvii, 1642 p. St. Louis, Missouri: Elsevier Mosby.

2 Smith, R.I.E. (2006). The blind cat or cat with retinal disease. In: *Problem-based Feline Medicine*, xiv, 1479 p. (ed. J. Rand). Edinburgh; New York: Saunders.

3 Tilley, L.P. and Smith, F.W.K. (2004). *The 5-Minute Veterinary Consult: Canine and Feline*, 3e. Philadelphia: Lippincott Williams & Wilkins.

4 Wasik, B. and Adkins, E. (2010). Canine anterior uveitis. *Compend. Contin. Educ. Vet.* 32 (11): E1.

5 Laminack, E.B., Myrna, K., and Moore, P.A. (2013). Clinical Approach to the canine red eye. *Today's Veterinary Practice* (May/June).

6 Ollivier, F.J. and Plummer, C.E. (2007). The eye examination and diagnostic procedures. In: *Veterinary Opthalmology* (ed. K.N. Gelatt), 438–483. Ames, Iowa: Blackwell.

7 Moore, P.A. (2001). Examination techniques and interpretation of ophthalmic findings. *Clin. Tech. Small Anim. Pract.* 16 (1): 1–12.

8 Gwin, R.M. (1988). Anterior uveitis - diagnosis and treatment. *Semin. Vet. Med. Surg.* 3 (1): 33–39.

9 Gelatt, K.N. (ed.) (2000). Diseases and surgery of the canine anterior uvea. In: *Essentials of Veterinary Ophthalmology*, 197–225. Philadelphia: Lippincott Williams & Wilkins.

10 Carastro, S.M., Dugan, S.J., and Paul, A.J. (1992). Intraocular dirofilariasis in dogs. *Compend. Cont. Educ. Pract.* 14 (2): 209–217.

11 Torrent, E., Leiva, M., Segales, J. et al. (2005). Myocarditis and generalised vasculitis associated with leishmaniosis in a dog. *J. Small Anim. Pract.* 46 (11): 549–552.

12 Ciaramella, P. and Corona, M. (2003). Canine leishmaniasis: clinical and diagnostic aspects. *Compend. Cont. Educ. Pract.* 25 (5): 358–369.

13 Dubielzig, R.R. (1990). Ocular neoplasia in small animals. *Vet. Clin. North Am. Small Anim. Pract.* 20 (3): 837–848.

14 Diters, R.W., Dubielzig, R.R., Aguirre, G.D., and Acland, G.M. (1983). Primary ocular melanoma in dogs. *Vet. Pathol.* 20 (4): 379–395.

15 Wilcock, B.P. and Peiffer, R.L. Jr. (1986). Morphology and behavior of primary ocular melanomas in 91 dogs. *Vet. Pathol.* 23 (4): 418–424.

16 Massa, K.L., Gilger, B.C., Miller, T.L., and Davidson, M.G. (2002). Causes of uveitis in dogs: 102 cases (1989–2000). *Vet. Ophthalmol.* 5 (2): 93–98.

17 Sapienza, J.S., Simo, F.J., and Prades-Sapienza, A. (2000). Golden retriever uveitis: 75 cases (1994–1999). *Vet. Ophthalmol.* 3 (4): 241–246.

18 Townsend, W.M. and Gornik, K.R. (2013). Prevalence of uveal cysts and pigmentary uveitis in Golden retrievers in three Midwestern states. *J. Am. Vet. Med. Assoc.* 243 (9): 1298–1301.

19 Grahn, B.H., Starrack, G., and Bauer, B. (2012). Diagnostic ophthalmology. *Can. Vet. J.* 53 (11): 1223–1224.

20 Blackwood, S.E., Barrie, K.P., Plummer, C.E. et al. (2011). Uveodermatologic syndrome in a rat terrier. *J. Am. Anim. Hosp. Assoc.* 47 (4): e56–e63.

21 Horikawa, T., Vaughan, R.K., Sargent, S.J. et al. (2013). Pathology in practice. Uveodermatologic syndrome. *J. Am. Vet. Med. Assoc.* 242 (6): 759–761.

22 Kern, T.J., Walton, D.K., Riis, R.C. et al. (1985). Uveitis associated with poliosis and vitiligo in six dogs. *J. Am. Vet. Med. Assoc.* 187 (4): 408–414.

23 Pye, C.C. (2009). Uveodermatologic syndrome in an Akita. *Can. Vet. J.* 50 (8): 861–864.

24 Sigle, K.J., McLellan, G.J., Haynes, J.S. et al. (2006). Unilateral uveitis in a dog with uveodermatologic syndrome. *J. Am. Vet. Med. Assoc.* 228 (4): 543–548.

25 Yamaki, K. and Ohono, S. (2008). Animal models of Vogt-Koyanagi-Harada disease (sympathetic ophthalmia). *Ophthalmic Res.* 40 (3–4): 129–135.

26 Baiker, K., Scurrell, E., Wagner, T. et al. (2011). Polymyositis following Vogt-Koyanagi-Harada-like syndrome in a Jack Russell terrier. *J. Comp. Pathol.* 144 (4): 317–323.

27 Greene, C.E. (2006). *Infectious Diseases of the Dog and Cat*, 3e. St. Louis: Saunders Elsevier.

28 Legendre, A.M. and Toal, R.L. (2000). Diagnosis and treatment of fungal disease of the respiratory system. In: *Kirk's Current Veterinary Therapy XIII* (ed. J.D. Bonagura), 815–819. Philadelphia: WB Saunders.

29 Leiva, M., Naranjo, C., and Pena, M.T. (2005). Ocular signs of canine monocytic ehrlichiosis: a retrospective study in dogs from Barcelona, Spain. *Vet. Ophthalmol.* 8 (6): 387–393.

30 Low, R.M. and Holm, J.L. (2005). Canine rocky mountain spotted fever. *Compend. Cont. Educ. Pract.* 27 (7): 530–538.

31 Martin, C.L. (1999). Ocular manifestations of systemic disease. In: *Veterinary Ophthalmology* (ed. K.N. Gelatt), 1401–1504. Philadelphia: Lippincott Williams & Wilkins.

32 Munger, R.J. (1990). Uveitis as a manifestation of Borrelia-Burgdorferi infection in dogs. *J. Am. Vet. Med. Assoc.* 197 (7): 811.

33 Neer, T.M., Breitschwerdt, E.B., Greene, R.T., and Lappin, M.R. (2002). Consensus statement on ehrlichial disease of small animals from the infectious disease study group of the ACVIM. American College of Veterinary Internal Medicine. *J. Vet. Intern. Med.* 16 (3): 309–315.

34 Neer, T.M. and Harrus, S. (2006). Canine monocytic ehrlichiosis and neorickettsiosis. In: *Infectious Diseases of the Dog and Cat* (ed. C.E. Greene), 203–217. St. Louis: Saunders Elsevier.

35 Schultze, A.E., Ring, R.D., Morgan, R.V., and Patton, C.S. (1998). Clinical, cytologic and histopathologic manifestations of prototothecosis in two dogs. *Vet. Ophthalmol.* 1 (4): 239–243.

36 Sessions, J.K. and Greene, C.E. (2004). Canine leptospirosis: treatment, prevention, and zoonosis. *Compend. Cont. Educ. Pract.* 26 (9): 700–706.

37 Strunck, E., Billups, L., and Avgeris, S. (2004). Canine prototothecosis. *Compend. Cont. Educ. Pract.* 26 (2): 96–102.

38 Townsend, W.M., Stiles, J., and Krohne, S.G. (2006). Leptospirosis and panuveitis in a dog. *Vet. Ophthalmol.* 9 (3): 169–173.

39 Greene, C.E. (ed.) (2006). Cryptococcosis. In: *Infectious Diseases of the Dog and Cat*, 584–598. St. Louis: Elsevier Saunders.

40 Bloom, J.D., Hamor, R.E., and Gerding, P.A. Jr. (1996). Ocular blastomycosis in dogs: 73 cases, 108 eyes (1985–1993). *J. Am. Vet. Med. Assoc.* 209 (7): 1271–1274.

41 Gelatt, K.N., Chrisman, C.L., Samuelson, D.A. et al. (1991). Ocular and systemic aspergillosis in a dog. *J. Am. Anim. Hosp. Assoc.* 27 (4): 427–431.

42 Gilger, B.C. (2000). Ocular manifestations of systemic infectious diseases. In: *Kirk's Current Veterinary Therapy XIII* (ed. J.D. Bonagura), 276–279. Philadeophia: WB Saunders.

18

Anisocoria

18.1   Introduction to the Pupil

The pupil is an intentional anatomical defect in the iris [1, 2].

Each species has a characteristic pupil shape. The canine pupil is always round, whether ambient light is strong or dim. The feline pupil takes on the shape of a vertical slit in everyday lighting, and rounds out as it dilates [1, 2]. (see Figures 18.1a–c).

The pupil is to the iris what an aperture is to a camera: it allows light into the system. How much light enters the eye depends upon the pupil's size. The iris controls the size of the pupil based upon the body's needs. As ambient lighting dims, pupils widen to increase the amount of light that enters the eye. This dilation of the pupils is called mydriasis, as compared to miosis, a state in which the pupils are constricted [1, 2].

Pupils also dilate in response to activation of the sympathetic nervous system as occurs during "fight or flight" [1, 2] (see Figures 18.2a–c).

Feline pupils are especially reactive to sympathetic tone. A stressed, startled, or scared cat is likely to have mydriatic pupils [1, 2].

When pupils are mydriatic, they do not always constrict in response to weak light sources such as a penlight. A stronger light source is often required to obtain a pupillary light reflex (PLR) [1].

Ambient lighting and state of mind are not the only determinant of pupil size. Certain medications also can cause mydriasis. Consider an anticholinergic drug, atropine, for example. When used in the injectable form, atropine acts as a pre-anesthetic medication to counter opioid-induced bradycardia [3]. Because it has parasympatholytic effects, atropine also causes mydriasis [3] (see Figure 18.3).

Because atropine causes mydriasis, it is also formulated as an ophthalmic solution. This can be applied directly to the eye to facilitate fundoscopy [3].

18.2   Introduction to Anisocoria

Normal pupils work in concert with each other. When one constricts, so should the other. When one dilates, the other should, too. Normal pupils are therefore symmetrical in shape and action [1, 2].

Anisocoria is the pathological condition by which pupils are asymmetrically shaped [1, 2]. Anisocoria can occur in both dogs and cats (see Figures 18.4a–c).

Anisocoria can be overt or subtle. Heterochromic irises can make it challenging to determine if the patient has true anisocoria or if it is imagined due to the differences in eye color (see Figures 18.5a, b).

18.3   Primary Causes of Anisocoria

Anisocoria can be the result of primary ocular disease or primary neurological disease [2, 4, 5].

18.3.1   Ocular Causes of Anisocoria

Ocular causes of anisocoria include the following [2–11]:

- Medications
- Bromide toxicosis
- Exposure to toxic plants
- Anterior uveitis
- Iris hypoplasia

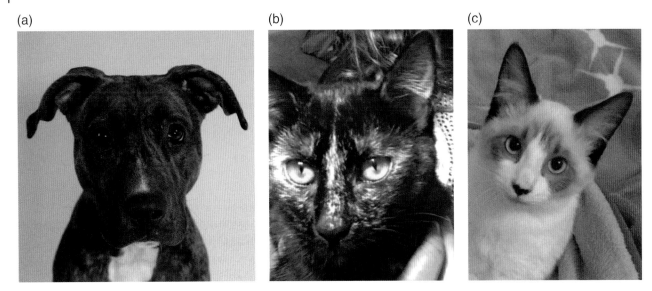

Figure 18.1 (a) The normal dog has a circular pupil, regardless of the strength of ambient lighting. *Source:* Courtesy of John A. Schwartz. (b) The normal cat has a pupil that is shaped like a vertical slit when ambient lighting is adequate and the patient is not in "fight or flight" mode. *Source:* Courtesy of Leigh Ann Howard, DVM. (c) When ambient lighting is dim or when the patient is in "fight or flight" mode, the cat's pupil becomes increasingly rounded. *Source:* Courtesy of Lydia McDaniel, DVM.

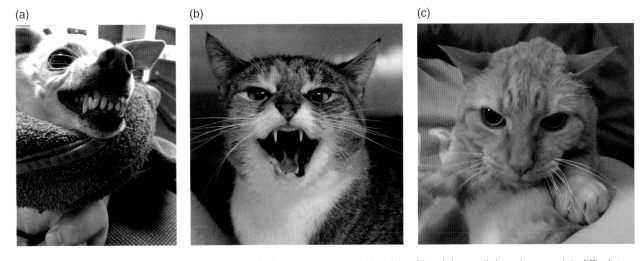

Figure 18.2 (a) This canine patient is reacting aggressively to veterinary care. Note how dilated the pupils have become. It is difficult to appreciate where the pupils begin and end. The eyes take on the appearance of black orbs. The iris has shrunken down to just a tiny rim. *Source:* Courtesy of Stefanie Perry. (b) This cat is becoming increasingly agitated by veterinary care. Note how the shape of both pupils is reflecting this state of mind. *Source:* Courtesy of Jennifer Lang. (c) This cat just endured a nail trim and is agitated. Note the extensive mydriasis. *Source:* Courtesy of Rachel A. Karner.

- Iris atrophy
- Posterior synechiae
- Feline spastic pupil syndrome

18.3.1.1 Medications

Atropine was discussed briefly in Section 18.1 as an anticholinergic drug with parasympatholytic properties. When administered topically to one eye, atropine will cause its pupil to become mydriatic. This can facilitate fundoscopy [3].

Incidentally, atropine is also used to temporarily reduce ciliary spasms in eyes that perpetuate painful conditions, such as anterior uveitis [10]. This improves the comfort of the affected eye(s) during medical treatment [10].

18.3.1.2 Bromide Toxicosis

Idiopathic epilepsy is a common neurological condition in companion animal medicine [1, 2]. Historically, epilepsy was managed by the administration of bromide salts or phenobarbital [11, 12]. More recently, potassium bromide has been prescribed in combination with phenobarbital to improve patient response when patients have been refractory to treatment with phenobarbital alone [13–20].

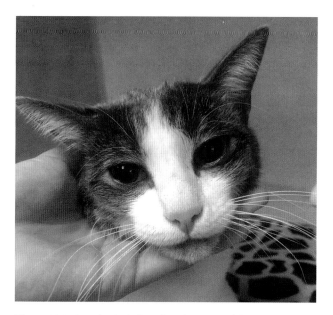

Figure 18.3 Anesthesia-induced mydriasis in a feline patient. *Source:* Courtesy of Sami Moon.

Unfortunately, an excess of bromide can result in toxicosis [11, 12, 21–23]. This toxicosis is called bromism [12]. Because bromide is eliminated through the urinary tract, bromism is more likely to occur in those patients that have pre-existing renal insufficiency [11, 12].

Bromism in human patients targets the integumentary, gastrointestinal, and nervous systems [12, 23]. In dogs with bromide toxicosis, neurological signs predominate [11, 12]. These include apparent muscular weakness, ataxia, and hyperexcitability [11, 17, 18, 21, 22]. In addition, patients may develop either bilateral mydriasis or anisocoria [11, 12].

History taking and medical record review play an important role in the diagnosis of bromism, particularly if an emergency clinician is seeing the patient for the very first time. Learning that the patient has been receiving bromide should raise the index of suspicion that bromism is possible. This presumptive diagnosis can be supported by serum bromide concentrations, or by the patient's clinical improvement after dose reduction [12].

(a)

(b)

(c)

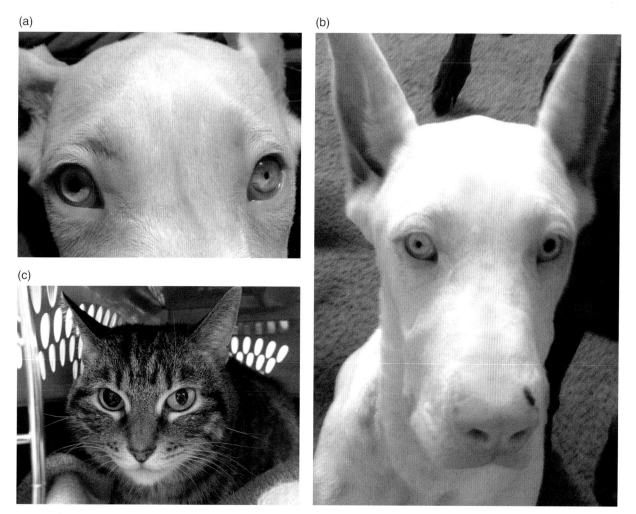

Figure 18.4 (a) Anisocoria in a canine patient. Note how the pupil that is associated with the left eye (OS) is miotic as compared to the right (OD). *Source:* Courtesy of Jetta Schirmer. (b) Anisocoria in a canine patient. Note how the pupil that is associated with the right eye (OD) is miotic as compared to the left (OS). *Source:* Courtesy of Jetta Schirmer. (c) Anisocoria in a feline patient. The pupil that is associated with the right eye (OD) is mydriatic compared to the left (OS). *Source:* Courtesy of the Media Resources Department at Midwestern University.

(a)

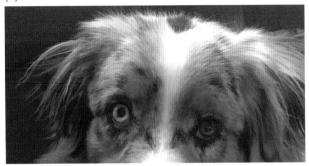

(b)

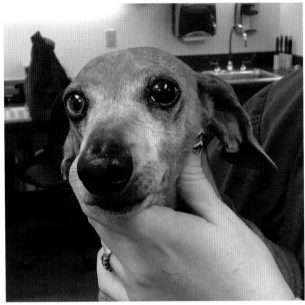

Figure 18.5 (a) Heterochromic irises in a canine patient. This patient does not have anisocoria. However, the different colored irises would make it difficult to appreciate subtle anisocoria. *Source:* Courtesy of Amanda Leigh Rappaport. (b) Heterochromic irises in a canine patient. This patient does have anisocoria. You can appreciate the challenges of comparing pupil size between the left and right eyes because the pupil of the left eye (OS) blends in with the dark brown color that is associated with the iris.

18.3.1.3 Toxic Plants

Certain toxins cause anisocoria when they come into direct contact with the eye. Consider, for example, the ornamental plant, *Datura stramonium*. Colloquially, this plant is known as jimsonweed, thorn apple, or the devil's snare. It is related to *Atropa belladonna*, deadly nightshade (see Figures 18.6a, b).

Since the sixteenth century, *D. stramonium* has been used in medicinal preparations and for its hallucinogenic properties [6]. Most recently, it has been used in human patients to reduce the bronchial spasms associated with asthma [6].

The active ingredients of *D. stramonium* include atropine, scopolamine, and hyoscyamine [6, 24–26].

When it is ingested, *D. stramonium* causes peripheral and central neuropathy. Its atropine results in tachycardia and bilateral mydriasis [6]. Cardiac and respiratory arrest are dose-dependent sequelae [6].

However, ingestion is not the only way that *D. stramonium* can cause adverse effects. Ocular contact with *D. stramonium* in humans as well as animals causes anisocoria [6, 27, 28]. This was experimentally proven in dogs by Hansen et al. in 2002 [6]. Dogs that had ocular contact with extract containing the crushed stems of *D. stramonium* experienced marked anisocoria [6]. Anisocoria also occurred after exposure to macerated leaves, but not after exposure to infusions of *Datura* flowers [6]. Stems contain more toxic alkaloids than seeds, and young plants contain the highest concentrations [29].

18.3.1.4 Anterior Uveitis

Anterior uveitis was previously discussed. Refer to Chapter 17, Section 17.3 to review the ocular changes associated with inflammation of the iris and ciliary body [30].

18.3.1.5 Iris Hypoplasia

Iris hypoplasia refers to an abnormal condition in which the iris does not develop properly or is abnormally thin [31]. In dogs, this may be inherited or secondary to inflammation of the iris itself.

Iris hypoplasia has been linked to the merle gene [31]. Color-dilute dogs or dogs that have albinotic coats are more likely to experience this condition.

Over time, iris hypoplasia progresses to the point that defects are visible [31]. If these defects are significant in terms of size, they may create the illusion of anisocoria. The pupil may appear larger because there is less iris to contain it.

These "holes" in the iris are called iris colobomas. They allow for unregulated entry of light into the eye. This may cause affected patients to squint because the light is too bright.

18.3.1.6 Iris Atrophy

Iris atrophy refers to the degeneration of the iris in adult or geriatric patients.

Iris atrophy is an expected age-related change. Affected patients may have irregular pupillary margins, and their PLRs may be slower than normal [31]. This so-called senile iris atrophy occurs commonly in Toy and Miniature Poodles, Chihuahuas, and Miniature Schnauzers [31]. Siamese cats may also be predisposed [31] (see Figures 18.7a, b).

Iris atrophy may also be secondary to chronic ocular disease, such as glaucoma and recurrent uveitis [31].

18.3.1.7 Synechiae

Adhesions between the iris and another ocular structure are termed synechiae.

(a)

(b)

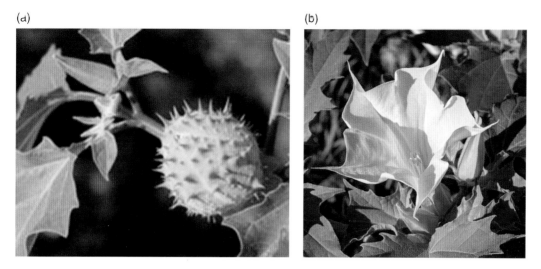

Figure 18.6 (a) The fruit associated with the ornamental plant, *Datura stramonium*. (b) The flower of *D. stramonium*.

(a)

(b)

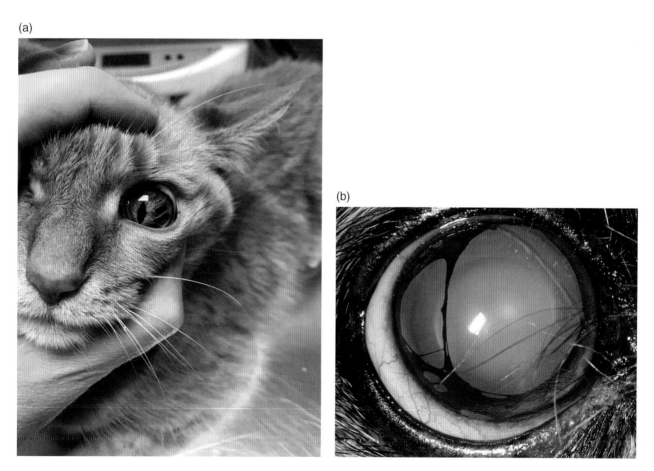

Figure 18.7 (a) Iris atrophy in a feline patient. *Source:* Courtesy of Elizabeth E. Ferguson, DVM. (b) Close-up of iris atrophy in a canine patient. *Source:* Courtesy of D.J. Haeussler, Jr., MS, DVM, DACVO.

Anterior synechiae are strands of tissue that adhere the iris to the cornea. These are associated with inflammation of the iris, and occur frequently in cases of uveitis. They may also result from corneal disease. The iris can be thought of as attempting to seal corneal lesions like a Band-Aid (see Figures 18.8a–c).

Posterior synechiae are strands of tissue that attach the iris to the lens capsule [7]. When this occurs, the central

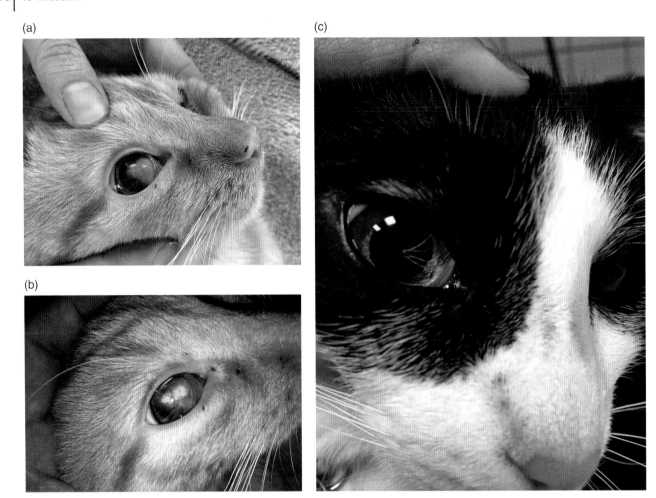

Figure 18.8 (a) Anterior synechiae in a feline patient with corneal disease. *Source:* Courtesy of Paul Ebner. (b). Anterior synechiae in a feline patient. *Source:* Courtesy of Paul Ebner, LVT. (c) Anterior synechiae in a feline patient. *Source:* Courtesy of Lauren Griggs, DVM.

aspect of the iris bends backward in space, creating a larger pupil in the affected eye [7]. The affected pupil may also appear to be misshapen [7].

18.3.1.8 Feline Spastic Pupil Syndrome

Feline spastic pupil syndrome is an unusual condition in which anisocoria occurs sporadically [32]. Pupils may alternate in terms of which appears mydriatic [32].

Patients with this condition should be screened for feline leukemia virus (FeLV) and feline immunodeficiency virus (FIV) [4, 9, 32].

These patients are likely to develop myeloproliferative disease, if they have not yet already done so [32].

18.3.2 Neurological Causes of Anisocoria

The most common neurological causes of anisocoria in companion animal medicine include the following:

- Head trauma
- Intracranial neoplasia
- Organophosphate toxicity

- Sympathetic denervation to the eye
- Parasympathetic denervation to the eye
- Concurrent sympathetic and parasympathetic denervation to the eye

18.3.2.1 Head Trauma

Head trauma may result in hemorrhage or increased intracranial pressure [7]. Both can compress the brain [7]. If the midbrain is compressed at the level of the third cranial nerve, the oculomotor (CN III), then parasympathetic dysfunction may result [7]. If trauma is symmetrical, then both pupils will be miotic [7]. If trauma is asymmetrical, then only the pupil on the affected side will be miotic, resulting in anisocoria [7].

If compression of the brain is not resolved, miotic pupils will become mydriatic and lose their PLRs [7]. This patient has a dire prognosis [7].

18.3.2.2 Intracranial Neoplasia

Meningiomas are the most common intracranial neoplasia in dogs and cats [7]. These may develop in the second cranial nerve, the optic (CN II), cerebrum, brainstem, and spinal cord [7]. Less common tumors include gliomas, lymphoma, and peripheral nerve sheath tumors [7].

All intracranial tumors can cause compression that leads to anisocoria in the same way that head trauma can [7].

18.3.2.3 Organophosphate Toxicity

Organophosphates are active ingredients in a number of insecticides and herbicides. When ingested, these compounds bind to and inactivate acetylcholinesterase so that acetylcholine persists at the neuromuscular junction [4]. Acute signs of intoxication include classic "SLUD" signs: excessive salivation, lacrimation, urination, and defecation [4].

Sometimes, patients present for muscle tremors or cervical ventroflexion [4].

Usually, both pupils are mydriatic [4]. However, anisocoria is possible [33].

History taking plays an important role in documenting organophosphate exposure [4]. Rapid treatment with pralidoxime, 2-pyridine aldoxime methyl chloride (2-PAM), is indicated [4].

18.3.2.4 Sympathetic Denervation to the Eye

The sympathetic pathway to the eye is responsible for dilation of the pupil [7].

Three neurons are involved in the pathway that provides sympathetic innervation to the eye [7, 34]:

- First order, upper motor neuron
- Second order, preganglionic neuron
- Third order, postganglionic neuron

The cell body of the first order neuron originates in the hypothalamus [7, 34]. Its axon travels through the brainstem and cervical spinal cord to the T1–T3 spinal segments [34].

Second order neurons arise within the T1–T3 spinal region [34]. Here, they extend their axons to become part of the vagosympathetic trunk [34]. The vagosympathetic trunk courses through the cranial thorax.

Axons of preganglionic neurons synapse with postganglionic neurons adjacent to the tympanic bulla, within the cranial cervical ganglion [34].

Axons of feline postganglionic neurons extend into the calvaria by passing through the tympanic bulla [34]. Axons of canine postganglionic neurons extend into the calvaria by passing near, rather than through, the tympanic bulla [34].

Ultimately, these axons terminate at the eye [34].

Any part of the aforementioned pathway can be compromised [34]. The resultant sympathetic denervation causes Horner Syndrome or Horner's syndrome, depending upon which article is referenced [4, 7, 34].

Horner's syndrome is characterized by miosis of the affected pupil [35]. In addition, patients with classic Horner's syndrome have three other presenting complaints with regard to the affected eye [35]:

- Ptosis of the upper eyelid
- Enophthalmos
- Prominent third eyelid or nictitans membrane (see Figures 18.9a, b)

(a)

(b)

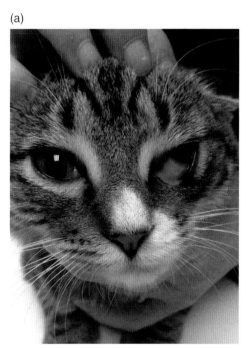
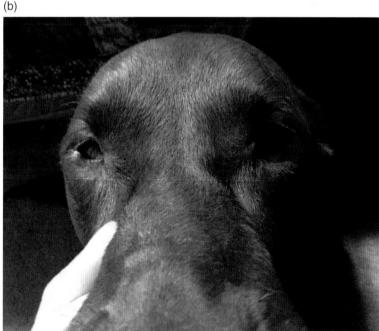

Figure 18.9 (a) Horner's syndrome in a feline patient. Note that the left eye (OS) is the affected eye. *Source:* Courtesy of Pamela Mueller, DVM. (b) Enophthalmos in a canine patient. *Source:* Courtesy of Jessica Darmofal.

Ptosis refers to droopiness of the eyelid. It occurs when the upper lid loses smooth muscle tone that is ordinarily provided by sympathetic fibers to keep the lid retracted and open [35].

Sympathetic innervation is also important in maintaining orbital smooth muscle tone [35]. In health, this tone maintains the spatial orientation and position of the globe [35]. When sympathetic innervation is compromised, orbital smooth muscle relaxes such that the globe retracts into the orbit [35]. This gives the appearance of a sunken-in globe [35].

When the globe retreats into the socket, the nictitans membrane becomes passively more prominent in both canine and feline patients [35].

Additionally, cats have smooth muscle within their third eyelids [35]. In health, this smooth muscle keeps the third eyelid retracted and out of view [35]. When sympathetic innervation is compromised in the cat, smooth muscle associated with the nictitans relaxes such that the membrane pops up and into view [35].

At least half of canine patients with Horner's syndrome have idiopathic dysfunction [7]. That is, the cause is never determined. Most recover on their own timetable, without treatment [7, 36, 37].

The known causes of Horner's syndrome in both cats and dogs include the following [7, 35, 38, 39]:

- Acute, asymmetrical, cervical spinal cord lesions
  - fibrocartilaginous emboli (FCE)
  - traumatic cervical disk extrusions
  - vertebral luxations
  - vertebral fractures
- Brachial plexus disease
  - Traumatic avulsion of the brachial plexus
  - Brachial plexus neuritis
  - Malignant nerve sheath tumor
- Soft tissue disease in the cervical region, within the proximity of the vagosympathetic trunk
  - Trauma secondary to jugular venipuncture [7]
  - Trauma associated with the use of choke chains [7]
  - Pharyngeal stick foreign bodies
  - Esophageal neoplasia
  - Chronic esophagitis
  - Chronic tracheitis
- Otitis media
- Nasopharyngeal polyps
- Complications of middle ear surgery, in particular, ventral bulla osteotomy in cats [40–43]

These are beyond the scope of this chapter; however, two of these will be touched upon further here because they present with concurrent signs that assist with diagnosis.

The first among these is brachial plexus disease. Brachial plexus disease impacts the second order neuron [35]. If

trauma to the brachial plexus has been sustained, then onset will be rapid; if brachial plexus disease is neoplastic, then onset will be progressive [35]. In either case, the patient will develop thoracic limb lameness or monoparesis [35]. This is evident on physical examination [35].

Horner's syndrome develops when brachial plexus neoplasia advances cranially [35]. The cutaneous trunci reflex on the side of the lesion may also be absent, with overlying muscle atrophy [35].

Nasopharyngeal polyps, in particular those involving the middle ear, also commonly result in Horner's syndrome in cats [2, 44]. Nasopharyngeal polyps represent a noninfectious cause of upper airway disease and tend to occur in young cats [2, 45–48].

Nasopharyngeal polyps cause upper airway obstruction during the inspiratory part of the respiratory cycle. As a result, affected patients typically present for stertor, a snoring sound. Stertor is typically pronounced when the patient is asleep; however, it may persist when the patient is awake [2].

An oropharyngeal examination under sedation may assist with the diagnosis of a nasopharyngeal polyp by allowing for manipulation of the soft palate; however, advanced imaging such as a CT scan may be indicated to better evaluate the upper airway sinuses for turbinate destruction and/or mass effect [45] (see Figure 18.10).

When nasopharyngeal polyps invade the middle ear, they are typically managed surgically. A common surgical approach is the ventral bulla osteotomy [49–52]. This involves opening up the middle ear and effectively scooping out the polyp [49–52] (see Figure 18.11).

Postoperative recurrence rate is low [49–52].

Because sympathetic nerve fibers pass through the tympanic bulla in the cat, a transient Horner's syndrome is a common adverse effect in the postoperative period [44] (see Figure 18.12).

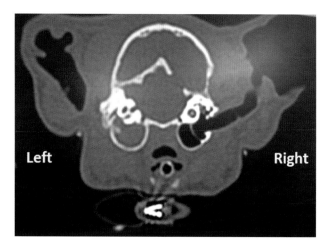

Figure 18.10 Transverse CT scan demonstrating appreciable fluid in the left tympanic bulla.

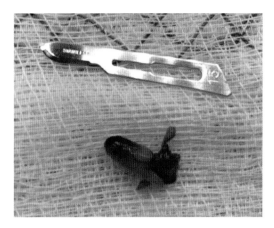

Figure 18.11 Nasopharyngeal polyp after surgical extraction.

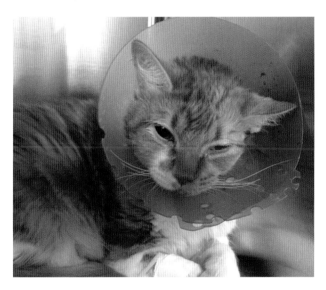

Figure 18.12 Postoperative ptosis and pronounced nictitating membrane OS in a feline patient that underwent ventral bulla osteotomy.

18.3.2.5 Parasympathetic Denervation to the Eye

The parasympathetic pathway to the eye is responsible for constriction of the pupil [7]. This is a two-neuron pathway that starts in the midbrain, when the parasympathetic nuclei of CN III extend preganglionic fibers to the eye [7]. These fibers synapse in the ciliary ganglion, from which postganglionic fibers extend to the iris sphincter muscle [7]. The iris sphincter muscle proceeds to constrict the pupil [7].

Dysfunction at any point along this pathway will prevent pupil constriction [7].

18.3.2.6 Concurrent Sympathetic and Parasympathetic Denervation to the Eye

When the patient experiences simultaneous sympathetic and parasympathetic denervation to the eye, it is said to have dysautonomia [7, 31]. The etiology of dysautonomia

is unknown; however, it results in an abnormally low number of neurons at autonomic ganglia [31].

Onset of disease is acute in young adults [31]. Historically, dysautonomia has been reported more often in cats than in dogs [31]. Among dogs, medium-to-large breeds tend to be at greater risk, particularly those that reside in rural areas [7, 53].

Patients typically present with bilateral mydriasis; however, pupils can exhibit anisocoria [7, 31]. PLRs are absent [7, 31].

In addition, affected patients exhibit ptosis of the upper eyelids and prominent nictitans membranes [7, 31].

Because the denervation in these patients is not limited to the eyes, these patients present with other systemic signs of dysfunction, including the following [7, 31]:

- Cardiovascular disturbances
  - Bradycardia
- Gastrointestinal disturbances
  - Anorexia
  - Megaesophagus with associated regurgitation
  - Delayed gastric emptying and associated vomiting
  - Fecal incontinence
- Urinary disturbances
  - Distended urinary bladder
  - Urinary incontinence
- Other disturbances
  - Lethargy
  - Tacky mucous membranes from lack of saliva
  - Keratoconjunctivitis sicca, otherwise known as "dry eye"

Prognosis in these patients is poor [7, 31]. There are no effective treatments [7, 31]. Euthanasia is considered to be a humane outcome for these cases [7, 31].

18.4 Diagnostic Tools for Lesion Localization

Anisocoria may be the result of one or more lesions within the visual, sympathetic, or parasympathetic pathways [7]. Lesion localization is important because it helps to narrow down the list of rule-outs, thereby facilitating diagnosis and treatment.

PLRs are one method to distinguish between sympathetic and parasympathetic lesions [7]. Although both sympathetic and parasympathetic lesions have normal menace responses and visual tracking, they differ in their ability to elicit PLRs. Sympathetic lesions do not alter PLRs, and affected patients should therefore have normal PLRs [7]. By contrast, PLRs are absent in patients with parasympathetic lesions [7].

Despite the clinician's best efforts, it is sometimes a challenge to localize the lesion. Pharmaceutical methods have been devised to differentiate between lesions within the sympathetic and parasympathetic pathways.

To document sympathetic denervation, dilute (1.0%) phenylephrine can be administered to both eyes [7]. If there is postganglionic sympathetic dysfunction, the affected eye(s) will dilate within 20 min of topical application [7].

If neither eye dilates, then the treatment is repeated with concentrated (10%) phenylephrine. If there is a preganglionic lesion, the affected eye(s) will dilate within 20–40 min. Patients with preganglionic sympathetic lesions should undergo body cavity imaging [54]. Specifically, cervical and thoracic radiographs are indicated to rule out cervical and mediastinal tumors [54].

If neither eye dilates with concentrated phenylephrine, then there is unlikely to be a sympathetic disturbance [7].

To document parasympathetic denervation, physostigmine (0.5%) is applied topically to the eyes [55]. As a cholinesterase inhibitor, physostigmine prevents the breakdown of acetylcholine at the neuromuscular junction [7, 55]. This indirectly enhances the effects of acetylcholine.

The normal pupil should constrict [55]. If there is a preganglionic lesion, the affected pupil(s) will constrict rapidly [55]. To be specific, the affected pupil will constrict 40–60 min before the normal pupil [55]. If there is a postganglionic lesion, then there is no pupil constriction [55].

A solution of 2% pilocarpine may also be used to test for parasympathetic denervation [55]. Pilocarpine is a direct parasympathomimetic agent [55]. If there is a parasympathetic lesion, the affected pupil will constrict sooner than the normal pupil [55].

When the eye is exposed to dilute solutions of pilocarpine (0.1–0.2%), the normal eye exhibits no change [55]. However, eyes with postganglionic parasympathetic lesions will constrict [55].

References

1 DeLahunta, A., Glass, E., and Kent, M. (2015). *Veterinary Neuroanatomy and Clinical Neurology*, 4e. St. Louis, MO: Elsevier/Saunders.

2 Englar, R.E. (2017). *Performing the Small Animal Physical Examination*. Hoboken, NJ: Wiley.

3 Mama K. (2014). Therapeutics Snapshot: Atropine. Veterinary Team Brief [Internet]; (September). https://www.veterinaryteambrief.com/sites/default/files/attachments/PTB_TS_Atropine.pdf.

4 Bagley, R.S. (2006). The cat with anisocoria or abnormally dilated or constricted pupils. In: *Problem-Based Feline Medicine* (ed. J. Rand), 870–889. Edinburgh; New York: Saunders.

5 Plummer CE. (2013). Anisocoria. Clinician's Brief [Internet]; (November):[20 p.]. https://www.cliniciansbrief.com/article/anisocoria.

6 Hansen, P. and Clerc, B. (2002). Anisocoria in the dog provoked by a toxic contact with an ornamental plant: Datura stramonium. *Vet. Ophthalmol.* 5 (4): 277–279.

7 Heller HB, Bentley E. (2016). The Practitioner's Guide to Neurologic Causes of Canine Anisocoria. Today's Veterinary Practice [Internet]; (January/February):[77–83 pp.]. https://todaysveterinarypractice.com/wp-content/uploads/sites/4/2016/05/TVP_2016-0102_OO-Anisocoria.pdf.

8 Otto CM. (2010). Head Trauma (Proceedings). DVM 360 [Internet]. http://veterinarycalendar.dvm360.com/head-trauma-proceedings.

9 Phillips, T.R., Prospero-Garcia, O., Puaoi, D.L. et al. (1994). Neurological abnormalities associated with feline immunodeficiency virus infection. *J. Gen. Virol.* 75 (Pt 5): 979–987.

10 Sandmeyer, L.S., Bauer, B.S., and Grahn, B.H. (2014). Diagnostic ophthalmology. *Can. Vet. J.* 55 (11): 1105–1106.

11 Yohn, S.E., Morrison, W.B., and Sharp, P.E. (1992). Bromide toxicosis (bromism) in a dog treated with potassium bromide for refractory seizures. *J. Am. Vet. Med. Assoc.* 201 (3): 468–470.

12 Rossmeisl, J.H. and Inzana, K.D. (2009). Clinical signs, risk factors, and outcomes associated with bromide toxicosis (bromism) in dogs with idiopathic epilepsy. *J. Am. Vet. Med. Assoc.* 234 (11): 1425–1431.

13 Pearce, L.K. (1990). Potassium bromide as an adjunct to phenobarbital for the management of uncontrolled seizures in dogs. *Prog. Vet. Neurol.* 1: 95–101.

14 Sisson, A. and LeCouteur, R.A. (1990). Potassium bromide as an adjunct to phenobarbital for the management of uncontrolled seizures in the dog (Letter). *Prog. Vet. Neurol.* 1: 114–116.

15 Podell, M. (1998). Antiepileptic drug therapy. *Clin. Tech. Small Anim. Pract.* 13 (3): 185–192.

16 Podell, M. and Fenner, W.R. (1993). Bromide therapy in refractory canine idiopathic epilepsy. *J. Vet. Intern. Med.* 7 (5): 318–327.

17 Podell, M. and Fenner, W.R. (1994). Use of bromide as an antiepileptic drug in dogs. *Comp. Cont. Educ. Pract.* 16 (6): 767–774.

18 March, P.A., Podell, M., and Sams, R.A. (2002). Pharmacokinetics and toxicity of bromide following high-dose oral potassium bromide administration in healthy Beagles. *J. Vet. Pharmacol. Ther.* 25 (6): 425–432.

19 Trepanier, L.A. (1995). Topics in drug-therapy – use of bromide as an anticonvulsant for dogs with epilepsy. *J. Am. Vet. Med. Assoc.* 207 (2): 163–166.

20 Trepanier, L.A., Van Schoick, A., Schwark, W.S., and Carrillo, J. (1998). Therapeutic serum drug concentrations in epileptic dogs treated with potassium bromide alone or in combination with other anticonvulsants: 122 cases (1992–1996). *J. Am. Vet. Med. Assoc.* 213 (10): 1449–1453.

21 Rosenblum, I. (1958). Bromide intoxication. I. Production of experimental intoxication in dogs. *J. Pharmacol. Exp. Ther.* 122 (3): 379–385.

22 Nichols, E.S., Trepanier, L.A., and Linn, K. (1996). Bromide toxicosis secondary to renal insufficiency in an epileptic dog. *J. Am. Vet. Med. Assoc.* 208 (2): 231–233.

23 James, L.P., Farrar, H.C., Griebel, M.L., and Bates, S.R. (1997). Bromism: intoxication from a rare anticonvulsant therapy. *Pediatr. Emerg. Care* 13 (4): 268–270.

24 Frohne, D. and Pfander, H.A. (1983). *Colour Atlas of Poisonous Plants*. London: Wolfe Science Books.

25 Gowdy, J.M. (1972). Stramonium intoxication: review of symptomatology in 212 cases. *JAMA* 221 (6): 585–587.

26 Smith, E.A., Meloan, C.E., Pickell, J.A., and Oehme, F.W. (1991). Scopolamine poisoning from homemade 'moon flower' wine. *J. Anal. Toxicol.* 15 (4): 216–219.

27 Bein, C. and Granier, M. (1999). Une cause rare de mydriase unilaterale. *La Presse Medicale* 28: 1070.

28 Savitt, D.L., Roberts, J.R., and Siegel, E.G. (1986). Anisocoria from Jimsonweed. *J. Am. Med. Assoc.* 255 (11): 1439–1440.

29 Miraldi, E., Masti, A., Ferri, S., and Barni Comparini, I. (2001). Distribution of hyoscyamine and scopolamine in Datura stramonium. *Fitoterapia* 72 (6): 644–648.

30 Wasik, B. and Adkins, E. (2010 (November)). Canine anterior uveitis. *Compend. Cont. Educ. Vet.* 32 (11): E1.

31 Maggs, D.J., Miller, P.E., and Ofri, R. (2013). *Slatter's Fundamentals of Veterinary Ophthalmology*. Philadelphia: Elsevier Saunders.

32 Davidson M. (2016). Comparative Neuro-Ophthalmology. https://cvm.ncsu.edu/wp-content/uploads/2016/06/01_Pupil-4-19-16-Compatibility-Mode.pdf.

33 Townsend, W., Bedford, P., and Jones, G. (2009). Small animal ophthalmology: a problem-oriented approach. In: *Small Animal Ophthalmology: A Problem-Oriented Approach*, 4e (ed. R.L. Peiffer and S.M. Petersen-Jones), 67–115. Edinburgh; New York: Saunders/Elsevier.

34 Troxel, M. (2014). Horner syndrome at a glance. *Clinician's Brief* (May): 25.

35 Penderis, J. (2015). Diagnosis of Horner's syndrome in dogs and cats. *In Pract.* 37 (3): 107–119.

36 Morgan, R.V. and Zanotti, S.W. (1984). Horner's syndrome in dogs and cats: 49 cases. (1980–1986). *J. Am. Vet. Med. Assoc.* 194 (8): 1096–1099.

37 Boydell, P. (2000). Idiopathic horner syndrome in the golden retriever. *J. Neuroophthalmol.* 20 (4): 288–290.

38 Boydell, P. (1995). Horner's syndrome following cervical spinal surgery in the dog. *J. Small Anim. Pract.* 36 (11): 510–512.

39 Garosi, L.S., Dennis, R., Penderis, J. et al. (2001). Results of magnetic resonance imaging in dogs with vestibular disorders: 85 cases (1996–1999). *J. Am. Vet. Med. Assoc.* 218 (3): 385–391.

40 Garosi, L.S., Lowrie, M.L., and Swinbourne, N.F. (2012). Neurological manifestations of ear disease in dogs and cats. *Vet. Clin. North Am. Small Anim. Pract.* 42 (6): 1143–1160.

41 Smeak, D.D. and Dehoff, W.D. (1986). Total ear canal ablation – clinical-results in the dog and cat. *Vet. Surg.* 15 (2): 161–170.

42 Williams, J.M. and White, R.A.S. (1992). Total ear canal ablation combined with lateral bulla osteotomy in the cat. *J. Small Anim. Pract.* 33 (5): 225–227.

43 Bacon, N.J., Gilbert, R.L., Bostock, D.E., and White, R.A. (2003). Total ear canal ablation in the cat: indications, morbidity and long-term survival. *J. Small Anim. Pract.* 44 (10): 430–434.

44 Baines, S.J. (2014). Pharynx. In: *Feline Soft Tissue and General Surgery* (ed. S.J. Langley-Hobbs, J. Demetriou and J.F. Ladlow), 617–633. Edinburgh; New York: Saunders/Elsevier.

45 Quimby, J. and Lappin, M.R. (2012). The upper respiratory tract. In: *The Cat: Clinical Medicine and Management* (ed. S.E. Little), 846–861. St. Louis: Saunders Elsevier.

46 Henderson, S.M., Bradley, K., Day, M.J. et al. (2004). Investigation of nasal disease in the cat–a retrospective study of 77 cases. *J. Feline Med. Surg.* 6 (4): 245–257.

47 Schmidt, J.F. and Kapatkin, A. (1990). Nasopharyngeal and ear canal polyps in the cat. *Feline Pract.* 18 (4): 16–19.

48 Kapatkin, A.S., Matthiesen, D.T., Noone, K.E. et al. (1990). Results of surgery and long-term follow-up in 31 cats with nasopharyngeal Polyps. *J. Am. Anim. Hosp. Assoc.* 26 (4): 387–392.

49 White, R.A. (2003). Middle ear. In: *Textbook of Small Animal Surgery* (ed. D.H. Slatter), 1760–1767. Philadelphia: WB Saunders.

50 Trevor, P.B. and Martin, R.A. (1993). Tympanic bulla osteotomy for treatment of middle-ear disease in cats: 19 cases (1984–1991). *J. Am. Vet. Med. Assoc.* 202 (1): 123–128.

51 Pope, E.R. (2000). Feline respiratory tract polyps. In: *Kirk's Current Veterinary Therapy XIII* (ed. J. Bonagura), 794–796. Philadelphia: WB Saunders.

52 Faulkner, J.E. and Budsberg, S.C. (1990). Results of ventral bulla osteotomy for treatment of middle-ear polyps in cats. *J. Am. Anim. Hosp. Assoc.* 26 (5): 496–499.

53 Berghaus, R.D., O'Brien, D.P., Johnson, G.C., and Thorne, J.G. (2001). Risk factors for development of dysautonomia in dogs. *J. Am. Vet. Med. Assoc.* 218 (8): 1285–1290.

54 van den Broek, A.H. (1987). Horner's syndrome in cats and dogs: a review. *J. Small Anim. Pract.* 28: 929–940.

55 Davidson M. (2016). Neuro-Ophthalmology. https://cvm.ncsu.edu/wp-content/uploads/2016/05/Davidson_2016-Neuroophthalmology-notes-4-19-16.pdf.

19

Abnormalities Associated with the Upper and Lower Palpebrae

19.1 Introduction to Periocular Anatomy

Both cats and dogs have upper and lower eyelids called palpebrae [1–5]. These are essentially folds of skin that are seated dorsal and ventral to the globe [1–5] (see Figures 19.1a, b).

When intrinsic muscular action causes these folds to be brought together, they essentially close off access to the eye [1, 3, 6] (see Figures 19.2a, b).

The space between the open upper and lower palpebrae is the palpebral fissure [3–5]. The medial and lateral canthi are the corners of the palpebral fissure where the upper and lower palpebrae meet [3–5].

Cats do not typically have eyelid cilia, otherwise known as eyelashes. Dogs typically only have lashes along the upper eyelids [7]. They may have two to four rows [8].

Lash length in dogs is breed- and coat-dependent. In general, short-coated dogs have shorter eyelashes, whereas long-coated dogs have longer lashes to keep their coats out of their eyes (see Figures 19.3a–c).

Unlike humans, cats and dogs also have a third eyelid, the nictitating membrane or the nictitans [3–6, 9, 10]. Abnormalities associated with this structure will be discussed in Chapter 20.

19.2 Clinical Presentations that Involve the Upper and/or Lower Palpebrae

There are four main clinical presentations that involve the upper and/or lower palpebrae:

- Eyelid agenesis
- Blepharitis
- Entropion
- Ectropion

19.2.1 Eyelid Agenesis

Eyelid agenesis is a developmental defect that occurs spontaneously in cats [11–14]. It may be partial or complete. When eyelid agenesis is partial, it tends to target the upper lid at the lateral canthus [12, 14] (see Figure 19.4).

Within domestic breeds, eyelid agenesis is most commonly seen in Burmese and Birman cats [12–14]. However, isolated case reports describe its occurrence in wild felids, including snow leopards and mountain lions [15, 16].

Eyelid agenesis is problematic. It predisposes the patient to exposure keratitis. Every time that eyelids come together in the basic action of blinking, they redistribute the tear film over the normal globe. When a portion or all of that lid is absent, the patient loses that protective function.

The upper lid is more mobile than the lower lid [1, 2]. Without that upper lid being intact, the lower lid cannot possible close the gap. A portion of the cornea is left open to the environment and it dessicates.

Over time, this leads to ocular discomfort. Humans with exposure keratitis report ocular pain, which triggers epiphora. Patients may also describe light sensitivity, blurred vision, and the sensation that there is a foreign body in their eye [17].

The gross appearance of the cornea will also change if the condition is not addressed. The patient is likely to develop corneal edema secondary to inflammation. Corneal ulcerations are common sequelae. These ulcerations will respond to medical management; however, they frequently scar. Recurrence is likely.

In addition, eyelid agenesis makes it possible for fur to make contact with the cornea. This so-called trichiasis promotes keratitis and associated corneal disease [12].

Eyelid agenesis requires reconstructive surgery to rebuild the missing lid [12, 18–21].

(a)

(b)

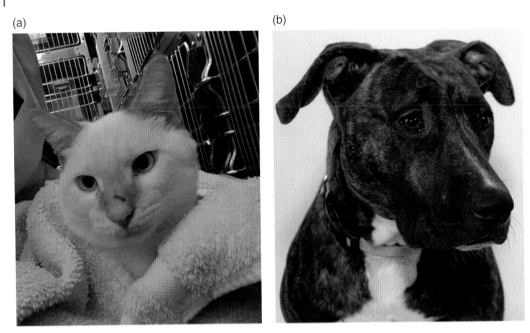

Figure 19.1 (a) Normal appearance associated with the upper and lower palpebrae in a feline patient, when both structures are open. *Source:* Courtesy of Danielle Cucuzella. (b) Normal appearance associated with the upper and lower palpebrae in a canine patient, when both structures are open. *Source:* Courtesy of John A. Schwartz.

(a)

(b)

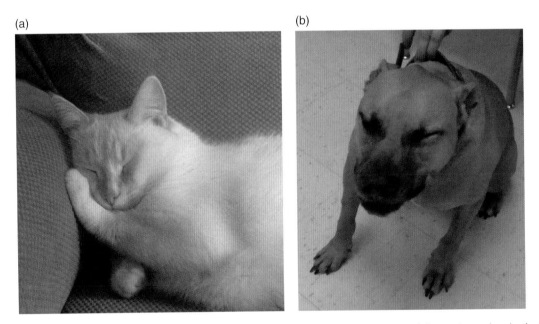

Figure 19.2 (a) Normal appearance associated with the upper and lower palpebrae in a feline patient, when both structures are closed. *Source:* Courtesy of Kathryn Knowles. (b) Normal appearance associated with the upper and lower palpebrae in a canine patient, when both structures are closed. *Source:* Courtesy of Patricia Bennett, DVM.

19.2.2 Blepharitis

Inflammation of the eyelids is called blepharitis [8, 22]. Inflammation may be diffuse or localized. Focal granulomatous swellings called chalazia are common and are associated with the Meibomian glands [8, 22] (see Figures 19.5a–c).

The eyelids may swell markedly [8, 22]. This is called blepharoedema and is often most visible from an aerial view (see Figure 19.6).

Other clinical signs may involve excessive tearing or epiphora, skin lesions, including ulcerations, secondary to moist dermatitis, and pruritus [8, 22] (see Figure 19.7a–c).

(a)

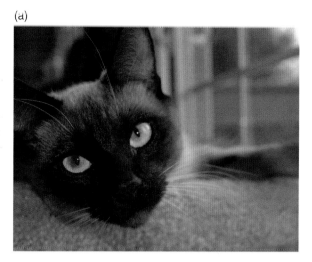

(b)   (c)

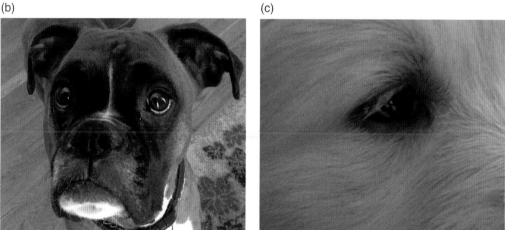

Figure 19.3 (a) Normal appearance of the eyelids in a feline patient. Note that there are no eyelashes. *Source:* Courtesy of Erika Olney, DVM. (b) Normal appearance of the eyelids in a Boxer dog. The eyelashes are very difficult to appreciate because they are so short, as is typical for short-coated dogs. *Source:* Courtesy of Symmantha Page. (c) Normal appearance of the eyelids in a Golden Retriever puppy. The eyelashes are much longer in this patient and are easier to appreciate.

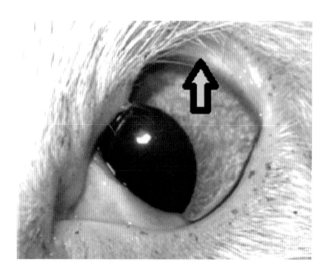

Figure 19.4 Partial eyelid agenesis in a feline patient. Note the absence of the upper lid at the level of the lateral canthus.

Blepharitis is typically bilateral [8, 23]. Blepharitis may occur in isolation of other ocular conditions. However, it is often associated with conjunctivitis or keratoconjunctivitis sicca (KCS) [22].

There are three main causes of blepharitis [8]:

- Bacterial infection
- Parasitic infestation
- Immune-mediated disease

Bacterial blepharitis is commonplace in canine medicine [8]. Cats appear to be resistant to the condition [22]. Although many species of bacteria can cause blepharitis, *Staphylococcus* and *Streptococcus* sp. are the most common isolates [8, 23].

Historically, treatment with antibiotics, anti-inflammatories, and/or eye-safe skin cleansers has been initiated based upon the patient's clinical appearance. However, the development of antibiotic resistance raises concerns

(a)　(b)

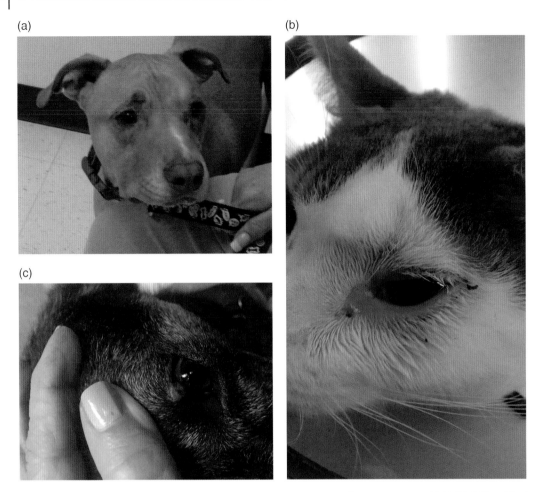

(c)

Figure 19.5 (a) Diffuse blepharitis in a canine patient. *Source:* Courtesy of Patricia Bennett, DVM. (b) Diffuse blepharitis in a feline patient. *Source:* Courtesy of Eric Stone. (c) Chalazion in a canine patient. *Source:* Courtesy of Blake and Danielle Tafoya.

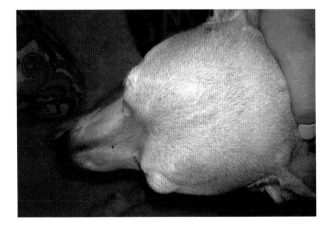

Figure 19.6 Severe blepharoedema in a canine patient. *Source:* Courtesy of Patricia Bennett, DVM.

about starting treatment without diagnostic confirmation. Impression smears of lesions affecting the eyelids are supportive of the diagnosis: intracellular cocci in the presence of neutrophilic inflammation confirm bacterial infection [8, 23, 24]. Subsequent culture and susceptibility testing should guide choice of treatment [8].

Parasitic blepharitis is typically the result of infestation with mange mites [8]. Although *Demodex canis* is the most common isolate, all *Demodex* and *Sarcoptes sp.* have the potential to induce blepharitis [25] (see Figure 19.8).

In affected patients, blepharitis is just one of many clinical signs that are suggestive of mange. Refer to Chapter 5, Section 5.8 for a description of clinical demodicosis and sarcoptic mange. Recall that positive skin scrapings will confirm the diagnosis. However, the false negative rate for *Sarcoptes* sp. is high. For this reason, it is possible that sarcoptic mange occurs with greater frequency than is diagnosed [26].

Pemphigus foliaceus, discoid lupus erythematosus, and uveodermatologic syndrome may cause immune-mediated blepharitis [8, 24, 25, 27, 28]. Refer to Chapter 12, Section 12.4 and Chapter 17, Section 17.3.1 to review other more common clinical presentations of pemphigus foliaceus and uveodermatologic syndrome.

(a)

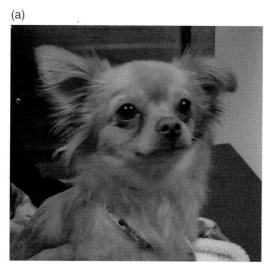

(b)   (c)

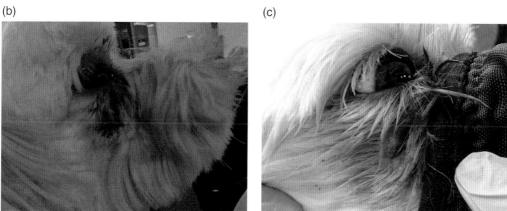

Figure 19.7 (a) Epiphora in a canine patient. *Source:* Courtesy of Patricia Bennett, DVM. (b) Accumulation of crusts associated with dried tears secondary to tear overflow. If these crusts remain, they are likely to irritate the underlying skin, resulting in dermatitis. *Source:* Courtesy of Patricia Bennett, DVM. (c) Moist dermatitis associated with tear overflow. This is what the periocular skin looked like after crusts associated with dried tears were removed. *Source:* Courtesy of Patricia Bennett, DVM.

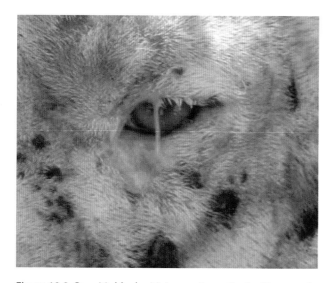

Figure 19.8 Parasitic blepharitis in a canine patient with sarcoptic mange. *Source:* Courtesy of Laura Polerecky, LVT.

Recall the role that biopsy plays in diagnosis of immune-mediated disease [8]. Histopathologic examination is essential for differentiation between the various types of pemphigus [8]. Histopathologic evaluation can also be confirmatory for cases of uveodermatologic syndrome. However, a presumptive diagnosis of uveodermatologic syndrome can be made based upon breed predisposition and presenting signs, such as concurrent anterior uveitis [8].

19.2.3 Entropion

Entropion involves the rolling in of one or both eyelids [29–31]. Think of it as the eyelid curling in toward the eye (see Figures 19.9a, b).

In cats, the lower eyelid is more likely to be involved, and typically just the central portion [29].

Affected patients may have a genetic or breed predisposition for entropion. Brachycephalic breeds are frequently

(a) (b)

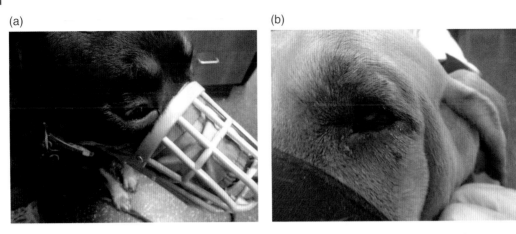

Figure 19.9 (a) Entropion associated with the lower eyelid of this canine patient. *Source:* Courtesy of Patricia Bennett, DVM. (b) Entropion associated with the upper eyelid of this canine patient. *Source:* Courtesy of Patricia Bennett, DVM.

cited in the veterinary medical literature, including English Bulldogs, Pugs, and the Pekingese [30, 32].

Brachycephalic cats are also more likely to develop entropion, in particular, the Persian and the Himalayan breeds [30, 31].

Brachycephalic skull shape is a predisposing factor because the foreshortened face places excessive tension on the medial palpebral ligament [30]. In addition, the abundance of nasal folds supports the curling in of the eyelids associated with the medial canthus [30]. The combination frequently results in entropion [30].

In addition, the toy and giant breeds are more likely to develop entropion [30]. So, too, are those with excessive skin folds, for example, the Chow Chow and Shar Pei dogs [30]. These patients have excessive laxity associated with the lateral palpebral ligament [30]. This tends to promote entropion at the lateral canthus [30].

Cats frequently develop entropion in response to pre-existing ocular conditions. Patients with oversized palpebral fissures, for example, are more likely to develop entropion because the tension on the lower eyelid is less than normal [29] (see Figure 19.10).

Cats in particular seem prone to entropion when they have enophthalmos (see Figure 19.11).

Enophthalmos may be the result of significant weight loss: loss of orbital fat causes the globe to sink into the socket [30]. Enophthalmos may also result from significant muscle atrophy [30].

Spastic entropion is also common in cats [33]. Entropion may develop in response to painful conditions that involve the eye, for example, ulcerative keratitis [33]. The concern is that resolution of the painful ocular condition does not always lead to resolution of entropion [33]. Entropion may persist.

Entropion is more than just an aesthetic condition. Entropion can lead to trichiasis in canine patients, in which the lashes of the upper eyelid are misdirected

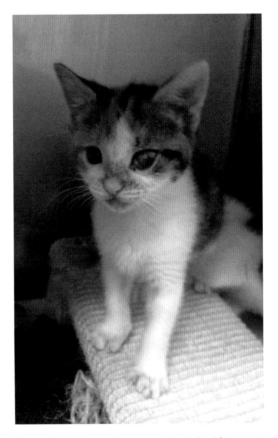

Figure 19.10 Larger-than-normal palpebral fissure associated with left eye (OS). This has predisposed the patient to subtle entropion of the lower lid that is pronounced at the medial canthus. *Source:* Courtesy of Kimberly Wallitsch.

toward and ultimately come into contact with the cornea. Even though cats lack lashes, they, too, can still develop corneal irritation when fur contacts the cornea after one or more lids have curled in or under [30, 31].

Trichiasis is uncomfortable. It may trigger blepharospasm and chronic ocular discharge, in response to the

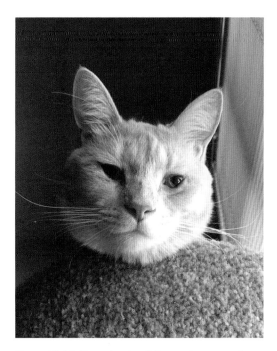

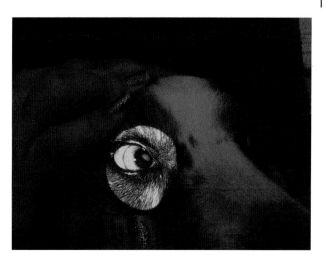

Figure 19.12 Positive (+) fluorescein stain in a canine patient. Note the area of fluorescein uptake. This uptake demonstrates corneal damage. *Source:* Courtesy of Daniel Foy, MS, DVM, DACVIM, DACVECC.

Figure 19.11 Entropion in a feline patient secondary to enophthalmos. Both sets of eyelids are affected, those associated with the right eye and those with the left. However, entropion of the left upper and lower lids is most pronounced. *Source:* Courtesy of Tiffany Li, DVM Candidate at Midwestern University Class of 2020.

persistence of a foreign body, fur or lashes, against the cornea [29]. Epiphora is common [29].

Trichiasis may also cause corneal abrasion and ulceration [29, 31]. Corneal ulcers are most easily detected using fluorescein stain. Fluorescein does not stain intact cornea. The orange dye adheres to damaged cornea and will fluoresce a brilliant green color under a blue light (see Figure 19.12).

The response to corneal ulceration by the adjacent limbus may be neovascularization [29].

Depending upon the severity of entropion, surgical correction may be advised to prevent these sequelae from occurring and reoccurring [30, 33–35]. Surgical approaches are varied and include eyelid wedge resection, the Hotz-Celsus procedure and Quickert-Rathbun technique [30, 33–35].

In addition, dogs with excessive skin folds may undergo stellate rhytidectomy to surgically excise those folds that are weighing down the upper eyelids [36] (see Figure 19.13).

19.2.4 Ectropion

Ectropion involves eversion of one or more of the eyelids [29, 37] (see Figure 19.14).

Affected patients are most likely to be dogs [29, 37]. Patients with loose facial skin are predisposed [37]. Consider bloodhounds, for example. In these patients,

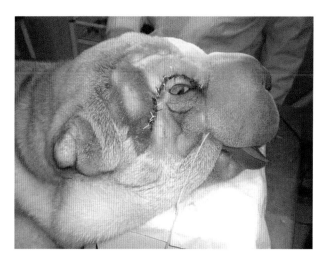

Figure 19.13 Shar Pei dog immediately following surgery to excise excessive skin folds overlaying the upper eyelids to alleviate the tendency of the eyelids to curl inwards and under. *Source:* Courtesy of Danielle Cucuzella.

the skin folds associated with the cheeks are heavy and drag down the lower lids, exposing the palpebral conjunctiva and/or the nictitans [37].

Some dogs may develop transient ectropion from fatigue [37]. Consider the sporting breeds, for instance, including spaniels, hounds, and retrievers.

When mild, ectropion may be purely aesthetic. However, tear drainage is often impacted [37]. Rather than tears draining through the nasolacrimal duct to the nose, they spill out over the eyelids and onto the face [37] (see Figure 19.15).

When ectropion is mild, only good hygiene is indicated; that is, taking care to wipe the face as needed to

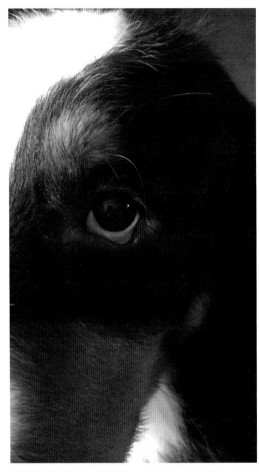

Figure 19.14 Ectropion associated with the lower eyelid of this canine patient. *Source:* Courtesy of Peggy Abramson, LVT.

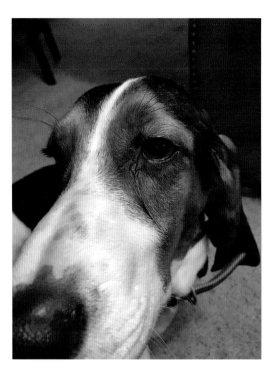

Figure 19.15 Tear overflow in a canine patient. This patient has very subtle ectropion of the lower lid. You can just barely see the pink sliver of the nictitans and the palpebral conjunctiva that collectively give the patient a droopy appearance. *Source:* Courtesy of Amber May.

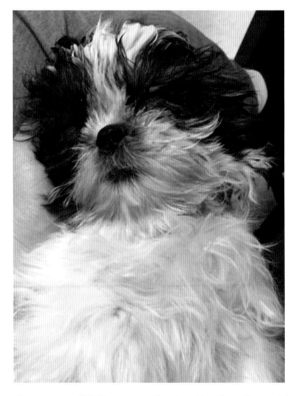

Figure 19.16 Shih Tzu puppy, sleeping. Note how the pup's long facial fur could very easily contact both corneas if this patient's eyes were open. Facial fur that makes corneal contact is an example of trichiasis. *Source:* Courtesy of Gail Nason.

remove accumulations of tears and crusting of dried tears, before they may cause moist dermatitis [37].

Mildly affected patients may also benefit from lubricating eye drops to keep the overexposed cornea from drying out [37]. Without lubrication, the cornea is prone to desiccation. Exposure keratitis is common in advanced cases of ectropion [38].

Affected patients may also develop conjunctivitis.

Surgical reconstruction is reserved for severe cases [37, 38].

19.3 Clinical Presentations that Involve Eyelid Cilia or Aberrant Fur that Contacts the Cornea

Trichiasis was discussed briefly in Sections 19.2.1 and 19.2.3 in the context of fur and/or eyelashes that, despite being in their normal anatomical position, contact the cornea. Trichiasis is commonly seen in patients with excessive nasal folds or in breeds with excessive facial fur [39] (see Figure 19.16).

Two additional clinical presentations involving eyelid cilia are relatively common in companion animal practice.

The first, distichiasis, occurs when cilia emerge from the Meibomian gland or any other abnormal location along the eyelid margin [39]. Distichia may also arise from the lower lid, even though dogs do not tend to have lower eyelid lashes [39]. Distichia may or may not be symptomatic [39]. Lid-splitting techniques were once advocated as a means of surgical correction in symptomatic patients; however, these are likely to predispose the patient to entropion [39]. Cryotherapy or electroepilation are preferred means of cilia removal [39].

Ectopic cilia arise from the underside of the eyelid; that is, they emerge from the palpebral conjunctival surface [39]. Ectopic cilia are more likely than distichia to be irritating to the patient because they are always in contact with the cornea [39]. Removal via cryotherapy is indicated in most cases to alleviate corneal contact and irritation [39]. However, clients need to be informed that ectopic cilia may recur [39]. Therefore, one procedure may not be sufficient. The patient may require additional treatments as new ectopic cilia arise [39].

One concern associated with cryotherapy is the potential for damage to the eyelids [39]. Cryotherapy requires advanced training and skill. Board-certified veterinary ophthalmologists should be consulted before this procedure is undertaken [39].

References

1 Sisson, S. (1910). *A Textbook of Veterinary Anatomy*, 3 p. l., 11-826 p. Philadelphia, London: W.B. Saunders Company.

2 Aspinall, V. and Capello, M. (2009). *Introduction to Veterinary Anatomy and Physiology*. New York: Elsevier.

3 Evans, H.E. and Miller, M.E. (2013). *Miller's Anatomy of the Dog*, 4e, xix, 850 p. St. Louis, Missouri: Elsevier.

4 Rijnberk, A. and FJv, S. (2009). *Medical History and Physical Examination in Companion Animals*, 2e, viii, 333 p. Edinburgh; New York: Saunders/Elsevier.

5 Englar, R.E. (2017). *Performing the Small Animal Physical Examination*. Hoboken, NJ: Wiley.

6 Konig, H.E. and Liebich, H.-G. (eds.). *Veterinary Anatomy of Domestic Mammals: Textbook and Colour Atlas*, 3e. Austria: Schattauer.

7 Yuill C. (2010). Distichia or Distichiasis in Dogs. https://vcahospitals.com/know-your-pet/distichia-or-distichiasis-in-dogs.

8 White BL, Belknap EB. (2015). Clinical Approach to Canine Eyelid Disease: Blepharitis. Today's Veterinary Practice [Internet]:[71–9 pp.]. https://todaysveterinarypractice.com/observations-in-ophthalmology-clinical-approach-to-canine-eyelid-disease-blepharitis/.

9 Maggs, D.J., Miller, P.E., and Ofri, R. (2013). *Slatter's Fundamentals of Veterinary Ophthalmology*. Philadelphia: Elsevier Saunders.

10 Hyman J. (2008). Ophthalmic anatomy for the veterinary technician (Proceedings). DVM 360 [Internet]: http://veterinarycalendar.dvm360.com/ophthalmic-anatomy-veterinary-technician-proceedings.

11 Narfstrom, K. (1999). Hereditary and congenital ocular disease in the cat. *J. Feline Med. Surg.* 1 (3): 135–141.

12 Hartley, C. (2010). Treatment of corneal ulcers: when is surgery indicated? *J. Feline Med. Surg.* 12 (5): 398–405.

13 Belhorn, R.W., Barnett, K.C., and Henkind, P. (1971). Ocular colobomas in domestic cats. *J. Am. Vet. Med. Assoc.* 159 (8): 1015–1021.

14 Koch, S.A. (1979). Congenital ophthalmic abnormalities in the Burmese cat. *J. Am. Vet. Med. Assoc.* 174 (1): 90–91.

15 Barnett, K.C. and Lewis, J.C. (2002). Multiple ocular colobomas in the snow leopard (Uncia uncia). *Vet. Ophthalmol.* 5 (3): 197–199.

16 Cutler, T.J. (2002). Bilateral eyelid agenesis repair in a captive Texas cougar. *Vet. Ophthalmol.* 5 (3): 143–148.

17 Rajaii F, Prescott C. (2014). Management of Exposure Keratopathy. EyeNet [Internet]. (April). https://www.aao.org/eyenet/article/management-of-exposure-keratopathy-2.

18 Roberts, S.R. and Bistner, S.I. (1968). Surgical correction of eyelid agenesis. *Mod. Vet. Pract.* 49: 40–43.

19 Wolfer, J.C. (2002). Correction of eyelid coloboma in four cats using subdermal collagen and a modified Stades technique. *Vet. Ophthalmol.* 5 (4): 269–272.

20 Munger, R.J. and Gourley, I.M. (1981). Cross lid flap for repair of large upper eyelid defects. *J. Am. Vet. Med. Assoc.* 178 (1): 45–48.

21 Esson, D. (2001). A modification of the Mustarde technique for the surgical repair of a large feline eyelid coloboma. *Vet. Ophthalmol.* 4 (2): 159–160.

22 Stiles, J. (2012). Ocular infections. In: *Infectious Diseases of the Dog and Cat*, 4e (ed. C.E. Greene), 974–991. St. Louis, Mo: Elsevier/Saunders.

23 Giuliano, E.A. (2013). Diseases and surgery of the canine lacrimal system. In: *Veterinary Ophthalmology* (ed. K.G. Gelatt, B.C. Gilger and T.J. Kern), 912–930. Ames, IA: Wiley.

24 Pena, M.A. and Leiva, M. (2008). Canine conjunctivitis and blepharitis. *Vet. Clin. North Am. Small Anim. Pract.* 38 (2): 233–249.

25 Miller, W.H., Griffin, C.E., and Campbell, K.L. (eds.) (2013). Diseases of eyelids, claws, anal sacs and ears. In: *Muller and Kirk's Small Animal Dermatology*, 110–125. Philadelphia: Elsevier-Saunders.

26 Pin, D., Bensignor, E., Carlotti, D.N., and Cadiergues, M.C. (2006). Localised sarcoptic mange in dogs: a retrospective study of 10 cases. *J. Small Anim. Pract.* 47 (10): 611–614.

27 Stades, F.C. and van der Woerdt, A. (2013). Diseases and surgery of the canine eyelid. In: *Veterinary Opthalmology*, 2e (ed. K.G. Gelatt, B.C. Gilger and T.J. Kern), 832–860. Ames, IA: Wiley.

28 Scott, D.W., Walton, D.K., Slater, M.R., and Smith, C.A. (1987). Immune-mediated dermatoses in domestic-animals – 10 years after 2. *Compend. Cont. Educ. Pract.* 9 (5): 539–551.

29 Bernays, M.E. (2006). The cat with abnormal eyelid appearance. In: *Problem-Based Feline Medicine* (ed. J. Rand), 1317–1329. Edinburgh; New York: Saunders.

30 Tilley, L.P. and Smith, F.W.K. (eds.) (2004). Entropion. In: *The 5-Minute Veterinary Consult: Canine and Feline*, 406–407. Philadelphia: Lippincott Williams & Wilkins.

31 Williams, D.L. and Kim, J.Y. (2009). Feline entropion: a case series of 50 affected animals (2003–2008). *Vet. Ophthalmol.* 12 (4): 221–226.

32 Krecny, M., Tichy, A., Rushton, J., and Nell, B. (2015). A retrospective survey of ocular abnormalities in pugs: 130 cases. *J. Small Anim. Pract.* 56 (2): 96–102.

33 Read, R.A. and Broun, H.C. (2007). Entropion correction in dogs and cats using a combination Hotz-Celsus and lateral eyelid wedge resection: results in 311 eyes. *Vet. Ophthalmol.* 10 (1): 6–11.

34 White, J.S., Grundon, R.A., Hardman, C. et al. (2012). Surgical management and outcome of lower eyelid entropion in 124 cats. *Vet. Ophthalmol.* 15 (4): 231–235.

35 Williams, D.L. (2004). Entropion correction by fornix-based suture placement: use of the Quickert-Rathbun technique in ten dogs. *Vet. Ophthalmol.* 7 (5): 343–347.

36 van der Woerdt, A. (2004). Adnexal surgery in dogs and cats. *Vet. Ophthalmol.* 7 (5): 284–290.

37 Tilley, L.P. and Smith, F.W.K. (eds.) (2004). Ectropion. In: *The 5-Minute Veterinary Consult: Canine and Feline*, 390–391. Philadelphia: Lippincott Williams & Wilkins.

38 Hamilton, H.L., McLaughlin, S.A., Whitley, R.D., and Swaim, S.F. (1998). Surgical reconstruction of severe cicatricial ectropion in a puppy. *J. Am. Anim. Hosp. Assoc.* 34 (3): 212–218.

39 Tilley, L.P. and Smith, F.W.K. (eds.) (2004). Eyelash disorders. In: *The 5-Minute Veterinary Consult: Canine and Feline*, 438–439. Philadelphia: Lippincott Williams & Wilkins.

20

Abnormal Presentations Involving the Nictitans

20.1 Introduction to the Nictitans

In addition to the upper and lower palpebrae, dogs and cats have a third eyelid [1, 2]. This structure is called the nictitans or nictitating membrane. Historically, it was known as the haw, and it was erroneously thought to be vestigial, like the appendix or wisdom teeth [3].

In actuality, the nictitans has important structural and functional roles. Located in the ventromedial orbit, it consists of a T-shaped hyaline cartilage [2]. This cartilage is like a windshield wiper [2]. With each blink, it glides across the surface of the cornea to spread tear film [2].

Movement of the nictitans is characteristically passive [2]. However, cats have some degree of active control over its movement [2].

The cartilage of the nictitans also serves as an additional protective barrier between the environment and the globe [2].

The nictitans is lined by conjunctiva on both sides: the palpebral conjunctiva, on the surface that faces the eyelids, and the bulbar conjunctiva, on the surface that faces the globe [2]. The bulbar surface contains lymphoid follicles [1, 2]. These pink-red structures are thought to play a role in ocular immunity [2].

There is also a seromucoid gland at the base of this cartilage [1, 2]. This gland produces anywhere from 25% to 50% of tears [1, 2, 4].

Operating as a single unit, the nictitans is typically out of sight (see Figures 20.1a, b).

The hidden position of the nictitans is maintained by the sympathetic tone of the orbital smooth muscles [1]. These muscles control where the nictitans sits relative to the globe [1]. When sympathetic tone is diminished or absent, as occurs in Horner's syndrome, the globe is displaced caudally, and the position of the nictitans becomes prominent [1].

Each nictitans should be evaluated at every veterinary visit [5]. In order to bring the nictitans into view, the veterinarian must manipulate the soft tissue over each orbit [5]. Pushing down gently, but firmly, over the upper palpebra will elevate the nictitans for visual inspection [5] (see Figures 20.2a–c).

Patients that present with ocular complaints may have prominent nictitating membranes that do not require the veterinarian's assistance to bring them into view [5].

A prominent nictitans may indicate systemic illness or generalized unthriftiness [5]. In young patients, particularly kittens, visible nictitans have been linked to severe cases of gastrointestinal parasitism [5].

More often, the prominent nictitating membrane reflects ocular pain or irritation, as from a corneal ulcer [6] (see Figure 20.3).

Nictitating membranes may also be prominent if there is a foreign body in the orbit [5]. Plant material, especially seeds, can lodge beneath the nictitans, causing inflammation of the conjunctival lining. This may make the nictitans puffy enough to visualize on its own. Additional concerns regarding foreign bodies include the potential for corneal abrasion and ulceration [5].

20.2 Primary Clinical Presentations that Involve the Nictitans

In addition to the aforementioned scenarios, there are three primary presentations in clinical practice that involve the nictitans:

- Horner's syndrome [7–10]
- Prolapse of the nictitans [2, 4, 11–15]
- Neoplasia of the nictitans [16–20]

20.2.1 Horner's Syndrome

Recall that Horner's syndrome results from sympathetic denervation to the eye, and is characterized by miosis, ptosis, enophthalmos, and elevation of the nictitans [7, 10, 21, 22].

Refer to Chapter 18, Section 18.3.2 for additional details.

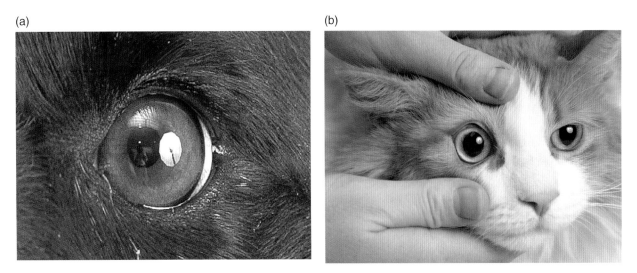

Figure 20.1 (a). Canine eye. Note that the nictitans is not apparent. It is hidden from view. *Source:* Courtesy of the Media Resources Department at Midwestern University. (b). Feline eyes during physical examination. Neither nictitans is visible. *Source:* Courtesy of the Media Resources Department at Midwestern University.

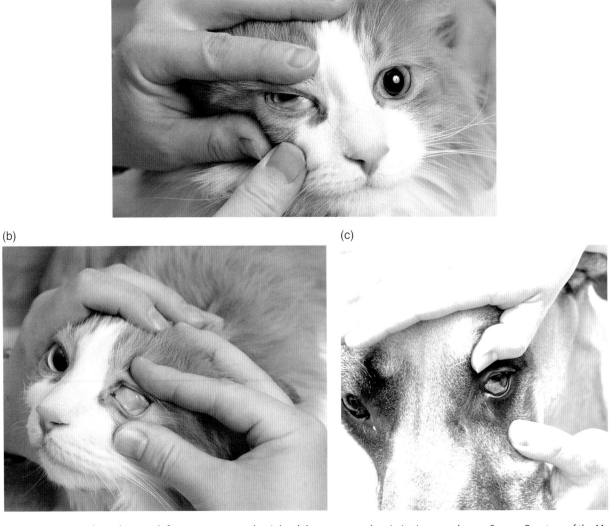

Figure 20.2 (a) Pushing down with firm pressure over the right globe to expose the nictitating membrane. *Source:* Courtesy of the Media Resources Department at Midwestern University. (b) The nictitating membrane associated with the left globe is now fully exposed. *Source:* Courtesy of the Media Resources Department at Midwestern University. (c). Evaluating the nictitans in a canine patient. *Source:* Courtesy of the Media Resources Department at Midwestern University.

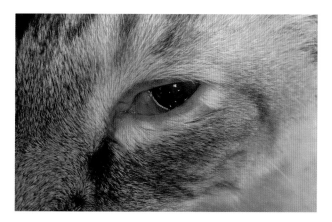

Figure 20.3 Prominent nictitans in a feline patient that has a corneal ulcer. In this case, the nictitans is elevated in response to ocular pain as a protective barrier between the external environment and the damaged cornea.

20.2.2 Prolapse of the Nictitans

The third eyelid can become dislodged from its normal resting position in the ventromedial orbit. This occurrence is known as a prolapse of the nictitans. Colloquially, this is referred to as "cherry eye" because the prolapsed gland looks like a cherry red mass bulging out from beneath the lower palpebra [1, 11, 23, 24] (see Figures 20.4a–d).

Although this prolapse can be initially transient, it frequently takes on a permanent abnormal position in which it is visible all the time. Over time, the smooth, shiny, moist surface of the nictitans dries out, and the gland may become secondarily infected [1, 11, 23].

The etiology is unknown [11]. However, certain canine breeds appear to be predisposed to this condition, including Cocker Spaniels, Boston Terriers, Pekingese, Beagles, Bassett Hounds, English Bulldogs, Lhasa Apsos, and Shih Tzus [13, 23–26]. Larger breeds that are over-represented include Great Danes, German Shepherds, Weimaraners, German Shorthaired Pointers, Irish Setters, and Newfoundland dogs [15, 27–31].

Patients with a breed predisposition often develop cherry eye as young adults. Frequently, they are less than two years of age at presentation [13, 24, 26].

One or both nictitating membranes may be involved. It is also possible that unilateral presentations will progress to bilateral ones [1, 11, 24].

Cats are less often afflicted [13, 14, 32–35]. Of the few cases that have been reported, the majority involve Burmese cats or kittens [12, 14, 34]. Isolated cases involving a British Blue, Persian, and Domestic Shorthaired cat also appear in the veterinary medical literature [12, 14].

Before the gland's role in tear film production was established, surgical correction of cherry eye classically involved excision of the gland. However, subsequent keratoconjunctivitis sicca (KCS) or "dry eye" was the most common sequelae. Since this association was made, surgical techniques have been revised to replace the gland to its normal anatomic position [13]. There is no one right method [13, 26, 32, 36–39]. One of the most commonly employed methods is the conjunctival pocket technique because the rate of postoperative recurrence is low [26].

Thermal cautery has recently been explored as an alternate approach [15]. The theory underlying this technique is that by reshaping the T-shaped hyaline cartilage, the nictitans may be more likely to drop back into its normal position [15]. Care must be taken not to inadvertently damage the gland associated with the third eyelid, or else KCS could still result [15].

20.2.3 Neoplastic Disease Involving the Nictitans

Neoplasia of the nictitans is uncommonly seen in companion animal practice [13, 16]. When it occurs, neoplastic disease at this location is typically malignant [13, 16, 40–43].

Older patients are most at risk [13].

Few studies explore breed predisposition to disease concerning neoplasia of the nictitans. However, a 2016 study by Dees et al. demonstrated greater frequency in mixed breed dogs, Labrador retrievers, Shih Tzus, Cocker Spaniels, Dachshunds, Beagles, and Golden Retrievers [17]. The same study reported more cases involving domestic short, medium, and longhaired breeds, Siamese, and Maine Coon cats [17].

In both dogs and cats, adenocarcinomas are most common [16, 42, 43]. These are much more concerning in the feline patient because they exhibit potential for metastatic disease, whereas in the dog, they tend to remain localized [16, 42, 43].

Other neoplasia that has been reported in dogs and cats include hemangiosarcoma, mast cell tumor, lymphoma, squamous cell carcinoma, hemangioma, fibrosarcoma, and malignant melanoma [17, 19, 44–51].

Because there is such variety in terms of tumor type, neoplasia of the nictitans does not have a classic appearance. However, in general, the neoplastic nictitans is more bulbous (see Figures 20.5a, b).

Neoplasia of the nictitans requires excision of the nictitating membrane as opposed to replacement of the gland within its anatomic pocket [13, 16, 17, 40, 41, 52].

Recurrence is possible, particularly because complete surgical removal of the nictitans is a challenge. It is difficult to obtain 5–10 mm of normal tissue margins [16]. Cryotherapy and/or radiation therapy may be indicated as adjunct therapy to reduce the risk of recurrence [16, 42, 53].

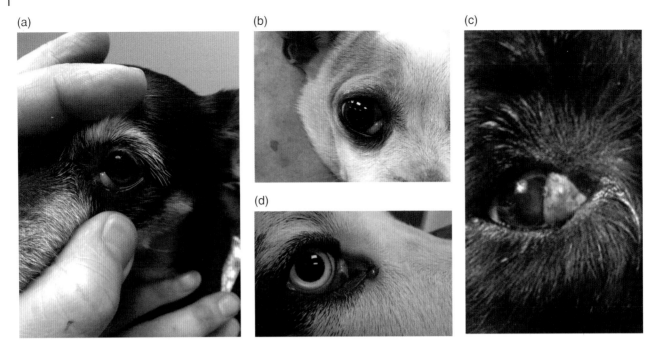

Figure 20.4 (a) Typical appearance of a prolapsed nictitans associated with the left eye (OS) of a canine patient. *Source:* Courtesy of the Frank Isom, DVM. (b) Typical appearance of a prolapsed nictitans associated with the right eye (OD) of a canine patient. *Source:* Courtesy of Samantha B. Thurman, DVM. (c). Prolapsed nictitans associated with the right eye (OD) of a canine patient. Note the appearance of the nictitans. It is dry due to chronic exposure. *Source:* Courtesy of Kathryn Knowles. (d) Everted T-shaped hyaline cartilage associated with the third eyelid. *Source:* Courtesy of Patricia Bennett, DVM.

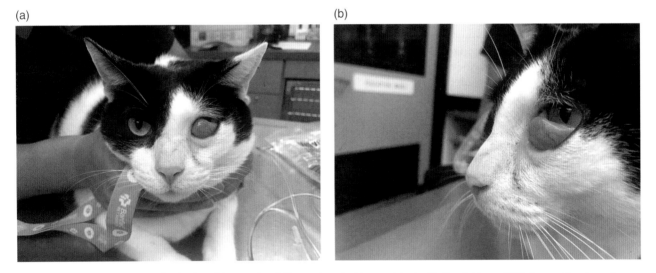

Figure 20.5 (a) Head-on view of a third eyelid tumor in a feline patient that is associated with the right eye (OD). *Source:* Courtesy of Brooke Wells Certa. (b) Side view of a third eyelid tumor in a feline patient. *Source:* Courtesy of Brooke Wells Certa.

References

1 Maggs, D.J. and Eyelid, T. (2013). *Slatter's Fundamentals of Veterinary Ophthalmology*, 5e (ed. D.J. Maggs, P.E. Miller, R. Ofri and D.H. Slatter), 151–156. St. Louis, Mo: Elsevier.

2 Brooks, D.E. (2005). Removal of the third eyelid. *NAVC Clinician's Brief* (January): 47–49.

3 Miller P. (2006). Why do cats have an inner eyelid as well as outer ones? Scientific American [Internet]: https://www.scientificamerican.com/article/why-do-cats-have-an-inner.

4 Gomez, J.B. (2012). Repairing nictitans gland prolapse in dogs. *Vet. Rec.* 171 (10): 244–245.

5 Englar, R.E. (2017). *Performing the Amall Animal Physical Examination*. Hoboken, NJ: Wiley.

6 Lim, C.C. (2015). *Small Animal Ophthalmic Atlas and Guide*, 1–168. Ames, Iowa: John Wiley & Sons, Inc.

7 Penderis, J. (2015). Diagnosis of Horner's syndrome in dogs and cats. *In Pract.* 37 (3).

8 Boydell, P. (1995). Horner's syndrome following cervical spinal surgery in the dog. *J. Small Anim. Pract.* 36 (11): 510–512.

9 Garosi, L.S., Dennis, R., Penderis, J. et al. (2001). Results of magnetic resonance imaging in dogs with vestibular disorders: 85 cases (1996–1999). *J. Am. Vet. Med. Assoc.* 218 (3): 385–391.

10 Heller HB, Bentley E. (2016). The Practitioner's Guide to Neurologic Causes of Canine Anisocoria. Today's Veterinary Practice [Internet]. (January/February): [77-83 pp.]. http://todaysveterinarypractice.navc.com/wp-content/uploads/2016/05/TVP_2016-0102_OO-Anisocoria.pdf.

11 Mazzucchelli, S., Vaillant, M.D., Weverberg, F. et al. (2012). Retrospective study of 155 cases of prolapse of the nictitating membrane gland in dogs. *Vet. Rec.* 170 (17): 443.

12 Williams, D., Middleton, S., and Caldwell, A. (2012). Everted third eyelid cartilage in a cat: a case report and literature review. *Vet. Ophthalmol.* 15 (2): 123–127.

13 Aquino, S.M. (2008). Surgery of the eyelids. *Top Companion Anim. Med.* 23 (1): 10–22.

14 Chahory, S., Crasta, M., Trio, S., and Clerc, B. (2004). Three cases of prolapse of the nictitans gland in cats. *Vet. Ophthalmol.* 7 (6): 417–419.

15 Allbaugh, R.A. and Stuhr, C.M. (2013). Thermal cautery of the canine third eyelid for treatment of cartilage eversion. *Vet. Ophthalmol.* 16 (5): 392–395.

16 Aquino, S.M. (2007). Management of eyelid neoplasms in the dog and cat. *Clin. Tech. Small Anim. Pract.* 22 (2): 46–54.

17 Dees, D.D., Schobert, C.S., Dubielzig, R.R., and Stein, T.J. (2016). Third eyelid gland neoplasms of dogs and cats: a retrospective histopathologic study of 145 cases. *Vet. Ophthalmol.* 19 (2): 138–143.

18 Galarza, R.M.R., Shrader, S.M., Koehler, J.W., and Abarca, E. (2016). A case of basal cell carcinoma of the nictitating membrane in a dog. *Clin. Case Rep.* 4 (12): 1161–1167.

19 Liapis, I.K. and Genovese, L. (2004). Hemangiosarcoma of the third eyelid in a dog. *Vet. Ophthalmol.* 7 (4): 279–282.

20 Wang, A.L. and Kern, T. (2015). Melanocytic ophthalmic neoplasms of the domestic veterinary species: a review. *Top. Companion Anim. Med.* 30 (4): 148–157.

21 Troxel, M. (2014). Horner syndrome at a glance. *Clinician's Brief* (May): 25.

22 Bagley, R.S. (2006). The cat with anisocoria or abnormally dilated or contricted pupils. In: *Problem-Based Feline Medicine. Edinburgh* (ed. J. Rand), 870–889. New York: Saunders.

23 Hendrix, D.V.H. (2007). Canine conjunctiva and nictitating membrane. In: *Veterinary Ophthalmology* (ed. K.S. Gelatt), 662–689. Blackwell Publishing.

24 Plummer, C.E., Kallberg, M.E., Gelatt, K.N. et al. (2008). Intranictitans tacking for replacement of prolapsed gland of the third eyelid in dogs. *Vet. Ophthalmol.* 11 (4): 228–233.

25 Dugan, S.J., Severin, G.A., Hungerford, L.L. et al. (1992). Clinical and histologic evaluation of the prolapsed third eyelid gland in dogs. *J. Am. Vet. Med. Assoc.* 201 (12): 1861–1867.

26 Morgan, R.V., Duddy, J.M., and Mcclurg, K. (1993). Prolapse of the gland of the 3rd-Eyelid in dogs – a retrospective study of 89 cases (1980 to 1990). *J. Am. Anim. Hosp. Assoc.* 29 (1): 56–60.

27 Martin, C.L. (1970). Everted membrana nictitans in German shorthaired pointers. *J. Am. Vet. Med. Assoc.* 157 (9): 1229–1232.

28 Moore, C.P. and Constantinescu, G.M. (1997). Surgery of the adnexa. *Vet. Clin. North Am. Small Anim. Pract.* 27 (5): 1011–1066.

29 Crispin, S. (1986). Treating the everted membrana nictitans in the dog. *In Pract.* 8 (2): 66–67.

30 Gelatt, K.N. (1972). Surgical correction of everted nictitating membrane in the dog. *Vet. Med. Small Anim. Clin.* 67 (3): 291–292.

31 Jensen, H.E. (1971). *Stereoscopic Atlas of Clinical Ophthalmology of Domestic Animals*, xi, 201 p. Saint Louis: Mosby.

32 Albert, R.A., Garrett, P.D., Whitley, R.D., and Thomas, K.L. (1982). Surgical correction of everted third eyelid in two cats. *J. Am. Vet. Med. Assoc.* 180 (7): 763–766.

33 Christmas, R. (1992). Surgical correction of congenital ocular and nasal dermoids and third eyelid gland prolapse in related Burmese kittens. *Can. Vet. J.* 33 (4): 265–266.

34 Koch, S.A. (1979). Congenital ophthalmic abnormalities in the Burmese cat. *J. Am. Vet. Med. Assoc.* 174 (1): 90–91.

35 Schoofs, S.H. (1999). Prolapse of the gland of the third eyelid in a cat: a case report and literature review. *J. Am. Anim. Hosp. Assoc.* 35 (3): 240–242.

36 Moore, C.P. (1983). Alternate technique for prolapsed gland of the third eyelid (replacement technique). In: *Current Techniques in Small Animal Surgery* (ed. M.J. Bojrab), 52–53. Philadelphia, P.A: Lea & Febiger.

37 Stanley, R.G. and Kaswan, R.L. (1994). Modification of the orbital rim Anchorage method for surgical replacement of the gland of the 3rd Eyelid in dogs. *J. Am. Vet. Med. Assoc.* 205 (10): 1412–1414.

38 Twitchell, M.J. (1984). Surgical repair of a prolapsed gland of the 3rd Eyelid in the dog. *Mod. Vet. Pract.* 65 (3): 223.

39 Kaswan, R.L. and Martin, C.L. (1985). Surgical-correction of 3rd Eyelid prolapse in dogs. *J. Am. Vet. Med. Assoc.* 186 (1): 83.

40 Gelatt, K.N. (1994). Surgery of the eyelids. In: *Small Animal Ophthalmic Surgery*, vol. 1 (ed. K.N. Gelatt and J.P. Gelatt), 60–125. Tarrytown, NY: Pergamon Veterinary Handbook Series.

41 Krohne, S. (2002). Ocular tumors of the dog and cat. In: *Cancer in Dogs and Cats: Medical and Surgical Management* (ed. W.B. Morrison), 701–726. Jackson, WY: Teton NewMedia.

42 Wilcock, B. and Peiffer, R. Jr. (1988). Adenocarcinoma of the gland of the third eyelid in seven dogs. *J. Am. Vet. Med. Assoc.* 193 (12): 1549–1550.

43 Komaromy, A.M., Ramsey, D.T., Render, J.A., and Clark, P. (1997). Primary adenocarcinoma of the gland of the nictitating membrane in a cat. *J. Am. Anim. Hosp. Assoc.* 33 (4): 333–336.

44 Roels, S. and Ducatelle, R. (1998). Malignant melanoma of the nictitating membrane in a cat (Felis vulgaris). *J. Comp. Pathol.* 119 (2): 189–193.

45 Buyukmihci, N. (1975). Fibrosarcoma of nictitating-membrane in a cat. *J. Am. Vet. Med. Assoc.* 167 (10): 934–935.

46 Peiffer, R.L. Jr., Duncan, J., and Terrell, T. (1978). Hemangioma of the nictitating membrane in a dog. *J. Am. Vet. Med. Assoc.* 172 (7): 832–833.

47 Larocca, R.D. (2000). Eosinophilic conjunctivitis, herpes virus and mast cell tumor of the third eyelid in a cat. *Vet. Ophthalmol.* 3 (4): 221–225.

48 Lavach, J.D. and Snyder, S.P. (1984). Squamous cell carcinoma of the third eyelid in a dog. *J. Am. Vet. Med. Assoc.* 184 (8): 975–976.

49 Hallstrom, M. (1970). Mastocytoma in the third eyelid of a dog. *J. Small Anim. Pract.* 11 (7): 469–472.

50 Multari, D., Vascellari, M., and Mutinelli, F. (2002). Hemangiosarcoma of the third eyelid in a cat. *Vet. Ophthalmol.* 5 (4): 273–276.

51 Williams, L.W., Gelatt, K.N., and Gwin, R.M. (1981). Ophthalmic neoplasms in the cat. *J. Am. Anim. Hosp. Assoc.* 17: 999–1008.

52 Willis, A.M. and Wilkie, D.A. (2001). Ocular oncology. *Clin. Tech. Small Anim. Pract.* 16 (1): 77–85.

53 Collins, B.K., Collier, R.R., and Miller, M.A. (1993). Biologic behavior and histologic characteristics of canine conjunctival melanoma. *Prog. Vet. Comp. Ophthalmol.* 3: 135–140.

21

Changes in Globe Position within the Orbit

21.1 Introduction to the Orbit as it Pertains to Normal Globe Position

The globe of the eye is essentially the eyeball. The canine and feline eyeballs are seated within incomplete bony orbits [1–3] (see Figures 21.1a, b).

Each orbit maintains isolation between the eye and the cranial vault [4]. Various foramina and fissures make vasculature and neuronal connections between the brain and the eye possible [4].

The skeletal aspects of the canine and feline orbit include the frontal, lacrimal, and zygomatic bones [1–3]. These bones provide structural support that is largely medial and ventral to the globe [1–3].

The orbital ligament provides the dorsolateral boundary of the orbit [1–3]. This ligament extends from the frontal process of the zygomatic bone to the zygomatic process of the frontal bone [4].

The remainder of the orbit consists of soft tissue structures, such as the periorbita [1, 4]. This layer of connective tissue encases the orbital contents, including the extraocular muscles [1, 4]. Between the periorbital and extraocular muscles, there is an orbital fat pad [4].

Additional support for the orbit is provided by the masticatory muscles [4]. Of these, the temporalis muscle surrounds the coronoid process of the mandible [1]. When the mouth opens, this action impinges on the periorbita [1]. In health, this does not cause pain. However, in diseased states, such as retrobulbar abscesses, it may become painful to open the jaw [1].

The canine and feline orbits have rostral positions within the skull, as compared to its position in grazers such as sheep and cattle [4]. This allows for greater binocular vision in dogs and cats [4].

Dogs and cats have a variety of skull shapes, including, for example [4–16]:

- Brachycephalic: a foreshortened skull in terms of length, such that the muzzle looks "pushed in"
- Mesocephalic: skull of intermediate length and width

- Dolichocephalic: skull that is markedly longer than it is wide (see Figures 21.2a–f)

Skull shape does not dramatically alter the size of the globe; however, it does impact where the globe sits within the orbit [1]. Dolichocephalic breeds have deeply seated globes as compared to brachycephalic breeds, the globes of which protrude [1]. Dogs and cats with protruding globes appear "bug-eyed" because their eyes protrude prominently beyond the orbital rim. Globe protrusion occurs because the orbits of brachycephalic breeds are appreciably shallow. This predisposes them to corneal injury [1].

21.2 Introduction to Abnormal Globe Position

In addition to breed-specific globe protrusion, there are two main clinical presentations that involve the abnormal positioning of one or both eyes:

- Enophthalmos
- Exophthalmos

21.2.1 Enophthalmos

Enophthalmos is a clinical presentation that is characterized by caudal displacement of the globe [17] (see Figures 21.3a, b).

Displacement of the globe in a caudal direction may occur if something rostral to the globe is encroaching upon the globe's space [17]. For example, a prominent nictitans may displace the globe caudally [17].

A prolapsed nictitans or a space-occupying mass may achieve the same effect (see Figures 21.4a–c).

Other potential etiologies for enophthalmos include the following [17, 18]:

- Ocular pain
- Dehydration
- Horner's syndrome

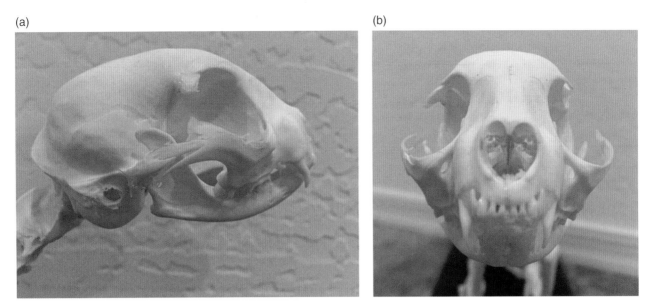

Figure 21.1 (a) Lateral aspect of a synthetic feline skull, demonstrating the incomplete bony orbit of the cat. (b) Head-on view of a synthetic feline skull, demonstrating the incomplete bony orbit of the cat.

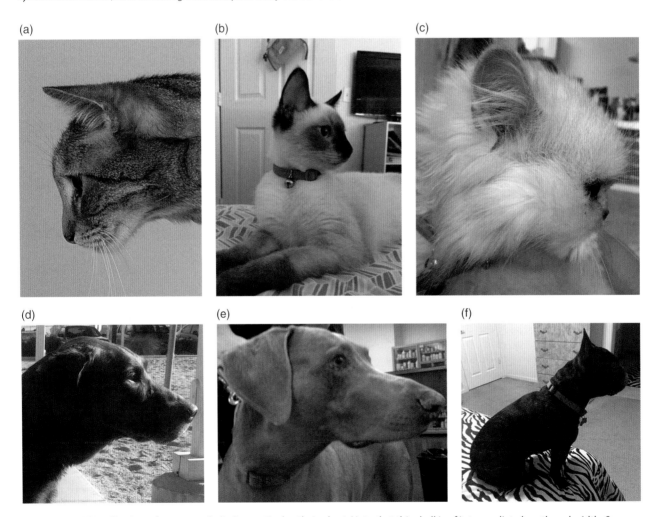

Figure 21.2 (a) Profile view of a mesocephalic Domestic shorthaired cat. Note that this skull is of intermediate length and width. *Source:* Courtesy of the Media Resources Department at Midwestern University. (b) Profile view of a dolichocephalic Siamese cat. Note that this skull is longer than it is wide. Other dolichocephalic cat breeds include the Abyssinian cat and the Balinese. *Source:* Courtesy of Nikalette Gros, Student Veterinarian 2019. (c) Profile view of a brachycephalic Persian cat. Note the foreshortened muzzle, which has a "pushed in" appearance. *Source:* Courtesy of Dr. Madison Skelton. (d) Profile view of a mesocephalic dog. Note that this skull is of intermediate length and width. *Source:* Courtesy of Jess Darmofal, DVM. (e) Profile view of a dolichocephalic Weimaraner. Note that this skull is longer than it is wide. Other dolichocephalic dog breeds include the Collie and the Greyhound. *Source:* Courtesy of Dr. Elizabeth Robbins. (f) Profile view of a brachycephalic French bulldog. Note the foreshortened muzzle, which has a "pushed in" appearance. Other brachycephalic dog breeds include the Pug and the Pekingese. *Source:* Courtesy of Cailin McElhenny.

(a) (b)

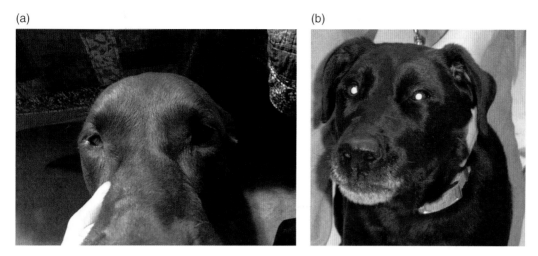

Figure 21.3 (a) The clinical appearance of enophthalmos associated with the right eye (OD) of a canine patient. Note how OD appears smaller. In this patient, the globe is not truly reduced in size. It has simply been displaced caudally. *Source:* Courtesy of Jess Darmofal, DVM. (b) The clinical appearance of enophthalmos in a canine patient with tetanus. Tetanus increases the retractor tone associated with the extraocular muscles, causing the globe to be pulled back into the socket. *Source:* Courtesy of Daniel Foy, MS, DVM, DACVIM, DACVECC.

(a) (b) (c)

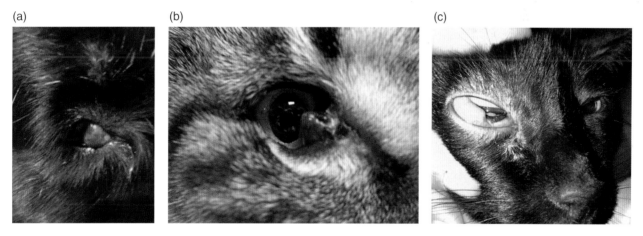

Figure 21.4 (a) Appreciate how this prolapsed nictitans or "cherry eye" has resulted in enophthalmos of the globe in this canine patient. *Source:* Courtesy of Kathryn Knowles. (b) Conjunctival mass associated with the right eye (OD) of a feline patient. The presence of this mass is causing enophthalmos of the globe. *Source:* Courtesy of Patricia Bennet, DVM. (c) Feline patient with epitheliotropic lymphoma. Note how the space-occupying lesion rostral to the right globe has resulted in caudal displacement of the globe. *Source:* Courtesy of Jill Macleese Barriteau, DVM.

- Collapse of the globe
- Orbital neoplasia [19]
- Reduced orbital volume
  - Loss of orbital fat
  - Extraocular muscle atrophy [20]
- Atrophy of the masticatory muscles
- Increased extraocular muscle retractor tone [18]
  - Tetanus
  - Strychnine poisoning
- Trauma sustained to the skull, as from a bite injury
  - Fracture of the zygomatic arch [21]

Retraction of the globe from ocular pain is common [22]. Many conditions can induce ocular pain, including keratitis and corneal ulceration, as from entropion.

Dehydration results in globe retraction only when severe. This is because there is a decrease in the volume of the globe, causing the globe to reduce in size. The smaller globe then settles deeper within the orbit. This creates a "sunken-in" appearance that is typical of enophthalmos.

Review Chapter 18, Section 18.3.2.4 to recall how Horner's syndrome, loss of sympathetic innervation to the orbit, results in enophthalmos [23].

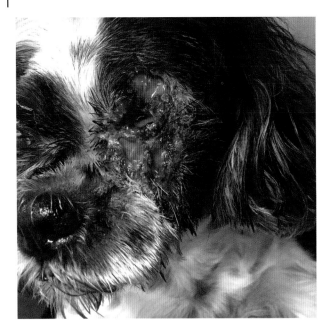

Figure 21.5 The patient depicted here had its eye washed out with hydrogen peroxide because the owner felt that the eye was infected. Contact dermatitis and keratitis resulted, with corneal ulceration. Although it is difficult to appreciate, this patient presented with subtle enophthalmos. This was likely due to ocular pain. *Source:* Courtesy of Stephanie Horwitz.

Because enophthalmos is typically the result of underlying disease, the diagnostic approach and/or treatment plan targets the primary problem. Consider, for example, a state of extreme dehydration. Restoring hydration will reverse enophthalmos.

Alternatively, consider the patient in Figure 21.5. This patient presented in a state of extreme ocular and periocular pain secondary to contact dermatitis and keratitis. Although this patient required extensive wound management, the provision of analgesia reduced the degree of enophthalmos while the patient was mending.

Consider a patient that presents with a space-occupying mass rostral to the globe. A diagnostic approach to this patient involves cytology at the least and ideally histopathologic examination of a biopsied specimen [17]. Identification of tumor type is critical to patient care and patient outcome. The tumor type dictates treatment recommendations. It also determines prognosis in terms of whether the lesion is expected to be locally invasive or metastasize.

Recall from Section 21.1 that dolichocephalic breeds have deeply seated globes [1]. Consider, for example, the Flat-Coated Retriever, the Collie, and the Rough Collie. These breeds are more likely to have conformational enophthalmos [24]. In these breeds, enophthalmos is not pathological; it is purely aesthetic. Cosmetic concerns may include the accumulation of mucoid ocular discharge or crusts at the palpebral fissure. The owner can manage these cosmetic issues quite readily by gently cleansing the eyelids daily with a moistened cloth.

21.2.2 Atraumatic Exophthalmos

Exophthalmos is a clinical presentation that is characterized by rostral displacement of the globe [17, 25].

Exophthalmos typically refers to atraumatic displacement as from space-occupying orbital disease [26–28].

Examples of space-occupying orbital disease that may result in exophthalmos include the following [17, 19, 25, 28–32]:

- Zygomatic salivary gland disease
- Infectious disease
- Orbital cellulitis
- Retrobulbar abscesses
- Myositis
- Retrobulbar tumors (see Figures 21.6a–f)

Patients with space-occupying orbital disease often present with decreased retropulsion [25, 33]. Retropulsion should be tested in every patient on every physical examination [34]. To test for retropulsion, the clinician applies even, firm pressure to the globe through closed eyelids [34]. The normal globe has some "give," meaning that it can be displaced ever so gently into the orbit via gentle ballottement [34]. Displacement occurs because there is nothing to obstruct the globe's caudally directed movement within the orbit [34]. As soon as the clinician lets up on the pressure, the globe "bounces" back to its normal anatomic position [34].

However, when there is a space-occupying orbital lesion, the globe's path is obstructed [34]. The globe cannot be gently displaced to a caudal position within the orbit because the mass blocks its path [34]. There will be palpable resistance to retropulsion [34].

Patients with space-occupying orbital lesions may also experience pain when the mouth is opened [25]. Owners may report a reduced appetite. This could be due to pain associated with chewing [25].

Finally, patients with space-occupying orbital lesions may develop strabismus, that is, the appearance of being cross-eyed [25]. Strabismus results if the lesions create pressure in such a way as a cause deviation of one or both globes [25, 31].

21.2.2.1 Zygomatic Salivary Gland Disease
The zygomatic salivary gland is adjacent to the orbit. Specifically, the zygomatic salivary gland contributes to the ventral border of the orbit, along with the medial pterygoid muscle [1–3]. Because of the close proximity of the zygomatic salivary gland to the orbit, any disease of this gland can result in orbital pain and swelling [17].

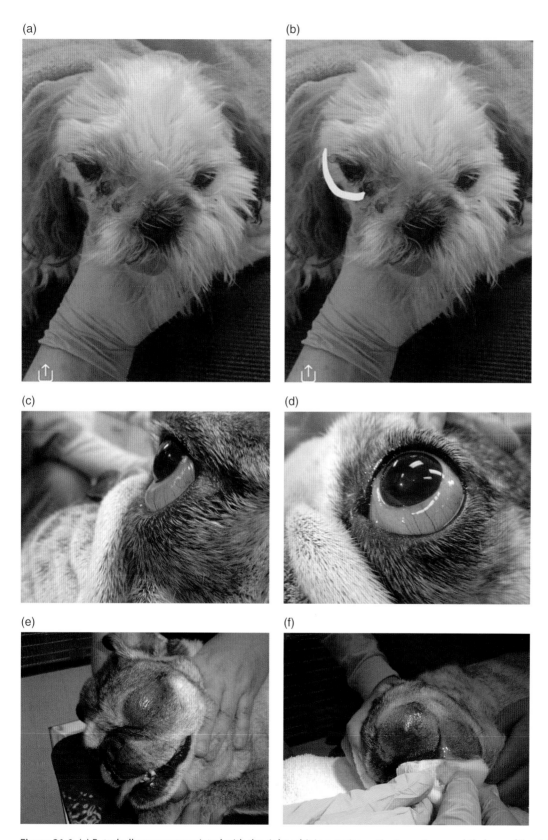

Figure 21.6 (a) Retrobulbar mass associated with the right orbit in a canine patient, causing exophthalmos of the right globe (OD). *Source:* Courtesy of Patricia Bennett, DVM. (b) Same patient as in Figure 21.6a, with yellow highlighting to emphasize the presenting complaint, exophthalmos. *Source:* Courtesy of Patricia Bennett, DVM. (c) Canine patient with scleral edema and a presumptive retrobulbar mass, causing subtle exophthalmos of the left globe (OS). *Source:* Courtesy of Jackie Kucskar, DVM. (d) Same patient as in Figure 21.6d, from a different angle to appreciate the subtle exophthalmos that is associated with OS. *Source:* Courtesy of Jackie Kucskar, DVM. (e) Left-sided orbital abscess in a canine patient that had previously undergone enucleation of the left globe (OS). *Source:* Courtesy of Daniel Foy, MS, DVM, DACVIM, DACVECC. (f) Same patient as in Figure 21.6e, from a different angle. *Source:* Courtesy of Daniel Foy, MS, DVM, DACVIM, DACVECC.

Zygomatic salivary gland disease is uncommon in both dogs and cats, and includes the following [25]:

- Salivary mucoceles
- Sialadenitis
- Salivary gland neoplasia

Salivary mucoceles are benign, cystic lesions in which mucoid saliva accumulates [27, 33, 35]. Salivary mucoceles develop in submucosal or subcutaneous tissues following inflammation or rupture of either the salivary gland capsule or duct. Salivary mucoceles are typically slow-growing as the reservoir of saliva builds. They are soft and fluctuant [27]. Affected patients may have mucosal swelling at the level of the maxillary molars on oral examination [27]. This occurs because the zygomatic salivary gland has one or more ducts that empty out opposite the first maxillary molar [3, 25]. In addition, the affected globe may deviate dorsally because of the ventral anatomic position of the zygomatic salivary gland relative to the globe. In most cases, surgical excision of the salivary mucocele is indicated [27].

Sialadenitis refers to inflammation of the salivary gland and is relatively uncommon in companion animal medicine [33, 36, 37]. It is more often identified during necropsy as an incidental finding than on physical examination as a presenting complaint. Inflammation of the salivary gland may result from immune-mediated disease or infection secondary to oral foreign bodies [33, 36]. It could potentially lead to the development of a salivary mucocele [38].

Salivary gland neoplasia is uncommonly seen in dogs and cats [25, 33]. When it occurs, carcinomas and adenocarcinomas are most likely [25]. Both are locally invasive and may metastasize [25]. As can be imagined, wide, clean surgical margins are difficult to obtain [25]. As a result, surgical excision is rarely curative. Adjunct therapy, such as radiation therapy, is indicated [25, 33].

21.2.2.2 Infectious Disease, Orbital Cellulitis, and Retrobulbar Abscess

Exophthalmos may occur secondary to orbital inflammation and/or infectious disease. Orbital cellulitis and/or retrobulbar abscesses may result from the following [25, 39–48]:

- Oropharyngeal trauma, as from the migration of wooden stick foreign bodies through the oral mucosa and/or palate [47, 48]
- Abscessation of maxillary molar(s)
- Spread of infection via the bloodstream and/or salivary gland
- Infection extending through the nasal cavity, sinuses, and/or bone

Several species of aerobic and anaerobic bacteria have been implicated, and mixed infections are common [25].

Staphylococcus, Escherichia, Pasteurella, Bacteroides, and *Clostridium* are frequent isolates [49].

Although bacterial infections are most common, fungi have also been isolated from retrobulbar abscesses, including *Aspergillus, Penicillium, Pythium,* and *Cryptococcus* [25, 40, 50–53].

As compared to zygomatic salivary gland disease, cases involving orbital cellulitis and/or retrobulbar abscesses tend to present more acutely [40]. Whereas salivary gland disease causes a slow progression of clinical signs, orbital cellulitis and retrobulbar abscesses are rapid in onset [40]. Patients are quick to develop pain upon opening of the mouth [40]. Owners often report reluctance to eat [54]. Prehension of food is painful. In addition, patients may become systemically ill [40, 54]. They may develop a fever and present for generalized malaise [40, 54].

When possible, retrobulbar abscesses may be lanced and flushed through the mouth, caudal to the last maxillary molar of the affected side [49, 55].

Systemic antibiotic and/or antifungal therapy is also indicated in cases involving retrobulbar abscess [25]. Although most bacterial infections will respond to cephalosporins, extended, spectrum penicillins, potentiated penicillins, and carbapenems, culture and susceptibility testing should guide the drug of choice [25, 49].

Occasionally, retrobulbar abscesses may be refractory to treatment [56]. This is likely due to the difficulty of accessing the retrobulbar space. Such circumstances require a more aggressive surgical approach than straightforward lancing and flushing via the oral cavity. Modified lateral orbitotomy may need to be performed, with or without a zygomatic osteotomy, to improve exposure [56].

21.2.2.3 Myositis

Myositis that results in exophthalmos may involve the muscles of mastication or the extraocular muscles [17, 57, 58].

Masticatory myositis is an immune-mediated condition that involves the temporalis, masseter, and pterygoideus muscles [57, 58]. It results in trismus, the inability to open the jaw [58, 59]. This may persist, even under anesthesia [58, 60, 61].

Masticatory myositis is a painful condition [59].

In acute phases of disease, patients may present with swelling associated with the muscles of mastication [59]. As the disease progresses and the jaw is underutilized, these muscles experience progressive atrophy [59].

Young-to-middle-aged German shepherds, Weimaraners, Doberman Pinschers, Golden Retrievers, and Labrador Retrievers are predisposed [57, 62].

Affected individuals develop autoantibodies against type II muscle fibers [59]. These can be detected via the 2M antibody blood test [59, 63]. In the acute phase of disease, a blood chemistry profile may also display an elevated level of creatine kinase (CK) [59]. As the disease progresses, CK values tend to normalize [59]. Therefore, a normal CK does not rule out a diagnosis of masticatory myositis [59].

Equivocal 2M antibody blood test results can be followed up with a biopsy of the temporalis or masseter muscle [63]. Histopathologic findings that are supportive of a diagnosis of masticatory myositis include atrophy and fibrosis of the muscle, as well as lymphocytic-plasmacytic cellular infiltrates [59, 63].

Treatment requires immunosuppressive doses of prednisone or an alternate immunosuppressive agent [59]. However, it is not uncommon for patients to relapse [59].

Extraocular myositis is rarely seen in companion animal practice [64]. A retrospective case analysis by Williams in 2008 evaluated 37 dogs, all of which presented for bilateral exophthalmos [64]. Many of these patients had a unique appearance that stemmed from prominent sclera [64]. This so-called "scleral show" made patients appear spooked, startled, or surprised [64]. Although scleral prominence was diffuse in some cases, most patients presented with either dorsally or ventrally prominent sclera [64].

Some, but not all of the patients, had concurrent chemosis and/or strabismus [64].

Over 50% of affected patients were Golden Retrievers, and 13.5% were Labrador Retrievers or Labrador crosses [64]. Most patients were young and female [64].

The clinical appearance of these patients is sufficient to make a presumptive diagnosis [64]. Rarely is histopathologic evaluation performed in suspects [64]. When it is, it mirrors those findings associated with masticatory myositis [64]. Medical management is also similar. Azathioprine has been used in lieu of prednisone in some cases [64].

21.2.2.4 Retrobulbar Tumors

Retrobulbar tumors are uncommon in dogs and cats [32, 65]. They may be primary or secondary, resulting from metastatic disease [65].

When they occur, retrobulbar tumors are immensely varied in terms of tumor type because any type of orbital tissue can be the source of the tumor [65].

The most commonly reported retrobulbar tumors include the following [32, 41, 65–79]:

- Meningiomas
- Nerve sheath tumors
- Fibromas
- Fibrosarcomas
- Lymphomas
- Mast cell tumors
- Osteosarcomas
- Osteochondrosarcomas
- Squamous cell carcinomas

Few retrospective studies appear in the veterinary medical literature, making it difficult to make generalizations about the epidemiological data [32, 65, 80, 81]. However, large breed dogs may be overrepresented [65].

Patients with retrobulbar tumors tend to present for unilateral exophthalmos [65]. In addition, the affected eye may develop lagophthalmos. This means that even during blinking, the eyelids of the affected eye cannot close over the entire cornea [17]. This predisposes patients to exposure keratitis secondary to corneal dessication [65].

Patients may be misdiagnosed as having glaucoma because exophthalmos and buphthalmos carry a similar appearance [26, 65]. However, exophthalmos and buphthalmos are distinct presentations [26].

The globe in a patient with exophthalmos is of the expected size [26]. It has simply been pushed forward in the orbit [26]. By contrast, the globe in a patient with buphthalmos is seated in its normal anatomic position; however, the buphthalmic globe is enlarged [26] (see Figure 21.7).

Imaging is typically required for patients with presumptive retrobulbar tumors [65]. Radiographs may be taken of the skull to evaluate for aggressive bony lesions [65]. Skull radiographs may also detect involvement of the sinuses, nasal cavity, and/or tooth roots [27].

However, there are limits to what skull radiography can discern [27, 28]. In a retrospective study by Attali-Soussay et al., four cases were identified in which advanced imaging was required [65].

Advanced imaging may involve ocular ultrasonography or computed tomography (CT) [28, 65]. CT scans of

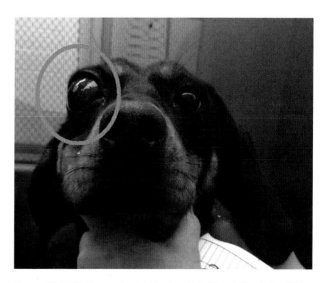

Figure 21.7 Canine patient with a buphthalmic right globe (OD) secondary to glaucoma. *Source:* Courtesy of Tradel Harris, DVM.

(a)

(b)

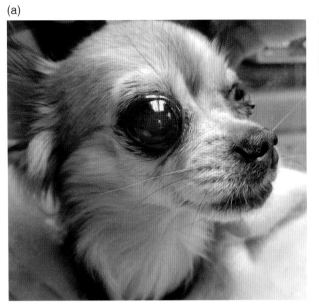
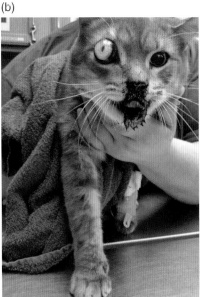

Figure 21.8 (a) Clinical appearance of a proptosed globe in a canine patient. *Source:* Courtesy of Kelli L. Crisfulli, RVT. (b) The clinical appearance of a proptosed globe in a feline patient. This patient was a hit by a car. *Source:* Courtesy of Kelli L. Crisfulli, RVT.

the skull are able to capture the orbit in exquisite detail [28]. Although expense, equipment availability, and the need for the patient to be in an anesthetic plane are limiting factors, CT scans provide important data regarding the extent of the retrobulbar mass and its relationship to other important structures [28]. CT also facilitates surgical planning [17, 28]. In addition to advanced imaging of the skull, survey films of the chest are also important to rule out pulmonary metastases [65].

The retrobulbar tumor may be debulked surgically via a lateral approach to the orbit as a palliative, globe-sparing measure [17]. Alternatively, the patient may undergo exenteration, in which all orbital contents, including the globe, are excised [17]. Given the limitations based upon location of the mass, the need for adjunct therapy in the form of radiation or chemotherapy is likely [17].

21.2.3 Traumatic Exophthalmos

Trauma may also force the globe to be displaced rostrally, without concurrent space-occupying orbital disease.

Consider, for example, fractures of the bony orbit or traumatic proptosis of the globe (see Figures 21.8a, b).

Proptosis is visually impressive and unmistakable. There is also usually a history of known trauma, such as an automobile accident or a bite injury [82].

Overaggressive restraint may also result in proptosis in brachycephalic canine breeds due to their shallow orbits [83]. By contrast, traumatic proptosis is much less likely to occur in cats because their orbits are deep [82, 84]. When traumatic proptosis occurs in the feline patient, the degree of tissue damage is significant [82].

Refer to Chapter 15, Section 15.5 and Chapter 16, Section 16.2.1 to recall other clinical signs that may result from proptosis.

Proptosed globes may be returned to the orbit through surgical manipulation; however, vision may or may not return, depending upon the degree to which the optic nerve was stretched [83]. For this reason, many patients undergo enucleation [83].

References

1 Dyce, K.M., Sack, W.O., and Wensing, C.J.G. (2010). *Textbook of Veterinary Anatomy*, 4e, xii, 834 p. St. Louis, Mo: Saunders/Elsevier.

2 Evans, H.E. and DeLahunta, A. (2004). *Guide to the Dissection of the Dog*, 6e, xiv, 378 p. St. Louis, Mo: Saunders.

3 Evans, H.E. and Miller, M.E. (2013). *Miller's Anatomy of the Dog*, 4e, xix, 850 p. St. Louis, Missouri: Elsevier.

4 Sisson, S., Grossman, J.D., and Getty, R. (1975). *Sisson and Grossman's: The Anatomy of the Domestic Animals*, 5e. Philadelphia: Saunders.

5 Holmstrom, S.E. and Holmstrom, S.E. (2013). *Veterinary Dentistry: A Team Approach*, 2e, viii, 434 p. St. Louis, Mo: Elsevier/Mosby.

6 Kunzel, W., Breit, S., and Oppel, M. (2003). Morphometric investigations of breed-specific features in feline skulls and considerations on their functional implications. *Anat. Histol. Embryol.* 32 (4): 218–223.

7 Christiansen, P. (2008). Evolution of skull and mandible shape in cats (Carnivora: Felidae). *PLoS One* 3 (7): e2807.

8 Biknevicius, A.R. and Van Valkenburgh, B. (1996). Design for killing: craniodental adaptations of predators. In: *Carnivore Behavior, Ecology, and Evolution*, vol. 2 (ed. J.L. Gittleman), 393–428. New York: Cornell University Press.

9 Christiansen, P. and Wroe, S. (2007). Bite forces and evolutionary adaptations to feeding ecology in carnivores. *Ecology* 88 (2): 347–358.

10 Monfared, A.L. (2013). Anatomy of the Persian cat's skull and its clinical value during regional anesthesia. *Global Vet.* 10 (5): 551–555.

11 Schoenebeck, J.J. and Ostrander, E.A. (2013). The genetics of canine skull shape variation. *Genetics* 193 (2): 317–325.

12 McGreevy, P., Grassi, T.D., and Harman, A.M. (2004). A strong correlation exists between the distribution of retinal ganglion cells and nose length in the dog. *Brain Behav. Evol.* 63 (1): 13–22.

13 Coppinger, R. and Schneider, R. (1995). Evolution of working dogs. In: *The Domestic Dog: Its Evolution, Behaviour, and Interactions with People* (ed. J. Serpell), 21–50. Cambridge; New York: Cambridge University Press.

14 Haworth, K.E., Islam, I., Breen, M. et al. (2001). Canine TCOF1; cloning, chromosome assignment and genetic analysis in dogs with different head types. *Mamm. Genome* 12 (8): 622–629.

15 Wayne, R.K. (1986). Cranial morphology of domestic and wild canids – the influence of development on morphological change. *Evolution* 40 (2): 243–261.

16 Young, A. and Bannasch, D. (2006). Morphological variation in the dog. In: *The Dog and Its Genome* (ed. E.A. Ostrander, U. Giger and K. Lindblad-Toh), 47–65. Cold Spring Harbor, NY: Cold Spring Harbor Laboratory Press.

17 Tilley, L.P., FWK, S., and Tilley, L.P. (eds.) (2007). Orbital diseases. In: *Blackwell's Five-Minute Veterinary Consult: Canine and Feline*, 4e, 940–941. Ames, Iowa: Blackwell.

18 Martin, C.L. (2009). *Ophthalmic Disease in Veterinary Medicine*. Boca Raton, FL: Taylor & Francis Group, LLC.

19 Pentlarge, V.W., Powell-Johnson, G., Martin, C.L. et al. (1989). Orbital neoplasia with enophthalmos in a cat. *J. Am. Vet. Med. Assoc.* 195 (9): 1249–1251.

20 Tilley, L.P. and Smith, F.W.K. (eds.) (2004). Entropion. In: *The 5-Minute Veterinary Consult: Canine and Feline*, 406–407. Philadelphia: Lippincott Williams & Wilkins.

21 Konrade, K.A., Clode, A.B., Michau, T.M. et al. (2009). Surgical correction of severe strabismus and enophthalmos secondary to zygomatic arch fracture in a dog. *Vet. Ophthalmol.* 12 (2): 119–124.

22 Slatter, D.H. (1995). *Pocket Companion to Textbook of Small Animal Surgery*, xxiii, 914 p. Philadelphia: Saunders.

23 Penderis, J. (2015). Diagnosis of Horner's syndrome in dogs and cats. *In Pract.* 37 (3).

24 Barnett, K.C. (1990). *Color Atlas of Veterinary Ophthalmology*. Baltimore: Williams & Wilkins. 184 p.

25 Betbeze, C. (2015). Management of orbital diseases. *Top. Companion Anim. Med.* 30 (3): 107–117.

26 Ofri, R. (2014). Differentiating exophthalmos, buphthalmos, & proptosis. *NAVC Clinician's Brief* (May): 29–31.

27 McDonald, J. and Knollinger, A. (2016). Diagnosing canine exophthalmos. *NAVC Clinician's Brief* (May): 75–78.

28 Boroffka, S.A.E.B. (1996). Exophthalmos in dogs: a challenge for diagnostic imaging. *Vet. Q.* 18: S56.

29 Caruso, K., Marrion, R., and Silver, G. (2002). What is your diagnosis? – MRI diagnosis – Retrobulbar mass indenting the inferior aspect of the right globe. The mass involved the optic nerve but did not appear to invade the cranial vault; the inferior aspect of the mass was less defined. *J. Am. Vet. Med. Assoc.* 221 (11): 1553–1554.

30 Haak, C.E., Breshears, M.A., and Lackner, P.A. (2007). What is your diagnosis? *J. Am. Vet. Med. Assoc.* 231 (6): 863–864.

31 van der Woerdt, A. (2008). Orbital inflammatory disease and pseudotumor in dogs and cats. *Vet. Clin. North Am. Small* 38 (2): 389–401.

32 Gilger, B.C., McLaughlin, S.A., Whitley, R.D., and Wright, J.C. (1992). Orbital neoplasms in cats: 21 cases (1974–1990). *J. Am. Vet. Med. Assoc.* 201 (7): 1083–1086.

33 Boland, L., Gomes, E., Payen, G. et al. (2013). Zygomatic salivary gland diseases in the dog: three cases diagnosed by MRI. *J. Am. Anim. Hosp. Assoc.* 49 (5): 333–337.

34 Englar, R.E. (2017). *Performing the Small Animal Physical Examination*. Hoboken, NJ: Wiley.

35 Bellenger, C.R. and Simpson, D.J. (1992). Canine sialocoeles – 60 clinical cases. *J. Small Anim. Pract.* 33 (8): 376–380.

36 Simison, W.G. (1993). Sialadenitis associated with periorbital disease in a dog. *J. Am. Vet. Med. Assoc.* 202 (12): 1983–1985.

37 Cannon, M.S., Paglia, D., Zwingenberger, A.L. et al. (2011). Clinical and diagnostic imaging findings in dogs with zygomatic sialadenitis: 11 cases (1990–2009). *J. Am. Vet. Med. Assoc.* 239 (9): 1211–1218.

38 Spangler, W.L. and Culbertson, M.R. (1991). Salivary gland disease in dogs and cats: 245 cases (1985–1988). *J. Am. Vet. Med. Assoc.* 198 (3): 465–469.

39 Halenda, R.M. and Reed, A.L. (1997). Ultrasound computed tomography diagnosis – Fungal, sinusitis and retrobulbar myofascitis in a cat. *Vet. Radiol. Ultrasoun.* 38 (3): 208–210.

40 Hamilton, H.L., Whitley, R.D., and McLaughlin, S.A. (2000). Exophthalmos secondary to aspergillosis in a cat. *J. Am. Anim. Hosp. Assoc.* 36 (4): 343–347.

41 Grahn, B.H., Szentimrey, D., Battison, A., and Hertling, R. (1995). Exophthalmos associated with frontal-sinus osteomyelitis in a puppy. *J. Am. Anim. Hosp. Assoc.* 31 (5): 397–401.

42 Kraijer-Huver, I.M.G., ter Haar, G., Djajadiningrat-Laanen, S.C., and Boeve, M.H. (2009). Peri- and retrobulbar abscess caused by chronic otitis externa, media and interna in a dog. *Vet Rec.* 165 (7): 209–211.

43 Tovar, M.C., Huguet, E., and Gomezi, M.A. (2005). Orbital cellulitis and intraocular abscess caused by migrating grass in a cat. *Vet. Ophthalmol.* 8 (5): 353–356.

44 Spiess, B.M. and Pot, S.A. (2013). Diseases and surgery of the canine orbit. In: *Veterinary Ophthalmology* (ed. K.N. Gelatt, B.C. Gilger and T.J. Kern), 793–831. Oxford: Wiley-Blackwell.

45 Ramsey, D.T., Marretta, S.M., Hamor, R.E. et al. (1996). Ophthalmic manifestations and complications of dental disease in dogs and cats. *J. Am. Anim. Hosp. Assoc.* 32 (3): 215–224.

46 Collins, B.K., Moore, C.P., Dubielzig, R.R., and Gengler, W.R. (1991). Anaerobic orbital cellulitis and septicemia in a dog. *Can. Vet. J.* 32 (11): 683–685.

47 O'Reilly, A., Beck, C., Mouatt, J.G., and Stenner, V.J. (2002). Exophthalmos due to a wooden foreign body in a dog. *Aust. Vet. J.* 80 (5): 268–271.

48 Hartley, C., McConnell, J.F., and Doust, R. (2007). Wooden orbital foreign body in a Weimaraner. *Vet. Ophthalmol.* 10 (6): 390–393.

49 Wang, A.L., Ledbetter, E.C., and Kern, T.J. (2009). Orbital abscess bacterial isolates and in vitro antimicrobial susceptibility patterns in dogs and cats. *Vet. Ophthalmol.* 12 (2): 91–96.

50 Wilkinson, G.T., Sutton, R.H., and Grono, L.R. (1982). Aspergillus Spp infection associated with orbital cellulitis and sinusitis in a cat. *J. Small Anim. Pract.* 23 (3): 127–131.

51 Peiffer, R.L., Belkin, P.V., and Janke, B.H. (1980). Orbital cellulitis, sinusitis, and pneumonitis caused by Penicillium Sp in a cat. *J. Am. Vet. Med. Assoc.* 176 (5): 449–451.

52 Gerds-Grogan, S. and Dayrell-Hart, B. (1997). Feline cryptococcosis: a retrospective evaluation. *J. Am. Anim. Hosp. Assoc.* 33 (2): 118–122.

53 Bissonnette, K.W., Sharp, N.J.H., Dykstra, M.H. et al. (1991). Nasal and retrobulbar mass in a cat caused by Pythium-insidiosum. *J. Med. Vet. Mycol.* 29 (1): 39–44.

54 Mccalla, T.L. and Moore, C.P. (1989). Exophthalmos in dogs and cats. Part II. *Compend. Cont. Educ. Pract.* 11 (8): 911–926.

55 Westermeyer, H.D. and Hendrix, D.V.H. (2012). Basic ophthalmic surgical procedures. In: *Veterinary Surgery Small Animal* (ed. K.M. Tobias and S.A. Johnston), 2116. Philadelphia, PA: Saunders Elsevier.

56 Tremolada, G., Milovancev, M., Culp, W.T.N., and Bleedorn, J.A. (2015). Surgical management of canine refractory retrobulbar abscesses: six cases. *J. Small Anim. Pract.* 56 (11): 667–670.

57 Morgan, R.V. (2008). *Handbook of Small Animal Practice*, 5e, xx, 1378 p. St. Louis, Mo: Saunders/Elsevier.

58 Czerwinski, S.L., Plummer, C.E., Greenberg, S.M. et al. (2015). Dynamic exophthalmos and lateral strabismus in a dog caused by masticatory muscle myositis. *Vet. Ophthalmol.* 18 (6): 515–520.

59 Purina Pro-Club. (2014). Early Diagnosis of Masticatory Muscle Myositis Is Needed for Treatment Success. Purina Pro-Club Updates [Internet]: https://www.purinaproclub.com/resource-library/pro-club-updates/early-diagnosis-of-masticatory-muscle-myositis-is-needed-for-treatment-success.

60 Shelton, G.D. (2007). From dog to man: the broad spectrum of inflammatory myopathies. *Neuromuscul. Disord.* 17 (9–10): 663–670.

61 Shelton, G.D., Cardinet, G.H. 3rd, and Bandman, E. (1987). Canine masticatory muscle disorders: a study of 29 cases. *Muscle Nerve* 10 (8): 753–766.

62 Thompson, M.S. (2014). *Small Animal Medical Differential Diagnosis: A Book of Lists*, 2e, xvi, 360 p. St. Louis, Missouri: Elsevier/Saunders.

63 Lorenz, M.D., Kornegay, J.N., and Oliver, J.E. (2004). *Handbook of Veterinary Neurology*, 4e, xi, 468 p. Philadelphia, PA: Saunders.

64 Williams, D.L. (2008). Extraocular myositis in the dog. *Vet. Clin. North Am. Small* 38 (2): 347–359.

65 Attali-Soussay, K., Jegou, J.P., and Clerc, B. (2001). Retrobulbar tumors in dogs and cats: 25 cases. *Vet. Ophthalmol.* 4 (1): 19–27.

66 Nerschbach, V., Eule, J.C., Eberle, N. et al. (2016). Ocular manifestation of lymphoma in newly diagnosed cats. *Vet. Comp. Oncol.* 14 (1): 58–66.

67 Mauldin, E.A., Deehr, A.J., Hertzke, D., and Dubielzig, R.R. (2000). Canine orbital meningiomas: a review of 22 cases. *Vet. Ophthalmol.* 3 (1): 11–16.

68 Dennis, R. (2008). Imaging features of orbital myxosarcoma in dogs. *Vet. Radiol. Ultrasoun.* 49 (3): 256–263.

69 Ralic, M., Vasic, J., Jovanovic, M., and Cameron, B. (2014). Retrobulbar chondrosarcoma in a dog. *Open Vet. J.* 4 (1): 51–55.

70 Barnett, K.C. and Grimes, T.D. (1972). Retrobulbar tumor and retinal-detachment in a dog. *J. Small Anim. Pract.* 13 (6): 315–319.

71 Barnett, K.C., Kelly, D.F., and Singleton, W.B. (1967). Retrobulbar and chiasmal meningioma in a dog. *J. Small Anim. Pract.* 8 (7): 391–394.

72 Abrams, K. and Toal, R.L. (1990). What is your diagnosis – Here is the diagnosis. *J. Am. Vet. Med. Assoc.* 196 (6): 951–952.

73 Buyukmihci, N. (1977). Orbital meningioma with intraocular invasion in a dog. Histology and ultrastructure. *Vet. Pathol.* 14 (5): 521–523.

74 Cottrill, N.B., Carter, J.D., Pechman, R.D. et al. (1987). Bilateral orbital parosteal osteoma in a cat. *J. Am. Anim. Hosp. Assoc.* 23 (4): 405–408.

75 McCalla, T.L., Moore, C.P., Turk, J. et al. (1989). Multilobular osteosarcoma of the mandible and orbit in a dog. *Vet. Pathol.* 26 (1): 92–94.

76 Groff, J.M., Murphy, C.J., Pool, R.R. et al. (1992). Orbital multilobular tumor of bone in a dog. *J. Small Anim. Pract.* 33 (12): 597–600.

77 Hayden, D.W. (1976). Squamous-cell carcinoma in a cat with intraocular and orbital metastases. *Vet. Pathol.* 13 (5): 332–336.

78 Knecht, C.D. and Greene, J.A. (1977). Osteoma of zygomatic arch in a cat. *J. Am. Vet. Med. Assoc.* 171 (10): 1077–1078.

79 Langham, R.F., Bennett, R.R., and Zydeck, F.A. (1971). Primary retrobulbar meningioma of the optic nerve of a dog. *J. Am. Vet. Med. Assoc.* 159 (2): 175–176.

80 Kern, T.J. (1985). Orbital neoplasia in 23 dogs. *J. Am. Vet. Med. Assoc.* 186 (5): 489–491.

81 Ruhli, M.B. and Spiess, B.M. (1995). Retrobulbar space-occupying lesions in dogs and cats: symptoms and diagnosis. *Tierarztl. Prax.* 23 (3): 306–312.

82 Gilger, B.C., Hamilton, H.L., Wilkie, D.A. et al. (1995). Traumatic ocular proptoses in dogs and cats: 84 cases (1980–1993). *J. Am. Vet. Med. Assoc.* 206 (8): 1186–1190.

83 Kennard G. (2009). Ocular emergencies: Presenting signs, initial exam and treatment (Proceedings). DVM360 [Internet]: http://veterinarycalendar. dvm360.com/ocular-emergencies-presenting-signs-initial-exam-and-treatment-proceedings.

84 Nasisse, M.P. (1991). Feline ophthalmology. In: *Veterinary Ophthalmology* (ed. K.N. Gelatt), 529–575. Philadelphia: Lea & Febiger.

22

Changes in Globe Size

22.1 Introduction to Globe Size

The canine and feline globe is sized to fit within an incomplete bony orbit for protection from the external environment [1–3]. Although there are differences in skull shape among the varied domestic dog and cat breeds, these variations do not drastically alter the size of the globe [1, 4–16]. Globe size is measured in terms of axial length, that is, the distance between the rostral and caudal poles of the eye [17]. In the canine eye, the mean axial length is 20.8 millimeters (mm) as compared to the feline eye, which has a mean axial length of 22.3 mm [17, 18].

The anterior and posterior segments of the eye are primarily responsible for axial length [1–3].

22.1.1 The Anterior Segment of the Eye and Aqueous Humor

The anterior segment consists of the anterior and posterior chambers. The anterior chamber is the fluid-filled space between the cornea and the iris. Its fluid contents are called aqueous humor. The posterior chamber is the fluid-filled space between the iris and the lens. It also contains aqueous humor [1–3].

Aqueous humor is produced by the ciliary body of the eye [19–21]. It circulates from the posterior to anterior chambers through the pupil of the eye [1–3, 19]. Aqueous humor production and flow maintains intraocular pressure (IOP) [19, 20]. Approximately 60–75% of aqueous humor production is dependent upon enzyme activity, specifically, carbonic anhydrase [19, 22, 23].

Once aqueous humor has flowed through the pupil, it ultimately leaves the eye [19]. This occurs via two pathways [19].

The conventional pathway is the primary means for aqueous humor outflow [19]. Aqueous humor flows from the base of the iris to the cornea, through the pectinate ligaments [24]. It then travels from the trabecular meshwork through angular plexus, and ultimately into the episcleral veins [24]. The efficient passage of aqueous

humor via this route is dependent upon the iridocorneal angle (ICA) [19].

The uveoscleral or nonconventional pathway is a secondary route by which aqueous humor exits the eye [19]. This pathway is responsible for conducting 15% of drainage in dogs and 3% in cats [19, 21, 25]. It relies upon hydrostatic pressure differences between the anterior chamber and suprachoroidal spaces to force aqueous humor into the adjacent sclera [19, 25].

22.1.2 The Posterior Segment of the Eye and Vitreous Humor

The posterior segment comprises the bulk of the eye, including every structure caudal to the lens. This includes the retina, choroid, and optic nerve. A gelatin-like material fills the space between the lens and the retina [1–3, 26]. This gel is called vitreous humor. It helps to maintain the shape of the eye [1–3].

22.1.3 Changes in Axial Length of the Eye Through Life

As is expected, the eye experiences growth in terms of axial length as puppies and kittens age [17]. This growth is rapid and is primarily the result of increasing posterior segment depth [17]. Between six months of age and seven years old, there is little to no change in the posterior segment depth of the canine eye [17]. In other words, axial length in a healthy eye is fairly static once the patient has matured.

22.1.4 Introduction to Pathological Variations in Size of the Globe

Ocular pathology is numerous; however, three distinct presentations are characterized by a distinct change in the size of the globe [27–29]:

- Buphthalmos
- Microphthalmos
- Phthisis bulbi

22.2 Introduction to Buphthalmos

Buphthalmos is the state of having an enlarged globe [27–30] (see Figures 22.1a–c).

Although the globe is seated within the orbit in its normal anatomic position, the fact that it is enlarged makes it appear as if it is bulging forward. This appearance is often mistaken for exophthalmos when in fact the exophthalmic globe is normal in size, but seated forward in the orbit [31].

Buphthalmos is the clinical presentation that occurs when there is an increase in IOP [27–29].

22.2.1 Introduction to IOP and Tonometry

IOP is determined primarily by aqueous humor production and flow [19]. However, additional variables for IOP include species, patient temperament and demeanor, corneal health, diurnal variation, exercise, and pharmaceutical agents [19, 27, 32–40]. Tropicamide, for example, is a mydriatic agent that can significantly raise IOP [41–43]. So, too, can corticosteroids [44].

Age is an important contributor to IOP in the cat. Geriatric cats typically have lower IOP than adolescent cats, which have higher IOP than adult cats, which have higher IOP than week-old kittens [44–47].

In addition, excessive patient restraint may artificially elevate readings, for example, through compression of the jugular vein(s) [19, 39, 40].

IOP is assessed via ocular tonometry [19, 48].

In veterinary medicine, there are two accepted techniques for determining IOP in companion animal practice [48, 49]:

- Applanation tonometry
- Rebound tonometry

(a)

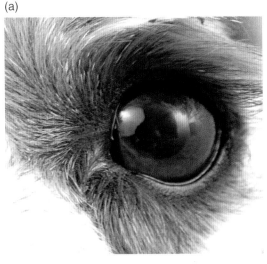

(b)   (c)

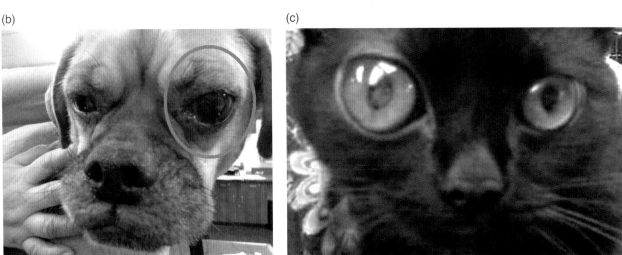

Figure 22.1 (a) Normal-sized globe in a canine patient. *Source:* Courtesy of the Media Resources Department at Midwestern University. (b) Canine patient with buphthalmos associated with the left globe (OS). *Source:* Courtesy of Dr. Elizabeth Robbins. (c) Feline patient with buphthalmos associated with the right globe (OD).

Applanation tonometry involves the use of portable, self-calibrating devices such as the Tono-Pen [48]. The Tono-Pen is gently tapped against the surface of a numbed cornea [48]. As the device comes into contact with the cornea, it flattens the cornea [48]. This is called applanation, hence the name of the technique (see Figure 22.2).

To achieve corneal flattening, a certain force is required. The Tono-Pen determines this force by averaging several readings, and offers a percentage error [48]. This force provides a rough estimate of IOP [48]. IOP can then be compared between eyes to determine if the pressures are similar. They should be.

One advantage of applanation tonometry is that the patient does not need to have its head positioned in any particular way to obtain an accurate reading [48]. In other words, the Tono-Pen is not position-dependent. This facilitates determination of IOP in wiggly or uncooperative patients.

Mean normal values of IOP as obtained through applanation tonometry vary from study to study. In the dog, normal IOP via applanation tonometry has been reported to be 12.9 mmHg ± 2.7 mmHg and 19.2 mmHg ± 5.5 mmHg [19, 50–52]. In the cat, normal IOP has been reported as 18.4 mmHg ± 0.67 mmHg [53].

Rebound tonometry is an alternate approach to the measurement of IOP and involves the use of portable devices such as the Tono-Vet [48]. This device has a lightweight probe that requires only momentary contact with the cornea to obtain a reading. The probe is magnetized via an induction coil [48]. The rebound of the probe upon corneal contact creates an induction current [48]. This allows the device to calculate the IOP [48].

One advantage is that this tool does not require the use of topical anesthetic [48]. However, the probe does require proper head positioning [48]. For the reading to be accurate, the probe must be directed horizontally [48].

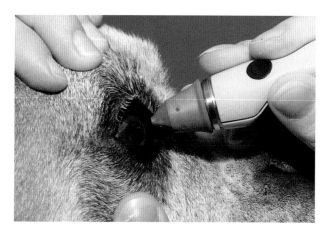

Figure 22.2 Using applanation tonometry to assess intraocular pressure (IOP) in a canine patient. *Source:* Courtesy of D.J. Haeussler, Jr., MS, DVM, DACVO.

Mean normal values of IOP as obtained through rebound tonometry also vary depending upon the study. In the dog, normal IOP via rebound tonometry has been reported to be 10.8 mmHg ± 3.1 mmHg and 9.1 mmHg ± 3.4 mmHg [19, 50, 51]. In the cat, normal IOP has been reported as 20 mmHg ± 0.48 mmHg [53].

22.2.2 Introduction to Glaucoma

As mentioned earlier, an increase in IOP results in the clinical presentation of buphthalmos [27–29]. Glaucoma is the name for the disease that underlies this clinical presentation [19].

Glaucoma may be congenital or acquired [19, 28, 54]. Congenital glaucoma is rare, and develops at birth or within a few weeks to months of life [19, 20, 49]. One or both globes may be affected. Patients present acutely for buphthalmos and corneal edema [49]. They often have concurrent pathology, including cataracts and retinal dysplasia [49]. The clinician should therefore make no assumption that congenital glaucoma is the only ocular pathology.

Acquired glaucoma occurs with greater frequency in companion animal practice and is typically bilateral; however, one eye may be affected before the other [19, 49].

Acquired glaucoma may be primary or secondary [19, 49]. Primary glaucoma occurs more often than secondary glaucoma in the dog [19, 39, 49]. Glaucoma in the cat is relatively rare [44].

22.2.2.1 Acquired Primary Glaucoma

Acquired primary glaucoma is inherited and results from misshapen pectinate ligaments and/or an improperly formed, narrowed ICA [49, 54]. When a narrowed ICA is involved, the condition is called primary closed-angle glaucoma (PCAG) [19]. The state of having misshapen pectinate ligaments is called goniodysgenesis [19].

Goniodysgenesis impairs the drainage of aqueous humor through the conventional pathway [49]. An abnormally narrow ICA achieves the same end result: a back-up of aqueous humor, thereby raising IOP [49].

American Cocker Spaniels and Basset Hounds are predisposed to closed-angle glaucoma [19, 20, 49, 55]. Boston Terriers and Shar Pei dogs are also overrepresented [49]. Females are more likely than males to develop glaucoma [55, 56]. Disease is most common in adults between the ages of 4 and 10 years old [19].

In addition to PCAG, Beagles and Norwegian Elkhounds may also develop primary open-angle glaucoma (POAG) [19]. Patients with this condition do not have an abnormally narrowed IGA. Instead, the flow of aqueous humor is compromised by goniodysgenesis and/or a loss of trabecular endothelia.

Cats are less likely to develop primary glaucoma [19]. However, certain breeds are overrepresented, including Siamese, Burmese, Persian, and Domestic Shorthaired cats [44, 49].

22.2.2.2 Acquired Secondary Glaucoma

Consider the flow of aqueous humor through the eye. When drainage is physically obstructed, acquired secondary glaucoma results [49]. Examples of obstructions that may occlude the pupil include posterior synechiae. Recall from Chapter 18, Section 18.3.1.7 that posterior synechiae attach the iris to the lens capsule [57]. Another example of a structure that could potentially block the pupil and thereby flow of aqueous humor is the lens, when it undergoes pathological luxation [49] (see Figure 22.3).

Hyphema and hypopyon may also impair aqueous humor flow and drainage from the eye [49]. Review Chapters 16 and 17 to explore the etiologies of both.

In cats, glaucoma is likely to be secondary to intraocular neoplasia [44, 45, 58–60]. Cases involving anterior uveal melanoma and lymphoma predominate [44, 45, 58–60]. Intraocular sarcomas have also been reported in cats months to years following trauma to the globe [44, 61, 62].

22.2.3 Additional Clinical Signs of Glaucoma

Patients with glaucoma, whether it is primary or secondary, acute or chronic, exhibit buphthalmos [19, 28, 29, 49]. In addition, they may present with these additional clinical signs [19, 20, 49]:

- "Red eye"
- Epiphora

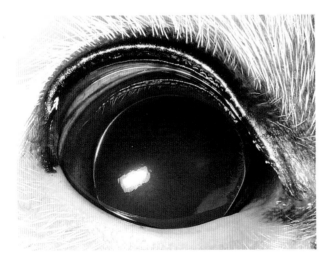

Figure 22.3 Anterior lens luxation in a canine patient. *Source:* Courtesy of D.J. Haeussler, Jr., MS, DVM, DACVO.

- Blindness
  - Absent menace response
- Blepharospasm
- Being head-shy
- Episcleral congestion
- Conjunctival hyperemia
- Corneal edema
- Mild mydriasis
- Prominent nictitans (see Figures 22.4a–d)

Blepharospasm, head-shyness, and the prominent nictitans are thought to reflect ocular pain [19, 49].

Dogs frequently present on emergency for apparent ocular discomfort and "red eye" [19]. Note that none of the aforementioned signs are pathognomonic for glaucoma, especially "red eye." "Red eye" is a generic descriptor that may be apparent in a variety of case presentations, including anterior uveitis, blepharitis, conjunctivitis, keratitis, scleritis, and episcleritis [29, 30].

As compared to dogs, the progression of glaucoma in cats is slow and insidious [19]. Feline patients may not be diagnosed until the disease has become chronic and corneal edema is pronounced [19].

22.2.4 Diagnostics Associated with Glaucoma

Patient history and clinical presentation set the stage for a presumptive diagnosis of glaucoma. The clinician's index of suspicion is then confirmed via tonometry [19]. Patients with glaucoma will have consistently elevated IOP as measured by tonometers. Early-stage glaucoma may result in mild increases in IOP, such as 25–30 mmHg [19]. However, spikes in IOP can be severe and range between 50 and 70 mmHg [19].

Care must be taken to reduce or eliminate external factors that may artificially elevate IOP [19, 27, 32–40]. For example, to avoid diurnal fluctuations in IOP, tonometry should be performed at the same time of day. Tonometry should also be performed in the same patient using the same technique. This is because applanation and rebound tonometry report slight differences in what constitutes canine and feline normal reference ranges for IOP [19, 50, 51, 53].

By demonstrating a consistently elevated IOP, tonometry is able to confirm the diagnosis of glaucoma. However, tonometry is unable to ascertain whether the patient has PCAG or POAP. Gonioscopy is indicated to visualize the ICA [19].

Fundoscopy is equally important to assess the patient for sequelae that are associated with chronic glaucoma. The chronicity of elevated IOP places the patient at great risk of developing retinal changes, including chorioretinal atrophy, diffuse retinal degeneration, optic nerve head degeneration, and cupping [19].

(a)
(b)
(c)
(d)

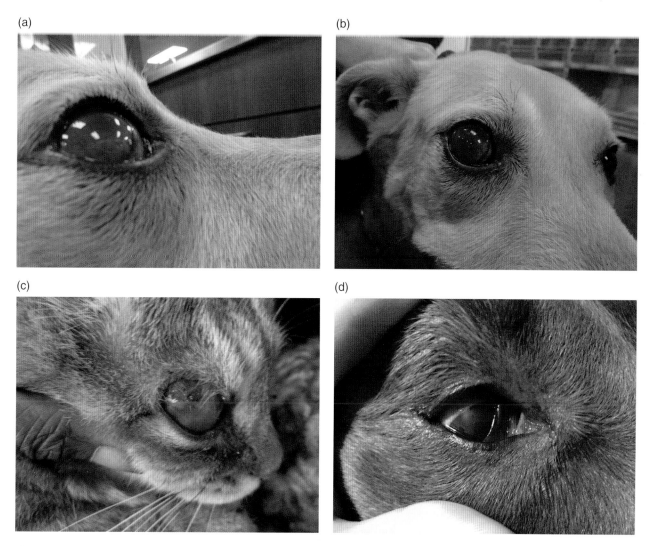

Figure 22.4 (a) "Red eye" in a canine patient with glaucoma. *Source:* Courtesy of Patricia Bennett, DVM. (b) Subtle corneal edema in a canine patient that is being medically managed for glaucoma. *Source:* Courtesy of Patricia Bennett, DVM. (c) Severe corneal edema in a feline patient that has glaucoma. *Source:* Courtesy of Patricia Bennett, DVM. (d) "Red eye" and corneal edema in a canine patient with glaucoma. *Source:* Courtesy of Jennifer Darmofal.

22.2.5 Management of Glaucoma

Glaucoma is painful [54]. Ocular pain increases as IOP increases [54]. Ocular pain is reduced as IOP is lowered [54].

Contrary to popular belief, non-steroidal anti-inflammatory drugs do not reduce pain. In fact, they can increase IOP, in effect worsening both the pain and the severity of glaucoma [54]. Some clinicians prescribe tramadol for pain; however, to the author's knowledge, its efficacy against glaucoma-induced pain has not been studied [54].

The mainstay of treatment is therefore reducing IOP to preserve what vision remains and decrease the likelihood of progressive retinal damage [19]. However, it is unclear which value of IOP is "safe" for patients with

overt glaucoma [19]. The target range for IOP in medically managed patients varies from study to study. That being said, it is generally agreed upon that IOP should not exceed 19–20 mmHg in the canine glaucoma patient [19].

The breadth and depth of medical and surgical treatment is beyond the scope of this textbook; however, in general, medical management typically addresses aqueous humor production and/or flow.

Historically, mannitol was used in emergency situations to increase extracellular fluid osmolality and effectively reduce the vitreous body [19, 49].

Mannitol is still used on occasion to manage emergency spikes in IOP; however, other rapid-acting agents have been developed that are equally effective. These agents include the prostaglandin analogs (PGAs), latanoprost, bimatoprost, and travoprost. These increase aqueous humor outflow by acting on ciliary body muscles. Miosis is a common side effect [19]. For this reason, PGAs are contraindicated in patients with anterior lens luxations. These patients already have experienced occlusion of the pupil. They do not benefit from additional pupil constriction, which may aggravate the obstruction [19].

Parasympathomimetic drugs, such as demecarium bromide, also increase aqueous humor outflow through a similar mechanism [19].

Both PGAs and parasympathomimetic drugs have the potential to damage the blood–ocular barrier [19]. Therefore, use of either drug class is ill-advised in patients with uveitis [19, 39].

Other drugs focus their efforts on reducing inflow. Consider, for example, carbonic anhydrase inhibitors (CAIs), such as topical dorzolamide and brinzolamide [19, 49, 63]. By inhibiting the enzyme that is responsible for the bulk of aqueous humor production in dogs and cats, these prescription drugs reduce aqueous humor production [19].

Topical CAIs are preferred to systemic therapy because the latter class of drugs may result in metabolic acidosis, gastrointestinal upset, panting, and lethargy [19]. Cats are particularly sensitive to the effects of hypokalemia, which may be caused by the systemic use of CAIs [19, 39].

Medical management may stabilize disease; however, it is important to remember that most cases of glaucoma progress [19]. Surgical management of glaucoma is expanding as techniques are developed to improve postoperative patient outcomes [19, 49]. These procedures selectively target the ciliary body to reduce aqueous humor production and improve outflow [19].

However, surgical failures are not uncommon [19]. Avisual patients may be managed appropriately via chemical ablation of the ciliary body with an intravitreal injection of gentamicin or cidofovir [19, 49].

Alternatively, enucleation or evisceration of one or both globes in the blind patient is a reasonable course of action [19, 21]. Either procedure improves the patient's quality of life by alleviating ocular discomfort [19].

22.3 Microphthalmos

Microphthalmos is the state of having a globe that is reduced in size as compared to the norm [27–29] (see Figures 22.5a, b).

Microphthalmos is typically not apparent until the eyelids open, approximately 10–14 days after birth. One or both eyes may be affected [64].

The affected eye may be only slightly smaller than normal or it may be a vestigial structure [64].

The palpebral fissure of the affected globe may also be reduced in size [27–29].

Microphthalmos may be the only ocular anomaly, or it may occur in combination with other ocular pathology.

In cats, microphthalmos may be inherited or linked to exposure to toxins [64]. Consider, for example, the

(a)

(b)

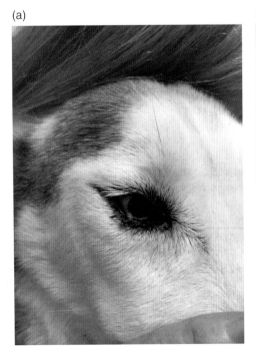
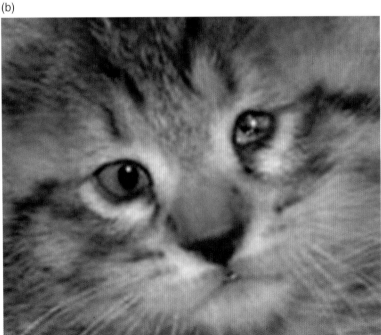

Figure 22.5 (a) Microphthalmos in a canine patient. *Source:* Courtesy of Samantha B. Thurman, DVM. (b) Unilateral microphthalmos in a kitten.

administration of griseofulvin to pregnant queens [65]. Affected kittens may have concurrent cyclopia and optic nerve aplasia [65]. Some kittens in the litter may even have anophthalmos, meaning that they are born without one or both globes [65].

In dogs, microphthalmos may be inherited, linked to exposure to toxins, or result from vitamin A deficiency [64, 66–68].

In certain dog breeds, microphthalmos is often linked to congenital cataracts. Consider, for example, Old English Sheepdogs, Akitas, Miniature Schnauzers, and Cavalier King Charles Spaniels [65, 69].

Microphthalmos and retinal dysplasia are developmentally linked in Beagles, Bedlington Terriers, and Labrador Retrievers [65].

Finally, microphthalmos is inherited as an autosomal recessive trait in Australian Shepherds and other dogs with merle coats, including Shetland Sheepdogs, Collies, Dachshunds, and Great Danes [65]. Patients are said to be affected with merle ocular dysgenesis [65, 70]. This means that they present with a constellation of ocular signs, not just microphthalmos. Additional ocular pathologies that have been reported in the affected population of patients include cataracts, retinal dysplasia, choroidal and/or optic nerve hypoplasia, retinal detachment, and persistent pupillary membranes [65].

There is no treatment for microphthalmos. Visually, clients may express aesthetic concerns, particularly if the patient has concurrent enophthalmos, and/or a prominent nictitans. These impact the outward appearance of the patient.

Aesthetics aside, the biggest concern for the patient is that its vision may be reduced or absent [27–29, 65].

Because most cases of microphthalmos are inherited, breeding management plays an essential role in reducing its prevalence [65].

22.4 Phthisis Bulbi

Phthisis bulbi is a clinical presentation in which a patient has one or both shrunken globes [27–29] (see Figure 22.6).

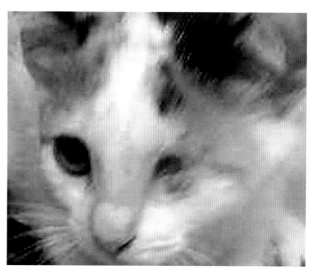

Figure 22.6 Unilateral phthisis bulbi in a kitten.

(a)

(b)

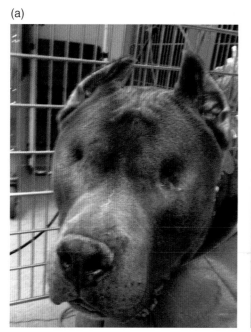
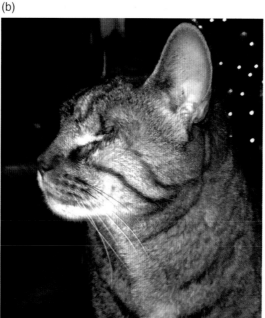

Figure 22.7 (a) Typical appearance of bilateral enucleated orbits in a canine patient. *Source:* Courtesy of Robert Eisemann. (b) Typical appearance of an enucleated orbit in a feline patient. *Source:* Courtesy of Robert Eisemann.

Phthisis bulbi may resemble microphthalmos in the early stages [71]. However, as the condition progresses, the globe may take on a caved-in appearance. Sometimes the surface even develops a prune-like appearance as the globe shrivels from sight.

Corneal edema is also more prominent in cases of phthisis bulbi as compared to microphthalmos [71].

Phthisis bulbi is the outcome of significant, sustained intraocular pathology, such as chronic inflammatory disease. Consider, for example, persistent uveitis [27].

A globe with phthisis bulbi is not capable of conveying vision to the patient.

Many owners elect not to surgically excise a globe with phthisis bulbi because of the sunken-in appearance of an enucleated orbit [71] (see Figures 22.7a, b).

However, feline patients should undergo enucleation. There is an apparent link between longstanding intraocular inflammation or globe-related trauma and the development of intraocular sarcoma [44, 61, 62, 71].

References

1 Dyce, K.M., Sack, W.O., and Wensing, C.J.G. (2010). *Textbook of Veterinary Anatomy*, 4e, xii, 834 p. St. Louis, Mo.: Saunders/Elsevier.

2 Evans, H.E. and DeLahunta, A. (2004). *Guide to the Dissection of the Dog*, 6e, xiv, 378 p. St. Louis, Mo.: Saunders.

3 Evans, H.E. and Miller, M.E. (2013). *Miller's Anatomy of the Dog*, 4e, xix, 850 p. St. Louis, Missouri: Elsevier.

4 Holmstrom, S.E. and Holmstrom, S.E. (2013). *Veterinary Dentistry: A Team Approach*, 2e, viii, 434 p. St. Louis, Mo.: Elsevier/Mosby.

5 Kunzel, W., Breit, S., and Oppel, M. (2003). Morphometric investigations of breed-specific features in feline skulls and considerations on their functional implications. *Anat. Histol. Embryol.* 32 (4): 218–223.

6 Sisson, S., Grossman, J.D., and Getty, R. (1975). *Sisson and Grossman's The Anatomy of the Domestic Animals*, 5e. Philadelphia: Saunders.

7 Christiansen, P. (2008). Evolution of skull and mandible shape in cats (carnivora: felidae). *PLoS One* 3 (7): e2807.

8 Biknevicius, A.R. and Van Valkenburgh, B. (1996). Design for killing: craniodental adaptations of predators. In: *Carnivore Behavior, Ecology, and Evolution*, vol. 2 (ed. J.L. Gittleman), 393–428. New York: Cornell University Press.

9 Christiansen, P. and Wroe, S. (2007). Bite forces and evolutionary adaptations to feeding ecology in carnivores. *Ecology* 88 (2): 347–358.

10 Monfared, A.L. (2013). Anatomy of the Persian cat's skull and its clinical value during regional anesthesia. *Global Veterinaria* 10 (5): 551–555.

11 Schoenebeck, J.J. and Ostrander, E.A. (2013). The genetics of canine skull shape variation. *Genetics* 193 (2): 317–325.

12 McGreevy, P., Grassi, T.D., and Harman, A.M. (2004). A strong correlation exists between the distribution of retinal ganglion cells and nose length in the dog. *Brain Behav. Evol.* 63 (1): 13–22.

13 Coppinger, R. and Schneider, R. (1995). Evolution of working dogs. In: *The Domestic Dog: Its Evolution, Behaviour, and Interactions with People* (ed. J. Serpell), 21–50. Cambridge; New York: Cambridge University Press.

14 Haworth, K.E., Islam, I., Breen, M. et al. (2001). Canine TCOF1; cloning, chromosome assignment and genetic analysis in dogs with different head types. *Mamm. Genome* 12 (8): 622–629.

15 Wayne, R.K. (1986). Cranial morphology of domestic and wild canids – the Influence of development on morphological change. *Evolution* 40 (2): 243–261.

16 Young, A. and Bannasch, D. (2006). Morphological variation in the dog. In: *The Dog and Its Genome* (ed. E.A. Ostrander, U. Giger and K. Lindblad-Toh), 47–65. Cold Spring Harbor, NY: Cold Spring Harbor Laboratory Press.

17 Mutti, D.O., Zadnik, K., and Murphy, C.J. (1999). Naturally occurring vitreous chamber-based myopia in the Labrador retriever. *Invest. Ophthalmol. Vis. Sci.* 40 (7): 1577–1584.

18 Vakkur, G.J. and Bishop, P.O. (1963). The schematic eye in the cat. *Vis. Res.* 61: 357–381.

19 Maggio, F. (2015). Glaucomas. *Top. Companion Anim. Med.* 30 (3): 86–96.

20 Reinstein, S., Rankin, A., and Allbaugh, R. (2009). Canine glaucoma: pathophysiology and diagnosis. *Compend. Contin. Educ. Vet.* 31 (10): 450–452; quiz 2–3.

21 Dietrich, U. (2005). Feline glaucomas. *Clin. Tech. Small Anim. Pract.* 20 (2): 108–116.

22 O'Rourke, J., Macri, F.J., and Berghoffer, B. (1969). Studies in uveal physiology. I. Adaptation of isotope clearance procedures for external monitoring of anterior uveal bloodflow and aqueous humor turnover in the dog. *Arch. Ophthalmol.* 81 (4): 526–533.

23 Shahidullah, M., Wilson, W.S., Yap, M., and To, C.H. (2003). Effects of ion transport and channel-blocking drugs on aqueous humor formation in isolated bovine eye. *Invest. Ophthalmol. Vis. Sci.* 44 (3): 1185–1191.

24 Samuelson, D.A. (2013). Chapter 2:Ophthalmic anatomy. In: *Veterinary Opthalmology* (ed. K.N. Gelatt, B.C. Gilger and T.J. Kern), 39–170. Ames, IA: Wiley-Blackwell.

25 Gum, G.G. and MacKay, E.O. (2013). Chapter 3: Physiology of the eye. In: *Veterinary Ophthalmology* (ed. K.N. Gelatt, B.C. Gilger and T.J. Kern), 171–207. Ames, IA: Wiley-Blackwell.

26 Meekins, J.M. (2015). Acute Blindness. *Top. Companion Anim. Med.* 30 (3): 118–125.

27 Aiello, S.E. and Moses, M.C. (2016). *Merck Veterinary Manual*. Whitehouse Station, NJ: Merck Sharp & Dohme Corp.

28 Côté, E. (2015). *Clinical Veterinary Advisor. Dogs and Cats*, 3e, xxxvii, 1642 p. St. Louis, Missouri: Elsevier Mosby.

29 Tilley, L.P., Smith, F.W.K., and Tilley, L.P. (2007). *Blackwell's Five-Minute Veterinary Consult: Canine and Feline*, 4e. Ames, Iowa: Blackwell.

30 Englar, R.E. (2017). *Performing the Small Animal Physical Examination*. Hoboken, NJ: Wiley.

31 Ofri, R. (2014). Differentiating exophthalmos, buphthalmos, & proptosis. *NAVC Clinician's Brief* (May): 29–31.

32 Brubaker, R.F. (1991). Flow of aqueous humor in humans [The Friedenwald Lecture]. *Invest. Ophthalmol. Vis. Sci.* 32 (13): 3145–3166.

33 Koskela, T. and Brubaker, R.F. (1991). The nocturnal suppression of aqueous humor flow in humans is not blocked by bright light. *Invest. Ophthalmol. Vis. Sci.* 32 (9): 2504–2506.

34 Liu, J.H. and Weinreb, R.N. (2011). Monitoring intraocular pressure for 24 h. *Br. J. Ophthalmol.* 95 (5): 599–600.

35 Drance, S.M. (1964). Effect of oral glycerol of intraocular pressure in normal and glaucomatous eyes. *Arch. Ophthalmol.* 72: 491–493.

36 Qureshi, I.A. (1995). Effects of mild, moderate and severe exercise on intraocular pressure of sedentary subjects. *Ann. Hum. Biol.* 22 (6): 545–553.

37 Patel, P.M., Patel, H.H., and Roth, D.M. (2011). General anesthetics and therapeutic gases. In: *Goodman & Gilman's: The Pharmacological Basis of Therapeutics* (ed. L. Brunton, B.A. Chabner and B. Knollman), 527–564. New York: The McGraw-Hill Companies, Inc.

38 Plumb, D.C. (2011). *Plumb's Veterinary Drug Handbook*, 7e, 1187 p. Stockholm, Wis. Ames, Iowa: PharmaVet; Distributed by Wiley.

39 Plummer, C.E., Regnier, A., and Gelatt, K.N. (2013). The canine glaucomas. In: *Veterinary Ophthalmology II* (ed. K.N. Gelatt, B.C. Gilger and T.J. Kern), 1050–1145. Ames, IA: Wiley-Blackwell.

40 von Spiessen, L., Karck, J., Rohn, K., and Meyer-Lindenberg, A. (2015). Clinical comparison of the TonoVet (R) rebound tonometer and the Tono-Pen Vet (R) applanation tonometer in dogs and cats with ocular disease: glaucoma or corneal pathology. *Vet. Ophthalmol.* 18 (1): 20–27.

41 Stadtbaumer, K., Frommlet, F., and Nell, B. (2006). Effects of mydriatics on intraocular pressure and pupil size in the normal feline eye. *Vet. Ophthalmol.* 9 (4): 233–237.

42 Stadtbaumer, K., Kostlin, R.G., and Zahn, K.J. (2002). Effects of topical 0.5% tropicamide on intraocular pressure in normal cats. *Vet. Ophthalmol.* 5 (2): 107–112.

43 Gomes, F.E., Bentley, E., Lin, T.L., and McLellan, G.J. (2011). Effects of unilateral topical administration of 0.5% tropicamide on anterior segment morphology and intraocular pressure in normal cats and cats with primary congenital glaucoma. *Vet. Ophthalmol.* 14 (Suppl 1): 75–83.

44 McLellan, G.J. and Teixeira, L.B. (2015). Feline glaucoma. *Vet. Clin. North Am. Small Anim. Pract.* 45 (6): 1307–1333, vii.

45 McLellan, G.J. and Miller, P.E. (2011). Feline glaucoma–a comprehensive review. *Vet. Ophthalmol.* 14 (Suppl 1): 15–29.

46 Adelman, S., GJ, M.L., and Ellinwood, N.M. (eds.) (2013). *Early life intraocular pressures in normal cats and cats with primary congenital glaucoma*. Puerto Rico: American College of Veterinary Ophthalmologists.

47 Kroll, M.M., Miller, P.E., and Rodan, I. (2001). Intraocular pressure measurements obtained as part of a comprehensive geriatric health examination from cats seven years of age or older. *J. Am. Vet. Med. Assoc.* 219 (10): 1406–1410.

48 Wilkie, D.A. (2013). Determining intraocular pressure. *NAVC Clinician's Brief* (February): 77–79.

49 Reinstein S. (2017). Under Pressure: Canine and Feline Glaucoma. Michigan Veterinary Medical Association [Internet]: https://michvma.org/resources/Documents/MVC/2017%20Proceedings/reinstein%2005.pdf.

50 Knollinger, A.M., La Croix, N.C., Barrett, P.M., and Miller, P.E. (2005). Evaluation of a rebound tonometer for measuring intraocular pressure in dogs and horses. *J. Am. Vet. Med. Assoc.* 227 (2): 244–248.

51 Leiva, M., Naranjo, C., and Pena, M.T. (2006). Comparison of the rebound tonometer (ICare) to the applanation tonometer (Tonopen XL) in normotensive dogs. *Vet. Ophthalmol.* 9 (1): 17–21.

52 Gelatt, K.N. and MacKay, E.O. (1998). Distribution of intraocular pressure in dogs. *Vet. Ophthalmol.* 1 (2–3): 109–114.

53 Rusanen, E., Florin, M., Hassig, M., and Spiess, B.M. (2010). Evaluation of a rebound tonometer (Tonovet) in clinically normal cat eyes. *Vet. Ophthalmol.* 13 (1): 31–36.

54 Colitz, C.M.H. (2010). Canine glaucoma. *NAVC Clinician's Brief* (March): 24–26.

55 Gelatt, K.N. and MacKay, E.O. (2004). Prevalence of the breed-related glaucomas in pure-bred dogs in North America. *Vet. Ophthalmol.* 7 (2): 97–111.

56 Slater, M.R. and Erb, H.N. (1986). Effects of risk factors and prophylactic treatment on primary glaucoma in the dog. *J. Am. Vet. Med. Assoc.* 188 (9): 1028–1030.

57 Heller HB, Bentley E. (2016). The Practitioner's Guide to Neurologic Causes of Canine Anisocoria. Today's Veterinary Practice [Internet]. (January/February):[77–83 pp.]. http://todaysveterinarypractice.navc.com/wp-content/uploads/2016/05/TVP_2016-0102_OO-Anisocoria.pdf.

58 Blocker, T. and Van Der Woerdt, A. (2001). The feline glaucomas: 82 cases (1995–1999). *Vet. Ophthalmol.* 4 (2): 81–85.

59 Walde, I. and Rapp, E. (1993). Feline glaucoma: Clinical and morphological aspects (a retrospective study of 38 cases). *Eur. J. Compan Anim. Pract.* 4: 87–105.

60 Wilcock, B.P., Peiffer, R.L. Jr., and Davidson, M.G. (1990). The causes of glaucoma in cats. *Vet. Pathol.* 27 (1): 35–40.

61 Dubielzig, R.R., Everitt, J., Shadduck, J.A., and Albert, D.M. (1990). Clinical and morphologic features of post-traumatic ocular sarcomas in cats. *Vet. Pathol.* 27 (1): 62–65.

62 Dubielzig, R.R. and Zeiss, C. (2004). Feline Post-traumatic ocular sarcoma: Three morphologic variants and evidence that some are derived from lens epithelial cells. *Invest. Ophthalmol. Vis. Sci.* 45: 3562.

63 Maslanka, T. (2015). A review of the pharmacology of carbonic anhydrase inhibitors for the treatment of glaucoma in dogs and cats. *Vet. J.* 203 (3): 278–284.

64 Dell, M. (2010). Severe bilateral microphthalmos in a Pomeranian pup. *Can. Vet. J.* 51 (12): 1405–1407.

65 Peterson, M.E. and Kutzler, M.A. (2011). *Small Animal Pediatrics: The First 12 Months of Life.* St. Louis, Mo.: Saunders/Elsevier.

66 Hyttel, P., Sinowatz, F., and Vejlsted, M. (2010). *Essentials of Domestic Animal Embryology.* New York: Saunders Elsevier.

67 Drew, M.N. and DeLahunta, A. (1985). *Embryology of Domestic Animals.* Baltimore: Williams & Wilkins.

68 Mellersh, C.S. (2014). The genetics of eye disorders in the dog. *Canine Genet. Epidemiol.* 1: 3.

69 Esson, D.W. (2015). *Clinical Atlas of Canine and Feline Ophthalmic Disease.* Chichester, UK: Wiley.

70 Bauer, B.S., Sandmeyer, L.S., and Grahn, B.H. (2015). Diagnostic ophthalmology. Microphthalmos and multiple ocular anomalies (MOA) OU consistent with merle ocular dysgenesis (MOD). *Can. Vet. J.* 56 (7): 767–768.

71 Martin, C.L. (2009). *Ophthalmic Disease in Veterinary Medicine.* Boca Raton, FL: Taylor & Francis Group.

23

Abnormal Alignment of One or Both Eyes

23.1 Introduction to Eye Alignment

Chapter 21 reviewed the normal anatomic position of the eye within the orbit, as compared to a globe that is pathologically too rostral or too caudal. Chapter 22 emphasized the normal size of the eye, as compared to a globe that is pathologically too large or too small.

The emphasis of this chapter is on proper alignment of the eyes.

At any given point, both eyes should be looking at the same place at the same time [1]. In order to maintain this alignment with one another, the patient requires functional and balanced extraocular muscles as well as functional cranial nerves [1].

There are three pairs of extraocular muscles of importance to companion animal patients [2–4]:

- Dorsal rectus and ventral rectus
- Medial rectus and lateral rectus
- Dorsal oblique and ventral oblique

These extraocular muscles establish alignment of the globes and control synergistic globe movement [2–4].

Just as flexor and extensor muscles of the distal limbs work to achieve opposite effects, so, too, do the extraocular muscles of each pair [5]. They act relative to one another in a reciprocal manner [5].

Each muscle is named according to the direction in which it moves the globe. Consider, for example, the dorsal and ventral rectus. These extraocular muscles work to elevate and depress the globe, respectively. Likewise, the medial rectus adducts the globe, as compared to the lateral rectus, which abducts the globe [2–4].

The dorsal and ventral oblique muscles create rotation of the globe. The dorsal oblique muscle rotates the dorsal aspect of the globe medially and ventrally, whereas the ventral oblique muscle rotates the ventral aspect of the globe medially and dorsally [2–4].

Innervation of the extraocular muscles is via specific cranial nerves [2–4, 6]. The third cranial nerve (CN III), the oculomotor nerve, innervates the dorsal, ventral, medial, and ventral oblique rectus muscles [2–4, 6]. The fourth cranial nerve (CN IV), the trochlear nerve, innervates the dorsal oblique muscle, and the sixth cranial nerve (CN VI), the abducens nerve, innervates the lateral rectus [2–4, 6].

23.2 Introduction to Strabismus

Primary muscular or neurological issues can create dysfunction in one or more of the extraocular muscles [7]. When this occurs, the extraocular muscle(s) become(s) uncoordinated, and there is a loss of controlled movement of one or both globes. The result is strabismus.

Strabismus is a clinical presentation in which one or both eyes deviate from the expected visual axis [1, 5, 7–12].

Mild strabismus may have little to no impact on visual acuity. However, moderate to severe strabismus may compromise binocular vision and depth perception [5, 13–15].

Historically, strabismus has been equated with having crossed eyes. However, eyes may or may not be crossed. Only in cases of bilateral esotropia, a type of strabismus, do both globes turn inward [16]. A synonym for this clinical presentation is convergent strabismus [16]. This yields the crossed eye appearance.

Other patients may have exotropia, in which one or both globes deviate outward [16]. A synonym for this clinical presentation is divergent strabismus [16].

Convergent and divergent strabismus are the most common clinical presentations in companion animal practice.

The following presentations are less common, but possible [16]:

- Hypertropia, a type of strabismus that is characterized as having one or both globes deviating upward
- Hypotropia, a type of strabismus that is characterized as having one or both globes deviating downward
- Incyclotorsion, a type of strabismus in which one or both globes deviate toward the top inward
- Excyclotorsion, a type of strabismus in which one or both globes deviate toward the top outward (see Figures 23.1a–e)

Common Clinical Presentations in Dogs and Cats, First Edition. Ryane E. Englar.
© 2019 John Wiley & Sons, Inc. Published 2019 by John Wiley & Sons, Inc.

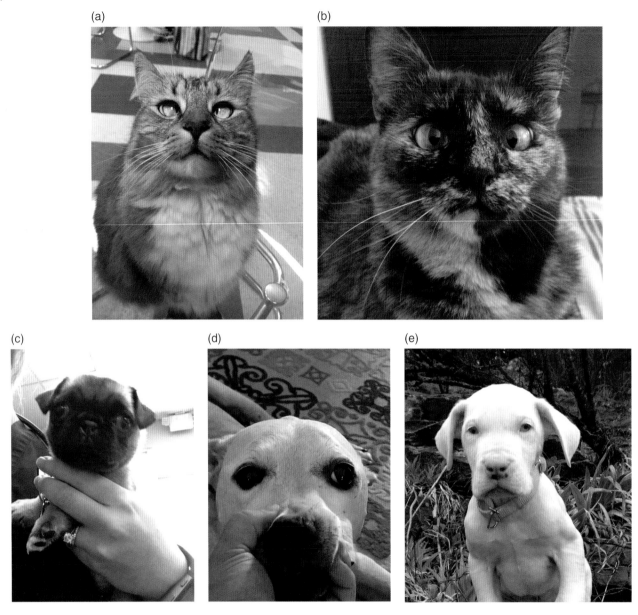

Figure 23.1 (a) Severe convergent strabismus or esotropia in a feline patient. *Source:* Courtesy of Benjamin J. Turner. (b) Moderate convergent strabismus or esotropia in a feline patient. *Source:* Courtesy of Shelby Newton. (c) Divergent strabismus or exotropia in a canine patient. (d) Divergent strabismus or exotropia in a canine patient. *Source:* Courtesy of Elizabeth E. Ferguson, DVM. (e) Unilateral hypotropia associated with the right globe (OD) in a canine patient. *Source:* Courtesy of Jetta Schirmer.

Strabismus is relatively rare in companion animal medicine as a clinical presentation [17].

When strabismus develops acutely, the burden falls upon the clinician to localize the lesion. Having a working knowledge of extraocular muscles, their actions, and their innervations facilitates lesion localization.

Consider, for example, a dog or cat with medial strabismus. Alignment of the globe in a horizontal plane is dependent upon the actions of the lateral and medial rectus. For the globe to point straight forward, both the lateral and medial rectus have to be equally engaged. If the lateral rectus is not engaged due to underlying pathology, the globe points medially. The root of the problem may be in the lateral rectus itself or it may be a primary neurological issue. Because CN VI innervates the lateral rectus, the abducens nerve also requires investigation [2–4, 6, 9].

Consider an alternate example in which a patient presents for ventrolateral strabismus. This clinical presentation may result from weakness in both the dorsal and medial rectus muscles and/or dysfunction in the cranial nerve that innervates them, CN III, the oculomotor nerve [2–4, 6, 18, 19].

Finally, consider rotatory strabismus. This may result from weakness in the dorsal oblique muscle and/or dysfunction in the cranial nerve that innervates it, CN IV, the trochlear nerve [2–4, 6].

It is also important to recognize that strabismus-inducing lesions are not limited to the extraocular muscles or the cranial nerves. Eye position, alignment, and movement require additional inputs from higher centers [20]. These include the cerebellum and the vestibular centers [20].

23.3 Congenital Strabismus

Strabismus may be congenital or acquired [20].

Among companion animals, brachycephalic dogs are predisposed to congenital strabismus [8]. In particular, English Bulldogs, Pugs, Boston Terriers, Shih Tzus, and Pekingese are more likely to exhibit congenital exotropia [8]. This may be unilateral or bilateral. It does not tend to progress with age, and does not appear to impact their vision [8].

Shar Pei dogs are predisposed to juvenile esotropia that is thought to be inherited [17, 21]. The medial rectus muscle is replaced with fibrous tissue [21].

Siamese and Himalayan cats are also predisposed to congenital strabismus. The clinical presentation for these breeds is typically esotropia [8, 20]. Esotropia is inherited as an autosomal recessive trait in these color-point breeds [8] (see Figures 23.2a, b).

Refer to Chapter 8, Section 8.2 for a review of the color-point coat patterns that are most notably seen in the Siamese, Burmese, Tonkinese, Balinese, and Himalayan breeds [22, 23].

Recall that color-point breeds, such as the Siamese, have darker faces and extremities than the torso. These regions of the body are said to be "pointed." Points are the result of a mutation of the albino gene [22, 24–26].

The effects of albinism are not limited to the coat. As early as the 1960s, it was recognized that albinism resulted in impaired visual acuity and poor binocular vision [27, 28]. In addition, patients with albinism were more likely to develop nystagmus [27, 28].

Because Siamese cats have a mutated albino gene, the effects of coat color on vision have been studied extensively in this breed [29–33]. The ratio of Y- to X-type retinal ganglion cells is lower in Siamese cats, as compared to other breeds [10, 27].

Siamese cats also have aberrant pathways for retino-geniculate fibers [29–33]. Fibers traverse to the lateral geniculate body on the side opposite that which is expected [34–36].

Although the visual cortex is able to functionally adapt, there are limitations [34–36]. For instance, visual cortex neurons must be bilaterally responsive in order to confer binocular vision and stereopsis, that is, depth perception [27]. Siamese cats do not have binocularly responsive visual cortex neurons [34–36]. Instead, their neurons are monocularly driven [34–36]. This means that affected cats have poor depth perception [37].

It has been theorized that perhaps esotropia is way for Siamese cats and related breeds to compensate for their visual deficits [8, 38].

(a)

(b)

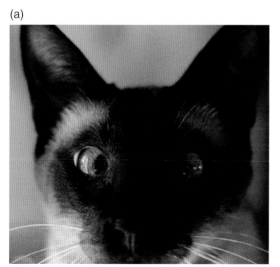
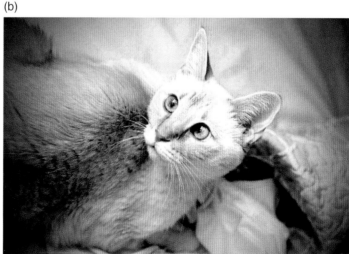

Figure 23.2 (a) Convergent strabismus or esotropia in a Siamese cat. (b) Unilateral esotropia associated with the left globe (OS) in a Siamese mix. *Source:* Courtesy of Heather N. Cornell, DVM.

23.4 Acquired Strabismus

Acquired strabismus may result from the following [7, 10, 11, 20, 39–43]:

- Traumatic injury to the globe and extraocular muscles
- Scar tissue from prior inflammatory disease that is now restrictive of extraocular muscle movement
- Orbital disease
- Cranial nerve dysfunction
- Vestibular disease

23.4.1 Proptosis

Proptosis is a common cause of acquired strabismus [10, 20, 44]. Recall from Chapter 21, Section 21.2.3 that proptosis results in traumatic exophthalmos. Review Figures 21.8a, b to appreciate the extent of the damage to the globe and orbital tissues.

Patients that experience traumatic exophthalmos sustain damage to the medial rectus muscle [10, 20]. This results in divergent strabismus.

23.4.2 Extraocular Myositis

Recall from Chapter 21, Section 21.2.2.3 that extraocular myositis is rare in companion animal practice [45]. Affected patients have bilateral exophthalmos and a startled appearance due to prominent sclera [45].

Although displaying the whites of the eyes, "scleral show," is the most memorable finding, extraocular myositis may also present with restrictive strabismus [17, 45].

Restrictive strabismus may be unilateral or bilateral [17]. Isolated case reports also demonstrate a variety of presentations for strabismus: ventral, ventromedial, or medial [17].

In all cases, strabismus is severe [17]. Most cases of hypotropia result in the absence of visible cornea [17]. The cornea is hidden beneath the lower palpebra, with only the conjunctiva readily apparent to the outside observer [17].

Globe position and alignment is relatively fixed [17]. It is very difficult to get the globe to move [17].

Because strabismus is extreme when it occurs in cases of extraocular myositis, patients are visually impaired [17].

Cases that are medically managed with corticosteroids do not develop strabismus. This supports the theory that the restrictive nature of the strabismus is due to fibrosis. Corticosteroids prevent the disease from reaching the fibrotic state [17].

With medical and/or surgical treatment, it is possible for globe deviation to be reduced and for the globe to be restored to its normal position and alignment [17].

23.4.3 Other Types of Orbital Disease

Extraocular myositis is a type of orbital disease. Other types of orbital disease include the following [46–53]:

- Zygomatic salivary gland disease
- Infectious disease
- Orbital cellulitis
- Retrobulbar abscesses
- Retrobulbar tumors

Recall from Chapter 21, Section 21.2.2 that orbital disease is typically associated with exophthalmos, rostral displacement of the globe [46, 49, 50, 54, 55].

Strabismus may result if lesions create sufficient pressure to deviate one or both globes [10, 20, 42, 43, 46, 51, 56].

23.4.4 Vestibular Disease

Vestibular disease is a condition in which the body's sense of balance is disturbed [40].

Balance is maintained in health by the vestibular system, in addition to inputs from the visual and general proprioceptive systems [40, 57–60]. A body that is balanced is able to coordinate body posture and eye position relative to where the head is positioned and how it moves through space [40, 61].

A functional vestibular system requires both central and peripheral components [40]. When one or both of these components exhibit dysfunction, body posture, head posture, eye position, eye movement, and gait are jeopardized [40, 57, 60].

The peripheral vestibular system is composed of the middle ear and inner ear, including the semicircular canals, the utricle and saccule, and the eighth cranial nerve, CN VIII, the vestibulocochlear nerve [3, 4, 62]. Inner ear disease is more likely to result in strabismus than middle ear disease, which is associated primarily with a head tilt [63].

The central vestibular system is composed of the brainstem, the cerebellum, and two caudal cerebellar peduncles [3, 4]. Within the brainstem, there are eight vestibular nuclei [3, 4]. These communicate, via the medial longitudinal fasciculus and the third, fourth, and sixth cranial nerves, with the spinal cord, the cerebrum, and the extraocular muscles [3, 4, 62].

23.4.4.1 Clinical Signs Associated with Vestibular Disease

When there is vestibular dysfunction, patients may exhibit one or more of the following signs [40, 57, 60, 61, 63–68]:

- Vestibular ataxia, with the patient falling toward the side of the lesion in unilateral disease.
- Circling with a tight-turning radius.

- Rolling.
- Head tilt:
  - Usually toward the side of the lesion in cases of peripheral vestibular disease.
  - To either side in cases of central vestibular disease.
- Pathologic nystagmus, meaning that there are distinct fast and slow phases:
  - Direction of nystagmus may be horizontal or rotary in cases of peripheral vestibular disease, with the fast phase typically away from the lesion.
  - Direction of nystagmus may be horizontal, vertical, or rotary in cases of central vestibular disease, and the direction may change as the head position changes in space.
- Crouched stance with wide, exaggerated, lateral excursions of the head in cases of bilateral peripheral vestibular disease. These patients tend to lack head tilts and pathologic nystagmus.
- Postural deficits ipsilateral to the lesion in cases of central vestibular disease.
- Conscious proprioception (CP) deficits, i.e. knuckling, ipsilateral to the lesion in cases of central vestibular disease.
- Altered consciousness in some, but not all, cases of central vestibular disease.
  Horner's syndrome.
  - Commonly seen in cases of peripheral vestibular disease.
  - Rare in cases of central vestibular disease.
- Vestibular strabismus.

Vestibular strabismus is also called positional strabismus [11, 40]. When the head and neck are extended, the patient experiences ventral to ventrolateral deviation of the globe [40]. This causes the sclera to be visible dorsally [40].

When the patient's head returns to a non-extended, relaxed position, the strabismus resolves [11, 40].

Positional strabismus may occur in dogs and cats, and with either central or peripheral vestibular disease [40, 61].

Positional strabismus is common in cases of vestibular disease [11].

However, positional strabismus is not pathognomonic for any root cause of vestibular disease, and the conditions that are reviewed below tend to present with much more consistent, striking signs. When it occurs, positional strabismus is noted, but secondary to a number of other clinical signs that point the clinician in the right direction of the presumptive diagnosis.

23.4.4.2 Causes of Peripheral Vestibular Disease

The most common cause of peripheral vestibular disease is otitis media or otitis interna [63]. This degree of inflammation typically stems from unresolved, persistent, and progressive otitis externa [40, 63]. Patients may present with non-neurologic signs such as head-shaking, aural discharge, temporomandibular pain, or pain over the affected bulla [40, 68, 69]. When these patients are examined, they frequently present with Horner's syndrome and have ipsilateral deficits associated with the facial (CN VII) and vestibulocochlear (CN VIII) nerves [40].

Otoscopy is an appropriate first step in the diagnostic work-up [40]. Myringotomy, with samples submitted for cytologic evaluation and culture, are important secondary steps [40]. *Staphylococcus* sp., *Pseudomonas, Streptococcus, Proteus, Candida,* and *Malassezia* are commonly cultured [40]. Culture and sensitivity panels are essential, particularly given the trend toward increasing multi-drug resistant *Pseudomonas* and *Staphylococcus* sp. [40].

In cats, middle and inner ear disease may also result from the presence of inflammatory polyps [40, 63]. Affected cats tend to be young and may have concurrent respiratory signs. The nasopharynx is the site of origin for many of these lesions [63].

Oropharyngeal and/or otoscopic examination are typically sufficient for presumptive diagnosis of nasopharyngeal polyps (see Figure 23.3).

Advanced imaging of the skull is indicated in patients with nasopharyngeal polyps to determine the extent of disease and bulla involvement [40].

Nasopharyngeal polyps can be removed orally, via traction polypectomy, or through the external ear if the tympanic cavity is not involved [40] (see Figures 23.4a–d).

Transient Horner's syndrome is common immediately following traction polypectomy (see Figure 23.5).

Thirty to forty percent of nasopharyngeal polyps recur after traction polypectomy [40].

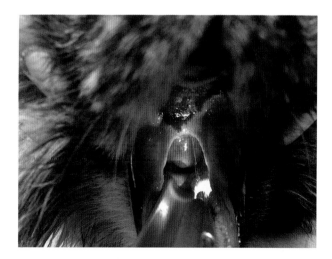

Figure 23.3 Oral exam of a feline patient with a nasopharyngeal polyp. *Source:* Courtesy of Daniel Foy, MS, DVM, DACVIM, DACVECC.

(a)

(b)

(c)

(d)

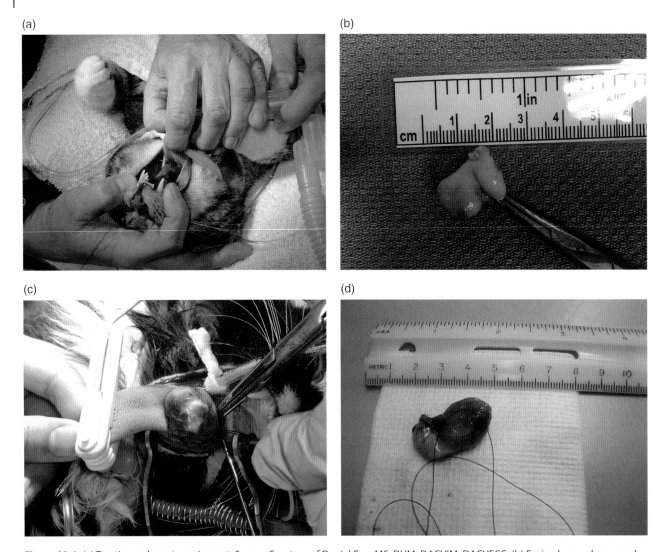

Figure 23.4 (a) Traction polypectomy in a cat. *Source:* Courtesy of Daniel Foy, MS, DVM, DACVIM, DACVECC. (b) Excised nasopharyngeal polyp. *Source:* Courtesy of Daniel Foy, MS, DVM, DACVIM, DACVECC. (c) Traction polypectomy in a cat. *Source:* Courtesy of Daniel Foy, MS, DVM, DACVIM, DACVECC. (d) Excised nasopharyngeal polyp. *Source:* Courtesy of Daniel Foy, MS, DVM, DACVIM, DACVECC.

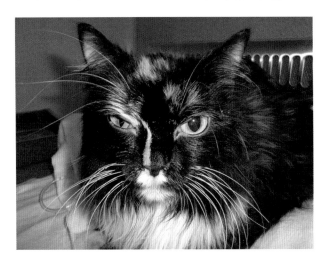

Figure 23.5 Horner's syndrome in a feline patient that just underwent traction polypectomy for a nasopharyngeal polyp. *Source:* Courtesy of Daniel Foy, MS, DVM, DACVIM, DACVECC.

In both dogs and cats, aural neoplasia may result in peripheral vestibular dysfunction [40]. Tumor types that are most commonly reported in this location include ceruminous adenomas and adenocarcinomas, sebaceous adenomas and adenocarcinomas, and squamous cell carcinomas [70, 71]. Feline aural lymphoma has also been reported [70, 71]. Approximately 85% and 60% of aural tumors in cats and dogs, respectively, are malignant [40, 70, 71]. Most can be visualized on otoscopic examination [40]. Occasionally, swellings external to the ear are palpable [40]. Advanced imaging is required to identify the extent of disease. Lysis of the bulla and/or petrous temporal bone is associated with neoplasia as compared to aural inflammatory disease [40].

Another common cause of peripheral vestibular disease in canine patients is idiopathic "old dog" vestibular disease [63]. The etiology of this condition remains unknown; however, clients frequently report that their dog had a "stroke" [63]. Onset is rapid, acute to peracute, and patients may develop gastrointestinal signs related to motion sickness [63]. Nausea and vomiting are common [63]. Patients typically respond to supportive care, although any head tilt that develops as a result of this condition may persist [63].

Cats may also develop idiopathic vestibular disease; however, young patients appear to be affected as often as seniors [72]. In other words, there is a bimodal distribution [72]. For reasons unknown to the author, seasonal changes may precipitate the development of this condition in cats [72]. Cats with idiopathic vestibular disease tend to have bilateral involvement [72].

Less common causes of peripheral vestibular disease include the following [40, 63]:

- Ototoxicity
- Vascular accident
- Hypothyroidism
- Neuromas or neurofibromas of CN VIII
- Trauma to the petrous temporal bone, which houses the semicircular canals, vestibule, and cochlea

Ototoxicity may result from topically or systemically administered agents [63]. The link between aminoglycosides and ototoxicity has been well established [63]. Vestibular signs are more likely to result from the use of streptomycin, whereas gentamycin and neomycin are more likely to be detrimental to the sense of hearing [63].

In addition, certain breeds have been reported to develop a congenital form of peripheral vestibular disease between birth and three months of age [63]. Those that classically exhibit unilateral disease include Siamese and Burmese cats as well as English Cocker Spaniels, Doberman Pinschers, and German Shepherds [63]. Beagles and Akitas are more apt to develop bilateral disease [63].

23.4.4.3 Causes of Central Vestibular Disease

There are many causes of central vestibular disease, including the following [63, 73–75]:

- Primary neoplasia
- Metastatic neoplasia
- Thiamine (vitamin B1) deficiency
- Inflammatory disease
- Toxicity
- Infectious disease
- Vascular accident
- Trauma

Meningiomas, choroid plexus tumors, and gliomas are the most common types of intracranial neoplasia in dogs and cats [40, 63]. Advanced imaging is required to document extent of disease and for either surgical or radiation planning [63]. Magnetic resonance imaging (MRI) is preferred to computed tomography (CT) in cases of presumptive intracranial neoplasia [40]. The latter modality causes an artifact that makes it challenging to identify small lesions within the cerebellum, pons, and medulla [40].

Thiamine deficiency in cats is typically due to an all-fish diet [63, 76–78]. Because raw fish contains thiaminase, patients become deficient [63, 78].

Deficiency develops rapidly, causing necrosis of brain tissue and hemorrhage within the gray matter [63, 73, 79]. The classic sign of thiamine deficiency in cats is ventroflexion of the cervical spine [63]. Strabismus is possible, but rare. More commonly, pupils are dilated, but aligned.

Thiamine may also be destroyed in cooked food due to heating [78].

Thiamine deficiency has been produced experimentally in dogs, and has been identified in clinical practice as a result of feeding sulfite-preserved meat [73, 74]. Sulfites render thiamine inactive [73, 75].

Granulomatous meningoencephalomyelitis (GME) is the most likely form of inflammatory disease in dogs [63]. It rarely occurs in cats [63]. Small breed dogs appear to be predisposed [63]. At onset, patients are typically young to middle-aged [63]. Cerebral spinal fluid (CSF) collection yields an inflammatory fluid that supports this diagnosis [63]. Biopsy is required, but rarely performed, for confirmation. Patients may initially respond to corticosteroids or other forms of anti-inflammatory and/or immunomodulatory drugs [63]. However, disease is progressive, and most succumb within three months to a year of diagnosis [63].

Infectious causes of central vestibular disease are varied; however, the most commonly implicated agents include the following [40, 63]:

- Viruses
  - Rabies virus
  - Canine distemper virus
  - Feline infectious peritonitis (FIP)
- Protozoa
  - Toxoplasmosis in cats and dogs
  - *Neospora caninum* in dogs
- Fungi
  - *Cryptococcus neoformans*
  - *Coccidioides immitis*
  - *Blastomycosis*
  - *Histoplasmosis*

Clinical signs associated with each of the above are beyond the scope of this text. An infectious disease text should be consulted to assess those cases in which there is a high index of suspicion.

Be aware that such cases will present with an array of clinical signs, not just strabismus.

References

1 Englar, R.E. (2017). *Performing the Small Animal Physical Examination*. Hoboken, NJ: Wiley.

2 Dyce, K.M., Sack, W.O., and Wensing, C.J.G. (2010). *Textbook of Veterinary Anatomy*, 4e, xii, 834 p. St. Louis, Mo.: Saunders/Elsevier.

3 Evans, H.E. and DeLahunta, A. (2004). *Guide to the Dissection of the Dog*, 6e, xiv, 378 p. St. Louis, Mo.: Saunders.

4 Evans, H.E. and Miller, M.E. (2013). *Miller's Anatomy of the Dog*, 4e, xix, 850 p. St. Louis, Missouri: Elsevier.

5 Maggs, D.J., Miller, P.E., Ofri, R., and Slatter, D.H. (2013). *Slatter's Fundamentals of Veterinary Ophthalmology*, 5e, x, 506 p. St. Louis, Mo: Elsevier.

6 Penderis, J. (2008). Recognition of Common Cranial Nerve Abnormalities in Dogs and Cats. ACVIM Proceedings [Internet]. https://www.vin.com/apputil/content/defaultadv1.aspx?id=3865564&pid=11262&print-1.

7 Tilley, L.P. and Smith, F.W.K. (2016). *Blackwell's Five-Minute Veterinary Consult. Canine and Feline*, 6e, lxix, 1622 p. Ames, Iowa, USA: Wiley.

8 Peterson, M.E. and Kutzler, M.A. (2011). *Small Animal Pediatrics: The First 12 Months of Life*, xvi, 526 p. St. Louis, Mo.: Saunders/Elsevier.

9 Delahunta, A. (1997). The neurological examination. *Vet. Q.* 19 (sup1): 6–8.

10 Gelatt, K.N. and Plummer, C.E. (2001). *Color Atlas of Veterinary Ophthalmology*. Ames, IA: Wiley-Blackwell.

11 Dewey, C.W. and Da Costa, R.C. (2016). *Practical Guide to Canine and Feline Neurology*, 3e, xi, 672 p. Chichester, West Sussex; Hoboken: Wiley-Blackwell.

12 Mitchell, N. (2006). Feline ophthalmology part I: examination of the eye. *Irish Vet. J.* 59 (3): 164–168.

13 Gunton, K.B., Wasserman, B.N., and DeBenedictis, C. (2015). Strabismus. *Prim. Care* 42 (3): 393–407.

14 Campos, E.C. (2008). Why do the eyes cross? A review and discussion of the nature and origin of essential infantile esotropia, microstrabismus, accommodative esotropia, and acute comitant esotropia. *J. AAPOS* 12 (4): 326–331.

15 Ketring, K.L. and Glaze, M.B. (2012). *Atlas of Feline Ophthalmology*, 2e, xviii, 172 p. Chichester, West Sussex, UK; Ames, Iowa: Wiley-Blackwell.

16 Rutstein, R.P. (2011). Care of the Patient with Strabismus: Esotropia and Exotropia. American Optometric Association [Internet]. https://www.aoa.org/documents/optometrists/CPG-12.pdf.

17 Allgoewer, I., Blair, M., Basher, T. et al. (2000). Extraocular muscle myositis and restrictive strabismus in 10 dogs. *Vet. Ophthalmol.* 3 (1): 21–26.

18 O'Neill, J.J., Kent, M., Glass, E.N. et al. (2013). Insertion of the dorsal oblique muscle in the dog: an anatomic

basis for ventral strabismus associated with oculomotor nerve dysfunction. *Vet. Ophthalmol.* 16 (6): 467–471.

19 Crispin, S.M. (2007). Examination of the feline eye and adnexa. *European Journal of Companion Animal Practice (EJCAP)* 17 (3): 1–15.

20 Chandler, E.A., Hilbery, A.D.R., and Gaskell, C.J. (1985). *British Small Animal Veterinary Association. Feline Medicine and Therapeutics*, ix, 405 p., 10 p. of plates p. Oxford; Boston: Blackwell Scientific Publications: USA, St Louis Blackwell Mosby Book Distributors.

21 Scagliotti, R.H. (1999). Comparative neuro-ophthalmology. In: *Veterinary Ophthalmology*, 3e (ed. K.N. Gelatt), 1307–1400. Philadelphia: Lippincott Williams & Wilkins.

22 Stokking, L.B. and Campbell, K.C. (2004). Disorders of pigmentation. In: *Small Animal Dermatology Secrets* (ed. K.C. Campbell), 352–355. Philadelphia: Hanley & Belfus.

23 Gebhardt, R.H., Pond, G., and Raleigh, I. (1979). *A Standard Guide to Cat Breeds*, 319 p. New York: McGraw-Hill.

24 Association CF. (1994–2004). Cat Colors FAQ: Cat Color Genetics [Available from: http://www.fanciers.com/other-faqs/color-genetics.html].

25 Lyons, L.A., Imes, D.L., Rah, H.C., and Grahn, R.A. (2005). Tyrosinase mutations associated with Siamese and Burmese patterns in the domestic cat (Felis catus). *Anim. Genet.* 36 (2): 119–126.

26 Ye, X.C., Pegado, V., Patel, M.S., and Wasserman, W.W. (2014). Strabismus genetics across a spectrum of eye misalignment disorders. *Clin. Genet.* 86 (2): 103–111.

27 Lennerstrand, G. (1979). Contractile properties of extraocular muscle in Siamese cat. *Acta Ophthalmol.* 57 (6): 1030–1038.

28 Duke-Elder, S. (1963). *System of Ophthalmology: Normal and Abnormal Development: Congenital Deformities*. St. Louis: Mosby.

29 Guillery, R.W., Casagrande, V.A., and Oberdorfer, M.D. (1974). Congenitally abnormal vision in Siamese cats. *Nature* 252 (5480): 195–199.

30 Guillery, R.W. and Kaas, J.H. (1971). Study of Normal and congenitally abnormal retinogeniculate projections in cats. *J. Comp. Neurol.* 143 (1): 73–100.

31 Guillery, R.W. (1969). An abnormal retinogeniculate projection in Siamese cats. *Brain Res.* 14 (3): 739–741.

32 Kalil, R.E., Jhaveri, S.R., and Richards, W. (1971). Anomalous retinal pathways in the Siamese cat: an inadequate substrate for normal bionocular vision. *Science* 174 (4006): 302–305.

33 Shatz, C. (1977). A comparison of visual pathways in Boston and Midwestern Siamese cats. *J. Comp. Neurol.* 171 (2): 205–228.

34 Cool, S.J. and Crawford, M.L. (1972). Absence of binocular coding in striate cortex units of Siamese cats. *Vis. Res.* 12 (11): 1809–1814.

35 Kaas, J.H. and Guillery, R.W. (1973). Transfer of abnormal visual-field representations from dorsal lateral geniculate nucleus to visual-cortex in siamese cats. *Brain Res.* 59 (Sep14): 61–95.

36 Hubel, D.H. and Wiesel, T.N. (1971). Aberrant visual projections in Siamese cat. *J. Physiol.* 218 (1): 33–62.

37 Packwood, J. and Gordon, B. (1975). Stereopsis in normal domestic cat, Siamese cat, and cat raised with alternating monocular occlusion. *J. Neurophysiol.* 38 (6): 1485–1499.

38 Rengstorff, R.H. (1976). Strabismus measurements in the Siamese cat. *Am. J. Optom. Physiol. Optic* 53 (10): 643–646.

39 August, J.R. (ed.) (2010). *Consultations in Feline Medicine*. St. Louis, MO: Saunders Elsevier.

40 Rossmeisl, J.H. Jr. (2010). Vestibular disease in dogs and cats. *Vet. Clin. North Am. Small Anim. Pract.* 40 (1): 81–100.

41 Troxel, M.T. (2016). Congenital hydrocephalus. *NAVC Clinician's Brief* (September): 26–30.

42 Regan, D.P., Kent, M., Mathes, R. et al. (2011). Clinicopathologic findings in a dog with a retrobulbar meningioma. *J. Vet. Diagn. Investig.* 23 (4): 857–862.

43 Aaroe, W.C. (2013). An eye on canine orbital disease: Causes, diagnostics, and treatment. DVM360 [Internet]. http://veterinarymedicine.dvm360.com/ eye-canine-orbital-disease-causes-diagnostics-and-treatment.

44 Gilger, B.C., Hamilton, H.L., Wilkie, D.A. et al. (1995). Traumatic ocular proptoses in dogs and cats: 84 cases (1980–1993). *J. Am. Vet. Med. Assoc.* 206 (8): 1186–1190.

45 Williams, D.L. (2008). Extraocular myositis in the dog. *Vet. Clin. North Am. Small* 38 (2): 347–359.

46 Betbeze, C. (2015). Management of Orbital Diseases. *Top. Companion Anim. Med.* 30 (3): 107–117.

47 Caruso, K., Marrion, R., and Silver, G. (2002). What is your diagnosis? – MRI diagnosis – Retrobulbar mass indenting the inferior aspect of the right globe. The mass involved the optic nerve but did not appear to invade the cranial vault; the inferior aspect of the mass was less defined. *J. Am. Vet. Med. Assoc.* 221 (11): 1553–1554.

48 Haak, C.E., Breshears, M.A., and Lackner, P.A. (2007). What is your diagnosis? *J. Am. Vet. Med. Assoc.* 231 (6): 863–864.

49 Tilley, L.P., FWK, S., and Tilley, L.P. (eds.) (2007). Orbital Diseases. In: *Blackwell's Five-Minute Veterinary Consult: Canine and Feline*, 4e, 940–941. Ames, Iowa: Blackwell.

50 Boroffka, S.A.E.B. (1996). Exophthalmos in dogs: a challenge for diagnostic imaging. *Vet. Q.* 18: 56.

51 van der Woerdt, A. (2008). Orbital inflammatory disease and pseudotumor in dogs and cats. *Vet. Clin. North Am. Small* 38 (2): 389–401.

52 Gilger, B.C., McLaughlin, S.A., Whitley, R.D., and Wright, J.C. (1992). Orbital neoplasms in cats: 21 cases (1974–1990). *J. Am. Vet. Med. Assoc.* 201 (7): 1083–1086.

53 Pentlarge, V.W., Powell-Johnson, G., Martin, C.L. et al. (1989). Orbital neoplasia with enophthalmos in a cat. *J. Am. Vet. Med. Assoc.* 195 (9): 1249–1251.

54 Ofri, R. (2014). Differentiating exophthalmos, buphthalmos, & proptosis. *NAVC Clinician's Brief* (May): 29–31.

55 McDonald, J. and Knollinger, A. (2016). Diagnosing canine exophthalmos. *NAVC Clinician's Brief* (May): 75–78.

56 Spiess, B.M. (2007). Diseases and surgery of the canine orbit. In: *Veterinary Ophthalmology* (ed. K.N. Gelatt), 539–562. Ames, IA: Blackwell Publishing.

57 DeLahunta, A., Glass, E., and Kent, M. (2015.). *Veterinary Neuroanatomy and Clinical Neurology*, 4e. St. Louis, MO: Elsevier.

58 Angelaki, D.E. and Cullen, K.E. (2008). Vestibular system: the many facets of a multimodal sense. *Annu. Rev. Neurosci.* 31: 125–150.

59 Brandt, T. and Strupp, M. (2005). General vestibular testing. *Clin. Neurophysiol.* 116 (2): 406–426.

60 Thomas, W.B. (2000). Vestibular dysfunction. *Vet. Clin. North Am. Small Anim. Pract.* 30 (1): 227–249, viii.

61 Troxel, M.T., Drobatz, K.J., and Vite, C.H. (2005). Signs of neurologic dysfunction in dogs with central versus peripheral vestibular disease. *J. Am. Vet. Med. Assoc.* 227 (4): 570–574.

62 Rylander, H. (2012). Vestibular syndrome: What's causing the head tilt and other neurologic signs? DVM360 [Internet]. http://veterinarymedicine.dvm360.com/ vestibular-syndrome-whats-causing-head-tilt-and-other-neurologic-signs.

63 LeCouteur, R.A. (2009). Vestibular disorders of dogs and cats. CVC Proceedings [Internet]. http://veterinarycalendar. dvm360.com/vestibular-disorders-dogs-and-cats-proceedings.

64 Sanders, S.G. and Bagley, R.S. (2003). Disorders of hearing and balance: the vestibulocochlear nerve (VIII) and associated structures. In: *A Practical Guide to Canine and Feline Neurology* (ed. C.W. Dewey), 213–240. Ames, IA: Iowa State Press.

65 LeCouteur, R.A. (2003). Feline vestibular diseases--new developments. *J. Feline Med. Surg.* 5 (2): 101–108.

66 LeCouteur, R.A. and Vernau, K.M. (1999). Feline vestibular disorders. Part I: anatomy and clinical signs. *J. Feline Med. Surg.* 1 (2): 71–80.

67 Schunk, K.L. (1988). Disorders of the vestibular system. *Vet. Clin. North Am. Small* 18 (3): 641–665.

68 Schunk, K.L. and Averill, D.R. (1983). Peripheral vestibular syndrome in the dog – a review of 83 cases. *J. Am. Vet. Med. Assoc.* 182 (12): 1354–1357.

69 Shell, L.G. (1988). Otitis media and otitis interna. Etiology, diagnosis, and medical management. *Vet. Clin. North Am. Small Anim. Pract.* 18 (4): 885–899.

70 Fan, T.M. and de Lorimier, L.P. (2004). Inflammatory polyps and aural neoplasia. *Vet. Clin. North Am. Small Anim. Pract.* 34 (2): 489–509.

71 London, C.A., Dubilzeig, R.R., Vail, D.M. et al. (1996). Evaluation of dogs and cats with tumors of the ear canal: 145 cases (1978–1992). *J. Am. Vet. Med. Assoc.* 208 (9): 1413–1418.

72 Pancotta, T. (ed.) (2016). *Central vs. Peripheral Vestibular Diseases*. CVC.

73 Singh, M., Thompson, M., Sullivan, N., and Child, G. (2005). Thiamine deficiency in dogs due to the feeding of sulphite preserved meat. *Aust. Vet. J.* 83 (7): 412–417.

74 Read, D.H. and Harrington, D.D. (1981). Experimentally induced thiamine deficiency in beagle dogs: clinical observations. *Am. J. Vet. Res.* 42 (6): 984–991.

75 Studdert, V.P. and Labuc, R.H. (1991). Thiamin deficiency in cats and dogs associated with feeding meat preserved with Sulphur dioxide. *Aust. Vet. J.* 68 (2): 54–57.

76 Jubb, K.V., Saunders, L.Z., and Coates, H.V. (1956). Thiamine deficiency encephalopathy in cats. *J. Comp. Pathol.* 66 (3): 217–227.

77 Loew, F.M., Martin, C.L., Dunlop, R.H. et al. (1970). Naturally-occurring and experimental thiamin deficiency in cats receiving commercial cat food. *Can. Vet. J.* 11 (6): 109–113.

78 Moon, S.J., Kang, M.H., and Park, H.M. (2013). Clinical signs, MRI features, and outcomes of two cats with thiamine deficiency secondary to diet change. *J. Vet. Sci.* 14 (4): 499–502.

79 Oliver, J.E., Hoerlein, B.F., and Mayhew, I.G. (1987). *Veterinary Neurology*. Philadelphia: Saunders.

24

Nystagmus

24.1 Introduction to Nystagmus and Associated Terminology

Chapter 23 reviewed the normal alignment of the eyes relative to each other and how coordination of extraocular eye muscles allows for conjugate eye movement. In health, both eyes move together smoothly to fixate on an object that falls within the patient's visual field. This requires input from cranial nerves, functional visual pathways, and higher centers that include the vestibular systems. Review Section 23.4.4 to recall the anatomy of the central and peripheral vestibular systems.

This chapter emphasizes altered movements of the globes such that one or both globes experience involuntary, rhythmic oscillations. This clinical presentation is called nystagmus [1–3]. To an observer, it may appear that the eyes are ricocheting back and forth without focusing.

Oscillations of the globes may be described in terms of their direction [4]:

- Vertical nystagmus involves oscillations that move the globe(s) in a dorsal-ventral (up/down) plane.
- Horizontal nystagmus involves oscillations that move the globe(s) in a side-to-side (left/right or right/left) plane.
- Rotary or torsional nystagmus involves oscillations along the globe's rostral-caudal axis.

Note that these directional terms are not necessarily exclusive. One type of directional nystagmus may be superimposed on another.

Nystagmus may also be described by its fluidity using the following terms [1, 3]:

- Pendular nystagmus
- Jerk nystagmus

Pendular nystagmus is characterized as being all slow-phase, fluid oscillations of equal velocity [3]. Contrast this presentation with that of jerk nystagmus. Jerk nystagmus is biphasic. In jerk nystagmus, one or both globes

move slowly in one direction, only to bounce back rapidly in the opposite direction [1, 3].

As expected, the so-called fast phase refers to the direction of rapid rebound.

Note that, for any given patient, the fast phase depends upon the underlying disease. Lesion localization is critical to facilitate diagnosis and case management.

Finally, nystagmus may also be described as [5]

- Physiologic
- Spontaneous
- Positional.

Physiologic nystagmus is normal and transient. It occurs with routine head position changes as long as the oculomotor nerve (CN III), the abducens (CN VI), and the vestibulocochlear (CN VIII) nerves are intact[6].

Physiologic nystagmus has a slow phase and a fast phase. The fast phase is in the direction of the head turn [4]. For example, if the patient turned its head to the left, both globes would be expected to display horizontal nystagmus. The globes would display a few tics, with the fast phase to the left [5].

Likewise, if the patient turned its head to the right, both globes would initially oscillate in that direction, with the fast phase to the right [5].

Once the head settles into its new position, physiologic nystagmus abates.

Clinicians may also induce physiologic nystagmus in normal animals by turning the patient's head instead of the patient executing the motion on its own [7]. Physiologic nystagmus will occur with head position changes that are up-down and side-to-side.

Spontaneous or resting nystagmus, on the other hand, occurs in the absence of head position changes [4, 5, 7, 8]. This is pathologic [7].

Positional nystagmus occurs only when head position is extremely unusual, such as upside down, as opposed to the typical everyday motions of up-down and side-to-side [5, 8].

24.2 Primary Causes of Pendular Nystagmus

Pendular nystagmus is much less frequently seen in clinical practice than jerk nystagmus [3]. When it occurs, pendular nystagmus is an indication that there is abnormal development of central visual pathways due to aberrant rerouting of axonal projections from the eye to the brain [9–18].

This congenital condition is common in imperfect albino cats [3, 10]. Because of their color-point coats, Siamese, Birmans, and Himalayans are predisposed [8–10].

Recall from Chapter 23, Section 23.3 that these breeds are also predisposed to esotropia [19, 20]. Esotropia and pendular nystagmus often present concurrently in the same cat [9, 10, 21].

24.3 Primary Causes of Jerk Nystagmus

Unlike pendular nystagmus, jerk nystagmus is typically acquired and most commonly results from vestibular disease [8]. Recall from Chapter 23, Section 23.4.4 that vestibular disease involves dysfunction of the balance centers of the body, and may have peripheral or central origins [22–25]. Compromise of one or both of these components leads to aberrant body and head posture, eye position, eye movement, and gait [22, 26–34].

Jerk nystagmus, in combination with a head tilt, indicates vestibular compromise [8].

In addition, patients with vestibular disease may develop ataxia, circling, and positional strabismus: head elevation may cause the globe on the affected side to deviate ventrally or ventrolaterally [8, 22, 26–34].

Head tilts and jerk nystagmus are typically extinguished in patients with bilateral disease [8]. These patients tend to crouch and move the head side-to-side in exaggerated, swaying movements [8].

Review Chapter 23, Section 23.4.4 to recall the most common causes of peripheral and central vestibular disease. This chapter will address select causes that were not previously explored.

24.3.1 Metronidazole Toxicity

Metronidazole is frequently prescribed in companion animal practice as an antibiotic and antidiarrheal agent [35, 36]. It has been used to treat giardiasis and *Helicobacter*-associated gastritis [35–39]. In addition, it may reduce neurologic signs in patients with hepatic encephalopathy by decreasing the amount of ammonia-producing bacteria in the colon [35, 36, 40–43].

Metronidazole toxicity is an established cause of central vestibular disease [31, 44–46]. Affected patients typically present after chronic use with ataxia and nystagmus, paresis, and/or seizures [31, 35, 36, 47–51].

Doses that exceed 60 mg/kg per day are considered toxic [31]. However, there is immense individual variability in terms of sensitivity, and cats as a species appear to be much more sensitive to metronidazole than dogs [36]. This is likely because their ability to use glucuronidation to metabolize metronidazole is diminished as compared to dogs [48].

Metronidazole should be immediately discontinued in patients that develop presumptive toxicity [48]. Supportive care and injectable diazepam may speed improvement of clinical signs [35, 48, 49, 52]. However, it may take two weeks for complete resolution [48].

24.3.2 Permethrin Toxicity

Permethrin is a pyrethroid [53, 54]. This is a synthetic insecticide. Its actions are intended to replicate those of the naturally occurring ester, pyrethrin, which is extracted from the flower of the *Chrysanthemum* [54] (see Figure 24.1).

In low doses, pyrethrins act as insect repellants. Higher doses target the nervous systems of insects. Specifically, pyrethrins target sodium channels, integral proteins through which ion transport of sodium into the cell is linked to the process of depolarization [54, 55].

In the absence of pyrethrin, these channels close after an action potential passes through a cell. In the presence of pyrethrin, these channels remain open [54, 55]. This allows for prolonged influx of sodium that results in the cell being repeatedly discharged. Hyperexcitation of nerve cells leads to loss of function, paralysis, and insect death.

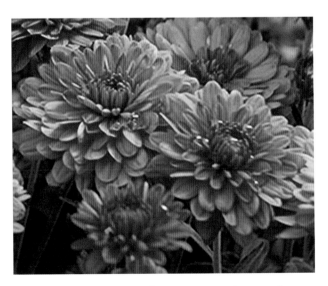

Figure 24.1 *Chrysanthemum* flowers as a natural source of insecticide.

If mammals are inadvertently exposed to pyrethroids, either through ingestion or dermal absorption, most are able to metabolize and excrete it rapidly without ill effect [54, 55]. Metabolism of these agents relies heavily upon hepatic glucuronidation [54, 56, 57]. Because cats are deficient in hepatic glucuronosyltransferase, the enzyme required for glucuronidation, they are extraordinarily sensitive to the effects of permethrin [54, 55]. Permethrin is exceptionally toxic because of its enhanced potency as compared to pyrethrin. In addition, pyrethroids are more stable in the environment, which means that they last longer. This combination has the potential to be lethal in feline patients [54, 55]. Nervous tissue readily takes up permethrin. It is not uncommon for permethrin concentration within the brain to reach 1.5–7.5 times the concentration of the blood [53, 58].

Cats are typically exposed to permethrin via spot-on flea preventative treatments [54]. Clients may inadvertently apply canine flea preventative to cats [54]. Canine products frequently contain permethrin.

Alternatively, cat owners may have purchased unsafe, over-the-counter feline flea preventative that contains permethrin.

Clinical signs are rapid in onset: most develop within minutes to hours of exposure [54, 55]. It is rare, but possible, to observe a delayed onset, meaning 24–72 h after topical application [54–56, 59].

Nystagmus is one of many clinical signs associated with permethrin toxicosis [53]. Clients may report mydriasis, ear flicking, paw shaking, shivering, twitching, tremoring, muscle fasciculations, and hyperesthesia [54, 55].

On presentation, patients may be febrile and/or ataxic [54, 55].

In addition, patients with oral exposure, for instance, those that may have licked the application site of a spot-on preventative treatment, may present with ptyalism [54]. Death may result from cardiac arrhythmias, tachypnea, and cardiac and/or respiratory arrest [54, 56, 60–63].

Treatment of affected patients emphasizes decontamination and supportive care [54].

24.3.3 Toxoplasmosis

Toxoplasmosis infects cats, dogs, humans, and most other mammals [64]. However, only members of the family, *Felidae*, are definitive hosts that excrete oocysts of the protozoan parasite, *Toxoplasma gondii* [64, 65]. Infection occurs through one of three primary routes [64]:

- Congenital transmission during pregnancy via placentitis
- Ingestion of food and/or water that has been contaminated with oocysts
- Ingestion of intermediate hosts whose central nervous system (CNS), muscle, and visceral organs contain cysts

Toxoplasmosis may also be spread through infected milk, blood transfusion, and organ transplantation [64].

Clinical toxoplasmosis is aggravated by stress and/or concurrent disease [64]. For example, canine distemper virus and ehrlichiosis have been linked to canine toxoplasmosis [64]. Immunosuppressive disease, such as feline leukemia virus (FeLV) and feline immunodeficiency virus (FIV), often are concurrent with clinical toxoplasmosis in cats [64]. Prolonged use of glucocorticoids in both dogs and cats may also precipitate clinical disease [64].

Consult an infectious disease text for details on the enteroepithelial and extraintestinal, asexual and sexual life cycles of *T. gondii* and its pathogenesis.

Recognize that *T. gondii* can induce a constellation of clinical signs, many of which are nonspecific [64]. Cats are more varied in their presentations than dogs: clinical toxoplasmosis in cats may result in pulmonary, CNS, hepatic, pancreatic, cardiac, and ocular syndromes [64]. Clinical disease in dogs, on the other hand, tends to limit itself to the respiratory, gastrointestinal, and neuromuscular systems [64].

Note that neurologic dysfunction is possible in both dogs and cats [64]. Ataxia, behavioral changes, tremors, and seizures are consistent findings in a patient that has been affected with neurologic disease [64]. However, nystagmus is possible and appears in isolated case reports [65, 66].

Serologic testing to detect antibodies against *T. gondii* is commonly employed as a diagnostic tool [64]. However, it is important to remember that the presence of antibodies cannot distinguish between exposure and active disease [64]. In the United States alone, nearly one in three cats has antibodies against *T. gondii* [64, 67].

24.3.4 Feline Infectious Peritonitis

Feline infectious peritonitis (FIP) is a systemic viral infection [3, 68].

Affected cats can be any age at time of onset; however, those less than two years old are most likely to present [68].

There are two primary clinical presentations for FIP [3, 68]:

- Effusive ("wet")
- Non-effusive ("dry")

Effusive FIP is associated with ascites and/or thoracic effusion [68]. Roughly 12% of affected patients develop neurological disease [68].

By contrast, non-effusive FIP is associated with the development of granulomatous-to-pyogranulomatous lesions throughout the body [68]. Lesions can be anywhere [68]. However, they tend to concentrate within abdominal organs, globes, lung surfaces, and the vasculature of the CNS [68]. One-fourth to one-third of cats with non-effusive FIP develop neurological signs [68].

When neurological signs develop as a result of FIP, ataxia is most commonly seen [68]. Nystagmus is the second most common presenting sign, followed by seizures [68–71].

Diagnosis of FIP without histologic examination is a challenge. FIP antibody tests cannot differentiate between exposure to feline coronavirus and active infection with FIP, and gross appearance of lesions in cases of non-effusive FIP at necropsy is highly variable [68]. Pyogranulomas and vasculitis are essential histopathologic changes to make the diagnosis [68]. The presence of the virus within affected tissues via immunohistochemistry is confirmatory [68].

Consult an infectious disease text for details on viral etiology and pathogenesis.

References

1   Côté, E. (2015). *Clinical Veterinary Advisor. Dogs and Cats*, 3e, xxxvii, 1642 p. St. Louis, Missouri: Elsevier Mosby.

2   Englar, R.E. (2017). *Performing the Small Animal Physical Examination*. Hoboken, NJ: Wiley.

3   Tilley, L.P., Smith, F.W.K., and Tilley, L.P. (2007). *Blackwell's Five-Minute Veterinary Consult: Canine and Feline*, 4e. Ames, Iowa: Blackwell.

4   Abramson, C.J. (ed.) (2009). *The Neurological Examination: How to Describe What you See & Know if it Is Normal*. Phoenix, AZ: American Animal Hospital Association.

5   Schubert T. (2018). Physical and Neurologic Examinations. Merck Vet Manual [Internet]. http://www.merckvetmanual.com/nervous-system/nervous-system-introduction/physical-and-neurologic-examinations.

6   Mitchell, N. (2006). Feline ophthalmology part I: examination of the eye. *Ir. Vet.* 59 (3): 164–168.

7   LeCouteur RA. (2009). Vestibular disorders of dogs and cats. DVM 360 [Internet]. http://veterinarycalendar.dvm360.com/vestibular-disorders-dogs-and-cats-proceedings.

8   Munana, K. (2013). Head tilt and nystagmus. In: *BSAVA Manual of Canine and Feline Neurology*, 4e (ed. S.R. Platt and N.J. Olby). Quedgeley, Gloucester: British Small Animal Veterinary Association.

9   Crispin, S.M. (2007). Examination of the feline eye and adnexa. *Eur. J. Companion Anim. Pract.* 17 (3): 1–15.

10   Tilley, L.P. and Smith, F.W.K. (2016). *Blackwell's Five-Minute Veterinary Consult. Canine and Feline*, 6e, lxix, 1622 p. Ames, Iowa, USA: Wiley.

11   Guillery, R.W., Casagrande, V.A., and Oberdorfer, M.D. (1974). Congenitally abnormal vision in Siamese cats. *Nature* 252 (5480): 195–199.

12   Guillery, R.W. and Kaas, J.H. (1971). Study of Normal and congenitally abnormal Retinogeniculate projections in cats. *J. Comp. Neurol.* 143 (1): 73–100.

13   Guillery, R.W. (1969). An abnormal retinogeniculate projection in Siamese cats. *Brain Res.* 14 (3): 739–741.

14   Kalil, R.E., Jhaveri, S.R., and Richards, W. (1971). Anomalous retinal pathways in the Siamese cat: an inadequate substrate for normal bioncular vision. *Science* 174 (4006): 302–305.

15   Shatz, C. (1977). A comparison of visual pathways in Boston and Midwestern Siamese cats. *J. Comp. Neurol.* 171 (2): 205–228.

16   Cool, S.J. and Crawford, M.L. (1972). Absence of binocular coding in striate cortex units of Siamese cats. *Vis. Res.* 12 (11): 1809–&.

17   Kaas, J.H. and Guillery, R.W. (1973). Transfer of abnormal visual-field representations from dorsal lateral geniculate nucleus to visual-cortex in Siamese cats. *Brain Res.* 59 (Sep14): 61–95.

18   Hubel, D.H. and Wiesel, T.N. (1971). Aberrant visual projections in Siamese cat. *J. Physiol. Lond.* 218 (1): 33–62.

19   Peterson, M.E. and Kutzler, M.A. (2011). *Small Animal Pediatrics: The First 12 Months of Life*, xvi, 526 p. St. Louis, Mo: Saunders/Elsevier.

20   Chandler, E.A., Hilbery, A.D.R., and Gaskell, C.J. (1985). *British Small Animal Veterinary Association. Feline Medicine and Therapeutics*, ix, 405 p., 10 p. of plates p. Oxford; Boston: Blackwell Scientific Publications: USA, St Louis Blackwell Mosby Book Distributors.

21   Johnson, B.W. (1991). Congenitally abnormal visual pathways of Siamese cats. *Compend. Cont. Educ. Pract.* 13 (3): 374–378.

22   Rossmeisl, J.H. Jr. (2010). Vestibular disease in dogs and cats. *Vet. Clin. North Am. Small Anim. Pract.* 40 (1): 81–100.

23   Rylander H. (2012). Vestibular syndrome: What's causing the head tilt and other neurologic signs? DVM360 [Internet]. http://veterinarymedicine.dvm360.com/vestibular-syndrome-whats-causing-head-tilt-and-other-neurologic-signs.

24   Evans, H.E. and DeLahunta, A. (2004). *Guide to the Dissection of the Dog*, 6e, xiv, 378 p. St. Louis, Mo: Saunders.

25   Evans, H.E. and Miller, M.E. (2013). *Miller's Anatomy of the Dog*, 4e, xix, 850 p. St. Louis, Missouri: Elsevier.

26 Thomas, W.B. (2000). Vestibular dysfunction. *Vet. Clin. North Am. Small Anim. Pract.* 30 (1): 227–249, viii.

27 DeLahunta, A., Glass, E., and Kent, M. (2015). *Veterinary Neuroanatomy and Clinical Neurology*, 4e. St. Louis, MO: Elsevier.

28 Troxel, M.T., Drobatz, K.J., and Vite, C.H. (2005). Signs of neurologic dysfunction in dogs with central versus peripheral vestibular disease. *J. Am. Vet. Med. Assoc.* 227 (4): 570–574.

29 Sanders, S.G. and Bagley, R.S. (2003). Disorders of hearing and balance: the vestibulocochlear nerve (VIII) and associated structures. In: *A Practical Guide to Canine and Feline Neurology* (ed. C.W. Dewey), 213–240. Ames, IA: Iowa State Press.

30 LeCouteur, R.A. (2003). Feline vestibular diseases–new developments. *J. Feline Med. Surg.* 5 (2): 101–108.

31 LeCouteur RA. (2009). Vestibular disorders of dogs and cats. CVC Proceedings [Internet]. http://veterinarycalendar.dvm360.com/vestibular-disorders-dogs-and-cats-proceedings.

32 LeCouteur, R.A. and Vernau, K.M. (1999). Feline vestibular disorders. Part I: anatomy and clinical signs. *J. Feline Med. Surg.* 1 (2): 71–80.

33 Schunk, K.L. (1988). Disorders of the vestibular system. *Vet. Clin. N. Am. Small Anim. Pract.* 18 (3): 641–665.

34 Schunk, K.L. and Averill, D.R. (1983). Peripheral vestibular syndrome in the dog – a review of 83 cases. *J. Am. Vet. Med. Assoc.* 182 (12): 1354–1357.

35 Plumb, D.C. (2015). *Plumb's veterinary drug handbook*, 8e, 11 unnumbered pages, 1279 p. Stockholm, Wisconsin Ames, Iowa: Pharma Vet Inc. Distributed by John Wiley & Sons.

36 Olson, E.J., Morales, S.C., McVey, A.S., and Hayden, D.W. (2005). Putative metronidazole neurotoxicosis in a cat. *Vet. Pathol.* 42 (5): 665–669.

37 Strauss-Ayali, D. and Simpson, K.W. (1999). Gastric helicobacter infection in dogs. *Vet. Clin. N. Am. Small Anim. Pract.* 29 (2): 397–414.

38 Papich, M.G. (1993). Antiulcer therapy. *Vet. Clin. N. Am. Small Anim. Pract.* 23 (3): 497–512.

39 Groman, R. (2000). Metronidazole. *Comp. Cont. Educ. Pract.* 22 (12): 1104–+.

40 Salgado, M. and Cortes, Y. (2013). Hepatic encephalopathy: diagnosis and treatment. *Compend. Contin. Educ. Pract.* 35 (6): E1–E9; quiz E10.

41 Taboada, J. and Dimski, D.S. (1995). Hepatic encephalopathy: clinical signs, pathogenesis, and treatment. *Vet. Clin. North Am. Small Anim. Pract.* 25 (2): 337–355.

42 Tyler, J.W. (1990). Hepatoencephalopathy. 2. Pathophysiology and treatment. *Comp. Cont. Educ. Pract.* 12 (9): 1260–&.

43 Tyler, J.W. (1990). Hepatoencephalopathy. 1. Clinical signs and diagnosis. *Compend. Educ. Pract.* 12 (8): 1069–&.

44 Bichsel P, Lyman R. (2004). Metronidazole: Uses, toxicity and management of neurologic sequellae. DVM 360 [Internet]. http://veterinarynews.dvm360.com/metronidazole-uses-toxicity-and-management-neurologic-sequllae.

45 Lee JA. (2014). Metronidazole Risks. Clinician's Brief [Internet]:[10–1 pp.]. https://www.cliniciansbrief.com/sites/default/files/attachments/WOC_Metronidazole_final.pdf.

46 Caylor, K.B. and Cassimatis, M.K. (2001). Metronidazole neurotoxicosis in two cats. *J. Am. Anim. Hosp. Assoc.* 37 (3): 258–262.

47 Khan, S.A. and Hooser, S.B. (2012). Common Toxicologic issues in small animals preface. *Vet. Clin. N. Am. Small.* 42 (2): Xi–Xii.

48 Lee, J.A. (2014). Metronidazole risks. *NAVC Clinician's Brief* (September): 10.

49 Fitzgerald, K.T. (2013). Metronidazole. In: *Small Animal Toxicology*, 3e (ed. M.E. Peterson, P.A. Talcott and M.E. Peterson), 653–658. St. Louis, Mo: Elsevier.

50 Dow, S.W., LeCouteur, R.A., Poss, M.L., and Beadleston, D. (1989). Central nervous system toxicosis associated with metronidazole treatment of dogs: five cases (1984–1987). *J. Am. Vet. Med. Assoc.* 195 (3): 365–368.

51 Hajek, I., Simerdova, V., Vavra, M., and Agudelo, C.F. (2017). Toxic encephalopathy associated with high-dose metronidazole therapy in a dog: a case report. *Vet. Med.* 62 (2): 105–110.

52 Evans, J., Levesque, D., Knowles, K. et al. (2003). Diazepam as a treatment for metronidazole toxicosis in dogs: a retrospective study of 21 cases. *J. Vet. Intern. Med.* 17 (3): 304–310.

53 Muley, V.D., Dighe, D.G., Velhankar, R.D. et al. (2009). Therapeutic Management of Permethrin Toxicity in a kitten – a case report. *Vet. Pract.* 10 (2): 157–158.

54 Boland, L.A. and Angles, J.M. (2010). Feline permethrin toxicity: retrospective study of 42 cases. *J. Feline Med. Surg.* 12 (2): 61–71.

55 Richardson, J.A. (2000). Permethrin spot-on toxicoses in cats. *J. Vet. Emerg. Crit. Care* 10: 103–106.

56 Linnett, P.J. (2008). Permethrin toxicosis in cats. *Aust. Vet. J.* 86 (1–2): 32–35.

57 Whittem, T. (1995). Pyrethrin and Pyrethroid insecticide intoxication in cats. *Compend. Cont. Educ. Pract.* 17 (4): 489–492.

58 Anadon, A., Martinezlarranaga, M.R., Diaz, M.J., and Bringas, P. (1991). Toxicokinetics of Permethrin in the rat. *Toxicol. Appl. Pharmacol.* 110 (1): 1–8.

59 Meyer, E.K. (1999). Toxicosis in cats erroneously treated with 45 to 65% permethrin products. *J. Am. Vet. Med. Assoc.* 215 (2): 198–203.

60 Hansen, S.R. and Buck, W.B. (1992). Treatment of adverse reactions in cats to flea control products containing Pyrethrin Pyrethroid insecticides. *Feline Pract.* 20 (5): 25–27.

61 Hansen, S.R., Stemme, K.A., Villar, D., and Buck, W.B. (1994). Pyrethrins and Pyrethroids in dogs and cats. *Compend. Cont. Educ. Pract.* 16 (6): 707–&.

62 Gray, A. (2000). Permethrin toxicity in cats. *Vet. Rec.* 147 (19): 556.

63 Sutton, N.M., Bates, N., and Campbell, A. (2007). Clinical effects and outcome of feline permethrin spot-on poisonings reported to the veterinary poisons information service (VPIS), London. *J. Feline Med. Surg.* 9 (4): 335–339.

64 Dubey, J.P. and Lappin, M.R. (2006). Toxoplasmosis and Neosporosis. In: *Infectious Diseases of the Dog and Cat*, 3e (ed. C.E. Greene), 755–775. St. Louis, MO: Saunders/Elsevier.

65 Czopowicz, M., Szalus-Jordanow, O., and Frymus, T. (2010). Cerebral toxoplasmosis in a cat. *Med. Weter.* 66 (11): 784–786.

66 Spellman, P.G. (1988). Toxoplasmosis in cats. *Vet. Rec.* 122 (13): 311.

67 DeFeo, M.L., Dubey, J.P., Mather, T.N., and Rhodes, R.C. (2002). Epidemiologic investigation of seroprevalence of antibodies to Toxoplasma gondii in cats and rodents. *Am. J. Vet. Res.* 63 (12): 1714–1717.

68 Addie, D.D. and Jarrett, O. (2012). Feline coronavirus infections. In: *Infectious Diseases of the Dog and Cat*, 4e (ed. C.E. Greene). St. Louis, Mo: Elsevier/Saunders.

69 Baroni, M. and Heinold, Y. (1995). A review of the clinical-diagnosis of feline infectious peritonitis viral Meningoencephalomyelitis. *Prog. Vet. Neurol.* 6 (3): 88–94.

70 Kline, K.L., Joseph, R.J., and Averill, D.R. (1994). Feline infectious peritonitis with neurologic involvement – clinical and pathological findings in 24 cats. *J. Am. Anim. Hosp. Assoc.* 30 (2): 111–118.

71 Kornegay, J.N. (1978). Feline infectious peritonitis – central nervous-system form. *J. Am. Anim. Hosp. Assoc.* 14 (5): 580–584.

25

Reflex Blepharospasm

25.1 Introduction to Terminology

The upper and lower eyelids of cats and dogs, the palpebrae, are the bodyguards of the globe [1–5]. They exist largely for protection. When they close, they prevent external access to the eye [1, 3, 6].

Blinking is a protective reflex. Although blinking also facilitates the distribution of tear film across the globe's surface, it is primarily a mechanical barrier to the outside world. Blinking protects the eyes from wind, dust, and other foreign objects. Consider the menace response. The clinician uses this test to assess the function of the optic (II) and facial (VII) cranial nerves [7, 8]. Recall from Chapter 15, Section 15.2 that in this test the clinician makes a sudden movement toward each eye with his hand [7, 8]. If the patient is visual, it will see the threat coming toward the eye and blink [7, 8]. This is a protective action. This is expected and normal.

Any abnormal contraction of the eyelids is called blepharospasm [9]. Colloquially, some clinicians refer to this action as squinting. Blepharospasm is similar to blinking in that the eyelids are drawn together to protect the globe. However, its effects last beyond what is typical for the blink reflex. In other words, blepharospasm results in sustained, forced, tight closure of the lids for minutes to hours.

There are two main types of blepharospasm [10]:

- Essential or primary blepharospasm
- Reflex blepharospasm

Essential blepharospasm is the result of a primary neuropathy [6, 11–16]. This presentation is more commonly seen in humans than in companion animals, and the etiology is unknown [10]. Stress and fatigue may be inciting factors.

Reflex blepharospasm is common in companion animal patients (see Figures 25.1a–e).

Reflex blepharospasm results from pain within or around the eye, including the following regions: the orbit, eyelids, cornea, conjunctiva, iris, and ciliary body [10]. The lens, vitreous, choroid, and retina do not appear to have pain receptors and are therefore unable to initiate this reflex [10].

Sensation of pain in the ocular region occurs via branches of the trigeminal nerve (CN V) [10]. The motor action of eyelid closure is mediated through the innervation of the orbicularis oculi muscle by the facial nerve (CN VII) [10].

Corneal pain may also be transmitted directly to the anterior uvea [10]. This causes a local release of histamine, prostaglandins, and acetylcholine, and compounds the inflammation [10].

25.2 Clinical Signs that May Accompany Reflex Blepharospasm

Patients that exhibit reflex blepharospasm are in pain [10]. In response to pain, the nictitans of the affected eye(s) may be prominent [17].

In addition, patients may also develop transient light sensitivity. They are thus said to be photophobic [18]. Photophobia is caused by spasms of the ciliary muscle in response to strong light [18].

Patients with reflex blepharospasm may or may not present with ocular discharge. Photophobia commonly triggers epiphora, that is, excessive lacrimation [18].

In addition to clear discharge, cloudy and colored discharge may be present as a clue to the underlying pathology.

When present, it is important that the color and consistency of ocular discharge be noted in the patient's medical record, as well as whether it is unilateral or bilateral. These details will assist the clinician with developing a list of rule-outs [5]. For example, clear ocular discharge may result from irritation, inflammation, allergies, or viral infection [5]. On the other hand, ocular discharge that is white, yellow, or green may indicate an underlying bacterial infection [5]. Refer to Chapter 26 for additional details surrounding ocular discharge.

In addition to what was noted above, patients with reflex blepharospasm may present with a myriad of

Common Clinical Presentations in Dogs and Cats, First Edition. Ryane E. Englar.
© 2019 John Wiley & Sons, Inc. Published 2019 by John Wiley & Sons, Inc.

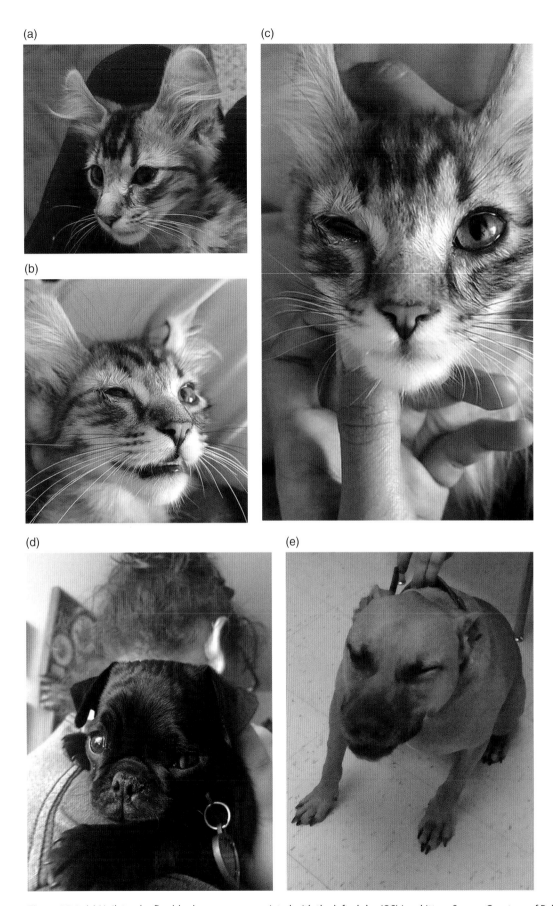

Figure 25.1 (a) Unilateral reflex blepharospasm associated with the left globe (OS) in a kitten. *Source:* Courtesy of Pallavi Sinha. (b) Unilateral reflex blepharospasm associated with the right globe (OD) in a kitten. Three-quarter/side view. *Source:* Courtesy of Pallavi Sinha. (c) Unilateral reflex blepharospasm associated with the right globe (OD) in a kitten. Head-on view. *Source:* Courtesy of Pallavi Sinha. (d) Unilateral reflex blepharospasm associated with the left globe (OS) in a Pug. The puppy had sustained a corneal ulcer after wrestling with another pet in the household. *Source:* Courtesy of Brenda Goodenberger. (e) Bilateral reflex blepharospasm in a canine patient.

clinical signs, depending upon the primary injury or disease process. These include the following [19–22]:

- Appearing to be "head shy"
- Scratching or pawing at the affected eye(s)
- Tear staining secondary to epiphora
- "Red eye"
- Scleral injection
- Scleritis or scleral edema
- Conjunctival edema or chemosis
- Conjunctival hyperemia
- Corneal edema (see Figures 25.2a–i)

Blepharospasm rarely occurs in isolation. More often, one or more of the aforementioned signs develop concurrently. Any of these signs in combination with blepharospasm indicate that eye inflammation or injury is likely. Even if just one globe is affected, examination of both eyes meticulously is critical to obtain a diagnosis [21]. If truly unaffected, the contralateral globe provides a comparison. Alternatively, the "unaffected" eye may well be affected, but lagging behind the contralateral globe in terms of disease presentation.

25.3 Diagnostic Work-Up for Reflex Blepharospasm

Blepharospasm is a clinical sign, not a diagnosis.

To obtain a diagnosis, history taking is indicated. When taking a history, the clinician should query the client about the duration and progression of the patient's reflex blepharospasm. It is also important to understand what, if anything, incited the issue. In addition, the clinician should ask whether the patient is indoor-only, indoor-outdoor, or outdoor-only. Lifestyle helps the clinician to determine what or who the patient may have been exposed to [5]. This may help the clinician to prioritize his list of rule-outs.

Finally, the veterinarian should inquire as to whether the presenting issue is a new complaint, a recurrent issue, or one that has persisted, meaning that it has never resolved [5, 23].

In addition to history taking, the patient should undergo a comprehensive physical examination, including ophthalmic evaluation [21]. The ophthalmic component involves gross examination of the eye as well as direct or indirect ophthalmoscopy to evaluate the fundus and other structures that lie within the caudal aspect of the globe [21] (see Figures 25.3a–c).

Consult an ophthalmology textbook to study how to appropriately perform the fundoscopic examination and to learn the science behind the appropriate techniques.

In addition to fundoscopy, the following three diagnostic tools should be considered for use in every patient, particularly those that present with blepharospasm and "red eye" [21]:

- Schirmer tear test (STT)
- Fluorescein staining
- Tonometry

25.3.1 The Schirmer Tear Test

The STT evaluates the patient for keratoconjunctivitis sicca or "dry eye" by evaluating tear production based upon the aqueous component [22, 24]. A commercial STT strip is folded at the notch, and then placed inside and under the lower eyelid. Proper placement of the strip is several millimeters medial to the lateral canthus. The strip is then left in place for 60 s. The reading is documented straightaway, before repeating the process in the contralateral eye [25] (see Figures 25.4a–b).

Reference texts differ in terms of what is considered the normal reference range in millimeters per minute (mm/min). Most agree that 15–20 mm/min in dogs is acceptable [25]. Patients with dry eye have diminished tear function and therefore score below this mark [22, 24]. Severe "dry eye" occurs when tear production is less than 5 mm/min [25].

Note, however, that there is age- and species-related variation in normal values. Geriatric dogs tend to produce fewer tears than young adult dogs, and cats tend to have very low to non-existent values in clinical settings, where they tend to be maximally stressed [25].

In addition, tear production is temporarily reduced by general anesthesia [26].

25.3.2 Fluorescein Staining

Recall from Chapter 19, Section 19.2.3 that fluorescein staining is most useful for the detection of corneal ulcers because the dye does not stain intact cornea. By contrast, damaged cornea allows the orange dye to adhere. Under a blue light, the adhered dye will fluoresce a brilliant green color. Review Chapter 19, Figure 19.12.

25.3.3 Tonometry

Tonometry measures intraocular pressure (IOP) [27–29]. Refer to Chapter 22, Section 22.2.1 to review applanation and rebound tonometry [28, 29].

Although IOP may vary between species and based upon extraocular factors such as patient temperament and demeanor, corneal health, diurnal variation, exercise, and pharmaceutical agents [27, 30–39], IOP is

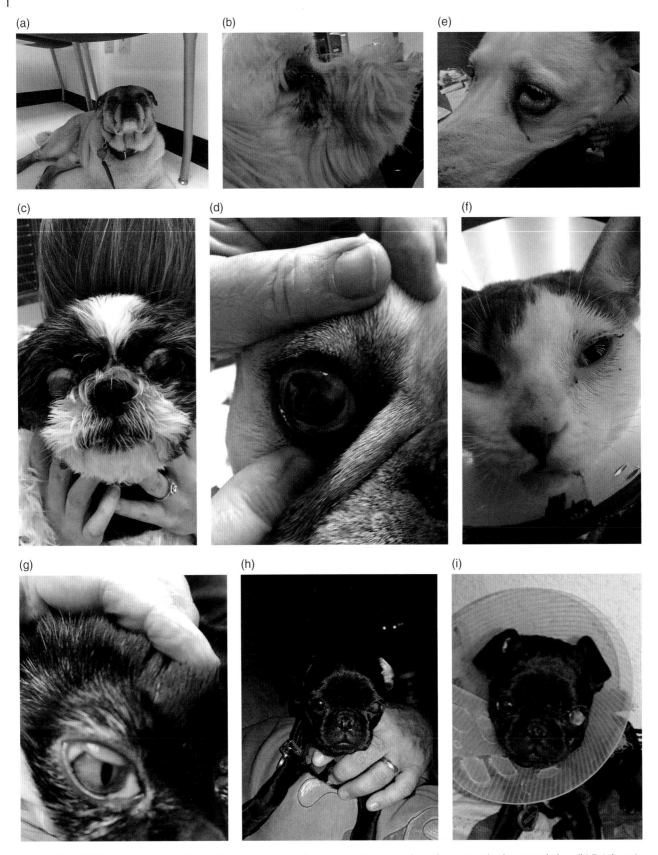

Figure 25.2 (a) "Head shy" canine patient, hiding underneath of an examination room chair. This patient had a corneal ulcer. (b) Epiphora in a canine patient with marked tear staining. *Source:* Courtesy of Patricia Bennett, DVM. (c) Severe bilateral "red eye" in a Shih Tzu dog. *Source:* Courtesy of Frank Isom, DVM. (d) Scleral injection in a Pug dog. *Source:* Courtesy of Pamela Mueller, DVM. (e) Scleral edema in a canine patient. (f) Conjunctivitis in a two-year-old cat. *Source:* Courtesy of Eric Stone. (g) Chemosis associated with the right globe (OD) of a feline patient. *Source:* Courtesy of Pamela Mueller, DVM. (h) Corneal edema in a canine patient with a corneal ulcer. *Source:* Courtesy of Brenda Goodenberger. (i) Worsening corneal edema in the same patient that is depicted in Figure 25.2h. *Source:* Courtesy of Brenda Goodenberger.

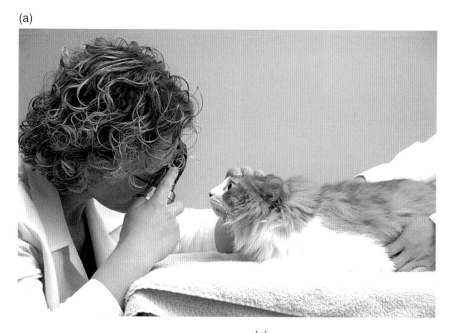

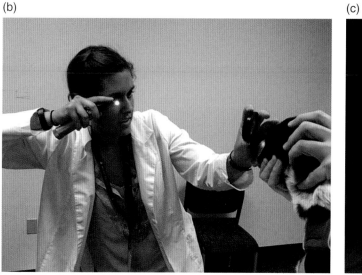

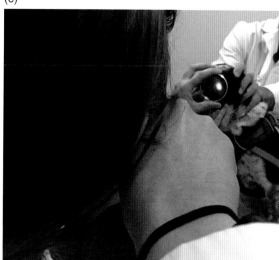

Figure 25.3 (a) Direct ophthalmoscopy of a feline patient. *Source:* Courtesy of the Media Resources Department at Midwestern University. (b) Indirect ophthalmoscopy of a canine patient. (c) Indirect ophthalmoscopy of a canine patient.

primarily determined by aqueous humor production and flow [27].

Increased IOP is a characteristic of glaucoma, whereas uveitis tends to result in decreased IOP [27, 40–42].

25.4 Primary Causes of Reflex Blepharospasm

There are innumerable causes of blepharospasm, of which the most common in companion animal practice include the following [19–22, 24, 43–50]:

- Blepharitis (refer to Chapter 19, Section 19.2.2)
- Entropion (refer to Chapter 19, Section 19.2.3)
- Conjunctivitis
- Corneal foreign body
- Corneal ulcer (refer to Chapter 19, Section 19.2.3)
- Keratoconjunctivitis sicca
- Anterior uveitis (refer to Chapter 17, Section 17.3)
- Glaucoma (refer to Chapter 22, Section 22.2.2)

In addition, there are iatrogenic causes of blepharospasm, including failure to apply eye lubricant to patients that are undergoing general anesthesia [43]. Because general anesthesia reduces tear production, there is a high risk for ocular irritation in those patients that forego lubrication [43]. These patients may awake from general anesthesia with blepharospasm secondary to exposure keratitis.

(a) (b)

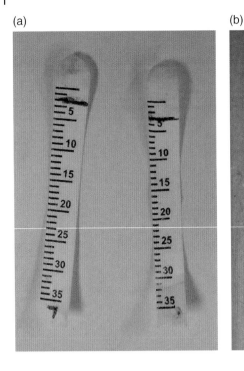

Figure 25.4 (a) Unused commercial STT strip. Note the presence of the notch, which will be folded so that it can be placed inside and under the lower eyelid. *Source:* Courtesy of Patricia Bennett, DVM. (b) Used commercial STT strip. Note the blue dye that has tracked up the strip of paper. This value is a reflection of the aqueous production of tear film and is stated as the number of millimeters (mm) per minute (min).

The primary causes of reflex blepharospasm will not be individually discussed as they were covered extensively elsewhere.

The most important aspect for clinicians to recognize about patients that present with reflex blepharospasm is to look deeper. They all have an underlying issue that has resulted in ocular pain. The issue may range the gamut from minor to severe, medical to surgical.

The importance of a comprehensive physical examination and ophthalmic evaluation cannot be understated. These diagnostic tools, in addition to the STT, fluorescein staining, and tonometry, will pave the way to a diagnosis.

References

1 Sisson, S. (1910). *A Textbook of Veterinary Anatomy*, 3 p. l., 11–826 p. Philadelphia, London: W.B. Saunders Company.

2 Aspinall, V. and Capello, M. (2009). *Introduction to Veterinary Anatomy and Physiology*. New York: Elsevier.

3 Evans, H.E. and Miller, M.E. (2013). *Miller's Anatomy of the Dog*, 4e, xix, 850 p. St. Louis, Missouri: Elsevier.

4 Rijnberk, A. and FJv, S. (2009). *Medical History and Physical Examination in Companion Animals*, 2e, viii, 333 p. Edinburgh; New York: Saunders/Elsevier.

5 Englar, R.E. (2017). *Performing the Small Animal Physical Examination*. Hoboken, NJ: Wiley.

6 Yen, M.T. (2018). Surgical Myectomy for essential Blepharospasm and Hemifacial spasm. *Int. Ophthalmol. Clin.* 58 (1): 63–70.

7 Englar, R.E. (2017). *Performing the Small Animal Physical Examination*. Hoboken, NJ: Wiley.

8 Chrisman CL. (2006). The Neurologic Examination. Clinician's Brief [Internet]. (January):[11–6 pp.]. https://www.cliniciansbrief.com/sites/default/files/sites/cliniciansbrief.com/files/7.pdf.

9 Studdert, V.P., Gay, C.C., and Blood, D.C. (2012). *Saunders Comprehensive Veterinary Dictionary*, 4e, xiii, 1325 p. Edinburgh; New York: Saunders Elsevier.

10 Gelatt, K.N. and Plummer, C.E. (2001). *Color Atlas of Veterinary Ophthalmology*. Ames, IA: Wiley-Blackwell.

11 Lee, S., Park, S., and Lew, H. (2018 February). Long-term efficacy of Botulinum neurotoxin-a treatment for essential Blepharospasm. *Korean J. Ophthalmol.* 32 (1): 1–7.

12 Digre, K.B. (2015). Benign essential Blepharospasm-there is more to it than just blinking. *J. Neuroophthalmol.* 35 (4): 379–381.

13 Evinger, C. (2013). Animal models for investigating benign essential Blepharospasm. *Curr. Neuropharmacol.* 11 (1): 53–58.

14 Evinger, C. (2015). Benign essential Blepharospasm is a disorder of neuroplasticity: lessons from animal models. *J. Neuroophthalmol.* 35 (4): 374–379.

15 Ozzello, D.J. and Giacometti, J.N. (2018). Botulinum toxins for treating essential Blepharospasm and Hemifacial spasm. *Int. Ophthalmol. Clin.* 58 (1): 49–61.

16 Weller, C. and Leyngold, I. (2018). The facial nerve and selective Neurectomy for treatment of benign essential Blepharospasm. *Int. Ophthalmol. Clin.* 58 (1): 89–95.

17 Lim, C.C. (2015). *Small Animal Ophthalmic atlas and Guide.* Wiley Blackwell. 168 p.

18 Gelatt, K.N. (2014). *Essentials of Veterinary Ophthalmology.* Ames, IA: Wiley.

19 Turner, S.M. (2008). *Saunders Solutions in Veterinary Practice: Small Animal Ophthalmology.* Philadelphia: Saunders Elsevier.

20 Turner, S. (2008). *Small Animal Ophthalmology,* ix, 370 p. Edinburgh; New York: Elsevier Saunders.

21 Brown, M.H. (2007). The red eye. *NAVC Clinician's Brief* (October): 14–18.

22 Clode, A. (2015). Canine keratoconjunctivitis siccca. *Clinician's Brief* (Decemeber): 81–85.

23 Rijnberk, A. and van Sluijs, F.S. (2009). *Medical History and Physical Examination in Companion Animals,* 333 p. The Netherlands: Elsevier Limited.

24 Best, L.J. and Ward, D.A. (2014). Diagnosis and treatment of keratoconjunctivitis sicca in dogs. *Today's Veterinary Practice* (July/August): 16–22.

25 Gionfriddo JR. (2010). Just Ask the Expert: What is a normal Schirmer tear test result?. DVM 360 [Internet]. http://veterinarymedicine.dvm360.com/just-ask-expert-what-normal-schirmer-tear-test-result.

26 Peche, N., Kostlin, R., Reese, S., and Pieper, K. (2015). Postanesthetic tear production and ocular irritation in cats. *Tierarztl. Prax. Ausg. K Klientiere Heimtiere* 43 (2): 75–82.

27 Maggio, F. (2015). Glaucomas. *Top. Companion Anim. Med.* 30 (3): 86–96.

28 Wilkie, D.A. (2013). Determining intraocular pressure. *NAVC Clinician's Brief* (February): 77–79.

29 Reinstein S. (2017). Under Pressure: Canine and Feline Glaucoma. Michigan Veterinary Medical Association [Internet]. https://michvma.org/resources/Documents/MVC/2017%20Proceedings/reinstein%2005.pdf.

30 Brubaker, R.F. (1991). Flow of aqueous humor in humans [the Friedenwald lecture]. *Invest. Ophthalmol. Vis. Sci.* 32 (13): 3145–3166.

31 Koskela, T. and Brubaker, R.F. (1991). The nocturnal suppression of aqueous humor flow in humans is not blocked by bright light. *Invest. Ophthalmol. Vis. Sci.* 32 (9): 2504–2506.

32 Liu, J.H. and Weinreb, R.N. (2011). Monitoring intraocular pressure for 24 h. *Br. J. Ophthalmol.* 95 (5): 599–600.

33 Drance, S.M. (1964). Effect of Oral glycerol of intraocular pressure in Normal and glaucomatous eyes. *Arch. Ophthalmol.* 72: 491–493.

34 Qureshi, I.A. (1995). Effects of mild, moderate and severe exercise on intraocular pressure of sedentary subjects. *Ann. Hum. Biol.* 22 (6): 545–553.

35 Aiello, S.E. and Moses, M.C. (2016). *Merck Veterinary Manual.* Whitehouse Station, NJ: Merck Sharp & Dohme Corp.

36 Brunton, L., Chabner, B.A., and Knollman, B. (2011). *General Anesthetics and Therapeutic Gases. Goodman & Gilman's: The Pharmacological Basis of Therapeutics,* 539. New York: The McGraw-Hill Companies, Inc.

37 Plumb, D.C. (2011). *Plumb's veterinary drug handbook,* 7e, 1187 p. Stockholm, Wis. Ames, Iowa: PharmaVet; Distributed by Wiley.

38 Plummer, C.E., Regnier, A., and Gelatt, K.N. (2013). The canine Glaucomas. In: *Veterinary Ophthalmology II* (ed. K.N. Gelatt, B.C. Gilger and T.J. Kern), 1050–1145. Ames, IA: Wiley-Blackwell.

39 von Spiessen, L., Karck, J., Rohn, K., and Meyer-Lindenberg, A. (2015). Clinical comparison of the TonoVet (R) rebound tonometer and the Tono-pen vet (R) applanation tonometer in dogs and cats with ocular disease: glaucoma or corneal pathology. *Vet. Ophthalmol.* 18 (1): 20–27.

40 Laminack, E.B., Myrna, K., and Moore, P.A. (2013). Clinical approach to the canine red eye. *Today's Veterinary Practice* (May/June).

41 Ollivier, F.J. and Plummer, C.E. (2007). The eye examination and diagnostic procedures. In: *Veterinary Opthalmology* (ed. K.N. Gelatt), 438–483. Ames, Iowa: Blackwell Publishing.

42 Moore, P.A. (2001). Examination techniques and interpretation of ophthalmic findings. *Clin. Tech. Small Anim. Pract.* 16 (1): 1–12.

43 Williams, D.L. and Kim, J.Y. (2009). Feline entropion: a case series of 50 affected animals (2003–2008). *Vet. Ophthalmol.* 12 (4): 221–226.

44 Sandmeyer, L.S., Breaux, C.B., and Grahn, B.H. (2010). Diagnostic ophthalmology. *Can. Vet. J.* 51 (7): 783–784.

45 Millichamp, N.J. (2010). Ocular diseases unique to the feline patient. *DVM 360.*

46 Pena, M.A. and Leiva, M. (2008). Canine conjunctivitis and blepharitis. *Vet. Clin. North Am. Small Anim. Pract.* 38 (2): 233–249, v.

47 Ofri, R. (2017). Conjunctivitis in dogs. *Clinician's Brief* (April): 89–93.

48 Hyman J. (2008). Current approaches to uveitis in the dog and cat. DVM 360 [Internet]. http://veterinarycalendar.dvm360.com/current-approaches-uveitis-dog-and-cat-proceedings.

49 Tilley, L.P. and Smith, F.W.K. (2004). *The 5-Minute Veterinary Consult: Canine and Feline,* 3e. Baltimore, MD: Lippincott Williams & Wilkins.

50 Côté, E. (2011). *Clinical Veterinary Advisor. Dogs and Cats,* 2e, xlv, 1738 p. St. Louis, Mo: Mosby.

26

Abnormal Tear Production and Other Ocular Discharge

26.1 Introduction to Tear Film as a Normal Ocular Secretion

The bony orbit was previously discussed in Chapter 21, Section 21.1 as being protective against external trauma [1–3].

In addition to surrounding itself with this skeletal structure, the globe carries additional defense mechanisms to prevent infection of the corneal surface with microorganisms [4, 5]. Although normal flora in the form of gram-positive *Staphylococcus* sp. and gram-negative *Neisseria* sp. is allowed to colonize the canine conjunctiva, the ocular surface itself is protected by the tear film [4, 6–9].

From its outermost surface moving inward, the tear film is a three-layered conglomerate of lipid, water, and mucus [4, 10–14]. In health, every companion animal patient produces tear film.

The outermost lipid layer is produced by the Meibomian glands [4, 12, 15]. These structures are located in the tarsal plates and function as modified sebaceous glands [4, 15]. The secretions of these glands, meibum, are the first layer of defense against debris that might contaminate the tear film [15]. In addition, meibum coats the middle aqueous layer, slowing its evaporation, and creates an even, regular optical surface [4, 15].

The middle aqueous layer is produced by a combination of efforts from the lacrimal and nictitans glands [11, 12, 16]. The former structure is a part of the periorbita and is seated dorsolateral to the globe [12]. It produces the majority of what we consider to be tears. The nictitans gland supplements this contribution by providing roughly one-fourth to one-third of the aqueous layer [11, 12].

The aqueous layer maintains the health of the globe by allowing oxygen and nutrients to reach the corneal surface [9, 12, 14]. In addition, the aqueous layer contributes to the defense of the globe by washing away surface debris [4, 8].

The aqueous layer, however, does far more than simply cleanse the ocular surface as a defensive mechanism [4]. Its contents include a host of antimicrobial substances, including the following [4, 14, 17–25]:

- Immunoglobulins IgA, IgG, and IgM
- Lysozyme
- α-lysin
- Lactoferrin

Of the aforementioned immunoglobulins, IgA contributes the greatest by way of concentration [17]. IgA is protective against many bacteria, viruses, and parasites [26]. Its mechanism of action is to coat microbes. This prevents them from attaching to and ultimately colonizing the corneal surface [4, 17, 27].

IgG and IgM are present in small amounts; however, the concentration of IgG in the tear film increases during inflammatory processes [17–20].

Lysozyme and α-lysin cause bacteriolysis [4, 23, 24, 28]. In addition, lysozyme has the potential to digest chitin and is therefore capable of acting as an antifungal agent [4, 17].

Lactoferrin sequesters iron, making it difficult for bacteria to harvest the resources necessary to sustain metabolism and growth [25].

Parasympathetic and sympathetic stimulation influence the lacrimal gland and therefore alter the amount of aqueous secretion in the tear film [29–31].

The innermost layer of the tear film is produced by conjunctival goblet cells [4, 12, 16]. This conglomerate of mucin, urea, salts, immunoglobulins, enzymes, glucose, and leukocytes is the final line of defense for the cornea [4]. The mucus ensnares bacteria for dispatch by IgA and other immune mechanisms [4, 27]. In addition, mucus allows the aqueous layer to spread over the hydrophobic cornea so that the corneal epithelium is lubricated [4, 32].

As a whole, the tear film represents an essential component of ocular health. An excess or reduction of one or more components can lead to significant pathology [4, 8].

Common Clinical Presentations in Dogs and Cats, First Edition. Ryane E. Englar.
© 2019 John Wiley & Sons, Inc. Published 2019 by John Wiley & Sons, Inc.

26.2 Reduction in Tear Film

Reduction of one or more components result in tear film instability and subsequent damage to the cornea [4, 33, 34]. For example, a diminished aqueous layer results in mucus clumping rather than even distribution over the corneal surface [4, 33–35]. Because the mucus adheres to itself rather than to the globe, there is a loss of protection with resultant damage to the cornea [4, 33, 34].

The aforementioned condition is called keratoconjunctivitis sicca (KCS) or "dry eye" [36, 37] (see Figures 26.1a, b).

"Dry eye" was discussed previously in Chapter 25, Section 25.3.1 relative to the Schirmer tear test (STT), as a quantitative means of assessing the aqueous component of the tear film [38, 39]. Recall that reference texts vary in terms of what they report to be the normal reference range for aqueous tear production in millimeters per minute (mm/min). Most agree that 15–20 mm/min in dogs is acceptable [40]. Patients with "dry eye" score below this mark on account of diminished tear production [38, 39]. Severe "dry eye" occurs when tear production is less than 5 mm/min [40].

Over time, "dry eye" results in mucoid to mucopurulent conjunctivitis [4, 38, 39, 41]. Conjunctivitis and secondary infection result from overgrowth of the normal flora of canine and feline conjunctiva [4]. Additional pathogenic microorganisms take up residence within the conjunctiva, including coagulase-positive *Staphylococcus* sp., beta-hemolytic *Streptococci* sp., and *Pseudomonas* sp. [4, 6].

In addition, the corneal irritation that is associated with KCS progresses to keratitis [4]. Potential sequelae include corneal ulceration and blindness [4, 42, 43].

Patients with presumptive KCS should undergo in-house testing via STT [11, 44]. Refer to Chapter 25, Section 25.3.1 to review the appropriate technique. The STT test strip acts as a topical irritant, which causes reflex tearing [11, 45]. This allows for quantitative assessment of aqueous tear production [11]. For reflex tearing to occur, the patient requires a functional ophthalmic branch of the trigeminal nerve, cranial nerve five (CN V), as well as the facial nerve, cranial nerve seven (VII) [11].

Recall that age plays a role in aqueous tear film production: it is not uncommon for older dogs to produce fewer tears than young adult dogs [40]. Recall also that the STT is less accurate for the diagnosis of KCS in cats because they tend to have very low to nonexistent values in clinical settings [40, 46].

(a)   (b)

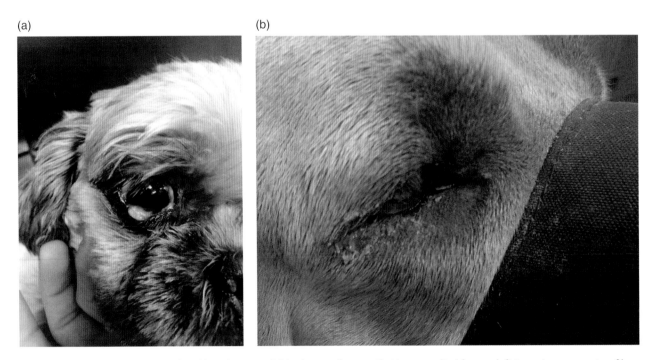

Figure 26.1 (a) KCS in a canine patient. Note the appreciable clumps of mucus that have resulted from a deficiency in aqueous tear film. *Source:* Courtesy of Andrew Weisenfeld, DVM. (b) KCS in a canine patient. Note the periocular irritation and the dried crusts from mucus that spilled over the edge of the lower palpebra. *Source:* Courtesy of Patricia Bennett, DVM.

26.3 Overproduction of the Aqueous Component of Tear Film

Underproduction of tears is not the only pathology of the lacrimal system that exists in companion animal medicine. Overproduction of the aqueous component of tear film can also occur. Epiphora is the appropriate medical term for excessive lacrimation and/or associated tear overflow [12, 36, 37, 44, 45, 47] (see Figure 26.2). Patients with epiphora present with wet eyes and moist periocular fur [12].

Epiphora is aesthetically unappealing to many owners, particularly those who own pets with light-colored coats [12]. When tears dry, they stain pale fur a rusty-brown [12]. If moisture is excessive such that periocular fur does not dry, it can result in moist dermatitis of the skin. This can lead to infection. Owners may also complain of a "wet dog" smell [12].

When epiphora occurs, it may be [44]

- Real
- Apparent
- Physiologic.

26.3.1 Real Epiphora

Real epiphora means that lacrimation is indeed increased. Increased lacrimation may be the result of ocular irritation, as from entropion, eyelid masses, distichiasis, or trichiasis [8, 36, 37, 44, 48] (see Figures 26.3a–c).

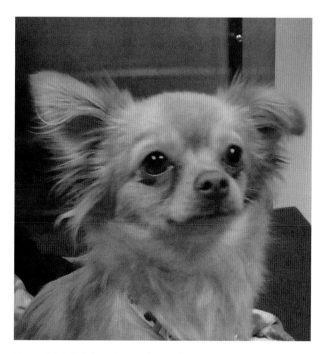

Figure 26.2 Epiphora in a canine patient.

26.3.2 Apparent Epiphora

Apparent epiphora involves an obstruction of nasolacrimal drainage [44].

Ordinarily, tears drain from the upper and lower nasolacrimal puncta [12, 16]. These two structures are located in the palpebral conjunctiva, adjacent to the medial canthus [12, 16]. Tears drain from the upper and lower puncta through the upper and lower canaliculi respectively, and to the lacrimal sac [12, 16]. The lacrimal sac is a dilation that funnels tears into the nasolacrimal duct [12, 16]. This duct narrows as it runs over the lacrimal bone to enter the maxillary bone [12, 16]. Ultimately, tears drain out into the nasal cavity [16].

When there is a partial or complete obstruction in the nasolacrimal duct, tears back up in the system [12, 16]. This back-up forces tears to exit the eye via an alternate route, the route of least resistance. Tears flow up and over the lower eyelid, giving the illusion of excessive lacrimation.

Causes of nasolacrimal duct obstruction include the following [12, 16, 44]:

- Foreign body
- Imperforate lacrimal puncta
- Skull shape and conformation
- Nictitans prolapse (refer to Chapter 20, Section 20.2.2)
- Dacryocystitis, inflammation of the lacrimal sac

Imperforate lacrimal puncta is a congenital condition in which there is no opening to the nasolacrimal duct [16]. Patients present at an early age with epiphora [16]. This is rare [16].

Skull shape and conformation more frequently play a role in epiphora. Consider, for example, brachycephalic breeds. Because of their cephalic index, these breeds have much shorter, tortuous nasolacrimal ducts that are more likely to become obstructed [12].

Dacryocystitis may result from chronic stimulation by debris, inflammation of surrounding tissues, such as conjunctivitis, or a mass effect [16].

26.3.3 Physiologic Epiphora

Physiologic epiphora is secondary to external stimulation that is temporary [44]. Consider, for example, an outdoor dog on a blustery day. The wind nipping at the eyes dries the corneas, causing reflex lacrimation. This transiently increases tear production to compensate for tears lost to the elements.

Another example of physiologic epiphora is strong lighting [47].

The patient who does not exhibit epiphora indoors, and only exhibits it outdoors, is likely to have physiologic epiphora [47]. Certain breeds appear to be predisposed to this sensitivity, including Chow Chows and Shar Peis [47].

(a)

(c)

(b)

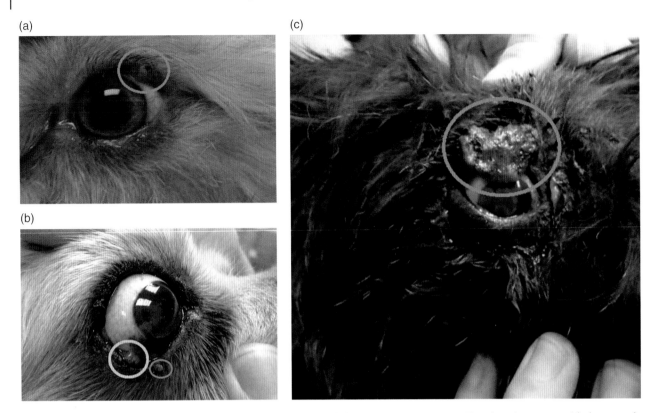

Figure 26.3 (a). Mass associated with the upper palpebra of the left globe (OS) in a canine patient. Note how its contact with the corneal surface is a trigger for real epiphora. *Source:* Courtesy of Patricia Bennett, DVM. (b) Two eyelid masses associated with the lower palpebra of the right globe (OD) in a canine patient. Note how the mass circled in yellow contacts the corneal surface. This contact is a trigger for real epiphora. *Source:* Courtesy of Patricia Bennett, DVM. (c) Ulcerative upper eyelid mass in a canine patient. Note how the mass contacts the corneal surface. This is likely to irritate the cornea and trigger reflex lacrimation. *Source:* Courtesy of Patricia Bennett, DVM.

26.3.4 Distinguishing Between the Types of Epiphora

It is important to differentiate real from apparent epiphora because case management is exceedingly different. In order to do so, the clinician must establish the patency of the nasolacrimal duct [44]. This can be achieved using fluorescein dye [44].

Fluorescein dye was first introduced in Chapter 19, Section 19.2.3 as a means of detecting corneal ulceration. However, it can also be added to the eye to track its path through the nasolacrimal duct. One drop of fluorescein dye is placed into the eye of the patient, followed by one to two drops of sterile eyewash [44].

In a patient that has a functional nasolacrimal apparatus, fluorescein dye will drain from the lacrimal puncta into the nasal cavity [44]. After two to five minutes, fluorescein dye will appear from the nares [44]. The use of a cobalt blue filter will facilitate detection of fluorescence [44].

A positive dye test confirms that the nasolacrimal apparatus is patent [44]. In this patient, epiphora is not apparent. It is real. Causes of lacrimal gland hypersecretion will need to be evaluated [47].

Note that brachycephalic breeds are notorious for failing the dye test in spite of a patent nasolacrimal system [44]. This has been theorized to be due to the tortuosity of their nasolacrimal ducts. It is possible that the fluorescein dye gets caught up in the twists and turns and there just is not enough dye to reach the end of the path. In this case, flushing the nasolacrimal duct may cause fluorescent fluid to appear through the nose [44].

Flushing is achieved by inserting a cannula into the nasolacrimal puncta following the administration of topical anesthetic [44]. One to two milliliters of sterile saline is then injected into the cannula to flush the duct [44].

Sometimes, fluid will not appear at the nose [44]. Occasionally, the duct opens in abnormal locations, causing fluid to flow elsewhere. Consider, for example, the patient that swallows or gags after nasolacrimal flushing [44]. This patient likely has a patent duct; however, the duct drained into the oropharynx rather than the nose [44]. The duct is still considered to be patent.

26.4 Ocular Discharge

In health, the periorbita produces the tear film. This creates the glossy, smooth appearance of the corneal surface of canine and feline globes (see Figures 26.4a, b).

As mentioned earlier, certain physiologic and pathologic states result in either too much or too little of one or more components of tear film. The result is ocular discharge, an abnormal secretion [36, 37].

Up until now, ocular discharge has been described as either serous, from epiphora, or mucoid, secondary to KCS. However, ocular discharge comes in many varieties.

Ocular discharge can also be mucopurulent, that is, it may contain mucus, leukocytes, and bacterial and/or

(a)

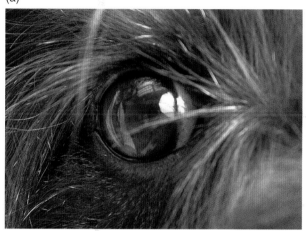

(b)

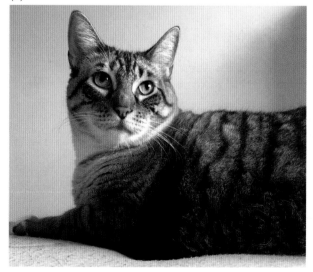

Figure 26.4 (a) Normal canine eyes. Note that a healthy tear film creates shiny corneal surfaces. (b) Normal feline eyes. Note how both corneal surfaces appear glossy. *Source:* Courtesy of Joshua Siegel.

fungal agents [36, 37]. The presentations of ocular discharge are varied (see Figures 26.5a–h).

As evident from Figures 26.5a–h, concurrent ocular and periocular pathology are common. In addition to those previously mentioned in relation to KCS and epiphora, some of the most common clinical presentations include the following [36, 37]:

- Conjunctivitis
- Blepharitis
- Blepharospasm
- Corneal ulceration
- Entropion
- Ectropion
- Distichiasis
- Ectopic cilia
- Trichiasis
- Anterior uveitis

Of those presentations listed above, conjunctivitis is quite common in feline practice and, as such, is frequently a cause of ocular discharge in cats [49].

In some patients with conjunctivitis, blepharospasm is quite pronounced (see Figure 26.6).

Conjunctivitis will be covered more thoroughly in Chapter 27; however, note that the most common causes of conjunctivitis in the cat are infectious [49]. Of these, the most common etiology in clinical practice is feline herpesvirus type-1 (FHV-1) [49].

Although canine conjunctivitis does occur, it is seen in clinical practice much less frequently than feline conjunctivitis [50]. Primary infectious disease, such as bacterial conjunctivitis, is uncommon [50].

When canine conjunctivitis occurs, it tends to result from allergic and immune-medicated disease, including atopy, the pemphigus complex of diseases, and lupus erythematosus [51]. Refer to Chapter 27 for additional information about these conditions.

26.5 The Diagnostic Work-Up for Ocular Discharge

Any time that ocular discharge of any sort is present, the following items should be determined during history taking and/or physical examination [36, 37]:

- Patient's age
- Patient's breed, to determine predispositions to disease
- Anatomic features that may predispose to disease, for example, entropion or ectropion
- Ocular discharge: its quality, quantity, and laterality
- The nature of the onset of the discharge: acute versus chronic

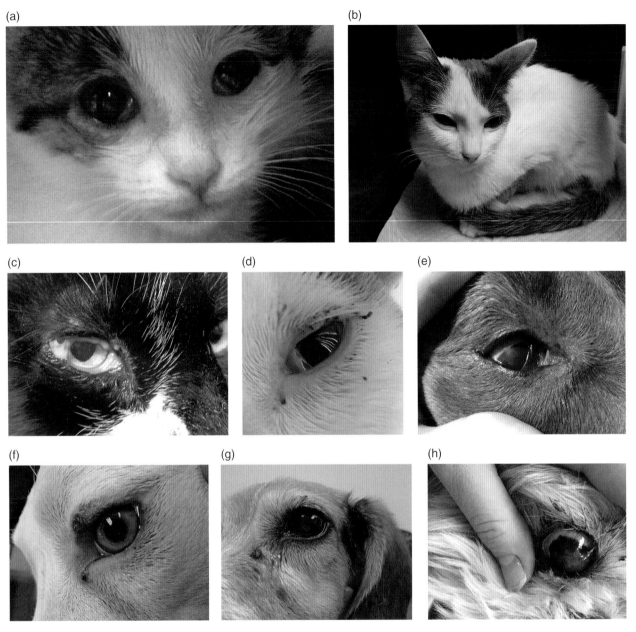

Figure 26.5 (a) Serous ocular discharge in a kitten. Note the apparent wetness of periocular fur bilaterally. *Source:* Courtesy of Karen Burks, DVM. (b) Serous ocular discharge in an adult cat. Note that the periocular fur is moist bilaterally. *Source:* Courtesy of "Axl" and Monica Chen. (c). Mucopurulent ocular discharge in a cat with conjunctivitis. *Source:* Courtesy of Patricia Bennett, DVM. (d) Crusty ocular discharge in a cat with conjunctivitis. Note concurrent blepharitis. *Source:* Courtesy of Eric Stone. (e) Serous ocular discharge in a canine patient. Note the apparent wetness of periocular fur. *Source:* Courtesy of Jess Darmofal, DVM. (f) Serous to mucoid ocular discharge with periocular crusting in a canine patient. Note concurrent blepharitis and periocular irritation. There is a periocular abrasion dorsomedially to the left globe (OS). (g) Mucoid to mucopurulent ocular discharge in a canine patient. *Source:* Courtesy of Patricia Bennett, DVM. (h) Mucoid to mucopurulent ocular discharge in a canine patient.

- The progression of the discharge: have any changes been noticed and, if so, what are they?
- Is the discharge a new finding or a recurrent issue?
- Is the ocular discharge present in a "red eye"?
- What, if any additional clinical signs are present?
- If the patient is in a multi-pet household, are any other animals showing clinical signs?
- Was the patient recently boarding, kenneled, or housed in close proximity to conspecifics?
- Does the patient have a history of underlying immunosuppressive disease?
- Is the patient receiving any immunosuppressive medications?
- Did the patient experience any recent stressful event, such as moving or rehoming?
- Are there any potential aggravating factors that the client has noticed, for example, the introduction of a new, dusty, or fragranced cat litter?

- STT (review Chapter 25, Section 25.3.1)
- Fluorescein staining to evaluate for corneal defects (review Chapter 25, Section 25.3.2)
- Fluorescein dye test to assess for patency of the nasolacrimal apparatus
- Tonometry (review Chapter 25, Section 25.3.3)

As a clinician, it is important to prioritize which tests are essential and to order them such that one test will not negate another's results. For example, it would be ill-advised to perform applanation tonometry prior to the STT because the former technique requires the administration of topical anesthetic. This application would artificially increase STT results.

Diagnostic tools are essential components of the work-up for ocular discharge because the list of differentials is vast [36, 37].

Treatment depends upon the underlying cause, and the only way to narrow one's list of rule-outs is via diagnostic testing [36, 37].

26.6 Ocular Discharge in Enucleated Patients

Enucleated patients occasionally present for evaluation of orbital swelling and/or tenderness (see Figure 26.7).

In theory, enucleated patients should have zero secretory tissue within the orbit. During enucleation, all such tissue, including the conjunctiva and the nictitans, are supposed to be excised. However, on occasion remnants of one or more of these secretory tissues are inadvertently left behind at the time of surgery [59].

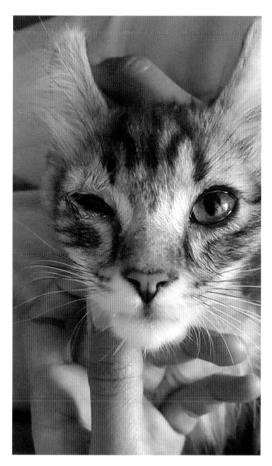

Figure 26.6 Blepharospasm associated with the right globe (OD) of a feline patient. *Source:* Courtesy of Pallavi Sinha.

A thorough ophthalmic examination should follow a comprehensive physical examination [36, 37]. Magnification of the eyelids may be required to observe distichia, trichiasis, or ectopic cilia [36, 37].

Conjunctival swabs or scrapes may help to characterize the ocular discharge microscopically and diagnose conjunctivitis [52, 53]. In addition, cytological analysis of swabs and scrapes may diagnose the underlying etiology. For example, infection of the feline patient with *Chlamydophila* or *Mycoplasma* can be determined microscopically [36, 37, 54].

Consult an ophthalmology textbook for appropriate technique for conjunctival swabs and scrapes.

Swabs may also be submitted from either the conjunctiva and/or the cornea, in cases of corneal ulceration, for culture [36, 37]. In addition, swabs can be tested via polymerase chain reaction (PCR) for certain infectious diseases, including FHV-1 [36, 37, 55]. However, keep in mind that cats may have a positive PCR test, indicating exposure, without active disease. Therefore, the utility of this test has been called into question.

In addition to examination of the whole patient as well as the eye, the following ophthalmic tests may be indicated [38–40, 56–58]:

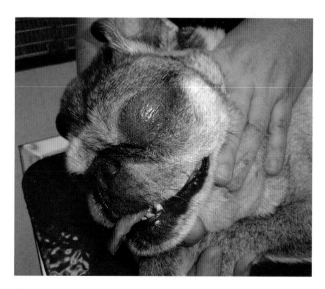

Figure 26.7 Orbital abscess in a canine patient that had previously undergone enucleation. *Source:* Courtesy of Daniel Foy, MS, DVM, DACVIM, DACVECC.

When such tissues remain in place, they continue to contribute to tear film production even in the absence of a globe to bathe with tears [59].

Tears may accumulate rapidly after surgery. Alternatively, tears may take months to accumulate in affected patients, particularly if the patient still has an intact nasolacrimal drainage system [59].

The transpalpebral approach to enucleation should lessen the risk of secretory tissue retention by removing the globe, conjunctiva, and nictitans en bloc [59].

References

1 Dyce, K.M., Sack, W.O., and Wensing, C.J.G. (2010). *Textbook of Veterinary Anatomy*, 4e, xii, 834 p. St. Louis, Mo: Saunders/Elsevier.

2 Evans, H.E. and DeLahunta, A. (2004). *Guide to the Dissection of the Dog*, 6e, xiv, 378 p. St. Louis, Mo: Saunders.

3 Evans, H.E. and Miller, M.E. (2013). *Miller's Anatomy of the Dog*, 4e, xix, 850 p. St. Louis, Missouri: Elsevier.

4 Davidson, H.J. and Kuonen, V.J. (2004). The tear film and ocular mucins. *Vet. Ophthalmol.* 7 (2): 71–77.

5 Lemp, M.A. and Blackman, H.J. (1981). Ocular surface defense mechanisms. *Ann. Ophthalmol.* 13 (1): 61–63.

6 SM, P.-J. (1997). Quantification of conjunctival sac bacteria in normal dogs and those suffering from keratoconjunctivitis sicca. *Vet. Comp. Ophthalmol.* 7: 29–35.

7 Gerding, P.A. Jr. and Kakoma, I. (1990). Microbiology of the canine and feline eye. *Vet. Clin. North Am. Small Anim. Pract.* 20 (3): 615–625.

8 MacLaren N. (2008). Management of tear film disorders in the dog and cat (Proceedings). DVM 360 [Internet]. http://veterinarycalendar.dvm360.com/management-tear-film-disorders-dog-and-cat-proceedings.

9 Dubielzig, R.R., Ketring, K.L., McLellan, G.J., and Albert, D.M. (2010). *Veterinary Ocular Pathology E-Book: A Comparative Review*. Saunders Ltd.

10 Wolff, E. (1951). *The Anatomy of the Eye and Orbit*. Philadelphia: Blakiston Co.

11 Vaden, S.L. (2009). *Blackwell's Five-Minute Veterinary Consult. Laboratory Tests and Diagnostic Procedures: Canine & Feline*, xliii, 763 p. Ames, Iowa: Wiley-Blackwell.

12 Turner, S. (2008). *Small Animal Ophthalmology*, ix, 370 p. Edinburgh; New York: Elsevier Saunders.

13 Turner, S.M. (2006). *Veterinary Ophthalmology: A Manual for Nurses and Technicians*, 206. Butterworth-Heinemann.

14 Grahn, B.H. and Storey, E.S. (2004). Lacrimostimulants and lacrimomimetics. *Vet. Clin. North Am. Small Anim. Pract.* 34 (3): 739–753.

15 Driver, P.J. and Lemp, M.A. (1996). Meibomian gland dysfunction. *Surv. Ophthalmol.* 40 (5): 343–367.

16 Gelatt KN. (2018). Nasolacrimal and Lacrimal Apparatus. Merck Veterinary Manual [Internet]. http://www.merckvetmanual.com/eye-and-ear/ophthalmology/nasolacrimal-and-lacrimal-apparatus.

17 Bron, A.J. and Seal, D.V. (1986). The defences of the ocular surface. *Trans. Ophthalmol. Soc. U. K.* 105 (Pt 1): 18–25.

18 German, A.J., Hall, E.J., and Day, M.J. (1998). Measurement of IgG, IgM and IgA concentrations in canine serum, saliva, tears and bile. *Vet. Immunol. Immunopathol.* 64 (2): 107–121.

19 Coyle, P.K. and Sibony, P.A. (1986). Tear immunoglobulins measured by ELISA. *Invest. Ophthalmol. Vis. Sci.* 27 (4): 622–625.

20 McClellan, B.H., Whitney, C.R., Newman, L.P., and Allansmith, M.R. (1973). Immunoglobulins in tears. *Am J. Ophthalmol.* 76 (1): 89–101.

21 Brightman, A.H., Wachsstock, R.S., and Erskine, R. (1991). Lysozyme concentrations in the tears of cattle, goats, and sheep. *Am. J. Vet. Res.* 52 (1): 9–11.

22 Banyard, M.R.C. and Mckenzie, H.A. (1982). The fractionation and characterization of bovine tear proteins, especially lactoferrin. *Mol. Cell. Biochem.* 47 (2): 115–124.

23 Eichenbaum, J.D., Lavach, J.D., Severin, G.A., and Paulsen, M.E. (1987). Immunology of the ocular surface. *Comp. Cont. Educ. Pract.* 9 (11): 1101–1109.

24 Ford, L.C., DeLange, R.J., and Petty, R.W. (1976). Identification of a nonlysozymal bactericidal factor (beta lysin) in human tears and aqueous humor. *Am J. Ophthalmol.* 81 (1): 30–33.

25 Selinger, D.S., Selinger, R.C., and Reed, W.P. (1979). Resistance to infection of the external eye – role of tears. *Surv. Ophthalmol.* 24 (1): 33–38.

26 Sullivan, D.A., Stern, M.E., Tsubota, K. et al. (2000). Third international conference on the lacrimal gland, tear film and dry eye syndromes: basic science and clinical relevance – Maui, Hawaii – November 15–18, 2000 - Preface. *Cornea* 19 (6): S49.

27 Chandler, J.W. and Gillette, T.E. (1983). Immunologic defense mechanisms of the ocular surface. *Ophthalmology* 90 (6): 585–591.

28 Repaske, R. (1956). Lysis of gram-negative bacteria by lysozyme. *Biochim. Biophys. Acta* 22 (1): 189–191.

29 Dartt, D.A., Hodges, R.R., and Zoukhri, D. (1998). Signal transduction pathways activated by cholinergic and alpha 1-adrenergic agonists in the lacrimal gland. *Adv. Exp. Med. Biol.* 438: 113–121.

30 Sullivan, D.A., Kelleher, R.S., Vaerman, J.P., and Hann, L.E. (1990). Androgen regulation of secretory component synthesis by lacrimal gland acinar cells in vitro. *J. Immunol.* 145 (12): 4238–4244.

31 Walcott, B., Cameron, R.H., and Brink, P.R. (1994). The anatomy and innervation of lacrimal glands. *Adv. Exp. Med. Biol.* 350: 11–18.

32 McKenzie, R.W., Jumblatt, J.E., and Jumblatt, M.M. (2000). Quantification of MUC2 and MUC5AC transcripts in human conjunctiva. *Invest. Ophthalmol. Vis. Sci.* 41 (3): 703–708.

33 Ashutosh, S. (1993). Energetics of corneal epithelial cell-ocular mucus-tear film interactions: some surface-chemical pathways of corneal defense. *Biophys. Chem.* 47: 87–99.

34 Adams, A.D. (1986). Conjunctival surface mucus. In: *The Preocular Tear Film in Health, Disease, and Contact Lens Wear* (ed. F. Holly), 677–687. Lubbock, TX: Dry Eye Institute, Inc.

35 Carrington, S.D., Bedford, P.G.C., Guillon, J.P., and Woodward, E.G. (1987). Polarized-light biomicroscopic observations on the pre-corneal tear film. 2. Keratoconjunctivitis Sicca in the dog. *J. Small Anim. Pract.* 28 (8): 671–680.

36 Côté, E. (2015). *Clinical Veterinary Advisor. Dogs and Cats*, 3e, xxxvii, 1642 p. St. Louis, Missouri: Elsevier Mosby.

37 Tilley, L.P. and Smith, F.W.K. (2004). *The 5-Minute Veterinary Consult: Canine and Feline*, 3e, lviii, 1487 p. Baltimore, MD: Lippincott Williams & Wilkins.

38 Best, L.J. and Ward, D.A. (2014). Diagnosis and treatment of keratoconjunctivitis sicca in dogs. *Today's Veterinary Practice* (July/August): 16–22.

39 Clode, A. (2015). Canine keratoconjunctivitis siccca. *Clinician's Brief* (December): 81–85.

40 Gionfriddo JR. (2010). Just Ask the Expert: What is a normal Schirmer tear test result?. DVM 360 [Internet]. http://veterinarymedicine.dvm360.com/just-ask-expert-what-normal-schirmer-tear-test-result.

41 Reinstein S. (2017). Dry Eye in Dogs: When Good Glands Go Bad. Veterinary Team Brief [Internet]. (January/February). https://www.veterinaryteambrief.com/sites/default/files/attachments/Dry%20Eye%20in%20Dogs_When%20Good%20Glands%20Go%20Bad_0.pdf.

42 Kaswan, R. (1994). Characteristics of a canine model of KCS: effective treatment with topical cyclosporine. *Adv. Exp. Med. Biol.* 350: 583–594.

43 Sansom, J., Barnett, K.C., and Long, R.D. (1985). Keratoconjunctivitis sicca in the dog associated with the administration of salicylazosulphapyridine (sulphasalazine). *Vet. Rec.* 116 (15): 391–393.

44 Ford, R.B. and Mazzaferro, E. (2011). *Kirk & Bistner's Handbook of Veterinary Procedures and Emergency Treatment*. St. Louis, MO: Elsevier Saunders.

45 Saito, A. and Kotani, T. (1999). Tear production in dogs with epiphora and corneal epitheliopathy. *Vet. Ophthalmol.* 2 (3): 173–178.

46 Sebbag, L., Kass, P.H., and Maggs, D.J. (2015). Reference values, intertest correlations, and test-retest repeatability of selected tear film tests in healthy cats. *J. Am. Vet. Med. Assoc.* 246 (4): 426–435.

47 Martin, C.L. (2009). *Ophthalmic Disease in Veterinary Medicine*. Boca Raton, FL: Taylor & Francis Group, LLC.

48 Williams, D.L. and Kim, J.Y. (2009). Feline entropion: a case series of 50 affected animals (2003–2008). *Vet. Ophthalmol.* 12 (4): 221–226.

49 Millichamp NJ. (2010). Ocular diseases unique to the feline patient. DVM 360 [Internet]. http://veterinarycalendar.dvm360.com/ocular-diseases-unique-feline-patient-proceedings.

50 Ofri, R. (2017). Conjunctivitis in dogs. *Clinician's Brief* (April): 89–93.

51 Pena, M.A. and Leiva, M. (2008). Canine conjunctivitis and blepharitis. *Vet. Clin. North Am. Small Anim. Pract.* 38 (2): 233–249, v.

52 Martin, C.L. (1973). Conjunctivitis. Differential diagnosis and treatment. *Vet. Clin. North. Am.* 3 (3): 367–383.

53 Brown, M.H. (2007). The red eye. *Clinician's brief* (October): 14–18.

54 Lavach, J.D., Thrall, M.A., Benjamin, M.M., and Severin, G.A. (1977). Cytology of normal and inflamed conjunctivas in dogs and cats. *J. Am. Vet. Med. Assoc.* 170 (7): 722–727.

55 Grahn, B.H. and Sandmeyer, L.S. (2010). Diagnostic Ophthalmology Ophtalmologie diagnostique. *Can. Vet. J.* 51 (3): 327.

56 Maggio, F. (2015). Glaucomas. *Top. Companion Anim. Med.* 30 (3): 86–96.

57 Wilkie, D.A. (2013). Determining intraocular pressure. *NAVC Clinician's Brief* (February): 77–79.

58 Reinstein S. (2017). Under Pressure: Canine and Feline Glaucoma. Michigan Veterinary Medical Association [Internet]. https://michvma.org/resources/Documents/MVC/2017%20Proceedings/reinstein%2005.pdf.

59 Ward, A.A. and Neaderland, M.H. (2011). Complications from residual adnexal structures following enucleation in three dogs. *J. Am. Vet. Med. Assoc.* 239 (12): 1580–1583.

27

Abnormal Appearances of the Conjunctiva

27.1 Introduction to the Conjunctiva

The conjunctiva is a thin, supportive mucous membrane that cushions the globe [1, 2]. Although it is one continuous structure, it is often considered as two distinct entities from an anatomical and clinical perspective [3, 4]:

- The palpebral conjunctiva lines the inner aspect of the upper and lower palpebrae, the eyelids
- The bulbar conjunctiva is the continuation of the palpebral conjunctiva onto the sclera

These structures collectively serve as an additional layer that protects the globe.

In health, the conjunctiva is moist and has a characteristic pink appearance [1, 5, 6]. It is also not typically obvious on gross examination of a healthy feline or canine patient, that is, one without conjunctivitis [1] (see Figures 27.1a, b).

Certain eyelid conformations may make the conjunctiva apparent without the clinician investigating further. Consider ectropion, for example. Recall from Chapter 19, Section 19.2.4 that ectropion refers to the eversion of one or more of the eyelids [7, 8]. Certain breeds of dogs are more likely to be affected, including hounds [7, 8]. Typically both lower palpebrae are involved. As these structures take on a droopy appearance, they expose the palpebral conjunctiva [7] (see Figure 27.2).

In patients without entropion, clinicians must raise or lower the eyelids in order to gain an appreciation for the palpebral conjunctiva (see Figures 27.3a, b).

27.2 Introduction to Terminology Associated with Conjunctival Pathology

In health, the conjunctiva is thin, smooth, and relatively transparent [4, 5]. When conjunctiva becomes edematous, particularly in cats, it takes on a billowy or "puffy" appearance [5, 6] (see Figures 27.4a, b).

The appropriate medical terminology to describe this clinical appearance is chemosis. Chemosis refers to conjunctival edema [9].

The conjunctiva is a vascularized structure; however, in health, the individual vessels are not typically apparent [4, 5]. Conjunctival pathology can result in intense hyperemia [1, 4, 5, 9]. Conjunctival hyperemia is redness associated with the conjunctiva due to increased blood supply, as from inflammatory processes [1, 9] (see Figures 27.5a, b).

Dilation of individual vessels may also result from conjunctival pathology. These vessels are now evident on gross inspection of the bulbar conjunctiva. The conjunctiva is said to be injected. Colloquially, this is referred to as having bloodshot eyes (see Figure 27.6).

Conjunctivitis is a condition that is characterized by inflammation of the conjunctiva. Patients with conjunctivitis typically present with one or more of the aforementioned clinical signs: chemosis, hyperemia, and/or injection.

Conjunctivitis may reflect underlying primary disease in the conjunctiva; however, it may also result secondary to other ocular and orbital diseases, including those involving the [9]

- Eyelid
- Cornea
- Orbit
  - Dental disease
  - Neoplasia
- Nasolacrimal apparatus.

Therefore, an examination of a patient with conjunctivitis should never be restricted to the conjunctiva only [9]. All associated structures must be examined to identify any and all potential rule-outs, including systemic disease.

27.3 Feline Infectious Conjunctivitis

Feline conjunctivitis is a common clinical presentation in companion animal practice [10]. When it occurs, it is most often the result of infectious disease [1, 11–18].

Common Clinical Presentations in Dogs and Cats, First Edition. Ryane E. Englar.
© 2019 John Wiley & Sons, Inc. Published 2019 by John Wiley & Sons, Inc.

(a)

(b)

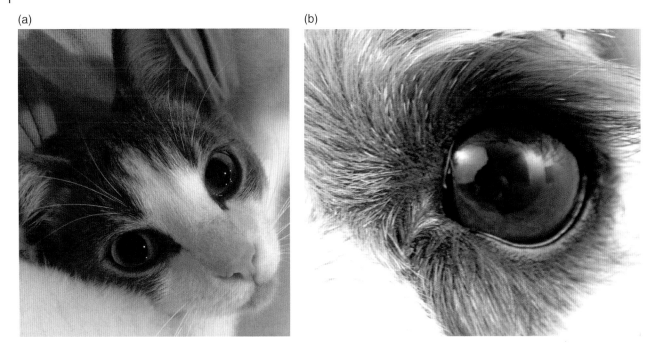

Figure 27.1 (a) Normal appearance of the globe in a cat without conjunctivitis. Note that the conjunctiva is not apparent on gross examination. *Source:* Courtesy of Sami Moon. (b) Normal appearance of the globe in a dog without conjunctivitis. Note that the conjunctiva is not apparent on gross examination. *Source:* Courtesy of the Media Resources Department at Midwestern University.

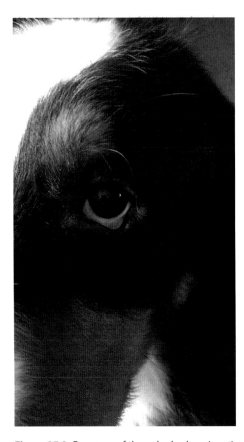

Figure 27.2 Exposure of the palpebral conjunctiva in a canine patient with bilateral ectropion. *Source:* Courtesy of Peggy Abramson, LVT.

The most common causes of infectious conjunctivitis in cats are the following [1, 10, 16]:

- Feline herpesvirus type-1 (FHV-1)
- *Chlamydophila felis*
- *Mycoplasma* spp.
- Feline calicivirus
- *Bordetella bronchiseptica*

27.3.1 FHV-1

FHV-1 is the most common cause of infectious conjunctivitis in cats [11, 17, 19].

FHV-1 is a host-specific herpesvirus that is ubiquitous [1, 12]. As many as 80% of cats in the world may be carriers of the virus, and 95 % are likely to have at one point in time been exposed [12, 15, 20–24].

Occasionally, FHV-1 is referred to in the veterinary medical literature as feline viral rhinotracheitis (FVR) [9].

The replication of FHV-1 within epithelial cells ultimately ends in cytolysis; however, the virus is able to persist within the trigeminal ganglion for the life of the host [11, 12, 25, 26]. This so-called latency is a feature that allows FHV-1 to reactivate. Reactivation may result in recurrence of clinical signs in the host and transmission to other naïve cats [11].

Within 2–10 days of exposure, newly infected hosts begin to display their own clinical signs [11]. Ocular, oropharyngeal, and nasal secretions are infectious, and

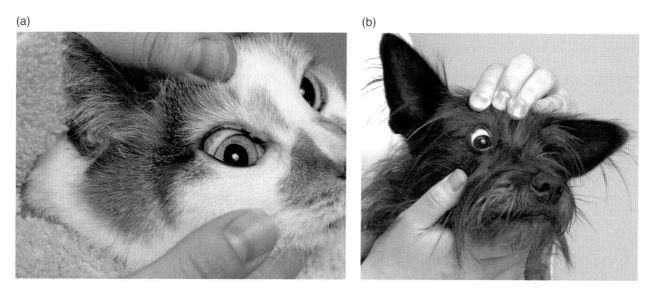

Figure 27.3 (a) Raising the upper eyelid in a feline patient to inspect the conjunctiva. Note that so doing also allows the clinician to inspect the sclera. *Source:* Courtesy of the Media Resources Department at Midwestern University. (b) Raising the upper eyelid in a canine patient to inspect the conjunctiva. *Source:* Courtesy of the Media Resources Department at Midwestern University.

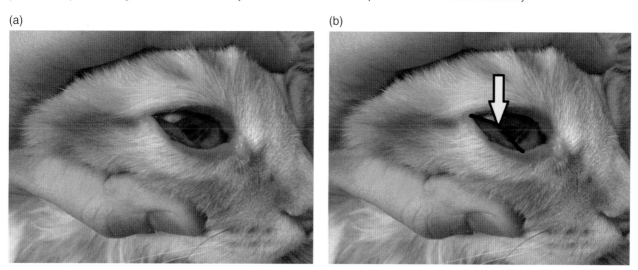

Figure 27.4 (a) The classic billowy appearance associated with the bulbar conjunctiva of a feline patient with conjunctivitis. *Source:* Courtesy of Dr. Elizabeth Robbins. (b) Same patient as in Figure 27.4a, with a yellow arrow pointing to the bulbar conjunctiva, which has also been outlined in black.

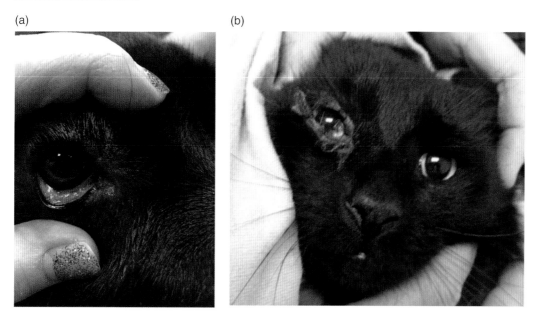

Figure 27.5 (a) Conjunctival hyperemia in a canine patient. (b) Conjunctival hyperemia and chemosis in a feline patient. *Source:* Courtesy of Patricia Bennett, DVM.

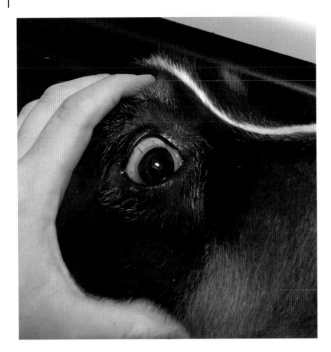

Figure 27.6 Injected conjunctiva in a canine patient. *Source:* Courtesy of Kimberly Wallitsch.

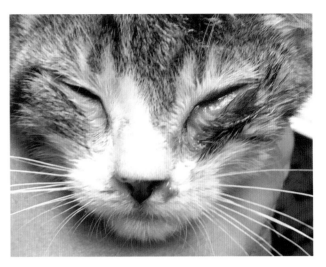

Figure 27.7 Systemic signs of infection in a kitten that has succumbed to feline herpesvirus type-1 (FHV-1). *Source:* Courtesy of Frank Isom, DVM.

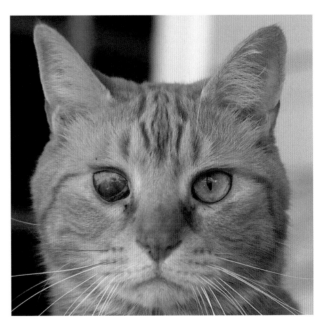

Figure 27.8 Symblepharon of the right globe (OD) of a feline patient. Symblepharon is a complication of severe conjunctivitis. *Source:* Courtesy of Jackie Kucskar, DVM.

viral shedding via these routes is prolonged [11]. It is not atypical for shedding to last for three weeks beyond the time of inoculation [11]. Because hosts remain carriers of FHV-1, they will continue to shed on and off throughout life [11].

Stressful events are more likely to reactivate FHV-1, causing disease to recrudesce [12, 23–25, 27]. For this reason, history taking is essential. FHV-1 should be on the differential list for any cat that presents with conjunctivitis that has recently undergone stressful change(s) in its life. These include, but are not limited to, changes in residence, ownership, the household itself, the members of the household (human or otherwise), or a change in physiologic state, such as pregnancy, parturition, or lactation [12, 25]. Chronic use of glucocorticoid therapy may also incite a flare-up of previously quiescent FHV-1 [12, 25, 28–30].

Clinical disease is typically self-limiting although secondary bacterial infection is possible [11]. Initial infection is typically bilateral, with a systemic component either in the form of general malaise or concurrent upper respiratory infection (URI) [11, 12]. Sneezing, nasal discharge, depression, fever, and decreased appetite are commonly seen in the early stages of infection, in addition to conjunctivitis [9, 12–15, 22, 31] (see Figure 27.7).

In severe cases, the conjunctiva may become attached to the cornea. This is called symblepharon [9, 16] (see Figure 27.8).

Hosts are susceptible to "flare-ups" of FHV-1 because local immunity that is triggered by the initial infection is not lifelong [9]. When "flare-ups" occur, they are more likely to cause unilateral disease, without systemic sequelae [9, 11] (see Figure 27.9).

Not all individuals with FHV-1 have the same response to infection, and not all individuals with FHV-1 latency experience clinical signs that are associated with recrudesce [11]. Severity of disease is highly individual [11]. However, in general, conjunctivitis is milder during subsequent attacks [11].

In addition to conjunctivitis, cats with FHV-1 may present with classic dendritic ulcers [11, 16, 27, 32]. These are linear and branching as opposed to global corneal ulcers that are expansive and overtake much of the cornea's surface [9, 11] (see Figure 27.10).

In addition to ulceration, corneal cloudiness may develop. This change in corneal translucency is indicative of keratitis (see Figures 27.11a, b).

Age, history, and clinical signs typically point the clinician to the presumptive diagnosis of FHV-1, and the patient is managed via supportive care [9]. Diagnostic investigations to obtain a definitive diagnosis are more commonly performed in catteries when a persistent problem exists [9].

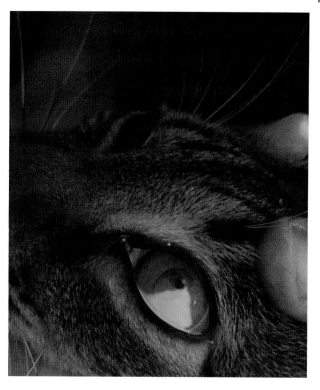

Figure 27.10 Expansive corneal ulcer in a feline patient. Note that this ulcer is not the typical dendritic or branching ulcer that is associated with feline herpesvirus type-1 (FHV-1). However, dendritic ulcers may coalesce to form larger, global ulcers such as this one. *Source:* Courtesy of Ben Turner.

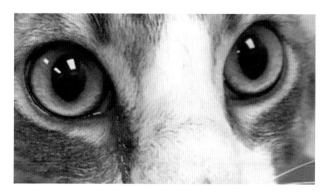

Figure 27.9 Ocular discharge in an adult cat with mild, unilateral conjunctivitis.

(a)   (b)

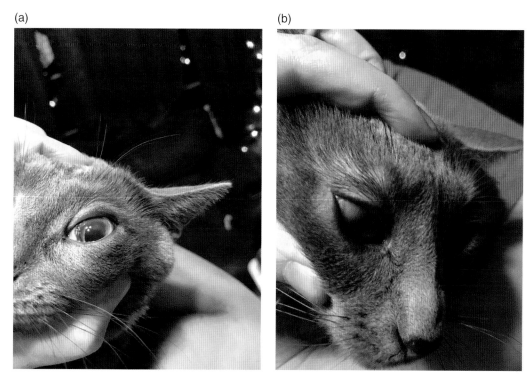

Figure 27.11 (a) Head-on view of corneal edema secondary to presumptive feline herpesvirus type-1 (FHV-1). *Source:* Courtesy of Erin M. Miracle. (b) Side view of corneal edema secondary to presumptive FHV-1. *Source:* Courtesy of Erin M. Miracle.

Polymerase chain reaction (PCR) may be performed on conjunctival swabs to test for FHV-1 [1, 25, 33, 34]. However, this diagnostic test is not without its frustrations. Subclinical, otherwise healthy patients may shed FHV-1, resulting in a false positive for clinical disease [12]. Alternatively, false negatives may occur during periods of recrudescence, when shedding is present, but low [12]. Finally, because FHV-1 is so prevalent, exposure to disease and the development of antibodies in response to vaccination may complicate test results [12]. Positives may occur in exposed, but not infected, patients [12].

27.3.2 Chlamydophila felis

C. felis is a gram-negative obligate intracellular bacteria that used to be called *Chlamydia psittaci var. felis* [1, 11, 35–37]. Its reclassification reflects its preference for cats as hosts [11]. In addition, the organism is far less likely to be zoonotic than *Chlamydia psittaci*, although the potential exists among the immunocompromised [11].

C. felis replicates in epithelial cells, like FHV-1, and causes so-called chlamydial conjunctivitis [38]. Chlamydial conjunctivitis is relatively common in kittens [35, 39–42]. Cats older than five years of age are rarely affected [12, 43]. It has been theorized that natural immunity develops as cats age [43].

C. felis may cause unilateral disease that becomes bilateral, or it remains unilateral [12].

Chlamydial conjunctivitis appears within a three- to five-day incubation period. Affected cats tend to become febrile and may develop submandibular lymphadenopathy [11, 35]. Chemosis tends to be much more severe in chlamydial conjunctivitis than in FHV-1 [12].

As opposed to FHV-1, concurrent respiratory signs are mild, if they are even present [11]. Infection may be severe; however, it is not lifelong [11]. Shedding is prolonged at approximately 60 days post infection, and cat-to-cat transmission is likely if in-contact cats are not treated [11].

C. felis should always be on the differential diagnosis list in cases of chronic disease or in those presentations that are characterized by marked chemosis [12, 13, 22, 44].

C. felis targets the conjunctiva primarily. However, its tissue preference is expansive as compared to FHV-1, and therefore it is more likely to infect additional tissues including the liver, spleen, lung, kidneys, and peritoneum [11]. For this reason, systemic therapy is often advised for infected cats, even in the absence of systemic disease.

Cytological diagnosis via conjunctival scrape is possible. Topical anesthetic is applied to the patient's globe [1]. The conjunctiva is then scraped, either with a cyto-brush or the blunt end of a scalpel handle [1].

Unfortunately, the yield for conjunctival scrapes is low in chronic cases [1]. What clinicians are looking for is one or more intracytoplasmic elementary bodies of *C. felis* within epithelial cells [12]. These bodies are not present during all stages of infection [12]. Their transience makes them difficult to detect [12].

More often, conjunctival swabs are submitted for testing via PCR for *C. felis* as well as for FHV-1 [1, 25, 33, 34]. PCR is highly sensitive, meaning that there are few false negatives [1, 11]. However, multiple strains of *C. felis* have since been discovered [11]. It appears that some of these microorganisms continue to go undetected [11]. It may be that a clinician has to rely upon history, clinical signs, and response to therapy for a presumptive, rather than definitive, diagnosis [11].

27.3.3 *Mycoplasma* spp.

Historically, the presence of *Mycoplasma* spp. among conjunctival tissues was considered an incidental finding in otherwise healthy cats [1, 12–15, 39–41]. However, in actuality, *Mycoplasma* appears to be an opportunist [1]. In fact, several types of *Mycoplasma* have been implicated as causative agents for feline conjunctivitis, including *Mycoplasma felis*, *Mycoplasma gatae*, and *Mycoplasma arginine* [1].

In addition to conjunctivitis, *Mycoplasma* can cause lower airway disease, particularly in immune-suppressed patients [1].

Unlike FHV-1, neither *Mycoplasma* nor *C. felis* targets the cornea [1]. Therefore, ulcerative keratitis is not seen in cases of either [1].

Diagnosis is also via PCR, and medical management against *C. felis* will also target *Mycoplasma* [1].

27.3.4 Feline Calicivirus

Feline calicivirus is yet another agent of feline conjunctivitis [1]. However, affected cats typically present with signs of systemic illness, including URI [1]. Feline calicivirus is also more likely than FHV-1 to cause ulcerations of oral and oropharyngeal mucosa [1, 11]. Calicivirus frequently causes oral ulceration and/or stomatitis, both of which are considered hallmark signs [1].

Like *Mycoplasma* and *C. felis*, feline calicivirus does not target the cornea, and therefore does not cause ulcerative keratitis [11].

27.3.5 Bordetella bronchiseptica

Recognize that *B. bronchiseptica* is not the first pathogen to consider in cases of feline conjunctivitis, but it certainly can induce and/or contribute to pre-existing disease [16].

B. bronchiseptica is more likely to cause URI in cats; however, it has been implicated in cases of chronic feline conjunctivitis [1, 16]. Therefore, patients with persistent disease may benefit from having a bacterial culture [1]. If a bacterial culture is performed, it is important to recognize that the conjunctiva has an established resident flora, which is considered to be normal [1, 16, 45]. This flora includes the following:

- *Staphylococcus aureus*
- *Staphylococcus epidermidis*
- *Streptococcus* spp.
- *Corynebacterium* spp.

If one of more of the aforementioned microorganisms are identified on culture, these should be considered commensal organisms until proved otherwise [16, 45].

27.4 Feline Noninfectious Conjunctivitis

Although infectious causes of conjunctivitis are most common in feline patients, feline conjunctivitis may also result from structural abnormalities, such as entropion, or feline eosinophilic conjunctivitis [1, 46–48]. This tends to target the lower lid [1, 49]. Eosinophils infiltrate the conjunctiva, causing swelling of the conjunctiva and adjacent structures, including the eyelid [1, 49]. In addition, there may be depigmentation and/or erosion of the lid margin [1, 49]. Affected eyes may be associated with a mucoid to mucopurulent ocular discharge [49]. Alternatively, a caseous exudate may develop [49].

Conjunctival scrapes of patients that demonstrate eosinophils and/or mast cells are supportive of a diagnosis of eosinophilic conjunctivitis [49, 50].

Eosinophilic conjunctivitis is responsive to topical or systemic anti-inflammatory drugs; however, recurrence is common [49].

Keratoconjunctivitis sicca (KCS) may also be associated with feline conjunctivitis. However, it is usually the result of conjunctivitis rather than its cause [12, 13, 22, 44].

27.5 Canine Conjunctivitis

Although canine conjunctivitis does occur in clinical practice, it is much less prevalent than feline conjunctivitis [2].

27.5.1 Canine Infectious Conjunctivitis

Primary infectious disease, such as bacterial or viral conjunctivitis, is uncommon among dogs [1, 2].

Overgrowth of *Staphylococcus* spp. and *Streptococcus* spp. may cause infectious conjunctivitis in dogs [2]. In addition, acute cases of canine distemper virus (CDV) have been associated with conjunctivitis in clinical

settings [2]. Canine herpesvirus type-1 (CHV-1) has caused conjunctivitis experimentally [1, 2].

27.5.2 Canine Noninfectious Conjunctivitis

When canine conjunctivitis occurs, it tends to result from some other primary, underlying disease [1, 2, 51]. The most common among these include [1, 2, 14, 51–55, the, following]:

- KCS (refer to Chapter 25, Section 25.3.1 and Chapter 26, Section 26.2)
- Abnormal eyelid conformations (refer to Chapter 19, Sections 19.2.3 and 19.2.4)
- Conjunctival foreign body
  Corneal disease (refer to Chapter 29)
  – Keratitis
  – Corneal ulceration(s)
- Uveitis (refer to Chapter 17, Section 17.3)
- Glaucoma (refer to Chapter 22, Section 22.2.2)
- Infection of the nasolacrimal apparatus (refer to Chapter 26, Section 26.3.2)
- Systemic leishmaniasis, causing ocular signs
  – Allergic and immune-mediated disease
  – Atopy (refer to Chapter 5, Section 5.8)
  – The pemphigus complex of diseases (refer to Chapter 3, Section 3.8.3 and Chapter 12, Section 12.4)
  – Lupus erythematosus (refer to Chapter 13, Section 13.1.2)

27.5.3 Conjunctival Foreign Bodies

Conjunctival foreign bodies are small, yet immensely irritating to the eye. Grass awns or seeds are exceptionally good at tucking behind the nictitans [1]. The resulting inflammation makes it easy for awns to disappear beneath the billowy connective tissue [1]. To facilitate diagnosis, the clinician needs to check for foreign bodies within the fornices of the conjunctiva [1]. This requires the application of topical anesthetic so that the patient may allow these regions to be explored using a moistened tip of a cotton-tipped applicator [1].

27.5.4 Pathology Associated with the Nasolacrimal Apparatus

An infection of the nasolacrimal apparatus will also cause conjunctivitis; however, an obstruction of the same route will cause epiphora [1]. Epiphora is often mistaken for conjunctivitis [1]. Patients that present with unilateral serous ocular discharge, in the absence of conjunctival inflammation, are more likely to have nasolacrimal duct dysfunction. These patients need to have the patency of the nasolacrimal system explored via the fluorescent dye test that was outlined in Chapter 26, Section 26.3.4 [56].

27.5.5 Allergic Conjunctivitis

Allergic, infectious, and immune-mediated conjunctivitis should only be considered when the other aforementioned differentials have been ruled out.

Patients with allergic conjunctivitis typically also exhibit facial and/or aural pruritus, with or without concurrent blepharitis [1]. In severe cases of facial rubbing, patients may present with self-inflicted traumatic wounds to the face [57, 58]. It is not uncommon for patients with intense pruritus to scratch at their face and/or ears to the point that they create curvilinear excoriations [5].

The presumptive diagnosis of allergic conjunctivitis is supported by the presence of eosinophils on a conjunctival scrape [1].

Treatment is aimed largely at increasing patient comfort. This may require the use of topical or oral steroids to resolve clinical signs before tapering down to the lowest effective dose [1].

27.6 Other Manifestations of Conjunctivitis in the Cat and Dog

The conjunctiva represents the third most common location of canine ocular tumors, immediately after the globe and the eyelid [59].

Conjunctival masses may take on any appearance (see Figures 27.12a, b).

Most common types of primary conjunctival neoplasia in cats and dogs include the following [59–61]:

- Melanomas
- Lymphomas
- Hemangiomas
- Hemangiosarcomas
- Squamous papillomas
- Squamous cell carcinomas
- Mast cell tumors
- Viral papillomas

Most conjunctival melanomas are malignant [59]. They have a high recurrence rate, but do not typically metastasize [59]. The bulbar conjunctiva is the most typical location for this tumor type [62]. Cats with conjunctival melanoma appear to have a worse prognosis than dogs with the same tumor type in the same location [62].

Ocular lymphoma in cats and dogs has been historically associated with hyphema, blindness, and/or anterior uveitis [60, 63–65]. Conjunctival lymphoma has also been described in the dog in relation to the conjunctiva that lines the nictitans [66]. Affected dogs typically have a bilateral presentation [60]. A 2013 study by Nerschbach et al. confirmed that conjunctival lymphoma occurs in cats as well and presents as chemosis [60].

For more information about individual types of conjunctival neoplasia, consult a veterinary ophthalmology, oncology and/or pathology textbook.

Recognize that conjunctival neoplasia can be diagnosed via biopsy [1]. Conjunctival biopsy is obtained by applying a topical anesthetic agent to the affected eye [1]. Because the conjunctiva is loosely adhered to the dorsolateral sclera, it can be snipped easily at this location to create a 3 × 3 mm specimen [1].

Biopsies play a critical role in establishing a definitive diagnosis. Conjunctival lymphoma, for instance, may be mistaken for non-neoplastic conjunctivitis without a biopsy [2].

(a)

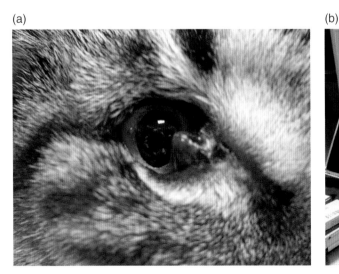

(b)

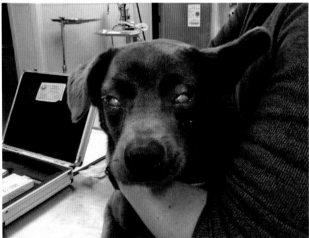

Figure 27.12 (a) Unilateral conjunctival mass in a feline patient. *Source:* Courtesy of Patricia Bennet, DVM. (b) Bilateral conjunctival masses in a canine patient. *Source:* Courtesy of Dr. Stephanie Harris.

References

1 Heinrich C. (2015). Assessing canine conjunctivitis. Vet Times [Internet]. www.vettimes.co.uk/app/uploads/wp-post-to-pdf-enhanced-cache/1/assessing-canine-conjunctivitis.pdf.

2 Ofri, R. (2017). Conjunctivitis in dogs. *NAVC Clinician's Brief* (April): 89–93.

3 Gelatt, KN. Disorders of the Conjunctiva in Cats. The Merck Manual [Internet]. https://www.merckvetmanual.com/cat-owners/eye-disorders-of-cats/disorders-of-the-conjunctiva-in-cats.

4 Dyce, K.M., Sack, W.O., and Wensing, C.J.G. (2010). *Textbook of Veterinary Anatomy*, 4e, xii, 834 p. St. Louis, MO: Saunders/Elsevier.

5 Englar, R.E. (2017). *Performing the Small Animal Physical Examination*. Hoboken, NJ: Wiley.

6 Lim, C.C. (2015). *Small Animal Ophthalmic Atlas and Guide*, xiii, 151 p. Chichester, West Sussex: Wiley.

7 Pickett, J.P. (2004). Ectropion. In: *The 5-Minute Veterinary Consult: Canine and Feline* (ed. L.P. Tilley and F.W.K. Smith), 390–391. Philadelphia: Lippincott Williams & Wilkins.

8 Bernays, M.E. (2006). The cat with abnormal eyelid appearance. In: *Problem-Based Feline Medicine* (ed. J. Rand), 1317–1329. Edinburgh; New York: Saunders.

9 Smith, R.I.E. (2006). The cat with ocular discharge or changed conjunctival appearance. In: *Problem-Based Feline Medicine* (ed. J. Rand), 1207–1232. Edinburgh; New York: Saunders.

10 Millichamp NJ. (2010). Ocular diseases unique to the feline patient (Proceedings). DVM 360 [Internet]. http://veterinarycalendar.dvm360.com/ocular-diseases-unique-feline-patient-proceedings.

11 Lim, C.C. and Maggs, D.J. (2012). Ophthalmology. In: *The Cat: Clinical Medicine and Management* (ed. S.E. Little), 807–845. St. Louis, Missouri: Saunders Elsevier.

12 Ofri, R. (2017). Conjunctivitis in cats. *NAVC Clinician's Brief* (April): 95–100.

13 Maggs, D.J. (2013). Conjunctiva. In: *Slatter's Fundamentals of Veterinary Opthalmology* (ed. D.J. Maggs, P.E. Miller and R. Ofri), 140–158. St. Louis, MO: Elsevier.

14 Aroch, I., Ofri, R., and Sutton, G. (2013). Ocular manifestations of systemic diseases. In: *Slatter's Fundamentals of Veterinary Ophthalmology* (ed. D.J. Maggs, P.E. Miller and R. Ofri), 184–219. St. Louis, MO: Elsevier.

15 Stiles, J. (2013). Feline ophthalmology. In: *Veterinary Ophthalmology* (ed. K.N. Gelatt, B.C. Gilger and T.J. Kern), 1477–1559. Ames, IA: Wiley-Blackwell.

16 Mitchell, N. (2006). Feline ophthalmology part 2: clinical presentation and aetiology of common ocular conditions. *Irish Vet. J.* 59 (4): 223–232.

17 Chandler, E.A., Gaskell, R.M., and Gaskell, C.J. (2008). *Feline Medicine and Therapeutics*. Ames, IA: Wiley.

18 Hartmann, K. and Levy, J. (2011). *Feline Infectious Diseases: Self-Assessment Color Review (Veterinary Self-Assessment Color Review Series)*. Boca Raton, FL: Taylor & Francis Group, LLC.

19 Reinstein, S. (ed.) (2017). *The Squinting Cat: Herpes Until Proven Otherwise*. Michigan: Michigan VMA.

20 Stiles, J. (2014). Ocular manifestations of feline viral diseases. *Vet. J.* 201 (2): 166–173.

21 Stiles, J. and Pogranichniy, R. (2008). Detection of virulent feline herpesvirus-1 in the corneas of clinically normal cats. *J. Feline Med. Surg.* 10 (2): 154–159.

22 Maggs, D.J. (2005). Update on pathogenesis, diagnosis, and treatment of feline herpesvirus type 1. *Clin. Tech. Small Anim. Pract.* 20 (2): 94–101.

23 Gould, D. (2011). Feline herpesvirus-1: ocular manifestations, diagnosis and treatment options. *J. Feline Med. Surg.* 13 (5): 333–346.

24 Westermeyer, H.D., Thomasy, S.M., Kado-Fong, H., and Maggs, D.J. (2009). Assessment of viremia associated with experimental primary feline herpesvirus infection or presumed herpetic recrudescence in cats. *Am. J. Vet. Res.* 70 (1): 99–104.

25 Grahn, B.H. and Sandmeyer, L.S. (2010). Diagnostic ophthalmology ophtalmologie diagnostique. *Can Vet. J.* 51 (3): 327.

26 Nasisse, M.P., Davis, B.J., Guy, J.S. et al. (1992). Isolation of feline herpesvirus 1 from the trigeminal ganglia of acutely and chronically infected cats. *J. Vet. Intern. Med.* 6 (2): 102–103.

27 Plummer, C.E. (2012). Herpetic keratoconjunctivitis in a cat. *NAVC Clinician's Brief* (January): 26–28.

28 Ellis, T.M. (1981). Feline respiratory virus carriers in clinically healthy cats. *Aust. Vet. J.* 57 (3): 115–118.

29 Gaskell, R.M. and Povey, R.C. (1977). Experimental induction of feline viral rhinotracheitis virus re-excretion in FVR-recovered cats. *Vet. Rec.* 100 (7): 128–133.

30 Nasisse, M.P., Guy, J.S., Davidson, M.G. et al. (1989). Experimental ocular herpesvirus infection in the cat. Sites of virus replication, clinical features and effects of corticosteroid administration. *Invest. Ophthalmol. Vis. Sci.* 30 (8): 1758–1768.

31 Nasisse, M.P., Guy, J.S., Stevens, J.B. et al. (1993). Clinical and laboratory findings in chronic conjunctivitis in cats: 91 cases (1983–1991). *J. Am. Vet. Med. Assoc.* 203 (6): 834–837.

32 Smith L. (2011). The dos and don'ts of treating ocular disease in cats (Proceedings). DVM 360 [Internet]. http://veterinarycalendar.dvm360.com/dos-and-donts-treating-ocular-disease-cats-proceedings.

33 Tilley, L.P. and Smith, F.W.K. (2004). *The 5-Minute Veterinary Consult: Canine and Feline*, 3e, lviii, 1487 p. Baltimore, MD: Lippincott Williams & Wilkins.

34 Côté, E. (2015). *Clinical Veterinary Advisor. Dogs and Cats*, 3e, xxxvii, 1642 p. St. Louis, Missouri: Elsevier Mosby.

35 Lappin, M.R. (2001). *Feline Internal Medicine Secrets*. Philadelphia: Hanley & Belfus, Inc.

36 Gruffydd-Jones T, editor. (2009). Chlamydial Infections of Cats. Proceedings of the 34th World Small Animal Veterinary Congress WSAVA 2009; Sao Paulo, Brazil.

37 Gruffydd-Jones, T., Addie, D., Belak, S. et al. (2009). Chlamydophila felis infection. ABCD guidelines on prevention and management. *J. Feline Med. Surg.* 11 (7): 605–609.

38 Shewen, P.E., Povey, R.C., and Wilson, M.R. (1978). Case report. Feline chlamydial infection. *Can. Vet. J.* 19 (10): 289–292.

39 Low, H.C., Powell, C.C., Veir, J.K. et al. (2007). Prevalence of feline herpesvirus 1, Chlamydophila felis, and Mycoplasma spp DNA in conjunctival cells collected from cats with and without conjunctivitis. *Am. J. Vet. Res.* 68 (6): 643–648.

40 Hartmann, A.D., Hawley, J., Werckenthin, C. et al. (2010). Detection of bacterial and viral organisms from the conjunctiva of cats with conjunctivitis and upper respiratory tract disease. *J. Feline Med. Surg.* 12 (10): 775–782.

41 Sandmeyer, L.S., Waldner, C.L., Bauer, B.S. et al. (2010). Comparison of polymerase chain reaction tests for diagnosis of feline herpesvirus, Chlamydophila fells, and Mycoplasma spp. infection in cats with ocular disease in Canada. *Can. Vet. J.–Revue Veterinaire Canadienne* 51 (6): 629–633.

42 Volopich, S., Benetka, V., Schwendenwein, I. et al. (2005). Cytologic findings, and feline herpesvirus DNA and Chlamydophila felis antigen detection rates in normal cats and cats with conjunctival and corneal lesions. *Vet. Ophthalmol.* 8 (1): 25–32.

43 Cullen, C.L. and Webb, A.A. (2013). Ocular manifestations of systemic disease. Part 2: the cat. In: *Veterinary Ophthalmology* (ed. K.N. Gelatt, B.C. Gilger and T.J. Kern), 1978–2036. Ames, IA: Wiley-Blackwell.

44 Maggs, D.J. (2013). Cornea and sclera. In: *Slatter's Fundamentals of Veterinary Ophthalmology* (ed. D.J. Maggs, P.E. Miller and R. Ofri), 184–219. St. Louis, MO: Elsevier.

45 Gerding, P.A. Jr. and Kakoma, I. (1990). Microbiology of the canine and feline eye. *Vet. Clin. North Am. Small Anim. Pract.* 20 (3): 615–625.

46 Pentlarge, V.W. and Riis, R.C. (1984). Proliferative keratitis in a cat – a case-report. *J. Am. Anim. Hosp. Assoc.* 20 (3): 477–480.

47 Paulsen, M.E., Lavach, J.D., Severin, G.A., and Eichenbaum, J.D. (1987). Feline eosinophilic keratitis – a review of 15 clinical cases. *J. Am. Anim. Hosp. Assoc.* 23 (1): 63–69.

48 Bedford, P.G.C. and Cotchin, E. (1983). An unusual chronic keratoconjunctivitis in the cat. *J. Small Anim. Pract.* 24 (2): 85–102.

49 Allgoewer, I., Schaffer, E.H., Stockhaus, C., and Vogtlin, A. (2001). Feline eosinophilic conjunctivitis. *Vet. Ophthalmol.* 4 (1): 69–74.

50 Ketring, K.L. and Glaze, M.B. (2012). *Atlas of Feline Ophthalmology*, 2e, xviii, 172 p. Chichester, West Sussex, UK; Ames, Iowa: Wileyl.

51 Maggs, D.J. (2013). Diagnostic techniques. In: *Slatter's Fundamentals of Veterinary Opthalmology* (ed. D.J. Maggs, P.E. Miller and R. Ofri), 79–109. St. Louis, MO: Elsevier.

52 Pena, M.A. and Leiva, M. (2008). Canine conjunctivitis and blepharitis. *Vet. Clin. North Am. Small Anim. Pract.* 38 (2): 233–249, v.

53 Lourenco-Martins, A.M., Delgado, E., Neto, I. et al. (2011). Allergic conjunctivitis and conjunctival provocation tests in atopic dogs. *Vet. Ophthalmol.* 14 (4): 248–256.

54 Furiani, N., Scarampella, F., Martino, P.A. et al. (2011). Evaluation of the bacterial microflora of the conjunctival sac of healthy dogs and dogs with atopic dermatitis. *Vet. Dermatol.* 22 (6): 490–496.

55 Freitas, J.C., Nunes-Pinheiro, D.C., Lopes Neto, B.E. et al. (2012). Clinical and laboratory alterations in dogs naturally infected by Leishmania chagasi. *Rev. Soc. Bras. Med. Trop.* 45 (1): 24–29.

56 Ford, R.B. and Mazzaferro, E. (2011). *Kirk & Bistner's Handbook of Veterinary Procedures and Emergency Treatment*. St. Louis, MO: Elsevier Saunders.

57 Stein, D.J., Dodman, N.H., Borchelt, P., and Hollander, E. (1994). Behavioral disorders in veterinary practice: relevance to psychiatry. *Compr. Psychiatry* 35 (4): 275–285.

58 Scott, D.W., Miller, W.H., and Erb, H.N. (2013). Feline dermatology at Cornell University: 1407 cases (1988–2003). *J. Feline Med. Surg.* 15 (4): 307–316.

59 Dubielzig R. (2014). Primary Tumors of the Canine Conjunctiva, Eyelids and Orbit. UW School of Veterinary Medicine [Internet]. https://www.vetmed.wisc.edu/pbs/dubielzig/pages/coplow/PowerPoints/CanineConjLidsOrbitSask2014.pdf.

60 Nerschbach, V., Eule, J.C., Eberle, N. et al. (2016). Ocular manifestation of lymphoma in newly diagnosed cats. *Vet. Comp. Oncol.* 14 (1): 58–66.

61 Ehrhart EJ, Gardiner D, Tancredi-Ballugera T, Gionfriddo JR. (2008). A challenging case: Conjunctival lymphoma in a cat. DVM 360 [Internet]. http://

veterinarymedicine.dvm360.com/challenging-case-conjunctival-lymphoma-cat.

62 Schobert, C.S., Labelle, P., and Dubielzig, R.R. (2010). Feline conjunctival melanoma: histopathological characteristics and clinical outcomes. *Vet. Ophthalmol.* 13 (1): 43–46.

63 Krohne, S.G., Henderson, N.M., Richardson, R.C., and Vestre, W.A. (1994). Prevalence of ocular involvement in dogs with multicentric lymphoma: prospective evaluation of 94 cases. *Vet. Comp. Ophthalmol.* 4: 127–135.

64 Gwin, R.M., Gelatt, K.N., and Williams, L.W. (1982). Ophthalmic neoplasms in the Dog. *J. Am. Anim. Hosp. Assoc.* 18 (6): 853–866.

65 Massa, K.L., Gilger, B.C., Miller, T.L., and Davidson, M.G. (2002). Causes of uveitis in dogs: 102 cases (1989–2000). *Vet. Ophthalmol.* 5 (2): 93–98.

66 Hong, I.H., Bae, S.H., Lee, S.G. et al. (2011). Mucosa-associated lymphoid tissue lymphoma of the third eyelid conjunctiva in a dog. *Vet. Ophthalmol.* 14 (1): 61–65.

28

Abnormal Appearances of the Sclera

28.1 Introduction to the Sclera

The sclera is a stiff, white, fibrous tissue that joins with the cornea, rostrally, to form the outermost layer of the globe [1, 2]. The sclera protects the globe by maintaining the shape of the eye. It also serves as a site of attachment for extraocular muscles.

The thickness of the sclera is not uniform. It varies depending upon location [1]. Scleral thickness is at its maximum of 1 mm near the limbus, which is the point at which the sclera and the cornea meet [1, 3].

Just as clinicians must raise or lower the eyelids to gain an appreciation for the palpebral conjunctiva, so, too, is the case for the sclera. The sclera is not normally visible when the patient is staring straight ahead (see Figures 28.1a, b).

Sometimes just a sliver of the sclera is visible in the healthy patient [4]. This sliver may increase as the patient becomes anxious or fearful [4]. When a large amount of the sclera is visible, the patient is said to have "whale eye" [4]. This may indicate fear and discomfort with the current situation [4] (see Figures 28.2a–d).

Note that the sclera is also prominent in brachycephalic breeds by virtue of their oversized palpebral fissures and very shallow orbits [5]. In these patients, the sclera is visible because of conformational issues rather than fear or discontent.

Although the sclera is typically white, certain dogs have limbal pigment [1, 3]. This pigment alters the color of the sclera from white to a dark-brown or black [3] (see Figure 28.3).

Scleral pigment, secondary to melanin deposition, may be focal, as evident in Figure 28.3, or it may be widespread [3]. The sclera may appear gray if melanin distribution is light and expansive [3].

The sclera has a blood supply, unlike the cornea [1, 4]. Scleral vessels are not typically prominent, although in some patients, the scleral venous plexus is visible as a ring adjacent to the limbus [1].

Because the sclera of kittens and puppies is thin, as compared to that of adults, the bluish color associated with scleral vasculature may shine through. This is considered normal in juvenile patients [1].

A normal sclera in both the juvenile and adult patient should be free of hyperemia, hemorrhage, icterus, and masses.

28.2 Abnormal Scleral Pigment

Pigment-associated changes to the sclera are typically shades of yellow and are reflective of icterus, otherwise referred to as jaundice [1, 4].

Icterus is the result of bile accumulating in the body [6]. This pigment can be detected throughout the body; however, it is easiest to identify at the following locations in dogs and cats [4]:

- Sclera
- Mucous membranes
- Peri-aural or pre-auricular skin in the feline patient, on account of species-associated focal hypotrichosis
- All other regions of skin, provided that the overlying fur has been parted (see Figures 28.4a–f)

Note that icteric mucous membranes may also be pale. Pallor and icterus are not necessarily mutually exclusive and may both be reflective of the same underlying disease process [6].

When it occurs, icterus results from one of three pathways [4, 6–9]:

- Pre-hepatic
- Hepatic
- Post-hepatic

28.2.1 Pre-Hepatic Icterus

Pre-hepatic icterus occurs in the face of extensive hemolysis [7, 8, 10]. Ordinarily, when erythrocytes rupture or are otherwise destroyed, their components are metabolized by the body [11]. Erythrocytes contain heme, which makes up hemoglobin. Enzyme activity facilitates the metabolic conversion of heme to

(a) (b)

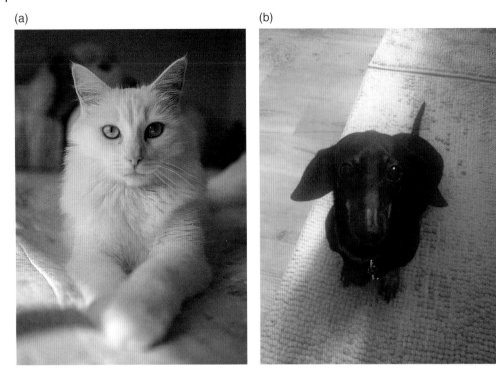

Figure 28.1 (a) The sclera is largely hidden from view in a normal, non-stressed, and healthy feline patient. *Source:* Courtesy of Kat Blincoe. (b) The sclera is largely hidden from view in a normal, non-stressed, and healthy canine patient. *Source:* Courtesy of Meghan Teixeira.

biliverdin, and biliverdin to unconjugated bilirubin [11]. Unconjugated bilirubin is subsequently conjugated within the liver to improve its solubility in water [11].

Conjugated bilirubin will either become a component of bile or colonic contents [11]. Within the colon, bacteria deconjugate bilirubin to its original form, which is then converted into urobilinogen [11]. The oxidation of urobilinogen creates urobilin, which is excreted by the kidneys, and stercobilin, which is excreted in the feces [11]. A small portion of urobilinogen returns to the bile via enterohepatic circulation so that the cycle can repeat [11].

Excessive breakdown of erythrocytes overwhelms the body's ability to metabolize and ultimately excrete bilirubin [11]. The buildup of unconjugated bilirubin in the bloodstream results in icterus [11].

Note that hemolysis may be the result of intrinsic defects within the erythrocytes themselves, or it may be due to external factors.

In the cat, the most common causes of pre-hepatic icterus include the following [7–16]:

- Adverse vaccine and/or drug reactions
  - Acetaminophen
  - New methylene blue
- Onion toxicity
- Infectious disease

  - Hemobartonellosis, as caused by *Mycoplasma haemofelis* (refer to Chapter 6, Section 6.4.5)
  - Cytauxzoonosis, as caused by *Cytauxzoon felis* (refer to Chapter 6, Section 6.5.8)
  - Feline immunodeficiency virus (FIV)
  - Feline leukemia virus (FeLV)
- Immune-mediated hemolytic anemia (IMHA)
- Transfusion reactions
- Neonatal isoerythrolysis

The dog may also experience IMHA and adverse drug reactions that precipitate pre-hepatic icterus [8]. The infectious disease, babesiosis, shares the same outcome [8].

Patients with pre-hepatic icterus may present for general malaise and weakness. A complete blood count (CBC) may reveal severe anemia, hemoglobinemia, and hemoglobinuria [8] (see Figures 28.5a, b).

28.2.1.1 Acetaminophen Toxicity

Acetaminophen, otherwise referred to as paracetamol, is a non-steroidal anti-inflammatory drug (NSAID) [17]. Its availability in over-the-counter formulations has led to a spike in reports of acetaminophen toxicity for people among companion animals [18]. Cats are particularly sensitive to the effects of acetaminophen because of their reduced ability to break it down into nontoxic metabolites [18–23].

(a)

(b)

(d)

(c)

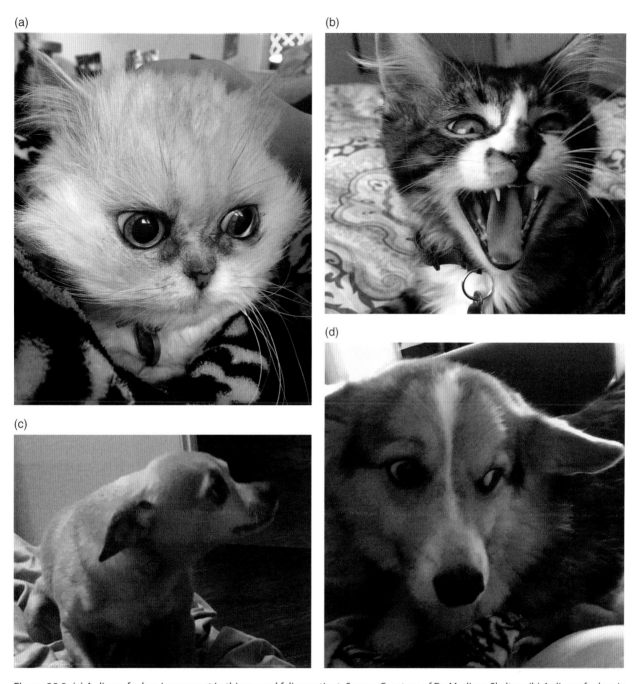

Figure 28.2 (a) A sliver of sclera is apparent in this normal feline patient. *Source:* Courtesy of Dr. Madison Skelton. (b) A sliver of sclera is apparent in this potentially fractious feline patient. *Source:* Courtesy of Hilary Lazarus, DVM. (c) A sliver of sclera is apparent in this timid canine patient. *Source:* Courtesy of Lydia McDaniel. (d) "Whale eye" in a frightened canine patient. *Source:* Courtesy of Cora Zenko.

Acetaminophen is metabolized by the liver [18, 23]. Conjugation with glucuronic acid is the primary pathway for metabolism [18, 23]. Conjugation with sulfate represents a secondary and minor pathway [18, 23]. The enzyme, glucuronyl transferase, mediates glucuronidation [18].

As compared to dogs, cats are deficient in this enzyme [18]. The result is that both glucuronidation and sulfation pathways become saturated [18]. When this happens, the toxic metabolite, N-acetyl-para-benzoquinone imine (NAPQI), accumulates [18, 19, 23–25].

Doses as low as 10 mg/kg have caused acetaminophen toxicosis in cats [23, 24]. Even one 80 mg tablet, as might be obtained in a children's over-the-counter formulation, is toxic to the average-sized cat [23].

NAPQI disrupts the integrity of cell membranes, causing cellular injury and death [23]. Hepatocytes and erythrocytes are significantly impacted [18, 19, 24].

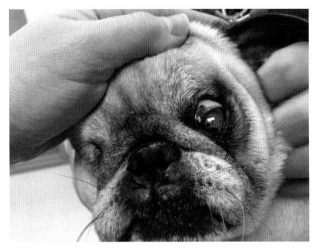

Figure 28.3 Normal variation of scleral pigment in a Pug dog. This patient has excessive limbal pigment.

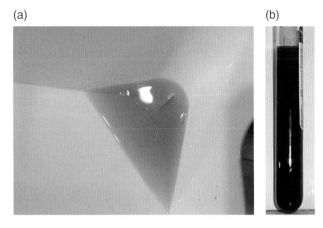

Figure 28.5 (a) Normal urine from a feline patient that inappropriately eliminated in a storage bin. *Source:* Courtesy of Stephanie Horwitz. (b) Hemoglobinuria in a canine patient with pre-hepatic icterus.

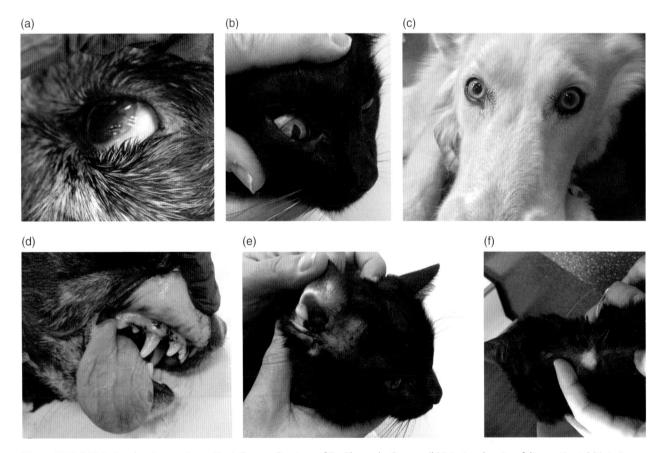

Figure 28.4 (a) Icteric sclera in a canine patient. *Source:* Courtesy of Dr. Alexandra Brower. (b) Icteric sclera in a feline patient. (c) Icteric sclera in a Husky dog. Because this dog's irises are pale blue, the yellow hue of icterus creates the illusion of a color change to lime green. *Source:* Courtesy of Dr. Stephanie Harris. (d) Icteric mucous membranes in a canine patient. *Source:* Courtesy of Dr. Alexandra Brower. (e) Peri-aural icterus in a feline patient. (f) Icterus associated with the skin at the base of the neck when fur has been parted by the clinician.

NAPQI oxidizes ferrous iron, Fe^{+2}, to ferric iron, Fe^{+3} [18]. The result is transformation of hemoglobin into methemoglobin, which is inefficient at transporting oxygen in systemic circulation [18, 19, 24]. If severe, methemoglobinemia results in a chocolate or muddy brown appearance to the mucous membranes and potentially pigmenturia [18, 23].

As hemoglobin undergoes oxidation, it is denatured [18]. Remnants of hemoglobin precipitate out onto erythrocyte surfaces [18]. These precipitations appear as bulges on the surfaces of erythrocytes. These bulges are called Heinz bodies [18, 26].

Heinz bodies are never normal occurrences in canine blood [26]. By contrast, in healthy cats, as many as 5–10% of erythrocytes may be affected by Heinz bodies [26]. Clinicians should become concerned when Heinz bodies in feline patients exceed this percentage.

Heinz bodies are visible on blood smears that have been prepared with commercial Romanowsky stains, such as Diff-Quik [18]. The use of a vital stain, such as 0.5% new methylene blue, will accentuate these morphological changes [18, 26] (see Figures 28.6a–c).

Heinz bodies target affected erythrocytes for premature removal from systemic circulation [26].

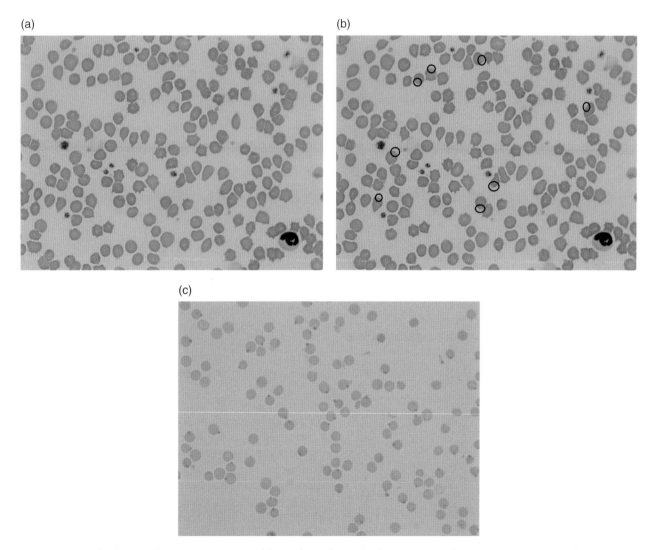

Figure 28.6 (a) Blood smear demonstrating appreciable numbers of Heinz bodies, 100× magnification. *Source:* Courtesy of Nora Springer, DVM, DACVP. (b) Same blood smear as in Figure 28.6a; however, some of the most obvious Heinz bodies have been circled with black. They appear like blisters or bulges on the surface of the erythrocytes. *Source:* Courtesy of Nora Springer, DVM, DACVP. (c) Blood smear stained with new methylene blue. Note that Heinz bodies stain deep blue.

Heinz bodies also induce instability of the erythrocyte population [18]. Because their fragility is increased, erythrocytes break apart [18]. The result is hemolytic anemia [18]. Hemolytic anemia causes icterus.

Patients may also present in respiratory distress due to poor oxygenation [18, 20, 23–25]. Facial and paw edema is also characteristic of acetaminophen toxicosis in cats [18, 20, 23, 24, 27]. However, the pathophysiology of this feature remains unknown [18].

28.2.1.2 Onion Toxicity

Onions are a member of the *Allium* genus, which is a category of flowering plants that includes leeks, garlic, and chives [28, 29]. These plants contain organosulfoxides [28, 29]. When these plants are chewed, organosulfoxides are converted into noxious sulfur-containing compounds that cause oxidative hemolysis.

Both dogs and cats can succumb to toxicosis; however, cats are two to three times more susceptible than dogs because of their low threshold for tolerating oxidative damage [28, 29]. It takes a mere 5 g of onions per kilogram of body weight to incite hemolysis in cats, as compared to 15–30 g/kg in dogs [28, 29].

As was true of acetaminophen toxicosis, *Allium* sp. cause anemia, methemoglobinemia, impaired oxygen transport, Heinz body formation, and increased erythrocyte fragility [28, 29].

Affected patients very often become icteric [28, 29].

Cooked *Allium* and spoiled *Allium* are no less toxic [28, 29].

History taking plays an important role in diagnosis [28–30]. Certain foods, such as the skin of commercially prepared rotisserie chickens, powdered soup mix, and jars of baby food, may contain *Allium*.

28.2.1.3 Immune-Mediated Hemolytic Anemia

IMHA is a disease in which the body's defense mechanisms turn self against self and attack erythrocytes [30, 31]. Erythrocytes are coated with antibodies and other proteins that collectively make up the complement system of immunity. This tags them for removal from systemic circulation, so that they can be destroyed within the spleen or liver. Alternatively, they may undergo cytolysis within the bloodstream itself [31]. The former scenario is called extravascular hemolysis as compared to the latter scenario, intravascular hemolysis [31].

IMHA may result from primary autoimmune disease [31].

Alternatively, IMHA may be triggered by the following [31]:

- Administration of certain drugs and, potentially, vaccinations
- Change in physiologic state, such as the onset of estrus and/or whelping

- Infectious organisms, such as *Babesia*, *Ehrlichia*, and *Leishmania* spp.
- Inflammatory disease, such as severe enteritis
- Neoplastic or myeloproliferative disease

Middle-aged to older dogs are at greater risk of developing IMHA [30, 31]. Within the United States, the Cocker Spaniel, Springer Spaniel, and Old English Sheepdog may be predisposed [31]. Females may also be at greater risk of developing IMHA [30].

IMHA may occur in conjunction with immune-mediated thrombocytopenia (IMTP), or it may occur alone [31].

Intravascular hemolysis results in hyperbilirubinemia [31]. Patients may also present with pallor due to reduced erythrocyte populations [30, 31]. Owners often report lethargy and exercise intolerance [30, 31]. These clinical signs stem from anemia [30, 31].

Severe cases will result in icterus [30, 31].

Blood smears may demonstrate classic changes that are supportive of a presumptive diagnosis of IMHA, including the following [31–33]:

- Spherocytes
- Polychromasia
- Ghost cells
- Nucleated erythrocytes

Spherocytes lack the biconcave shape of erythrocytes [32, 33]. They are sphere shaped; hence, the name.

On a blood smear, normal-shaped erythrocytes have a lighter center and a darker periphery that reflects their biconcavity [32]. This is particularly true in dogs [32].

By contrast, spherocytes are more compact due to lack of biconcavity [32, 33]. This gives them a smaller-than-normal, denser appearance, without central pallor [32, 33] (see Figures 28.7a, b).

Note that spherocytes are not pathognomonic for IMHA. This cell type may also be present in patients with splenic disease, hypophosphatemia, or zinc toxicosis [30, 34, 35].

The erythrocytes of patients with IMHA may also exhibit polychromasia in their erythrocytes on blood smears [32, 33]. Polychromasia is a characteristic of reticulocytes in circulation [32, 33]. Reticulocytes are immature erythrocytes [32, 33]. Because these contain more RNA in the form of ribosomes than mature erythrocytes and because RNA appears bluer than the red of hemoglobin, reticulocytes appear purple [32, 33] (see Figure 28.8).

In health, reticulocytes are released into circulation, where they lose RNA to complete the maturation process [32, 33]. It is normal to see <1.5% of the erythrocyte population on blood smear as reticulocytes in healthy dogs and cats. However, if that percentage is significantly

(a)

(b)

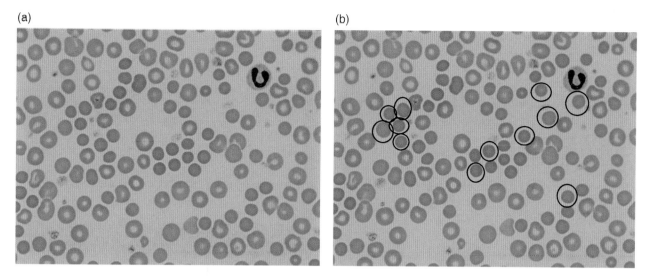

Figure 28.7 (a) Blood smear demonstrating spherocytes, 100× magnification. *Source:* Courtesy of Nora Springer, DVM, DACVP. (b) Same blood smear as in Figure 28.6a; however, some spherocytes have been circled with black. Their lack of central pallor makes them appear flat rather than three-dimensional. *Source:* Courtesy of Nora Springer, DVM, DACVP.

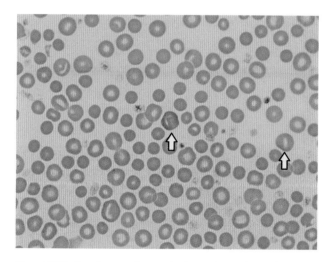

Figure 28.8 Blood smear demonstrating spherocytes and polychromasia. Cells displaying polychromasia are indicated by yellow arrows, outlined in black, 100× magnification. *Source:* Courtesy of Nora Springer, DVM, DACVP.

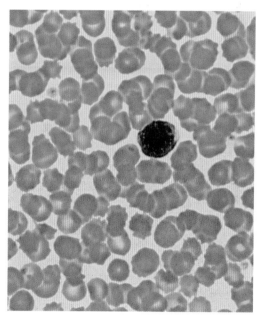

Figure 28.9 Blood smear, demonstrating nucleated erythrocyte, 100× magnification. *Source:* Courtesy of Nora Springer, DVM, DACVP.

increased, the patient is likely experiencing regenerative anemia [32, 33]. One reason for this is to compensate for erythrocytes that have undergone hemolysis as a result of IMHA [32, 33].

In cases of strongly regenerative anemia, nucleated erythrocytes may even be seen in circulation. These indicate that the body is under immense pressure to compensate for erythrocyte loss by releasing new cells into the circulation, even if they are not mature enough to perform their function [32, 33] (see Figure 28.9).

Ghost cells may also be present on blood smears from patients that have IMHA [32, 33]. Ghost cells are ruptured erythrocytes [32, 33]. Without hemoglobin, they appear as just a faded membrane [32, 33]. They result from intravascular hemolysis [32, 33] (see Figures 28.10a, b).

Note that intravascular hemolysis could be due to IMHA; however, the presence of ghost cells could also be artifactual [32, 33]. For example, if the sample was collected or handled incorrectly, ghost cells may develop. If patients were not fasted and their samples are lipemic, then ghost cell formation as an artifact is more likely.

The presence of ghost cells is therefore not pathognomonic for IMHA. The savvy clinician must act as a

(a)

(b)

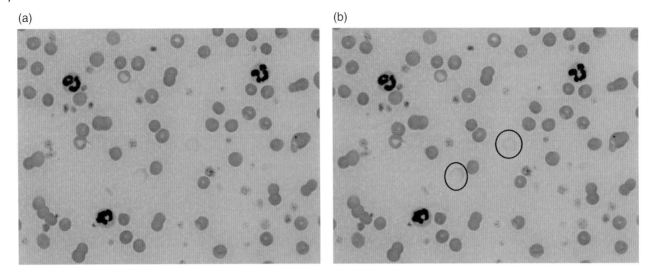

Figure 28.10 (a) Blood smear, demonstrating ghost cells, 100× magnification. *Source:* Courtesy of Nora Springer, DVM, DACVP. (b) Same blood smear as in Figure 28.10a, but with ghost cells circled in black. *Source:* Courtesy of Nora Springer, DVM, DACVP.

detective and consider ghost cells as one of many factors that could support a presumptive diagnosis. The patient with ghost cells secondary to poor handling of the blood, for example, freezing blood samples, will never develop hemoglobinuria, whereas the patient with IMHA is likely to.

Patients with IMHA may also develop spontaneous autoagglutination [31–33]. This refers to abnormal clumping of erythrocytes, and may be grossly evident along the sides of an EDTA blood collection tube (see Figure 28.11).

For patients that are suspected of having IMHA, clinicians may perform an in-house saline agglutination test [10, 30–33].

EDTA-anticoagulated blood is placed as a single droplet onto a slide, and is mixed with saline [30, 32, 33]. Typically one to two drops of saline are added to canine blood, as compared to three to four drops of saline for feline blood. This is because cats have a tendency to develop rouleaux formation, in which erythrocytes adhere to each other, but without an underlying immune-based cause [32, 33].

The slide mixture of blood and saline is initially observed for macroagglutination [30, 32, 33] (see Figure 28.12).

The slide may also be evaluated for microagglutination using light microscopy [30, 32, 33]. Microagglutination will appear cytologically as clumps of erythrocytes that appear in clusters like grapes, as compared to rouleaux formation, which has more of a stacked appearance, like coins [32, 33] (see Figure 28.13).

Healthy cats may have rouleaux formation; however, it is commonly seen in cats with systemic illness [32, 33]. Dogs do not typically demonstrate rouleaux formation [32, 33].

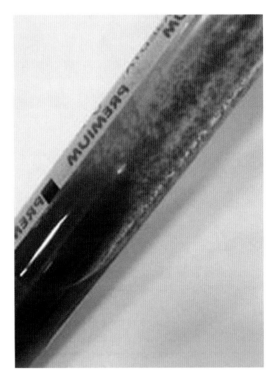

Figure 28.11 Spontaneous autoagglutination of blood within an EDTA blood collection tube. Note how the clumped erythrocytes adhere to the side of the tube. This is abnormal and is considered macroagglutination because it is visible to the naked eye.

Note that a positive in-house saline autoagglutination test is supportive of IMHA [10]. However, a negative test is insufficient to rule it out. This is because autoagglutination only occurs when anti-erythrocyte antibodies are very high in circulation. Lower levels of antibodies are incapable of inducing autoagglutination, even though IMHA may be present [32, 33].

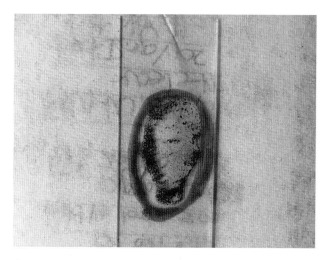

Figure 28.12 Positive in-house saline autoagglutination test. Note that macroagglutination is present. Clumps of erythrocytes are visible to the naked eye. *Source:* Courtesy of Dr. Lisa Keenan.

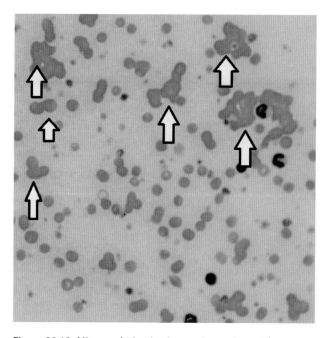

Figure 28.13 Microagglutination in a canine patient with immune-mediated hemolytic anemia (IMHA). Note how erythrocytes appear as clusters rather than "stacks of coins." *Source:* Courtesy of Nora Springer, DVM, DACVP.

Consult a clinical pathology reference to explore additional diagnostic testing that may confirm the diagnosis, including the Coombs test, antinuclear antibody test (ANA), and flow cytometry [30, 31].

28.2.2 Hepatic Icterus

Hepatic icterus results from liver disease [8]. Liver disease may be primary or secondary [8]. The differential list for both is extensive [8].

The most commonly implicated primary liver diseases that result in icterus include the following [7–9, 11, 36, 37]:

- Portosystemic shunts
  - Congenital
  - Acquired
- Infections
  - Toxoplasmosis, as caused by *Toxoplasma gondii*
  - Feline infectious peritonitis (FIP)
  - Leptospirosis
- Hepatic lipidosis
- Hepatitis
  - Copper-associated hepatitis, an inherited defect
- Cholangiohepatitis
  - Lymphocytic
  - Suppurative or neutrophilic
  - Fluke-associated
- Hepatic abscessation
- Neoplasia
  - Lymphoma
  - Biliary cystadenoma or cystadenocarcinoma
  - Hepatocellular or biliary carcinoma

The most commonly implicated secondary liver diseases that result in icterus include the following [7–9, 11, 36]:

- Drugs and toxins
  - Acetaminophen
  - Diazepam
  - Ketoconazole
  - Methimazole
  - Phenols
  - Aflatoxins
- Sepsis
- Metastatic neoplasia

Note that acetaminophen can cause both pre- and hepatic icterus.

The details of each of the aforementioned conditions are beyond the scope of this text.

Consult internal medicine, infectious disease, oncology, and toxicology references for more information as needed to facilitate next steps for diagnostic tools and case management.

28.2.2.1 Hepatic Lipidosis

Hepatic lipidosis is seen more commonly in cats than dogs. Hepatic lipidosis may be idiopathic; however, the majority of patients have an underlying reason for its development [38].

Anorexia is a trigger for hepatic lipidosis, particularly in obese, indoor-only cats [8]. Recent, stressful events are additional risk factors [8].

Anorexia triggers the body to mobilize peripheral fat as an energy source [38]. The liver is initially able to create energy from fat by means of β-oxidation. However, over time the amount of mobilized fat overwhelms the liver. The efficiency of β-oxidation decreases, and triglycerides are not exported from the liver as rapidly as they should be [38].

Hepatocytes begin to stockpile triglycerides in the form of vacuoles [38]. As their cytosol becomes distended on account of growing fat reserves, hepatocytes encroach upon bile canaliculi [38].

The compression of canaliculi results in severe cholestasis. Cholestasis is when the flow of bile is halted. Bile backs up because it cannot reach the duodenum, and hepatocellular damage results.

Icterus is one of many clinical signs that patients with hepatic lipidosis will present with, including weight loss, dehydration, generalized malaise, intermittent vomiting, and/or diarrhea [8, 38, 39].

Treatment is largely supportive and relies upon jump-starting the patient's appetite, as well as correcting dehydration and electrolyte imbalances [38]. Feeding tube placement may be necessary if the patient is averse to food and unwilling to reinitiate appetite on its own [38].

Once stable, patients may need to undergo exploratory laparotomy for abdominal organ biopsies to establish a definitive diagnosis that explains what led to hepatic lipidosis [38]. Greater than 85% of cats with hepatic lipidosis have underlying pathology [38].

Consult an internal medicine reference for additional information.

28.2.2.2 Additional Causes of Cholestasis

Hepatic lipidosis is not the only cause of cholestasis. Cholestasis may also result from additional sources of intrahepatic compression of the bile duct including the following [8, 37, 40]:

- Inflammatory infiltrates around the portal triad and/ or biliary tree
- Hepatocellular swelling secondary to corticosteroid hepatopathy in dogs
- Cirrhosis, that is, scarring of the liver with fibrosis
- Parasitic infestation, as from the liver fluke, *Platynosomum concinnum*

28.2.2.3 Suppurative Cholangiohepatitis

Suppurative cholangiohepatitis is pyogenic infection of the biliary tract. It is more common in cats than in dogs. The most common bacterial species to be involved include the following [38]:

- *Escherichia coli*
- *Enterobacter*
- *Enterococcus*
- *Β-hemolytic Streptococcus*

- *Klebsiella*
- *Actinomyces*
- *Clostridia*
- *Bacteroides*

Salmonella, Campylobacter, and *Leptospira* spp. are more frequently isolated in dogs with suppurative cholangiohepatitis [38].

T. gondii has also been implicated in feline presentations [38].

Consult an infectious disease textbook for additional details.

28.2.2.4 Poikilocytes and Liver Disease

The liver plays an essential role in lipid metabolism and cholesterol production [41, 42]. This impacts the lipid composition of erythrocyte membranes [41, 42]. When the liver is not functioning appropriately, changes are often seen in erythrocyte membranes that distort erythrocyte size and, in particular, shape [41, 42].

When patients have liver disease, poikilocytes are commonly seen on cytological examination of blood smears [40–42]. Poikilocytes are abnormally shaped erythrocytes [40]. They may be flat, elongated, crescent-, or tear-shaped. They may also develop pointy projections. There are different names for these cytological appearances. Refer to a clinical pathology text for appropriate nomenclature (see Figure 28.14).

Poikilocytes more frequently appear in feline than canine blood [38]. However, when they are detected, it is wise for the clinician to investigate the liver as a potential source [38].

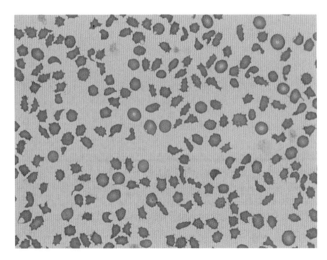

Figure 28.14 Poikilocytosis on a feline blood smear. *Source:* Courtesy of Nora Springer, DVM, DACVP.

28.2.3 Post-Hepatic Icterus

Post-hepatic icterus is due to common bile duct obstruction [8].

The common bile duct extends from the liver to the duodenum. It represents a shared route for both the cystic and hepatic ducts [43, 44].

There are important species differences relative to the anatomy of the biliary system [43, 44].

In dogs, the major duodenal papilla is where the common bile duct enters the duodenum. At the point of entry, it is adjacent to, but not conjoined with the pancreatic duct. The pancreatic duct empties its contents into the duodenum at a separate location, the minor duodenal papilla [43, 44].

Cats are unique in that the common bile duct and pancreatic ducts both empty into the major duodenal papilla [43, 44]. For this reason, cats are much more prone to the development of pancreatitis. Any pathology that affects the major duodenal papilla has the potential to create ascending inflammation or infection through the pancreas [43, 44].

Common bile duct obstruction in both the dog and cat results in cholestasis involving extrahepatic sources, including the following [8, 40]:

- Choleliths
- Pancreatitis
- Gall bladder mucocoeles
- Pancreatic, biliary, or duodenal neoplasia

Any of the above can cause post-hepatic icterus.

Consult an internal medicine reference for additional information.

28.3 Prominent Scleral Vasculature

In addition to assessing the sclera for changes in pigment, the clinician should assess the sclera for alterations in vasculature. Scleral vessels are typically not prominent, although the scleral venous plexus may be visible in some patients [1].

There are normally four vessels, the vortex or vorticose veins, which drain the choroid and aqueous humor [43].

For unknown reasons, one or more of these may be engorged and prominent on physical examination [4] (see Figure 28.15).

This is considered a variation of normal and should not be concerning to either the clinician or the client.

By contrast, episcleritis is not a normal presentation [45]. Episcleritis is an inflammatory condition that involves the episclera [38, 46]. The episclera is the outermost layer of the sclera [4, 43]. It sits in between the

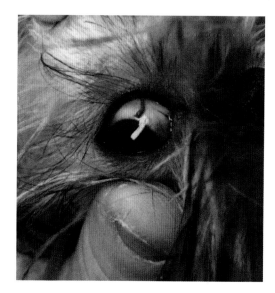

Figure 28.15 Prominent vortex vein as a variation of normal in this canine patient.

conjunctiva and the scleral stroma, which are bathed by the superficial and deep episcleral vessels [43].

Episcleritis may present as one of two forms:

- Nodular
- Diffuse

Nodular episcleritis appears as a focal, 2–3 mm, pink-tan elevation within the episclera itself [38, 46]. This form of episcleritis appears most often in collie breeds and often appears in the veterinary medical literature as nodular granulomatous episclerokeratitis (NGE) [47].

Diffuse episcleritis occurs with greater frequency in clinical practice and involves generalized redness and/or the engorgement of superficial episcleral vessels [46]. The affected globe(s) appear(s) bloodshot. Therefore, episcleritis is yet another rule-out for "red eye" (see Figures 28.16a–c).

Episcleritis may be immune-mediated [46–50]. Certain breeds, including American Cocker Spaniels and Golden Retrievers, appear to be predisposed to this clinical presentation [46–49, 51].

Other etiologies for episcleritis include the following [38, 46, 47]:

- Infectious disease
  - *Ehrlichia canis*
- Inflammatory disease
  - Glaucoma
  - Keratitis
  - Uveitis
- Parasitic infestations
  - *Onchocerca* spp.
- Neoplasia

(a)

(c)

(b)

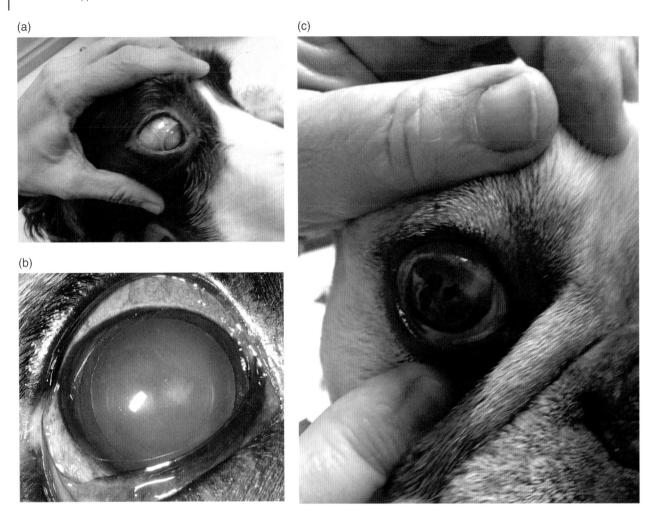

Figure 28.16 (a) Episcleritis in a canine patient. *Source:* Courtesy of Patricia Bennett, DVM. (b) Episcleritis in a canine patient. *Source:* Courtesy of D.J. Haeussler, Jr., MS, DVM, DACVO. (c) Episcleritis in a canine patient that has a corneal ulcer. *Source:* Courtesy of Pamela Mueller, DVM.

(a)

(b)

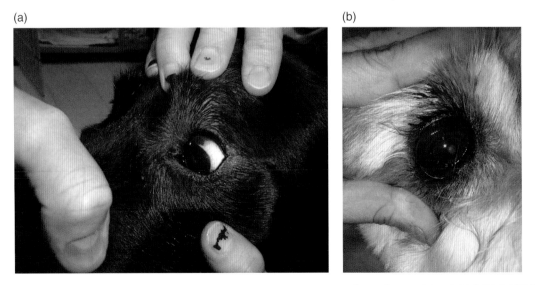

Figure 28.17 (a) Scleral hemorrhage in a canine patient. *Source:* Courtesy of Daniel Foy, MS, DVM, DACVIM, DACVECC. (b) Subconjunctival hemorrhage in a canine patient.

- Ocular trauma
  - Penetrating foreign bodies
  - Ocular surgery

Episcleritis is typically self-limiting.

Diffuse episcleritis tends to respond well to topical anti-inflammatory therapy [38, 46]. Recurrence is possible, but progression to scleritis is unlikely [46].

Nodular episcleritis may require oral immunosuppressive agents and/or intralesional corticosteroid therapy [46].

28.4 Scleral Hemorrhage

Blunt force trauma to the globe can result in appreciable damage to ocular structures [38, 39, 52]. Trauma may result in subconjunctival or scleral hemorrhage, and scleral rupture. These pathologies are visually apparent sequelae (see Figures 28.17a, b).

Scleral foreign bodies are also potential culprits [53]. Advanced imaging in the form of ocular ultrasonography, orbital radiographs, and/or computed tomography (CT) may facilitate detection of a foreign body [38, 53].

28.5 Scleral Masses

It is difficult to differentiate primary episcleritis from secondary neoplasia without a biopsy [47]. A biopsy of the former should yield a mixed population of inflammatory cells [47]. Biopsy results for a neoplastic mass depend upon the tumor type. For example, a biopsied scleral mast cell tumor (MCT) should yield mast cells

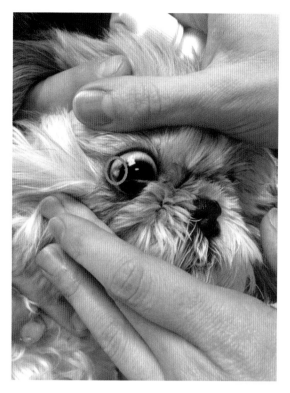

Figure 28.18 Scleral mast cell tumor (MCT) in a canine patient. *Source:* Courtesy of Amanda Maltese, DVM.

on cytological and histopathologic examination (see Figure 28.18).

Consult an oncology textbook for details as to the most likely scleral tumor types for canine and feline patients.

References

1 Boeve, M.H., Stades, F.C., and Djajadiningrat-Laanen, S.C. (2009). Eyes. In: *Medical History and Physical Examination in Companion Animals* (ed. A. Rijnberk and F.J. van Sluijs), 175–201. China: Elsevier Limited.

2 Gelatt, K.N. (2016). Eye structure and function in cats. In: *The Merck Veterinary Manual*, 11e (ed. S.E. Aiello and M.A. Moses). Whitehouse Station, N.J.: Merck & Co.

3 Gionfriddo, J.R. (2011). Just Ask the Expert: Can a smoky sclera be normal?. DVM 360 [Internet]. http://veterinarymedicine.dvm360.com/just-ask-expert-can-smoky-sclera-be-normal.

4 Englar, R.E. (2017). *Performing the Small Animal Physical Examination*. Hoboken, NJ: Wiley.

5 Packer, R.M., Hendricks, A., and Burn, C.C. (2015). Impact of facial conformation on canine health: corneal ulceration. *PLoS One* 10 (5): e0123827.

6 Schaer, M. (2008). Icterus. *NAVC Clinician's Brief* (September): 8.

7 Wray, J. (2017). *Canine Internal Medicine: What's Your Diagnosis?* Hoboken, NJ: Wiley.

8 Schaer, M. The Icteric Dog and Cat. Delaware Valley Academy of Veterinary Medicine [Internet]. http://www.delawarevalleyacademyvm.org/pdfs/may10/Icteric.pdf.

9 Lappin, M. (2001). *Feline Internal Medicine Secrets*. Philadelphia: Hanley & Belfus, Inc.

10 Schaer, M. (2010). Immune-mediated hemolytic anemia. *NAVC Clinician's Brief* (March): 78.

11 Gordon, J. (2011). Clinical approach to icterus in the cat (Proceedings). DVM 360 [Internet]. http://veterinarycalendar.dvm360.com/clinical-approach-icterus-cat-proceedings.

12 Caruso, K. (2004). Feline erythroparasites. *NAVC Clinician's Brief* (June): 36–38.

13 Fry, J.K. and Burney, D.P. (2012). Feline cytauxzoonosis. *NAVC Clinician's Brief* (July): 85–89.

14 Haber, M. (2005). Icterus & pancytopenia in a cat. *NAVC Clinician's Brief* (July): 21–23.

15 Bowles, M. (2017). Identifying and treating 3 tick-borne diseases in dogs. DVM 360 [Internet]. http://veterinarymedicine.dvm360.com/identifying-and-treating-3-tick-borne-diseases-dogs.

16 Colleran, E. (2017). Tick-borne disease in cats: two to watch for. DVM 360 [Internet]. http://veterinarynews.dvm360.com/tick-borne-disease-cats-two-watch.

17 Plumb, D.C. (2018). *Plumb's Veterinary Drug Handbook*, 9e, 11 unnumbered pages, 1279 p. Stockholm, Wisconsin, Ames, Iowa: Wiley-Blackwell.

18 Allen, A.L. (2003). The diagnosis of acetaminophen toxicosis in a cat. *Can. Vet. J.* 44 (6): 509–510.

19 Sellon, R.K. (2001). Acetaminophen. In: *Small Animal Toxicology* (ed. M.E. Peterson and P.A. Talcott), 388–395. Toronto: WB Saunders.

20 Aronson, L.R. (1996). Acetaminophen toxicosis in 17 cats. *J. Vet. Emerg. Crit. Care* 6: 65–69.

21 Jones, R.D., Baynes, R.E., and Nimitz, C.T. (1992). Nonsteroidal anti-inflammatory drug toxicosis in dogs and cats: 240 cases (1989–1990). *J. Am. Vet. Med. Assoc.* 201 (3): 475–477.

22 Court, M.H. (2001). Acetaminophen UDP-glucuronosyltransferase in ferrets: species and gender differences, and sequence analysis of ferret UGT1A6. *J. Vet. Pharmacol. Ther.* 24 (6): 415–422.

23 Steenbergen, V. (2003). Acetaminophen and cats – a dangerous combination. *Vet. Tech.* 24 (1): 43–45.

24 Richardson, J.A. (2000). Management of acetaminophen and ibuprofen toxicoses in dogs and cats. *J. Vet. Emerg. Crit. Care* 10: 285–291.

25 Rumbeiha, W.K., Lin, Y.S., and Oehme, F.W. (1995). Comparison of N-acetylcysteine and methylene blue, alone or in combination, for treatment of acetaminophen toxicosis in cats. *Am. J. Vet. Res.* 56 (11): 1529–1533.

26 Caruso, K. (2003). Applied cytology: case study of the mouth. *NAVC Clinician's Brief* (February): 42–43.

27 Meadows, I. and Gwaltney-Brant, S. (2006). The 10 most common toxicoses in dogs. *Vet. Med. US* 101 (3): 142–148.

28 Cope, R.B. (2005). Toxicology Brief: Allium species poisoning in dogs and cats. DVM 360 [Internet]. http://veterinarymedicine.dvm360.com/toxicology-brief-allium-species-poisoning-dogs-and-cats.

29 Cope, R.B. (2005). Allium species poisoning in dogs and cats. *Vet. Med. US* 100 (8): 562–566.

30 Shaw, N. (2008). IMHA: Diagnosing and treating a complex disease. DVM 360 [Internet]. http://veterinarymedicine.dvm360.com/imha-diagnosing-and-treating-complex-disease.

31 Day, M.J. (2012). Canine immune-mediated hemolytic anemia. *NAVC Clinician's Brief* (October): 53–57.

32 Latimer, K.S. (2011). *Duncan and Prasse's Veterinary Laboratory Medicine: Clinical Pathology*. Ames, IA: Wiley.

33 Stockham, S.L. (2008). *Fundamentals of Veterinary Clinical Pathology*. Ames, IA: Blackwell Publishing.

34 Giger, U. (2005). Regenerative anemias caused by blood loss or hemolysis. In: *Textbook of Veterinary Internal Medicine* (ed. S.J. Ettinger and E.C. Feldman), 1886–1907. St. Louis, MO: Elsevier CO.

35 Weinkle, T.K., Center, S.A., Randolph, J.F. et al. (2005). Evaluation of prognostic factors, survival rates, and treatment protocols for immune-mediated hemolytic anemia in dogs: 151 cases (1993–2002). *J. Am. Vet. Med. Assoc.* 226 (11): 1869–1880.

36 Norsworthy, G.D. (2011). The icteric cat: a case study. DVM 360 [Internet]. http://veterinarycalendar.dvm360.com/icteric-cat-case-study-proceedings.

37 Webb, C. (2013). Liver conditions in dogs. *NAVC Clinician's Brief* (May): 85–87.

38 Tilley, L.P. and Smith, F.W.K. (2004). *The 5-Minute Veterinary Consult: Canine and Feline*, 3e, lviii, 1487 p. Baltimore, MD: Lippincott Williams & Wilkins.

39 Côté, E. (2015). *Clinical Veterinary Advisor. Dogs and Cats*, 3e, xxxvii, 1642 p. St. Louis, Missouri: Elsevier Mosby.

40 ECLIN PATH. (2013). Available from: http://www.eclinpath.com/chemistry/liver/cholestasis.

41 Morse, E.E. (1990). Mechanisms of hemolysis in liver disease. *Ann. Clin. Lab. Sci.* 20 (3): 169–174.

42 Owen, J.S., Bruckdorfer, K.R., Day, R.C., and McIntyre, N. (1982). Decreased erythrocyte membrane fluidity and altered lipid composition in human liver disease. *J. Lipid Res.* 23 (1): 124–132.

43 Evans, H.E. and Miller, M.E. (2013). *Miller's Anatomy of the Dog*, 4e, xix, 850 p. St. Louis, Missouri: Elsevier.

44 Singh, B. and Dyce, K.M. (2018). *Dyce, Sack, and Wensing's Textbook of Veterinary Anatomy*, 5e. St. Louis, Missouri: Saunders.

45 Laminack, E.B., Myrna, K., and Moore, P.A. (2013). Clinical approach to the canine red eye. *Today's Veterinary Practice* (May/June): 12–41.

46 Grahn, B.H. and Sandmeyer, L.S. (2008). Canine episcleritis, nodular episclerokeratitis, scleritis, and necrotic scleritis. *Vet. Clin. North Am. Small Anim. Pract.* 38 (2): 291–308, vi.

47 Sandmeyer, L.S. and Grahn, B.H. (2008). Diagnostic ophthalmology. *Can. Vet. J.–Revue Veterinaire Canadienne* 49 (11): 1141–1142.

48 Deykin, A.R., Guandalini, A., and Ratto, A. (1997). A retrospective histopathologic study of primary episcleral and scleral inflammatory disease in dogs. *Prog. Vet. Comp. Ophthalmol.* 7: 245–258.

49 Paulsen, M.E., Lavach, J.D., and Snyder, S.P. (1987). Nodular granulomatous episcleritis in dogs: 19 cases (1973–1985). *J. Am. Vet. Med. Assoc.* 190: 1581–1587.

50 Breaux, C.B., Sandmeyer, L.S., and Grahn, B.H. (2007). Immunohistochemical investigation of canine episcleritis. *Vet. Ophthalmol.* 10 (3): 168–172.

51 Grahn, B.H. and Peiffer, R.L. (2007). Fundamentals of veterinary ophthalmic pathology. In: *Veterinary Ophthalmology* (ed. K.N. Gelatt), 355–437. Ames, IA: Blackwell Publishing.

52 Rampazzo, A., Eule, C., Speier, S. et al. (2006). Scleral rupture in dogs, cats, and horses. *Vet. Ophthalmol.* 9 (3): 149–155.

53 Welihozkiy, A., Pirie, C.G., and Pizzirani, S. (2011). Scleral and suprachoroidal foreign body in a dog – a case report. *Vet. Ophthalmol.* 14 (5): 345–351.

29

Abnormal Appearances of the Cornea

29.1 Introduction to the Cornea

The cornea and the sclera together form the outermost tunic, or layer, or the eye [1–5]. This layer is fibrous and maintains the shape of the globe [5]. The sclera forms the bulk of this outer tunic [5]. Refer to Chapter 28, Section 28.1 for a brief discussion of the anatomy and function of the sclera.

The cornea comprises one-fourth of the fibrous tunic [6, 7]. It is the most rostral aspect of the globe [6, 7]. In addition to shaping the eye, the cornea refracts incoming light [3, 8]. This is its primary function relative to the special sense of vision [8].

The cornea is multilayered [3]. The corneal epithelium is the outermost layer [3]. This layer is relatively thin. The stroma sits beneath the epithelium [3]. This layer is acellular and is largely supportive [3]. Beneath the stroma is Descemet's membrane [3]. Underneath this membrane is a single layer of endothelium [3].

In health, the stroma of the cornea is maintained in a dehydrated state [8]. The process by which this dehydration occurs is called deturgescence [8]. It requires corneal endothelial cells to pump fluid out of the cornea. Deturgescence is essential for maintaining the clarity of the cornea. Clarity impacts the cornea's ability to serve as a refractive surface.

In addition to lacking hydration, the cornea lacks a blood supply [5, 8, 9]. Vessels at the limbus are responsible for nourishing the cornea [5]. Additional nutrient delivery to the cornea is via the lacrimal fluid and aqueous humor [5].

Despite being avascular, the cornea is highly sensitized [5, 8]. Free nerve endings are present throughout the surface of the cornea [5]. These are extensions of the long ciliary nerves [5]. When the cornea is contacted by a foreign body, these nerve endings are responsible for triggering the corneal reflex [5]. This causes the eyelids to close protectively, thereby limiting corneal contact.

The cornea is composed of connective tissue fibers. These fibers are arranged in lamellar form, in such a way as to maintain corneal transparency [5, 8, 9] (see Figures 29.1a, b).

29.2 Corneal Opacities

Transparency of the cornea is essential for it to function as a refractive surface [9]. The development of corneal opacities impairs this function [8] (see Figures 29.2a, b).

Corneal opacities are common in clinical practice [3]. There are six primary causes of corneal opacities [8, 10]:

- Edema
- Infiltration of inflammatory cells
- Deposition of lipid or mineral
- Fibrosis
- Melanosis
- Neovascularization

Each pathological process has a classic appearance [8] (see Figures 29.3a–f).

29.2.1 Corneal Edema

Corneal edema causes the affected eye(s) to appear blue [8]. "Blue eye" may occur focally, as from blunt-force corneal trauma, or diffusely, as in the patient depicted in Figure 29.3a, due to endothelial degeneration [8, 10].

Age-related endothelial degeneration is relatively common in certain breeds of dog, including Boston Terriers, Dachshunds, and Chihuahuas [8, 11]. This condition results from the damage that is sustained by the corneal endothelium over time [11]. These cells do not regenerate easily [11]. As they age, they become less proficient at maintaining a state of deturgescence [8, 11]. This results in eventual "blue eye." This cause of "blue eye" does not cause pain.

On the other hand, if corneal edema is diffuse and the patient is in pain, then intraocular disease, such as uveitis or glaucoma, is likely [2, 8, 12].

Unlike dogs, cats do not typically develop age-related endothelial degeneration [8]. When diffuse edema is present in cats, it is more likely due to severe corneal disease [8]. Young cats are predisposed [8] (see Figure 29.4).

Feline patients with diffuse corneal edema may spontaneously rupture their globe [8].

(a)

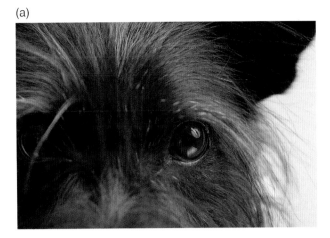

(b)

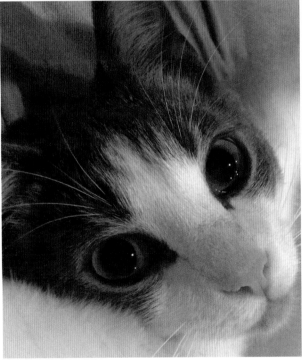

Figure 29.1 (a) Normal canine eye. Appreciate that the cornea is transparent. *Source:* Courtesy of the Media Resources Department at Midwestern University. (b) Normal feline eye. Appreciate that the cornea is transparent. *Source:* Courtesy of Sami Moon.

29.2.2 Corneal Inflammation

Infiltration with inflammatory cells imparts a yellow-green or creamy-tan appearance to the stroma [8]. This discoloration suggests that leukocytes are present. Their presence is typically in response to infectious keratitis [8].

Infectious keratitis is most often bacterial [8]. Beta-hemolytic *Streptococcus* spp. and *Pseudomonas* are commonly implicated [8]. Aerobic bacterial culture will help to guide therapy [8, 9].

Infectious keratitis may also be mycotic in origin [8]. Fungal cultures may be advisable if the patient is not responding to antibacterial therapy [8].

Sometimes, leukocytes associate with fibrin to form keratic precipitates [8]. These are deposited along the inner aspect of the corneal endothelium as pinpoint specks [8]. Although they may appear anywhere along the endothelial surface, they tend to precipitate out ventrally due to gravity [8]. Keratic precipitates are a sign that the patient may have underlying uveitis [8].

In any case of infectious keratitis, leukocyte infiltration may be accompanied by stromal "melting" [8]. Keratomalacia means that the cornea has softened to the point of oozing beyond the borders of its normal curvature. This is due to the digestion of corneal collagen by leukocyte and bacterial collagenases [8, 9, 13]. This is a medical emergency.

29.2.3 Corneal Lipid and/or Mineral Deposition

Lipid or mineral deposits may result from breed-related corneal dystrophies, age-related corneal degeneration, or inflammatory disease, such as keratitis [8].

Corneal dystrophies have been described in the dog more so than the cat as inherited defects in one or more layers of the cornea [14]. Corneal dystrophies are named by the primary region that is affected. Boxers and Shetland Sheepdogs are more likely to develop epithelial dystrophy, as compared to Airedale Terriers and Siberian Huskies, which tend to develop stromal dystrophies [14]. The American Cocker Spaniel, Boston Terrier, and Chihuahua are more likely to develop endothelial dystrophy [14].

Of these three categories, stromal dystrophies are more often associated with lipid deposition [14] (see Figure 29.5).

Chronic use of topical corticosteroids may also result in lipid accumulation [8].

Lipid deposits are typically cholesterol, whereas mineral deposits are typically calcium [8].

29.2.4 Corneal Fibrosis

Fibrosis of the cornea is essentially corneal scarring [8]. Corneal scars are typically gray-white [8]. They may appear wispy as opposed to solid, and these lesions are typically permanent [8]. Although scars may lessen in size with time, particularly in young patients, persistent lesions, particularly those that are extensive, impact vision [8].

29.2.5 Corneal Melanosis

Corneal melanosis occurs when melanin deposits on the surface of the cornea [8]. Sometimes, this deposition is

(a)

(b)

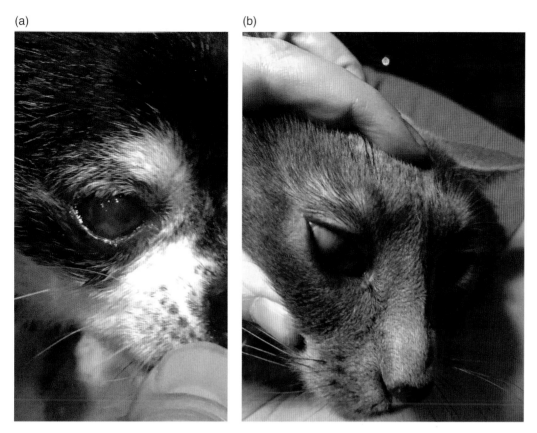

Figure 29.2 (a) Corneal opacity in a canine patient. Note how the cornea appears opaque. *Source:* Courtesy of Frank Isom, DVM. (b) Corneal opacity in a feline patient. Note how the cornea appears opaque. *Source:* Courtesy of Erin M. Miracle.

referred to as pigmentary keratitis because it most often results from chronic irritation of the cornea. This irritation may be due to a poor blink reflex that allows the corneal surface to dry out. Patients that sleep with their eyelids ajar may develop corneal melanosis for similar reasons [8].

Other sources of irritation include chronic rubbing of nasal fold fur against the cornea, entropion, or keratoconjunctivitis sicca (KCS), so-called "dry eye."

Pigment is likely to continue to deposit unless the underlying cause is removed.

29.2.6 Corneal Neovascularization

Corneal neovascularization is always pathological. The cornea is intentionally avascular to facilitate its transparency as a refractive surface [5, 8]. When vessels invade the corneal surface, they are typically responding to inflammation [15]. Angiogenesis is encouraged by the production of vascular endothelial growth factor (VEGF) and fibroblast growth factors from inflammatory cells [15, 16]. These mediators stimulate endothelial cells to create branches from pre-existing vessels [15].

Vessels may be superficial or deep [8].

When there is superficial ocular disease, conjunctival vessels at the limbus respond. These vessels create new branches that cross the limbus onto the cornea in "tree-shaped" patterns [8]. Refer to Figure 29.3f to appreciate this branching appearance.

Deep corneal blood vessels typically form in response to intraocular disease, including uveitis and glaucoma [8]. Rather than branching, these vessels are densely clustered. This gives them the appearance that they collectively form the stroke of a paintbrush or a thick marker at the limbus [8].

Note that corneal neovascularization is typically a response to chronic as opposed to acute inflammation [8]. New vessel formation takes, on average, three to five days [8]. Once established, vessels continue to grow at the rate of 1 mm/day [8]. Therefore, acute corneal injuries, such as superficial corneal ulcers, are unlikely to present with vessel formation [8]. If vessels are present in the face of acute injury, then they were likely there prior to the lesion for which the patient is actually presenting [8]. On the other hand, when a corneal ulcer is chronic or non-healing, then neovascularization is to be expected [8].

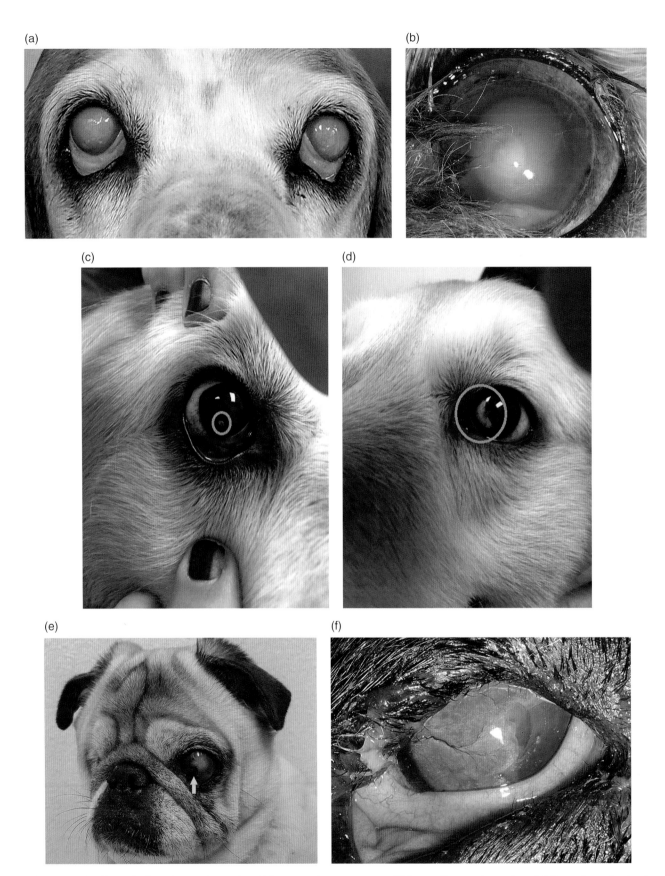

(a)

(b)

(c)

(d)

(e)

(f)

Figure 29.3 (a) Corneal edema in a canine patient. This creates the appearance of "blue eye" in a canine patient. (b) Corneal opacity due to inflammatory cell infiltration. This canine patient has a corneal ulcer. Note how the corneal stroma appears yellow-green. *Source:* Courtesy of D.J. Haeussler, Jr., MS, DVM, DACVO. (c) Focal lipid deposit, most likely cholesterol, in a canine patient. The result is a silvery or white opacity. Mineral deposits result in the same opacity, but are typically due to calcium. (d) More extensive lipid deposit in a canine patient. (e) Corneal opacity due to melanosis in a canine patient. The orange arrow points to melanin deposition. Note that the same patient also has a lens opacity, a cataract. Cataracts will be discussed in a subsequent chapter. *Source:* Courtesy of Ashley Parker. (f) Corneal neovascularization in a canine patient. *Source:* Courtesy of D.J. Haeussler, Jr., MS, DVM, DACVO.

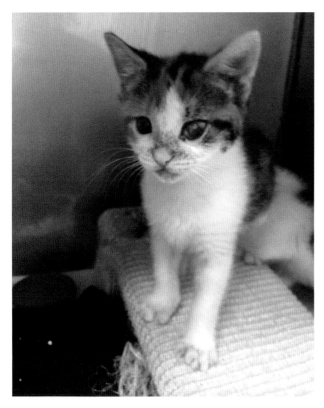

Figure 29.4 Diffuse corneal edema associated with the left globe (OS) of a kitten. *Source:* Courtesy of Kimberley Wallitsch.

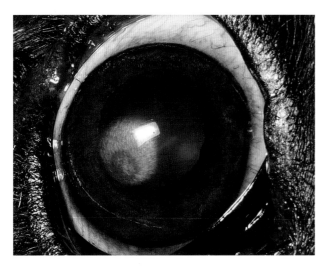

Figure 29.5 Corneal dystrophy in a canine patient. *Source:* Courtesy of D.J. Haeussler, Jr., MS, DVM, DACVO.

29.3 Corneal Ulcers

Corneal ulcers disrupt the corneal epithelium. They can be thought of as sores that begin on the rostral aspect of the globe.

Corneal ulcers are a frequent occurrence in companion animal practice [9]. They most often result from

trauma [9]. Corneas may become scratched by claws in fights or by objects in the environment, such as plant material, that inadvertently scrape the eye.

Infection at time of injury is uncommon; however, bacterial contaminants may rapidly take hold of the cornea [9, 17–22].

Corneal ulcer depth depends upon the extent of the initial trauma as well as progression of disease [9]. Corneal ulcers may be superficial, stromal, or perforating [9, 18, 19, 23].

29.3.1 Superficial Corneal Ulcers

Superficial corneal ulcers are surface-dwelling sores that typically heal rapidly without scarring [9]. Treatment is largely supportive. Topical prophylaxis with antibiotic therapy is often advised to guard against secondary infection during the healing phase [9, 19, 24, 25].

Ciliary muscle spasms secondary to corneal ulceration may result in ocular pain. This can be managed through the prescription of the mydriatic agent, atropine [9].

Recurrent superficial ulcers may require additional therapy, including, but not limited to, debridement and/or grid keratectomies to reinitiate healing [9, 18, 19, 23, 25–30].

Boxer dogs are prone to delays in corneal healing, and are therefore likely to require prolonged therapy, even in the face of a superficial corneal ulcer [27].

29.3.2 Stromal or Deep Corneal Ulcers

Stromal or deep ulcers are more likely to be infected and/or progress to keratomalacia [9]. Non-progressive corneal ulcers may be treated in the same manner as outlined above for superficial ulcers [9]. However, they could potentially benefit from a conjunctival graft or flap [9]. Either procedure would provide additional protection.

When stromal ulcers are progressive, the risk is permanent loss of vision [9]. Aggressive therapy is indicated if the goal of the clinician and client is to preserve a functional globe [9].

29.3.3 Descemetoceles

A descemetocele is the severest form of corneal ulcer [9]. In this scenario, the stroma has thinned such that only Descemet's membrane remains intact (see Figures 29.6a, b).

If Descemet's membrane erodes, then the integrity of the globe is lost.

Note that any corneal ulcer may rapidly decline if treatment is not initiated rapidly [9]. Diagnosis is critical to have the best chance of securing a successful patient outcome [9, 17, 18, 26, 31].

(a)

(b)

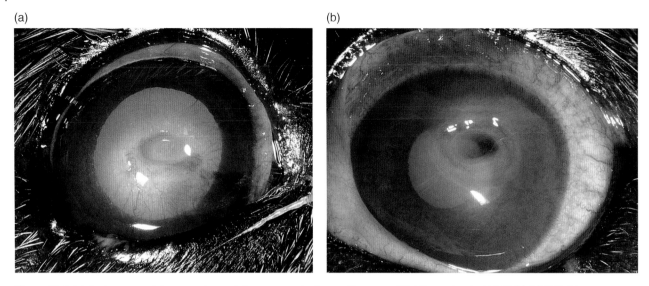

Figure 29.6 (a) Canine corneal degeneration and descemetocele. *Source:* Courtesy of D.J. Haeussler, Jr., MS, DVM, DACVO. (b) Descemetocele in a canine patient. *Source:* Courtesy of D.J. Haeussler, Jr., MS, DVM, DACVO.

29.3.4 Diagnosis of Corneal Ulcers

Diagnosis is facilitated through the use of fluorescein stain [9].

Recall from Chapter 26, Section 26.3.4 that fluorescein stain can be used to establish the patency of the nasolacrimal duct [32]. However, it is more commonly used to detect defects in the corneal epithelium [9]. The orange dye adheres to a damaged cornea and will fluoresce a brilliant green color under a cobalt blue light [1, 9, 18, 31] (see Figures 29.7a–c).

Fluorescein is purchased either as a solution or as a paper strip [9, 31, 33]. The former is applied topically to the eye [9]. To use the latter, the examiner must first moisten it with 0.9% saline [9]. The moistened, impregnated strip can then be gently tapped against the dorsal bulbar conjunctiva [9]. The examiner then manually closes the patient's eyelids to spread fluorescein across the surface of the globe [9]. It is best to flush the eye with sterile saline flush afterward to eliminate any excess dye [9]. Stromal uptake of fluorescein will be undisturbed by flushing, whereas excess stain will be rinsed off [9].

An alternate technique is to place the impregnated strip in a syringe that contains 0.9% saline [9]. This creates a solution of fluorescein that can then be applied to the cornea through the syringe.

29.3.5 Corneal Cytology

Corneal cytology may be advised while the results of culture and sensitivity testing are pending, particularly in the face of progressing and/or melting ulcers [9, 18]. A variety of techniques, involving a gamut of tools, have been described [9]. Among these are cotton swabs.

Cotton swabs are often used because they cause less trauma than the blunt edge of a sterile scalpel blade [9]. Once a sample has been retrieved by rolling the swab across the surface of the ulcer, the sample is transferred onto a glass slide to be heat- or chemical-fixed [9]. Romanowsky, Giemsa, and/or Gram stains will facilitate identification of inflammatory cells and organisms, including bacteria [9, 18, 34]. Although these results will not have the same degree of sensitivity that cultures have, they facilitate the initiation of medical therapy that is more likely to be a better fit for the patient [9]. After all, medical care can be tailored to the population of organisms that are identified on cytological examination.

29.3.6 Corneal Cultures

It is rare that a culture would be performed for a superficial corneal ulcer [9]. However, cultures and sensitivity testing are essential when the patient presents for a deep, progressing, or melting ulcer [9]. Samples should be taken prior to initiating medical therapy, by rolling a sterile moistened swab over the area of interest [9, 35].

Note that not all bacteria that reside at the corneal surface are pathogenic. Several species comprise the normal corneal flora, particularly those of the Gram positive variety [9]. These include the following [9]:

- *Staphylococcus* spp.
- *Streptococcus* spp.
- *Corynebacterium* spp.
- *Bacillus* spp.
- *Pseudomonas aeruginosa*
- *Escherichia coli*
- *Klebsiella*

(a)

(b)

(c)

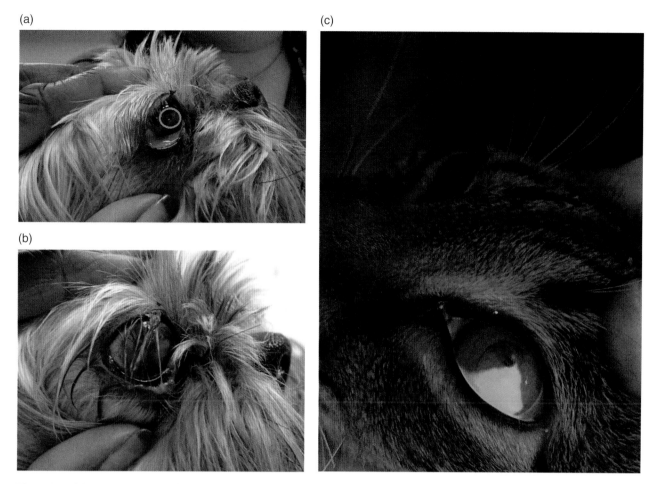

Figure 29.7 (a) Gross appearance of a corneal epithelial defect in a canine patient. *Source:* Courtesy of Patricia Bennett, DVM. (b) Same patient as depicted in Figure 29.6b, after fluorescein staining. Note how fluorescein is retained by the damaged stroma, causing visible fluorescence. This fluorescence is intensified when examined under a cobalt blue light. *Source:* Courtesy of Patricia Bennett, DVM. (c) Positive fluorescein staining in a feline patient. The uptake of stain signifies that there is a corneal epithelial defect. *Source:* Courtesy of Ben Turner.

In dogs, but not in cats, the following two anaerobes may also be present as part of the normal flora [9, 33, 34]:

- *Neisseria* spp.
- *Fusobacterium* spp.

Pathogenic bacteria that have been implicated in corneal disease include [9]

- *Staphylococcus aureus*
- *B-hemolytic Streptococcus*
- *P. aeruginosa*.

Note that some of the above are part of the normal flora that can become opportunistic invaders when corneal integrity is breached [9].

29.4 Corneal Dermoids

Although corneal opacities occur frequently in companion animal practice, other less common clinical presentations of the cornea may be observed by the astute clinician. One such presentation is the corneal dermoid.

A dermoid is an accumulation of normal epithelial tissue in an abnormal place [36]. Because this misplaced tissue contains ectodermal and mesodermal elements, it often includes fur, nerves, sebaceous glands, and blood vessels in addition to keratinized epithelium [36, 37].

Dermoids can occur anywhere in the body. Concerning the eye and periorbital tissue, dermoids have been reported in association with the eyelids, conjunctiva, nictitans, and cornea [36, 38–42].

Dogs are more likely to develop dermoids than cats [36, 43, 44]. Large breeds of dogs, such as Saint Bernards and German Shepherds, may be predisposed, along with short-legged dogs like the Welsh Corgi, Dachshund, and Bassett Hound [41]. Domestic shorthaired (DSH), Burmese, and Birman cats are also overrepresented [2, 36, 40].

Corneal dermoids are present at birth; however, they may not be immediately noticed until they irritate the globe [36, 45]. Excessive lacrimation and corneal ulceration are common sequelae that result when dermoid-associated fur chronically scrapes up against the surface of the affected cornea [36, 41, 46, 47]. As mentioned earlier, the use of fluorescein stain facilitates detection of corneal ulceration.

In addition to keratitis, reflex uveitis and conjunctival hyperemia may develop in the affected globe [36].

Corneal dermoids that cause chronic irritation can be surgically excised [36, 41, 48]. Surgical excision may result in a corneal opacity; however, corneal scarring should resolve with time [41].

29.5 Chronic Superficial Keratitis

Chronic superficial keratitis, otherwise referred to as pannus, is an immune-mediated condition to which German Shepherd dogs and Greyhounds are predisposed [39, 49, 50]. Although any age group may be affected, patients are typically young adults at time of onset [49].

The environment also seems to play a role in development of disease. Patients that are exposed to high altitude and ultraviolet radiation appear to be most susceptible [50].

Patients present for a grossly observable, pink-red, fleshy, cobblestone mass along the corneal surface of the affected eye(s) [49, 50] (see Figure 29.8).

Lesions tend to become symmetrical and progress over time as plasma cells, lymphocytes, and blood vessels infiltrate the affected corneas [49]. Pigment may be laid down in response to chronic corneal irritation [49, 50]. Corneal fibrosis is also quite common [49, 50].

Without treatment, pannus is likely to overtake the entire cornea [49]. Because corneal transparency is lost and the cornea can no longer function as a refractive surface, the patient will become avisual [49, 50].

The nictitans of patients with pannus may develop concurrent lesions [50]. These take the form of nodules [50]. The nictitans may also lose pigment along its leading edge [50].

Medical management is essential to reverse corneal damage and to preserve vision [49]. Treatment most typically involves topical administration of corticosteroid, cyclosporine, or tacrolimus [49]. Some patients require combinations of these drugs, which are designed to control pannus rather than cure it [49, 50].

29.6 Feline Corneal Sequestra

Corneal sequestra are specific to feline, ophthalmology [51]. These represent plaques of discolored tissue along the corneal surface.

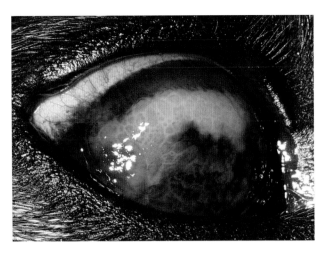

Figure 29.8 Pannus in a canine patient. *Source:* Courtesy of D.J. Haeussler, Jr., MS, DVM, DACVO.

Classically, these lesions are black and opaque, hence their alternate name of corneal nigrum [51–53]. The black color results from degeneration and eventual necrosis of stromal collagen [51, 54]. In actuality, corneal sequestra exhibit a range of transparencies and colors, including amber [53].

Certain breeds are predisposed [52]. These include Persian, Himalayan, Siamese, Burmese, and DSH cats [52, 55–60]. It has been theorized that the facial conformation of brachycephalic breeds causes exposure keratitis, which precipitates sequestra formation [52, 60–62].

In addition to breed, the following patient-related factors have been implicated in the formation of corneal sequestra [51, 52, 55–57, 59, 63–65]:

- KCS
- Structural abnormalities
  – Entropion
  – Trichiasis
- Traumatic keratitis
  – Ocular trauma
  – Prior grid keratotomies
- Ulcerative keratitis
- Viral keratitis
  – Feline herpesvirus-1 (FHV-1)

Chlamydophila felis and *Toxoplasma gondii* may also be causative agents [59, 66, 67].

Corneal sequestra are irritating to the eye and can be a source of ocular pain [52]. Patients often exhibit epiphora and blepharospasm [52]. Surgical management of corneal sequestra is often advised to improve patient comfort [52].

Superficial lesions may be cured via keratectomy [65]. However, deep lesions may require conjunctival grafting or corneoconjunctival transposition [51, 52, 54, 59, 65].

References

1 Englar, R.E. (2017). *Performing the Small Animal Physical Examination*. Hoboken, NJ: Wiley.

2 Gelatt, K.N. (2014). *Essentials of Veterinary Ophthalmology*. Ames, IA: Wiley.

3 Gelatt KN. (2018). Cornea Merck Veterinary Manual [Internet]. https://www.merckvetmanual.com/eye-and-ear/ophthalmology/cornea.

4 Evans, H.E. and Miller, M.E. (1993). *Miller's Anatomy of the Dog*, 3e, xvi, 1113 p. Philadelphia: W.B. Saunders.

5 Singh, B. and Dyce, D.K.M. (2018). *Sack, and Wensing's Textbook of Veterinary Anatomy*, 5e. St. Louis, Missouri: Saunders.

6 Boeve, M.H., Stades, F.C., and Djajadiningrat-Laanen, S.C. (2009). Eyes. In: *Medical History and Physical Examination in Companion Animals* (ed. A. Rijnberk and F.J. van Sluijs), 175–201. China: Elsevier Limited.

7 Gelatt, K.N. (2016). Eye structure and function in cats. In: *The Merck Veterinary Manual* (ed. S.E. Aiello and M.A. Moses). Merck.

8 Strom, A.R. and Maggs, D.J. (2015). Corneal Opacities in Dogs & Cats. *Today's Veterinary Practice* (May/June): 105–113.

9 Ollivier, F.J. (2003). Bacterial corneal diseases in dogs and cats. *Clin. Tech. Small Anim. Pract.* 18 (3): 193–198.

10 Gelatt, K.N., Gilger, B.C., and Kern, T.J. (2013). *Veterinary Ophthalmology*. Wiley-Blackwell.

11 Northwest Animal Eye Specialists. (2010). Corneal Endothelial Degeneration. Northwest Animal Eye Specialists [Internet]. http://www.northwestanimaleye.com/corneal-endothelial-degeneration.pml.

12 Townsend, W.M. (2008). Canine and feline uveitis. *Vet. Clin. North Am. Small Anim. Pract.* 38 (2): 323–346, vii.

13 Wang, L., Pan, Q.S., Xue, Q. et al. (2008). Evaluation of matrix metalloproteinase concentrations in precorneal tear film from dogs with Pseudomonas aeruginosa-associated keratitis. *Am. J. Vet. Res.* 69 (10): 1341–1345.

14 Cooley, P.L. and Dice, P.F. 2nd (1990). Corneal dystrophy in the dog and cat. *Vet. Clin. North Am. Small Anim. Pract.* 20 (3): 681–692.

15 Chiang HH, Hemmati HD. (2013). Treatment of Corneal Neovascularization. EyeNet Magazine [Internet]. https://www.aao.org/eyenet/article/treatment-of-corneal-neovascularization.

16 Papathanassiou, M., Theodoropoulou, S., Analitis, A. et al. (2013). Vascular endothelial growth factor inhibitors for treatment of corneal neovascularization: a meta-analysis. *Cornea* 32 (4): 435–444.

17 Bistner, S. (1981). Clinical diagnosis and treatment of infectious keratitis. *Compend. Contin. Educ. Pract. Vet.* 3: 1056–1066.

18 Slatter, D. (1990). *Fundamentals of Veterinary Ophthalmology*. Philadelphia: Saunders.

19 Whitley, R.D. (2000). Canine and feline primary ocular bacterial infections. *Vet. Clin. North Am. Small Anim. Pract.* 30 (5): 1151–1167.

20 Nasisse, M.P. (1986). Canine ulcerative keratitis. *Compend. Contin. Educ. Pract. Vet.* 7: 686–701.

21 Kern, T.J. (1990). Ulcerative keratitis. *Vet. Clin. North Am. Small Anim. Pract.* 20 (3): 643–666.

22 Koch, S.A. (1973). Ulcerative keratitis. *Vet. Clin. North Am.* 3 (3): 385–406.

23 Whitley, R.D. and Gilger, B.C. (1999). Diseases of the canine cornea and sclera. In: *Veterinary Ophthalmology* (ed. K.N. Gelatt), 635–671. Philadelphia: Lippincott Williams & Wilkins.

24 Slatter, D.H. and Dietrich, U. (1985). Cornea and sclera. In: *Textbook of Small Animal Surgery* (ed. D.H. Slatter), 1368–1369. Philadelphia: W.B. Saunders.

25 Regnier, A. (1999). Antimicrobials, anti-inflammatory agents, and antiglaucoma drugs. In: *Veterinary Ophthalmology* (ed. K.N. Gelatt), 297–336. Philadelphia: Lippincott Williams & Wilkins.

26 Severin, G.A. (1976). *Veterinary Ophthalmology Notes*. Fort Collins, CO: Colorado State University.

27 Gelatt, K.N. and Samuelson, D.A. (1982). Recurrent corneal erosions and epithelial dystrophy in the boxer dog. *J. Am. Anim. Hosp. Assoc.* 18 (3): 453–460.

28 Kirschner, S.E., Brazzell, R.K., Stern, M.E., and Baird, L. (1991). The use of topical epidermal growth-factor for treatment of nonhealing corneal erosions in dogs. *J. Am. Anim. Hosp. Assoc.* 27 (4): 449–452.

29 Swank, A. and Hosgood, G. (1996). Corneal wound healing and the role of growth factors. *Comp. Cont. Educ. Pract.* 18 (9): 1007–1017.

30 Champagne, E.S. and Munger, R.J. (1992). Multiple punctate keratotomy for the treatment of recurrent epithelial erosions in dogs. *J. Am. Anim. Hosp. Assoc.* 28 (3): 213–216.

31 Strubbe, T.D. and Gelatt, K.N. (1999). Ophthalmic examination and diagnostic procedures. In: *Veterinary Ophthalmology* (ed. K.N. Gelatt), 427–466. Philadelphia: Lippincott Williams & Wilkins.

32 Ford, R.B. and Mazzaferro, E. (2011). *Kirk & Bistner's Handbook of Veterinary Procedures and Emergency Treatment*. St. Louis, MO: Elsevier Saunders.

33 Moore, C.P. and Nasisse, M.P. (1999). Clinical microbiology. In: *Veterinary Ophthalmology* (ed. K.N. Gelatt), 259–290. Philadelphia: Lippincott, Williams, & Wilkins.

34 Gerding, P.A., McLaughlin, S.A., and Troop, M.W. (1988). Cytology of normal and inflamed conjunctivas in dogs and cats. *J. Am. Vet. Med. Assoc.* 193: 242–244.

35 Ward, D. (1999). Ocular pharmacology. In: *Veterinary Ophthalmology* (ed. K.N. Gelatt), 336–354. Philadelphia: Lippincott Williams & Wilkins.

36 LoPinto, A.J., Pirie, C.G., Huynh, T., and Beamer, G. (2016). Dorsally located corneal dermoid in a cat. *JFMS Open Rep.* 2 (1): 2055116916641970.

37 Grahn, B.H. and Peiffer, R.L. (2013). Veterinary ophthalmic pathology. In: *Veterinary Ophthalmology* (ed. K.N. Gelatt), 456–457. Ames, IA: Wiley.

38 Latimer, C.A. and Wyman, M. (1985). Neonatal ophthalmology. *Vet. Clin. North Am. Equine Pract.* 1 (1): 235–259.

39 Labelle P. (2016). Pathology of the Cornea and Sclera. NC State College of Veterinary Medicine [Internet]. https://cvm.ncsu.edu/wp-content/uploads/2016/06/Labelle_Cornea-sclera-2016c.pdf.

40 Hendy-Ibbs, P.M. (1985). Familial feline epibulbar dermoids. *Vet. Rec.* 116 (1): 13–14.

41 Choudhury, M. and Kalita, D. (2016). Surgical management of sclero-corneal dermoid in a dog. *Intas Polivet* 16 (2): 478–479.

42 Magrane, W.G. and Helper, L.C. (1989). *Magrane's Canine Ophthalmology*, 4e, xi, 297 p. Philadelphia: Lea & Febiger.

43 Stiles, J. (2013). Feline ophthalmology. In: *Veterinary Ophthalmology* (ed. K.N. Gelatt, B.C. Gilger and T.J. Kern), 1500–1501. Ames, IA: Wiley.

44 Priester, W.A. (1972). Congenital ocular defects in cattle, horses, cats, and dogs. *J. Am. Vet. Med. Assoc.* 160 (11): 1504–1511.

45 Moore, P.A. (2005). Feline corneal disease. *Clin. Tech. Small Anim. Pract.* 20: 83–93.

46 Dubielzig, R. (2010). Diseases of the eyelids and conjunctiva. In: *Veterinary Ocular Pathology: A Comparative Review* (ed. R. Dubielzig, K. Ketring and G. McLellan), 143–199. St. Louis, MO: Saunders Elsevier.

47 Maggs, D.J. (2008). Conjunctiva. In: *Slatter's Fundamentals of Veterinary Ophthalmology* (ed. D.J. Maggs, P. Miller and R. Ofri), 148–149. St. Louis, MO: Elsevier.

48 Ledbetter, E.C. and Gilger, B.C. (2013). Diseases and surgery of the canine cornea and sclera. In: *Veterinary Ophthalmology* (ed. K.N. Gelatt, B.C. Gilger and T.J. Kern), 983–986. Ames, IA: Wiley.

49 Collins BK. (2009). Canine corneal diseases: treatment for transparency greater than the federal stimulus. DVM 360 [Internet]. http://veterinarycalendar.dvm360.com/canine-corneal-diseases-treatment-transparency-greater-federal-stimulus-proceedings.

50 Gunderson E. (2013). Canine non-ulcerative corneal diseases. Southeastern Wisconsin Veterinary Medical Association [Internet]. http://sewvma.org/files/october_2013_meeting/note_canine_non_ulcerative_corneal_diseases_dr_eg.pdf.

51 Graham, K.L., White, J.D., and Billson, F.M. (2017). Feline corneal sequestra: outcome of corneoconjunctival transposition in 97 cats (109 eyes). *J. Feline Med. Surg.* 19 (6): 710–716.

52 Andrew, S.E., Tou, S., and Brooks, D.E. (2001). Corneoconjunctival transposition for the treatment of feline corneal sequestra: a retrospective study of 17 cases (1990–1998). *Vet. Ophthalmol.* 4 (2): 107–111.

53 Glaze, M.B. and Gelatt, K.N. (1999). Feline ophthalmology. In: *Veterinary Ophthalmology* (ed. K.N. Gelatt), 997–1052. Philadelphia: Lippincott Williams & Wilkins.

54 Featherstone, H.J. and Sansom, J. (2004). Feline corneal sequestra: a review of 64 cases (80 eyes) from 1993 to 2000. *Vet. Ophthalmol.* 7 (4): 213–227.

55 Blogg, J.R., Stanley, R.G., and Dutton, A.G. (1989). Use of conjunctival pedicle grafts in the management of feline keratitis nigrum. *J. Small Anim. Pract.* 30 (12): 678–684.

56 Morgan, R.V. (1994). Feline corneal sequestration – a retrospective study of 42 cases (1987–1991). *J. Am. Anim. Hosp. Assoc.* 30 (1): 24–28.

57 Pentlarge, V.W. (1989). Corneal sequestration in cats. *Comp. Cont. Educ. Pract.* 11 (1): 24–32.

58 Souri, E. (1975). Feline corneal nigrum. *Vet. Med. Small Anim. Clin.* 70 (5): 531–534.

59 Laguna, F., Leiva, M., Costa, D. et al. (2015). Corneal grafting for the treatment of feline corneal sequestrum: a retrospective study of 18 eyes (13 cats). *Vet. Ophthalmol.* 18 (4): 291–296.

60 Startup, F.G. (1988). Corneal necrosis and sequestration in the cat – a review and record of 100 cases. *J. Small Anim. Pract.* 29 (7): 476–486.

61 Gelatt, K.N., Peiffer, R.L., and Stevens, J. (1973). Chronic ulcerative keratitis and sequestrum in the domestic cat. *J. Am. Anim. Hosp. Assoc.* 9: 204–213.

62 Gelatt, K.N. (1971). Corneal sequestration in a cat. *Vet. Med. Small Anim. Clin.* 66 (6): 561–562.

63 Nasisse, M.P. (1990). Feline herpesvirus ocular disease. *Vet. Clin. North Am. Small Anim. Pract.* 20 (3): 667–680.

64 Nasisse, M.P., Glover, T.L., Moore, C.P., and Weigler, B.J. (1998). Detection of feline herpesvirus 1 DNA in corneas of cats with eosinophilic keratitis or corneal sequestration. *Am. J. Vet. Res.* 59 (7): 856–858.

65 Bentley, E. and Telle, M.R. (2017). Feline Corneal Sequestra. *Clinician's Brief* (November): 44.

66 Cullen, C.L., Wadowska, D.W., Singh, A., and Melekhovets, Y. (2005). Ultrastructural findings in feline corneal sequestra. *Vet. Ophthalmol.* 8 (5): 295–303.

67 Volopich, S., Benetka, V., Schwendenwein, I. et al. (2005). Cytologic findings, and feline herpesvirus DNA and Chlamydophila felis antigen detection rates in normal cats and cats with conjunctival and corneal lesions. *Vet. Ophthalmol.* 8 (1): 25–32.

30

Abnormal Appearances of the Iris

30.1 Introduction to the Iris

The iris is one of several structures that comprises the uvea, or middle layer of the eye [1]. The iris is essentially flattened tissue that sits between the cornea and the lens [2]. It remains in place because of the pectinate ligament, which anchors it to the sclera, and the ciliary body, which sits just behind it [2].

At the center of the iris is an intentional anatomical defect, the pupil [3, 4]. Recall from Chapter 18, Section 18.1 that the pupil is akin to an aperture of a camera: it allows light into the system. How much light enters the eye depends upon the size of the pupil [3, 4].

It is the job of the iris to control pupil size [3, 4]. As lighting becomes dim, pupils widen to increase the amount of light that enters the eye [3, 4]. This so-called mydriasis is the result of dilator muscle in the iris [2]. The fibers of this muscle are arranged radially [2]. When they contract, the pupil widens [2].

The pupil narrows when the smooth sphincter muscle contracts [2]. The constricted or miotic pupil allows less light into the eye [2].

30.2 Normal Variations in Iris Color

Veterinary clients are perhaps most familiar with the iris as the colored part of the eye [2–4]. Iris color is an important aesthetic quality for many cat and dog owners, and neither cats nor dogs disappoint in terms of the great variety of colors that exist among the general population. Colors range from copper-yellow and green to brilliant blue in cats, and browns to light blues in dogs [4] (see Figures 30.1a–m).

The color of the iris depends ultimately on how many pigmented cells are present in the stroma and what type of pigment they contain [2]. Melanin-containing cells confer the color brown to the iris when cells are tightly packed. Yellow-colored irises result when melanin-containing cells are present, but less abundant [2].

Albino patients lack pigment altogether [2]. The result is that blood flowing through capillaries is now visible to the outside observer. This creates the illusion that the iris is red-pink [2].

Both irises typically share the same shade or color. That is, both irises may be solid blue or solid green. However, irises may also differ in color, within the same eye, or between eyes. When this occurs, they are said to be heterochromic [5, 6].

There are two types of heterochromic irises [6]:

- Heterochromia iridium
  – Pigment varies within the iris of the same eye.
- Heterochromia iridis
  – Pigment differs between irises.

Both heterochromia iridium and heterochromia iridis are considered normal in companion animal patients [6] (see Figures 30.2a–d).

Heterochromia iridis occurs with greater frequency in dogs than cats [4]. It is most common in dogs that carry the merle gene [4]. This gene suppresses melanocytes. The iris that contains the least pigment-producing cells will be blue [2].

There is an association between congenital deafness and blue-eyed, white-coated cats [4, 6]. Congenital deafness also occurs with greater frequency in those with heterochromic irises [5, 7]. In particular, the following breeds are overrepresented [6]:

- Australian Cattle Dog
- Boston Terrier
- Dalmatian
- English Bulldog
- English Setter
- Old English Sheepdog

30.3 Iris Nevus

An iris nevus is a focal spot of hyperpigmentation [6]. It is sometimes referred to as an iris freckle [4, 8]. This freckle may be congenital or acquired [8]. It is typical

Common Clinical Presentations in Dogs and Cats, First Edition. Ryane E. Englar.
© 2019 John Wiley & Sons, Inc. Published 2019 by John Wiley & Sons, Inc.

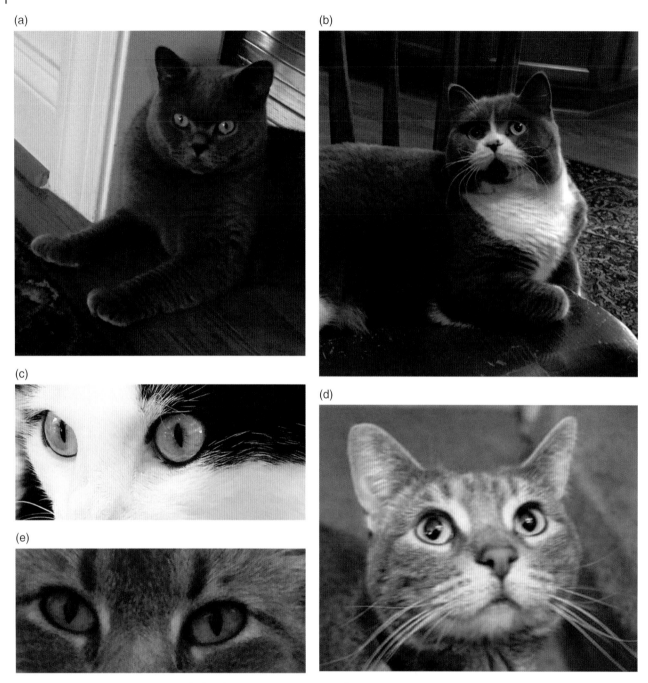

Figure 30.1 (a) Copper irises in a British Shorthair cat. *Source:* Courtesy of Richard, Jill, and Gwen Englar. (b) Hazel irises in a British Shorthair cat. *Source:* Courtesy of Richard, Jill, and Bliss Englar. (c) Yellow irises in cat. *Source:* Courtesy of Kelly Chappell. (d) Yellow-green irises in a cat. *Source:* Courtesy of Ann Marie Wronkowski. (e) Green irises in a cat. *Source:* Courtesy of Rozalyn Donner. (f) Pale blue irises in a cat. *Source:* Courtesy of Danielle Cucuzella. (g) Blue-green irises in a cat. *Source:* Courtesy of Heather N. Cornell, DVM. (h) Blue irises in a cat. *Source:* Courtesy of Arielle Hatcher. (i) Caribbean blue irises in a cat. *Source:* Courtesy of Samantha Rudolph, DVM. (j) Deep brown irises in a dog. *Source:* Courtesy of Zabzoo Services. (k) Medium-brown irises in a dog. *Source:* Courtesy of the Media Resources Department at Midwestern University. (l) Hazel irises in a chocolate Labrador retriever. *Source:* Courtesy of Jackie Kucskar, DVM. (m) Blue irises in a dog.

(f)

(g)

(h)

(i)

(j)

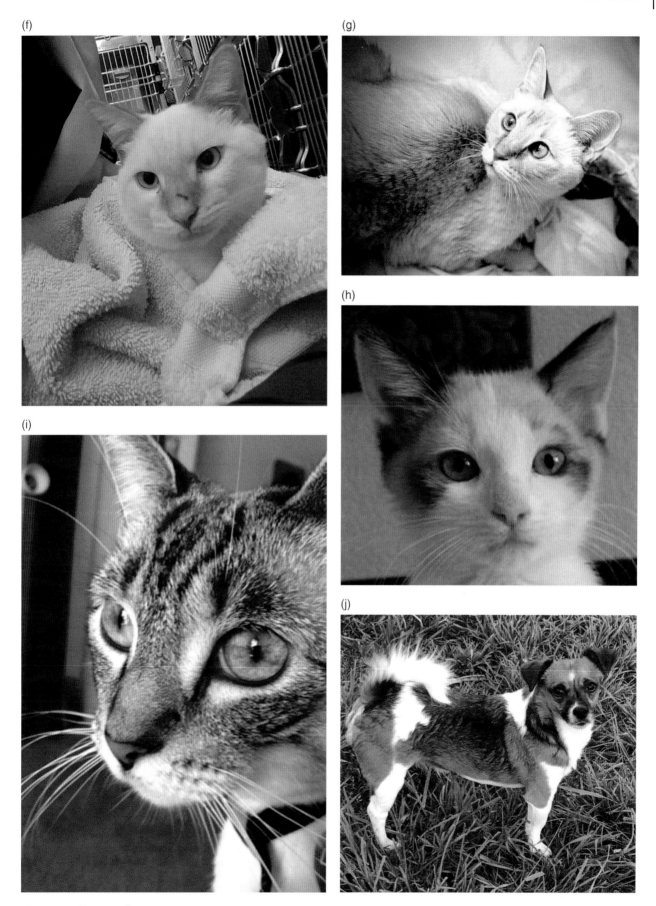

Figure 30.1 (Continued)

(k)

(l)

(m)

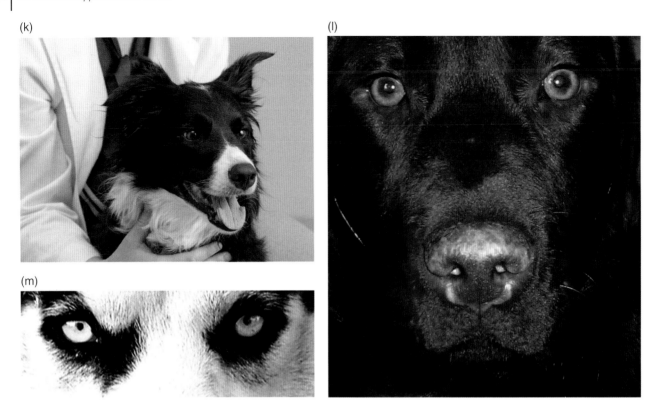

Figure 30.1 (Continued)

to see increased numbers of iris nevi in patients as they age [5, 6, 8].

Iris nevi are in and of themselves benign; however, they have the potential to transform into iris melanoma, particularly in cats [4, 6, 8] (see Figures 30.3a, b).

Both lesions may progress, meaning that the size of an iris nevus does not necessarily indicate malignant transformation.

30.4 Iris Melanoma

Melanomas are common intraocular tumors of both dogs and cats [8–15]. When cats develop iris melanomas, they tend to develop in patches that grow into one another [8]. The result is diffuse iris melanoma [8]. Its clinical presentation is typically unilateral [8, 15].

Diffuse iris melanoma in the cat presents as flatter lesions than in the dog, which develops raised nodules [8]. Feline diffuse iris melanoma may also have a velvety appearance [8].

Diffuse iris melanoma may alter pupil shape and size as the stroma is invaded by abnormal cells [8, 11]. Progression of disease may also distort the iridocorneal angle, causing secondary glaucoma [8, 12]. Refer to Chapter 22, Section 22.2.2 for a description of clinical signs and sequelae.

Iris melanoma in the dog typically represents localized disease [8, 9]. However, in the cat, iris melanoma is more likely to metastasize [8, 9]. Studies in the veterinary literature vary drastically, but metastatic rates of up to 63% have been reported [8, 12, 16–18]. Metastatic bone lesions are uncommon [8, 11, 19]. More likely, secondary lesions develop in the lymph nodes, lungs, liver, and spleen [8, 12, 14, 18, 19].

Histopathologic examination of the affected tissue is required to make a definitive diagnosis [8]. However, uveal biopsies are not routinely performed [8]. A presumptive diagnosis is more often made based upon clinical presentation and documentation of progression [8]. Raised, velvety lesions increase the index of suspicion [8].

Although photoablation of small lesions with a laser is possible, new lesions are likely to form [8, 11]. Enucleation is preferred to prevent progression of disease beyond the iris stroma [8, 12, 17]. Unfortunately, metastasis is not always apparent until necropsy [8]. This presents a clinical dilemma in terms of when to recommend enucleation to a veterinary client. The recommendation to enucleate may be premature. The lesion may be mistaken for melanoma when in fact it is benign melanosis [8]. Client communication is key to an acceptable outcome for all who are involved in patient care.

(a)

(b)

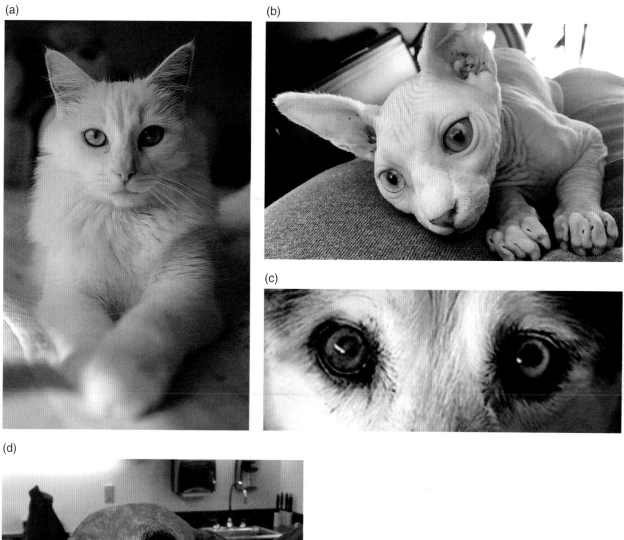

(c)

(d)

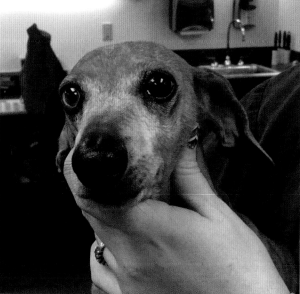

Figure 30.2 (a) Heterochromia iridis in a feline patient. *Source:* Courtesy of Kat Blincoe. (b) Heterochromia iridis in a feline patient. *Source:* Courtesy of Jennifer Urda and "Newt." (c) Heterochromia iridis in a canine patient. (d) Heterochromia iridis and heterochromia iridium in a canine patient. Note how the iris of the left eye (OD) is a solid brown, whereas the iris of the right eye (OS) is not a solid shade of blue. There is instead a central core of deep blue-gray against a backdrop of light blue.

(a)

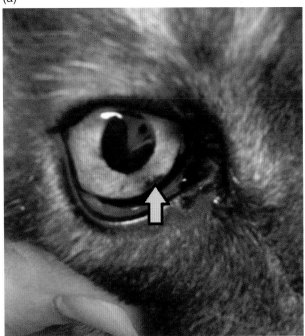

(b)

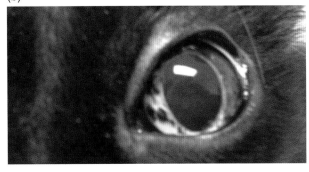

Figure 30.3 (a) Presumptive iris nevus in a feline patient. *Source: Courtesy of Patricia Bennett, DVM.* (b) Presumptive iris melanoma in a feline patient.

30.5 Synechiae

Synechiae are adhesions that involve the iris. These adhesions may be congenital or acquired. Acquired synechiae occur with greater frequency in companion animal practice.

There are two main types of synechiae [4, 20, 21]:

- Anterior
- Posterior

Anterior synechiae are adhesions that bridge the cornea and the iris [4] (see Figures 30.4a, b).

As is evident in Figures 30.4a, b, anterior synechiae may result from corneal disease. They may also develop secondary to uveitis. Refer to Chapter 17, Section 17.3

to review uveitis in terms of its clinical presentation and varied etiologies.

Posterior synechiae are adhesions between the iris and the lens [4, 20–22]. These adhesions may cause the affected portion(s) of the iris to bend backward in space, creating a larger pupil in the affected eye [22]. The affected pupil may also appear to be misshapen [22].

Posterior synechiae often result from ocular injury and associated hyphema [21]. Refer to Chapter 16 to review the causes of hyphema and the implications for the health of the globe.

Recall from Chapter 22, Section 22.2.2 that synechiae represent more than just aesthetic changes in the uvea. Posterior synechiae in particular may block the pupil. This obstructs the flow of aqueous humor, in effect inducing glaucoma [23].

30.6 Persistent Pupillary Membranes

In the embryo, a vascular network runs through the pupillary region [6]. The purpose of this network is to provide nutrition to the developing lens [6].

As fetal development progresses, this vasculature is supposed to regress so that, by two to three months of age, the pupil of the pediatric dog or cat is a wide-open aperture [6].

Occasionally, one or more remnants fail to regress [4, 6]. The persistence of one or more bands of tissue is visually apparent as a web from one edge of the iris to another [4, 6]. These webs or bridges of tissue are called persistent pupillary membranes (PPMs) [4, 6].

As long as PPMs only involve the iris, there is no adverse impact on vision [6]. However, vision will potentially be reduced if there is corneal or lens involvement [6].

PPMs occur more commonly in dogs than cats. The trait is inherited in Basenjis [6].

30.7 Iris Atrophy

Iris atrophy refers to degeneration of the iris [24] (see Figures 30.5a, b).

Iris atrophy may be age-related or secondary to inflammatory ocular disease, such as glaucoma or uveitis [24].

Refer to Chapter 18, Section 18.3.1.6 to review the details of this condition. Recall that, as the iris degenerates, it may impact the size and shape of the pupil. Anisocoria is a common finding in those patients with unilateral or asymmetrical iris atrophy [24] (see Chapter 18, Figures 18.7a, b).

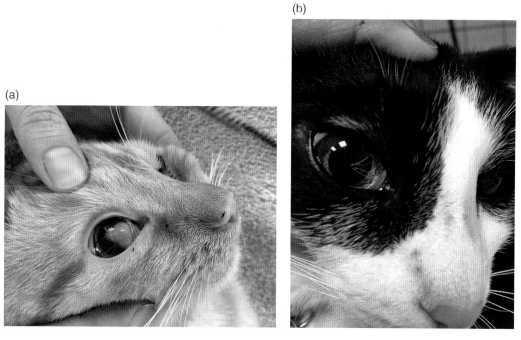

Figure 30.4 (a) Anterior synechiae in a feline patient with corneal disease. Note that the anterior synechiae connect the iris to the cornea. They can be thought of as a Band-Aid, attempting to seal the corneal defect. *Source:* Courtesy of Paul Ebner, LVT. (b) Anterior synechiae in a feline patient. *Source:* Courtesy of Dr. Lauren Griggs.

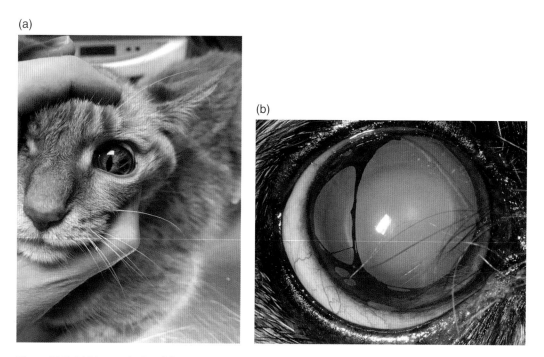

Figure 30.5 (a) Iris atrophy in a feline patient. *Source:* Courtesy of Elizabeth E. Ferguson, DVM. (b) Close-up of iris atrophy in a canine patient. *Source:* Courtesy of D.J. Haeussler, Jr., MS, DVM, DACVO.

References

1 Wasik, B. and Adkins, E. (2010). Canine Anterior Uveitis. *Compend. Contin. Educ. Pract.* 32 (11): E1–E11.

2 Singh, B. and Dyce, K.M. (2014). *Dyce, Sack, and Wensing's Textbook of Veterinary Anatomy*, 5e. St. Louis, Missouri: Saunders.

3 DeLahunta, A., Glass, E., and Kent, M. *Veterinary Neuroanatomy and Clinical Neurology*, 4e. St. Louis, Missouri: Saunders.

4 Englar, R.E. (2017). *Performing the Small Animal Physical Examination*. Hoboken, NJ: Wiley.

5 Martin, C.L. (2005). Anterior uvea and anterior chamber. In: *Ophthalmic Disease in Veterinary Medicine* (ed. C.L. Martin), 298–336. London, UK: Manson Publishing, Inc.

6 Maggs, D., Miller, P., and Ofri, R. (2012). *Slatter's Fundamentals of Veterinary Ophthamology*. St. Louis, MO: Elsevier Saunders.

7 Strain, G.M. (2012). Canine deafness. *Vet. Clin. Small Anim.* 42: 1209–1224.

8 Sandmeyer, L.S., Leis, M.L., Bauer, B.S., and Grahn, B.H. (2017). Diagnostic ophthalmology. *Can. Vet. J.* 58 (7): 757–758.

9 Newbold, G.M. and Hendrix, D. (2018). Common ophthalmic neoplasms in dogs and cats. *NAVC Clinician's Brief* (February): 30–33.

10 Hendrix, D. (2013). Diseases and surgery of the canine anterior uvea. In: *Veterinary Ophthalmology* (ed. K.N. Gelatt, B.C. Gilger and T.J. Kern), 1179. Ames, IA: Wiley-Blackwell.

11 Stiles, J.S. (2013). Feline ophthalmology. In: *Veterinary Ophthalmology* (ed. K.N. Gelatt, B.C. Gilger and T.J. Kern), 1477–1559. Ames, IA: Wiley-Blackwell.

12 Wiggans, K.T., Reilly, C.M., Kass, P.H., and Maggs, D.J. (2016). Histologic and immunohistochemical predictors of clinical behavior for feline diffuse iris melanoma. *Vet. Ophthalmol.* 19 (Suppl 1): 44–55.

13 Day, M.J. and Lucke, V.M. (1995). Melanocytic neoplasia in the cat. *J. Small Anim. Pract.* 36 (5): 207–213.

14 Patnaik, A.K. and Mooney, S. (1988). Feline melanoma: a comparative study of ocular, oral, and dermal neoplasms. *Vet. Pathol.* 25 (2): 105–112.

15 Boydell, P. and Enache, A. (2012). Approach to feline iris melanoma. *Vet. Pract.* 8: 18–21.

16 Wilcock, B.P. and Peiffer, R.L. Jr. (1986). Morphology and behavior of primary ocular melanomas in 91 dogs. *Vet. Pathol.* 23 (4): 418–424.

17 Kalishman, J.B., Chappell, R., Flood, L.A., and Dubielzig, R.R. (1998). A matched observational study of survival in cats with enucleation due to diffuse iris melanoma. *Vet. Ophthalmol.* 1 (1): 25–29.

18 Duncan, D.E. and Peiffer, R.L. (1991). Morphology and prognostic indicators of anterior uveal melanomas in cats. *Prog. Vet. Comp. Ophthalmol.* 1: 25–32.

19 Planellas, M., Pastor, J., Torres, M.D. et al. (2010). Unusual presentation of a metastatic uveal melanoma in a cat. *Vet. Ophthalmol.* 13 (6): 391–394.

20 Nelson, R.W. and Couto, C.G. (2009). Disorders of hemostasis. In: *Small Animal Internal Medicine* (ed. R.W. Nelson and C.G. Couto), 1242–1259. Missouri: Mosby Elsevier.

21 Carter RT. (2009). Feline uveitis: a review of its causes, diagnosis, and treatment. DVM 360 [Internet]. http://veterinarymedicine.dvm360.com/feline-uveitis-review-its-causes-diagnosis-and-treatment.

22 Heller HB, Bentley E. (2016). The Practitioner's Guide to Neurologic Causes of Canine Anisocoria. Today's Veterinary Practice [Internet]. (January/February):[77–83 pp.]. https://todaysveterinarypractice.com/observations-ophthalmologythe-practitioners-guide-neurologic-causes-canine-anisocoria.

23 Reinstein S. (2017). Under Pressure: Canine and Feline Glaucoma. Michigan Veterinary Medical Association [Internet]. https://michvma.org/resources/Documents/MVC/2017%20Proceedings/reinstein%2005.pdf.

24 Maggs, D.J., Miller, P.E., and Ofri, R. (2013). *Slatter's Fundamentals of Veterinary Ophthalmology*. Philadelphia: Elsevier Saunders.

31

Abnormal Appearances of the Lens

31.1 Introduction to the Lens

The lens is the transparent part of the eye [1–5]. Positioned caudal to the iris and pupil, it refracts light so that light falls upon the retina for visual processing [1–4, 6]. To achieve this end, the lens is elastic [3]. It adjusts its shape to facilitate accommodation, that is, a change in optical power to allow objects that are both near and far to come into focus [3, 5].

The lens provides the bulk of the refractive power of the eye in companion animal patients [6]. A canine eye has 60 diopters (D) of refractive power in total [6]. Two-thirds is provided by the lens [6].

When the lens is not functional due to disease, the patient's vision suffers tremendously. Aphakic vision, that is, vision without contributions from the lens, is estimated to be 20/800 [6, 7]. The equivalent of this poor acuity would be a person who is seated 20 feet away from the Snellen eye chart and who is unable to see the large "E" [6].

The lens is biconvex, with anterior and posterior poles [1–5]. The anterior pole is shielded by one to two layers of epithelium and a relatively thick capsule, as compared to the posterior pole, which is thinner and lacks an epithelial cushion [3, 4].

The equator of the lens is where the anterior and posterior poles meet. Here, the zonular fibers that form the suspensory apparatus of the lens attach [3, 4]. These secure the lens to the ciliary processes of the ciliary body [3, 4]. This design allows the lens to be suspended in space.

The lens capsule is under tension [3]. If this tension were unopposed, the lens would be inclined to take on a spherical shape [3]. Instead, the zonular fibers counter this tendency by exerting a radial pull on the equator [5]. This creates the normal resting shape of the lens as a biconvex structure [1–4]. This is how the lens is shaped to bring distant objects into focus [3]. This is also how the lens is shaped when the canine or feline patient is at rest or asleep [3].

When the focus needs to shift onto near objects, the ciliary body muscle contracts [3]. This brings the ciliary processes of the ciliary body nearer to the lens, thus relaxing the zonular fibers [3]. With the zonular fibers disengaged, the lens is released from opposing tension in such a way that it now can round out [3]. When the lens takes on this more spherical shape, it is able to bring near objects into focus [3].

The process of accommodation is present in companion animal patients [5]. However, it is less refined than in the human [3, 5]. The ciliary muscle is less developed in dogs and cats, and therefore both companion species are somewhat limited in their ability to adjust focus based upon spatial relationships [3].

The lens is a layered solid [3, 4]. It is estimated to contain 22,000 layers [6]. Yet the lens is compact. A typical lens in a dog is just 10 mm in diameter and 7 mm thick [6, 8]. The lens of a cat is slightly larger than that of a dog, with a diameter of 9 to 12 mm [5, 9].

Lens fibers are laid down in concentric sheets, in an onion-like pattern [3, 4, 6]. These sheets surround the central lens nuclei [4].

Lens fibers are soft in the peripheral, or the so-called cortical, lens [3]. They become increasingly firm as they track toward the central, or the so-called nuclear, lens [3].

Fibers loop from anterior to posterior surfaces [3]. Within each sheet, fibers connect to each other at each other's ends [6]. The junctions of these fibers, otherwise known as suture lines, form a three-pointed star [3, 4]. When viewed head-on, the suture lines in the anterior lens appear as an upright "Y" [4, 5]. The "Y" appears inverted in the posterior lens [4, 5] (see Figure 31.1).

Y-shaped suture lines are not visible to the observer's naked eye in normal, healthy adult patients. They may become visible when patients develop cataracts. A cataract is focal or diffuse cloudiness within the lens due to increased turbidity within the lens fibers [3, 4].

Y-shaped suture lines may also be visible when viewed through the slit lamp microscope in puppies and kittens [3].

Common Clinical Presentations in Dogs and Cats, First Edition. Ryane E. Englar.
© 2019 John Wiley & Sons, Inc. Published 2019 by John Wiley & Sons, Inc.

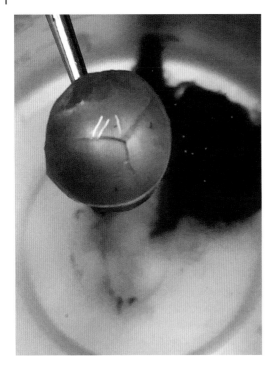

Figure 31.1 Y-shaped suture lines in a lens that has been removed from a patient that underwent cataract surgery. *Source:* Courtesy of Paul Ebner.

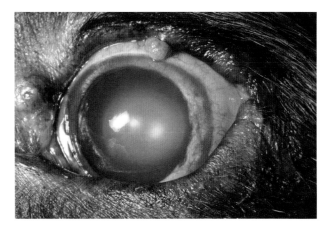

Figure 31.2 Nuclear sclerosis in a canine patient. This age-related process confers a hazy appearance to the lens. Note the unrelated, incidental finding of a papilloma associated with the upper eyelid. *Source:* Courtesy of D.J. Haeussler Jr., BS, MS, DVM, DACVO.

Transparency is just as important to the lens as it is to the cornea for both to function as refractive surfaces [4–6, 10]. To maintain its transparency, the lens is avascular [4–6]. The hyaloid artery, which nourished the lens in embryonic life, degenerates shortly after birth [3, 5]. Thereafter, the lens receives nutrients indirectly from the aqueous humor, via diffusion [3, 5, 6, 11].

Occasionally, a remnant of the hyaloid artery is visible, microscopically, attached to the posterior capsule [3].

In addition to lacking a blood supply, the lens lacks innervation [4].

In health, the lens should not be visible to the observer macroscopically. It should be perfectly clear and therefore invisible to the naked eye.

Various pathologies cause the lens to come into view. The most common among these are described here.

31.2 Nuclear Sclerosis

The lens is not a static structure. Not only does its shape change for the purpose of accommodation, its size changes, too, throughout life. The lens grows as the patient ages [5, 12]. New cells are produced within the cortical lens [12]. This forces older cells inward. [12] As this occurs, the lens nucleus becomes increasingly compact [5, 6, 12, 13].

As mentioned earlier, the nuclear lens is already more firm than the cortical lens. This becomes even more

pronounced with age [5]. Age-related denseness of the lens is called lenticular sclerosis or, because it pertains to the nuclear lens, nuclear sclerosis [4, 5, 13]. Nuclear sclerosis creates a physiologic haziness that is visible to the observer [12] (see Figure 31.2).

The haziness that is associated with nuclear sclerosis occurs because the compressed lens fibers scatter light [12]. In addition, the patient may have an age-related increase in insoluble proteins that contribute to the cloudiness [12].

Nuclear sclerosis occurs in both dogs and cats [12]. Middle-aged to older adults are most commonly affected. Nuclear sclerosis tends to start at or around seven years of age [12, 14].

At this time, there do not appear to be breed or sex predispositions to the development of nuclear sclerosis [12]. However, excessive exposure to sunlight may accelerate the process [12].

After dilation of the pupils with a mydriatic agent and transillumination of the eye, nuclear sclerosis appears within the nuclear lens as a gray-blue translucence [5]. The cortical lens remains clear [5].

Unlike cataracts, nuclear sclerosis does not appreciably impair vision [5, 12]. Nuclear sclerosis also does not prevent the tapetal reflection or obstruct fundoscopy [5, 14].

31.3 Cataracts

Nuclear sclerosis is often mistaken for cataracts by veterinary clients and clinicians alike [5, 12].

Cataracts are opacities of the lens or lens capsule [2–6]. Unlike nuclear sclerosis, which appears as an opalescent, smooth opacity, cataracts seem chunky. They have been described as taking on a crushed ice appearance [12] (see Figure 31.3a, b).

There are several ways to classify cataracts, including the following [2, 5, 6]:

- Etiology
  - Inherited
  - Secondary to trauma, radiation, drugs, nutrition, or toxins
  - Secondary to underlying disease
    o Uveitis
    o Diabetes mellitus
    o Retinal degeneration
- Age of onset
  - Congenital
  - Juvenile
  - Senile
- Position within the lens
  - Nuclear
  - Cortical
  - Capsular
  - Subcapsular
  - Equatorial
- Stage of development
  - Incipient
  - Immature
  - Mature
  - Hypermature

31.3.1 Inherited Cataracts in the Dog

Cataracts are inherited more often in dogs than cats [15–17]. Based upon data from the Canine Eye Registry

Foundation (CERF), it is believed that over 90 canine breeds have heritable cataracts [18–21].

Although the mode of inheritance remains unclear in most, several breeds are known to develop early-onset cataracts that are assumed to be inherited [16, 17]. These breeds include, but are not limited to the following [16–20, 22–40]:

- Afghan Hound
- Australian Shepherd
- Bearded Collie
- Bichon Frise
- Boston Terrier
- Brussels Griffon
- Chesapeake Bay Retriever
- Chow Chow
- Cocker Spaniel
- French Bulldog
- German Shepherd
- Golden Retriever
- Havanese
- Japanese Chin
- Labrador Retriever
- Miniature Poodle
- Miniature Schnauzer
- Old English Sheepdog
- Silky Terrier
- Springer Spaniel
- Staffordshire Bull Terrier
- Standard Poodle
- Toy Poodle
- West Highland White Terrier

(a)
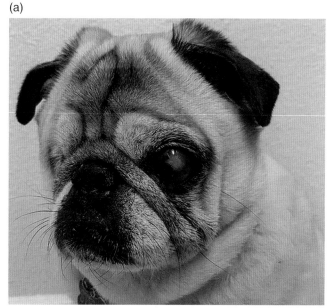
(b)
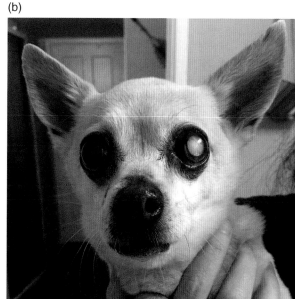

Figure 31.3 (a) Cataract in a Pug dog. *Source:* Courtesy of Ashley Parker. (b) Cataract in a Chihuahua. *Source:* Courtesy of Lai-Ting Torres.

Prevalence of cataracts varied by breed in a 2005 study by Gelatt et al., with most breeds listed above ranking between 5 and 12% [18]. Prevalence in purebreds was significantly higher than in mixed breeds. Mutts had a prevalence of 1.61% [18].

In addition to breed, age appears to be a factor when it comes to cataract development [18]. Patients are at greater risk of developing cataracts after four to seven years of age [18, 39, 41].

On the other hand, cataracts do not seem to prefer one sex to another. An apparent exception to the rule is the American Cocker Spaniel, in which females seem to develop cataracts with greater frequency than males [18]. By contrast, males are overrepresented among the Brussels Griffon, Japanese Chin, and Bearded Collie [18].

31.3.2 Cataracts in the Dog Secondary to Diabetes Mellitus

As mentioned earlier, genetics plays an important role in the development of cataracts in the canine patient [16, 39].

Another common cause of cataracts in dogs is diabetes mellitus [6, 39, 42–44].

The lens relies upon anaerobic glycolysis for energy [6, 45]. Glucose is acted upon by three enzymes within the lens itself [46]:

- Hexokinase
- Aldose reductase
- Glucose dehydrogenase

Hexokinase catalyzes the conversion of glucose to glucose 6-phosphate and adenosine diphosphate (ADP) [46].

There are low levels of hexokinase in the lens. Patients with diabetes mellitus are chronically hyperglycemic. It does not take much glucose to overwhelm the system. Hexokinase easily reaches saturation [6, 46]. As a result, glucose is metabolized through an alternate pathway: it is converted into sorbitol by aldose reductase [6, 44]. Sorbitol dehydrogenase then catalyzes the transformation of sorbitol into fructose [6, 44].

Neither sorbitol nor fructose can cross the lens capsule [6]. Because these are osmotic agents and their presence within the lens has established a concentration gradient, water is drawn into the lens from the aqueous humor [6, 44].

Overhydrating the lens ruptures lens fibers [6, 42, 44]. Over time, the damage that is sustained by the crystalline lens promotes cataract formation [42].

Cataracts are common sequelae of diabetes mellitus in dogs: it is typical for cataracts to form within 6 to 12 months of being diagnosed as diabetic [6, 43, 47]. Cataracts are typically bilateral when they occur secondary to diabetes mellitus [14].

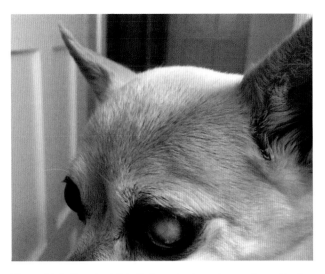

Figure 31.4 Grossly visible Y-shaped sutures in a canine patient that has been diagnosed with a cataract. *Source:* Courtesy of Lai-Ting Torres.

Often, owners report that the eyes clouded over, overnight. [47] These patients may present as acutely blind [47, 48].

The Y-shaped sutures are often visible due to appreciable swelling of the lens fibers [47] (see Figure 31.4).

Affected patients are at risk of widespread globe inflammation or rupture of the lens capsule, and secondary phacolytic uveitis [6, 47, 49].

In health, the normal lens release small amounts of crystallins [6, 50]. Crystallins are lens-associated proteins [19]. These are considered foreign substances by the body because lens proteins are sequestered away from the immune system during both embryonic life and postnatal development [19]. Small amounts of crystallins are tolerated by T-cells [47]. However, when lenses develop cataracts, they release greater amounts of crystallins [47]. This release, particularly the α–crystallins, overwhelms the body's tolerance. The body responds with both humoral and cell-mediated immune reactions [19].

Significant inflammation ensues [47]. This may involve one or more parts of the globe, including, but not limited to, the conjunctiva, sclera, cornea, and uvea [47].

31.3.3 Other Causes of Secondary Cataracts in the Dog

Environmental factors may also contribute to cataract development [6]. For example, dogs that are exposed to excessive ultraviolet radiation are more likely to develop cataracts [6, 51]. Similarly, inadvertent exposure of the eyes to an irradiated field during radiation therapy is likely to result in cataracts within 6 to 12 months [47, 52].

Traumatic injury to the eye, particularly sharp objects, such as cat claws and plant thorns, may result in cataracts [47].

Commercial milk replacers that are deficient in amino acids have been linked to cataract formation in puppies of both domestic dogs and timber wolves [47, 53].

Electrocution, as from being struck by lightning or chewing wires, are rare events; yet these, too, can result in cataracts [47].

Finally, age-related cataract formation is possible in dogs, just as it is in humans [47]. When this occurs, it is difficult to distinguish from genetic cataracts [47]. However, in general, patients of toy-to-small breeds that are 10 years of age or older when they present with lens opacities are likely to have developed cataracts on account of age rather than genes [47].

31.3.4 Inherited Cataracts in the Cat

Unlike dogs, cats do not typically present for primary cataracts [5, 15, 54]. When they do, the following breeds have been described in the veterinary literature [5, 15, 36, 55–60]:

- Bengal
- Birman
- Himalayan
- Russian blue
- British shorthair
- Persian, particularly blue-smoke Persian cats

31.3.5 Secondary Cataracts in the Cat

More often, cats develop cataracts secondary to external factors, such as trauma, or underlying disease, especially uveitis [5, 15, 16, 36, 61, 62].

Diabetes cataracts do occur in cats; however, the incidence is less so than in diabetic dogs [5, 54, 63].

Nutrition has also been implicated in cataract formation in kittens [5]. As was the case for pups, kittens that have been fed certain brands of commercially available milk replacers have been prone to cataract formation [5, 47, 62]. These products were suspected to be deficient in arginine [5].

Cataracts have also been described in two case reports of kittens with [5, 64, 65]

- Primary hypoparathyroidism, hypocalcemia, and hyperphosphatemia
- Nutritional secondary hyperparathyroidism and hypocalcemia.

Hypocalcemia secondary to metabolic disease tends to result in a classic "field of stars" appearance within the lens [47]. That is, several white specks develop within the lens as a multifocal cataract rather than one diffuse lesion.

31.3.6 Cataract Location

When a cataract is diagnosed on physical examination, it is important to determine its location within the lens [47, 66]. Location is one indication as to the likelihood of cataract progression [47, 66].

As cataracts progress, they may become more extensive [47, 66]. Being able to track cataract location over time provides a record of cataract progression [47, 66]. This may be helpful to the veterinary client, who has a voice in determining whether to initiate medical or surgical management.

As mentioned earlier, nuclear cataracts arise from within the central core of the lens [47]. These are typically present at birth or develop in the neonate [47]. Progression is unlikely [47]. If the patient was intended for breeding later in life, this may need to be reconsidered as there are a number of congenital cataracts that are inherited.

Cortical cataracts arise outside of the lens nucleus [47]. These may develop within the anterior cortex, posterior cortex, or both [47].

Capsular cataracts arise from the capsule itself, whereas subcapsular cataracts sit just beneath the capsule [47]. As with cortical cataracts, subcapsular cataracts may be situated in the anterior or posterior lens [47]. Many of these are inherited. [47] They may or may not progress [47].

Cataracts that are equatorial arise nearest the zonular fibers, which attach the lens to the ciliary body [3, 4]. Because the equator is where growth of the lens is most active, equatorial cataracts tend to be progressive [47]. Most diabetic cataracts also start at this location [47].

31.3.7 Cataracts at Various Stages of Development

Cataract location within the lens is straightforward. [47] However, cataract classification by stage of development is not necessarily as intuitive.

Incipient cataracts are the smallest of cataracts [6, 47]. They may be congenital or acquired [6]. Those that are congenital do not tend to progress [6].

When incipient cataracts are acquired, they often occur secondary to retinal or uveal disease [16, 43, 47, 65, 67–73]. It is important that the clinician complete a thorough ophthalmoscopic evaluation in order to rule out underlying ocular diseases such as uveitis [6].

In addition, the finding of one or more incipient cataracts warrants deeper investigation into the potential roots of the problem. Incipient cataracts often result from systemic disease [16, 43, 47, 65, 67–73]. Adverse effects of chronically administered medications, such as ketoconazole, have also been implicated in their development [67].

Because incipient cataracts represent less than 15% of lens volume, they do not typically obstruct vision [6] (see Figure 31.5).

Incipient cataracts do not tend to limit the clinician's view of deeper ocular structures via fundoscopy [6, 47].

Immature cataracts are larger than incipient ones, but they do not take up the entire lens volume, as do mature cataracts [6, 47] (see Figures 31.6a, b).

Immature cataracts may still have regions of clear lens fibers [6]. These allow for tapetal reflection to persist [6, 47]. Depending upon the location and the expansiveness, vision may be compromised [6, 47].

Immature cataracts may cause the lens to become edematous [47]. This may create the appearance of a fragmented lens [11].

Intumescence is the condition by which there is extreme swelling of the lens [6]. If this occurs, immature cataracts may leak excessive amounts of crystallins, thus triggering uveitis [6, 74]. In addition, intumescent lenses may obstruct the flow of aqueous humor through the pupil [6, 75]. Secondary glaucoma results [6].

Ideally, cataracts should undergo surgical management prior to this stage, when they are immature, but before they become intumescent [6, 8].

As cataracts mature, meaning that they now take up 100% of lens volume, cataract surgery is less efficacious at restoring vision [6, 47]. The patient is also more likely to experience intra- and/or postoperative complications [8, 76].

Without intervention, patients with mature cataracts are blind [47]. There is no tapetal reflex [6]. If the retina is still functional, pupillary light reflexes (PLRs) and the dazzle reflex will be intact, but the patient will be avisual [47].

Hypermature cataracts are those that have started to undergo resorption [47]. As cataracts progress, lens fibers break apart and release crystallins [6]. Their release triggers phacolytic uveitis [6].

Subsequent autolysis of the lens reduces its volume. The lens essentially shrinks in size [6, 16]. Because the capsule remains the same size, it becomes wrinkled as it envelops the smaller-than-normal lens [6, 16, 47].

The interior of the hypermature lens takes on a rather milky appearance. Increased density within the cataract itself causes it to become sparkly [14] (see Figure 31.7).

Although hypermature cataracts may still be operated on, capsules are predisposed to tearing [6]. This may prevent the insertion of artificial lenses [6, 8]. Patients are therefore less likely to have a positive surgical outcome when cataracts have advanced to the hypermature stage [6].

If a veterinary client is serious about pursuing cataract surgery, referral to a board-certified ophthalmologist

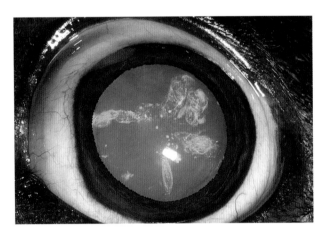

Figure 31.5 Incipient cataract in a canine patient. *Source:* Courtesy of D.J. Haeussler Jr., BS, MS, DVM, DACVO.

(a)

(b)

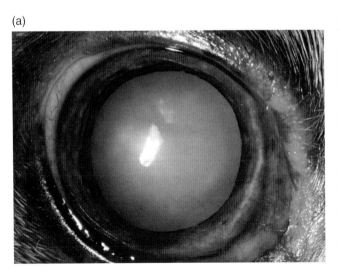
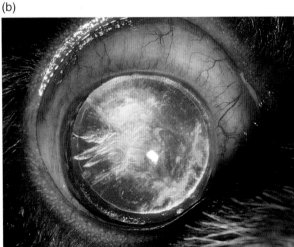

Figure 31.6 (a) Mature cataract in a canine patient. *Source:* Courtesy of D.J. Haeussler Jr., BS, MS, DVM, DACVO. (b) Advanced mature cataract in a canine patient. *Source:* Courtesy of D.J. Haeussler Jr., BS, MS, DVM, DACVO.

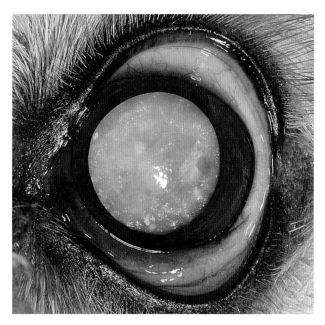

Figure 31.7 Hypermature cataract in a canine patient. *Source:* Courtesy of D.J. Haeussler Jr., BS, MS, DVM, DACVO.

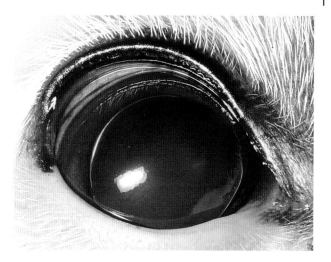

Figure 31.8 Anterior lens luxation in a canine patient. *Source:* Courtesy of D.J. Haeussler Jr., BS, MS, DVM, DACVO.

should occur as early in the disease process as possible [6]. Cataracts that are less advanced are more amenable to surgical management [6].

Phacoemulsification, followed by the implantation of an artificial lens, is considered the standard procedure for the surgical management of cataracts [6, 77].

31.4 Lens Luxation

The lens is suspended in space by its connection to the ciliary body via zonular fibers [3, 4]. When the lens capsule separates from these zonules, it loses its anchor. The lens is essentially dislocated.

31.4.1 Anterior Lens Luxation

An anterior lens luxation occurs when the lens migrates through the pupil into the anterior chamber of the eye [36, 78, 79] (see Figure 31.8).

When anterior lens luxation is acute, it is extremely painful, as evidenced by blepharospasm, epiphora, and/or pawing at the eye [78]. The cornea may become edematous, and intraocular pressure (IOP) may increase [78].

Primary anterior lens luxation is associated with certain breeds. In the dog, the following breeds may be predisposed [16, 78, 79]:

- Border Collie
- German Shepherd Dog

- Shar-Pei
- Terriers

Note that affected patients tend to have a unilateral presentation [78].

Age at presentation is highly variable among dogs, but tends to range from three to nine years old [78]. Cats with primary anterior lens luxation are less likely to present as young adults [36]. They tend to be seven to nine years of age, and are more likely to be Siamese [36, 78, 80, 81].

Although transcorneal reduction of the lens has been described to manage cases of anterior lens luxation, surgical removal of the lens is more typically performed [78, 82].

Anterior lens luxation in both dogs and cats may also occur secondary to chronic ocular disease [5, 78]. Glaucoma and cataracts have both been linked to the development of canine anterior lens luxation [78] (see Figure 31.9).

In cats, anterior lens luxation is most often secondary to glaucoma or uveitis [78, 80].

Lens removal is not advised in cases involving glaucomatous eyes [5]. This approach is likely to worsen glaucoma without restoring vision to the affected eye(s) [5].

31.4.2 Posterior Lens Luxation

The lens may also luxate into the posterior chamber, in which it will become fully bathed in the vitreous [83].

Posterior lens luxations tend to be less painful than anterior ones unless the lens blocks the flow of aqueous humor [5].

Unlike anterior lens luxations, posterior lens luxations may be difficult to appreciate grossly with the naked eye. The clinician's index of suspicion may be raised if the iris takes on a flat appearance. Fundoscopy or ocular ultrasonography may be indicated for confirmation [83].

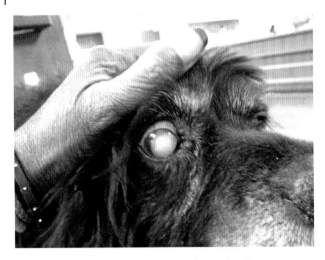

Figure 31.9 Anterior lens luxation in a dog with a diabetic cataract.

31.5 Intraocular Trauma

Corneal trauma was discussed in Chapter 29 as a common cause of ulcerations in companion animal practice [10]. Fights between patients that involve claws may end with one or more corneal scratches and/or punctures. Objects in the environment may also accidentally scrape the eye.

When corneal trauma is sustained, the cornea may not be the only part of the globe that is affected. The lens may also suffer collateral damage [78].

It is therefore critical to be thorough when performing the ophthalmic examination so that assumptions do not result in failure to diagnosis additional lesions. For instance, a positive fluorescein stain may be confirmatory for a corneal ulcer; however, the positive stain does not mean that a corneal ulcer is the only form of damage that the eye sustained.

Always be on the lookout for additional areas of concern. Comprehensive evaluations of the globe, particularly when trauma is involved, is essential to patient outcomes.

It is also important to note that cats with histories of ocular trauma are more likely to develop intraocular sarcomas [5, 84]. These may occur months to years after the injury was sustained [84, 85]. Patients as old as 15 years of age have been reported in the veterinary literature [86].

References

1 Evans, H.E. and Miller, M.E. (2013). *Miller's Anatomy of the Dog*, 4e, xix, 850 p. St. Louis, Missouri: Elsevier.

2 Englar, R.E. (2017). *Performing the Small Animal Physical Examination*. Hoboken, NJ: Wiley.

3 Singh, B. and Dyce, K.M. (2018). *Dyce, Sack, and Wensing's Textbook of Veterinary Anatomy*, 5e. St. Louis, Missouri: Saunders.

4 Boeve, M.H., Stades, F.C., and Djajadningrat-Laanen (2009). Eyes. In: *Medical History and Physical Examination in Companion Animals* (ed. A. Rijnberk and F.J. van Sluijs), 175–201. Elsevier Limited.

5 Sapienza, J.S. (2005). Feline lens disorders. *Clin. Tech. Small Anim. Pract.* 20 (2): 102–107.

6 Croix, N.L. (2008). Cataracts: when to refer. *Top. Companion Anim. Med.* 46–50.

7 Miller, P.E. and Murphy, C.J. (1995). Vision in dogs. *J. Am. Vet. Med. Assoc.* 207 (12): 1623–1634.

8 Adkins, E.A. and Hendrix, D.V.H. (2003). Cataract evaluation and treatment in dogs. *Compend. Contin. Educ. Pract.* 25 (11): 812–824.

9 Barnett, K.C. and Crispin, S.M. (eds.) (1998). Lens. In: *Feline Ophthalmology: An Atlas and Text*, 112–121. London: WB Saunders.

10 Ollivier, F.J. (2003). Bacterial corneal diseases in dogs and cats. *Clin. Tech. Small Anim. Pract.* 18 (3): 193–198.

11 Dziezyc, J. and Brooks, D.E. (1983). Canine cataracts. *Compend. Contin. Educ. Pract.* 5 (2): 81–90.

12 Giresi JC. (2005). Cataracts: How to uncover the imposter lenticular sclerosis. DVM 360 [Internet]. http://veterinarynews.dvm360.com/cataracts-how-uncover-imposter-lenticular-sclerosis.

13 Tobias, G., Tobias, T.A., and Abood, S.K. (2000). Estimating age in dogs and cats using ocular lens examination. *Compend. Contin. Educ. Pract.* 22 (12): 1085–1091.

14 Reinstein, S.L. (2016). The hazy lens: cataracts and nuclear sclerosis in dogs. *NAVC Clinician's Brief* (February): 48–50.

15 Nygren, K., Jalomaki, S., Karlstam, L., and Narfstrom, K. (2018). Hereditary cataracts in Russian blue cats. *J. Feline Med. Surg.* 20 (12): 1105–1109.

16 Davidson, M.G. and Nelms, S.R. (2013). Diseases of the lens and cataract formation. In: *Veterinary Ophthalmology* (ed. K.N. Gelatt, B.C. Gilger and T.J. Kern), 1199–1233. Ames, IA: Wiley-Blackwell.

17 Kristiansen, E., Revold, T., Lingaas, F. et al. (2017). Cataracts in the Norwegian Buhund-current prevalence and characteristics. *Vet. Ophthalmol.* 20 (5): 460–467.

18 Gelatt, K.N. and Mackay, E.O. (2005). Prevalence of primary breed-related cataracts in the dog in North America. *Vet. Ophthalmol.* 8 (2): 101–111.

19 Slatter, D. (2001). *Fundamentals of Veterinary Ophthalmology*. Philadelphia: W.B. Saunders.

20 Rubin, L.F. (1989). *Inherited Eye Diseases in Purebred Dogs*. Baltimore: Williams & Wilkins.

21 CERF (ed.) (1996). *Ocular Disorders Presumed to be Inherited in Purebred Dogs*. West Lafayette, IN: Purdue University.

22 Mellersh, C.S., Graves, K.T., McLaughlin, B. et al. (2007). Mutation in HSF4 associated with early but not late-onset hereditary cataract in the Boston terrier. *J. Hered.* 98 (5): 531–533.

23 Mellersh, C.S., Pettitt, L., Forman, O.P. et al. (2006). Identification of mutations in HSF4 in dogs of three different breeds with hereditary cataracts. *Vet. Ophthalmol.* 9 (5): 369–378.

24 Barnett, K.C. (1980). Hereditary cataract in the Welsh Springer spaniel. *J. Small Anim. Pract.* 21 (11): 621–625.

25 Barnett, K.C. (1985). Hereditary cataract in the miniature schnauzer. *J. Small Anim. Pract.* 26 (11): 635–644.

26 Barnett, K.C. (1986). Hereditary cataract in the German-shepherd dog. *J. Small Anim. Pract.* 27 (6): 387–395.

27 Barnett, K.C. and Startup, F.G. (1985). Hereditary cataract in the standard poodle. *Vet. Rec.* 117 (1): 15–16.

28 Curtis, R. (1984). Late-onset cataract in the Boston terrier. *Vet. Rec.* 115 (22): 577–578.

29 Curtis, R. and Barnett, K.C.A. (1989). Survey of cataracts in Golden and Labrador retrievers. *J. Small Anim. Pract.* 30 (5): 277–286.

30 Gelatt, K.N. (1972). Cataracts in golden retriever dog. *Vet. Med. Sm. Anim. Clin.* 67 (10): 1113–1115.

31 Gelatt, K.N., Samuelson, D.A., Barrie, K.P. et al. (1983). Biometry and clinical characteristics of congenital cataracts and microphthalmia in the miniature schnauzer. *J. Am. Vet. Med. Assoc.* 183 (1): 99–102.

32 Gelatt, K.N., Samuelson, D.A., Bauer, J.E. et al. (1983). Inheritance of congenital cataracts and microphthalmia in the miniature schnauzer. *Am. J. Vet. Res.* 44 (6): 1130–1132.

33 Gelatt, K.N., Whitley, R.D., Lavach, J.D. et al. (1979). Cataracts in Chesapeake Bay Retrievers. *J. Am. Vet. Med. Assoc.* 175 (11): 1176–1178.

34 Koch, S.A. (1972). Cataracts in interrelated old English sheepdogs. *J. Am. Vet. Med. Assoc.* 160 (3): 299–301.

35 Narfstrom, K. (1981). Cataract in the West Highland white terrier. *J. Small Anim. Pract.* 22 (7): 467–471.

36 Narfstrom, K. (1999). Hereditary and congenital ocular disease in the cat. *J. Feline Med. Surg.* 1 (3): 135–141.

37 Roberts, S.R. and Helper, L.C. (1972). Cataracts in afghan hounds. *J. Am. Vet. Med. Assoc.* 160 (4): 427–432.

38 Rubin, L.F. (1974). Cataract in Golden Retrievers. *J. Am. Vet. Med. Assoc.* 165 (5): 457–458.

39 Adkins, E.A. and Hendrix, D.V. (2005). Outcomes of dogs presented for cataract evaluation: a retrospective study. *J. Am. Anim. Hosp. Assoc.* 41 (4): 235–240.

40 Collins, B.K., Collier, L.L., Johnson, G.S. et al. (1992). Familial cataracts and concurrent ocular anomalies in chow chows. *J. Am. Vet. Med. Assoc.* 200 (10): 1485–1491.

41 Williams, D.L., Heath, M.F., and Wallis, C. (2004). Prevalence of canine cataract: preliminary results of a cross-sectional study. *Vet. Ophthalmol.* 7 (1): 29–35.

42 Basher, A.W. and Roberts, S.M. (1995). Ocular manifestations of diabetes mellitus: diabetic cataracts in dogs. *Vet. Clin. North Am. Small Anim. Pract.* 25 (3): 661–676.

43 Beam, S., Correa, M.T., and Davidson, M.G. (1999). A retrospective-cohort study on the development of cataracts in dogs with diabetes mellitus: 200 cases. *Vet. Ophthalmol.* 2 (3): 169–172.

44 Schermerhorn, T. (2008). Treatment of diabetes mellitus in dogs and cats. *NAVC Clinician's Brief* (January): 35–37.

45 Kinoshita, J.H. (1965). Pathways of glucose metabolism in the lens. *Investig. Ophthalmol.* 4: 619–628.

46 Pottinger, P.K. (1967). A study of three enzymes acting on glucose in the lens of different species. *Biochem. J.* 104 (2): 663–668.

47 Mancuso, L. and Hendrix, D. (2016). Cataracts in dogs. *NAVC Clinician's Brief* (August): 79–91.

48 Huang, A. (2012). Canine diabetes mellitus. *NAVC Clinician's Brief* (November): 47–50.

49 van der Woerdt, A., Nasisse, M.P., and Davidson, M.G. (1992). Lens-induced uveitis in dogs: 151 cases (1985–1990). *J. Am. Vet. Med. Assoc.* 201 (6): 921–926.

50 Denis, H.M., Brooks, D.E., Alleman, A.R. et al. (2003). Detection of anti-lens crystallin antibody in dogs with and without cataracts. *Vet. Ophthalmol.* 6 (4): 321–327.

51 Williams, D.L. (2006). Oxidation, antioxidants and cataract formation: a literature review. *Vet. Ophthalmol.* 9 (5): 292–298.

52 Roberts, S.M., Lavach, J.D., Severin, G.A. et al. (1987). Ophthalmic complications following megavoltage irradiation of the nasal and paranasal cavities in dogs. *J. Am. Vet. Med. Assoc.* 190 (1): 43–47.

53 Ranz, D., Gutbrod, F., Eule, C., and Kienzle, E. (2002). Nutritional lens opacities in two litters of Newfoundland dogs. *J. Nutr.* 132 (6 Suppl 2): 1688S–1689S.

54 Williams, D.L. and Heath, M.F. (2006). Prevalence of feline cataract: results of a cross-sectional study of 2000 normal animals, 50 cats with diabetes and one hundred cats following dehydrational crises. *Vet. Ophthalmol.* 9 (5): 341–349.

55 Peiffer, R.L. and Gelatt, K.N. (1975). Congenital cataracts in a Persian kitten (a case report). *Vet. Med. Small Anim. Clin.* 70 (11): 1334–1335.

56 Schwink, K. (1986). Posterior nuclear cataracts in 2 Birman kittens. *Feline Pract.* 16 (4): 31–33.

57 Rubin, L.F. (1986). Hereditary cataract in Himalayan cats. *Feline Pract.* 16 (1): 14–15.

58 Collier, L.L., Bryan, G.M., and Prieur, D.J. (1979). Ocular manifestations of the Chediak-Higashi-syndrome in 4 species of animals. *J. Am. Vet. Med. Assoc.* 175 (6): 587–590.

59 Irby NI, editor. (1983). Hereditary cataracts in the British shorthair cat. American College of Veterinary Ophthalmology Genetics Workshop.

60 Bourguet, A., Chaudieu, G., Briatta, A. et al. (2018). Cataracts in a population of Bengal cats in France. *Vet. Ophthalmol.* 21 (1): 10–18.

61 Stiles, J. (2013). Feline ophthalmology. In: *Veterinary Ophthalmology* (ed. K.N. Gelatt, B.C. Gilger and T.J. Kern), 1477–1559. Ames, IA: Wiley-Blackwell.

62 Remillard, R.L., Pickett, J.P., Thatcher, C.D., and Davenport, D.J. (1993). Comparison of kittens fed queen's milk with those fed milk replacers. *Am. J. Vet. Res.* 54 (6): 901–907.

63 Salgado, D., Reusch, C., and Spiess, B. (2000). Diabetic cataracts: different incidence between dogs and cats. *Schweiz. Arch. Tierheilkd.* 142 (6): 349–353.

64 Stiles, J. (1991). Cataracts in a kitten with nutritional secondary hyperparathyroidism. *Prog. Vet. Comp. Ophthalmol.* 4: 296–298.

65 Bassett, J.R. (1998). Hypocalcemia and hyperphosphatemia due to primary hypoparathyroidism in a six-month-old kitten. *J. Am. Anim. Hosp. Assoc.* 34 (6): 503–507.

66 Gelatt, K.N. (2013). Diseases of the lens and cataract formation. In: *Veterinary Ophthalmology* (ed. K.N. Gelatt, B.C. Gilger and T.J. Kern), 1199–1233. Ames, IA: Wiley.

67 da Costa, P.D., Merideth, R.E., and Sigler, R.L. (1996). Cataracts in dogs after long-term ketoconazole therapy. *Vet. Comp. Ophthalmol.* 6: 176–180.

68 Sapienza, J.S., Simo, F.J., and Prades-Sapienza, A. (2000). Golden Retriever uveitis: 75 cases (1994–1999). *Vet. Ophthalmol.* 3 (4): 241–246.

69 Gionfriddo JR. (2007). A challenging case: an unusual cause of blindness ion a Siberian husky. DVM360 [Internet]. http://veterinarymedicine.dvm360.com/challenging-case-unusual-cause-blindness-siberian-husky?id=&pageID=1&sk=&date.

70 Grahn, B. and Wolfer, J. (1995). Diagnostic ophthalmology. *Can. Vet. J. Rev. Vet. Can.* 36 (11): 722–723.

71 Kornegay, J.N., Greene, C.E., Martin, C. et al. (1980). Idiopathic hypocalcemia in 4 dogs. *J. Am. Anim. Hosp. Assoc.* 16 (5): 723–734.

72 Blocker, T. and van der Woerdt, A. (2000). What is your diagnosis? Cataract, retinal detachment, and a large mass protruding into the vitreous cavity. *J. Am. Vet. Med. Assoc.* 217 (1): 23–24.

73 Ching, S.V., Gillette, S.M., Powers, B.E. et al. (1990). Radiation-induced ocular injury in the dog – a histological study. *Int. J. Radiat. Oncol.* 19 (2): 321–328.

74 Ramsey DT, editor. (2002). Cataracts: which and when to refer. Proc North Am Vet Conf.

75 Wilkie, D.A., Gemensky-Metzler, A.J., Colitz, C.M. et al. (2006). Canine cataracts, diabetes mellitus and spontaneous lens capsule rupture: a retrospective study of 18 dogs. *Vet. Ophthalmol.* 9 (5): 328–334.

76 Biros, D.J., Gelatt, K.N., Brooks, D.E. et al. (2000). Development of glaucoma after cataract surgery in dogs: 220 cases (1987–1998). *J. Am. Vet. Med. Assoc.* 216 (11): 1780–1786.

77 Lim, C.C., Bakker, S.C., Waldner, C.L. et al. (2011). Cataracts in 44 dogs (77 eyes): a comparison of outcomes for no treatment, topical medical management, or phacoemulsification with intraocular lens implantation. *Can. Vet. J.* 52 (3): 283–288.

78 Colitz, C.M. and O'Connell, K. (2015). Lens-related emergencies: not always so clear. *Top. Companion Anim. Med.* 30 (3): 81–85.

79 Grahn, B.H., Storey, E., and Cullen, C.L. (2003). Diagnostic ophthalmology. Congenital lens luxation and secondary glaucoma. *Can. Vet. J.* 44 (5): 427, 9–30.

80 Olivero, D.K., Riis, R.C., Dutton, A.G. et al. (1991). Feline lens displacement: a retrospective analysis of 345 cases. *Prog. Vet. Comp. Ophthalmol.* 1: 239–244.

81 Payen, G., Hanninen, R.L., Mazzucchelli, S. et al. (2011). Primary lens instability in ten related cats: clinical and genetic considerations. *J. Small Anim. Pract.* 52 (8): 402–410.

82 Brown, M.H. (2006). Lens conditions. *NAVC Clinician's Brief* (September): 23–24.

83 Curtis, R. (1990). Lens luxation in the dog and cat. *Vet. Clin. North Am. Small Anim. Pract.* 20 (3): 755–773.

84 Dubielzig, R.R. (1984). Ocular sarcoma following trauma in three cats. *J. Am. Vet. Med. Assoc.* 184 (5): 578–581.

85 Southwick J. (2012). Feline ocular post-traumatic sarcoma in ten cats that had intraocular lens surgery. https://www.vetmed.wisc.edu/pbs/dubielzig/pages/coplow/PowerPoints/PostOpPTSCat.pdf.

86 Zeiss, C.J., Johnson, E.M., and Dubielzig, R.R. (2003). Feline intraocular tumors may arise from transformation of lens epithelium. *Vet. Pathol.* 40 (4): 355–362.

32

Abnormal Appearances of the External Ear

32.1 Introduction to the External Ear

As the outermost subdivision of the vestibulocochlear organ, the external ear is grossly visible on canine and feline physical examination and should always be examined [1].

The external ear consists of two parts [1–4]:

- The pinna, or auricle
- The external acoustic meatus, or external ear canal

32.1.1 The Two Pinnae

Both pinnae are cartilaginous flaps of tissue that branch off from the head to form what the veterinary client considers the ears.

In most cat breeds, the pinnae are erect because of stiff, auricular cartilage [1, 2, 5] (see Figures 32.1a, b).

An exception is the Scottish Fold breed, in which those cats with a dominant gene mutation develop abnormal cartilage that cannot support erect ears that stand up. Instead, the ears of affected cats bend forward and down, giving them a rounded appearance (see Figure 32.2).

The pinnae of most dog breeds are also erect; however, there are a greater number of button-eared or floppy-eared breeds [2] (see Figures 32.3a–e).

Both pinnae are typically symmetrical. However, the left pinna of cats may be surgically altered in a process that is called eartipping [2, 6] (see Figure 32.4).

Eartipping is a common procedure that is performed with the patient under anesthesia during routine elective ovariohysterectomy or orchiectomy [6]. A straight hemostat is placed perpendicular to the long axis of the ear to expose approximately three-eighths of an inch of tissue at the ear tip. The tip is then excised [6].

This ear tip or notch is a universal sign among trap-neuter-release (TNR) programs that a feral cat has been surgically sterilized [6]. Although this form of visual identification permanently alters the appearance of

the cat, it prevents the cat from being trapped a second time for a surgery that has already been performed [6].

The outer surfaces of both pinnae are typically furred [5]. However, the concave aspects are sparsely furred, if at all [5]. This is considered normal (see Figures 32.5a–d).

Both pinnae move independently of one another so that each can focus on different sounds [1, 5]. This is made possible by a number of auricular muscles that the facial nerve (CN VII) innervates [1, 5].

In any breed, the pinna acts as a funnel to receive sound [1].

Sound that is received by the pinna is ultimately funneled down through the external acoustic meatus to the tympanic membrane, or eardrum [1].

32.1.2 The External Acoustic Meatus

The external acoustic meatus is composed of two structures [1, 3, 5]:

- The vertical canal
- The horizontal canal

The distal end of the vertical canal directly contacts the pinna. The proximal end of the vertical canal feeds into the horizontal canal, which meets the tympanum, or eardrum [1, 3, 5]. The tympanum is a membranous separation between the external and middle ear [3].

As a whole, the external acoustic meatus is a curvilinear structure that begins as cartilage and ends as osseous tissue [1, 3, 5]. The vertical canal tracks ventro-rostrally before making a turn medially into the horizontal canal [3]. This junction between vertical and horizontal ear canals is angled at approximately 75° [7].

Both the vertical and horizontal aspects of the external ear canal are lined with sebaceous glands and ceruminous glands, which produce cerumen, or ear wax [1].

Some cats, particularly aged Siamese and Persians, produce an excess of cerumen naturally [8]. This is considered normal for them and is not of concern unless the

(a)

(b)

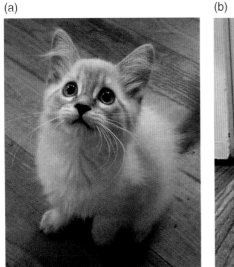
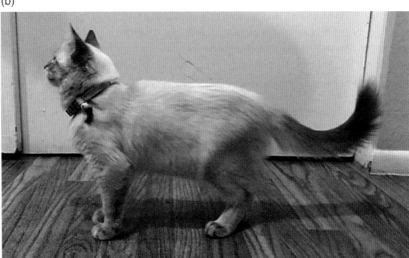

Figure 32.1 (a) Erect ears in a typical Domestic Medium-Haired (DMH) cat. *Source:* Courtesy of Kim Alvarez. (b) Profile view of erect ears in a typical DMH cat. *Source:* Courtesy of Kim Alvarez.

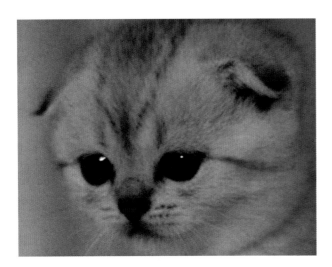

Figure 32.2 The classic appearance of bent ears in a Scottish Fold kitten. The bend is caused by mutated gene that involves cartilage. Note that affected cats may have abnormal cartilage in other regions of the body, not just limited to the ears.

patient presents with signs of otitis externa: malodorous aural discharge, head shaking, ear scratching, curvilinear excoriations along the affected pinna, stenosis of the entrance of the external ear canal, and aural pain [8, 9].

At birth, the external acoustic meatus is primitive and is functionally closed [1] (see Figures 32.6a, b).

The external acoustic meatus typically becomes patent 10–14 days after birth, at which point the patient is able to physically hear and process sounds [1, 2].

In cats, the entrance to the external ear canal has little to no fur. The same holds true for most dog breeds. Exceptions to this general rule include

Poodles, Schnauzers, and Rough-Coated Terriers [5] (see Figures 32.7a–c).

In both dogs and cats, the entrance to the external ear canal should not be occluded by discharge [2, 5].

There should also not be a strong odor associated with the ear canal itself [2, 5].

32.2 Abnormal Swelling of One or Both Pinnae

Auricular cartilage is the foundation of the pinna [3]. The apex of each pinna is essentially flat due to close apposition between the perichondrium of this cartilage, the overlying skin, and the vascular supply, which is via the caudal auricular artery [1, 3, 10]. This artery subdivides into lateral, intermediate, and medial vessels that course along the outer surface of the pinnae [3].

Both dogs and cats may present with abnormal swelling of one or both pinnae. In these classic presentations, the apex appears to be puffed up as opposed to maintaining its characteristic flat shape (see Figures 32.8a, b).

Note from Figure 32.8b that swelling of the pinna may be partial. Swelling may also begin as partial involvement of the pinna only to progress over time.

The swelling that is appreciated in Figures 32.8a, b is clinically referred to as an aural hematoma [11]. This is the accumulation of blood between the skin and auricular cartilage, forming a visible, palpable, and fluctuant pocket of fluid [3].

If left untouched, granulation tissue forms [3]. This causes pinnal fibrosis [3]. Ultimately, the affected pinna contracts [3]. This gives the pinna a thickened appearance

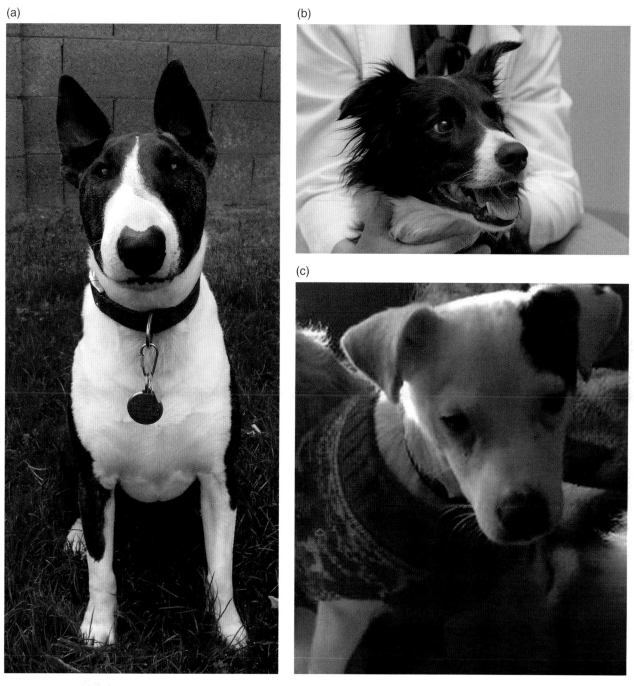

Figure 32.3 (a) Erect ears in a Bull Terrier. *Source:* Courtesy of Danielle Cucuzella. (b) This Border Collie is demonstrating the cocked or semi-pricked ear carriage that is typical for the breed. *Source:* Courtesy of the Media Resources Department at Midwestern University. (c) Button-ears in a terrier breed. (d) Natural ear carriage in a Boxer dog. The ears have not been cropped. *Source:* Courtesy of Symmantha Page. (e) Natural ear carriage in a Doberman Pinscher dog. The ears have not been cropped. *Source:* Courtesy of Michael and Naomi Englar. (f) Breed-characteristic floppy ears in a Bassett Hound puppy.

and a deformed "cauliflower" or "crinkle" shape [2] (see Figure 32.9).

Aural hematomas may be caused by continuous head shaking, as triggered by intense irritation of the pinna or external ear canal [3, 11]. It has been suggested that the

force of the pinna flapping against the body fractures the auricular cartilage and disrupts the vasculature [3].

When blood vessels that supply the ear burst, the resultant hemorrhage pools between the skin and auricular cartilage [3]. If the underlying cause of

(d)

(f)

(e)

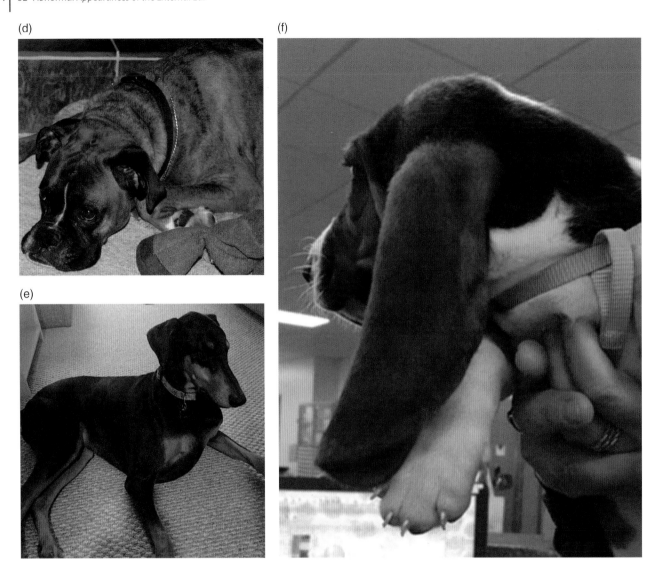

Figure 32.3 (Continued)

the head shaking is unresolved and head shaking persists, the pool of blood deepens [3]. This further separates the skin from the cartilage, creating a larger pocket [3].

In order to maintain an aesthetic appearance for the pinna, the hematoma needs to be drained [3]. For the best possible cosmetic outcome, drainage must occur before fibrosis has begun [3, 11].

In acute cases, drainage via needle aspiration may be effective [3]. However, chronic cases will routinely refill [3]. In these cases, the placement of a temporary drain, teat cannula, or vacuum-assisted device is indicated [3, 12–16] (see Figures 32.10a, b).

Alternatively, incisional drainage may be achieved under general anesthesia, followed by the placement of mattress sutures parallel to aural vasculature [3, 11]. The purpose of these sutures is to re-oppose the skin and aural cartilage [3]. Without a physical gap between the two, there is no space for fluid to accumulate, and the tissue is forced to heal, provided that the pinna is immobilized so as to guard against further trauma [3]. This immobilization is typically achieved by bandaging the ear over the top of the head or, if possible, along the neck [3].

Note the importance of addressing the primary problem that led to formation of the aural hematoma in the first place.

There is no substitute for a thorough otoscopic examination of the ear in any patient that presents for aural swelling [2, 3]. Refer to a primary care resource, such as *Performing the Small Animal Physical Examination* or Craig Griffin's *Otitis Techniques to Improve Practice*, for

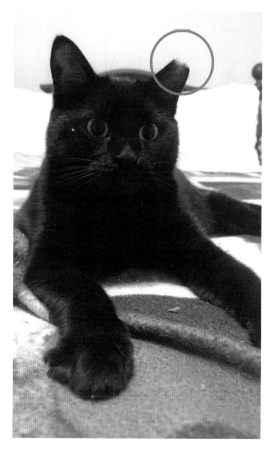

Figure 32.4 The cosmetic appearance of a cat that underwent eartipping of the left ear. *Source:* Courtesy of Pam Longenecker.

details regarding how best to perform otoscopy [2, 4]. Otoscopy also allows the clinician to assess the integrity of the tympanic membrane, which, if ruptured, has additional implications for patient management.

If the primary problem is not explored with measures taken to resolve it, then the aural hematoma is likely to recur.

32.3 Abnormal Aural Discharge

Cerumen is a waxy, yellow substance that is normally produced by a healthy ear canal [1, 7]. Some patients produce more or less earwax than others. Recall that aged Siamese and Persian cats tend to overproduce cerumen [8]. In addition, the Sphynx is also known for excessive cerumen production [2]. This is considered normal for the breed.

Aural discharge may also be abnormal for the patient based upon amount, color, consistency, or odor [7]. For example, consider a patient that typically does not have much, if any, visible cerumen. If this patient now

presents with an abundance of cerumen, this represents a change in the patient's norm.

All changes should be investigated, particularly in a patient that is exhibiting one or more of the following signs [8, 9]:

- Malodor
- Aural pain
- Head-shaking
- Pawing at ears
- Scratching at ears
- Whimpering when scratching at ears
- Occluded entrance to the external ear canal
- Reluctance to allow examiner to evaluate ears

The patient may also have visible excoriations or scratch wounds. Self-trauma is a common sign that the external ear is bothersome to the patient (see Figure 32.11).

All of the above signs are consistent with otitis externa, that is, inflammation associated with the external ear [8, 9].

Aural discharge is a common complaint in companion animal practice. Its presentation is also immensely varied in terms of the following [2, 7]:

- Malodor
  - "Yeasty"
  - Pungent
  - Rancid
- Color of discharge
  - White or cream
  - Yellow
  - Yellow-green
  - Green
  - Dark brown
  - Black
- Consistency of discharge
  - Gritty "coffee grounds"
  - Dry and flaky
  - Greasy
  - Goopy or gelatinous (see Figures 32.12a–i)

Historically, clinicians have made presumptive diagnoses based upon the aforementioned characteristics of the aural discharge [7]. For example, ear mite infestations have classically been reported to have dark brown-black, "coffee ground" debris that is gritty and dry [2, 7]. Light honey or brown, waxy exudate with a sweet "yeasty" odor has classically been associated with *Malassezia* overgrowth, whereas slimy, mucopurulent debris has been associated with bacterial infections [2, 17].

Although these characteristics may be used to heighten suspicions, they are not as consistent or as reliable as they were once thought [7, 18–23].

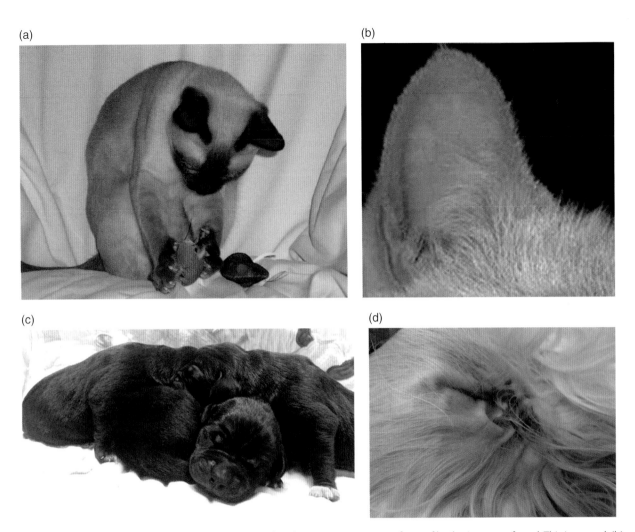

Figure 32.5 (a) Young adult Tonkinese cat. Appreciate that the convex, or outer, surfaces of both pinnae are furred. This is normal. (b) Young adult cat. Appreciate that the concave, or inner, surfaces of both pinnae are less densely furred. (c) Litter of puppies. Appreciate that the convex, or outer, surfaces of both pinnae are furred. This is normal. *Source:* Courtesy of Genevieve LaFerriere, DVM. (d) Adult dog. Appreciate that the concave, or inner, surfaces of both pinnae are less densely furred.

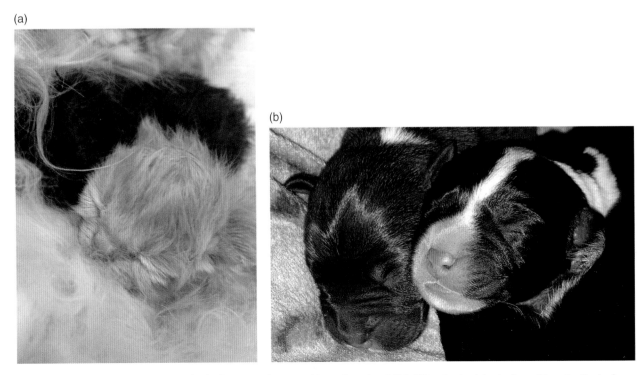

Figure 32.6 (a) One-day-old kitten. At birth, the external ear canal is not functional. This kitten is physiologically and transiently deaf. *Source:* Courtesy of Aimee Wong. (b) One-day-old puppies. Given their age, these puppies are also considered physiologically and transiently deaf. *Source:* Courtesy of Tara Beugel.

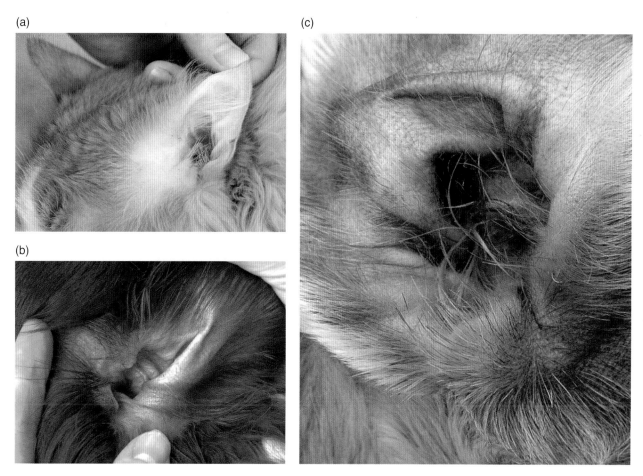

Figure 32.7 (a) Entrance to the external ear canal in a cat. Note that the entrance is devoid of fur. This is normal for cats. *Source:* Courtesy of the Media Resources Department at Midwestern University. (b) Entrance to the external ear canal in a dog. Note that the entrance is devoid of fur. This is normal for most dogs. *Source:* Courtesy of the Media Resources Department at Midwestern University. (c) Excessive fur coverage at the entrance to the external ear canal of this Miniature schnauzer dog. This is considered typical for the breed. *Source:* Courtesy of the Media Resources Department at Midwestern University.

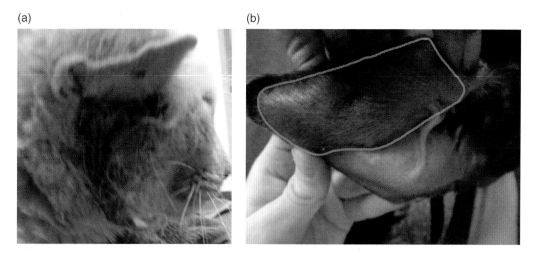

Figure 32.8 (a) Swelling of the entire right pinna in a feline patient. *Source:* Courtesy of Patricia Bennett, DVM. (b) Partial swelling of the pinna in a canine patient. The region of swelling has been outlined in orange. *Source:* Courtesy of Patricia Bennett, DVM.

32.3.1 Introduction to Aural Cytology

Cytology is the preferred tool for evaluation of aural debris [7, 19, 20, 23–27].

The most useful samples for cytology are taken from within the horizontal canal or, at least, the junction between the vertical and horizontal canals [7, 18, 28].

Both ears should be swabbed and evaluated microscopically, even if the patient is only presenting with grossly unilateral disease [7]. It may be that the appar-

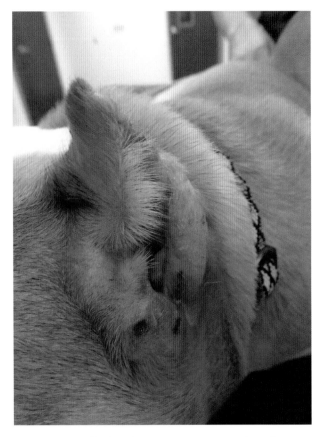

Figure 32.11 Self-induced traumatic excoriations along the outer aspect of the left pinna in a canine patient. This dog was subsequently diagnosed with otitis externa. *Source:* Courtesy of Kara Thomas, DVM, CVMA.

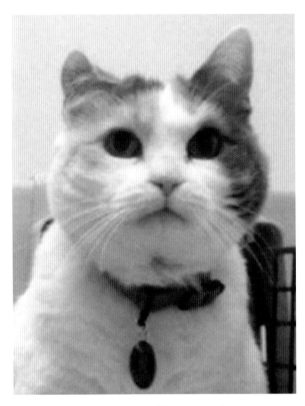

Figure 32.9 Pinnal fibrosis in a feline patient. *Source:* Courtesy of Patricia Bennett, DVM.

(a) (b)

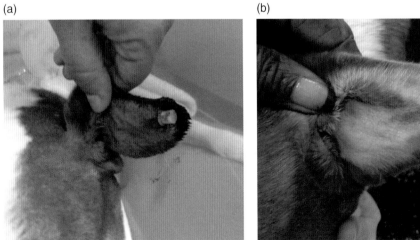
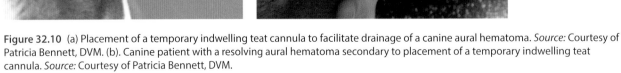

Figure 32.10 (a) Placement of a temporary indwelling teat cannula to facilitate drainage of a canine aural hematoma. *Source:* Courtesy of Patricia Bennett, DVM. (b). Canine patient with a resolving aural hematoma secondary to placement of a temporary indwelling teat cannula. *Source:* Courtesy of Patricia Bennett, DVM.

ently healthy ear is microscopically abnormal [7]. Bacterial or yeast overgrowth may be present that went undetected by the naked eye [7]. There may also be two infected ears, with different bacterial populations to manage [7, 28, 29].

Independent evaluation of both ears is essential so that medical management is tailored to the patient and each ear's individual needs [7].

Once a sample of each ear is obtained, the sample is rolled onto its own clean glass slide [7].

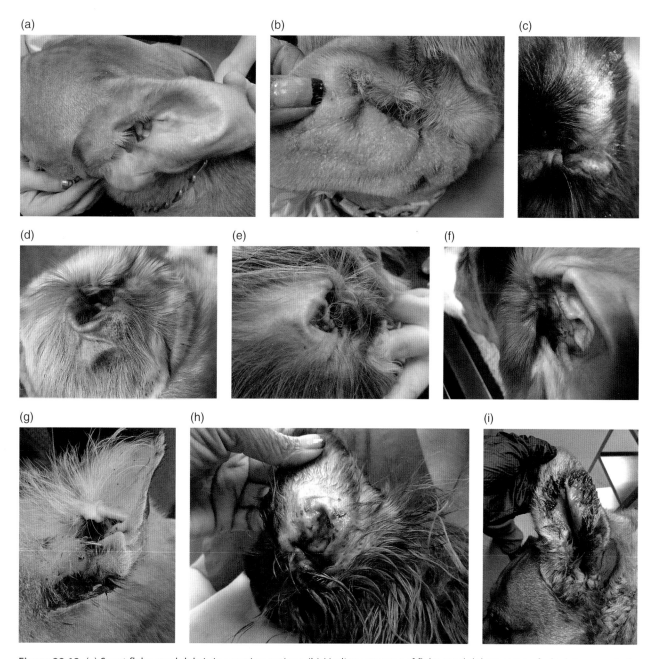

Figure 32.12 (a) Scant flaky aural debris in a canine patient. (b) Medium amount of flaky aural debris, some of which is encrusted on the inner aspect of the pinna. The pinna itself is hyperemic. *Source:* Courtesy of Patricia Bennett, DVM. (c) Large flakes of yellow crusty aural debris, some of which is adhered to the fur. (d) Scant amount of dark brown ceruminous aural debris. *Source:* Courtesy of Amber May. (e) Moderate amount of medium brown ceruminous aural debris coating the excessive hair at the entrance to the external ear canal. (f) Dark brown ceruminous debris. *Source:* Courtesy of Amber May. (g) Dark brown debris in a feline patient with curvilinear excoriations at the base of the pinna. (h) Mixed aural debris. There is a gelatinous layer of mucopurulent slime coating the inner surface of the pinna, in addition to a dark brown layer of ceruminous debris. (i) A second example demonstrating mixed aural debris. *Source:* Courtesy of Dr. Stephanie Harris.

(a)

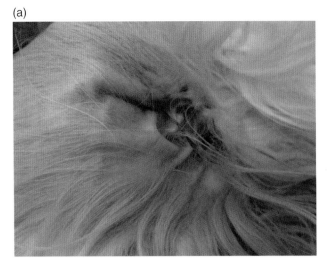

(b)

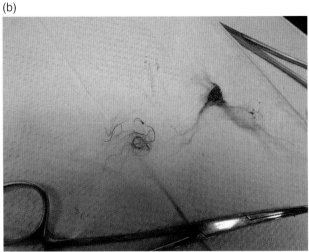

Figure 32.13 (a) Excessive hair at the entrance to the external ear canal may create favorable conditions for bacterial and/or yeast overgrowth. *Source:* Courtesy of Patricia Bennett, DVM. (b) Manual plucking of hair from the entrance to the external ear canal may predispose some patients to bacterial and/or yeast overgrowth. *Source: Source:* Courtesy of Patricia Bennet, DVM.

There is some debate as to whether or not the sample should be heat-fixed. Those who advocate for heat fixing do so because cerumen is largely lipid and is therefore more likely to wash away during the staining process. Using heat fixes the sample to the slide [7].

Modified Wright's stain, or Diff-Quik, is used frequently in-house to assist with the identification of leukocytes, bacteria, and yeast on aural cytology [7, 30]. Gram staining is rarely performed as an add-on procedure because most aural cocci will be Gram-positive (+) and most aural rods will be Gram-negative [7].

Following staining with Diff-Quik, the slide is air-dried, then examined by light microscopy. Low magnification is used initially to scan the field for an area of interest [7]. Regions with thinly spread debris are preferred to thick sheets because they offer improved visualization [7]. Cerumen and preparations of otic ointments do not take up stain and do not offer much by way of evaluation [7].

Once an area of interest is identified, magnification is increased. Magnification ×400, using the high-dry, ×40 objective, is sufficient for evaluation of large bacteria, yeast, erythrocytes, leukocytes, and cornified epithelium [7]. Magnification ×1000, using the oil immersion, ×100 objective, is necessary for identification of smaller bacteria [7].

The clinician should examine an average of five to ten high-powered fields, and document a rough estimate of the number of bacteria and yeast in each [7]. If bacterial, yeast, or mixed otitis externa is present and medical management is instituted, this information is vital to tracking response to treatment [7].

32.3.2 Cytology of the Normal Ear

Swabs of normal, healthy ears are likely to contain one or more of the following [7, 9, 22, 31, 32]:

- Non-staining cerumen
- Sheets of cornified squamous epithelial cells that stain blue due to keratin
- Resident bacteria
- Resident yeast

The resident bacteria of healthy ears tend to be cocci-shaped and include [7, 9, 19, 31]

- Coagulase-positive and coagulase-negative *Staphylococcus* spp.
- β-hemolytic *Streptococcus*.

Rod-shaped bacteria are not typically part of the normal flora of the canine or feline ear, with the exception of *Corynebacterium* spp. [7, 17, 19, 31].

The normal flora of the ear also includes basophilic yeast [7, 22, 32, 33]. These may or may not exhibit unipolar budding [7]. This creates the classic "footprint," "peanut," or "snowman" shape [7].

Aural swabs of healthy ears do not typically contain leukocytes [7, 18, 19, 28, 30].

32.3.3 Cytology of the Abnormal Ear

Although yeast and certain bacterial species normally reside within the external ear canal, they may exhibit overgrowth and become opportunistic pathogens if conditions are favorable [7]. These conditions include the following [9, 26, 27]:

- Long, droopy ears that prevent aeration of the external ear canal
- Excessive amounts of hair that occlude the entrance to the external ear canal
- Other forms of obstructive ear canal disease, including polyps
- Excessive moisture within the external ear canal, as from swimming or bathing
- The use of irritating ear rinse solutions, such as those containing high concentrations of alcohol
- Traumatic removal of hair from the external ear canal, inciting an inflammatory response (see Figures 32.13a, b)

In addition to overgrowth of normal flora, the following bacterial pathogens are most frequently isolated from diseased ears [9, 19, 29, 34, 35]:

- *Escherichia coli*
- *Enterococcus* spp.
- *Pseudomonas aeruginosa*
- *Proteus mirabilis*
- *Staphylococcus intermedius* (see Figure 32.14)

It has been suggested that greater than 14 bacteria per high-powered field, in cats, and 25, in dogs, indicates an abnormally increased bacterial population [7].

Of the bacterial species listed above, *P. aeruginosa* is most concerning. It is a common cause of otitis externa in canine patients, and frequently exhibits multi-drug resistance on drug susceptibility profiles [36, 37].

Cocker Spaniels may be predisposed to infection because of their atypical aural anatomy [37]. Rather than having simple hair follicles, the ear canals of Cocker spaniels contain densely arranged, compound follicles [37]. This alters their response to inflammation [37].

In response to inflammation, Cocker spaniels develop hyperplastic ceruminous glands [37]. This contributes to a hairy, narrowed environment that is well suited for inhabitation by *Pseudomonas* species [37].

Yeast overgrowth is also common among canine and feline patients in clinical practice. There are many species of *Malassezia*; however, among these, *Malassezia pachydermatis* is most common [9, 19, 33, 38–40] (see Figures 32.15a, b).

Candida spp. may also be isolated from the ears of those with otitis externa [19, 29, 34, 35].

It has been suggested by Ginel et al. that over 5 and 12 yeast per high-powered field in dogs and cats, respectively, is abnormal [7, 41]. However, this rubric is intended as a guideline [7].

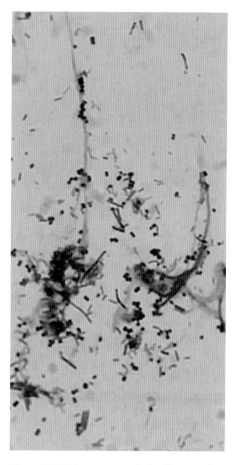

Figure 32.14 An example of mixed bacterial populations observed on aural cytology from a canine patient with otitis externa. Note the presence of cocci, diplococci, individual rods, and rods that are linked to one another like a necklace.

The decision to treat or not to treat must ultimately depend upon a combination of factors, including past pertinent history and presenting complaint(s) [7].

The presence of leukocytes on aural cytology confirms that some degree of otitis is present [7, 18, 19, 28, 30, 41]. Inflammation allows cells such as neutrophils and macrophages to access the lumen of the external ear canal [7].

In addition, dogs and cats with otitis externa may have increased numbers of cornified squamous epithelial cells on cytology [27].

32.3.4 The Additive Value of Bacterial Culture

When cocci are observed on cytology, they are most likely to be either *Staphylococcus* or *Streptococcus* spp. [7]. Cytology alone cannot differentiate between the two [7]. Cytology also cannot determine whether pre-existing bacteria are susceptible to certain classes of antibiotics

(a)

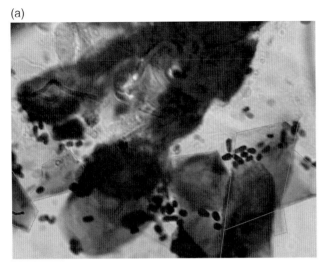

(b)

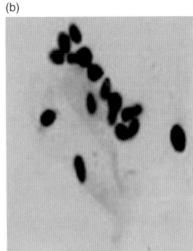

Figure 32.15 (a) Yeast overgrowth observed on aural cytology from a canine patient. Note that some of the yeast appears to be in budding. Cornified squamous epithelial cells have been outlined in orange. (b) Cytological demonstration of yeast overgrowth.

[7]. The additive value of bacterial culture is that it provides this additional information. This information, in combination with cytological findings, collectively guides the therapeutic plan for the patient [7].

Cultures are particularly essential when cytological findings include rod-shaped bacteria [37]. Given the tendency for rods to be multi-drug resistant, it is critical to determine the susceptibility profile of the pathogenic organism(s) [37, 42].

Other reasons to culture include the following [19, 20, 23, 40, 43, 44]:

- Chronic otitis
- Recurrent otitis
- Involvement of the middle ear
- Lack of response to current treatment

32.3.5   Potential Disadvantages of Bacterial Culture

Although bacterial culture and susceptibility profiles are intended to facilitate medical management, these diagnostic tools cannot distinguish resident from pathogenic organisms, or bacterial overgrowth from overt infection [7].

It is the responsibility of the clinician to understand which organisms are commensals and do not require consideration when devising the patient's management plan, even if diagnostic laboratory reports list susceptibility data for all organisms [7].

Culture is also not to be used in lieu of cytology [7]. Serial cytology is essential to tracking patient response to treatment [7].

32.4   Underlying Causes of Otitis Externa

Bacterial and fungal otitis externa may represent primary disease. However, more often, they are secondary to an underlying issue [8].

When otitis externa is unilateral, it is likely the result of [8, 9]

- Trauma
- Foreign bodies, particularly foxtails
- An aural polyp or other tumor.

By contrast, bilateral otitis externa is most likely due to the following [8, 9, 26, 27, 45, 46]:

- Allergic skin disease (refer to Chapters 11 and 12)
    - Contact allergy
    - Food hypersensitivity
    - Atopic dermatitis
- Autoimmune disease (refer to Chapter 3, Section 3.8.3)
    - Pemphigus foliaceus
    - Systemic lupus erythematosus (SLE)
- Other immune-mediated disease
    - Vasculitis
    - Erythema multiforme
- Metabolic imbalances (refer to Chapter 5, Section 5.7 and Chapter 9, Section 9.3.2)
    - Hypothyroidism
    - Hyperadrenocorticism
    - Alterations in sex hormones
- Keratinization disorders (refer to Chapter 13)
    - Seborrhea
    - Sebaceous adenitis

- Parasitic infestation
  - *Otodectes cynotis*
  - *Demodex canis*, in dogs
  - *Demodex cati*, in cats

32.4.1 *Otodectes cynotis*

O. cynotis is the ear mite [2, 7, 9, 19, 28, 47]. Although ear mites are not species-specific, they more frequently cause otitis externa in the cat [7–9, 48–52].

The preferred habitat for ear mites is the external ear canal, where they cause local irritation and inflammation [53]. As infestation progresses, affected patients accumulate aural debris [53]. Classically, this debris has been described as resembling "coffee grounds," that is, it is dark brown-to-black and gritty [53]. It is a combination of cerumen, dried blood, and mite feces [53].

However, as was previously discussed, gross appearance of aural discharge is not always reliable [7, 18–23]. As infestations with ear mites persist, patients may develop secondary bacterial or fungal otitis [9]. This results in a change in debris. Debris becomes less like "coffee grounds" and more purulent or ceruminous [9].

In addition to developing aural debris, patients with ear mite infestations may develop intense pruritus as a hypersensitivity reaction to mite antigen [2, 7, 53].

Ear mites are best seen via light microscopy using a mineral oil preparation for the slide [2, 7]. Low magnification using a 4× objective may reveal adult, eight-legged mites; six-legged larva; and eggs [7]. Identification of one or more of these stages is diagnostic for infestation with *O. cynotis* [7] (see Figure 32.16).

32.4.2 *Demodex* spp.

D. canis and *D. cati* have also been implicated as causes of ceruminous otitis externa [7, 9, 54].

Review Chapter 3, Section 3.8.1, Chapter 5, Section 5.1, and Chapter 6, Section 6.6 concerning demodicosis.

Recall that demodicosis may result in localized or generalized skin disease [55–60]. Because *Demodex* spp. are follicular mites, they may affect any hair follicles throughout the body, including those adjacent to or within the external ear canal [7].

If *Demodex* spp. are identified on otic preparations, then the patient should undergo a full dermatologic examination with skin scrapings to rule out systemic disease [7].

Common skin lesions in patients with demodicosis include erythema, hypotrichosis or alopecic patches with or without a papulopustular rash, folliculitis, or furunculosis, scaling, and follicular casts, pododermatitis, and/or paronychia [61–63]. The face and forelimbs are often involved.

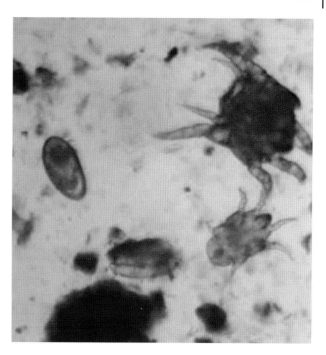

Figure 32.16 *Otodectes cynotis* adult mites, larva, and eggs as seen through light microscopy.

Refer to Chapter 3, Figures 3.12a–d and Chapter 5, Figures 5.21a–c for examples of clinical presentations.

Recall that deep skin scrapings are required to unearth the cigar-shaped *D. canis* and *D. cati* from hair follicles (see Figure 32.17).

This is in stark contrast to *Demodex gatoi,* which is a surface dweller.

32.5 Aural Polyps

The most common external ear canal mass in the cat is a nasopharyngeal polyp [3].

Recall from Chapter 18, Section 18.3.2.4 that nasopharyngeal polyps are benign, yet persistent masses that develop from the mucosa of the nasopharynx, auditory tube, or eardrum [3, 8]. They tend to occur in young cats and may be associated with noninfectious upper airway disease [2, 3, 8, 64–67]. Clinical signs include nasal discharge, sneezing, and stertor [2, 3].

If the external ear is involved, polyps may cause otitis, head shaking, and pruritus [3, 8]. This is evident on otoscopic examination, whether or not the polyp can be visualized in the external ear canal of the awake patient [3]. A more thorough examination under anesthesia will facilitate discovery of the polyp and/or advanced imaging studies to track the extent of the mass through the middle ear [3, 8].

Secondary bacterial or fungal infection is common when the external ear canal is involved [3, 9]. This is

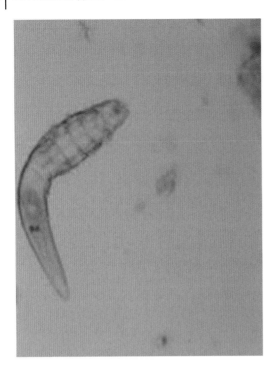

Figure 32.17 *Demodex canis* as seen through light microscopy.

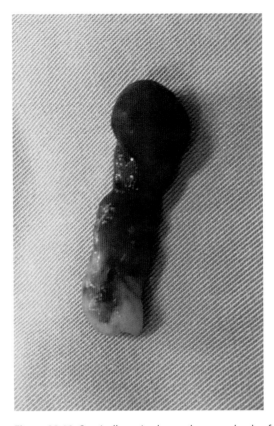

Figure 32.18 Surgically excised nasopharyngeal polyp from a nine-month-old cat. *Source:* Courtesy of Rodolfo O. Leal, DVM, PhD, Dipl. ECVIM-CA (Internal Medicine).

because the polyp is obstructive tissue that prevents drainage of exudate within the external ear [9].

Polyps are variable in terms of appearance. They may be fixed or mobile, smooth or nodular [3]. Polyps also frequently have a stalk-like attachment to underlying tissue [3] (see Figure 32.18).

This stalk facilitates their surgical removal; however, it may predispose them to recurrence if the stalk is not fully removed [3].

32.6 Parasites that Affect the Pinnae

Whereas *O. cynotis*, *D. canis*, and *D. cati* may contribute to otitis externa, skin parasites such as *Sarcoptes scabiei* and *Notoedres cati* are more likely to cause skin lesions associated with the pinnae [7].

Review Chapter 3, Figure 3.15, Chapter 5, Section 5.1, and Chapter 6, Section 6.6 and Figure 6.30, for more information on both mange mites. Recall that sarcoptic mange is more common in the dog, as compared to notoedric mange, which is more common in the cat.

Dogs infested with *S. scabiei* tend to present with lesions on the bridge of the nose, feet, claws, and tail [68–70].

N. cati causes facial crusts and scale, as well as paronychia [53, 71].

Both *Sarcoptes* and *Notoedres* cause pinnal lesions [53, 68–71]. These tend to take the form of crusts along the pinnal edge or margin.

Superficial skin scrapes confirm the diagnosis of both mange mites, although yield of mites is low, and false negatives are common [70, 72].

Humans in direct contact with the infested dog or cat may also develop mange because, unlike *Demodex* spp. and *O. cynotis*, both *Sarcoptes* and *Notoedres* mites are zoonotic [71, 73].

Historically, the pinnal-pedal reflex has also been used to diagnose canine scabies [74, 75]. One at a time, the suspect's ear flap is vigorously rubbed for 5 s. A response is considered positive if the patient initiates scratching at the ear with the ipsilateral hind leg.

Recently, the value of this test has been examined. As reported by Mueller et al., 82% of dogs with scabies demonstrate a positive pinnal-pedal reflex [74, 75]. This percentage climbs to 90 in dogs with both pinnal dermatitis and sarcoptic mange. However, dogs without scabies may also demonstrate a positive pinnal-pedal reflex [75].

According to Mueller, the specificity of testing for scabies by the pinnal-pedal scratch reflex is 93.8%, compared to a sensitivity of 81.8% [75]. The test's positive predictive value is 0.57, as compared to its negative predictive value of 0.98 [75].

In other words, the pinnal-pedal reflex is an important, but imperfect diagnostic tool.

32.7 Tumors that Affect the Pinnae

Pinnal neoplasia is uncommon in companion animal practice [8]. When it occurs, the diagnosis is most often squamous cell carcinoma (SCC). White-coated cats are more likely to develop SCC of the pinnae [3, 76]. In fact, their risk is estimated to be 13.4 times greater than cats with pigmented coats [76]. It is thought to be due to chronic overexposure of the skin to ultraviolet radiation [76].

Other common sites for SCC include the nasal planum, peri-auricular skin, and eyelids [3, 76].

SCC of one or both pinnae typically presents as crusts or erosions at or around the ears. The appearance of SCC varies; however, the pinnae may become flaky, scaly, or erythematous.

SCC of the pinnae is aggressive locally; however, local lymph nodes and the lungs seem to be spared [3, 77, 78].

Lesions are painful, erosive, and cosmetically challenging [3]. Pinnectomy or cryosurgery, for smaller lesions, is the common means by which to manage pinnal SCC [3].

Radiation therapy is yet another promising modality; however, its use up to now has been primarily to manage lesions on the nasal planum as opposed to the pinnae [3, 78, 79].

References

1 Singh, B. and Dyce, K.M. (2018). *Dyce, Sack, and Wensing's Textbook of Veterinary Anatomy*, 5e. St. Louis, Missouri: Saunders.

2 Englar, R.E. (2017). *Performing the Small Animal Physical Examination*. Hoboken, NJ: Wiley.

3 Lanz, O.I. and Wood, B.C. (2004). Surgery of the ear and pinna. *Vet. Clin. North Am. Small Anim. Pract.* 34 (2): 567–599, viii.

4 Griffin, C.E. (2006). Otitis techniques to improve practice. *Clin. Tech. Small Anim. Pract.* 21 (3): 96–105.

5 Venker-van Haagen, A.J. (2009). Ears. In: *Medical History and Physical Examination in Companion Animals* (ed. A. Rijnberk and F.J. van Sluijs), 202–206. Saunders Elsevier.

6 Alley Cat Allies. (2017). Feral Cat Protocol: Eartipping. https://www.alleycat.org/resources/feral-cat-protocol-eartipping.

7 Angus, J.C. (2004). Otic cytology in health and disease. *Vet. Clin. North Am. Small Anim. Pract.* 34 (2): 411–424.

8 Kennis, R.A. (2013). Feline otitis: diagnosis and treatment. *Vet. Clin. North Am. Small Anim. Pract.* 43 (1): 51–56.

9 Rosser, E.J. Jr. (2004). Causes of otitis externa. *Vet. Clin. North Am. Small Anim. Pract.* 34 (2): 459–468.

10 Evans, H.E. and Miller, M.E. (2013). *Miller's Anatomy of the Dog*, 4e, xix, 850 p. St. Louis, Missouri: Elsevier.

11 MacPhail, C. (2016). Current treatment options for auricular hematomas. *Vet. Clin. North Am. Small Anim. Pract.* 46 (4): 635–641.

12 Swaim, S.F. and Bradley, D.M. (1996). Evaluation of closed-suction drainage for treating auricular hematomas. *J. Am. Anim. Hosp. Assoc.* 32 (1): 36–43.

13 Romatowski, J. (1994). Nonsurgical treatment of aural hematomas. *J. Am. Vet. Med. Assoc.* 204 (9): 1318.

14 Wilson, J.W. (1983). Treatment of auricular hematoma, using a teat tube. *J. Am. Vet. Med. Assoc.* 182 (10): 1081–1083.

15 Kagan, K.G. (1983). Treatment of canine aural hematoma with an indwelling drain. *J. Am. Vet. Med. Assoc.* 183 (9): 972–974.

16 Pavletic, M.M. (2015). Use of laterally placed vacuum drains for management of aural hematomas in five dogs. *J. Am. Vet. Med. Assoc.* 246 (1): 112–117.

17 Kowalski, J.J. (1988). The microbial environment of the ear canal in health and disease. *Vet. Clin. North Am. Small Anim. Pract.* 18 (4): 743–754.

18 Harvey, R.G., Harari, J., and Delauche, A.J. (eds.) (2001). Diagnostic procedures. In: *Ear Diseases of the Dog and Cat*, 43–80. Ames, IA: Iowa State University Press.

19 Scott, D.W., Miller, W.H., and Griffin, C.E. (eds.) (2000). Diseases of eyelids, claws, anal sacs, and ears. In: *Muller and Kirk's Small Animal Dermatology*, 1185–1235. Philadelphia: WB Saunders.

20 Jacobson, L.S. (2002). Diagnosis and medical treatment of otitis externa in the dog and cat. *J. S. Afr. Vet. Assoc.* 73 (4): 162–170.

21 Little, C. (1996). A clinician's approach to the investigation of otitis externa. *In Pract.* 18: 9–16.

22 Morris, D.O. (1999). Malassezia dermatitis and otitis. *Vet. Clin. North Am. Small Anim. Pract.* 29 (6): 1303–1310.

23 Rosychuk, R.A. (1994). Management of otitis externa. *Vet. Clin. North Am. Small Anim. Pract.* 24 (5): 921–952.

24 Little, C. (1996). Medical treatment of otitis externa in the dog and cat. *In Pract.* 18: 66–71.

25 Rosser, E.J. Jr. (1988). Evaluation of the patient with otitis externa. *Vet. Clin. North Am. Small Anim. Pract.* 18 (4): 765–772.

26 Gotthelf, L.N. (2004). Diagnosis and treatment of otitis media in dogs and cats. *Vet. Clin. North Am. Small Anim. Pract.* 34 (2): 469–487.

27 Thomas, J.S. (2004). Otitis externa. *NAVC Clinician's Brief* (July): 33–35.

28 Chickering, W.R. (1988). Cytologic evaluation of otic exudates. *Vet. Clin. North Am. Small Anim. Pract.* 18 (4): 773–782.

29 Cole, L.K., Kwochka, K.W., Kowalski, J.J., and Hillier, A. (1998). Microbial flora and antimicrobial susceptibility patterns of isolated pathogens from the horizontal ear canal and middle ear in dogs with otitis media. *J. Am. Vet. Med. Assoc.* 212 (4): 534–538.

30 Cole, L.K. and Schwassmann, M. (2002). Antibiotic use in chronic otitis externa. In: *Advances in Veterinary Dermatology* (ed. K.L. Thoday, C.S. Foil and R. Bond), 212–223. Oxford: Blackwell Science.

31 Harvey, R.G., Harari, J., and Delauche, A.J. (2001). The normal ear. In: *Ear Diseases of the Dog and cat*, 9–42. Ames, IA: Iowa State University Press.

32 Guillot, J. and Bond, R. (1999). *Malassezia pachydermatis*: a review. *Med. Mycol.* 37 (5): 295–306.

33 Scott, D.W., Miller, W.H., and Griffin, C.E. (2000). Fungal skin diseases. In: *Muller and Kirk's Small Animal Dermatology*, 336–422. Philadelphia: WB Saunders.

34 Blue, J.L. and Wooley, R.E. (1977). Antibacterial sensitivity patterns of bacteria isolated from dogs with otitis externa. *J. Am. Vet. Med. Assoc.* 171 (4): 362–363.

35 Graham-Mize, C.A. and Rosser, E.J. Jr. (2004). Comparison of microbial isolates and susceptibility patterns from the external ear canal of dogs with otitis externa. *J. Am. Anim. Hosp. Assoc.* 40 (2): 102–108.

36 Moriello, K.A. (2014). Tris-EDA & otitis in dogs. *NAVC Clinician's Brief* (March): 56.

37 Paterson, S. (2010). Pseudomonas otitis. *NAVC Clinician's Brief* (June): 35–39.

38 Bond, R., Saijonmaa-Koulumies, L.E., and Lloyd, D.H. (1995). Population sizes and frequency of *Malassezia pachydermatis* at skin and mucosal sites on healthy dogs. *J. Small Anim. Pract.* 36 (4): 147–150.

39 Crespo, M.J., Abarca, M.L., and Cabanes, F.J. (2002). Occurrence of Malassezia spp. in the external ear canals of dogs and cats with and without otitis externa. *Med. Mycol.* 40 (2): 115–121.

40 Greene, C.E. (ed.) (2006). Otitis externa. In: *Infectious Diseases of the Dog and Cat*, 815–823. Philadelphia: WB Saunders.

41 Ginel, P.J., Lucena, R., Rodriguez, J.C., and Ortega, J. (2002). A semiquantitative cytological evaluation of normal and pathological samples from the external ear canal of dogs and cats. *Vet. Dermatol.* 13 (3): 151–156.

42 Hariharan, H., Coles, M., Poole, D. et al. (2006). Update on antimicrobial susceptibilities of bacterial isolates from canine and feline otitis externa. *Can. Vet. J.* 47 (3): 253–255.

43 Chester, D.K. (1988). Medical management of otitis externa. *Vet. Clin. North Am. Small Anim. Pract.* 18 (4): 799–812.

44 Griffin, C.E. (2000). Pseudomonas otitis therapy. In: *Kirk's Current Veterinary Therapy XIII* (ed. J.D. Bonagura), 586–588. Philadelphia: WB Saunders.

45 Paterson, S. (2010). Chronic otitis externa. *NAVC Clinician's Brief* (January): 65–67.

46 Paterson, S. (2016). Topical ear treatment- options, indications, and limitations of current therapy. *J. Small Anim. Pract.* 57: 668–678.

47 August, J.R. (1988). Otitis externa. A disease of multifactorial etiology. *Vet. Clin. North Am. Small Anim. Pract.* 18 (4): 731–742.

48 Becskei, C., Reinemeyer, C., King, V.L. et al. (2017). Efficacy of a new spot-on formulation of selamectin plus sarolaner in the treatment of Otodectes cynotis in cats. *Vet. Parasitol.* 238 (Suppl 1): S27–S30.

49 Perego, R., Proverbio, D., De Giorgi, G.B. et al. (2014). Prevalence of otitis externa in stray cats in northern Italy. *J. Feline Med. Surg.* 16 (6): 483–490.

50 Nardoni, S., Ebani, V.V., Fratini, F. et al. (2014). Malassezia, mites and bacteria in the external ear canal of dogs and cats with otitis Externa. *Slov. Vet. Res.* 51 (3): 113–118.

51 Taenzler, J., de Vos, C., Roepke, R.K. et al. (2017). Efficacy of fluralaner against Otodectes cynotis infestations in dogs and cats. *Parasit. Vectors* 10 (1): 30.

52 Roy, J., Bedard, C., and Moreau, M. (2011). Treatment of feline otitis externa due to Otodectes cynotis and complicated by secondary bacterial and fungal infections with Oridermyl auricular ointment. *Can. Vet. J.* 52 (3): 277–282.

53 Arther, R.G. (2009). Mites and lice: biology and control. *Vet. Clin. North Am. Small Anim. Pract.* 39 (6): 1159–1171, vii.

54 Van Poucke, S. (2001). Ceruminous otitis externa due to *Demodex cati* in a cat. *Vet. Rec.* 149 (21): 651–652.

55 Taffin, E.R., Casaert, S., Claerebout, E. et al. (2016). Morphological variability of *Demodex cati* in a feline immunodeficiency virus-positive cat. *J. Am. Vet. Med. Assoc.* 249 (11): 1308–1312.

56 Neel, J.A., Tarigo, J., Tater, K.C., and Grindem, C.B. (2007). Deep and superficial skin scrapings from a feline immunodeficiency virus-positive cat. *Vet. Clin. Pathol.* 36 (1): 101–104.

57 Frank, L.A., Kania, S.A., Chung, K., and Brahmbhatt, R. (2013). A molecular technique for the detection and

differentiation of Demodex mites on cats. *Vet. Dermatol.* 24 (3): 367–369, e82–3.

58 Cordero, A.M., Sheinberg-Waisburd, G., Romero Nunez, C., and Heredia, R. (2018). Early onset canine generalized demodicosis. *Vet. Dermatol.* 29 (2): 173.

59 Bowden, D.G., Outerbridge, C.A., Kissel, M.B. et al. (2017). Canine demodicosis: a retrospective study of a veterinary hospital population in California, USA (2000–2016). *Vet. Dermatol.*

60 Mueller, R.S. (2012). An update on the therapy of canine demodicosis. *Compend. Contin. Educ. Vet.* 34 (4): E1–E4.

61 Mueller, R.S., Bensignor, E., Ferrer, L. et al. (2012). Treatment of demodicosis in dogs: 2011 clinical practice guidelines. *Vet. Dermatol.* 23 (2): 86–96, e20–1.

62 Rouben, C. (2016). Claw and claw bed diseases. *Clinician's Brief* (April): 35–40.

63 Manning, T.O. (1983). Cutaneous diseases of the paw. *Clin. Dermatol.* 1 (1): 131–142.

64 Quimby, J. and Lappin, M.R. (2012). The upper respiratory tract. In: *The Cat: Clinical Medicine and Management* (ed. S.E. Little), 846–861. St. Louis: Saunders Elsevier.

65 Henderson, S.M., Bradley, K., Day, M.J. et al. (2004). Investigation of nasal disease in the cat--a retrospective study of 77 cases. *J. Feline Med. Surg.* 6 (4): 245–257.

66 Schmidt, J.F. and Kapatkin, A. (1990). Nasopharyngeal and ear canal polyps in the cat. *Feline Pract.* 18 (4): 16–19.

67 Kapatkin, A.S., Matthiesen, D.T., Noone, K.E. et al. (1990). Results of surgery and long-term follow-up in 31 cats with nasopharyngeal polyps. *J. Am. Anim. Hosp. Assoc.* 26 (4): 387–392.

68 Huang, H.P. and Lien, Y.H. (2013). Feline sarcoptic mange in Taiwan: a case series of five cats. *Vet. Dermatol.* 24 (4): 457–459, e104–5.

69 Malik, R., Stewart, K.M., Sousa, C.A. et al. (2006). Crusted scabies (sarcoptic mange) in four cats due to *Sarcoptes scabiei* infestation. *J. Feline. Med. Surg.* 8 (5): 327–339.

70 Hawkins, J.A., McDonald, R.K., and Woody, B.J. (1987). *Sarcoptes scabiei* infestation in a cat. *J. Am. Vet. Med. Assoc.* 190 (12): 1572–1573.

71 Sivajothi, S., Sudhakara Reddy, B., Rayulu, V.C., and Sreedevi, C. (2015). *Notoedres cati* in cats and its management. *J. Parasit. Dis.* 39 (2): 303–305.

72 Pin, D., Bensignor, E., Carlotti, D.N., and Cadiergues, M.C. (2006). Localised sarcoptic mange in dogs: a retrospective study of 10 cases. *J. Small Anim. Pract.* 47 (10): 611–614.

73 Aydingoz, I.E. and Mansur, A.T. (2011). Canine scabies in humans: a case report and review of the literature. *Dermatology* 223 (2): 104–106.

74 Rees C. (2008). Differential diagnoses for the itchy and scratchy. DVM 360 [Internet]. http://veterinarycalendar.dvm360.com/differential-diagnoses-itchy-and-scratchy-proceedings.

75 Mueller, R.S., Bettenay, S.V., and Shipstone, M. (2001). Value of the pinnal-pedal reflex in the diagnosis of canine scabies. *Vet. Rec.* 148 (20): 621–623.

76 Dorn, C. (1976). Epidemiology of canine and feline tumors. *J. Am. Anim. Hosp. Assoc.* 12: 307–312.

77 Hargis, A.M. (1981). A review of solar induced lesions in domestic animals. *Compend. Contin. Educ. Pract. Vet.* 3: 287–294.

78 Lana, S.E., Ogilvie, G.K., Withrow, S.J. et al. (1997). Feline cutaneous squamous cell carcinoma of the nasal planum and the pinnae: 61 cases. *J. Am. Anim. Hosp. Assoc.* 33 (4): 329–332.

79 Ruslander, D., Kaser-Hotz, B., and Sardinas, J.C. (1997). Cutaneous squamous cell carcinoma in cats. *Compend. Contin. Educ. Pract. Vet.* 19 (10): 1119–1129.

Part Four

The Respiratory System

33

Nasal Discharge

33.1 Introduction to the Upper Airway

The airway of the companion animal patient consists of the upper and lower respiratory tracts. The emphasis of this chapter is on one clinical presentation that is specific to the upper airway.

The upper respiratory tract can be thought of as all airway parts that are, in their entirety, positioned outside of the thoracic cavity. These include the following [1–7]:

- The nares, or nostrils
- The nasal alae, or wings of rounded tissue on either side of the nostrils
- The nasal planum, or flattened, front surface of the nose
- Paired nasal cavities, divided by the nasal septum
  - Vascularized conchae, or scroll-shaped, bony turbinates
    - o Dorsal conchae
    - o Middle conchae
    - o Ventral conchae
  - Nasal passages
    - o Dorsal nasal meatus
    - o Medial nasal meatus
    - o Ventral nasal meatus
  - Associated sinuses
    - o Frontal sinus
    - o Maxillary sinus
- Pharynx
- Larynx

As the external opening of the upper airway, the nose is the first visible respiratory structure to be observed on physical examination [2].

Although the external nose is anchored in bone, its cranial aspect is cartilaginous [1]. This allows the nose to be somewhat pliable as a structure.

In health, the nasal planum has a characteristic cobblestone appearance [1, 2] (see Figures 33.1a, b).

The nares should be open and symmetrical, to allow for maximal air flow into the nasal cavities. However, many brachycephalic breeds have stenotic nares as a consequence of their foreshortened facial structure, which causes the nose to be very short [1, 2] (see Figure 33.2).

The nares and nasal cavities contribute to olfaction. However, from the standpoint of respiratory function, their larger responsibility is to be a conduit for air to move from the external environment into the lower airway.

As incoming air moves through the nasal cavities, it passes over the nasal mucosa [5]. The nasal mucosa varies in thickness [5]. It is thickest ventrally, where it is heavily vascularized [5]. The addition of cavernous spaces that can be filled with blood, contributes to this thickness [5]. During times of vascular congestion, air flow is appreciably impeded [5]. This is what causes humans with head colds to feel "stuffy" [5].

Incoming air is modified in several ways as it moves through the nasal passageways [5]. The vascular mucosa warms the air, and vaporized tears and nasal secretions add moisture [5]. The mucus that lines the nasal passageways also removes particulate matter from the air by ciliary action, thereby cleansing it [5]. Particulate matter that has been trapped within mucus is unconsciously pushed toward the pharynx, where it is ultimately swallowed [5].

33.2 Normal Nasal Discharge

In health, the nasal planum is somewhat moist [1, 2].

The normal dog and cat may also have occasional serous discharge from one or both nostrils [1, 2]. Serous discharge is clear and watery [8]. When viewed on cytological preparations, cellular content is scant to none [8].

33.3 Abnormal Nasal Discharge

A common clinical presentation in companion animal practice is abnormal nasal discharge from one or both nares.

Common Clinical Presentations in Dogs and Cats, First Edition. Ryane E. Englar.
© 2019 John Wiley & Sons, Inc. Published 2019 by John Wiley & Sons, Inc.

(a)
(b)

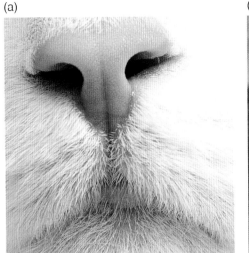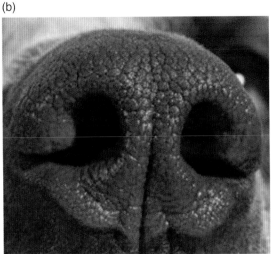

Figure 33.1 (a) Normal cobblestone appearance of the feline nasal planum. (b) Normal cobblestone appearance of the canine nasal planum.

As can be said of ocular discharge, nasal discharge is highly variable and may be described by both the client and in the medical record based upon the following:

- Distribution
  - Unilateral
  - Bilateral
- Onset
  - Acute
  - Chronic
- Gross appearance
  - Color
  - Transparency
- Consistency

- Thin and watery
- Thick and gelatinous
- Progression

33.3.1 Serous Nasal Discharge

Although small amounts of serous nasal discharge can be normal, larger amounts and/or its persistence may be indicative of the following [8]:

- Brewing viral infection
- Early inflammation within the nasal cavity

Copious serous discharge should be investigated further, particularly if it is persistent (see Figure 33.3).

Allergic rhinitis is an example of a condition that causes serous nasal discharge.

Figure 33.2 Stenotic nares in a brachycephalic dog. *Source:* Courtesy of Rodolfo Oliveira Leal, DVM (Portugal), PhD, Dipl. ECVIM-CA (Internal Medicine).

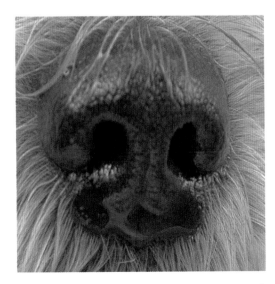

Figure 33.3 Serous nasal discharge in a dog. *Source:* Courtesy of the Media Resources Department at Midwestern University.

33.3.2 Other Types of Abnormal Nasal Discharge

The following types of abnormal nasal discharge have been described in dogs and cats [1, 2, 9]:

- Mucoid
- Mucopurulent
- Purulent
- Serohemorrhagic
- Hemorrhagic (see Figures 33.4a–g)

Nasal discharge that is mucoid is white-to-yellow in color [8]. It has the consistency of mucus, that is, it is slimy. It tends to be associated with chronic inflammation [8]. Like serous nasal discharge, mucoid nasal discharge has minimal cellular content [8].

On the other hand, nasal discharge that is purulent has high cellular content [8]. If cytology were performed, samples would demonstrate large populations of degenerate neutrophils and bacteria [8]. Intracellular bacteria support a diagnosis of infectious disease. In

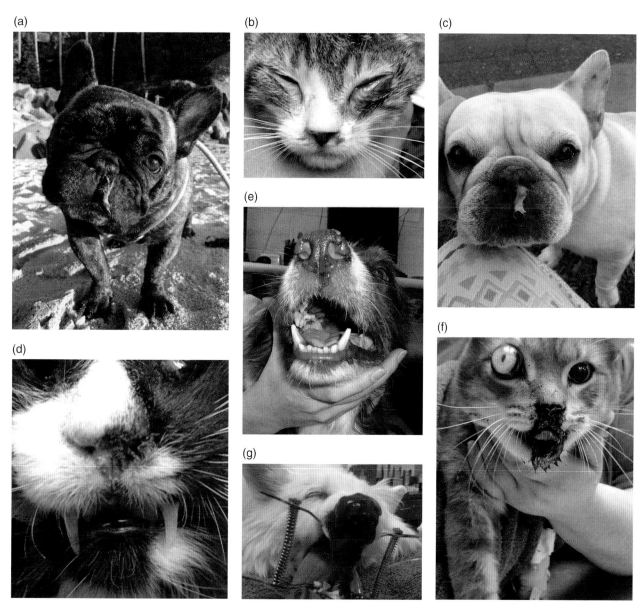

Figure 33.4 (a) Unilateral mucoid nasal discharge in a French bulldog. *Source:* Courtesy of Heather Hanna. (b) Mucopurulent nasal discharge in a kitten with an upper respiratory infection (URI). *Source:* Courtesy of Frank Isom, DVM. (c) Unilateral mucopurulent nasal discharge in a French bulldog. *Source:* Courtesy of Heather Hanna. (d) Dried purulent discharge in a cat. *Source:* Courtesy of Samantha Thurman. (e) Serohemorrhagic nasal discharge in a canine patient with nasal aspergillosis. *Source:* Courtesy of Daniel Foy, MS, DVM, DACVIM, DACVECC. (f) Hemorrhagic nasal discharge and extensive ocular and oral trauma in a feline patient that survived being hit by a car. *Source:* Courtesy of Kelli L. Crisfulli, RVT. (g) Hemorrhagic nasal discharge in a canine patient. *Source:* Courtesy of Dr. Elizabeth Robbins.

particular, purulent nasal discharge is consistent with bacterial upper respiratory infections (URIs) [8].

When patients have hemorrhagic or sanguinous nasal discharge, they are said to present for epistaxis, that is, a nosebleed [1, 2]. Hemorrhagic nasal discharge implies the presence of erythrocytes on cytology [8]. Erythrocytes are indicative that the vasculature has been compromised, meaning that vessel wall integrity is damaged [8].

Epistaxis may result from local disease, that is, disease concentrated within the upper airway [8]:

- Trauma
- Fungal infections
- Neoplasia

Epistaxis may also result from systemic disease, including the following [8–10]:

- Coagulopathies
- Thrombocytopenia
- Vasculitis
- Hypertension

Several systemic infectious diseases have been linked to epistaxis in dogs, including the following [11–14]:

- Bartonellosis
- Ehrlichiosis
- Leishmaniasis

Refer to Chapter 16, Section 16.2.2 for additional details regarding bleeding disorders.

33.4 The Role of Signalment and History in Evaluating Nasal Discharge

The patient's signalment is invaluable to the clinician when s/he prioritizes the list of differential diagnoses for nasal discharge [7].

The signalment is a descriptive statement for each patient that characterizes the patient's age, sex, sexual status, breed, and species. The following are examples of patient signalment as might be relayed orally, during clinic case rounds, or in writing, in the medical record:

- "Lowell is a seven-year-old, intact male, Fox terrier dog."
- "Juniper is a six-year-old spayed female, Himalayan cat."
- "Eric is a five-year-old castrated male, Bloodhound dog."
- "Bella is a four-year-old, intact female, Persian cat."

In general, younger patients are more likely to develop nasal discharge because of the following [8, 15]:

- Congenital disease, such as cleft palates
- Foreign bodies
- Infectious disease, such as feline herpesvirus-1 (FHV-1) or aspergillosis

By contrast, older patients are more likely to develop neoplastic nasal cavity disease. This is particularly true of dolichocephalic breeds, like Collies, or mesocephalic breeds, such as Golden Retrievers [8, 9, 16].

Breed is often a contributing factor when it comes to disease and risk assessment. Brachycephalic breeds, for example, are rarely diagnosed with nasal neoplasia [8]. German Shepherd Dogs, on the other hand, are more often diagnosed with nasal aspergillosis [8].

Being able to recognize patterns is important because more often than not, the clinician acts as a detective. Rarely is it possible in clinical practice to work-up every case for every potential differential the first time that the patient presents. Therefore, it is critical for the clinician to use sound judgment and critical thinking skills to prioritize which conditions are most likely and need to be evaluated first.

Likewise, a comprehensive history is an indispensable diagnostic tool [7, 9]. As technology in healthcare evolves, it is tempting to trade a comprehensive health history for diagnostic tests and test results. However, there is diagnostic value to every patient history [17]. In fact, roughly two-thirds of diagnoses can be made in human healthcare based upon patient history alone [18].

The following aspects of patient history are most critical to the clinical approach to nasal discharge [8, 9]:

- Acquisition of patient
  - Adopted from shelter, rescue, or other household?
  - Purchased from breeder or cattery?
- Onset
  - Acute versus chronic?
  - When did clinical signs develop?
    ○ After playing fetch with a stick
    ○ After undergoing dental extractions
  - Have clinical signs progressed?
- Laterality?
  - Is only one nostril or nasal passageway involved?
  - Are both nostrils or nasal passageways involved?
- Are other tissues or organs involved?
  - Is there concurrent ocular discharge?
  - Is there ulceration of the nasal planum?
  - Is the nasal planum or bridge of the nose deformed?
  - Is there bruising or bleeding in any other region of the body?
- Past pertinent history
  - Is this a new problem?
  - Is this a recurrent problem?
    ○ If so, is the problem seasonal?

– Does the patient have a history of rickettsial disease, including, but not limited to *Ehrlichia canis* or *Rickettsia rickettsia*?
– Does this patient have a recent history of trauma?
– Does this patient have a history of ingesting rodenticide?
– Does this patient have a history of immune-mediated disease?
- Lifestyle
  – Indoor
  – Outdoor
  – Indoor-outdoor
  – Is the patient housed in a rural, suburban, or urban environment?
  – Has the patient recently been to a groomer?
  – Has the patient recently been kenneled?
  – Has the patient recently experienced stress?
- Exposure to conspecifics, particularly those that are unvaccinated
- Exposure to other species, particularly those that are unvaccinated
- Travel history
  – In which state or region of the country does the patient typically reside?
  – Does the patient routinely visit other states or regions of the country?
  – Does the patient travel outside of the country?
- Vaccination history

33.5 Infectious Disease as a Cause of Nasal Discharge

Infectious disease is a common cause of nasal discharge in companion animal practice [19]. Examples include the following [8, 20–34]:

- Bacterial infectious disease
  – *Actinomyces* spp.
  – *Bordetella bronchiseptica* (refer to Chapter 27, Section 27.3.5 for feline conjunctivitis)
  – *Chlamydophila felis*, the causative agent of chlamydiosis (refer to Chapter 27, Section 27.3.2 for feline conjunctivitis)
    ○ *Mycoplasma felis*
    ○ *Mycoplasma gatae*
- Mycotic disease
  – *Aspergillus* spp. (refer to Chapter 9, Section 9.5.2 for skin depigmentation)
  – Coccidioidomycosis, so-called Valley Fever
  – *Cryptococcus neoformans*
  – *Cryptococcus gattii*
- Viral infectious disease
  – Canine infectious respiratory disease (CIRD) (refer to Section 33.5.1, below)

– Feline calicivirus (refer to Chapter 27, Section 27.3.4)
– FHV-1 (refer to Chapter 27, Section 27.3.1)
- Parasitic infectious disease
  – *Capillaria aerophila*
  – *Cuterebra* spp. (refer to Chapter 6, Section 6.3 for ectoparasite review)

An in-depth analysis of each of the above is beyond the scope of this chapter. Only the most common agents will be discussed in brief. For more information on those not highlighted here, please consult an infectious disease text.

33.5.1 Canine Infectious Respiratory Disease

CIRD is a complex syndrome that causes outbreaks of respiratory disease in canine populations [35–38].
CIRD includes the following pathogens [38]:
- Bacterial
  – *B. bronchiseptica*
  – *Mycoplasma* spp.
  – *Streptococcus equi*, subspecies *zooepidemicus*
- Viral
  – Canine adenovirus-2 (CAV-2)
  – Canine distemper virus (CDV)
  – Canine herpesvirus
  – Canine influenza (H3N8)
  – Canine parainfluenza
  – Canine respiratory coronavirus

The following characteristics or qualities increase patients' susceptibility to disease [36, 38–41]:

- Young
- Stressed
- Immune-compromised
- In close contact with conspecifics
- Housed in crowded conditions, such as pet shops, shelters, or kennel environments

Clinical signs include nasal discharge [36, 42]. In addition, patients may develop lethargy and reduced appetite [36, 42]. It has been suggested that post-nasal drips are irritating to the oropharynx and that a sore throat may be responsible for reluctance to swallow food.

Mortality tends to be low in cases involving CIRD, particularly among those receiving veterinary medical care [38]. However, CIRD can be serious. Patients may succumb to respiratory distress [42]. If untreated, CIRD can result in pneumonia and, potentially, death [38].

CIRD is highly contagious [36]. The incubation period depends upon the causative agent; however, most agents involve a period of 2–14 days, with active shedding for about the same amount of time post-infection [36, 43, 44].

Prevalence of causative agents varies depending upon which population is evaluated. For example, prevalence of H3N8 among shelter dogs that outwardly appear to have respiratory disease may reach 50%, whereas prevalence in dogs without signs of respiratory disease is typically 0.5–3% [38, 40, 45, 46].

Patients are often treated supportively and symptomatically with the presumptive diagnosis of CIRD. This presumption is based upon clinical signs and history, particularly if the history reveals the patient to have been at increased risk of exposure [38].

Swabs taken from the nose, mouth, or oropharynx are poor samples for submission for aerobic culture, given that resident bacteria will grow [38]. This makes it nearly impossible to differentiate the causative agent(s) from normal flora [38].

Because this syndrome is associated more with tracheobronchitis, or "kennel cough," it will be explored in greater depth in Chapter 35 [35, 36, 38].

A definitive diagnosis is more easily made in cases involving tracheobronchitis, in that appropriate samples of airway secretions can be collected from transtracheal wash, endotracheal wash, or bronchoalveolar lavage [38].

33.5.2   Nasal Aspergillosis

Sinorhinitis in dogs is often caused by *Aspergillus fumigatus*, the causative agent of aspergillosis [47–49].

Dogs with sinonasal aspergillosis tend to have chronic nasal discharge that is mucoid, mucopurulent, or hemorrhagic [50–52]. In addition, they tend to develop crusting of the external nares [49]. These lesions frequently become ulcerative [49]. Affected patients resent palpation of the face and associated structures [49]. Patients may also develop depigmentation of the nose, particularly the nasal planum or the alar folds [49–52]. Refer to Chapter 9, Figures 9.15a–c.

Dogs become infected via inhalation of spores, which are ubiquitous in the environment [50, 53–58]. Nasal trauma may also facilitate infection by allowing spores easier access to the nasal passageways [49]. The same could be said of destructive neoplastic disease [49].

Sinonasal aspergillosis is in and of itself destructive. Nasal turbinates are destroyed as the disease progresses [50, 59]. This may result in grossly apparent deformation of the face, particularly if the cribriform plate, nasal bones, and orbit are damaged [49, 50, 60, 61].

Long-snouted dogs are overrepresented, particularly German Shepherds and Rottweilers [49]. Most patients are young adults to middle-aged at the time of diagnosis [48].

Cats may also develop sinonasal and sino-orbital aspergillosis as a result of infection with, most notably, *A. fumigatus* and *Aspergillus felis* [62–71].

In stark contrast to the predisposition of dolichocephalic dog breeds, cats may be more susceptible if they are brachycephalic [72–74]. Increased rates of disease have been reported in Himalayans, Persians, and Exotic Shorthairs [72–74]. In a follow-up study by Barrs et al. [62], British Shorthairs and Scottish Shorthairs were overrepresented [62].

Feline sinonasal aspergillosis is also destructive as canine [62]. Lytic changes typically involve the cribriform plate, paranasal bone, and orbital lamina, as evident on advanced imaging [62]. Computed tomography (CT) scans are helpful because they document the extent of disease by way of bone destruction [75]. Rhinoscopy allows for direct observation of fungal granulomas and sample collection [3, 32]. Refer to Chapter 9, Figure 9.16.

33.5.3   Cryptococcosis

Feline cryptococcosis is a systemic fungal infection that takes root when spores from a contaminated environment are inhaled [76].

Environments that favor growth of *Cryptococcus* spp. include soils rich in avian guanos [76]. In particular, pigeon droppings facilitate fungal reproduction [76, 77].

Pigeons are also carriers for *C. neoformans* [76]. They inadvertently carry the organism on their bodies, contributing to the spread of this fungus worldwide [76, 78].

Disruption of the soil, as through logging, also increases the risk for patient development of cryptococcosis among those who reside within a 10 km radius [77].

Once the fungus is within the respiratory tract, it can take on one or more forms [76]. In mammalian hosts, the yeast form tends to predominate [76, 79, 80].

Most cats that are infected by *C. neoformans* or *C. gattii* are asymptomatic [76, 81]. However, clinical disease may occur [76].

When it occurs, clinical disease in the cat concentrates within the upper respiratory tract [76]. The ethmoid bone may allow for spread of disease to the cat's central nervous system, although this is a rare occurrence [76, 82]. Immunocompromised patients are at greater risk for nervous system involvement [82].

Cats with sinonasal cryptococcosis develop chronic nasal discharge [76]. Between patients, the discharge varies in color, transparency, and consistency [76]. It may be serous, mucoid, mucopurulent, or bloody [76].

In addition, affected patients frequently develop a so-called Roman nose due to swelling along the bridge of the nose [76]. Lesions may develop in this region of nasofacial swelling [76]. These lesions tend to ulcerate and drain [76]. Patients may be in pain on account of these lesions. They may also develop dyspnea because of airway occlusion secondary to progressive facial deformity [76, 83].

Direct inoculation of spores into wounds can also occur [76]. This causes a cutaneous form of disease [76].

Cat-to-cat transmission does not occur [76].

Cats are affected by disease five or six times more so than their canine counterparts [76, 84].

When dogs are affected, they tend to have multi-organ involvement [85]. Nervous system signs are particularly prominent in canine patients and may include the following [85]:

- Ataxia
- Seizures
- Paralysis
- Hyperesthesia

Based upon a limited number of case reports, there are apparent breed predispositions [86]. Among cats, Siamese, Birmans, and Ragdolls appear more often in the literature, whereas Doberman Pinschers, Great Danes, German Shepherds, and Cocker Spaniels are overrepresented among dogs [25, 85, 87, 88].

Age and activity are additional risk factors: younger, more active dogs and cats are more likely to develop disease [85].

Definitive diagnosis is via cytology or culture [85]. Tissue and nasal swabs are appropriate samples [85].

33.5.4 Feline Herpesvirus-1

FHV-1 was introduced in Chapter 27, Section 27.3.1 as the most common cause of conjunctivitis, particularly in kittens [89–91]. Conjunctivitis is often paired with an URI [90, 92]. Sneezing and nasal discharge are frequent clinical signs [92–98].

Because FHV-1 persists within the trigeminal ganglion for the life of the host and reactivates during times of stress, recurrent bouts of upper airway disease may occur well into adulthood [34, 90, 92, 99–102].

Some of these affected cats become "chronic snufflers" [20, 21]. These are cats that develop persistent rhinitis or rhinosinusitis despite being otherwise systemically healthy [20]. This can be a source of frustration for veterinary clients because the clinical signs of sneezing and nasal discharge do not abate [20].

33.5.5 Feline Calicivirus

Feline calicivirus was introduced in Chapter 27, Section 27.3.4 as another common cause of feline conjunctivitis [103]. However, much like FHV-1, feline calicivirus may also be associated with systemic illness, including URI [103].

Although feline calicivirus does not exhibit the potential for viral latency that is seen with FHV-1, it can also result in a "chronic snuffler" state [21, 23].

33.6 Inflammatory Disease as a Cause of Nasal Discharge

Inflammatory disease is a common cause of nasal discharge in companion animal practice. Examples include the following [8]:

- Allergic rhinitis
- Lymphoplasmacytic rhinitis (LPR) or chronic inflammatory rhinitis
- Nasopharyngeal polyp (refer to Chapter 18, Section 18.3.2.4 and Chapter 32, Section 32.5)

Rhinitis refers to inflammation of the nasal mucosa.

When rhinitis occurs in dogs and cats, it is not always apparent what has caused it [104].

Allergic rhinitis is documented extensively in human patients [104]. However, it appears in the veterinary medical literature infrequently as a cause of nasal discharge in dogs and cats, with the exception of experimental induction in dogs [104–110].

Typically, rhinitis among companion animal patients is idiopathic and poorly responsive to antihistamines [107, 111]. When such rhinitis is chronic, it is referred to as LPR.

Patients with LPR have persistent nasal discharge [104, 112–115]. Nasal discharge may be clear, purulent, bloody, or a mixture [104, 112–115]. Most often, nasal discharge is mucopurulent, yet free of bacterial growth when cultured [104, 107, 111].

It is thought that the mucopurulence of the nasal discharge is a reflection of chronicity of infection rather than infection [107]. This is supported by the fact that patients with LPR tend not to respond well to long-term antibiotic therapy [104, 107]. Short-term trials of antibiotics may curb overgrowth of normal flora and/or secondary infection; however, the response is transient at best [104].

At the time of presentation, nasal discharge is typically unilateral [107]. However, when advanced imaging studies are performed on affected patients, most have bilateral disease [104].

CT scans also reveal that LPR is a destructive disease, just like neoplasia or aspergillosis [104]. This is surprising because LPR was once thought to be a relatively benign disease [107]. Instead, affected patients are at risk of sustaining significant damage to nasal turbinates [107]. In addition, patients with LPR also often have frontal sinus involvement [107].

Rhinoscopy demonstrates changes consistent with an inflammatory response: hyperemia and edema [107, 111]. In addition, tissue is subjectively more fragile and lined by amorphous debris [107, 113, 116].

Histopathologic examination of nasal mucosa in patients with LPR demonstrates plasma cell and lymphocytic infiltration [107, 111, 117].

Patients with LPR respond poorly to glucocorticoids [104]. It is therefore unlikely to be strictly an immune-mediated disease [104].

More research is needed to establish the cause of LPR as well as therapeutic guidelines that produce positive patient outcomes.

33.7 Neoplasia as a Cause of Nasal Discharge

Neoplasia of the nasal cavity may also cause nasal discharge in companion animal practice. Malignancies of particular concern include the following [8, 23, 85, 118, 119]:

- Adenocarcinomas
  - More common in dogs
- Other carcinomas
  - Squamous cell carcinoma (SCC)
  - Transitional cell carcinoma
  - Undifferentiated carcinoma
- Lymphomas
  - More common in cats
- Sarcomas
  - Chondrosarcoma
  - Fibrosarcoma
  - Osteosarcomas
  - Hemangiosarcomas
- Mast cell tumor
- Melanoma
- Plasma cell tumor

Neoplasia should be suspected in any case of persistent nasal discharge, particularly when there is decreased airflow from one or both nares [9, 120]. Patency of airflow is an easy, inexpensive in-house diagnostic tool [9, 121].

A clean glass slide can be placed in front of each of the nares [121]. Airflow through the nares will result in the glass slide fogging over [121].

Note that nasopharyngeal polyps may also reduce airflow [121].

Alternatively, a tuft of cotton wool can be placed in front of each of the nares [121]. Airflow will move the tuft of cotton through space as it is held before the nares by the tester [121].

The patient's face should also be observed head-on and from the profile view for symmetry, as well as palpated for pain or subtle deformity [9, 121]. If tumors are destructive, they may reshape the nasal passageways as they grow, causing an observable or palpable structural change.

Nasal discharge of neoplastic origin is typically unilateral at first [9]. However, as tumors expand, they may destroy the nasal septum. This causes nasal discharge to progress in terms of laterality [9]. Many nasal tumors ultimately result in bilateral discharge [9].

CT scans of the skull are preferred to magnetic resonance imaging (MRI) because they provide better detail of bony structures [118]. Presumptive nasal tumors are frequently lytic. CT imaging allows for examination of nasal turbinates and the cribriform plate [118]. It is possible to detect if the tumor has invaded the olfactory bulb of the brain via CT scan [118].

Biopsies are performed after imaging rather than before [118]. The process of taking biopsies is likely to cause bleeding. Bleeding will make it difficult to appreciate fine details and tissue architecture on CT scan [118].

The most common nasal tumor in the dog is carcinoma [118]. Of all carcinoma subtypes, adenocarcinoma occurs most frequently among dogs [118].

Sarcomas are the second most common nasal tumor in the dog [118].

Lymphoma is the most common nasal tumor in cats [23, 119, 122]. Most of these are of B-cell origin [119]. The metastatic rate appears to be low [119, 123]. There also does not appear to be a link between feline leukemia virus (FeLV) or feline immunodeficiency virus (FIV) and nasal lymphoma [119, 123].

Nasal carcinomas, sarcomas, and lymphomas are routinely managed via radiation therapy [118, 123]. Radiation therapy aims to target tumor tissue maximally while sparing as much normal tissue as possible [118]. Despite this, the eyes are frequently exposed to radiation due to mass location. This exposure is likely to result in radiation-induced cataracts within 6–12 months post radiation therapy [118].

Surgical debulking is sometimes paired with radiation therapy [120]. Although this may improve airflow, it is unlikely to extend life [120]. Debulking also requires radical amputation of a large percentage, if not all, of the nose [120]. This is likely to raise both aesthetic and quality of life concerns for the veterinary client [120].

The use of non-steroidal anti-inflammatory drugs (NSAIDs) such as piroxicam is controversial in that there is ongoing debate as to whether or not it prolongs survival [120]. NSAIDs have been suggested as an aim of treatment because 80% of canine nasal carcinomas express COX-2, which NSAIDs target [120].

Without treatment, prognosis for dogs with nasal tumors is poor [120, 124, 125]. Median survival time is on average of 88–95 days [120].

Eight to fifteen months is the estimated median survival time for dogs with carcinomas [118]. Unfortunately, radiation therapy does not always reduce or eliminate nasal discharge. In many cases, nasal discharge persists due to the extent of nasal cavity damage [118].

33.8 Cleft Palates and Nasal Discharge

Clefts are splits in tissue. There are two main types of clefts in companion animal practice [126]:

- Clefts of the primary palate
- Clefts of the secondary palate

The primary palate is the first stage of developmental separation between the nasal and oral cavities [126]. It involves migration of maxillary and nasal processes toward midline, to form the nose and upper lip [126].

Clefts of the primary palate that involve the lip only are primarily cosmetic; however, clefts of the primary palate may also affect nostril formation [126]. Both are beyond the scope of this chapter.

The secondary palate is the hard palate [126]. This forms secondary to the primary palate [126].

A cleft of the secondary palate is an abnormal opening along the roof of the mouth [126]. There is abnormal communication between the oral and nasal cavities [126] (see Figure 33.5).

All clefts are congenital malformations that have been described in dogs and cats, among other species [127–131]. They occur, on average, once every one thousand canine births [127, 132].

Genetics plays a contributing role in the development of clefts [126, 133–138].

Certain pharmaceutical agents may also contribute to cleft formation if there is fetal exposure [126]. These adverse drug effects have been studied in greater depth in humans than in companion animals; however, aspirin has been linked to teratogenic effects in the dog [139–141].

Clefts of the primary palate are obvious at birth [126]. By contrast, clefts of the secondary palate are not grossly apparent unless the neonate's mouth is opened.

Inexperienced breeders may not assess the oral cavity of newborns. They may instead present the affected pup(s) or kitten(s) for unusual nasal discharge.

Clients may report that milk drips out of the nose during nursing.

As the patient is transitioned onto solid foods, solid foods will also emerge from the nose during feeding.

An oral examination, with emphasis on the integrity of the roof of the mouth, is indicated for any patient with a similar history [1, 2].

Surgical repair of cleft palate is indicated to close the roof of the mouth to eliminate the abnormal connection between oral and nasal cavities (see Figure 33.6).

Wound dehiscence is a potential complication in the immediate postoperative period [126].

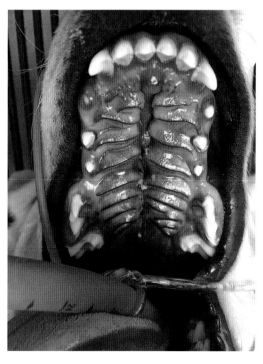

Figure 33.5 Cleft palate in a five-month-old, spayed female, Labrador retriever dog. *Source:* Courtesy of Jackie Kucskar, DVM.

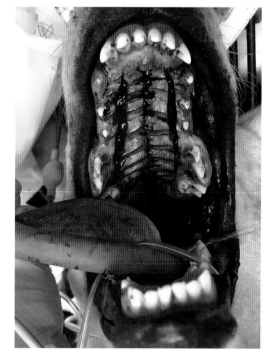

Figure 33.6 Cleft palate repair in the same Labrador retriever dog that was pictured in Figure 33.5. *Source:* Courtesy of Jackie Kucskar, DVM.

33.9 Oronasal Fistulas and Nasal Discharge

Oronasal fistulas are another type of abnormal connection between the mouth and nasal cavity [2]. Unlike cleft palates, oronasal fistulas are typically acquired [2, 142, 143].

The most common cause is periodontal destruction surrounding the maxillary canine tooth [142]. This typically involves the palatal aspect of the tooth [142]. Because the maxillary canine tooth's root sits next to the nasal cavity, a fistula through normal tissue causes oral cavity contents to spill over into the airway [142] (see Figure 33.7).

Affected patients experience chronic rhinitis because saliva, food, and water continue to access the nasal cavity via the mouth [142]. Oral bacteria also can seed the upper airway, causing secondary infection [142].

Oronasal fistulas may also result from [142]

- Traumatic avulsion of the maxillary canine tooth
- Severe overbite
- Iatrogenic causes.

Overbites are sometimes referred to, colloquially, as "parrot mouth." Patients with "parrot mouth" have a shorter-than-normal mandible relative to the maxilla. In severe cases, mandibular incisors come into contact with and ultimately penetrate the hard palate.

Dental extractions represent an iatrogenic cause of oronasal fistula [142].

Oronasal fistulas occur with greater frequency in certain breeds, including Dachshunds, Yorkshire Terriers, Poodles, and Schnauzers [142]. When they occur, they are often bilateral [142].

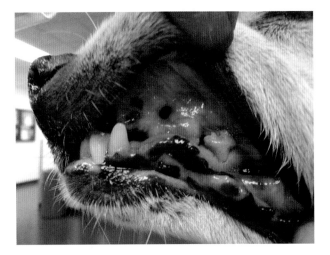

Figure 33.7 Oronasal fistula associated with the left maxillary arcade in a canine patient. *Source:* Courtesy of Patricia Bennett, DVM.

Gross appearance and consistency or nasal discharge varies, depending upon the patient's stage of disease. For example, patients with secondary URIs are more likely to display purulent nasal discharge, whereas a patient with extraction-induced oronasal fistula is more likely to develop acute epistaxis [142].

A thorough oral examination with dental radiography is an important diagnostic tool that assists with assessment of periodontal disease [142, 143]. Periodontal probing under general anesthesia also helps to establish the extent of disease, particularly when deep periodontal pockets are present that may or may not be associated with an oronasal fistula [142, 143].

Surgical repair of the oronasal fistula is achieved by extracting any associated teeth and creating a mucoperiosteal flap [142].

Serosanguinous-to-hemorrhagic nasal discharge is expected in the immediate postoperative period [142].

33.10 Other Abnormal Connections Between the Oral and Nasal Cavities

Clefts and oronasal fistulas are not the only two ways to obtain an abnormal connection between the oral and nasal cavity. The following etiologies are possible [143]:

- Neoplasia
- Bite wound
- Gunshot or pellet wound
- Automobile-associated trauma
- Penetrating foreign body (see Figures 33.8a–c)

33.11 Clinical Approach to Investigating Nasal Discharge

As evident from this chapter, the causes of nasal discharge are vast.

Although in theory every potential cause for nasal discharge in every patient should be explored, that is not the reality of clinical practice. More often than not, time and financial constraints present limits on what can be done, how often, and in what order. What, then, is the clinician to do in terms of prioritizing patient care and how does s/he make important decisions about where to begin in the diagnostic work-up?

Signalment and history taking are the foundation of the clinical approach to narrow the list of potential differentials into most versus least likely.

The physical examination provides important additional clues, some of which have already been touched upon [2].

(a)
(b)

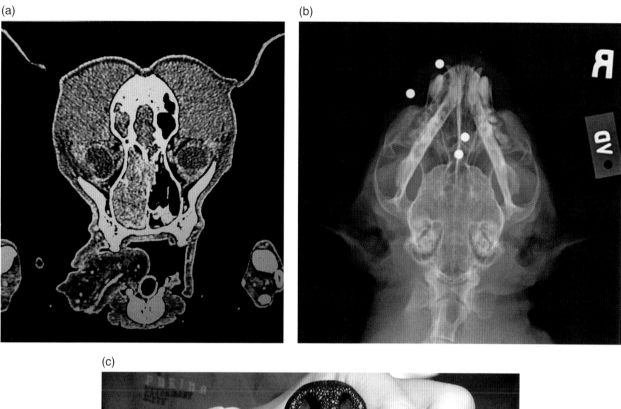

(c)

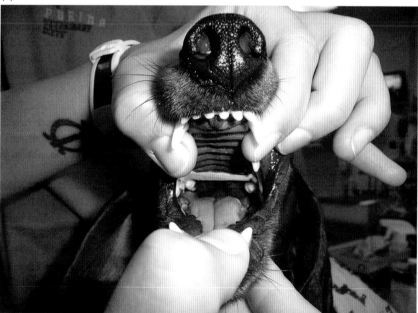

Figure 33.8 (a) Computed tomography (CT) scan demonstrating a nasal tumor in a feline patient. *Source:* Courtesy of Vicky Grossman. (b) Ventro-dorsal (V/D) radiograph of a stray cat, confirming bullets lodged within its skull and the soft tissue structures that are associated with the face. One can appreciate that the path of the bullet is through the palate. The cat survived. *Source:* Courtesy of Joseph Onello, DVM of Central Mesa Veterinary Hospital. (c) Wooden foreign body lodged within the oral cavity. Although this foreign body is not penetrating the hard palate at this time, one can imagine how easy it would be for a dog chasing a stick to have that stick pierce straight through the palate and into the nasal cavity. *Source:* Courtesy of Daniel Foy, MS, DVM, DACVIM, DACVECC.

To review [121]:

- The neonate with food or drink dribbling from the nose is more likely to have a congenital defect, such as a cleft palate.

- The patient with depigmentation of the nasal planum is more likely to have aspergillosis.
- The patient with a grossly observable or palpable distortion in facial structure is more likely to have neoplasia.

- The patient with reduced flow of air through one or both nares is more likely to have nasal cavity obstruction, as from a nasopharyngeal polyp or tumor.
- The feline patient with concurrent conjunctivitis is more likely to have infectious disease, such as FHV-1 or calicivirus, particularly if that patient is pediatric.
- The patient with dental disease, particularly periodontal disease, is more likely to have a tooth root abscess or oronasal fistula.
- The patient with epistaxis may have an underlying systemic bleeding disorder or may have been exposed to rodenticide.

An examination under general anesthesia may be necessary to thoroughly explore the oral cavity [121]. Pre-anesthetic hematology and biochemistry panels are considered standard of care. These tests may also provide important insight as to the presence of systemic or concurrent disease, although they are unlikely to reveal the cause of nasal discharge [121].

Viral testing for FeLV and FIV are important add-ons in feline practice [121]. Affected patients are more likely to be immunocompromised, which puts them at risk of other diseases, including cryptococcosis [121].

The saline agglutination test and add-on coagulation panels are essential for anemic patients with petechiations or ecchymoses.

Oropharyngeal swabs may be used for viral isolation to rule out FHV-1 and feline calicivirus, or FHV-1 may be detected by polymerase chain reaction (PCR), for instance, on conjunctival swabs [99, 103, 144, 145].

However, recall that FHV-1 is ubiquitous worldwide: as many as 81% of cats in the world may be carriers of the virus, and 95% are likely to have at one point in time been exposed [92, 96, 97, 101–103, 146, 147]. False positives are likely if subclinical patients are shedding FHV-1 [92]. Positives may also occur in exposed, but not infected, patients [92].

Fungal serology may be performed to evaluate patients for *Aspergillus*, *Cryptococcus*, and coccidioidomycosis [121]. The test sensitivity and specificity of each panel are important considerations when evaluating patient test results [121]. For example, serological testing for *Cryptococcus* in cats is highly sensitive and specific [121]. Therefore, false positives and false negatives are unlikely.

Culture of nasal discharge is unlikely to be of diagnostic aid, given that there will be appreciable contamination by resident flora [121]. It is also important to recall that positive bacterial cultures in chronic cases more accurately reflect secondary bacterial infection and that without identifying or addressing the primary case of disease, recurrence is almost guaranteed [121].

Imaging is particularly critical in cases involving chronic nasal discharge. Skull radiographs are the least sensitive imaging test; however, they are readily available in general practice [121]. They may demonstrate a change in opacity within the nasal cavities [121]. Instead of being air-filled, the nasal cavities may take on the opacity of soft tissue. This so-called mass effect heightens the index of suspicion that there is underlying neoplastic disease [121].

CT scans provide additional detail not afforded by traditional skull radiographs [15]. Lytic changes and the extent of disease are both more readily apparent [75].

Rhinoscopy allows for direct, gross observation of the nasal passageways, along with any fungal granulomas that may be present. Rhinoscopy also facilitates sample collection, although samples may also be collected blindly from the nasal cavity using approaches that are beyond the scope of this text [3, 32]. Iatrogenic damage can be done to the cribriform plate if the biopsy tool advances beyond the medial canthus [121].

Note that the use of ancillary diagnostic testing is prioritized based upon the likelihood of finding disease [148].

References

1 Stokhof, A.A. and Venker-van Haagen, A.J. (2009). Respiratory system. In: *Medical History and Physical Examination in Companion Animals* (ed. A. Rijnberk and F.J. van Sluijs), 63–74. Philadephia: Saunders Elsevier.

2 Englar, R.E. (2017). *Performing the Small Animal Physical Examination*. Hoboken, NJ: Wiley.

3 Elie, M. and Sabo, M. (2006). Basics in canine and feline rhinoscopy. *Clin Tech. Small Anim. Pract.* 21 (2): 60–63.

4 Grandage, J. (2003). Functional anatomy of the respiratory system. In: *Textbook of Small Animal Surgery* (ed. D.H. Slatter), 763–780. Philadelphia, PA: Saunders.

5 Singh, B. and Dyce, K.M. (2018). *Dyce, Sack, and Wensing's Textbook of Veterinary Anatomy*, 5e. St. Louis, Missouri: Saunders.

6 Evans, H.E. and Miller, M.E. (1993). *Miller's Anatomy of the Dog*, 3e, xvi, 1113 p. Philadelphia: W.B. Saunders.

7 Labuc R, editor. (2017). The approach to nasal discharge in the dog. The 8th Annual Vet Education International Online Veterinary Conference.

8 Gordon J. (2011). Clinical approach to nasal discharge. DVM 360 [Internet]. http://veterinarycalendar.dvm360.com/clinical-approach-nasal-discharge-proceedings.

9 Cohn, L.A. (2014). Canine nasal disease. *Vet. Clin. North Am. Small Anim. Pract.* 44 (1): 75–89.

10 Chartier, M. (2015). Canine primary (idiopathic) immune-mediated thrombocytopenia. *NAVC Clinician's Brief* (September): 82–86.

11 Mylonakis, M.E., Saridomichelakis, M.N., Lazaridis, V. et al. (2008). A retrospective study of 61 cases of spontaneous canine epistaxis (1998 to 2001). *J. Small Anim. Pract.* 49 (4): 191–196.

12 Petanides, T.A., Koutinas, A.F., Mylonakis, M.E. et al. (2008). Factors associated with the occurrence of epistaxis in natural canine leishmaniasis (Leishmania infantum). *J. Vet. Intern. Med.* 22 (4): 866–872.

13 Neer, T.M. (2003). Ehlichiosis in dogs. *NAVC Clinician's Brief* (May): 28–32.

14 Breitschwerdt, E.B. (2010). Canine bartonellosis. *NAVC Clinician's Brief* (July): 13–17.

15 Plickert, H.D., Tichy, A., and Hirt, R.A. (2014). Characteristics of canine nasal discharge related to intranasal diseases: a retrospective study of 105 cases. *J. Small Anim. Pract.* 55 (3): 145–152.

16 Reif, J.S., Bruns, C., and Lower, K.S. (1998). Cancer of the nasal cavity and paranasal sinuses and exposure to environmental tobacco smoke in pet dogs. *Am. J. Epidemiol.* 147 (5): 488–492.

17 Rich, E.C., Crowson, T.W., and Harris, I.B. (1987). The diagnostic value of the medical history. Perceptions of internal medicine physicians. *Arch. Intern. Med.* 147 (11): 1957–1960.

18 Lichstein, P.R. (1990). The Medical Interview. In: *Clinical Methods: The History, Physical, and Laboratory Examinations* (ed. H.K. Walker, W.D. Hall and J.W. Hurst). Boston: Butterworths.

19 Dye, J.A. (2008). Diagnosing feline respiratory disease. *NAVC Clinician's Brief* (July): 9–12.

20 Sharp, C.R. (2012). Feline rhinitis and upper respiratory disease. *Today's Veterinary Practice* (July/August): 14–20.

21 Van Pelt, D.R. and Lappin, M.R. (1994). Pathogenesis and treatment of feline rhinitis. *Vet. Clin. North Am. Small Anim. Pract.* 24 (5): 807–823.

22 Lamb, C.R., Richbell, S., and Mantis, P. (2003). Radiographic signs in cats with nasal disease. *J. Feline Med. Surg.* 5 (4): 227–235.

23 Henderson, S.M., Bradley, K., Day, M.J. et al. (2004). Investigation of nasal disease in the cat – a retrospective study of 77 cases. *J. Feline Med. Surg.* 6 (4): 245–257.

24 Binns, S.H., Dawson, S., Speakman, A.J. et al. (1999). Prevalence and risk factors for feline *Bordetella bronchiseptica* infection. *Vet. Rec.* 144 (21): 575–580.

25 Malik, R., Krockenberger, M., and O'Brien, C. (2006). Cryptococcosis. In: *Infectious Diseases of the Dog and Cat* (ed. C.E. Greene), 584–598. St. Louis: Elsevier Saunders.

26 Speakman, A.J., Dawson, S., Binns, S.H. et al. (1999). *Bordetella bronchiseptica* infection in the cat. *J. Small Anim. Pract.* 40 (6): 252–256.

27 Bradley, R.L. (1984). Selected oral, pharyngeal, and upper respiratory conditions in the cat. Oral tumors, nasopharyngeal and middle ear polyps, and chronic rhinitis and sinusitis. *Vet. Clin. North Am. Small Anim. Pract.* 14 (6): 1173–1184.

28 Cape, L. (1992). Feline Idiopathic Chronic Rhinosinusitis – a Retrospective Study of 30 Cases. *J. Am. Anim. Hosp. Assoc.* 28 (2): 149–155.

29 Ford, R.B. and Levy, J.K. (1994). Infectious diseases of the respiratory tract. In: *The Cat: Diseases and Clinical Management* (ed. R.G. Sherding), 489–500. New York: Churchill Livingstone.

30 Malik, R., Wigney, D.I., Muir, D.B. et al. (1992). Cryptococcosis in cats: clinical and mycological assessment of 29 cases and evaluation of treatment using orally administered fluconazole. *J. Med. Vet. Mycol.* 30 (2): 133–144.

31 Mochizuki, M., Kawakami, K., Hashimoto, M., and Ishida, T. (2000). Recent epidemiological status of feline upper respiratory infections in Japan. *J. Vet. Med. Sci.* 62 (7): 801–803.

32 Moore, A.H. (2007). Evaluation of chronic nasal disease in dogs: rhinoscopy in context. *NAVC Clinician's Brief* (May): 17–19.

33 Moore, L.E. (2003). Feline chronic respiratory disease. *NAVC Clinician's Brief* (August): 41–42.

34 Plummer, C.E. (2012). Herpetic keratoconjunctivitis in a cat. *NAVC Clinician's Brief* (January): 26–28.

35 Hurley K. (2010). Canine infectious respiratory disease complex: management and prevention in canine populations. DVM 360 [Internet]. http://veterinarycalendar.dvm360.com/canine-infectious-respiratory-disease-complex-management-and-prevention-canine-populations-proceedin.

36 Joffe, D.J., Lelewski, R., Weese, J.S. et al. (2016). Factors associated with development of Canine Infectious Respiratory Disease Complex (CIRDC) in dogs in 5 Canadian small animal clinics. *Can. Vet. J.* 57 (1): 46–51.

37 Chalker, V.J., Toomey, C., Opperman, S. et al. (2003). Respiratory disease in kennelled dogs: serological responses to *Bordetella bronchiseptica* lipopolysaccharide do not correlate with bacterial isolation or clinical respiratory symptoms. *Clin. Diagn. Lab. Immunol.* 10 (3): 352–356.

38 Nafe, L.A. (2014). Dogs infected with *Bordetella bronchiseptica* and Canine influenza virus (H3N8). *Today's Veterinary Practice* (July/August): 30–36.

39 Priestnall, S.L., Mitchell, J.A., Walker, C.A. et al. (2014). New and emerging pathogens in canine infectious respiratory disease. *Vet. Pathol.* 51 (2): 492–504.

40 Holt, D.E., Mover, M.R., and Brown, D.C. (2010). Serologic prevalence of antibodies against canine influenza virus (H3N8) in dogs in a metropolitan animal shelter. *J. Am. Vet. Med. Assoc.* 237 (1): 71–73.

41 Radhakrishnan, A., Drobatz, K.J., Culp, W.T., and King, L.G. (2007). Community-acquired infectious pneumonia in puppies: 65 cases (1993–2002). *J. Am. Vet. Med. Assoc.* 230 (10): 1493–1497.

42 Weese, J.S. and Stull, J. (2013). Respiratory disease outbreak in a veterinary hospital associated with canine parainfluenza virus infection. *Can. Vet. J.* 54 (1): 79–82.

43 Ellis, J.A. and Krakowka, G.S. (2012). A review of canine parainfluenza virus infection in dogs. *J. Am. Vet. Med. Assoc.* 240 (3): 273–284.

44 Erles, K., Toomey, C., Brooks, H.W., and Brownlie, J. (2003). Detection of a group 2 coronavirus in dogs with canine infectious respiratory disease. *Virology* 310 (2): 216–223.

45 Serra, V.F., Stanzani, G., Smith, G., and Otto, C.M. (2011). Point seroprevalence of canine influenza virus H3N8 in dogs participating in a flyball tournament in Pennsylvania. *J. Am. Vet. Med. Assoc.* 238 (6): 726–730.

46 Anderson, T.C., Crawford, P.C., Dubovi, E.J. et al. (2013). Prevalence of and exposure factors for seropositivity to H3N8 canine influenza virus in dogs with influenza-like illness in the United States. *J. Am. Vet. Med. Assoc.* 242 (2): 209–216.

47 Epstein, S. and Hardy, R. (2011). Clinical resolution of nasal aspergillosis following therapy with a homeopathic remedy in a dog. *J. Am. Anim. Hosp. Assoc.* 47 (6): e110–e115.

48 Sharp, N.J. (1998). Canine nasal aspergillosis-penicilliosis. In: *Infectious Diseases of the Dog and Cat*, 2e (ed. C. Greene), 404–409. Philadelphia: W.B. Saunders, Co.

49 Benitah, N. (2006). Canine nasal aspergillosis. *Clin. Tech. Small Anim. Pract.* 21 (2): 82–88.

50 Magro, M., Sykes, J., Vishkautsan, P., and Martinez-Lopez, B. (2017). Spatial patterns and impacts of environmental and climatic factors on canine sinonasal aspergillosis in northern California. *Front. Vet. Sci.* 4: 104.

51 Day, M.J. (2009). Canine sino-nasal aspergillosis: parallels with human disease. *Med. Mycol.* 47 (Suppl 1): S315–S323.

52 Sharp, N.J. and Harvey, C.E. (1991). Aspergillosis: report on diagnosis and treatment. *Tijdschr. Diergeneeskd.* 116 (Suppl 1): 35S–37S.

53 Mullins, J., Harvey, R., and Seaton, A. (1976). Sources and incidence of airborne *Aspergillus fumigatus* (Fres). *Clin. Allergy* 6 (3): 209–217.

54 Warris, A., Klaassen, C.H., Meis, J.F. et al. (2003). Molecular epidemiology of *Aspergillus fumigatus* isolates recovered from water, air, and patients shows two clusters of genetically distinct strains. *J. Clin. Microbiol.* 41 (9): 4101–4106.

55 Curtis, L., Cali, S., Conroy, L. et al. (2005). Aspergillus surveillance project at a large tertiary-care hospital. *J. Hosp. Infect.* 59 (3): 188–196.

56 Haines, J. (1995). Aspergillus in compost – straw man or fatal flaw. *Biocycle* 36 (4): 32–35.

57 Streifel, A.J., Lauer, J.L., Vesley, D. et al. (1983). Aspergillus-fumigatus and other thermotolerant fungi generated by hospital building demolition. *Appl. Environ. Microbol.* 46 (2): 375–378.

58 Ren, P., Jankun, T.M., Belanger, K. et al. (2001). The relation between fungal propagules in indoor air and home characteristics. *Allergy* 56 (5): 419–424.

59 Zonderland, J.L., Stork, C.K., Saunders, J.H. et al. (2002). Intranasal infusion of enilconazole for treatment of sinonasal aspergillosis in dogs. *J. Am. Vet. Med. Assoc.* 221 (10): 1421–1425.

60 Sharp, N.J.H., Harvey, C.E., and Obrien, J.A. (1991). Treatment of canine nasal aspergillosis penicilliosis with fluconazole (UK-49,858). *J. Small Anim. Pract.* 32 (10): 513–516.

61 Saunders, J.H., Zonderland, J.L., Clercx, C. et al. (2002). Computed tomographic findings in 35 dogs with nasal aspergillosis. *Vet. Radiol. Ultrasound* 43 (1): 5–9.

62 Barrs, V.R., Beatty, J.A., Dhand, N.K. et al. (2014). Computed tomographic features of feline sino-nasal and sino-orbital aspergillosis. *Vet. J.* 201 (2): 215–222.

63 Barrs, V.R. and Talbot, J.J. (2014). Feline aspergillosis. *Vet. Clin. North Am. Small Anim. Pract.* 44 (1): 51–73.

64 Barachetti, L., Mortellaro, C.M., Di Giancamillo, M. et al. (2009). Bilateral orbital and nasal aspergillosis in a cat. *Vet. Ophthalmol.* 12 (3): 176–182.

65 Kano, R., Itamoto, K., Okuda, M. et al. (2008). Isolation of Aspergillus udagawae from a fatal case of feline orbital aspergillosis. *Mycoses* 51 (4): 360–361.

66 Wilkinson, G.T., Sutton, R.H., and Grono, L.R. (1982). Aspergillus spp infection associated with orbital cellulitis and sinusitis in a cat. *J. Small Anim. Pract.* 23 (3): 127–131.

67 Declercq, J., Declercq, L., and Fincioen, S. (2012). Unilateral sino-orbital and subcutaneous aspergillosis in a cat. *Vlaams Diergen. Tijds.* 81 (6): 357–362.

68 Furrow, E. and Groman, R.P. (2009). Intranasal infusion of clotrimazole for the treatment of nasal aspergillosis in two cats. *J. Am. Vet. Med Assoc.* 235 (10): 1188–1193.

69 Giordano, C., Gianella, P., Bo, S. et al. (2010). Invasive mould infections of the naso-orbital region of cats: a case involving *Aspergillus fumigatus* and an aetiological review. *J. Feline Med. Surg.* 12 (9): 714–723.

70 Karnik, K., Reichle, J.K., Fischetti, A.J., and Goggin, J.M. (2009). Computed tomographic findings of fungal rhinitis and sinusitis in cats. *Vet. Radiol. Ultrasound* 50 (1): 65–68.

71 Smith, L.N. and Hoffman, S.B. (2010). A case series of unilateral orbital aspergillosis in three cats and treatment with voriconazole. *Vet. Ophthalmol.* 13 (3): 190–203.

72 Barrs, V.R., Halliday, C., Martin, P. et al. (2012). Sinonasal and sino-orbital aspergillosis in 23 cats: aetiology, clinicopathological features and treatment outcomes. *Vet. J.* 191 (1): 58–64.

73 Tomsa, K., Glaus, T.M., Zimmer, C., and Greene, C.E. (2003). Fungal rhinitis and sinusitis in three cats. *J. Am. Vet. Med. Assoc.* 222 (10): 1380–1384, 65.

74 Whitney, J., Beatty, J.A., Martin, P. et al. (2013). Evaluation of serum galactomannan detection for diagnosis of feline upper respiratory tract aspergillosis. *Vet. Microbiol.* 162 (1): 180–185.

75 Chapman, P. (2015). Nasal discharge in a labrador retriever. *Veterinary Team Brief* (September).

76 Pennisi, M.G., Hartmann, K., Lloret, A. et al. (2013). Cryptococcosis in cats: ABCD guidelines on prevention and management. *J. Feline Med. Surg.* 15 (7): 611–618.

77 Duncan, C.G., Stephen, C., and Campbell, J. (2006). Evaluation of risk factors for *Cryptococcus gattii* infection in dogs and cats. *J. Am. Vet. Med. Assoc.* 228 (3): 377–382.

78 Pal, M. (1989). *Cryptococcus neoformans* var. neoformans and munia birds. *Mycoses* 32 (5): 250–252.

79 Alspaugh, J.A., Davidson, R.C., and Heitman, J. (2000). Morphogenesis of *Cryptococcus neoformans*. *Contrib. Microbiol.* 5: 217–238.

80 Lin, X. and Heitman, J. (2006). The biology of the *Cryptococcus neoformans* species complex. *Annu. Rev. Microbiol.* 60: 69–105.

81 Malik, R., Wigney, D.I., Muir, D.B., and Love, D.N. (1997). Asymptomatic carriage of *Cryptococcus neoformans* in the nasal cavity of dogs and cats. *J. Med. Vet. Mycol.* 35 (1): 27–31.

82 Martins, D.B., Zanette, R.A., Franca, R.T. et al. (2011). Massive cryptococcal disseminated infection in an immunocompetent cat. *Vet. Dermatol.* 22 (2): 232–234.

83 Malik, R., Martin, P., Wigney, D.I. et al. (1997). Nasopharyngeal cryptococcosis. *Aust. Vet. J.* 75 (7): 483–488.

84 McGill, S., Malik, R., Saul, N. et al. (2009). Cryptococcosis in domestic animals in Western Australia: a retrospective study from 1995–2006. *Med. Mycol.* 47 (6): 625–639.

85 Norton, R. and Burney, D.P. (2012). Cryptococcosis. *NAVC Clinician's Brief* (December): 39–42.

86 Trivedi, S.R., Sykes, J.E., Cannon, M.S. et al. (2011). Clinical features and epidemiology of cryptococcosis in cats and dogs in California: 93 cases (1988–2010). *J. Am. Vet. Med. Assoc.* 239 (3): 357–369.

87 O'Brien, C.R., Krockenberger, M.B., Wigney, D.I. et al. (2004). Retrospective study of feline and canine cryptococcosis in Australia from 1981 to 2001: 195 cases. *Med. Mycol.* 42 (5): 449–460.

88 Malik, R., Dill-Macky, E., Martin, P. et al. (1995). Cryptococcosis in dogs: a retrospective study of 20 consecutive cases. *J. Med. Vet. Mycol.* 33 (5): 291–297.

89 Chandler, E.A., Gaskell, R.M., and Gaskell, C.J. (2008). *Feline Medicine and Therapeutics*. Ames, IA: Wiley.

90 Lim, C.C. and Maggs, D.J. (2012). Ophthalmology. In: *The Cat: Clinical Medicine and Management* (ed. S.E. Little), 807–845. St. Louis, Missouri: Saunders Elsevier.

91 Reinstein, S. (ed.) (2017). *The Squinting Cat: Herpes Until Proven Otherwise*. Michigan: Michigan VMA.

92 Ofri, R. (2017). Conjunctivitis in cats. *NAVC Clinician's Brief* (April): 95–100.

93 Smith, R.I.E. (2006). The cat with ocular discharge or changed conjunctival appearance. In: *Problem-Based Feline Medicine* (ed. J. Rand), 1207–1232. Edinburgh; New York: Saunders.

94 Maggs, D.J. (2013). Conjunctiva. In: *Slatter's Fundamentals of Veterinary Opthalmology* (ed. D.J. Maggs, P.E. Miller and R. Ofri), 140–158. St. Louis, MO: Elsevier.

95 Aroch, I., Ofri, R., and Sutton, G. (2013). Ocular manifestations of systemic diseases. In: *Slatter's Fundamentals of Veterinary Ophthalmology* (ed. D.J. Maggs, P.E. Miller and R. Ofri), 184–219. St. Louis, MO: Elsevier.

96 Stiles, J. (2013). Feline ophthalmology. In: *Veterinary Ophthalmology* (ed. K.N. Gelatt, B.C. Gilger and T.J. Kern), 1477–1559. Ames, IA: Wiley-Blackwell.

97 Maggs, D.J. (2005). Update on pathogenesis, diagnosis, and treatment of feline herpesvirus type 1. *Clin. Tech. Small Anim. Pract.* 20 (2): 94–101.

98 Nasisse, M.P., Guy, J.S., Stevens, J.B. et al. (1993). Clinical and laboratory findings in chronic conjunctivitis in cats: 91 cases (1983–1991). *J. Am. Vet. Med. Assoc.* 203 (6): 834–837.

99 Grahn, B.H. and Sandmeyer, L.S. (2010). Diagnostic ophthalmology ophtalmologie diagnostique. *Can. Vet. J.* 51 (3): 327.

100 Nasisse, M.P., Davis, B.J., Guy, J.S. et al. (1992). Isolation of feline herpesvirus 1 from the trigeminal ganglia of acutely and chronically infected cats. *J. Vet. Intern. Med.* 6 (2): 102–103.

101 Gould, D. (2011). Feline herpesvirus-1: ocular manifestations, diagnosis and treatment options. *J. Feline Med. Surg.* 13 (5): 333–346.

102 Westermeyer, H.D., Thomasy, S.M., Kado-Fong, H., and Maggs, D.J. (2009). Assessment of viremia associated with experimental primary feline herpesvirus infection or presumed herpetic recrudescence in cats. *Am. J. Vet. Res.* 70 (1): 99–104.

103 Heinrich C. (2015). Assessing conjunctivitis in cats. Vet Times [Internet]. https://www.vettimes.co.uk/

app/uploads/wp-post-to-pdf-enhanced-cache/1/
assessing-conjunctivitis-in-cats.pdf.

104 Windsor, R.C. and Johnson, L.R. (2006). Canine
chronic inflammatory rhinitis. *Clin. Tech. Small Anim.
Pract.* 21 (2): 76–81.

105 Willemse, A. (1984). Canine atopic disease:
investigations of eosinophils and the nasal mucosa.
Am. J. Vet. Res. 45 (9): 1867–1869.

106 Patterson, R. and Harris, K.E. (1999). Rush
immunotherapy in a dog with severe ragweed and
grass pollen allergy. *Ann. Allergy Asthma Immunol.* 83
(3): 213–216.

107 Windsor, R.C., Johnson, L.R., Herrgesell, E.J., and De
Cock, H.E. (2004). Idiopathic lymphoplasmacytic
rhinitis in dogs: 37 cases (1997–2002). *J. Am. Vet.
Med. Assoc.* 224 (12): 1952–1957.

108 Rudolph, K., Bice, D.E., Hey, J.A., and McLeod, R.L.
(2003). A model of allergic nasal congestion in dogs
sensitized to ragweed. *Am. J. Rhinol.* 17 (4): 227–232.

109 Tiniakov, R.L., Tiniakova, O.P., McLeod, R.L. et al.
(2003). Canine model of nasal congestion and
allergic rhinitis. *J. Appl. Physiol. (1985)* 94 (5):
1821–1828.

110 Cardell, L.O., Agusti, C., and Nadel, J.A. (2000). Nasal
secretion in ragweed-sensitized dogs: effect of
leukotriene synthesis inhibition. *Acta Otolaryngol.*
120 (6): 757–760.

111 Lobetti, R. (2014). Idiopathic lymphoplasmacytic
rhinitis in 33 dogs. *J. S. Afr. Vet. Assoc.* 85 (1): 1151.

112 McCarthy, T.C. and McDermaid, S.L. (1990).
Rhinoscopy. *Vet. Clin. North Am. Small Anim. Pract.*
20 (5): 1265–1290.

113 Tasker, S., Knottenbelt, C.M., Munro, E.A. et al.
(1999). Aetiology and diagnosis of persistent nasal
disease in the dog: a retrospective study of 42 cases.
J. Small Anim. Pract. 40 (10): 473–478.

114 Sullivan, M. (1998). Nasal discharge in the dog. In:
Canine Medicine and Therapeutics (ed. N.T. Gorman),
341–352. England: Oxford: Wiley-Blackwell.

115 Norris, A.M. and Laing, E.J. (1985). Diseases of the
nose and sinuses. *Vet. Clin. North Am. Small Anim.
Pract.* 15 (5): 865–890.

116 Russo, M., Lamb, C.R., and Jakovljevic, S. (2000).
Distinguishing rhinitis and nasal neoplasia by
radiography. *Vet. Radiol. Ultrasound* 41 (2):
118–124.

117 Mackin, A.J. (2004). Lymphoplasmacytic rhinitis. In:
Respiratory Diseases in Dogs and Cats (ed. L.G. King),
305–310. Philadelphia: W.B. Saunders.

118 Kent, M.S. (2009). Nasal discharge in a dog. *NAVC
Clinician's Brief* (September): 25–26.

119 Little, L., Patel, R., and Goldschmidt, M. (2007). Nasal
and nasopharyngeal lymphoma in cats: 50 cases
(1989–2005). *Vet. Pathol.* 44 (6): 885–892.

120 Mazzaferro, E.M. (2011). Nasal discharge and
epistaxis in a German shorthaired pointer. *Today's
Veterinary Practice* (November/December): 68–73.

121 Burrow RD, editor. (2008). Approach to Investigation
of Nasal Disease. British Small Animal Veterinary
Congress.

122 Mukaratirwa, S., van der Linde-Sipman, J.S.,
and Gruys, E. (2001). Feline nasal and paranasal
sinus tumours: clinicopathological study,
histomorphological description and diagnostic
immunohistochemistry of 123 cases. *J. Feline Med.
Surg.* 3 (4): 235–245.

123 Wooten SJ. (2016). When it comes to nasal tumors,
the nose knows. DVM 360 [Internet]. http://
veterinarynews.dvm360.com/when-it-comes-nasal-
tumors-nose-knows.

124 LaDue, T.A., Dodge, R., Page, R.L. et al. (1999).
Factors influencing survival after radiotherapy of
nasal tumors in 130 dogs. *Vet. Radiol. Ultrasound* 40
(3): 312–317.

125 Rassnick, K.M., Goldkamp, C.E., Erb, H.N. et al.
(2006). Evaluation of factors associated with survival
in dogs with untreated nasal carcinomas: 139 cases
(1993–2003). *J. Am. Vet. Med. Assoc.* 229 (3): 401–406.

126 Fiani, N., Verstraete, F.J., and Arzi, B. (2016).
Reconstruction of congenital nose, cleft primary
palate, and lip disorders. *Vet. Clin. North Am. Small
Anim. Pract.* 46 (4): 663–675.

127 Peralta, S., Fiani, N., Kan-Rohrer, K.H., and Verstraete,
F.J.M. (2017). Morphological evaluation of clefts of the
lip, palate, or both in dogs. *Am. J. Vet. Res.* 78 (8):
926–933.

128 Bleicher, N., Sloan, R.F., Gault, I.G., and Ashley, F.L.
(1965). Cleft Palate in a Dog. *Cleft Palate J.* 45:
56–61.

129 Calnan, J. (1961). The comparative anatomy of cleft lip
and palate. I. Classification of cleft lip and palate in
dogs. *Br. J. Plast. Surg.* 14: 180–184.

130 Dreyer, C.J. and Preston, C.B. (1974). Classification of
cleft lip and palate in animals. *Cleft Palate J.* 11:
327–332.

131 Mulvihill, J.J., Mulvihill, C.G., and Priester, W.A.
(1980). Cleft palate in domestic animals:
epidemiologic features. *Teratology* 21 (1):
109–112.

132 Nemec, A., Daniaux, L., Johnson, E. et al. (2015).
Craniomaxillofacial abnormalities in dogs with
congenital palatal defects: computed tomographic
findings. *Vet. Surg.* 44 (4): 417–422.

133 Senders, C.W., Eisele, P., Freeman, L.E., and
Sponenberg, D.P. (1986). Observations about the
normal and abnormal embryogenesis of the canine lip
and palate. *J. Craniofac. Genet. Dev. Biol. Suppl.*
2: 241–248.

134 Natsume, N., Miyajima, K., Kinoshita, H., and Kawai, T. (1994). Incidence of cleft lip and palate in beagles. *Plast. Reconstr. Surg.* 93 (2): 439.

135 Kemp, C., Thiele, H., Dankof, A. et al. (2009). Cleft lip and/or palate with monogenic autosomal recessive transmission in pyrenees shepherd dogs. *Cleft Palate Craniofac. J.* 46 (1): 81–88.

136 Moura, E., Cirio, S.M., and Pimpao, C.T. (2012). Nonsyndromic cleft lip and palate in boxer dogs: evidence of monogenic autosomal recessive inheritance. *Cleft Palate Craniofac. J.* 49 (6): 759–760.

137 Richtsmeier, J.T., Sack, G.H. Jr., Grausz, H.M., and Cork, L.C. (1994). Cleft palate with autosomal recessive transmission in Brittany spaniels. *Cleft Palate Craniofac. J.* 31 (5): 364–371.

138 Wolf, Z.T., Brand, H.A., Shaffer, J.R. et al. (2015). Genome-wide association studies in dogs and humans identify ADAMTS20 as a risk variant for cleft lip and palate. *PLoS Genet.* 11 (3): e1005059.

139 Robertson, R.T., Allen, H.L., and Bokelman, D.L. (1979). Aspirin: teratogenic evaluation in the dog. *Teratology* 20 (2): 313–320.

140 Elwood, J.M. and Colquhoun, T.A. (1997). Observations on the prevention of cleft palate in dogs by folic acid and potential relevance to humans. *N. Z. Vet. J.* 45 (6): 254–256.

141 Inoyama, K. and Meador, K.J. (2015). Cognitive outcomes of prenatal antiepileptic drug exposure. *Epilepsy Res.* 114: 89–97.

142 Peak, R.M. (2007). Inapparent Oronasal Fistula & Periodontal Disease. *NAVC Clinician's Brief* 11–14.

143 Kressin D. (2010). What are oronasal or oroantral fistulas? DVM 360 [Internet]. http://veterinarynews. dvm360.com/print/304293?page=full.

144 Tilley, L.P. and Smith, F.W.K. (2004). *The 5-minute Veterinary Consult: Canine and Feline*, 3e, lviii, 1487 p. Baltimore, MD: Lippincott Williams & Wilkins.

145 Côté, E. (2015). *Clinical Veterinary Advisor. Dogs and Cats*, 3e, xxxvii, 1642 p. St. Louis, Missouri: Elsevier Mosby.

146 Stiles, J. (2014). Ocular manifestations of feline viral diseases. *Vet. J.* 201 (2): 166–173.

147 Stiles, J. and Pogranichniy, R. (2008). Detection of virulent feline herpesvirus-1 in the corneas of clinically normal cats. *J. Feline Med. Surg.* 10 (2): 154–159.

148 Meler, E., Dunn, M., and Lecuyer, M. (2008). A retrospective study of canine persistent nasal disease: 80 cases (1998–2003). *Can. Vet. J.* 49 (1): 71–76.

34

Stertor and Stridor

34.1 Introduction to Abnormal, Obstructive, Upper Airway Sounds

Chapter 33 reviewed the conduction of air from the external environment through the upper airway. Recall that air enters the nares and travels into paired nasal cavities, where it is cleansed, warmed, and humidified en route to the lower airway [1–8]. In the normal patient, this process is relatively silent.

Upper airway disease, specifically *obstructive* upper airway disease, creates abnormal sounds that are audible without a stethoscope [9–13]. These sounds are the result of turbulent airflow through narrowed spaces [9, 10].

In order to take in the amount of air that is necessary to sustain life, the patient must work harder [9]. Respiratory effort in patients with obstructive airways is greater [9, 14, 15].

Obstruction worsens as the speed of airflow through the system increases in an attempt to get more air into narrowed spaces, and tissues and their associated secretions vibrate with intensity [9]. This raises the amplitude of the sound that is produced [9].

In addition, the resultant inflammation within the airway itself perpetuates obstructive disease [9]. Edema exacerbates the obstruction, forcing the patient to work even harder [9].

The harder the patient works, the more the airway inflames and the louder the associated sounds become [9].

Stertor and stridor are the primary abnormal sounds that result from airway resistance secondary to obstructive disease [1, 9, 10, 12, 13, 15–18]. They may occur simultaneously within the same patient, or they may occur in isolation from one another, in different patients.

Note that stertor and stridor are not strictly inspiratory sounds [1]. Either may be inspiratory or expiratory depending upon the location and the severity of the obstruction [1].

In the author's experience, stertor and stridor are frequently confused by the veterinary student and so should be addressed here. Although both are due to

obstructive airway disease, the sounds that result from each have a distinct pitch and originate from a different set of vibrations [9].

34.1.1 Definition of Stertor

Stertor results from vibrations of flaccid tissues or secretions [9]. When these vibrate, they create a classic low-pitched snoring sound [9, 10]. This snore is most typically the result of airway obstruction within the nose itself or the pharynx [9–11].

34.1.2 Definition of Stridor

Stridor occurs when rigid tissues vibrate [9]. This creates a harsh, high-pitched sound [9–11]. This sound may occur because of nasal obstruction. More typically, clinicians associate stridor with laryngeal narrowing, as from laryngeal paralysis, or tracheal collapse [1, 9–11].

34.1.3 Open-Mouth Breathing as a Potential Sign of Upper Airway Obstruction

Although dogs can breathe through both their nose and mouth, they typically prefer the former for oxygenation and the latter for panting. Panting in dogs is a normal physiologic action intended to regulate core body temperature [19–22]. Panting works by encouraging evaporative cooling from the respiratory tract [19–22].

Dogs will also open-mouth breathe when there is a nasal or nasopharyngeal obstruction. When bilateral nasal obstruction prevents airflow through the upper respiratory tract or when there is an obstruction at the level of the nasopharynx, airflow will take an alternate route through the oral cavity.

Panting is atypical in cats and ordinarily only occurs during times of extreme excitement or stress. The cat that persistently open-mouth breathes should undergo diagnostic work-up for nasopharyngeal disease as this patient is likely to be in a state of respiratory distress [11, 23] (see Figures 34.1a, b).

(a)

(b)

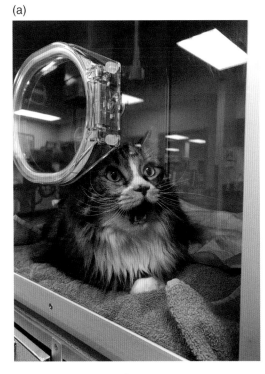 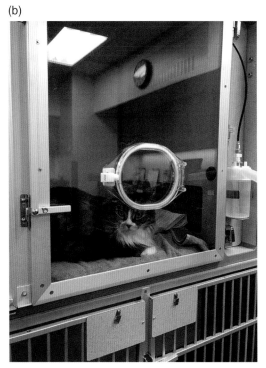

Figure 34.1 (a) Feline patient in respiratory distress. Note that the patient is open-mouth breathing. The patient was immediately placed in an oxygen cage. *Source:* Courtesy of Bianca J. Hartrum, DVM. (b) Same feline patient as in Figure 34.1a after receiving supplemental oxygen via oxygen cage for 30–60 min. Note that open-mouth breathing has resolved. The patient is more stable for diagnostic work-up. *Source:* Courtesy of Bianca J. Hartrum, DVM.

Respiratory distress is a medical emergency in any species [8, 12, 15, 17, 24]. Cats are particularly fragile and can decompensate rapidly [17].

34.1.4 Assessing for Nasal Airflow

Recall from Chapter 33, Section 33.7 that nasal airflow can be assessed in-house using rudimentary supplies. All that is necessary is a clean glass slide or a tuft of cotton wool [11].

Either tool is placed in front of each of the nares [25]. Airflow through the nares will result in the glass slide fogging over or the tuft of cotton moving through space as it is held before the nares by the tester [25].

34.1.5 Additional Signs of Obstructive Respiratory Disease

Depending upon the severity of the obstruction, upper respiratory disease may handicap the body's ability to cool itself [12, 13, 15, 24]. The affected patient may develop significant hyperthermia [12, 13, 15, 24].

In addition, patients that experience upper respiratory obstruction routinely become cyanotic [9, 26]. Cyanotic mucous membranes have blue-purple undertones that

result from an excess of deoxygenated hemoglobin in the circulation [9] (see Figures 34.2a, b).

34.2 Causes of Stertor and Stridor

The primary causes of stertor and stridor in the companion animal patient include the following [8–11, 13, 15, 17, 24, 27–37]:

- Congenital
  - Cleft palate
- Foreign body (refer to Chapter 33, Section 33.10)
  - ○ Plant material, particularly grass awns
- Infectious disease (refer to Chapter 33, Section 33.5)
  - Chronic rhinitis and sinorhinitis
    - ○ Secondary bacterial infection
    - ○ Opportunistic fungal infection
- Inflammatory disease (refer to Chapter 33, Section 33.6).
  - Idiopathic or lymphoplasmacytic rhinitis (LPR)
    - ○ Secondary bacterial infection
    - ○ Opportunistic fungal infection
- Mechanical obstruction
  - Brachycephalic airway syndrome
  - Laryngeal paralysis

(a)

(b)

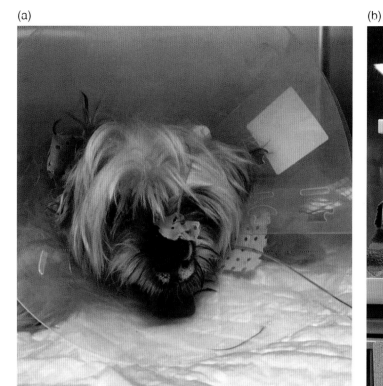
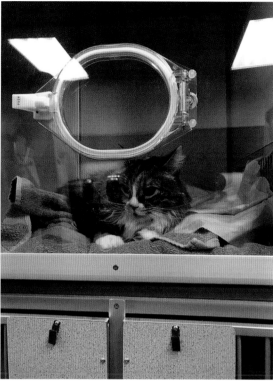

Figure 34.2 (a) Cyanotic canine patient. Note its appreciably purple tongue. *Source:* Courtesy of Rodolfo Oliveira Leal, DVM (Portugal), PhD, Dipl. ECVIM-CA (Internal Medicine). (b) Same feline patient as in Figures 34.1a and b. Note the color of the tongue that is peaking out of the cat's mouth. It is cyanotic. *Source:* Courtesy of Bianca J. Hartrum, DVM.

    – Nasopharyngeal polyp
    – Tracheal collapse
• Neoplasia (refer to Chapter 33, Section 33.6)
• Trauma
    – Nasal fractures
    – Oronasal fistula (refer to Chapter 33, Section 33.9)

The most common differential diagnoses will be discussed in greater depth here: brachycephalic syndrome, laryngeal paralysis, and tracheal collapse [8, 12]. Consult internal medicine textbooks for additional information on the other syndromes as needed.

34.3 Skull Shape, Cephalic Index, and Brachycephalic Syndrome

Skull shape varies immensely between canine and feline breeds [2]. A ratio of skull width-to-length, the so-called cephalic index (CI), facilitates comparisons between dogs and cats [2].

The higher the CI, the wider the skull as compared to skull length [2]. This is the most characteristic feature of the brachycephalic breeds [2, 38–46].

Common brachycephalic canine breeds include the following [2, 9, 26, 29, 39, 45, 47–49]:

• Boston Terriers
• Boxers
• Brussels Griffons
• Bull Mastiffs
• Chinese Shar-Peis
• Dogue de Bordeaux
• English Bulldogs
• French Bulldogs
• King Charles Cavalier Spaniels
• Lhasa apsos
• Pekingese
• Pugs
• Shih Tzus

Common brachycephalic feline breeds include [2, 9]

• Himalayans
• Persians.

All brachycephalic breeds have distinct facial morphology [2, 29]. The foreshortened face gives them a characteristic "pushed in" appearance [2, 40, 41]. In addition, they have shallow orbits and "bug-eyed" globes [2].

These bulgy eyes are also spaced further apart than in a dolichocephalic breed, that is, one with a skull that is longer than it is wide [2].

The combined appearance yields a child-like face that is popular among breed enthusiasts.

Unfortunately, the cosmetic appearance of brachycephalic breeds has underlying structural consequences.

Although the length of the skull is short, the associated soft tissue structures are not proportionally reduced [9, 18, 38]. The result is excessive tissue that bulges into the airway lumen, exacerbating airway obstruction [9].

Other potential structural defects that collectively comprise so-called brachycephalic airway syndrome include the following [2, 9, 18, 26, 50–52]:

- Abnormal conchae
- Elongated soft palate
- Everted laryngeal saccules
- Laryngeal collapse
- Laryngeal edema
- Stenotic nares

Some consider hypoplastic trachea to be a part of brachycephalic airway syndrome; others consider it a separate entity [24, 42, 53, 54] (see Figure 34.3a–c).

Note that affected dogs and cats do not require all of the above structural issues to be diagnosed with brachycephalic airway syndrome.

34.3.1 Compressed Nasal Passages and Stenotic Nares

The foreshortened skull results in compressed nasal passageways among those affected with brachycephalic airway syndrome [39, 41]. In addition, many patients with brachycephalic airway syndrome have stenotic nares. Stenotic nares are narrower than would be expected. This is evident on gross inspection of the nostrils (see Figures 34.4a–d).

Stenotic nares are the most common structural defect associated with brachycephalic airway syndrome in cats [9].

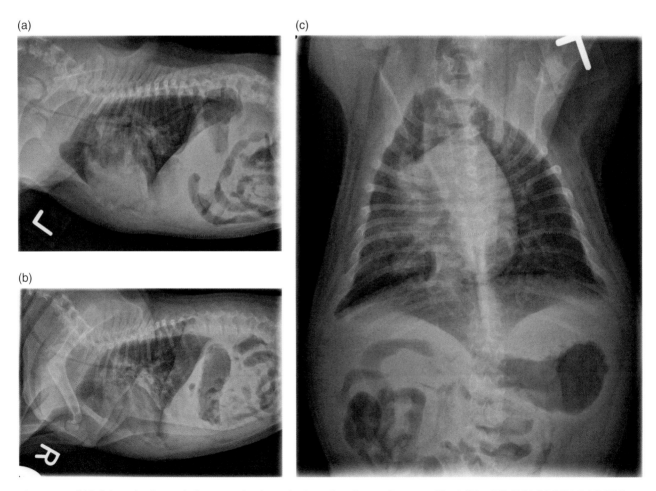

Figure 34.3 (a) Left lateral radiograph demonstrating hypoplastic trachea. *Source:* Courtesy of Daniel Foy, MS, DVM, DACVIM, DACVECC.
(b) Right lateral radiograph demonstrating hypoplastic trachea. *Source:* Courtesy of Daniel Foy, MS, DVM, DACVIM, DACVECC.
(c) Ventrodorsal (V/D) thoracic radiograph demonstrating hypoplastic trachea. *Source:* Courtesy of Daniel Foy, MS, DVM, DACVIM, DACVECC.

(a)

(b)

(c)

(d)

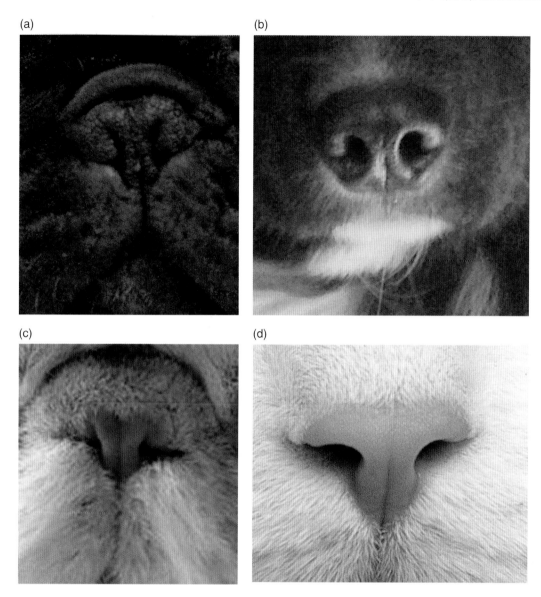

Figure 34.4 (a) Stenotic nares in a Bulldog. (b) Contrast the stenotic nares of the canine patient in Figure 34.4a with this image of normal nares. Appreciate the difference in airflow capacity through this normal dog's upper airway. (c) Stenotic nares in a Persian cat. (d). Contrast the stenotic nares of the feline patient in Figure 34.4c with this image of normal nares. Appreciate the difference in airflow capacity between cats. Recognize that the air flow would be greater through this cat's upper airway.

Stenotic nares are also common among dogs. They are present in approximately 50% of those affected with brachycephalic airway syndrome [9].

Stenotic nares vary in terms of severity. They can be so extreme as to be reduced to just a slit [39].

Regardless of severity, stenotic nares force patients to work harder during inspiration [42]. Taking in air through stenotic nares requires an increase in negative pressure during the inspiratory half of the respiratory cycle [42, 55, 56].

This increase in pressure has an impact on surrounding soft tissue structures [42]. For example, it may cause tissue to become edematous over time [42]. Inflamed tonsillar tissue is common [42].

It is possible for stenotic nares to worsen other components of brachycephalic airway syndrome [42]. For instance, the increase in negative pressure that results from stenosis may exacerbate an already elongated soft palate [42].

Increases in negative pressure may also cause laryngeal saccules to evert or laryngeal cartilages to weaken [42]. Any of these changes further narrow the lumen of the airway [42]. This increases resistance to airflow, which makes the patient have to work even harder to get air into the system [42].

Surgical reconstruction is advised in pediatric patients as early as three or four months of age to reduce the nares' contribution to upper airway pathology [43–45, 53, 57, 58].

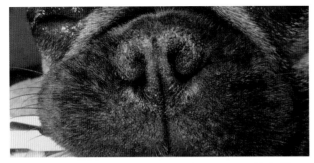

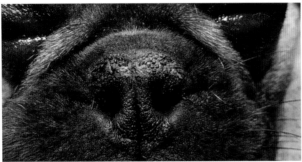

Figure 34.5 Before and after photographs of a Bulldog that underwent wedge resection as surgical management of stenotic nares. *Source:* Courtesy of Frank Isom, DVM.

Resection techniques are beyond the scope of this textbook; however, various wedge approaches have been described in the veterinary medical literature with successful cosmetic and functional outcomes [44, 57, 59] (see Figure 34.5).

34.3.2 Elongated Soft Palate

The soft palate is a normal mucosal structure [5, 40]. Anatomically, it represents the continuation of the hard palate [5, 40]. When the patient swallows, the soft palate shifts position. This functionally closes the nasopharynx so that ingesta cannot accidentally enter the airway [5, 40].

In a normal patient, with the tongue in a neutral position, the soft palate reaches the epiglottis [5, 26, 40, 60]. This can be appreciated with an anesthetized patient that has an endotracheal tube in place [57].

Many patients with brachycephalic airway syndrome have an elongated soft palate [26, 39, 42, 49, 50, 57, 61]. In other words, the structure is too large to fit within the space allotted for it. With nowhere else to stretch out, the elongated soft palate extends beyond the tip of the epiglottis [26]. This overriding structure obstructs the airway, creating increased resistance to airflow [9]. The resultant stertor can be quite loud.

Surgical management involves trimming the elongated soft palate [57]. Trimming is a trade-off between taking enough tissue to effect a change in the patient's respiratory status while not taking so much as to cause rhinitis,

sinusitis, or potentially even aspiration pneumonia [44, 45, 57–59].

Various surgical instruments and approaches have been described in the veterinary medical literature. These are beyond the scope of this textbook. Techniques typically either rely upon the traditional approach, using a scalpel blade or Metzenbaum scissors, or carbon dioxide (CO_2) laser [44, 57, 62].

Crushing and/or electrocautery are no longer advised [57]. These methods promote too much swelling in the postoperative period [44, 57, 63, 64].

34.3.3 Everted Laryngeal Saccules

Laryngeal saccules, otherwise known as laryngeal ventricles, are normal laryngeal structures in dogs [5, 40]. They sit between the lateral larynx and the vocal folds [5, 40].

In health, they are tucked up out of the way and largely hidden from view, even on a comprehensive oropharyngeal examination [42, 57].

However, the laryngeal saccules evert in approximately 50% of dogs with brachycephalic airway syndrome [42, 49, 58, 61].

Eversion of the laryngeal saccules occurs in these patients because they have developed excessive negative airway pressure in response to increased airway resistance [9]. This forces the saccules out into the airway lumen.

On oropharyngeal examination, everted saccules are whitish pink and shiny, convex pieces of tissue [18, 26, 42, 49, 57–60, 65]. These abnormally positioned structures vibrate throughout the respiratory cycle, contributing to stertor [9].

Surgical management is via resection [57]. Gentle pressure is enough to stop what minimal bleeding occurs [44, 45, 57, 58]. Wound closure is via second intention [57].

34.3.4 The Impact of Obesity on Patients with Brachycephalic Airway Syndrome

Upper respiratory obstruction caused by brachycephalic syndrome is intensified by obesity [9, 26]. This has been studied more extensively in humans; however, there is no reason to believe that a similar link does not exist in companion animal medicine [26, 66, 67].

34.3.5 The Impact of the Environment on Patients with Brachycephalic Airway Syndrome

Upper respiratory obstruction caused by brachycephalic syndrome is intensified by hot, humid weather [9, 18, 68]. This type of weather causes canine patients to pant more. These patients are already predisposed to hyperthermia on account of airway compromise [12, 13, 15,

24]. Panting may worsen airway edema, thus exacerbating resistance to airflow [9].

34.3.6 The Impact of Anxiety on Patients with Brachycephalic Airway Syndrome

Canine patients that are anxious are more likely than feline patients to pant. Because these patients have a compromised airway in terms of airflow, panting is an inefficient mechanism [12, 13, 15, 24].

Anxious patients will respond in the same way as overheated patients. They will pant to the point of respiratory distress if anxiety is not reduced or resolved.

Anxious patients are at extreme risk of worsening airway edema, and maximizing resistance to airflow [9, 29].

34.3.7 The Impact of Exercise on Patients with Brachycephalic Airway Syndrome

Exercise in moderation is beneficial to all companion animal patients. However, exercise to the point of overexertion is concerning in those patients with brachycephalic airway syndrome for the same reasons outlined above [18, 68]. These patients are ill-equipped to maximize the potential for evaporative cooling through panting. Thus, they overheat [12, 13, 15, 24].

34.4 Laryngeal Paralysis

Laryngeal paralysis is a condition in which one or both of the laryngeal arytenoid cartilages fail to abduct during the inspiratory part of the respiratory cycle [31].

Although laryngeal paralysis appears to be inherited in Siberian Huskies, Husky mixes, Dalmatians, Rottweilers, and Bouvier des Flandres, it is most often acquired later in life [9, 31]. Trauma, neoplasia, and iatrogenic nerve damage may also cause laryngeal paralysis, but these represent an isolated number of cases [31].

Acquired laryngeal paralysis is the most common form of disease that is seen in clinical practice [31]. Older large-breed dogs, such as Irish Setters, Golden Retrievers, and Labrador Retrievers, are overrepresented [8, 31, 69–73].

It is thought that affected patients have an underlying polyneuropathy [31, 70, 71, 74]. One of the sequelae includes degeneration of the recurrent laryngeal nerve, which innervates abductors of the arytenoid cartilages [31]. Without receiving the signal to contract, the cricoarytenoideus dorsalis muscle remains flaccid [31]. This causes the arytenoid cartilages to bow out into the airway lumen, where they result in obstructive airway disease.

Because the recurrent laryngeal nerve innervates other structures in the body, its degeneration is unlikely to result just in respiratory signs [31, 70, 71]. Patients may develop abnormal esophageal motility and dysphagia [31, 70, 71]. Megaesophagus and laryngeal paralysis often develop within the same patient. In these patients particularly, the potential for developing aspiration pneumonia is a significant concern [31].

In addition, affected patients may have difficulty rising from a seated position and/or have abnormal proprioception [31, 70, 71]. These neurological deficits may not be present initially, when patients present for respiratory distress [31]. However, they typically develop within one to three years of patients being diagnosed with laryngeal paralysis because degeneration of the recurrent laryngeal nerve is progressive [31].

Diagnosis is through gross observation of the larynx [31, 75]. This inspection requires a light plane of anesthesia in order for the patient to tolerate displacement of the epiglottis via laryngoscope for visualization of the larynx [31].

One concern about anesthesia is that it can potentially create false positives [31]. Anesthetic planes that are inadvertently too deep will not allow for complete abduction of the arytenoid cartilages. This may result in an erroneous diagnosis of laryngeal paralysis [31].

Watching for gag and swallowing reflexes are helpful ways of determining that the patient is in the correct plane of anesthesia to make a clinical assessment [31].

If the patient is taking shallow breaths, then the arytenoid cartilages will not naturally abduct to their maximal potential. This can make diagnosing true laryngeal paralysis challenging. Administration of doxapram in these shallow breathers may be necessary to stimulate maximum respiration [31, 76]. If under the influence of doxapram the patient is still not abducting the arytenoid cartilages, then laryngeal paralysis is real as opposed to artifactual.

Patients with laryngeal paralysis often present on emergency for stridor and/or cyanosis [31]. Up until the acute episode, patients may have appeared to be stable [31]. It is often excitement, exercise, or heat stress that causes decompensation [8, 31].

Sedation is critical to the management of laryngeal paralysis patients that present in acute crisis [8]. Some patients may benefit from anesthesia with propofol in order for them to become eupneic [8]. However, not all patients can be extubated and recovered safely without relapsing back into crisis [8]. These patients benefit from a tracheostomy to bypass upper airway obstruction [8, 31]. A tracheostomy is when a stoma, that is, a surgically created hole, is inserted into the trachea to create an alternate route for airflow.

Long-term management of laryngeal paralysis involves surgical manipulation of the larynx. Although many procedures have been described, unilateral arytenoid lateralization is commonly performed [32, 36]. This involves suturing the caudodorsal cricoid cartilage to the muscular process of the arytenoid cartilage.

This strategic placement of suture aims to make up for the dysfunctional cricoarytenoideus dorsalis muscle [32]. Although the suture cannot open and close the airway as would a fully functioning cricoarytenoideus dorsalis muscle, it does maintain patency of the airway lumen by keeping one arytenoid cartilage permanently rotated laterally [32].

Aspiration pneumonia is a potential surgical complication that could result from this procedure [32].

Depending upon the study that is consulted, as many as one in four patients may develop postoperative aspiration pneumonia [32, 72, 76–78]. The risk for aspiration pneumonia persists throughout the patient's life [32].

Because bilateral cricoarytenoid lateralization would potentiate the risk for aspiration pneumonia, only unilateral cricoarytenoid lateralization is typically pursued [32].

Cats may also develop laryngeal paralysis [34]. The same approach to treatment can be employed [34].

34.5 Tracheal Collapse

The trachea, or windpipe, is the link between the upper and lower airways, the larynx and the lungs [5, 40]. It can be thought of as a flexible, yet sturdy tube.

Tracheal patency is maintained by 35–45 C-shaped cartilaginous rings [5, 40, 79–81]. Dorsally, these rings are connected by the trachealis muscle [5, 40, 79–81].

In health, these C-shaped rings prop the trachea open [5, 40].

Tracheal collapse occurs when there is increased laxity of the trachealis muscle [79]. This can occur focally, or it may involve the entire length of the trachea [79].

At the affected site(s), the tracheal lumen loses its shape with each breath [79]. Because the disease is progressive, over time the C-shaped rings become ovoid [79]. In addition, because the rings lose their connection to each other through the trachealis muscle, their spacing becomes compromised [79]. They start to spread out.

Ring shape continues to be altered until the affected rings flatten out dorsoventrally [79]. Eventually, there is no shape left to maintain, and the trachea collapses [79]. If the trachea remains fully collapsed, the patient will develop acute respiratory distress [79].

Small-to-toy canine breeds, such as Pomeranians, Yorkshire Terriers, Chihuahuas, and Toy Poodles, are overrepresented in the veterinary medical literature [79]. Although less commonly reported, cats may also develop tracheal collapse [79].

The etiology of tracheal collapse is unknown [79]. Affected dogs have abnormally low cell counts within the affected cartilaginous rings [82–84]. There is likely to be a genetic component [79, 80].

Obesity may predispose patients to or aggravate tracheal collapse [79].

Environmental factors, such as pollution, allergens, and a history of canine infectious respiratory disease, have also been considered as potential contributing factors [79, 80, 82, 85].

(a)

(b)

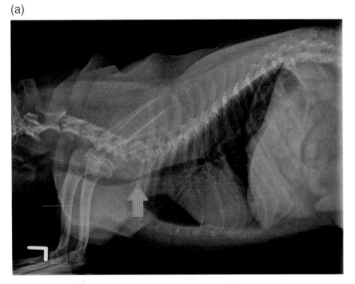
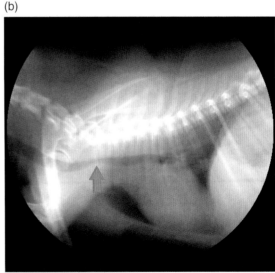

Figure 34.6 (a) This lateral radiograph is confirmatory for a diagnosis of tracheal collapse. *Source:* Courtesy of Daniel Foy, MS, DVM, DACVIM, DACVECC. (b) Confirmation of tracheal collapse via fluoroscopy. *Source:* Courtesy of Daniel Foy, MS, DVM, DACVIM, DACVECC.

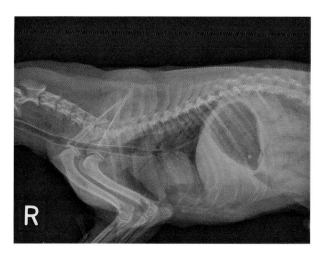

Figure 34.7 Canine patient with a tracheal stent. Lateral thoracic radiograph provided. *Source:* Courtesy of Daniel Foy, MS, DVM, DACVIM, DACVECC.

Patients classically present for an intermittent cough that sounds like a "goose honk" [79]. Clients may report that the cough worsens with excitement, activity, eating, drinking, and any form of tracheal pressure, such as pulling against a collar and leash [79].

This cough may be elicited on physical examination by tracheal palpation [79].

Imaging is required to obtain a definitive diagnosis [79]. Survey radiography with orthogonal views of the thorax, including the cervical region, is a typical starting point in clinical practice [79]. Fluoroscopy is more likely to be available in referral hospitals [79]. Either modality is appropriate (see Figures 34.6a, b).

During inspiration, tracheal collapse is more readily apparent in the cervical region; during expiration, tracheal collapse is more readily apparent in the thoracic region [79].

Tracheoscopy is considered the gold standard for diagnosis; however, availability is limited, and general anesthesia is required [79].

Medical management of tracheal collapse is typically pursued, at least initially [79]. This may involve combination therapy including, but not limited to the following [30]:

- Antitussives, such as hydrocodone, butorphanol, or codeine
- Bronchodilators, such as theophylline, in patients with concurrent bronchitis
- Sedatives, such as acepromazine, as needed, but not in patients with concurrent heart disease
- Systemic steroid therapy, such as prednisone, to reduce tracheal mucosal irritation
- Systemic antibiotic therapy for secondary, opportunistic bacterial infections

Antibiotic therapy is commonplace in patients with tracheal collapse because their abnormal tracheal structure impairs mucociliary clearance of pathogens [30].

In the event that medical management fails, the trachea may undergo surgical placement of extraluminal prosthetic support rings or intraluminal stents [33, 79, 86–88] (see Figure 34.7).

Consult a surgical textbook for the advantages and disadvantages of each approach.

34.6 Tracheostomy as an Intervention for Upper Airway Obstruction

The concept of a tracheostomy was first introduced as a temporary means of dealing with acute respiratory crisis in patients with laryngeal paralysis [8, 31]. The advantage of a tracheostomy is that it allows the patient to bypass upper airway obstruction and achieve lower resistance to airflow [89].

In addition to their use in cases of laryngeal paralysis, temporary tracheostomies are appropriate when traumatic injuries or space-occupying lesions occlude the upper airways [15, 80, 89–94].

There are select cases when tracheostomies may need to become permanent. This may be due to progressing neoplasia or severely affected patients with brachycephalic airway syndrome [89]. These patients can lead fully functional lives once they heal (see Figures 34.8a–d).

Patients with tracheostomies have only one lifestyle change that is a must: they cannot go swimming. The stoma will allow water unrestricted access to the airway. The patient would, in effect, drown.

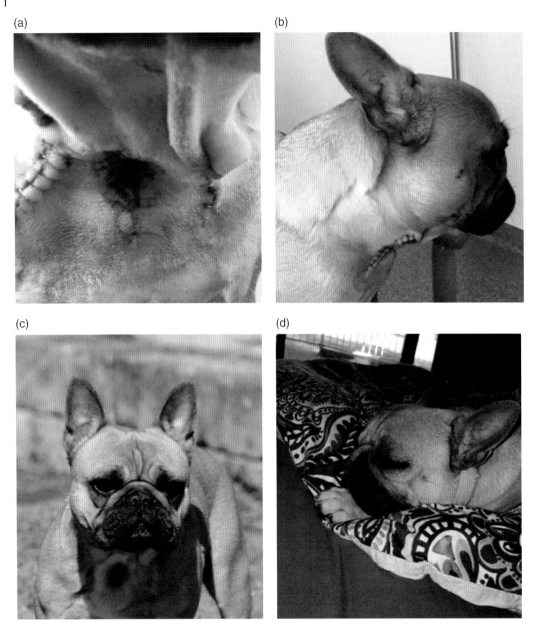

Figure 34.8 (a) Canine patient in the immediate postoperative period following permanent tracheostomy. (b) Side view of canine patient in the immediate postoperative period following permanent tracheostomy. (c) Canine patient fully healed, following permanent tracheostomy. (d) Canine patient fully healed, following permanent tracheostomy. According to the patient's owner, the tracheostomy site does not adversely impact the dog's comfort.

References

1 Stokhof, A.A. and Venker-van Haagen, A.J. (2009). Respiratory system. In: *Medical History and Physical Examination in Companion Animals* (ed. A. Rijnberk and F.J. van Sluijs), 63–74. Philadelphia: Saunders Elsevier.

2 Englar, R.E. (2017). *Performing the Small Animal Physical Examination*. Hoboken, NJ: Wiley.

3 Elie, M. and Sabo, M. (2006). Basics in canine and feline rhinoscopy. *Clin. Tech. Small Anim. Pract.* 21 (2): 60–63.

4 Grandage, J. (2003). Functional anatomy of the respiratory system. In: *Textbook of Small Animal Surgery* (ed. D.H. Slatter), 763–780. Philadelphia, PA: Saunders.

5 Singh, B. and Dyce, K.M. (2018). *Dyce, Sack, and Wensing's Textbook of Veterinary Anatomy*, 5e. St. Louis, Missouri: Saunders.

6 Evans, H.E. and Miller, M.E. (1993). *Miller's Anatomy of the Dog*, 3e, xvi, 1113 p. Philadelphia: W.B. Saunders.

7 Labuc R, editor. (2017). The approach to nasal discharge in the dog. The 8th Annual Vet Education International Online Veterinary Conference.

8 Rozanski, E. and Chan, D.L. (2005). Approach to the patient with respiratory distress. *Vet. Clin. North Am. Small Anim. Pract.* 35 (2): 307–317.

9 Tilley, L.P. and Smith, F.W.K. (2004). *The 5-minute Veterinary Consult: Canine and Feline*, 3e. Baltimore, MD: Lippincott Williams & Wilkins.

10 Rand, J. and Mason, R.A. (2006). The cat with stridor or stertor. In: *Problem-based Feline Medicine* (ed. J. Rand), 32–46. Philadelphia: Elsevier Limited.

11 Lappin, M.R. (2001). *Feline Internal Medicine Secrets*. Philadelphia: Hanley & Belfus, Inc.

12 Sharp, C.R. and Rozanski, E.A. (2013). Physical examination of the respiratory system. *Top. Companion Anim. Med.* 28 (3): 79–85.

13 King L. (2008). Managing upper airway obstruction in dogs. DVM 360 [Internet]. http://veterinarycalendar.dvm360.com/managing-upper-airway-obstruction-dogs-proceedings.

14 Sigrist, N.E., Adamik, K.N., Doherr, M.G., and Spreng, D.E. (2011). Evaluation of respiratory parameters at presentation as clinical indicators of the respiratory localization in dogs and cats with respiratory distress. *J. Vet. Emerg. Crit. Care (San Antonio)* 21 (1): 13–23.

15 Sumner, C. and Rozanski, E. (2013). Management of respiratory emergencies in small animals. *Vet. Clin. North Am. Small Anim. Pract.* 43 (4): 799–815.

16 Defarges, A. (2015). The physical examination. *NAVC Clinician's Brief* (September): 73–80.

17 Starybrat, D. and Tappin, S. (2016). Approaching the dysnoeic cat in the middle of the night. *Vet. Ir. J.* 6 (1): 37–43.

18 Fasanella, F.J., Shivley, J.M., Wardlaw, J.L., and Givaruangsawat, S. (2010). Brachycephalic airway obstructive syndrome in dogs: 90 cases (1991–2008). *J. Am. Vet. Med. Assoc.* 237 (9): 1048–1051.

19 Crawford, E.C. Jr. (1962). Mechanical aspects of panting in dogs. *J. Appl. Physiol.* 17: 249–251.

20 Schmidt-Nielsen, K., Bretz, W.L., and Taylor, C.R. (1970). Panting in dogs: unidirectional air flow over evaporative surfaces. *Science* 169 (3950): 1102–1104.

21 Blatt, C.M., Taylor, C.R., and Habal, M.B. (1972). Thermal panting in dogs: the lateral nasal gland, a source of water for evaporative cooling. *Science* 177 (4051): 804–805.

22 Goldberg, M.B., Langman, V.A., and Taylor, C.R. (1981). Panting in dogs: paths of air flow in response to heat and exercise. *Respir. Physiol.* 43 (3): 327–338.

23 Allen, H.S., Broussard, J., and Noone, K. (1999). Nasopharyngeal diseases in cats: a retrospective study of 53 cases (1991–1998). *J. Am. Anim. Hosp. Assoc.* 35 (6): 457–461.

24 Sharp, C.R. (2015). Approach to respiratory distress in dogs and cats. *Today's Veterinary Practice* (November/December): 53–60.

25 Burrow RD, editor. (2008). Approach to investigation of nasal disease. British Small Animal Veterinary Congress.

26 Miller, J. and Gannon, K. (2015). Perioperative management of brachycephalic dogs. *NAVC Clinician's Brief* (April): 54–59.

27 Klocke E. (2014). CVC highlight: The hunt for grass awns. DVM 360 [Internet]. http://veterinarymedicine.dvm360.com/cvc-highlight-hunt-grass-awns.

28 Ford RB, editor. (2005). Upper respiratory diseases in dogs. World Small Animal Veterinary Association World Congress Proceedings.

29 Phillips, H. (2016). Brachycephalic syndrome. *NAVC Clinician's Brief* (September).

30 Linklater, A. (2018). Tracheal collapse in dogs. *Plumb's Therapeutics Brief* (February): 46–57.

31 Mankin, K.T. (2015). Laryngeal paralysis diagnosis. *NAVC Clinician's Brief* (December): 67–71.

32 Mankin, K.T. (2015). Laryngeal paralysis surgery. *NAVC Clinician's Brief* (December): 73–79.

33 Moritz, A., Schneider, M., and Bauer, N. (2004). Management of advanced tracheal collapse in dogs using intraluminal self-expanding biliary wallstents. *J. Vet. Intern. Med.* 18 (1): 31–42.

34 Hardie, R.J., Gunby, J., and Bjorling, D.E. (2009). Arytenoid lateralization for treatment of laryngeal paralysis in 10 cats. *Vet. Surg.* 38 (4): 445–451.

35 Johnson, L.R. and Pollard, R.E. (2010). Tracheal collapse and bronchomalacia in dogs: 58 cases (7/2001-1/2008). *J. Vet. Intern. Med.* 24 (2): 298–305.

36 Nelissen, P. and White, R.A. (2012). Arytenoid lateralization for management of combined laryngeal paralysis and laryngeal collapse in small dogs. *Vet. Surg.* 41 (2): 261–265.

37 Sharp, C.R. (2012). Feline rhinitis and upper respiratory disease. *Today's Veterinary Practice* (July/August): 14–20.

38 Wykes, P.M. (1991). Brachycephalic airway obstructive syndrome. *Probl. Vet. Med.* 3 (2): 188–197.

39 Dupre, G. and Heidenreich, D. (2016). Brachycephalic syndrome. *Vet. Clin. North Am. Small Anim. Pract.* 46 (4): 691–707.

40 Evans, H.E. and Miller, M.E. (2013). *Miller's Anatomy of the Dog*, 4e, xix, 850 p. St. Louis, Missouri: Elsevier.

41 Schuenemann, R. and Oechtering, G.U. (2014). Inside the brachycephalic nose: intranasal mucosal contact points. *J. Am. Anim. Hosp. Assoc.* 50 (3): 149–158.

42 Trappler, M. and Moore, K. (2011). Canine brachycephalic airway syndrome: pathophysiology, diagnosis, and nonsurgical management. *Compend. Contin. Educ. Vet.* 33 (5): E1-4; quiz E5.

43 Hedlund, C.S. (1998). Brachycephalic syndrome. In: *Current Techniques in Small Animal Surgery* (ed. M.J. Bojrab), 357–362. Philadelphia: Williams & Wilkins.

44 Hedlund, C.S. (2002). Stenotic nares. In: *Small Animal Surgery* (ed. T.W. Fossum), 727–730. St. Louis: Mosby.

45 Hendricks, J.C. (1992). Brachycephalic airway syndrome. *Vet. Clin. North Am. Small Anim. Pract.* 22 (5): 1145–1153.

46 Hobson, H.P. (1995). Brachycephalic syndrome. *Semin. Vet. Med. Surg.* 10 (2): 109–114.

47 Asher, L., Diesel, G., Summers, J.F. et al. (2009). Inherited defects in pedigree dogs. Part 1: disorders related to breed standards. *Vet. J.* 182 (3): 402–411.

48 Meola, S.D. (2013). Brachycephalic airway syndrome. *Top. Companion Anim. Med.* 28 (3): 91–96.

49 Riecks, T.W., Birchard, S.J., and Stephens, J.A. (2007). Surgical correction of brachycephalic syndrome in dogs: 62 cases (1991–2004). *J. Am. Vet. Med. Assoc.* 230 (9): 1324–1328.

50 Ginn, J.A., Kumar, M.S.A., McKiernan, B.C., and Powers, B.E. (2008). Nasopharyngeal turbinates in brachycephalic dogs and cats. *J. Am. Anim. Hosp. Assoc.* 44 (5): 243–249.

51 Koch, D.A., Arnold, S., Hubler, M., and Montavon, P.M. (2003). Brachycephalic syndrome in dogs. *Compend. Contin. Educ. Pract.* 25 (1): 48–55.

52 Findji, L. and Dupre, G. (2013). Brachycephalic syndrome: innovative surgical techniques. *NAVC Clinician's Brief* (June): 79–85.

53 Huck, J.L., Stanley, B.J., and Hauptman, J.G. (2008). Technique and outcome of nares amputation (Trader's technique) in immature shih tzus. *J. Am. Anim. Hosp. Assoc.* 44 (2): 82–85.

54 Coyne, B.E. and Fingland, R.B. (1992). Hypoplasia of the trachea in dogs: 103 cases (1974–1990). *J. Am. Vet. Med. Assoc.* 201 (5): 768–772.

55 Aron, D.N. and Crowe, D.T. (1985). Upper airway obstruction. General principles and selected conditions in the dog and cat. *Vet. Clin. North Am. Small Anim. Pract.* 15 (5): 891–917.

56 Robinson, N.E. (1992). Airway physiology. *Vet. Clin. North Am. Small Anim. Pract.* 22 (5): 1043–1064.

57 Trappler, M. and Moore, K. (2011). Canine brachycephalic airway syndrome: surgical management. *Compend. Contin. Educ. Vet.* 33 (5): E1-7; quiz E8.

58 Poncet, C.M., Dupre, G.P., Freiche, V.G. et al. (2005). Prevalence of gastrointestinal tract lesions in 73 brachycephalic dogs with upper respiratory syndrome. *J. Small Anim. Pract.* 46 (6): 273–279.

59 Monnet, E. (2003). Brachycephalic airway syndrome. In: *Textbook of Small Animal Surgery* (ed. D. Slatter), 808–813. Philadelphia: WB Saunders.

60 Harvey, C.E. (1982). Upper airway obstruction surgery: everted laryngeal saccule surgery in brachycephalic dogs. *J. Am. Anim. Hosp. Assoc.* 18: 545–547.

61 Torrez, C.V. and Hunt, G.B. (2006). Results of surgical correction of abnormalities associated with brachycephalic airway obstruction syndrome in dogs in Australia. *J. Small Anim. Pract.* 47 (3): 150–154.

62 Davidson, E.B., Davis, M.S., Campbell, G.A. et al. (2001). Evaluation of carbon dioxide laser and conventional incisional techniques for resection of soft palates in brachycephalic dogs. *J. Am. Vet. Med. Assoc.* 219 (6): 776–781.

63 Clark, G.N. and Sinibaldi, K.R. (1994). Use of a carbon dioxide laser for treatment of elongated soft palate in dogs. *J. Am. Vet. Med. Assoc.* 204 (11): 1779–1781.

64 Bjorling, D., McAnulty, J., and Swainson, S. (2000). Surgically treatable upper respiratory disorders. *Vet. Clin. North Am. Small Anim. Pract.* 30 (6): 1227–1251, vi.

65 Ellison, G.W. (2004). Alapexy: an alternative technique for repair of stenotic nares in dogs. *J. Am. Anim. Hosp. Assoc.* 40 (6): 484–489.

66 Patil, S.P., Schneider, H., Schwartz, A.R., and Smith, P.L. (2007). Adult obstructive sleep apnea: pathophysiology and diagnosis. *Chest* 132 (1): 325–337.

67 Schwartz, A.R., Patil, S.P., Laffan, A.M. et al. (2008). Obesity and obstructive sleep apnea: pathogenic mechanisms and therapeutic approaches. *Proc. Am. Thorac. Soc.* 5 (2): 185–192.

68 Bach, J.F., Rozanski, E.A., Bedenice, D. et al. (2007). Association of expiratory airway dysfunction with marked obesity in healthy adult dogs. *Am. J. Vet. Res.* 68 (6): 670–675.

69 Monnet, E. and Tobias, K.M. (2012). Larynx. In: *Small Animal Veterinary Surgery* (ed. K.M. Tobias and S.A. Johnson), 1724–1731. Elsevier Saunders: St. Louis, MO.

70 Stanley, B.J., Hauptman, J.G., Fritz, M.C. et al. (2010). Esophageal dysfunction in dogs with idiopathic laryngeal paralysis: a controlled cohort study. *Vet. Surg.* 39 (2): 139–149.

71 Thieman, K.M., Krahwinkel, D.J., Sims, M.H., and Shelton, G.D. (2010). Histopathological confirmation of polyneuropathy in 11 dogs with laryngeal paralysis. *J. Am. Anim. Hosp. Assoc.* 46 (3): 161–167.

72 Bahr, K.L., Howe, L., Jessen, C., and Goodrich, Z. (2014). Outcome of 45 dogs with laryngeal paralysis treated by unilateral arytenoid lateralization or bilateral ventriculocordectomy. *J. Am. Anim. Hosp. Assoc.* 50 (4): 264–272.

73 von Pfeil, D.J., Edwards, M.R., and Dejardin, L.M. (2014). Less invasive unilateral arytenoid lateralization: a modified technique for treatment of idiopathic laryngeal paralysis in dogs: technique description and outcome. *Vet. Surg.* 43 (6): 704–711.

74 Jeffery, N.D., Talbot, C.E., Smith, P.M., and Bacon, N.J. (2006). Acquired idiopathic laryngeal paralysis as a prominent feature of generalised neuromuscular disease in 39 dogs. *Vet. Rec.* 158 (1): 17.

75 Jackson, A.M., Tobias, K., Long, C. et al. (2004). Effects of various anesthetic agents on laryngeal motion during laryngoscopy in normal dogs. *Vet. Surg.* 33 (2): 102–106.

76 MacPhail, C.M. and Monnet, E. (2001). Outcome of and postoperative complications in dogs undergoing surgical treatment of laryngeal paralysis: 140 cases (1985–1998). *J. Am. Vet. Med. Assoc.* 218 (12): 1949–1956.

77 Hammel, S.P., Hottinger, H.A., and Novo, R.E. (2006). Postoperative results of unilateral arytenoid lateralization for treatment of idiopathic laryngeal paralysis in dogs: 39 cases (1996–2002). *J. Am. Vet. Med. Assoc.* 228 (8): 1215–1220.

78 Snelling, S.R. and Edwards, G.A. (2003). A retrospective study of unilateral arytenoid lateralisation in the treatment of laryngeal paralysis in 100 dogs (1992–2000). *Aust. Vet. J.* 81 (8): 464–468.

79 Deweese, M.D. and Tobias, K.M. (2014). Tracheal collapse in dogs. *NAVC Clinician's Brief* (May): 83–87.

80 Sura, P. and Durant, A. (2012). Trachea and bronchi. In: *Veterinary Surgery: Small Animal* (ed. K.M. Tobias and S.A. Johnson), 1734–1750. St. Louis: Saunders Elsevier.

81 Ettinger, S.J. (2010). Diseases of the trachea and upper airways. In: *Textbook of Veterinary Internal Medicine* (ed. S.J. Ettinger and E.C. Feldman), 1066. St. Louis: Saunders Elsevier.

82 White, R.A.S. and Williams, J.M. (1994). Tracheal collapse in the dog – is there really a role for surgery – a survey of 100 cases. *J. Small Anim. Pract.* 35 (4): 191–196.

83 Dallman, M.J. and Brown, E.M. (1984). Statistical-analysis of selected tracheal measurements in normal dogs and dogs with collapsed trachea. *Am. J. Vet. Res.* 45 (5): 1033–1037.

84 Dallman, M.J., Mcclure, R.C., and Brown, E.M. (1988). Histochemical-study of normal and collapsed tracheas in dogs. *Am. J. Vet. Res.* 49 (12): 2117–2125.

85 Oskouizadeh, K., Selk-Ghafari, M., and Zahraei-Salehi, T. (2011). Isolation of Bordetella bronchiseptica in a dog with tracheal collapse. *Comp. Clin. Path.* 20: 527–529.

86 Buback, J.L., Boothe, H.W., and Hobson, H.P. (1996). Surgical treatment of tracheal collapse in dogs: 90 cases (1983–1993). *J. Am. Vet. Med. Assoc.* 208 (3): 380–384.

87 Tangner, C.H. and Hobson, H.P. (1982). A retrospective study of 20 surgically managed cases of collapsed trachea. *Vet. Surg.* 11 (4): 146–149.

88 Chisnell, H.K. and Pardo, A.D. (2015). Long-term outcome, complications and disease progression in 23 dogs after placement of tracheal ring prostheses for treatment of extrathoracic tracheal collapse. *Vet. Surg.* 44 (1): 103–113.

89 Caron, A. (2016). Temporary tracheostomy in dogs. *NAVC Clinician's Brief* (April): 18–24.

90 Pink, J.J. (2006). Intramural tracheal haematoma causing acute respiratory obstruction in a dog. *J. Small Anim. Pract.* 47 (3): 161–164.

91 Jordan, C.J., Halfacree, Z.J., and Tivers, M.S. (2013). Airway injury associated with cervical bite wounds in dogs and cats: 56 cases. *Vet. Comp. Orthop. Traumatol.* 26 (2): 89–93.

92 Jakubiak, M.J., Siedlecki, C.T., Zenger, E. et al. (2005). Laryngeal, laryngotracheal, and tracheal masses in cats: 27 cases (1998–2003). *J. Am. Anim. Hosp. Assoc.* 41 (5): 310–316.

93 Guenther-Yenke, C.L. and Rozanski, E.A. (2007). Tracheostomy in cats: 23 cases (1998–2006). *J. Feline Med. Surg.* 9 (6): 451–457.

94 Nicholson, I. and Baines, S. (2012). Complications associated with temporary tracheostomy tubes in 42 dogs (1998 to 2007). *J. Small Anim. Pract.* 53 (2): 108–114.

35

Sneezing and Coughing

35.1 Introduction to Sneezing and Coughing as Protective Reflexes

Sneezing is an involuntary, audible action that causes air to be exhaled forcefully through the nose. Sneezing is typically triggered by irritation of the nasal passageways, specifically the nasal mucosa [1]. Irritation can be secondary to particulate matter, such as dust, that settles into the upper airway [1]. Irritation can also be the result of chemical stimulation or inflammation [1].

Sneezing is a protective mechanism, designed to expel the source of the irritation from the upper airway [1–3].

When sneezing occurs, it may be dry or it may be paired with nasal discharge [1]. Review Chapter 33, Sections 33.2 and 33.3 to recall normal versus abnormal classifications of nasal discharge.

Coughing is also an audible, forceful expelling of air, only it occurs through the glottis rather than the nose [1, 4, 5]. Immediately preceding a cough, the patient reflexively inspires [1, 4, 5]. The glottis then closes, allowing intrathoracic pressure to raise [1, 4, 5]. Now the glottis opens and the cough commences [1, 4, 5]. This creates a powerful exhalation that is designed to expel foreign material from the upper airway [1–5].

The coughing reflex is typically triggered by either those nerve fibers associated with the glossopharyngeal or vagus nerves [1]. The former are located within the pharynx itself, whereas the latter reside within the larynx, trachea, and large bronchi [1, 6].

A cough that originates in the larynx may be associated with gagging or retching [1, 3].

Coughs may be further characterized as being wet or dry [3]. Wet coughs are associated with excessive amounts of airway secretions, such as mucus [3]. They are also often productive coughs, that is, they are more likely to produce sputum [3].

Tracheal and bronchial coughs tend to be dry in the initial, acute phase [3]. However, if these coughs become chronic, then they are more likely to become productive [3].

Sputum is not always visible to the veterinary client or clinician [3]. More often than not, it is swallowed as soon as it is coughed up [3].

35.2 Introduction to Reverse Sneezing

Reverse sneezing is an unusual phenomenon that occurs primarily in the dog [3]. In the author's experience, it is seen more frequently in clinical practice in brachycephalic breeds.

Sometimes, reverse sneezing is referred to as backward sneezing or paroxysmal respiration. It describes a respiratory event that is best characterized as a pharyngeal spasm [3]. The patient exhibits repeated, rapid inspiratory attempts that may be accompanied by stertor. The patient may extend its head and neck as if dyspneic [3].

The cycle may last seconds to minutes [3]. A veterinary client who has never before witnessed such an event may become alarmed that the patient has developed respiratory distress [7].

The cycle may be interrupted by massaging the patient's throat, blowing air gently in the patient's face, or gently occluding the dog's nostrils [3]. These actions encourage the patient to swallow, which short-circuits the cycle of reverse sneezing.

Patients that have one episode of reverse sneezing are prone to having more throughout life.

Particulate matter is likely to trigger an episode [7]. Other causes of reverse sneezes include the following [7–11]:

- Foreign bodies, such as grass awns
- Growths associated with the nasal passageways, including nasal polyps
- Nasal parasitism by such organisms as capillarid nematodes, *Capillaria boehmi*

35.2.1 Nasal Polyps in Dogs

Nasopharyngeal polyps were previously discussed concerning their frequent occurrence in young adult cats. Refer to Chapter 18, Section 18.3.2.4, Chapter 32, Section 32.5, and Chapter 33, Section 33.6.

Nasal polyps are less common in dogs, and may or may not be associated with mycotic airway disease [8, 12–16]. However, these thickenings of the canine nasal mucosa act as mechanical obstructions to airflow [8]. Affected patients often present for repeated bouts of reverse sneezing, with or without nasal discharge [8]. Patients may also demonstrate stertor and intermittent epistaxis [8]. Physical examination may reveal reduced airflow through the affected nare(s), but this is not a consistent finding among affected patients [8].

Soft tissue lesions are evident on computed tomography (CT) [8]. They may be focal or expansive. Rhinotomy is indicated for symptomatic patients; however, recurrence is possible [8, 17].

35.2.2 Nasal Capillariosis in Dogs

Capillaria boehmi is one of several capillarid nematodes that reside in the nasal turbinates and sinus cavities of North American and European foxes and wolves [9, 18–21].

Capillaria boehmi occurs sporadically in domestic dogs [9, 20–25]. That being said, the incidence appears to be on the rise [9–11].

Although some dogs develop subclinical infections, nasal capillariosis more typically induces rhinitis secondary to nasal turbinate damage [9]. Clinical signs that are associated with nematode-induced rhinitis include nasal discharge and reverse sneezing [9–11].

Dogs may also present with client complaints about their diminished sense of smell [9, 20, 21, 24–26].

Diagnosis is via detection of *Capillaria boehmi* eggs on fecal cytology and/or *Capillaria boehmi* DNA via polymerase chain reaction (PCR) analysis of rhinoscopy-obtained nasal biopsies [9].

Spot-on formulations, including imidacloprid/moxidectin combination therapy, appear to be effective against nasal capillariosis; however, this currently represents an off-label use [9–11].

35.3 Introduction to Diseases that Cause Sneezing

Although sneezing is the body's reflexive mechanism to cleanse the airway of debris, sneezing is also a clinical sign that may be associated with upper airway pathology [1, 3, 27].

Although it is not exhaustive, the following list represents the most common pathological causes of sneezing in companion animal medicine [1, 3, 27–48]:

- Allergic rhinitis (refer to Chapter 33, Section 33.6)
- Chronic inflammatory rhinitis or lymphoplasmacytic rhinitis (LPR) (refer to Chapter 33, Section 33.6)
- Congenital defect
  - Cleft palate (refer to Chapter 33, Section 33.8)
- Epistaxis (refer to Chapter 33, Section 33.3.2)
  - Coagulopathy
  - Hypertension
  - Thrombocytopenia
  - Vasculitis
- Foreign body obstruction, partial or complete
  - Grass awn
  - Other plant material
- Infectious disease (refer to Chapter 33, Section 33.5)
  - Bacterial
    - Actinomyces spp.
    - Bordetella bronchiseptica (refer to Chapter 27, Section 27.3.5 for feline conjunctivitis)
    - Chlamydophila felis, the causative agent of chlamydiosis (refer to Chapter 27, Section 27.3.2 for feline conjunctivitis)
    - Mycoplasma felis
    - Mycoplasma gatae
  - Viral
    - Canine infectious respiratory disease (CIRD) (refer to Chapter 33, Section 33.5.1)
    - Feline calicivirus (refer to Chapter 27, Section 27.3.4)
    - Feline herpesvirus-1 (FHV-1) (refer to Chapter 27, Section 27.3.1)
  - Fungal
    - Aspergillosis
    - Coccidioidomycosis
    - Cryptococcosis
- Nasal neoplasia (refer to Chapter 33, Section 33.7)
  - Adenocarcinoma
  - Lymphoma
  - Sarcoma
  - Mast cell tumor
  - Melanoma
  - Plasma cell tumor
- Nasal parasites
  - Cuterebriasis (refer to Chapter 6, Section 6.3)
  - *Linguatula serrata*, feline
  - Nasal capillariasis (refer to Section 35.2.2)
  - Pneumonyssoides, canine
- Polypoid mass
  - Nasal polyp, canine (refer to Section 35.2.1)
  - Nasopharyngeal polyp, feline (refer to Chapter 18, Section 18.3.2.4, Chapter 32, Section 32.5, and Chapter 33, Section 33.6)

Two etiologies will be discussed in detail here, in light of their morbidity and the frequency with which they occur in clinical practice.

The rest of these differential diagnoses have been previously addressed. For more information, please refer to the aforementioned sections and supplement the material as needed with an internal medicine and/or infectious disease text.

35.3.1 Bordetella bronchiseptica

Recall from Chapter 33, Section 33.5.1 that CIRD is a complex of bacterial and viral entities that individually or collectively create airway pathology [49–52].

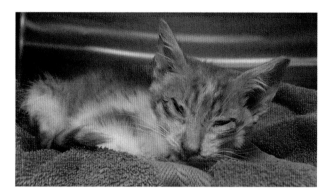

Figure 35.1 Pediatric feline patient with severe conjunctivitis and URI. Secondary infection with *Bordetella bronchiseptica* must be considered as a differential diagnosis. *Source:* Courtesy of Genevieve LaFerriere, DVM.

CIRD most often impacts those patients that are young, stressed, or immune-compromised [50, 52–55]. Other risk factors include close contact with conspecifics [50, 52–55].

All agents capable of inducing CIRD can result in nasal discharge, lethargy, and/or reduced appetite [50, 56].

In addition, one of these agents, *B. bronchiseptica*, is perhaps best known for inciting infectious tracheobronchitis (ITB), otherwise referred to as "kennel cough" [49, 50, 52].

B. bronchiseptica was first discussed in Chapter 27, Section 27.3.5 concerning its role in chronic feline conjunctivitis and concurrent upper respiratory infections (URIs) [57, 58] (see Figure 35.1).

However, "kennel cough" is by far more commonly experienced in clinical practice among canine patients.

B. bronchiseptica is a gram-negative, aerobic bacterium that often co-infects those with canine parainfluenza virus or canine adenovirus-2 (CAV-2) [59]. Effects of concurrent disease are cumulative; that is, patients develop significant clinical disease [59].

The incubation period for *B. bronchiseptica* is brief [59]. Within six days, *B. bronchiseptica* attaches to respiratory mucosa and produces toxins that inhibit mucociliary clearance [59]. This enables the bacteria to establish persistence within the airway [59]. It is not uncommon for the host to take three or more months to clear an infection with *B. bronchiseptica* from the respiratory tract [59].

(a)

(b)

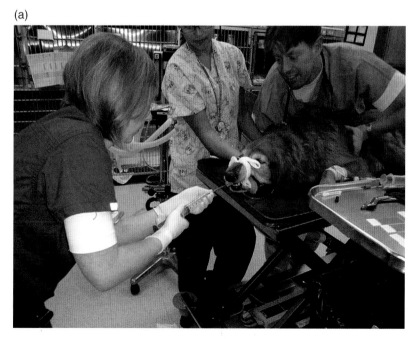

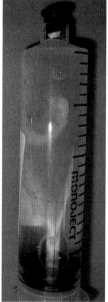

Figure 35.2 (a) Performing a transtracheal wash in a canine patient. *Source:* Courtesy of Daniel Foy, MS, DVM, DACVIM, DACVECC. (b) Sample obtained by transtracheal wash. *Source:* Courtesy of Daniel Foy, MS, DVM, DACVIM, DACVECC.

Rhinitis, nasal discharge, sneezing, and a "honking" cough are the most typical clinical signs to be associated with *B. bronchiseptica* infection [59]. However, if damage to the tracheal mucosa is severe, pneumonia may result [59].

A presumptive diagnosis is typically made based upon clinical history and response to therapy [59]. Nasopharyngeal swabs are not helpful in differentiating primary pathogens from resident flora or opportunistic invaders [59].

For diagnostic purposes, more appropriate samples may be collected from transtracheal aspirates, endotracheal or bronchoalveolar lavage for bacterial culture and susceptibility profiles [59] (see Figures 35.2a, b).

Antibiotic therapy may be prescribed out of consideration that "kennel cough" may precipitate bronchopneumonia [59]. However, the use of antibiotics is typically not necessary in uncomplicated cases, though they may shorten the duration of coughing [59].

Patients may or may not be prescribed antitussives [59]. Clients may appreciate that these medications alleviate cough, but suppressing a protective mechanism may potentially create harm [59]. Cough is an attempt by the body to discharge bacteria and associated secretions from the airway [59]. Stifling the cough reflex results in retention of those products, with potentially increased risk for bronchopneumonia [59].

Patients with excessive bronchial and tracheal secretions may benefit from aerosol therapy [59]. Nebulization with mucolytic agents, such as acetylcysteine, is no longer advised because it can worsen airway irritation [59]. However, nonabsorbable antibiotics, such as gentamicin and polymyxin B, effectively reduce bacterial populations [59].

Once recovered, patients appear to develop a natural immunity to reinfection for at least six months [59].

Prevention is not foolproof, but involves vaccination of canine patients. A number of products are available today, mostly as combination immunizations, via injectable, intranasal, and oral routes [59]. Puppies that are vaccinated by both parenteral and intranasal routes are better protected than those vaccinated by one or the other [59].

The efficacy of adult vaccinations based upon route of administration is less clear. Some argue that parenteral immunizations of adult, seropositive dogs are more protective than intranasal ones, whereas others find that intranasal vaccinations provide superior local and systemic immunity [59]. The verdict is still out.

What is agreed upon is that vaccination before potential exposures, such as kenneling, is ideal, if the timeline is logical. For example, intranasal vaccinations can be administered at least five days before exposure to see effect; however, vaccinating against "kennel cough" the day before boarding is unlikely to be effective [59].

35.3.2 Canine Influenza

Influenza is a potent respiratory virus with many types and subtypes. Canine influenza typically involves two specific varieties of influenza type A [60]:

- H3N8
- H3N2

The "H" portion of the subtype refers to the viral hemagglutinin receptor; the "N" portion refers to the viral neuraminidase receptor [60].

H3N8 was first introduced in Chapter 33, Section 33.5.1 concerning the prevalence of upper respiratory disease among sick shelter dogs versus those without clinical signs [52, 54, 61, 62].

H3N8 originated in horses, whereas H3N2 originated in birds [60]. The former was first identified in dogs in Florida, and the latter, in dogs in Korea [60, 63, 64].

With the exception of H3N2, which is capable of spreading from dogs to cats, both H3N8 and H3N2 are generally restricted to infected dogs [60].

Infection of ferrets with both strains has occurred experimentally [60, 65, 66]. Once ferrets are infected, infection can continue to spread horizontally [60, 65, 66].

Zoonosis does not appear to be a concern at this time [60, 67, 68].

Canine patients that are most at risk of contracting influenza are those at either extremes of age, the young and old, as well as those that are immunocompromised [60]. Additional risk factors include exposure to conspecifics and, in particular, overcrowding [60, 69].

Transmission is primarily via aerosol [60]. However, contact with fomites also results in spread of disease [60]. Infected patients often shed virus before they demonstrate clinical signs [60, 70].

Clinical signs include lethargy, with or without anorexia, sneezing, nasal discharge, mild cough, and fever [60].

Disease is typically mild and self-limiting [60]. Most patients respond well to supportive care, although secondary bacterial infections are common [60].

Patients may also develop pneumonia [60]. Tachypneic and/or dyspneic patients need to be watched carefully as they can decline rapidly.

Diagnosis is via viral isolation and virus-specific PCR [60]. Deep nasal, nasopharyngeal, and oropharyngeal swabs provide appropriate samples [60].

Canine vaccinations are available against H3N8 and H3N2 [60]. They may reduce clinical signs and viral shedding, which can collectively work to keep the spread of disease low among susceptible populations [60].

Note that other forms of influenza type A can cause respiratory disease in dogs, including H1N1, H3N1, H3N2, H5N1, H5N2, H5N6, H6N1, and H9N2 [60, 65, 71–77]. Whether these may become significant concerns for clinical practice in years to come remains to be determined.

35.4 Introduction to Diseases that Cause Coughing

Like sneezing, coughing is the body's reflexive mechanism to cleanse the airway of debris. Coughing is also a clinical sign that may be associated with upper or lower airway pathology [1].

Although it is not exhaustive, the following list represents the most common pathological causes of coughing in companion animal medicine [1, 78–97]:

- Upper respiratory tract diseases
  - Foreign body obstruction, partial or complete
    - ○ Nasopharyngeal
    - ○ Laryngeal
    - ○ Tracheal
  - Inhalation of irritants
    - ○ Dust particles
    - ○ Gas
    - ○ Hair
    - ○ Litter (cats)
    - ○ Pollen
    - ○ Smoke
  - ITB (refer to Section 35.3.1 above)
  - Laryngeal paralysis (refer to Chapter 34, Section 34.4)
  - Neoplasia
    - ○ Nasopharyngeal
    - ○ Laryngeal
    - ○ Tracheal
  - Polypoid mass
    - ○ Nasal polyp, canine (refer to Section 35.2.1 above)
    - ○ Nasopharyngeal polyp, feline (refer to Chapter 18, Section 18.3.2.4, Chapter 32, Section 32.5, and Chapter 33, Section 33.6)
  - Rhinitis and sinorhinitis with post-nasal drip
  - Tracheal collapse (refer to Chapter 34, Section 34.5)
- Lower respiratory tract diseases
  - Feline asthma/bronchitis complex
  - Bronchitis
  - Foreign body obstruction, partial or complete
    - ○ Bronchial

- ITB (refer to Section 35.3.1 above)
- Neoplasia
  - ○ Primary lung tumor
  - ○ Metastatic lung tumor
- Parasitic
  - ○ Feline heartworm-associated respiratory disease (HARD)
  - ○ Lungworms
- Pleuritis or other pleural space disease
  - ○ Pleural effusions
- Pneumonia
  - ○ Aspiration
  - ○ Bacterial
  - ○ Fungal
  - ○ Viral
- Pulmonary edema, non-cardiogenic
  - ○ Fluid overload
- Pulmonary embolism
- Pulmonary fibrosis
- Pulmonary infiltrates with eosinophils (PIE)

Coughing may also be associated with non-respiratory pathology [1, 79, 93, 98–100]:

- Cardiac
  - Congestive heart failure (CHF)
    - ○ Pulmonary venous dilation leads to pulmonary infiltrate
  - Dilated cardiomyopathy (DCM)
    - ○ Marked left atrial dilation leads to left mainstem bronchial compression
  - Parasitic
    - ○ Heartworm disease (HWD)
  - Pulmonary edema, cardiogenic
    - ○ Gastrointestinal
  - Gastroesophageal reflux disease (GERD)
  - Megaesophagus

A review of all of the aforementioned etiologies is beyond the scope of this chapter. The most common among these will be discussed here, given the likelihood that an entry-level veterinarian will encounter one or more of them in clinical practice.

Cardiac causes of cough will be covered in Part Five of the text.

Gastrointestinal causes of cough will be covered in Part Six of the text.

35.4.1 Feline Asthma/Bronchitis Complex

Just as in humans, asthma in cats refers to chronic inflammation within the bronchi and bronchioles [1, 78, 101]. Inflammation results in edematous mucosa and increased airway secretions [1, 78, 92, 101]. These narrow the lower airway lumens [1, 78, 101]. Narrowed airspace is compounded by bronchoconstriction [1, 78, 101].

Affected cats present for recurrent coughing episodes and wheezing [1, 78, 101].

Clients may also report exercise intolerance [1, 78, 101]. This may seem peculiar in that we do not often associate cats with exercise. However, more likely what it is that they are referring to is that asthmatic cats have difficulty sustaining play. This is because airway narrowing appreciably reduces airflow [101]. Consider, for example, an airway that has been reduced to 50% of its expected diameter [101]. This narrower tube has a 16-fold reduction in airflow [101]. This reduction cannot handle bursts of activity [101]. An attempt to play may be short-lived in an asthmatic cat, or the cat may quickly resort to panting [101].

Severe episodes may escalate beyond open-mouth breathing. Patients may become cyanotic [1, 92].

Young to middle-aged cats are more likely to be diagnosed with feline asthma [1, 92]. Siamese cats are also overrepresented [1, 92]. This breed predisposition suggests that there is an underlying genetic factor related to the development of asthma in cats; however, specific genes have not yet been identified [92].

Certain triggers may aggravate pre-existing disease. These are thought to include scented or dusty cat litter, cigarette smoke, hair spray, scented candles, and air fresheners [1]. Many of these are extrapolated from what is known about triggers in human asthmatics [92].

A presumptive diagnosis is often made based upon clinical history, once other causes of cough, such as lungworms, have been ruled out via fecal flotation, sedimentation, and/or the Baermann technique [1]. A positive response to treatment, corticosteroids, supports this diagnosis [92, 101].

Patients may appear to be clinically normal on physical examination, or they may have increased bronchovesicular lung sounds on thoracic auscultation [92]. Expiratory wheezes are suggestive of asthma [92]. Wheezing will be discussed in greater detail in Chapter 37. Wheezing is an adventitious lung sound that results when airways are obstructed by secretions [1].

Asthmatic cats may have evidence of peripheral eosinophilia on complete blood count (CBC) [1].

Thoracic radiographs support the diagnosis when they demonstrate diffuse thickening of the bronchial walls [1]. This thickening creates the illusion of a "donut" [92, 102]. Each bronchus is outlined by a thicker-than-normal circle of black [102]. This is referred to as peri-bronchial

cuffing [92]. Such cuffing is indicative of airway inflammation (see Figures 35.3a–f).

Airways may appear hyperinflated on thoracic radiography [1]. The diaphragm may also appear flatter than normal [1].

Note that radiographs can support a diagnosis of asthma; however, they cannot definitively discern the cause of lower airway disease. Lungworms may result in a similar radiographic appearance.

Communication plays a critical role in helping clients to understand the importance of sequentially ruling out other causes of cough. In this regard, feline asthma is a diagnosis of exclusion.

Once the diagnosis has been established, medical management is aimed at reducing clinical signs in a disease that is lifelong and progressive [1].

Historically, oral prednisolone was administered for life, to medically manage asthma.

Currently, oral prednisolone may be used to initiate treatment; however, it is advisable to transition from oral to inhalant therapy to reduce systemic side effects [101].

Inhalant corticosteroids, such as fluticasone propionate, are now the mainstay of therapy [1, 101].

These prescriptions are administered by fitting a metered dose inhaler into a spacer that has been outfitted with a feline-friendly facemask (see Figure 35.4).

The spacer is primed with the medication before the facemask is placed over the cat's mouth and nose. The cat is observed to breathe 7–10 times before the treatment is said to be complete [101].

Albuterol sulfate is considered a "rescue inhaler" [92, 94, 95, 101]. It is used as needed when a patient is in crisis to encourage bronchodilation [92, 94, 95, 101]. Its delivery is via the same method outlined above, for fluticasone [92, 94, 95, 101].

Status asthmaticus is a medical emergency for which parenteral terbutaline may be useful [92, 101].

35.4.2 Canine Bronchitis

Like feline asthma, canine bronchitis is a chronic inflammatory disease of the lower airway [90]. It is persistent and progressive [1]. Over time, chronic irritation leads to airway changes that are irreversible [1]. These include edema and epithelial metaplasia [1]. Airways become thickened [1]. Airway lumens are further narrowed by excessive mucus that is produced in response to mucosal irritation [1]. Collectively, these changes result in increased resistance to airflow and decreased ability to exhale with ease [1].

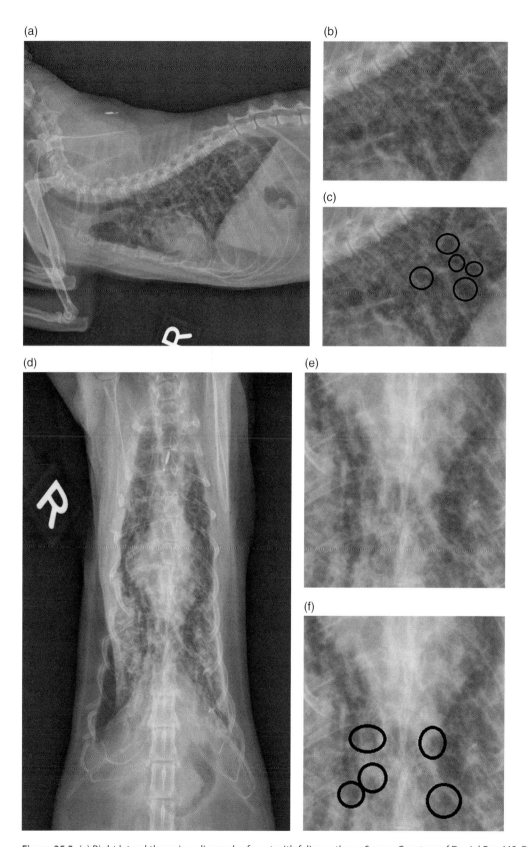

Figure 35.3 (a) Right lateral thoracic radiograph of a cat with feline asthma. *Source:* Courtesy of Daniel Foy, MS, DVM, DACVIM, DACVECC. (b) Close-up of right lateral thoracic radiograph of a cat with feline asthma. *Source:* Courtesy of Daniel Foy, MS, DVM, DACVIM, DACVECC. (c) Close-up of right lateral thoracic radiograph of a cat with feline asthma, with the classic "donut" bronchial pattern identified. *Source:* Courtesy of Daniel Foy, MS, DVM, DACVIM, DACVECC. (d) Ventrodorsal (V/D) thoracic radiograph of a cat with feline asthma. *Source:* Courtesy of Daniel Foy, MS, DVM, DACVIM, DACVECC. (e) Close-up of ventrodorsal (V/D) thoracic radiograph of a cat with feline asthma. *Source:* Courtesy of Daniel Foy, MS, DVM, DACVIM, DACVECC. (f) Close-up of ventrodorsal (V/D) thoracic radiograph of a cat with feline asthma, with the classic "donut" bronchial pattern identified. *Source:* Courtesy of Daniel Foy, MS, DVM, DACVIM, DACVECC.

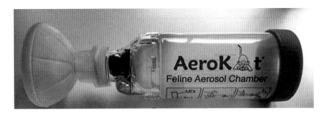

Figure 35.4 Example of a commercial device for delivery of inhalant medications to asthmatic cats.

Canine bronchitis is a diagnosis of exclusion [90, 91]. Other causes of cough must be ruled out, including the following [90, 91]:

- Cardiac
- Infectious
- Neoplastic
- Parasitic

Many of these causes of cough may predispose patients to canine bronchitis, particularly if they experience relapses or recurrent disease [1, 90].

Middle-aged to older patients are at increased risk for development of canine bronchitis [1, 90]. Small and toy breeds are overrepresented, especially Cocker Spaniels, Poodles, Pomeranians, and West Highland White Terriers [1, 90, 91].

Among large-breed dogs, German Shorthaired Pointers may be predisposed [91].

Affected patients typically present with a two-month history, or greater, of chronic cough that is best described as dry [1, 91].

A post-cough gag is common [1]. Some clients will not recognize this as being associated with a cough. They may believe that the dog is trying to vomit [1].

On physical examination, the trachea is typically sensitive, meaning that palpation is likely to elicit a cough and/or a gag [1].

Thoracic auscultation may reveal increased bronchovesicular lung sounds [1]. Wheezes are supportive of increased expiratory effort [1]. The observant clinician may also notice an expiratory abdominal push, evidence that the patient is working harder to expel air despite being at rest [1].

Obesity exacerbates clinical signs [1].

Radiographic changes are consistent with what has been described for feline asthma: the "donut" pattern and hyperinflation are commonly identified [1, 90]. In addition, thoracic radiographs may demonstrate bronchiectasis, middle lung lobe consolidation, or atelectasis [1, 90].

Additional imaging studies, such as CT or bronchoscopy, may provide additional details and, in the case of the latter, opportunities for sample collection [90, 91, 103]. Transtracheal washes are also appropriate for sample collection in medium-to-large-sized dogs, as compared to endotracheal washes, which are preferred in smaller patients [90].

Treatment largely focuses upon minimizing patient exposure to inciting factors [91]. Just as certain scents and particulate matter are thought to trigger an asthmatic attack, it is thought that airborne pollutants may aggravate chronic bronchitis [1, 90–92].

Home remodels should be performed without the patient present, if at all possible, to avoid exposure to noxious fumes [90]. Rehoming the dog temporarily is preferred. In cases where this is not possible, limiting the dog's access to the site of construction by confining it to one or more rooms is acceptable [90].

Weight loss should be encouraged in patients that are overweight [90].

The use of in-room humidifiers may help to mobilize airway secretions [91].

Tracheal irritation may be reduced by switching from a collar and leash to a harness [90, 91]. This will reduce the incidence of pulling at the neck.

Affected patients should limit exposure to conspecifics in settings that are considered high risk for respiratory disease [90]. Boarding kennels and grooming facilities, for example, are more likely to expose the patient to respiratory infection and should be avoided whenever possible [90].

Oral glucocorticoids may be used to initiate treatment; however, it is advisable to transition from oral prednisone to inhalant fluticasone propionate to reduce systemic side effects [90, 91]. These include polyuria and polydipsia (PU/PD), house soiling, polyphagia, and weight gain [91].

Inhalants are administered by fitting a metered dose inhaler into a spacer that has been outfitted with a canine-friendly facemask.

In addition, bronchodilators are commonly prescribed. These include albuterol sulfate and oral theophylline, which facilitates mucociliary clearance and decreases diaphragmatic fatigue [90, 91].

Because cough perpetuates a vicious cycle of inflammation–cough–inflammation–cough, antitussives are often prescribed [90]. These agents short-circuit the cycle of cough, thereby improving quality of life for patients and clients alike [90].

Medical management is lifelong, and patients often require dose adjustments as the disease progresses [90].

35.4.3 Feline Heartworm-Associated Respiratory Disease

HWD is caused by a filarial nematode, *Dirofilaria immitis* [78, 87, 100, 104–108] (see Figure 35.5).

Cats are infected with heartworms less easily than dogs, which are the usual definitive hosts [100]. Accordingly, infections within cats typically involve six or less heartworms. The lifespan of these worms is also shorter: roughly two to three years in cats as compared to five to seven years in dogs [78, 107, 109–111].

Infection occurs when an infected mosquito transmits third-stage larvae (L3) to the cat [78, 87, 100, 104–108]. Once within the cat, larvae migrate to the pulmonary arteries [78, 87, 100, 104–108]. This journey takes on average three to four months [78, 87, 100, 104–108].

Molting takes place during migration [78, 87, 100, 104–108].

Aberrant migration of fourth-stage larvae (L4) is more typical of cats than dogs [107]. Ectopic heartworms have been documented in body cavities and even within the central nervous system of cats [107, 112].

By the time they reach the pulmonary vasculature, larvae have transitioned into immature heartworms (L5) [78, 87, 100, 104–108].

Cats are unique as compared to dogs in their presentation for HWD [105].

Whereas dogs typically present for coughing, exercise intolerance, labored breathing, and/or syncope, many cats present for vomiting [113, 114]. Many are also misdiagnosed with asthma [1, 107]. This is because HWD in cats causes HARD [87, 100, 104–108].

Dogs may also develop HARD; however, this occurs much less frequently in canine than feline patients.

HARD is characterized by severe inflammation within the pulmonary vasculature [108]. This inflammation is

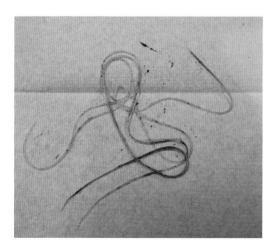

Figure 35.5 Adult heartworm, *Dirofilaria immitis*. *Source:* Courtesy of Laura Polerecky.

triggered by the heartworms themselves [108]. An additive effect is that when heartworms die, they occlude lumens of vessels [108]. They essentially act as thromboembolisms [108]. This can be fatal [108]. Sudden death is not uncommon in cats with HWD [100, 104, 105, 107, 112, 115–119].

Diagnosis of feline HWD and HARD can be challenging, given that cats typically have low worm burdens and, accordingly, low levels of antigen [107, 120]. A combination of tests is typically required to determine that feline HWD is likely [107]. These tests include the following [107]:

- Heartworm antigen test
- Heartworm antibody test
- Thoracic radiography
- Echocardiography
- Necropsy

No one test is perfect.

Antigen tests detect protein from the reproductive tract of the female nematode [107].

If an antigen test tests positive, then it is likely to be true: false-positive antigen tests are unusual [107].

However, false-negative results are common [107]. Cats with all-male infections will test negative [107]. Even cats with female *D. immitis* may test negative, given that infections in cats typically involve very few, if any, adult worms [107].

Antibody tests may be helpful for screening cats; however, these detect past or present exposure to *D. immitis*, rather than an active infection [107]. Patients with prior disease will test positive, even though they no longer have active disease [107].

False-negative antibody tests are also less rare than was once thought [107, 121–124].

Thoracic radiographs may demonstrate the following changes that are consistent with a diagnosis of feline HWD [78, 107, 125, 126]:

- Cardiomegaly
  - Right ventricular enlargement, based upon subjective inspection of the films
  - As determined by a value greater than expected for a normal vertebral heart score
- Enlarged, dilated, and/or tortuous pulmonary arteries
  - Based upon subjective inspection of the films
  - As determined by a mean ratio of >1.6 for the width of the right pulmonary artery to the width of the ninth rib, as compared on a dorsoventral (D/V) or ventrodorsal (V/D) view
- Pulmonary infiltrates
  - Mild and patchy
  - Severe and alveolar

Note that not all feline patients with HWD demonstrate these characteristic radiographic changes [107]. Unremarkable thoracic radiographs do not rule out a diagnosis of HWD [107, 125].

Echocardiography may be advantageous in cats that are suspected of having HWD, yet produced negative heartworm antigen test results [107, 127, 128]. Heartworms appear in cross section as parallel linear densities or "train tracks," and are more likely to be visualized in the pulmonary arteries, right ventricle, right atrium, and caudal vena cava [107]. However, this imaging modality is highly user-dependent: an inexperienced ultrasonographer may mistake reflections from the wall of the pulmonary artery for heartworms [78, 107, 129].

Necropsy may provide a definitive diagnosis in feline patients that experienced sudden death [107]. However, this method of gross inspection is likely to miss ectopic infections [107, 112].

Microfilarial tests are not typically helpful in cats because microfilaremia is transient, if it is present at all [78].

Despite the challenges associated with diagnosis, the astute clinician should consider HWD as a rule-out for any feline patient that is presenting with asthmatic signs. The successful clinician is able to assimilate the results of the various patient tests into a working diagnosis.

Symptomatic patients must be stabilized prior to medical management. Stabilization is achieved via supplemental oxygenation, glucocorticoids, and bronchodilators [1, 78, 107].

The use of adulticide therapy, melarsomine, is not advocated for use in feline patients [1]. Cats react adversely to adulticidal agents [107]. Fatal pulmonary thromboembolism is common [107].

Because curative medical management is unsafe in cats, therapies are therefore aimed at improving clinical signs and quality of life in those patients with advanced HARD [107].

Alternatively, heartworms may be removed surgically when their presence is confirmed via echocardiography [107]. Surgical extraction is typically achieved through transjugular catheterization [107, 130, 131]. However, it is not without risk [107].

35.4.4 Lungworms

Lungworms are respiratory parasites [86, 87, 89, 97]. Historically, *Aelurostrongylus abstrusus* has been most commonly recognized as infecting cats [97]. However, *A. abstrusus* is not the only feline lungworm. Additional species of importance to feline medicine include the following [89, 97, 132–135]:

- *Capillaria aerophila* or *Eucoleus aerophilus*
- *Paragonimus kellicotti*
- *Troglostrongylus brevior*

Cats are not the only domestic species to be affected by lungworms. Lungworms of the following species may also affect dogs [86, 132, 136–138]:

- *Angiostrongylus vasorum*
- *C. aerophila* or *E. aerophilus*
- *Crenosoma vulpis*
- *Eucoleus boehmi*
- *Filaroides hirthi*
- *Filaroides milksi*
- *Oslerus osleri*
- *P. kellicotti*

The life cycles of these helminth parasites of the respiratory tract are beyond the scope of this text.

What is important to highlight here is that lungworm infection creates clinical signs that are indistinguishable from asthma and other bronchial diseases [97, 133].

Coughing and wheezing are the most commonly reported signs associated with *A. abstrusus* infection [97, 133, 139, 140]. Sneezing, with nasal discharge, is also frequent [97, 133, 139, 140]. Young, debilitated, or immunosuppressed patients may experience respiratory distress [97]. These patients may present with tachypnea, dyspnea, or open-mouth breathing [141]. Sudden death is possible [141].

Diagnosis of lungworm infection is challenging in that their presentations are so similar to other causes of bronchial disease [97].

Consider, for example, that the radiographic appearance of lungworm-associated respiratory pathology is identical to that of feline asthma [97, 142, 143] (see Figures 35.6a–f).

The yield from direct fecal smears and routine in-house fecal flotation methods is low [97]. The solutions that are classically used are so concentrated that osmotic damage to larvae makes their observation unlikely [97, 139, 144].

The preferred technique for larval identification is the Baermann migration method [97, 133, 144, 145]. This technique requires patience in that samples may not test positive until 12–48 h after setup [97, 133, 144, 145].

Observers also have to be taught how to discriminate between the various species of lungworms based upon slight morphological appearances [97, 133, 144, 145] (see Figure 35.7a, b).

In addition to fecal analysis, cytological examination of transtracheal aspirates and samples obtained from bronchoalveolar lavage can be positive for lungworms [97]. However, these are rare finds [97].

Affected patients may or may not have peripheral eosinophilia [86, 87].

More recently, PCR has been developed to detect feline aelurostrongylosis and troglostrongylosis [97,

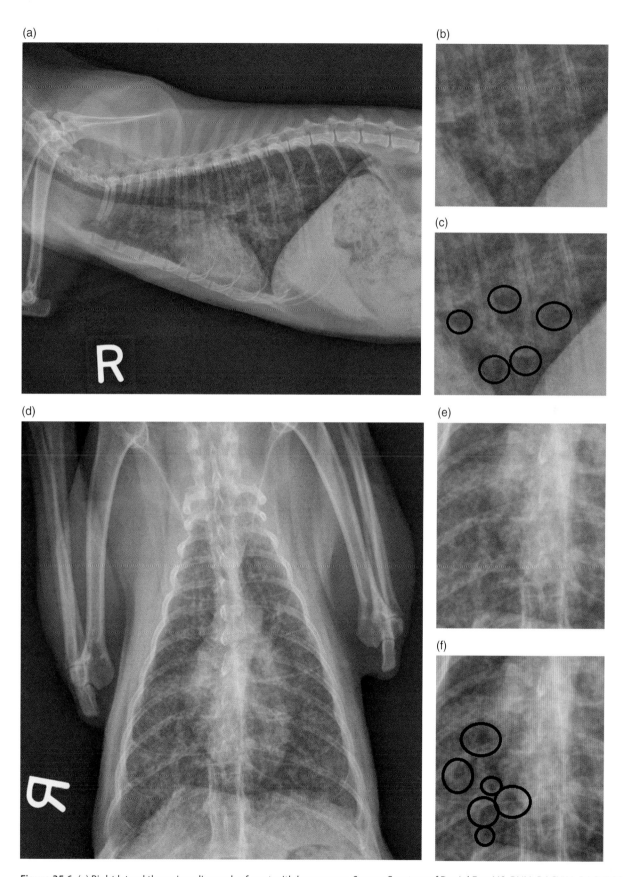

Figure 35.6 (a) Right lateral thoracic radiograph of a cat with lungworms. *Source:* Courtesy of Daniel Foy, MS, DVM, DACVIM, DACVECC. (b) Close-up of right lateral thoracic radiograph of a cat with lungworms. *Source:* Courtesy of Daniel Foy, MS, DVM, DACVIM, DACVECC. (c) Close-up of right lateral thoracic radiograph of cat with lungworms, with the classic "donut" bronchial pattern identified. *Source:* Courtesy of Daniel Foy, MS, DVM, DACVIM, DACVECC. (d) Ventrodorsal (V/D) thoracic radiograph of a cat with lungworms. *Source:* Courtesy of Daniel Foy, MS, DVM, DACVIM, DACVECC. (e) Close-up of ventrodorsal (V/D) thoracic radiograph of a cat with lungworms. *Source:* Courtesy of Daniel Foy, MS, DVM, DACVIM, DACVECC. (f) Close-up of ventrodorsal (V/D) thoracic radiograph of a cat with lungworms, with the classic "donut" bronchial pattern identified. *Source:* Courtesy of Daniel Foy, MS, DVM, DACVIM, DACVECC.

(a)

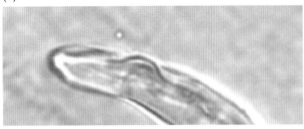

(b)

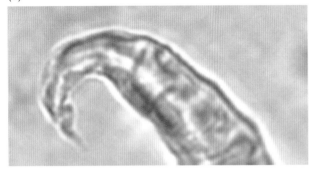

Figure 35.7 (a) The anterior end of the first-stage larvae (L1) of *Aelurostrongylus abstrusus* is rounded. (b) Note the kinked tail that is also characteristic of first-stage larvae (L1) of *Aelurostrongylus abstrusus*.

146–149]. This technique offers promise in being able to detect infection among cats that had negative fecal tests [150].

A similar assay has made detection of *C. aerophila* possible [22].

Treatments against lungworms are varied and most of what has been described constitutes off-label use [97]. For example, ivermectin repeatedly appears in the literature for use against aelurostrongylosis [151–153]. However, its efficacy is variable [151–153].

In the United States, fenbendazole is licensed to treat *A. abstrusus* [97].

Experimentally, selamectin and formulations involving both milbemycin oxime/praziquantel, and imidacloprid/moxidectin also show promise in resolving clinical signs [97].

References

1 Tilley, L.P. and Smith, F.W.K. (2016). *Blackwell's Five-Minute Veterinary Consult. Canine and Feline*, 6e, lxix, 1622 p. Ames, Iowa, USA: Wiley.

2 Reece, W.O. (ed.) (2012). *Dukes' Physiology of Domestic Animals*, 12e. Ithaca, NY: Cornell University Press.

3 Stokhof, A.A. and Haagen, V.-v. (2012). Respiratory system. In: *Medical History and Physical Examination in Companion Animals* (ed. A. Rijnberk and F.J. van Sluijs), 63–74. Philadelphiaq: Saunders Elsevier.

4 Newhouse, M., Sanchis, J., and Bienenstock, J. (1976). Lung defense mechanisms (second of two parts). *N. Engl. J. Med.* 295 (19): 1045–1052.

5 Newhouse, M., Sanchis, J., and Bienenstock, J. (1976). Lung defense mechanisms (first of two parts). *N. Engl. J. Med.* 295 (18): 990–998.

6 Widdicombe, J.G. (1980). Mechanism of cough and its regulation. *Eur. J. Respir. Dis. Suppl.* 110: 11–20.

7 Primm K. (2016). The essence of a reverse sneeze. DVM 360 [Internet]. http://www.dvm360.com/sites/default/files/images/pdfs-for-alfresco-articles/Reverse_sneeze_handout.pdf.

8 Holt, D.E. and Goldschmidt, M.H. (2011). Nasal polyps in dogs: five cases (2005–2011). *J. Small Anim. Pract.* 52 (12): 660–663.

9 Veronesi, F., Morganti, G., Di Cesare, A. et al. (2014). A pilot trial evaluating the efficacy of a 10% imidacloprid/2.5% moxidectin spot-on formulation in the treatment of natural nasal capillariosis in dogs. *Vet. Parasitol.* 200 (1–2): 133–138.

10 Adolph, C. (2014). Treating nasal capillariasis in dogs. *NAVC Clinician's Brief* (October): 38.

11 Adolph, C. (2015). No sneezing matter: capillaria boehmi. *NAVC Clinician's Brief* (February): 50.

12 Allison, N., Willard, M.D., Bentinck-Smith, J., and Davis, K. (1986). Nasal rhinosporidiosis in two dogs. *J. Am. Vet. Med. Assoc.* 188 (8): 869–871.

13 Easley, J.R., Meuten, D.J., Levy, M.G. et al. (1986). Nasal rhinosporidiosis in the dog. *Vet. Pathol.* 23 (1): 50–56.

14 Fox, S.M. (1986). Surgical extirpation for Rhinosporidiosis in a dog. *Compend. Contin. Educ. Pract.* 8 (3): 152–110.

15 Hoff, B. and Hall, D.A. (1986). Rhinosporidiosis in a dog. *Can. Vet. J.* 27 (6): 231–232.

16 Mosier, D.A. and Creed, J.E. (1984). Rhinosporidiosis in a dog. *J. Am. Vet. Med. Assoc.* 185 (9): 1009–1010.

17 Harvey, C.E. (1983). Surgery of the nasl cavity and sinuses. In: *Current Techniques in Small Animal Surgery* (ed. M.J. Bojrab), 253–257. Philadelphia: Lea & Febiger.

18 Sreter, T., Szell, Z., Marucci, G. et al. (2003). Extraintestinal nematode infections of red foxes (Vulpes vulpes) in Hungary. *Vet. Parasitol.* 115 (4): 329–334.

19 Schoning, P., Dryden, M.W., and Gabbert, N.H. (1993). Identification of a nasal nematode (Eucoleus boehmi) in greyhounds. *Vet. Res. Commun.* 17 (4): 277–281.

20 Baan, M., Kidder, A.C., Johnson, S.E., and Sherding, R.G. (2011). Rhinoscopic diagnosis of Eucoleus boehmi infection in a dog. *J. Am. Anim. Hosp. Assoc.* 47 (1): 60–63.

21 Campbell, B.G. and Little, M.D. (1991). Identification of the eggs of a nematode (Eucoleus boehmi) from the nasal mucosa of North American dogs. *J. Am. Vet. Med. Assoc.* 198 (9): 1520–1523.

22 Di Cesare, A., Castagna, G., Otranto, D. et al. (2012). Molecular detection of *Capillaria aerophila*, an agent of canine and feline pulmonary Capillariosis. *J. Clin. Microbiol.* 50 (6): 1958–1963.

23 Magi, M., Guardone, L., Prati, M.C. et al. (2012). First report of Eucoleus Boehmi (Syn. Capillaria Boehmi) in dogs in north-western Italy, with scanning electron microscopy of the eggs. *Parasite* 19 (4): 433–435.

24 Piperisova, I., Neel, J.A., and Tarigo, J. (2010). What is your diagnosis? Nasal discharge from a dog. *Vet. Clin. Pathol.* 39 (1): 121–122.

25 Veronesi, F., Lepri, E., Morganti, G. et al. (2013). Nasal eucoleosis in a symptomatic dog from Italy. *Vet. Parasitol.* 195 (1–2): 187–191.

26 Evinger, J.V., Kazacos, K.R., and Cantwell, H.D. (1985). Ivermectin for treatment of nasal capillariasis in a dog. *J. Am. Vet. Med. Assoc.* 186 (2): 174–175.

27 Rand, J. The cat with acute sneezing or nasal discharge. In: *Problem-Based Feline Medicine* (ed. J. Rand), 5–18. Philadelphia: Elsevier Saunds.

28 Gordon J. (2011). Clinical approach to nasal discharge. DVM 360 [Internet]. http://veterinarycalendar. dvm360.com/clinical-approach-nasal-discharge-proceedings.

29 Norton, R. and Burney, D.P. (2012). Cryptococcosis. *NAVC Clinician's Brief* (December): 39–42.

30 Kent, M.S. (2009). Nasal discharge in a dog. *NAVC Clinician's Brief* (September): 25–26.

31 Henderson, S.M., Bradley, K., Day, M.J. et al. (2004). Investigation of nasal disease in the cat – a retrospective study of 77 cases. *J. Feline Med. Surg.* 6 (4): 245–257.

32 Little, L., Patel, R., and Goldschmidt, M. (2007). Nasal and nasopharyngeal lymphoma in cats: 50 cases (1989–2005). *Vet. Pathol.* 44 (6): 885–892.

33 Cohn, L.A. (2014). Canine nasal disease. *Vet. Clin. North Am. Small Anim. Pract.* 44 (1): 75–89.

34 Chartier, M. (2015). Canine primary (idiopathic) immune-mediated thrombocytopenia. *NAVC Clinician's Brief* (September): 82–86.

35 Sharp, C.R. (2012). Feline rhinitis and upper respiratory disease. *Today's Veterinary Practice* (July/August): 14–20.

36 Van Pelt, D.R. and Lappin, M.R. (1994). Pathogenesis and treatment of feline rhinitis. *Vet. Clin. North Am. Small Anim. Pract.* 24 (5): 807–823.

37 Lamb, C.R., Richbell, S., and Mantis, P. (2003). Radiographic signs in cats with nasal disease. *J. Feline Med. Surg.* 5 (4): 227–235.

38 Binns, S.H., Dawson, S., Speakman, A.J. et al. (1999). Prevalence and risk factors for feline *Bordetella bronchiseptica* infection. *Vet. Rec.* 144 (21): 575–580.

39 Malik, R., Krockenberger, M., and O'Brien, C. (2006). Cryptococcosis. In: *Infectious Diseases of the Dog and Cat* (ed. C.E. Greene), 584–598. St. Louis: Elsevier Saunders.

40 Speakman, A.J., Dawson, S., Binns, S.H. et al. (1999). *Bordetella bronchiseptica* infection in the cat. *J. Small Anim. Pract.* 40 (6): 252–256.

41 Bradley, R.L. (1984). Selected Oral, pharyngeal, and upper respiratory conditions in the cat. Oral tumors, nasopharyngeal and middle ear polyps, and chronic rhinitis and sinusitis. *Vet. Clin. North Am. Small Anim. Pract.* 14 (6): 1173–1184.

42 Cape, L. (1992). Feline idiopathic chronic Rhinosinusitis – a retrospective study of 30 cases. *J. Am. Anim. Hosp. Assoc.* 28 (2): 149–155.

43 Ford, R.B. and Levy, J.K. (1994). Infectious diseases of the respiratory tract. In: *The Cat: Diseases and Clinical Management* (ed. R.G. Sherding), 489–500. New York: Churchill Livingstone.

44 Malik, R., Wigney, D.I., Muir, D.B. et al. (1992). Cryptococcosis in cats: clinical and mycological assessment of 29 cases and evaluation of treatment using orally administered fluconazole. *J. Med. Vet. Mycol.* 30 (2): 133–144.

45 Mochizuki, M., Kawakami, K., Hashimoto, M., and Ishida, T. (2000). Recent epidemiological status of feline upper respiratory infections in Japan. *J. Vet. Med. Sci.* 62 (7): 801–803.

46 Moore, A.H. (2007). Evaluation of chronic nasal disease in dogs: rhinoscopy in context. *NAVC Clinician's Brief* (May): 17–19.

47 Moore, L.E. (2003). Feline chronic respiratory disease. *NAVC Clinician's Brief* (August): 41–42.

48 Plummer, C.E. (2012). Herpetic keratoconjunctivitis in a cat. *NAVC Clinician's Brief* (January): 26–28.

49 Hurley K. (2010). Canine infectious respiratory disease complex: management and prevention in canine populations. DVM 360 [Internet]. http://veterinarycalendar. dvm360.com/canine-infectious-respiratory-disease-complex-management-and-prevention-canine-populations-proceedin.

50 Joffe, D.J., Lelewski, R., Weese, J.S. et al. (2016). Factors associated with development of canine infectious respiratory disease complex (CIRDC) in dogs in 5 Canadian small animal clinics. *Can. Vet. J.* 57 (1): 46–51.

51 Chalker, V.J., Toomey, C., Opperman, S. et al. (2003). Respiratory disease in kennelled dogs: serological responses to *Bordetella bronchiseptica* lipopolysaccharide do not correlate with bacterial isolation or clinical respiratory symptoms. *Clin. Diagn. Lab. Immunol.* 10 (3): 352–356.

52 Nafe, L.A. (2014). Dogs infected with *Bordetella bronchiseptica* and Canine influenza virus (H3N8). *Today's Veterinary Practice* (July/August): 30–36.

53 Priestnall, S.L., Mitchell, J.A., Walker, C.A. et al. (2014). New and emerging pathogens in canine infectious respiratory disease. *Vet. Pathol.* 51 (2): 492–504.

54 Holt, D.E., Mover, M.R., and Brown, D.C. (2010). Serologic prevalence of antibodies against canine influenza virus (H3N8) in dogs in a metropolitan animal shelter. *J. Am. Vet. Med. Assoc.* 237 (1): 71–73.

55 Radhakrishnan, A., Drobatz, K.J., Culp, W.T., and King, L.G. (2007). Community-acquired infectious pneumonia in puppies: 65 cases (1993–2002). *J. Am. Vet. Med. Assoc.* 230 (10): 1493–1497.

56 Weese, J.S. and Stull, J. (2013). Respiratory disease outbreak in a veterinary hospital associated with canine parainfluenza virus infection. *Can. Vet. J.* 54 (1): 79–82.

57 Heinrich C. (2015). Assessing conjunctivitis in cats. Vet Times [Internet]. www.vettimes.co.uk/app/uploads/wp-post-to-pdf-enhanced-cache/1/assessing-conjunctivitis-in-cats.pdf.

58 Mitchell, N. (2006). Feline ophthalmology part 2: clinical presentation and aetiology of common ocular conditions. *Irish Vet. J.* 59 (4): 223–232.

59 Ford, R.B. (2006). Canine infectious tracheobronchitis. In: *Infectious Diseases of the Dog and Cat* (ed. C.E. Greene), 54–63. St. Louis: Elsevier, Inc.

60 Hanson, J.M., Dunn, D., and Yeuroukis, C.K. (2016). Canine influenza. *NAVC Clinician's Brief* (September): 97–103.

61 Serra, V.F., Stanzani, G., Smith, G., and Otto, C.M. (2011). Point seroprevalence of canine influenza virus H3N8 in dogs participating in a flyball tournament in Pennsylvania. *Javma-J. Am. Vet. Med. A.* 238 (6): 726–730.

62 Anderson, T.C., Crawford, P.C., Dubovi, E.J. et al. (2013). Prevalence of and exposure factors for seropositivity to H3N8 canine influenza virus in dogs with influenza-like illness in the United States. *J. Am. Vet. Med. Assoc.* 242 (2): 209–216.

63 Crawford, P.C., Dubovi, E.J., Castleman, W.L. et al. (2005). Transmission of equine influenza virus to dogs. *Science* 310 (5747): 482–485.

64 Song, D., Kang, B., Lee, C. et al. (2008). Transmission of avian influenza virus (H3N2) to dogs. *Emerg. Infect. Dis.* 14 (5): 741–746.

65 Kim, H., Song, D., Moon, H. et al. (2013). Inter- and intraspecies transmission of canine influenza virus (H3N2) in dogs, cats, and ferrets. *Influenza Other Respir. Viruses* 7 (3): 265–270.

66 Lee, Y.N., Lee, D.H., Park, J.K. et al. (2013). Experimental infection and natural contact exposure of ferrets with canine influenza virus (H3N2). *J. Gen. Virol.* 94 (Pt 2): 293–297.

67 Krueger, W.S., Heil, G.L., Yoon, K.J., and Gray, G.C. (2014). No evidence for zoonotic transmission of H3N8 canine influenza virus among US adults occupationally exposed to dogs. *Influenza Other Respir. Viruses* 8 (1): 99–106.

68 Lyoo, K.S., Kim, J.K., Kang, B. et al. (2015). Comparative analysis of virulence of a novel, avian-origin H3N2 canine influenza virus in various host species. *Virus Res.* 195: 135–140.

69 Hong, M., Kang, B., Na, W. et al. (2013). Prolonged shedding of the canine influenza H3N2 virus in nasal swabs of experimentally immunocompromised dogs. *Clin. Exp. Vaccine Res.* 2 (1): 66–68.

70 Crawford, P.C. and Spindel, M. (2009). Canine influenza. In: *Infectious Disease Management in Animal Shelters* (ed. L. Miller and K. Hurley), 173–180. Ames, IA: Wiley-Blackwell.

71 Song, D., Moon, H.J., An, D.J. et al. (2012). A novel reassortant canine H3N1 influenza virus between pandemic H1N1 and canine H3N2 influenza viruses in Korea. *J. Gen. Virol.* 93 (Pt 3): 551–554.

72 Song, D.S., An, D.J., Moon, H.J. et al. (2011). Interspecies transmission of the canine influenza H3N2 virus to domestic cats in South Korea, 2010. *J. Gen. Virol.* 92 (Pt 10): 2350–2355.

73 Song, Q.Q., Zhang, F.X., Liu, J.J. et al. (2013). Dog to dog transmission of a novel influenza virus (H5N2) isolated from a canine. *Vet. Microbiol.* 161 (3–4): 331–333.

74 Songserm, T., Amonsin, A., Jam-on, R. et al. (2006). Fatal avian influenza A H5N1 in a dog. *Emerg. Infect. Dis.* 12 (11): 1744–1747.

75 Zhan, G.J., Ling, Z.S., Zhu, Y.L. et al. (2012). Genetic characterization of a novel influenza a virus H5N2 isolated from a dog in China. *Vet. Microbiol.* 155 (2–4): 409–416.

76 Lin, D., Sun, S., Du, L. et al. (2012). Natural and experimental infection of dogs with pandemic H1N1/2009 influenza virus. *J. Gen. Virol.* 93 (Pt 1): 119–123.

77 Lin, H.T., Wang, C.H., Chueh, L.L. et al. (2015). Influenza A(H6N1) Virus in Dogs, Taiwan. *Emerg. Infect. Dis.* 21 (12): 2154–2157.

78 Mason, R.A. and Rand, J. (2006). The coughing cat. In: *Problem-Based Feline Medicine* (ed. J. Rand), 90–108. Philadelphia: Elsevier Saunders.

79 Hawkins EC. (2007). Coughing dogs: determining why. NAVC Clinician's Brief [Internet]. https://www.

cliniciansbrief.com/column/category/column/capsules/coughing-dogs-determining-why.

80 Johnson, L.R. (2006). Chronic cough. *NAVC Clinician's Brief* (July): 51–52.

81 Ellis J. (2008). Chronic cough in a puppy. NAVC Clinician's Brief [Internet]. https://www.cliniciansbrief.com/article/chronic-cough-puppy.

82 Clercx, C. and Roels, E. (2015). Exercise intolerance and chronic cough in a geriatic dog. *NAVC Clinician's Brief* (December).

83 Grobman, M. and Reinero, C. (2016). Investigation of Neurokinin-1 receptor antagonism as a novel treatment for chronic bronchitis in dogs. *J. Vet. Intern. Med.* 30 (3): 847–852.

84 Dye, J. (2008). Cough in cats. *NAVC Clinician's Brief* (July): 17.

85 Deweese, M.D. and Tobias, K.M. (2014). Tracheal collapse in dogs. *NAVC Clinician's Brief* (May): 83–87.

86 Palma, D. (2016). Common pulmonary diseases in dogs. *NAVC Clinician's Brief* (October): 77–109.

87 Palma, D. (2017). Common pulmonary diseases in cats. *NAVC Clinician's Brief* (March): 107–115.

88 Fry, J.K. and Burney, D.P. (2012). Canine infectious respiratory disease. *NAVC Clinician's Brief* (November): 34–38.

89 Conboy, G. (2009). Helminth parasites of the canine and feline respiratory tract. *Vet. Clin. North Am. Small Anim. Pract.* 39 (6): 1109–1126, vii.

90 Kumrow, K.J. (2012). Canine chronic bronchitis: A review and update. *Today's Veterinary Practice* (November/December): 12–17.

91 Carey, S.A. (ed.) (2018). *Current Therapy for Canine Chronic Bronchitis*. Michigan Veterinary Medical Association.

92 Padrid, P. (2005). Feline asthma and bronchitis. *NAVC Clinician's Brief* (October): 37–40.

93 Byers, C.G. and Dhupa, N. (2005). Feline asthma and heartworm disease – reply. *Compend. Contin. Educ. Pract.* 27 (8): 573.

94 Byers, C.G. and Dhupa, N. (2005). Feline bronchial asthma: pathophysiology and diagnosis. *Compend. Contin. Educ. Pract.* 27 (6): 418–425.

95 Byers, C.G. and Dhupa, N. (2005). Feline bronchial asthma: treatment. *Compend. Contin. Educ. Pract.* 27 (6): 426–431.

96 Little S. (2010). Coughing and wheezing cats: diagnosis and treatment of feline asthma. DVM 360 [Internet]. http://veterinarycalendar.dvm360.com/coughing-and-wheezing-cats-diagnosis-and-treatment-feline-asthma-proceedings.

97 Traversa, D. and Di Cesare, A. (2016). Diagnosis and management of lungworm infections in cats: cornerstones, dilemmas and new avenues. *J. Feline Med. Surg.* 18 (1): 7–20.

98 Miller, M.W. (2007). Canine cough. *NAVC Clinician's Brief* (September): 27.

99 Miller, M.W. and Gordon, S.G. (2007). Canine congestive heart failure. *NAVC Clinician's Brief* (September): 31–35.

100 Lee, A.C.Y. and Kraus, M.S. (2012). Coughing cat: could it be heartworm? *NAVC Clinician's Brief* (June): 91–95.

101 Padrid P. (2011). Diagnosing and treating feline asthma (including the use of inhalants). DVM 360 [Internet]. http://veterinarycalendar.dvm360.com/diagnosing-and-treating-feline-asthma-including-use-inhalants-proceedings.

102 Englar, R.E. (2017). *Performing the Small Animal Physical Examination*. Hoboken, NJ: Wiley.

103 Padrid, P.A., Hornof, W.J., Kurpershoek, C.J., and Cross, C.E. (1990). Canine chronic bronchitis. A pathophysiologic evaluation of 18 cases. *J. Vet. Intern. Med.* 4 (3): 172–180.

104 Dillon, A.R., Blagburn, B.L., Tillson, M. et al. (2017). The progression of heartworm associated respiratory disease (HARD) in SPF cats 18 months after *Dirofilaria immitis* infection. *Parasit. Vectors* 10 (Suppl 2): 533.

105 Dillon, A.R., Blagburn, B.L., Tillson, M. et al. (2017). Heartworm-associated respiratory disease (HARD) induced by immature adult *Dirofilaria immitis* in cats. *Parasit. Vectors* 10 (Suppl 2): 514.

106 Litster, A., Atkins, C., and Atwell, R. (2008). Acute death in heartworm-infected cats: unraveling the puzzle. *Vet. Parasitol.* 158 (3): 196–203.

107 Litster, A.L. and Atwell, R.B. (2008). Feline heartworm disease: a clinical review. *J. Feline Med. Surg.* 10 (2): 137–144.

108 Nelson, C.T. (2007). Heartworm-associated respiratory disease in cats. *NAVC Clinician's Brief* (May): 15.

109 Brown, W., Paul, A., Venco, L. et al. (1999). Feline heartworm disease – part 3. *Feline Pract.* 27 (3): 14–20.

110 Brown, W., Paul, A., Venco, L. et al. (1999). Feline heartworm disease part 1. *Feline Pract.* 27 (1): 6–9.

111 Venco, L., McCall, J., Paul, A. et al. (1999). Feline heartworm disease – part 2. *Feline Pract.* 27 (2): 6–13.

112 Atkins, C.E., DeFrancesco, T.C., Coats, J.R. et al. (2000). Heartworm infection in cats: 50 cases (1985–1997). *J. Am. Vet. Med. Assoc.* 217 (3): 355–358.

113 Tams TR. (2009). Diagnosis and management of acute and chronic vomiting in dogs and cats. DVM 360 [Internet]. http://veterinarycalendar.dvm360.com/diagnosis-and-management-acute-and-chronic-vomiting-dogs-and-cats-proceedings.

114 Tams TR. (2009). Diagnosis of acute and chronic vomiting in dogs and cats. DVM 360 [Internet]. http://veterinarycalendar.dvm360.com/diagnosis-and-

management-acute-and-chronic-vomiting-dogs-and-cats-proceedings.

115 Bowman, D.D. and Atkins, C.E. (2009). Heartworm biology, treatment, and control. *Vet. Clin. North Am. Small Anim. Pract.* 39 (6): 1127–1158, vii.

116 Genchi, C., Venco, L., Ferrari, N. et al. (2008). Feline heartworm (*Dirofilaria immitis*) infection: a statistical elaboration of the duration of the infection and life expectancy in asymptomatic cats. *Vet. Parasitol.* 158 (3): 177–182.

117 Evans, E.A., Litster, A.L., Gunew, M.N.M., and Menrath, V.H. (2000). Forty-five cases of feline heartworm in Australia (1990–1998). *Aust. Vet. Pract.* 30 (1): 11–16.

118 Holmes, R.A. (1993). Feline heartworm disease. *Compend. Contin. Educ. Pract.* 15 (5): 687–695.

119 Ralston, S.L., Stemme, K., and Guerrero, J. (1998). Preventing feline heartworm disease. *Feline Pract.* 26 (3): 18–22.

120 Atkins, C. (1999). The diagnosis of feline heartworm infection. *J. Am. Anim. Hosp. Assoc.* 35 (3): 185–187.

121 Venco, L., Calzolari, D., Mazzocchi, D. et al. (1998). The use of echocardiography as a diagnostic tool for detection of feline heartworm (*Dirofilaria immitis*) infections. *Feline Pract.* 26 (3): 6–9.

122 Atkins, C.E., DeFrancesco, T.C., Miller, M.W. et al. (1998). Prevalence of heartworm infection in cats with signs of cardiorespiratory abnormalities. *J. Am. Vet. Med. Assoc.* 212 (4): 517–520.

123 Kalkstein, T.S., Kaiser, L., and Kaneene, J.B. (2000). Prevalence of heartworm infection in healthy cats in the lower peninsula of Michigan. *J. Am. Vet. Med. Assoc.* 217 (6): 857–861.

124 Berdoulay, P., Levy, J.K., Snyder, P.S. et al. (2004). Comparison of serological tests for the detection of natural heartworm infection in cats. *J. Am. Anim. Hosp. Assoc.* 40 (5): 376–384.

125 Schafer, M. and Berry, C.R. (1995). Cardiac and pulmonary-artery mensuration in feline heartworm disease. *Vet. Radiol. Ultrasound.* 36 (6): 499–505.

126 Holmes RA, Clark JN, Casey HW, Henk W, Plue RE, editors. (1992). Histopathologic and radiographic studies of the development of heartworm pulmonary vascular disease in experimentally infected cats. Proceedings of the Heartworm Symposium; Austin, Texas: American Heartworm Society.

127 DeFrancesco, T.C., Atkins, C.E., Miller, M.W. et al. (2001). Use of echocardiography for the diagnosis of heartworm disease in cats: 43 cases (1985–1997). *J. Am. Vet. Med. Assoc.* 218 (1): 66–69.

128 Genchi C, Kramer L, Venco L, Prieto G, Simon F, editors. (1998). Comparison of antibody and antigen testing with echocardiography fo the detection of heartworm (*Dirofilaria immitis*) in cats. Proceedings of the Heartworm Symposium; Tampa, Florida: American Heartworm Society.

129 Atwell R, editor. (2001). Feline dirofilariosis: epidemiology and diagnostics over 20 years in S.E. Queensland and Sydney, Australia. Proceedings of the Heartworm Symposium; San Antonio, Texas: American Heartworm Society.

130 Atwell, R.B. and Litster, A.L. (2002). Surgical extraction of transplanted adult *Dirofilaria immitis* in cats. *Vet. Res. Commun.* 26 (4): 301–308.

131 Borgarelli, M., Venco, L., Piga, P.M. et al. (1997). Surgical removal of heartworms from the right atrium of a cat. *J. Am. Vet. Med. Assoc.* 211 (1): 68–69.

132 Pechman, R.D. (1994). Respiratory parasites. In: *The Cat: Diseases and Clinical Management* (ed. R.G. Sherding), 613–622. New York: Churchill Livingstone.

133 Traversa, D. and Di Cesare, A. (2013). Feline lungworms: what a dilemma. *Trends Parasitol.* 29 (9): 423–430.

134 Brianti, E., Giannetto, S., Dantas-Torres, F., and Otranto, D. (2014). Lungworms of the genus Troglostrongylus (Strongylida: Crenosomatidae): neglected parasites for domestic cats. *Vet. Parasitol.* 202 (3–4): 104–112.

135 Bowman, D.D., Hendrix, C.M., and Lindsay, D.S. (2002). *Feline Clinical Parasitology*, 262–272, 338–50. Ames, IA: Iowa State University Press.

136 Herman, L.H. and Helland, D.R. (1966). Paragonimiasis in a Cat. *J. Am. Vet. Med. Assoc.* 149 (6): 753–757.

137 Pechman, R.D. (1976). Radiographic features of pulmonary Paragonimiasis in dog and cat. *J. Am. Vet. Radiol. Soc.* 17 (5): 182–191.

138 Pechman, R.D. (1980). Pulmonary Paragonimiasis in dogs and cats – review. *J. Small Anim. Pract.* 21 (2): 87–95.

139 Traversa, D., Di Cesare, A., Milillo, P. et al. (2008). *Aelurostrongylus abstrusus* in a feline colony from Central Italy: clinical features, diagnostic procedures and molecular characterization. *Parasitol. Res.* 103 (5): 1191–1196.

140 Traversa, D., Lia, R.P., Iorio, R. et al. (2008). Diagnosis and risk factors of *Aelurostrongylus abstrusus* (Nematoda, Strongylida) infection in cats from Italy. *Vet. Parasitol.* 153 (1–2): 182–186.

141 Pechman, R.D. Jr. (1984). Newer knowledge of feline bronchopulmonary disease. *Vet. Clin. North Am. Small Anim. Pract.* 14 (5): 1007–1019.

142 Losonsky, J.M., Thrall, D.E., and Prestwood, A.K. (1983). Radiographic evaluation of pulmonary abnormalities after *Aelurostrongylus abstrusus* inoculation in cats. *Am. J. Vet. Res.* 44 (3): 478–482.

143 Mahaffey, M.B. (1979). Radiographic-pathologic findings in experimental Aelurostrongylus-Abstrusus infection in cats. *J. Am. Vet. Radiol. Soc.* 20 (2): 81.

144 Traversa, D., Di Cesare, A., and Conboy, G. (2010). Canine and feline cardiopulmonary parasitic nematodes in Europe: emerging and underestimated. *Parasit. Vectors* 3: 62.

145 Lacorcia, L., Gasser, R.B., Anderson, G.A., and Beveridge, I. (2009). Comparison of bronchoalveolar lavage fluid examination and other diagnostic techniques with the Baermann technique for detection of naturally occurring *Aelurostrongylus abstrusus* infection in cats. *J. Am. Vet. Med. Assoc.* 235 (1): 43–49.

146 Annoscia, G., Latrofa, M.S., Campbell, B.E. et al. (2014). Simultaneous detection of the feline lungworms *Troglostrongylus brevior* and *Aelurostrongylus abstrusus* by a newly developed duplex-PCR. *Vet. Parasitol.* 199 (3–4): 172–178.

147 Di Cesare, A., Veronesi, F., Frangipane di Regalbono, A. et al. (2015). Novel molecular assay for simultaneous identification of neglected lungworms and heartworms affecting cats. *J. Clin. Microbiol.* 53 (9): 3009–3013.

148 Di Cesare, A., di Regalbono, A.F., Tessarin, C. et al. (2014). Mixed infection by *Aelurostrongylus abstrusus* and *Troglostrongylus brevior* in kittens from the same litter in Italy. *Parasitol. Res.* 113 (2): 613–618.

149 Di Cesare, A., Iorio, R., Crisi, P. et al. (2015). Treatment of *Troglostrongylus brevior* (Metastrongyloidea, Crenosomatidae) in mixed lungworm infections using spot-on emodepside. *J. Feline Med. Surg.* 17 (2): 181–185.

150 Traversa, D., Iorio, R., and Otranto, D. (2008). Diagnostic and clinical implications of a nested PCR specific for ribosomal DNA of the feline lungworm *Aelurostrongylus abstrusus* (Nematoda, Strongylida). *J. Clin. Microbiol.* 46 (5): 1811–1817.

151 Foster, S.F. and Martin, P. (2011). Lower respiratory tract infections in cats: reaching beyond empirical therapy. *J. Feline Med. Surg.* 13 (5): 313–332.

152 Foster, S.F., Martin, P., Allan, G.S. et al. (2004). Lower respiratory tract infections in cats: 21 cases (1995–2000). *J. Feline Med. Surg.* 6 (3): 167–180.

153 Scott, D.W. (1973). Current knowledge of aelurostrongylosis in the cat. Literature review and case reports. *Cornell Vet.* 63 (3): 483–500.

36

Changes in Respiratory Rates and Patterns

36.1 Introduction to the Respiratory Cycle and Normal Resting Respiratory Rate

The respiratory cycle refers to the sequence of events that occurs during one complete breath [1, 2]. It consists of an active inspiratory phase, followed by passive exhalation [1, 2].

Inspiration is a mechanical process that results from the coordinated contraction of the diaphragm and the intercostal muscles [1, 2]. During inhalation, the rib cage shifts rostrally, ventrally, and laterally to expand the thoracic cavity [1, 2].

It takes effort to draw air into the respiratory tract [1, 2].

Think of the rib cage as storing up potential energy that is then released during exhalation, when the diaphragm and rib cage spring back to their default position [1, 2].

In order for this process to be effective, the thoracic cage must be flexible, and the lungs must be elastic [1, 2].

At rest, the body also unconsciously engages in abdominal breathing [2]. That is, every time the diaphragm contracts, the chest rises and the abdomen expands [2]. This expansion is visible to the outside observer [2].

With every exhalation, the abdomen recoils [2]. This, too, is outwardly apparent [2].

Readers may be more familiar with the term diaphragmatic or deep breathing than abdominal breathing. This technique is often introduced to people in exercise or yoga classes that center on the art of breathing for relaxation. Our veterinary patients do this naturally, at rest.

The veterinary patient that breathes in this matter is considered eupnic. Eupnea refers to the natural state of breathing in relaxed animals.

The normal respiratory rate of dogs and cats varies depending upon which reference is consulted as well as the activity level of the patient.

Sleeping cats and dogs have lower resting respiratory rates than if they were awake [1, 2]. Cats average 16–25 breaths per minute as compared to dogs, at 18–25 [2].

Awake patients require more breaths per minute [1]. The respiratory rate for a normal awake cat ranges from 20–40 breaths per minute, as compared to 20–30 in a dog [1, 3].

The size of the canine patient is inversely proportional to the respiratory rate [1]. Large-breed dogs tend to have lower respiratory rates than toy breeds [1].

In addition to body size, several other intrinsic and extrinsic factors affect respiratory rate, including the following [2, 4]:

- Age
- Ambient temperature
- Digestive tract
- Excitement
- Pregnancy

The respiratory rate is higher in neonates than in adults [2].

The respiratory rate increases as the ambient temperature rises [2].

Anything that increases abdominal contents, such as a pregnant uterus or a full digestive tract, limits diaphragmatic movement when the patient inhales [2]. To maintain adequate ventilation, the patient compensates by increasing the respiratory rate [2].

36.2 Introduction to Abnormal Respiratory Rates and Patterns

Appropriate medical terminology defines when respiratory rates stray from the normal reference range [1, 2]:

- Bradypnea: Abnormally slow breathing, resulting in a lower-than-normal respiratory rate
- Tachypnea: Abnormally rapid breathing, resulting in a higher-than-normal respiratory rate

Common Clinical Presentations in Dogs and Cats, First Edition. Ryane E. Englar.
© 2019 John Wiley & Sons, Inc. Published 2019 by John Wiley & Sons, Inc.

In addition, the following medical descriptors have been borrowed from the human medical field to express changes in respiratory sensations based upon client perception [2, 5]:

- Orthopnea: The feeling of being unable to breathe when in a recumbent position
- Dyspnea: Difficulty or discomfort with breathing

Orthopnea, in particular, is difficult to extrapolate to veterinary patients because they cannot verbalize this experience during the consultation. However, patients with orthopnea are reluctant to lay down on their sides and are more likely to stand with their head and neck held in extension, as if trying to maximize air intake. This presentation in particular makes this rather subjective word choice appropriate.

Dyspnea is easier to recognize on physical examination. Breathing is visibly labored, and respiratory movements are forced [2, 5].

Note that dyspnea is not always pathologic: patients that have just endured strenuous activity may be dyspneic, particularly if they are overweight or in poor physical condition [5].

Dyspnea may also result from additional physiological causes, such as the following [4, 6–10]:

- Anxiety
- Fear
- Hyperactivity
- Hyperthermia
- Pain

36.3 Pathological Causes of Dyspnea

Dyspnea results from difficulty getting air in, getting air out, or both [1, 11].

A narrowed upper airway is the source of inspiratory dyspnea [1, 11]. The patient with inspiratory dyspnea has difficulty getting air into the body [1]. Inspiration takes more effort than is typical. The body may have to rely upon the accessory respiratory muscles, the scalenus and the sternocephalicus, to complete the process [1]. These patients may flare the nostrils or retract the lip folds to maximize air intake [1].

Expiratory dyspnea results from inelastic lungs, that is, lungs that do not recoil. Alternate causes of expiratory dyspnea include a noncompliant rib cage or narrowed bronchi [1]. Abdominal and intrathoracic pressures are increased against a closed glottis in an attempt to forcibly expel air [1].

Although this is intended to facilitate respiration, it is ultimately counterproductive [1]. The process itself is akin to trying to exhale forcibly through a straw. Patients with narrowed bronchi cannot get more air out faster [1]. Their respiratory distress is thus intensified [1].

Patients can also develop both inspiratory and expiratory dyspnea [1, 11].

The list of differential diagnoses for dyspnea is extensive. The most common among these include the following [1, 4, 12–31]:

- Cardiomyopathy
  - Congestive heart failure (CHF)
  - Hypertrophic cardiomyopathy (HCM)
  - Valvular disease
- Heatstroke [32, 33]
- Lower airway disease
  - Bronchial disease (refer to Chapter 35)
    o Asthma (see Chapter 35, Section 35.4.1)
    o Bronchopneumonia
    o Chronic bronchitis (see Chapter 35, Section 35.4.2)
  - Foreign body
  - Neoplasia
  - Other pulmonary parenchymal disease
  - Tracheal disease
    o Tracheal collapse (see Chapter 34, Section 34.5)
  - Tracheobronchial disease
    o Infectious tracheobronchitis (ITB)
- Metabolic disease
  - Hyperadrenocorticism
  - Hyperthyroidism
  - Metabolic acidosis
- Restrictive airway disease
  - Ascites
  - Diaphragmatic hernia
  - Heartworm-associated respiratory disease (HARD) (see Chapter 35, Section 35.4.3)
  - Intra-abdominal mass
  - Lungworms (see Chapter 35, Section 35.4.4)
  - Peritoneopericardial diaphragmatic hernia (PPDH)
  - Pectus excavatum
  - Pericardial effusion
  - Pleural effusion
    o Chylothorax
    o Hemothorax
    o Pyothorax
  - Pneumothorax
  - Pulmonary contusion
  - Pulmonary edema
  - Pulmonary embolism
  - Morbid obesity (Pickwickian Syndrome)
  - Severe gastric distension
- Shock
  - Hypovolemic
  - Septic

- Toxicosis
  - Acetaminophen
  - Anticoagulant rodenticides
  - Ethylene glycol
  - Onions and garlic
- Trauma
  - Head trauma
  - Cervical trauma
- Upper airway disease (refer to Chapter 34)
  - Brachycephalic airway syndrome (see Chapter 34, Section 34.3)
  - Foreign body
  - Nasal disease
    - ○ Nasal neoplasia
    - ○ Stenotic nares (see Chapter 34, Section 34.3.1)
  - Nasopharyngeal disease
    - ○ Elongated soft palate (see Chapter 34, Section 34.3.2)
    - ○ Everted laryngeal saccules (see Chapter 34, Section 34.3.3)
  - Laryngeal disease
    - ○ Laryngeal edema
    - ○ Laryngeal neoplasia
    - ○ Laryngeal paralysis (see Chapter 34, Section 34.4)

An exhaustive review of each of the above is beyond the scope of this text. However, several of the more common differentials will be discussed here as they pertain to dyspnea.

36.3.1 Morbid Obesity (Pickwickian Syndrome)

A dog or cat is overweight when its body weight is 10% more than what is optimal, based upon its breed and frame [1, 34–36]. A patient is said to be obese when its body weight is 15% or more [1, 34–36].

Obesity is common among companion animal patients [1, 29, 37, 38]. At least one out of every three dogs that presents to the veterinarian for a consultation is obese [38] (see Figures 36.1a–c).

Although certain canine breeds, such as Greyhounds, rarely experience obesity, others are more likely to become overweight [29, 35, 37, 39–41]:

- Basset Hound
- Beagle
- Boxer
- Cairn Terrier
- Cocker Spaniel
- Dachshund
- King Charles Cavalier Spaniel
- Labrador Retriever
- Scottish Terrier
- Shetland Sheepdog

Dogs are not alone in their tendency to put on extra weight. Most cats are estimated to have at least 50% body fat, if not higher [1, 42, 43].

The rising incidence of obesity among pets mirrors the same trend in the human population within the Western hemisphere [37, 38, 44–47].

Obesity is not without risk to patient health [37].

Obese dogs are predisposed to cardiovascular disease, osteoarthritis, insulin resistance, and diabetes mellitus [38, 48–56]. They also, on average, live for two years less than their lean counterparts [54, 57]. This reduction in lifespan is thought to be the result of an increased risk of cancer.

The link between obesity and cancer in humans has been established for colorectal carcinoma [58], postmenopausal breast adenocarcinoma [59], esophageal-gastric adenocarcinoma [60, 61], and hepatocellular carcinoma [62]. More research is needed to establish this link in companion animal patients.

Obesity also impacts the respiratory system and the body's oxygenation status [63]. Decreased tidal volume, increased airway reactivity, and increased respiratory rates can be appreciated in obese dogs [63]. Obesity thereby impairs respiratory function [63].

The negative impact of obesity on respiration is referred to as Pickwickian Syndrome [29, 37, 63, 64]. The name of this syndrome is borrowed from a portly character in *The Pickwick Papers*, a novel by Charles Dickens [63]. Dickens' character, Mr. Pickwick, demonstrated the excessive strain that obesity can place upon a person's health [63].

Indeed, the strain of obesity on the respiratory tract is significant. Because the respiratory muscles are surrounded by fat, the heart, lungs, and diaphragm have to work harder to maintain cardiopulmonary function [63].

Dyspnea is a common clinical sign of Pickwickian Syndrome [12, 65].

Because patients with Pickwickian Syndrome are unable to take in sufficient air for ventilation, they become hypoxic [29, 64].

Canine patients respond to hypoventilation and hypoxemia by stimulating the bone marrow to produce more erythrocytes [64]. The resultant polycythemia results in increased levels of circulating erythropoietin; however, blood oxygen (O_2) saturation levels remain low [64].

This response is assumed to occur in cats as well; however, it has not yet been documented in the veterinary medical literature [64].

36.3.2 Heatstroke

Recall from Section 36.1 that ambient temperature is one of many factors that affects the respiratory rate [2, 4]. As ambient temperature rises, so, too, does respiration. This is an attempt by the body to thermoregulate [2].

(a)

(b)

(c)

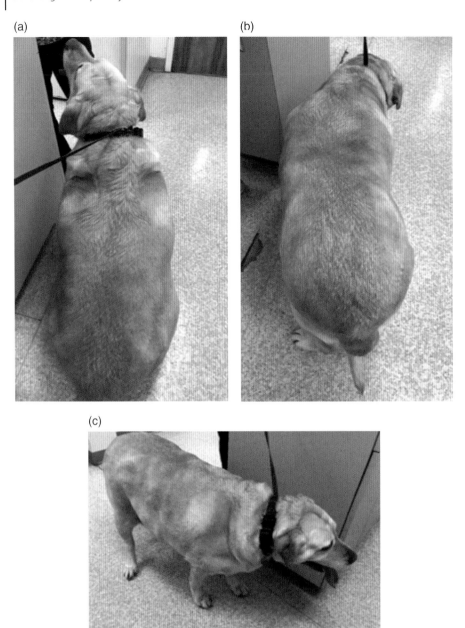

Figure 36.1 (a) Morbidly obese canine patient, in a seated position. *Source:* Courtesy of Pamela Mueller, DVM. (b) Morbidly obese canine patient, in a standing position. *Source:* Courtesy of Pamela Mueller, DVM. (c) Morbidly obese canine patient, panting after minimal exertion. It is easy to see how patients such as this one can become dyspneic. *Source:* Courtesy of Pamela Mueller, DVM.

If increasing the respiratory rate is insufficient, dogs are likely to pant as a form of evaporative cooling [2, 24, 66–69]. As the ambient humidity rises, panting becomes increasingly less efficient [24].

Unlike dogs, panting is not typical in cats. A panting cat is either very stressed or in a state of respiratory distress [70, 71].

Heatstroke occurs when the body is unable to effectively and efficiently dissipate heat [24]. In other words, there is a glitch in the body's thermostat. The body's core temperature has significantly exceeded the normal reference range. Now the patient cannot get its core temperature to drop below 106–109 °F [24].

Young and old patients are at greater risk for developing heatstroke [24]:

In addition, the following conditions increase the risk of heatstroke either because they prevent proper dissipation of heat or because they generate heat [24]:

- Brachycephalic airway syndrome
- Central nervous system (CNS) disease
- Fever

- Hyperthyroidism
- Laryngeal paralysis
- Obesity
- Severe muscle fasciculation
- Status epilepticus
- Tracheal collapse
- Upper airway obstruction

In the initial phases of heatstroke, the dog may continue to pant [32, 72]. Dyspnea is commonly reported by human patients who have suffered from heatstroke. The same action is observed in veterinary patients [72].

Initially, the patient's mucous membranes are flushed or hyperemic, in spite of the patient being dyspneic, and pulses are strong [72].

However, as heatstroke progresses, the patient experiences pooling of splanchnic blood [72]. This decreases circulating blood volume [72]. Decreased blood volume results in hypotension [72].

Peripheral vasodilation, in combination with hypovolemia, causes cardiac output to fall [72].

Reduced cardiac output leads to inadequate tissue perfusion [72].

In advanced stages, there is thermal-induced cerebral edema in addition to poor tissue perfusion. This combination suppresses patient mentation as well as the panting reflex [24, 72]. The respiratory rate falls. Respiratory arrest is possible [72].

Thermal damage to tissue extends beyond just the cerebrum [24]. The endothelium also suffers extensive damage that results in breaks within the vasculature [24]. Coagulopathies are common [24].

Hemorrhage may arise from any and every orifice, and includes the following [24]:

- The mouth, in the form of hemoptysis
- The nose, in the form of epistaxis
- The skin, in the form of petechiae and ecchymoses
- The stool, in the form of hematochezia
- The urine, in the form of hematuria
- The vomit, in the form of hematemesis

Hemorrhage may also be hidden internally [24].

Thrombocytopenia contributes to coagulopathy, and disseminated intravascular coagulation (DIC) is a significant concern [24, 72].

36.3.3 Cardiogenic Pulmonary Edema

Pulmonary edema is the condition in which fluid builds up within the air sacs, or alveoli, of the lungs [73]. This fluid layer interferes with gas exchange and may result in eventual respiratory failure.

Fluid buildup may result from capillary hydrostatic pressure that exceeds what is considered normal [73].

This excess of force tips the balance in favor of fluid buildup within the interstitial space [73]. Alternatively, lower-than-normal capillary oncotic pressure may cause pulmonary edema because what fluid is forced out of the vasculature with each cardiac cycle is not sufficiently drawn back in [73].

Pulmonary edema can be further classified based upon whether it is caused by primary heart disease or by primary respiratory disease [73].

Cardiogenic pulmonary edema is the result of left-sided CHF [73–75]. The left ventricle of the heart is responsible for pumping blood through the aorta and into the systemic circulation [2, 75]. When it fails as a pump, the left ventricle experiences backflow of blood into the left atrium [2, 75]. From the left atrium, blood backs up into the pulmonary vasculature, causing congestion of the lungs [73]. This congestion is visible on thoracic radiographs [73].

The most common causes of left-sided CHF in companion animal practice include the following [26, 27, 73, 76, 77]:

- Chronic valvular heart disease (CVHD)/myxomatous valve degeneration/endocardiosis
  - Mitral regurgitation (MR)
- Dilated cardiomyopathy (DCM)
- HCM

Cardiomyopathy is common in dogs, with several well-established breed predispositions to disease [78–81].

For example, acquired mitral valve disease (MVD) and associated MR are more likely to occur in older, small breeds such as the Chihuahua, Dachshund, King Charles Cavalier spaniel, Maltese, Miniature Schnauzer, and Toy Poodle [26, 27, 77, 81, 82]. This condition is the direct result of a degenerating mitral valve [27]. In health, the mitral valve exists to ensure forward flow of blood from the left atrium to the left ventricle and out to systemic circulation [27]. In MVD, the mitral valve steadily loses its ability to serve as a closed door to the left atrium during left ventricular contraction [27, 82]. The door, in a sense, remains ajar.

Depending upon the severity of disease, patients with MVD experience varying degrees of regurgitation of blood into the left atrium every time the heart beats [27, 81, 82]. As disease progresses, the amount of blood that flows into the aorta with each cardiac cycle reduces [27, 82]. Over time, the backflow of blood into the pulmonary vasculature causes pulmonary edema [27, 82].

DCM is another cause of left-sided CHF that is diagnosed in clinical practice. Among dogs, DCM is more commonly seen in Doberman Pinschers and Irish Wolfhounds, particularly males [26, 77, 78].

DCM in cats, on the other hand, has been primarily linked to taurine deficiency [83].

DCM is characterized by progressive left ventricular and atrial dilation [77]. Over time, ventricular contractility is compromised [77]. The heart is enlarged, yet flaccid. Its contractions are inefficient, and outgoing blood velocity is significantly reduced [77]. Blood backs up from the left ventricle into the left atrium, and ultimately the pulmonary vasculature. Ventricular arrhythmias are common, as is sudden death among those that acquire this disease [78].

HCM is the most common form of cardiomyopathy in the cat [1, 84, 85].

Patients with CHF are typically tachypneic and in respiratory distress [73]. On physical examination, they often have moderate to high-grade cardiac murmurs [73].

If there is bilateral involvement of the heart in CHF, the patient also experiences backflow of blood from the right ventricle, to the right atrium, and ultimately into the systemic circuit [73]. This buildup of fluid systemically may result in distension of the jugular vein or ascites [73]. Ascites is the accumulation of fluid within the peritoneal cavity. This results in a pot-bellied appearance. If buildup is sufficient, then a fluid wave is often palpable within the abdomen [1].

Radiographic evidence that supports a diagnosis of CHF includes the following changes on thoracic films [26, 73, 86]:

- Cardiomegaly, particularly left atrial
- Pulmonary venous distension
- Pulmonary infiltrate

Coughing is common among canine patients with left-sided CHF and results from a combination of pulmonary edema and compression of the mainstem bronchus by an enlarged left atrium [86].

Pulmonary infiltrate is typically interstitial to alveolar in appearance [73]. In canine patients, it tends to develop first at the perihilar region [73]. As the disease expands, infiltrate may fill the entire lung parenchyma [73] (see Figures 36.2a, b).

CHF requires lifelong medical management, which aims to reduce fluid buildup and improve oxygenation status through diuresis [73–75, 86, 87]. Furosemide is the most commonly prescribed diuretic among patients with CHF [73, 75].

Vasodilation is also key to treatment and is routinely managed by angiotensin-converting enzyme (ACE)

(b)

(a)

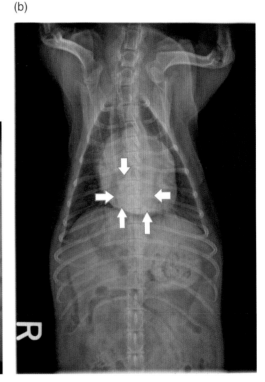

Figure 36.2 (a). Lateral thoracic radiograph of a canine patient with MVD that has resulted in left-sided congestive heart failure (CHF). Note the blue-outlined, white-filled arrows denoting an enlarged left atrium. Note the dark blue-outlined, orange-filled arrow depicting compression of the mainstem bronchus. This compression is likely to cause the patient to cough intermittently. *Source:* Courtesy of Daniel Foy, MS, DVM, DACVIM, DACVECC. (b) Orthogonal view of the same patient in Figure 13.1a. Note the blue-outlined, white-filled arrows denoting an enlarged left atrium. *Source:* Courtesy of Daniel Foy, MS, DVM, DACVECC.

inhibitors [74, 87]. ACE functions in the body to catalyze the conversion of angiotensin I into angiotensin II [74]. Angiotensin II acts as a potent vasoconstrictor [74]. In health, this pathway is under tight regulation: that is, the pathway is not always turned on.

However, in certain disease states, including CHF, the renin-angiotensin-aldosterone system (RAAS) is in overdrive [74]. Chronic stimulation causes vasoconstriction that, over time, induces systemic hypertension [74]. In the short term, this represents the body's attempt to help itself: hypertension is an attempt to improve cardiac output to maintain adequate tissue perfusion [74].

This is unsustainable [74]. The increased cardiac workload damages the myocardium [74]. This creates a vicious cycle. The increasingly damaged heart becomes increasingly dysfunctional, which means that it has to work even harder to perfuse tissues [74]. Venous pressure continues to rise, along with the rest of the vasculature. This ultimately dumps even more fluid into the alveoli. Pulmonary congestion steadily worsens, and the patient declines.

ACE inhibitors, such as enalapril and benazepril, reduce the workload on the heart by encouraging vasodilation [74].

Recently, the drug pimobendan was approved for use in dogs with valve-associated CHF, for example, MVD [74]. This drug increases the efficiency of the heart through the inhibition of phosphodiesterase and by sensitizing the heart to calcium [74]. This improves cardiac contractility [74].

36.3.4 Iatrogenic, Cardiogenic Pulmonary Edema

Overaggressive fluid therapy can potentially result in iatrogenic, cardiogenic pulmonary edema [73]. For this reason, fluid therapy must be tailored to the individual patient, and hospitalized patients that are receiving fluid therapy must be carefully observed for changes in respiratory rate that could indicate fluid overload.

One sign of fluid overload that typically precedes overt respiratory distress is the development of bilaterally symmetrical, serous, nasal discharge [1]. This is a patient that needs to be re-examined immediately.

36.3.5 Non-Cardiogenic Pulmonary Edema

Pulmonary edema is often, but not always related to failure of the heart as a pump. There are also non-cardiac causes of pulmonary edema. These include the following [1, 20, 73, 88, 89]:

- Accidental electrocution from the chewing of electric cords
- Near drowning

- Sepsis and acute respiratory distress syndrome (ARDS)
- Upper airway obstruction

Patients with non-cardiogenic pulmonary edema are typically tachypneic at time of presentation and in respiratory distress [73].

Unlike patients with primary heart disease, patients with non-cardiogenic pulmonary edema tend to have a normal heart rate [73]. In other words, they are not tachycardic [73]. They also tend not to have murmurs. If they do, they are incidental and unrelated.

Puppies that present in acute respiratory distress should have their oral cavities thoroughly examined once they have been stabilized [73]. It is important that they be assessed for lingual burns and other forms of oral lesions that might have been caused by chewing electric cords [73].

Thoracic radiographs typically demonstrate changes within the caudodorsal lung fields, whereas those patients with cardiogenic pulmonary edema have increased interstitial or alveolar opacity that is concentrated in the perihilar region [90]. Patients with non-cardiogenic pulmonary edema will also lack cardiomegaly [73] (see Figures 36.3a, b).

Oxygen therapy and rest are the mainstay of treatment for these patients [73, 91–95].

36.3.6 Pleural Effusion

Compared to pulmonary edema, which is the result of fluid buildup within the alveoli of the lungs, pleural effusion refers to fluid buildup within the chest cavity itself.

A membrane, the pleura, lines the chest cavity, or pleural space [96]. In health, there is only a small amount of fluid within the pleural space [96]. This fluid, approximately five milliliters or so, lubricates the pulmonary parenchyma [96].

Pathology occurs where there is buildup of fluid within this space. This buildup can result from an excess of fluid production or insufficient fluid absorption by the pleura [96].

When an excess of fluid is present in the pleural space, it restricts the ability of the lungs to expand [13]. Patients struggle to take in sufficient air. They present with inspiratory dyspnea, tachypnea, and/or open mouth breathing [13]. These patients prefer not to lie down. Their default position is sternal recumbency [13].

Breaths tend to be rapid and shallow [97].

Physical examination may reveal muffled lung sounds, especially ventrally [13]. However, these patients are critical and may decline rapidly. Immediate stabilization must be prioritized over thoracic radiography to lessen the chance of respiratory arrest.

Thoracocentesis, a "chest tap," is a necessary procedure in patients that are suspected of having pleural effusion

(b)

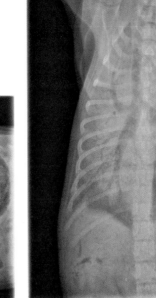

(a)

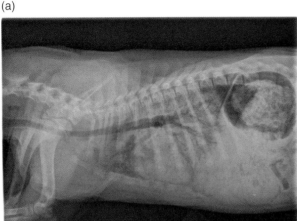

Figure 36.3 (a) Lateral radiograph of patient with non-cardiogenic pulmonary edema. Courtesy of Daniel Foy, MS, DVM, DACVIM, DACVECC. (b) Orthogonal radiographic view of the same patient that is depicted in Figure 36.3a. *Source:* Courtesy of Daniel Foy, MS, DVM, DACVIM, DACVECC.

[13]. Tapping the chest requires the insertion of a needle through the skin, intercostal muscles, and body wall to enter into the pleural space [98]. This allows fluid to be extracted from the pleural space [98].

Contraindications to thoracocentesis include coagulopathies and thrombocytopenia [98].

Refer to an emergency text or internal medicine reference for a description of the procedure itself and tips for obtaining diagnostic fluid.

Thoracocentesis is therapeutic because it improves restrictive airway disease in patients with pleural effusion [13].

Thoracocentesis is also an important diagnostic test. It provides the clinician with a fluid sample that can be evaluated grossly as well as cytologically [13].

Diagnostic testing of pleural fluid is important because there are many types of effusions, each of which has its own unique pathophysiology.

It is also important to recognize that pleural effusion is not in and of itself a diagnosis [13]. It is a condition caused by underlying disease(s) [13]. Without identifying the underlying disease, thoracocentesis is unlikely to be curative; that is, pleural fluid is likely to refill. Addressing the primary problem is the most important

aspect of any patient plan. This requires a diagnostic investigation into the source of the fluid.

There is more than one type of pleural effusion. Classification of the effusion is routinely based upon gross appearance, protein concentration, and nucleated cell content [13].

Grossly, there are hemorrhagic, purulent, and chylous effusions [13, 98]. These are the result of hemothorax, pyothorax, and chylothorax, respectively [98]. Pyothorax is synonymous with empyema, a term that is used with frequency in human medical texts [25, 96].

Hemorrhagic effusions are, expectedly, blood red in color (see Figure 36.4).

Older effusions may darken in terms of color to more of a dark red or rust brown.

Grossly, fluid from a pyothorax is said to take on the consistency of thickened "tomato soup." [96]. The color may range from strawberry-red to yellowish-green to a latte-like beige-brown [96].

Chyle is produced, in health, in the small intestine. It is a by-product of lipid digestion. Once formed, it enters into special lymphatics called lacteals. Lacteals combine into larger lymphatics that ultimately empty out into the thoracic duct. In health, the thoracic duct

ᅳᅳᅳᅳᅳ

ᅳᅳᅳᅳᅳᅳ

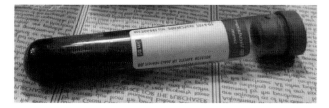

Figure 36.4 Hemorrhagic effusion.

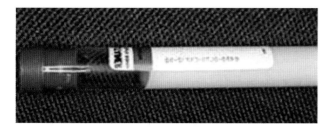

Figure 36.5 Chylous effusion.

transports chyle back into systemic circulation at the level of the vena cava.

Chyle accumulates within the pleural cavity if the thoracic duct is obstructed or if it has ruptured. Chyle is irritating to the pleural space in and of itself and often incites an inflammatory response [99].

When chylous effusions are extracted by thoracocentesis, they are typically milky white [99] (see Figure 36.5).

Effusions may be further described based upon clarity [100]. Turbid or opaque samples are more likely to be proteinaceous and/or highly cellular [100].

Note that appearance of the effusion alone is not diagnostic: not all effusions follow the textbook in terms of color. Further analysis is indicated to evaluate effusions based upon the following characteristics [13, 25, 96]:

- Cellularity
  - Highly cellular
  - Moderately cellular
  - Scant cellular content
  - Acellular
- Cell count differential: the percentage of cells that are
  - Erythrocytes
  - Leukocytes
- Protein content
  - High protein
  - Moderate protein
  - Low protein
- Triglyceride content
  - High triglyceride content
  - Low triglyceride content

Effusions with triglyceride concentrations that measure greater than 100 mg/dl are diagnostic for chyle [100].

If the triglyceride concentration of the sample is less than this value, but is more than double the value of serum triglycerides, then the effusion is also said to be chyle [100].

The protein and cellular content of effusions is particularly helpful in prioritizing differential diagnoses in clinical cases [13]. These categories collectively define effusions as being one of the following types [13, 25, 100, 101]:

- Pure transudate
  - Protein <3.0 g/dl
  - Nucleated cell count <1000/μl
- Modified transudate
  - Protein: 3.0–3.5 g/dl
  - Nucleated cell count: 1000–5000/μl
- Non-septic exudate
  - Protein: >3.0 g/dl
  - Nucleated cell count: >5000/μl
- Septic exudate
  - Protein: > 3.0 g/dl
  - Nucleated cell count: >50 000/μl

As indicated above, transudates are low-protein effusions [13, 100, 101]. These may result from pre-hepatic or portal hypertension [101]. Hypertension creates an excess of hydrostatic pressure at these sites that promotes leakage of lymph [101].

High-protein exudates are more likely to result from hepatic sinusoidal or post-sinusoidal hypertension, and CHF [101].

The cellular content of effusions may also provide clues [13, 96, 99–101]. For example, chylous effusions tend to have variable nucleated cell counts; however, the majority of cells are small lymphocytes [101]. In addition, non-degenerate neutrophils, macrophages, and lipid droplets may be appreciated [101]. As the effusion becomes chronic, lymphocyte counts remain elevated, but neutrophil counts significantly spike [101].

Pyothorax is confirmed by cytological identification of degenerate neutrophils and bacteria within the effusion [96]. Intracellular bacteria are commonly seen, and mixed bacterial infections occur with frequency [96]. Pyothorax is typically the result of bite wounds to the chest or pulmonary abscesses [96]. Pyothorax may also be iatrogenic, for example, if thoracocentesis is not performed under sterile conditions [96].

Neoplastic effusions are characterized by the presence of neoplastic cells [13].

Thoracic radiography is a helpful imaging modality that can confirm effusions; however, the dyspneic patient should not be imaged before attempts are made to stabilize it. Dyspneic patients are at extreme risk of respiratory arrest.

Radiographic changes that are supportive of pleural space disease include the following [63, 102]:

- Inability to differentiate where the cardiac silhouette ends and the diaphragm begins, when the film is taken with the patient in sternal recumbency
  - Fluid sinks ventrally and surrounds the heart
  - Fluid abuts the diaphragm
  - Because the heart, diaphragm, and effusion share the same opacity, they blur together as one indistinguishable structure
  - This is called border effacement
- Pleural fissure lines
- Rounded costophrenic angles
- Scalloped lung margins
- Separation of the lungs from the body wall
- Uniformly elevated trachea (see Figures 36.6a–d)

36.3.7 Pneumothorax

Pleural space disease may be caused by air instead of fluid [6, 103]. The condition by which air accumulates within the pleural space is pneumothorax [104].

There are three primary causes of pneumothorax [104]:

- Traumatic
- Spontaneous
- Iatrogenic

The most common cause of pneumothorax in companion animal practice is thoracic trauma [6, 103–110].

Younger, intact male dogs are at increased risk of sustaining thoracic trauma [104, 106, 111].

Thoracic trauma in turn may lead to either [104–106]

- Closed pneumothorax, in which the thoracic cavity sustains blunt force trauma without actually sustaining a wound
- Open pneumothorax, in which a wound extends from the outside environment into the thoracic cavity.

Traumatic, closed pneumothorax is more common than traumatic, open pneumothorax [104–106]. Vehicular injury is frequently implicated in the development of closed pneumothorax [104]. When the chest cavity is struck by an automobile, the likelihood of lung parenchyma rupturing is high [104, 107, 108]. This causes air to leak into the pleural space [104, 107, 108].

Lung damage can also be sustained if ribs fracture and pierce lung lobes [104].

As compared to closed pneumothorax, open pneumothorax is caused by a physical wound that enters the chest, creating a path between the thoracic cavity and the outside world [104]. Bite wounds, gunshots, and stab wounds can achieve this effect [104].

Spontaneous pneumothorax infrequently occurs [104, 105, 111–114]. When it does, it is more typical of deep-chested, large-breed dogs, particularly Siberian Huskies [104, 105, 115–117].

Spontaneous pneumothorax results from the rupture of bullae that develop when airway obstruction damages alveoli [105, 111, 112, 114, 116, 117]. More than one lung lobe can be involved; however, if only one lung lobe is involved, it is most commonly the right middle [117, 118].

Other causes of spontaneous pneumothorax include the following [104, 111, 112, 114, 117, 119–126]:

- Feline asthma
- Infection with heartworms, *Dirofilaria immitis*
- Migration of grass awns
- Migration of porcupine quills
- Neoplasia
- Pneumonia

Iatrogenic pneumothorax results from tracheal perforation secondary to over-inflation of the endotracheal cuff during intubation or removal of the endotracheal tube without deflating the cuff [97, 109, 127, 128].

Tracheal laceration may also occur secondary to faulty attempts at jugular venipuncture, or secondary to mechanical ventilation [104, 107].

Regardless of the cause, pneumothorax is a type of restrictive airway disease.

Air outside of the lungs restricts their ability to expand [13]. Patients cannot ventilate appropriately. They present much like patients with pleural effusion, that is, with inspiratory dyspnea, tachypnea, and/or open mouth breathing [13, 14].

Breaths tend to be rapid and shallow [97].

On physical examination, patients may have diminished lung sounds dorsally [6].

Patients with tracheal tears are also likely to have developed subcutaneous emphysema, that is, air beneath the skin [97, 104].

Patients in respiratory distress are unstable and require immediate intervention [6]. There is a pressing need to perform thoracocentesis in order to lessen the degree of restrictive airway disease [6].

Radiography is confirmatory for pneumothorax, but should be performed secondary to stabilization, rather than before [6, 104].

Radiographic changes that are supportive of a diagnosis include the following [104]:

- Loss of contact between the cardiac silhouette and the sternum: The heart essentially looks like it is floating in space
- Lung lobe atelectasis, or collapse
  - Affected lungs are more radiopaque than is typical of normal lung tissue
  - Affected lungs appear to peel away from the pleura (see Figures 36.7a, b)

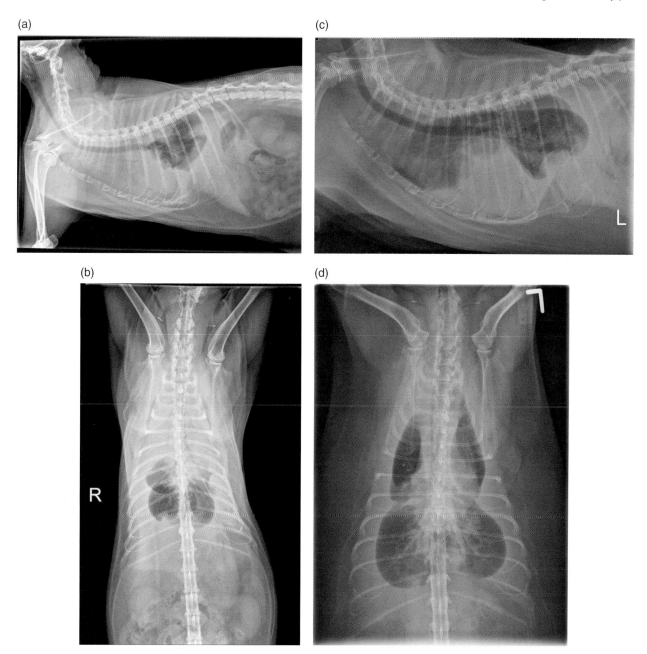

Figure 36.6 (a) Lateral radiograph of a feline patient with pleural effusion. Note the scalloped lung margins. This cat presented for dyspnea. (b) Orthogonal radiographic view of the feline patient that is depicted in Figure 36.6a. (c) Second example of a patient with pleural effusion. *Source:* Courtesy of Daniel Foy, MS, DVM, DACVIM, DACVECC. (d) Orthogonal radiographic view of the patient that is depicted in Figure 36.6c. *Source:* Courtesy of Daniel Foy, MS, DVM, DACVIM, DACVECC.

36.3.8 Mass Effect Within the Pleural Space

Section 36.3.6 reviewed how fluid within the pleural space can restrict the lungs' ability to expand on inspiration, and Section 36.3.7 reviewed how air can achieve the same outcome. However, fluid and air are not the only fillers to take up room within the pleural space. Pleural space disease may also take the form of solid tissue [1].

Solid tissue of any kind within the pleural space restricts lung expansion [1, 129].

Solid tissue may include [1, 6, 130–138]

- The contents of a diaphragmatic hernia
- Neoplasia.

36.3.8.1 Diaphragmatic Hernia
The diaphragm is a muscular barrier between the thoracic and abdominal cavities [1]. It plays a major role in respiration [1].

(a)

(b)

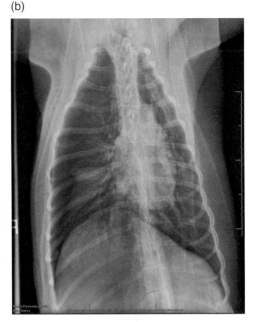

Figure 36.7 (a) Lateral radiograph of a patient with traumatic pneumothorax. *Source:* Courtesy of Daniel Foy, MS, DVM, DACVIM, DACVECC. (b) Orthogonal, dorsal-ventral (D/V) radiographic view of the feline patient that is depicted in Figure 36.7a. *Source:* Courtesy of Daniel Foy, MS, DVM, DACVIM, DACVECC.

A diaphragmatic hernia is an abnormal connection between both body cavities, resulting in the migration of abdominal organs into the thorax [1, 28].

Diaphragmatic hernias may be [1]

- Traumatic
- Congenital.

Traumatic events, such as the blunt force associated with automobile injuries, may cause a rent in the diaphragm.

Other patients have a thoracic-abdominal connection at the time of birth. The most common type among these is the PPDH [139–142]. PPDH is the condition by which the pericardial sac communicates with the peritoneal cavity [139–142] (see Figures 36.8a, b).

Patients with PPDH often have concurrent skeletal abnormalities, including abnormal numbers of sternebrae and vertebrae, or pectus excavatum [141].

Patients with PPDH may or may not have additional non-skeletal congenital anomalies, including heart-related conditions, such as atrial septal defect, or eyelid atresia and microphthalmia [141].

Note that not all patients are clinical for PPDH [143]. The size of the defect may be very small [143]. In some cases, only the omentum herniates [143].

In more significant cases, entire organs herniate from the abdominal cavity into the thorax [143]. The liver and/or gall bladder are most commonly involved [143]. However, the stomach, small intestines, and spleen are also capable of herniation [143].

If patients are clinical for disease, their signs typically pertain to the respiratory and/or digestive tracts [143]. Concerning respiration, patients are frequently tachypneic or dyspneic [143]. Owners may complain that they tire easily [143].

Concerning gastrointestinal signs, the patient may develop nausea, vomiting, or diarrhea [143]. The patient may also lose weight [143].

Surgical correction is advised [143].

36.3.8.2 Pleural Space Neoplasia

Neoplasia may also occur anywhere within the pleural space, including the cranial mediastinum. Cranial mediastinal masses include the following [144–147]:

- Ectopic thyroid carcinoma
- Lymphoma
- Thymoma
- Thymolipoma
- Thymic cyst

The presence of a cranial mediastinal mass may be suspected in the feline patient if the thorax exhibits reduced compressibility on palpation [1].

Thoracic radiographs support a diagnosis of cranial mediastinal mass [147]. The following changes on lateral thoracic films are suggestive [147]:

- Increased radiopacity cranial to the heart
- Tracheal elevation and/or compression
- Displacement of the heart caudally

(b)

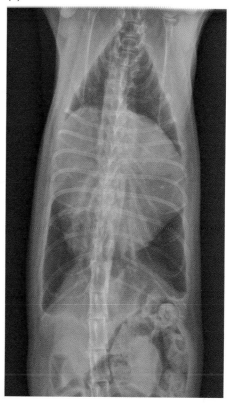

(a)

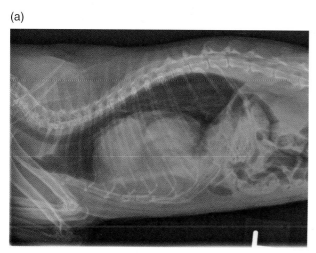

Figure 36.8 (a) Left lateral thoracic radiograph of a cat with peritoneopericardial hernia (PPDH), a congenital abnormality that improperly allows communication between the thoracic and abdominal cavities. *Source:* Courtesy of Daniel Foy, MS, DVM, DACVIM, DACVECC. (b) Ventrodorsal (V/D) thoracic radiograph of the same cat with PPDH. *Source:* Courtesy of Daniel Foy, MS, DVM, DACVIM, DACVECC.

- Displacement of the carina caudal to the sixth intercostal space
- Silhouetting of the mass with the heart

On orthogonal views, that is, the dorsoventral (D/V) or ventrodorsal (V/D), the cranial mediastinum typically appears wider than normal on account of the mass [147]. The cranial lung lobes may also be caudally displaced [147] (see Figures 36.9a, b).

Note that a mass effect within the pleural space may also be caused by enlarged sternal and cranial mediastinal lymph nodes [147] (see Figures 36.10a–c).

36.3.9 Pulmonary Neoplasia

Lung tumors may also compromise the ability of a patient to engage in effective, efficient respiration.

Lung tumors may be primary or metastatic.

36.3.9.1 Primary Lung Tumors

Primary lung tumors are relatively rare in companion animal practice, particularly in cats [148–154].

The most common primary lung tumors in dogs and cats are carcinomas, specifically adenocarcinomas [148,

150, 151, 153–158]. Squamous cell, bronchial gland, or alveolar cell carcinomas may also occur [148, 150, 157].

The impact of primary lung tumors on clinical signs and patient presentation depends upon their location within the thoracic cavity as well as their extensiveness [148].

Cough is the most common sign of a primary lung tumor in dogs [150, 151, 158]. Dyspnea is more likely to occur when the tumor is extensive, meaning that it involves a significant portion of one or more lung lobes [148]. Hemoptysis, that is, bloody sputum, is appreciated on occasion in dogs with primary lung tumors [148].

Dyspnea is more commonly reported in feline patients, regardless of tumor size, whereas cough is rarely appreciated [148].

Weight loss, anorexia, lethargy, and weakness are commonly reported in both cats and dogs [148].

As many as one in four cats with primary lung tumors present with lameness [148]. The potential for cats to develop lung-digit syndrome is a valid concern [148]. This is a condition in which the primary lung tumor metastasizes to the digits [148]. One or more digits may be affected. Affected digits may be swollen. They may develop alopecia. They may also develop ulcerative lesions (see Figures 36.11a, b).

(a)

(b)

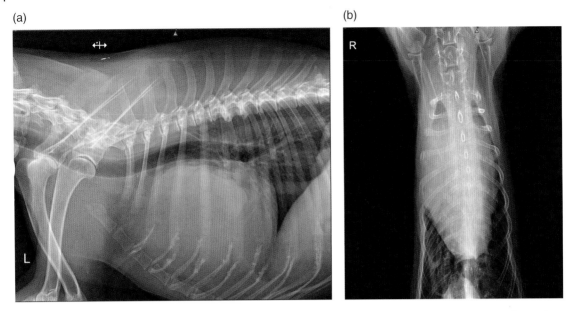

Figure 36.9 (a) Left lateral thoracic radiograph of a patient with a cranial mediastinal mass. *Source:* Courtesy of Daniel Foy, MS, DVM, DACVIM, DACVECC. (b) Orthogonal thoracic radiographic view of the same patient depicted in Figure 36.9a. *Source:* Courtesy of Daniel Foy, MS, DVM, DACVIM, DACVECC.

Primary lung tumors are visible in thoracic radiographs [148]. They may involve one or more lung lobes [148] (see Figures 36.12a–c).

Lung-digit syndrome does not appear to be common in dogs [148].

Computed tomography (CT) is able to detect tracheobronchial lymph node involvement with greater accuracy than radiography [148]. Dogs with tracheobronchial lymph node involvement have a poorer prognosis [148, 152, 158–160].

Ultrasound-guided fine-needle aspiration is a diagnostic tool that is a valuable starting point in the diagnostic work-up of the patient [148]. Fluoroscopy can also help with sampling, in lieu of ultrasonography [148, 161]. A good correlation exists between cytologic and histologic results [148, 161, 162].

Pneumonectomy, that is, partial or complete surgical removal of a lung lobe, is the treatment of choice for a primary lung tumor [148]. A synonym for this procedure is lung lobectomy.

The surgical approach for a lung lobectomy has historically been via thoracotomy [148]. However, thoracoscopy is gaining ground in both human and veterinary medicine because it results in less tissue trauma and reduced morbidity [148].

Depending upon clinical staging of the patient and histologic findings, adjuvant chemotherapy may be indicated [148]. Consult an oncology reference for more information on chemotherapy protocols that are typical for postoperative management of primary lung tumors.

36.3.9.2 Metastatic Lung Tumors

Tumors may also arise within the lungs as metastatic lesions from distant sites [149, 163].

Neoplastic cells spread to the lung through three main routes [163]:

- By direct extension of tumor cells
- Through the bloodstream
- Via lymphatic drainage

Not all tumors metastasize, and not all metastasize to the lungs.

Of those that do, not all share the same incidence of pulmonary metastasis. The types of cancer that frequently metastasize to the lungs of companion animal patients include the following [149, 163]:

- Hemangiosarcoma
- Mammary adenocarcinoma
- Oral melanoma
- Osteosarcoma

Patients that have metastatic lung tumors typically present with tachypnea and/or dyspnea [149, 163]. Cough is less likely to be seen in cases of pulmonary metastasis than primary lung tumors.

Pulmonary metastasis is evident on thoracic radiographs when lesions reach a certain size [149, 163]. When evaluating any patient for evidence of metastasis, it is common to take three radiographic views of the thorax. These consist of a right and left lateral thoracic radiograph, as well as one orthogonal view. Collectively, these make up the standard "met check"

(a)

(b)

(c)

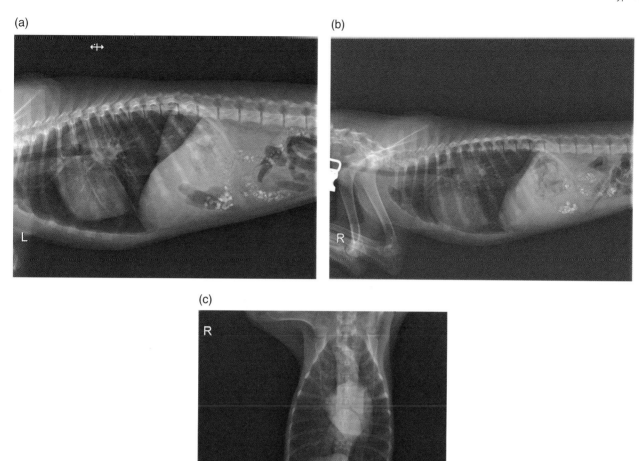

Figure 36.10 (a) Left lateral thoracic radiograph of a patient with tracheobronchial lymph node enlargement. *Source:* Courtesy of Daniel Foy, MS, DVM, DACVIM, DACVECC. (b) Right lateral thoracic radiograph of a patient with tracheobronchial lymph node enlargement. *Source:* Courtesy of Daniel Foy, MS, DVM, DACVIM, DACVECC. (c) V/D thoracic radiograph of a patient with tracheobronchial lymph node enlargement. *Source:* Courtesy of Daniel Foy, MS, DVM, DACVIM, DACVECC.

that is performed with frequency in clinical practice (see Figures 36.13a, b).

Note that lesions less than 3 mm in diameter may be missed [149, 163].

36.4 Bradypnea

Recall that bradypnea refers to abnormally slow breathing. The bradypneic patient has a lower-than-normal respiratory rate [1, 2].

Bradypnea is less likely to be appreciated in clinical practice than tachypnea or dyspnea.

When it occurs, bradypnea may be the result of [22, 31, 164–166]

- Drugs
- Hypothermia.

Bradypnea may be mild. However, bradypnea can potentially cause respiratory depression and apnea [167, 168]. Extreme cases can result in patient hypoxemia, respiratory acidosis, and death [167, 168].

(a)   (b)

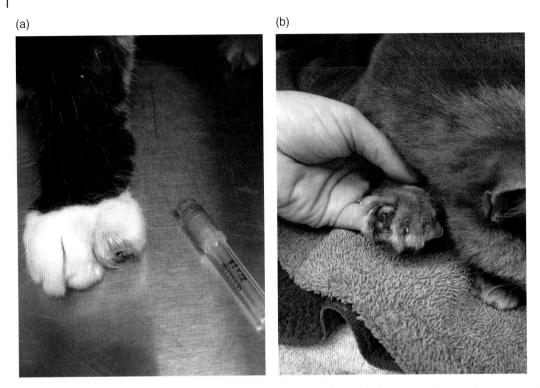

Figure 36.11 (a) Grossly swollen, alopecic digit in a feline patient with lung-digit syndrome. *Source:* Courtesy of Beki Cohen Regan, DVM, DACVIM (Oncology). (b) Ulcerated digit in a feline patient with lung-digit syndrome. *Source:* Courtesy of Beki Cohen Regan, DVM, DACVIM (Oncology).

36.4.1 Drug-Induced Respiratory Depression

Drug-induced respiratory depression (DIRD) is a common problem in human patients, particularly in the postoperative setting [164]. DIRD has been recognized in veterinary patients as well [30]. In both humans and animals, DIRD is often the direct result of medications that have been prescribed for analgesia or sedation [164].

36.4.1.1 Opioids
The administration of opioids may result in bradypnea [30]. Opioid-induced respiratory depression results from activation of the μ receptor [30]. One effect is a diminished response by the patient to carbon dioxide partial pressures (PCO_2). That is, when PCO_2 rises, the natural response of the body is to increase ventilation.

This response to rising levels of CO_2 is muted in patients that receive opioids [30]. The degree to which the response is reduced depends upon the dose [30]. The higher the dose, the greater the impact [30].

Dogs and cats are more resistant to this adverse effect than humans; however, concurrent anesthesia may increase the chance that respiratory depression will occur [30].

Neonatal patients are also more likely to become bradypneic when they receive opioids, so close monitoring is essential [30].

In addition to neonates, fetuses are susceptible to DIRD when drugs are capable of crossing the placenta [30]. This includes opioids [30].

36.4.1.2 Propofol
Propofol is a common induction agent in companion animal practice that works by enhancing the inhibitory effects of γ-aminobutyric acid [31, 167]. Cardiovascular and respiratory depression are common adverse events that, like opioids, are dose-dependent [31, 167, 169–171].

The risk of apnea appears to be greatest in dogs when the dose exceeds 14 mg/kg [31].

Administering doses slowly rather than as a bolus minimizes the risk of apnea [31]. Titrate dose to effect.

36.4.2 Hypothermia

Hypothermia is a condition by which core body temperature is lower than normal. Hypothermia may occur as a result of environmental extremes. Consider, for example, a patient that is exposed to wintry weather with inappropriate shelter. Alternatively, hypothermia may result due to an unexpected emergency, such as cold-water near drowning [165, 172]. Both of these circumstances represent situations involving primary hypothermia, as opposed to secondary hypothermia.

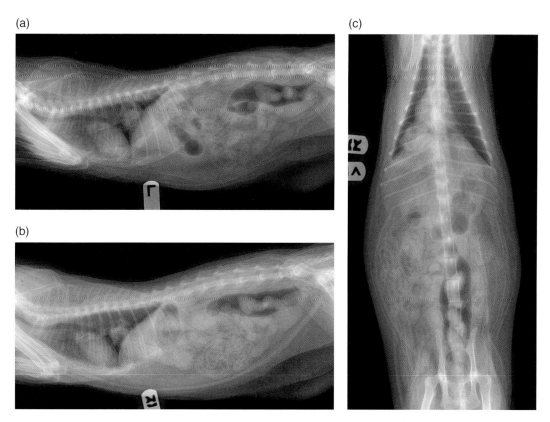

Figure 36.12 (a) Left lateral thoracic radiograph demonstrating a primary lung tumor. *Source:* Courtesy of Daniel Foy, MS, DVM, DACVIM, DACVECC. (b) Right lateral thoracic radiograph demonstrating a primary lung tumor. *Source:* Courtesy of Daniel Foy, MS, DVM, DACVIM, DACVECC. (c) Orthogonal view of the same patient depicted in Figures 36-12a and 36-12b, demonstrating an isolated primary lung tumor. *Source:* Courtesy of Daniel Foy, MS, DVM, DACVIM, DACVECC.

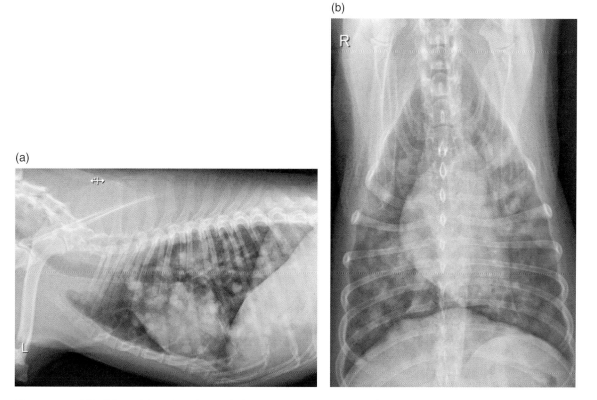

Figure 36.13 (a) Left lateral thoracic radiograph demonstrating metastasis to the lungs. *Source:* Courtesy of Daniel Foy, MS, DVM, DACVIM, DACVECC. (b) Orthogonal radiographic view of the thorax, demonstrating metastasis to the lungs. *Source:* Courtesy of Daniel Foy, MS, DVM, DACVIM, DACVECC.

Secondary hypothermia results from an underlying disease or disease process, such as peripheral vasodilation [165, 172].

Anesthesia-induced hypothermia is a common perioperative concern [166, 173–175].

Patients at extremes of age are most susceptible to hypothermia [165, 166, 172, 176, 177]. These patients are not typically effective at thermoregulation [165, 172]. Neonates, for instance, have a high body surface area to mass ratio [165, 172]. This causes them to lose heat rapidly [165, 172].

Hypothermia varies in terms of severity [165]. For classification purposes, primary hypothermia may be considered [165]:

- Mild
  - 90°–99°F (32°–37°C)
- Moderate
  - 82°–90°F (28°–32°C)
- Severe
  - 68°–82°F (20°–28°C)
- Profound
  - <68°F (<20°C)

Any of the above changes in temperature may result in bradycardia, CNS depression, and bradypnea [165]. The lower the core body temperature drops, the more profound the physiological and pathological changes [165, 172].

References

1 Englar, R.E. (2017). *Performing the Small Animal Physical Examination*. Hoboken, NJ: Wiley.

2 Reece, W.O., Erickson, H.H., Goff, J.P., and Uemura, E.E. (2015). *Dukes' Physiology of Domestic Animals*, 13e, xii, 748 p. Ames, Iowa, USA: Wiley Blackwell.

3 Stokhof, A.A. and Venker-van Haagen, A.J. (2009). Respiratory system. In: *Medical History and Physical Examination in Companion Animals* (ed. A. Rijnberk and F.J. van Sluijs), 63–74. Philadelphia: Saunders Elsevier.

4 Gough, A. and Murphy, K. (2015). *Differential Diagnosis in Small Animal Medicine*. Ames, IA: Wiley.

5 Mukerji, V. (1990). Dyspnea, orthopnea, and paroxysmal nocturnal dyspnea. In: *Clinical Methods: The History, Physical, and Laboratory Examinations* (ed. H.K. Walker, W.D. Wall and J.W. Hurst). Boston: Butterworths.

6 King, L. and Clarke, D. (2010). Emergency care of the patient with acute respiratory distress. *Vet. Focus* 20 (2): 36–43.

7 Horwitz, D.F. (2010). Hyperactivity in dogs. *NAVC Clinician's Brief* (April): 25–27.

8 Curtis TM. (2013). How to recognize and treat anxious dogs and cats. Veterinary Team Brief [Internet]. https://www.veterinaryteambrief.com/article/how-recognize-and-treat-anxious-dogs-and-cats.

9 Levine, E.D. (2008). Feline fear and anxiety. *Vet. Clin. North Am. Small Anim. Pract.* 38 (5): 1065–1079, vii.

10 Mazzaferro EM. (2012). The case: breathing difficulty in a "well" cat. NAVC Clinician's Brief [Internet]. https://www.cliniciansbrief.com/article/case-breathing-difficulty-well-cat.

11 Autran de Morais H. (2011). Why is this patient dyspneic (Proceedings). DVM 360 [Internet]. http://veterinarycalendar.dvm360.com/why-patient-dyspneic-proceedings.

12 Miller, M.W. (2004). Diagnostic tree: dyspnea. *NAVC Clinician's Brief* (May): 54.

13 Dowers K. (2011). Working up pleural effusions in cats. DVM 360 [Internet]. http://veterinarycalendar.dvm360.com/working-pleural-effusions-cats-proceedings.

14 Rozanski E. (2011). Pulmonary contusions and other thoracic trauma (Proceedings). DVM 360 [Internet]. http://veterinarycalendar.dvm360.com/pulmonary-contusions-and-other-thoracic-trauma-proceedings.

15 Rishniw M. (2006). Dyspnea in a cat. NAVC Clinician's Brief [Internet]. https://www.cliniciansbrief.com/article/dyspnea-cat.

16 Statz G. (2014). The Case: Acute respiratory distress. NAVC Clinician's Brief [Internet]. https://www.cliniciansbrief.com/article/case-acute-respiratory-distress.

17 Hawkins, E.C. (2015). Bacterial pneumonia. *NAVC Clinician's Brief* (August): 69–75.

18 Lee, J.A. (2015). Top 5 clinical situations that can't wait. *NAVC Clinician's Brief* (June): 27–29.

19 Davis, A., Khorzad, R., and Whelan, M. (2013). Dynamic upper airway obstruction secondary to severe feline asthma. *J. Am. Anim. Hosp. Assoc.* 49 (2): 142–147.

20 Pachtinger, G.E. (2015). Septic shock. *NAVC Clinician's Brief* (March): 13–16.

21 Richardson, J.A. and Gwaltney-Brant, S.M. (2003). Consultant on call: ethylene glycol toxicosis in dogs and cats. *NAVC Clinician's Brief* (January): 13–19.

22 Sueda, K.L.C. and Cho, J. (2016). Trazodone. *Therapeutics Plumb's Briefs* (July): 55–57.

23 Pachtinger, G.E. and King, L. (2010). Fever of unknown origin. *NAVC Clinician's Brief* (March): 29–32.

24 Powell, L.L. (2008). Canine heatstroke. *NAVC Clinician's Brief* (August): 13–16.

25 Gorris F, Faut S, S. Daminet, de Rooster H, Saunders JH, Paepe D. (2017). Pyothorax in cats and dogs. Vlaams Diergeneeskundig Tijdschrift [Internet]. http://vdt.ugent.be/sites/default/files/Dutchart07.pdf.

26 Hogan, D.F. (2004). Congestive heart failure in the dog. *NAVC Clinician's Brief* (September): 16–19.

27 Boswood, A. (2010). Chronic valvular disease in the dog. *NAVC Clinician's Brief* (December): 17–21.

28 Bright, R.M. (2005). Diaphragmatic hernia. *NAVC Clinician's Brief* (April): 59–60.

29 Byers CG. (2011). Obesity in dogs, Part 1: Exploring the causes and consequences of canine obesity. DVM 360 [Internet]. http://veterinarymedicine.dvm360.com/obesity-dogs-part-1-exploring-causes-and-consequences-canine-obesity.

30 Riviere, J.E. and Papich, M.G. (2017). *Veterinary Pharmacology and Therapeutics*, 10e. Hoboken, NJ: Wiley.

31 Muir, W.W. 3rd and Gadawski, J.E. (1998). Respiratory depression and apnea induced by propofol in dogs. *Am. J. Vet. Res.* 59 (2): 157–161.

32 Holowaychuk, M.K. (2016). Heatstroke in dogs. *NAVC Clinician's Brief* (June): 99–101.

33 Rainey, A. and Odunayo, A. (2015). Traumatic brain injury. *NAVC Clinician's Brief* (October): 69–72.

34 Laflamme, D.P. (2001). Challenges with weight-reduction studies. *Compend. Contin. Educ. Pract. Vet.* 23: 45–50.

35 Gosselin, J., Wren, J.A., and Sunderland, S.J. (2007). Canine obesity: an overview. *J. Vet. Pharmacol. Ther.* 30 (Suppl 1): 1–10.

36 Mason, E. (1970). Obesity in pet dogs. *Vet. Rec.* 86 (21): 612–616.

37 Zoran, D.L. (2010). Obesity in dogs and cats: a metabolic and endocrine disorder. *Vet. Clin. North Am. Small Anim. Pract.* 40 (2): 221–239.

38 German, A.J. (2006). The growing problem of obesity in dogs and cats. *J. Nutr.* 136 (7 Suppl): 1940S–1946S.

39 Diez, M. and Nguyen, P. (2006). The epidemiology of canine and feline obesity. *Waltham Focus* 16 (2): 2–8.

40 Meyer, H., Drochner, W., and Weidenhaupt, C. (1978). A contribution to the occurrence and treatment of obesity in dogs. *Dtsch. Tierarztl. Wochenschr.* 85 (4): 133–136.

41 Edney, A.T. and Smith, P.M. (1986). Study of obesity in dogs visiting veterinary practices in the United Kingdom. *Vet. Rec.* 118 (14): 391–396.

42 Bjornvad, C.R., Nielsen, D.H., Armstrong, P.J. et al. (2011). Evaluation of a nine-point body condition scoring system in physically inactive pet cats. *Am. J. Vet. Res.* 72 (4): 433–437.

43 German, A.J., Holden, S.L., Moxham, G.L. et al. (2006). A simple, reliable tool for owners to assess the body condition of their dog or cat. *J. Nutr.* 136 (7): 2031s–2033s.

44 Sandoe, P., Palmer, C., Corr, S. et al. (2014). Canine and feline obesity: a one health perspective. *Vet. Rec.* 175 (24): 610–616.

45 Day, M.J. (2010). One health: the small animal dimension. *Vet. Rec.* 167 (22): 847–849.

46 Wynn, S.G., Witzel, A.L., Bartges, J.W. et al. (2016). Prevalence of asymptomatic urinary tract infections in morbidly obese dogs. *PeerJ* 4: e1711.

47 Nijland, M.L., Stam, F., and Seidell, J.C. (2010). Overweight in dogs, but not in cats, is related to overweight in their owners. *Public Health Nutr.* 13 (1): 102–106.

48 White, G.A., Hobson-West, P., Cobb, K. et al. (2011). Canine obesity: is there a difference between veterinarian and owner perception? *J. Small Anim. Pract.* 52 (12): 622–626.

49 German, A.J. (2010). Obesity in companion animals. *companion anim. pract.* 32: 42–50.

50 Lund, E.M., Armstrong, P.J., Kirk, C.A., and Klausner, J.S. (2006). Prevalence and risk factors for obesity in adult dogs from private U.S. veterinary practices. *Int. J. Appl. Res. Vet. Med.* 4: 177–186.

51 Markwell, P.J., Vanerk, W., Parkin, G.D. et al. (1990). Obesity in the dog. *J. Small Anim. Pract.* 31 (10): 533–537.

52 Yam, P.S., Butowski, C.F., Chitty, J.L. et al. (2016). Impact of canine overweight and obesity on health-related quality of life. *Prev. Vet. Med.* 127: 64–69.

53 Weeth, L.P., Fascetti, A.J., Kass, P.H. et al. (2007). Prevalence of obese dogs in a population of dogs with cancer. *Am. J. Vet. Res.* 68 (4): 389–398.

54 Kealy, R.D., Lawler, D.F., Ballam, J.M. et al. (2002). Effects of diet restriction on life span and age-related changes in dogs. *J. Am. Vet. Med. Assoc.* 220: 1315–1320.

55 Mattheeuws, D., Rottiers, R., Kaneko, J.J., and Vermeulen, A. (1984). Diabetes mellitus in dogs: relationship of obesity to glucose tolerance and insulin response. *Am. J. Vet. Res.* 45 (1): 98–103.

56 Thengchaisri, N., Theerapun, W., Kaewmokul, S., and Sastravaha, A. (2014). Abdominal obesity is associated with heart disease in dogs. *BMC Vet. Res.* 10: 131.

57 Lawler, D.F., Larson, B.T., Ballam, J.M. et al. (2008). Diet restriction and ageing in the dog: major observations over two decades. *Br. J. Nutr.* 99 (4): 793–805.

58 Wei, E.K., Giovannucci, E., Wu, K. et al. (2004). Comparison of risk factors for colon and rectal cancer. *Int. J. Cancer* 108 (3): 433–442.

59 van den Brandt, P.A., Spiegelman, D., Yaun, S.S. et al. (2000). Pooled analysis of prospective cohort studies on height, weight, and breast cancer risk. *Am. J. Epidemiol.* 152 (6): 514–527.

60 Crew, K.D. and Neugut, A.I. (2004). Epidemiology of upper gastrointestinal malignancies. *Semin. Oncol.* 31 (4): 450–464.

61 Forman, D. (2004). Review article: oesophago-gastric adenocarcinoma – an epidemiological perspective. *Aliment. Pharmacol. Ther.* 20 (Suppl 5): 55–60; discussion 1–2.

62 Wang, X.J., Yuan, S.L., Lu, Q. et al. (2004). Potential involvement of leptin in carcinogenesis of hepatocellular carcinoma. *World J. Gastroenterol.* 10 (17): 2478–2481.

63 Schaer, M. (2003). *Clinical Medicine of the Dog and Cat*, 576 p. Ames, Iowa: Iowa State Press.

64 Rand, J. and Litster, A. (2006). The cat with polycythemia. In: *Problem-Based Feline Medicine* (ed. J. Rand), 568. St. Louis: Elsevier Limited.

65 Armstrong, P.J. (2004). Respiratory distress in a pug. *NAVC Clinician's Brief* (June): 9.

66 Crawford, E.C. Jr. (1962). Mechanical aspects of panting in dogs. *J. Appl. Physiol.* 17: 249–251.

67 Schmidt-Nielsen, K., Bretz, W.L., and Taylor, C.R. (1970). Panting in dogs: unidirectional air flow over evaporative surfaces. *Science* 169 (3950): 1102–1104.

68 Blatt, C.M., Taylor, C.R., and Habal, M.B. (1972). Thermal panting in dogs: the lateral nasal gland, a source of water for evaporative cooling. *Science* 177 (4051): 804–805.

69 Goldberg, M.B., Langman, V.A., and Taylor, C.R. (1981). Panting in dogs: paths of air flow in response to heat and exercise. *Respir. Physiol.* 43 (3): 327–338.

70 Allen, H.S., Broussard, J., and Noone, K. (1999). Nasopharyngeal diseases in cats: a retrospective study of 53 cases (1991–1998). *J. Am. Anim. Hosp. Assoc.* 35 (6): 457–461.

71 Lappin, M.R. (2001). *Feline Internal Medicine Secrets*. Philadelphia: Hanley & Belfus, Inc.

72 Stanley SM. (1980). A study of heat stroke and heat exhaustion in the dog. Iowa State University Digital Repository [Internet]. 42(1). https://lib.dr.iastate.edu/cgi/viewcontent.cgi?article=2978&context=iowastate_veterinarian.

73 Rozanski E. (2009). Pulmonary edema. DVM 360 [Internet]. http://veterinarycalendar.dvm360.com/print/328751?page=full.

74 Spier A. (2007). Congestive heart failure: approaches to care. NAVC Clinician's Brief [Internet]. https://www.cliniciansbrief.com/article/congestive-heart-failure-approaches-care.

75 Estrada, A. (2014). Heart disease: diagnosis & treatment. *NAVC Clinician's Brief* (March): 91–95.

76 Atkins, A. (2011). Finding a consensus on canine CVHD. *NAVC Clinician's Brief* (July): 53–57.

77 Saunders AB, Gordon SG. (2015). 6 Practical tips from cardiologists: heart failure in dogs. Today's Veterinary Practice [Internet]. (July/August). http://todaysveterinarypractice.navc.com/wp-content/uploads/2016/06/T1507F02.pdf.

78 Oyama, M.A. (2008). Canine cardiomyopathy. In: *Manual of Canine and Feline Cardiology*, 4e (ed. L.P. Tilley, S. FWK, M.A. Oyama and M.M. Sleeper), 139–150. Philadelphia: W.B. Saunders.

79 Chandler, M.L. (2016). Impact of obesity on cardiopulmonary disease. *Vet. Clin. North Am. Small Anim. Pract.* 46 (5): 817–830.

80 Meurs, K.M. (2010). Myocardial disease; canine. In: *Textbook of Veterinary Internal Medicine*, 7e (ed. S.J. Ettinger and E.C. Feldman), 1320–1327. St. Louis: Saunders Elsevier.

81 Rishniw, M. (2011). Canine heart murmur. *NAVC Clinician's Brief* (May): 49–52.

82 Mama, K. and Ames, M. (2016). Anesthesia for dogs with myxomatous mitral valve disease. *NAVC Clinician's Brief* (August): 99–105.

83 Kienle, R.D. (2008). Feline cardiomyopathy. In: *Manual of Canine and Feline Cardiology*, 4e (ed. L.P. Tilley, F.W.K. Smith, M.A. Oyama and M.M. Sleeper), 151–175. Philadelphia: W.B. Saunders.

84 Fuentes, V.L. (2006). Cardiomyopathy: establishing a diagnosis. In: *Consultations in Feline Internal Medicine*, 5e (ed. J.R. August), 301–310. St. Louis: Saunders Elsevier.

85 Ferasin, L., Sturgess, C.P., Cannon, M.J. et al. (2003). Feline idiopathic cardiomyopathy: a retrospective study of 106 cats (1994-2001). *J. Feline Med. Surg.* 5 (3): 151–159.

86 Hoskins JD. (2008). Keys to managing end-stage heart failure. DVM 360 [Internet]. http://veterinarynews.dvm360.com/print/316908?page=full.

87 DeFrancesco, T. (2015). Mitral valve disease in a dog. *Plumb's Therapeutics Briefs* (May): 13–16.

88 Slatter, D.H. (1985). *Textbook of Small Animal Surgery*. Philadelphia: W.B. Saunders.

89 Goldkamp, C.E. and Schaer, M. (2008). Canine drowning. *Compend. Contin. Educ. Vet.* 30 (6): 340–352; quiz 52.

90 Pachtinger, G.E. (2013). Noncardiogenic pulmonary edema. *NAVC Clinician's Brief* (June): 86–87.

91 Modell, J.H. (1993). Drowning. *N. Engl. J. Med.* 328 (4): 253–256.

92 Modell, J.H., Moya, F., Newby, E.J. et al. (1967). The effects of fluid volume in seawater drowning. *Ann. Intern. Med.* 67 (1): 68–80.

93 Orlowski, J.P., Abulleil, M.M., and Phillips, J.M. (1989). The hemodynamic and cardiovascular effects of near-drowning in hypotonic, isotonic, or hypertonic solutions. *Ann. Emerg. Med.* 18 (10): 1044–1049.

94 Tabeling, B.B. and Modell, J.H. (1983). Fluid administration increases oxygen delivery during continuous positive pressure ventilation after freshwater near-drowning. *Crit. Care Med.* 11 (9): 693–696.

95 Giammona, S.T. and Modell, J.H. (1967). Drowning by total immersion. Effects on pulmonary surfactant of distilled water, isotonic saline, and sea water. *Am. J. Dis. Child.* 114 (6): 612–616.

96 Rozanski E. (2011). Pyothorax in cats and dogs. DVM 360 [Internet]. http://veterinarycalendar.dvm360.com/pyothorax-cats-and-dogs-proceedings.

97 Mitchell, S.L., McCarthy, R., Rudloff, E., and Pernell, R.T. (2000). Tracheal rupture associated with intubation in cats: 20 cases (1996–1998). *J. Am. Vet. Med. Assoc.* 216 (10): 1592–1595.

98 Wong, C. (2008). Thoracocentesis. *NAVC Clinician's Brief* (June): 75–78.

99 Scruggs, J.L. and Jesty, S.A. (2013). Chylous effusion in a cat. *NAVC Clinician's Brief* (July): 8–10.

100 Beatty, S.S.K. and Wamsley, H.L. (2012). Body cavity effusions. *NAVC Clinician's Brief* (November): 84–85.

101 Ettinger, S.J., Feldman, E.C., and Côté, E. (2017). *Textbook of Veterinary Internal Medicine: Diseases of the Dog and the Cat*, 8e, 2 volumes (lviii, 2181, I–90 pages) p. St. Louis, Missouri: Elsevier.

102 Berry CR. (2010). Small animal thoracic radiology: Pulmonary edema vs. pleural effusion (lines and buckets) (Proceedings). http://veterinarycalendar.dvm360.com/small-animal-thoracic-radiology-pulmonary-edema-vs-pleural-effusion-lines-and-buckets-proceedings?id=&sk=&date=&%0A%09%09%09&pageID=3.

103 Sumner, C. and Rozanski, E. (2013). Management of respiratory emergencies in small animals. *Vet. Clin. North Am. Small Anim. Pract.* 43 (4): 799–815.

104 Maritato, K.C., Colon, J.A., and Kergosien, D.H. (2009). Pneumothorax. *Compend. Contin. Educ. Vet.* 31 (5): 232–242; quiz 42.

105 Puerto, D.A., Brockman, D.J., Lindquist, C., and Drobatz, K. (2002). Surgical and nonsurgical management of and selected risk factors for spontaneous pneumothorax in dogs: 64 cases (1986–1999). *J. Am. Vet. Med. Assoc.* 220 (11): 1670–1674.

106 Monnet, E. (2003). Pleura and pleural space. In: *Textbook of Small Animal Surgery* (ed. D.H. Slatter), 387–405. Philadelphia: Saunders.

107 Brockman, D.J. and Puerto, D.A. (2003). Pneumomediastinum and pneumothorax. In: *Textbook of Respiratory Diseases of Dogs and Cats*. (ed. L. King), 616–624. Phildelphia: Saunders.

108 Fossum, T.W. (ed.) (2002). Surgery of the lower respiratory system. In: *Small Animal Surgery*, 788–820. St. Louis: Mosbye.

109 Hardie, E.M., Spodnick, G.J., Gilson, S.D. et al. (1999). Tracheal rupture in cats: 16 cases (1983–1998). *J. Am. Vet. Med. Assoc.* 214 (4): 508–512.

110 Johnson-Neitman, J.L., Huber, M.L., and Amann, J.F. (2006). What is your diagnosis?: Pneumomediastinum and pneumopericardium. *J. Am. Vet. Med. Assoc.* 229 (3): 359–360.

111 Yoshioka, M.M. (1982). Management of spontaneous pneumothorax in 12 dogs. *J. Am. Anim. Hosp. Assoc.* 18 (1): 57–62.

112 Valentine, A., Smeak, D., Allen, D. et al. (1996). Spontaneous pneumothorax in dogs. *Compend. Contin. Educ. Pract.* 18 (1): 53.

113 Tamas, P.M., Paddleford, R.R., and Krahwinkel, D.J. (1985). Thoracic trauma in dogs and cats presented for limb fractures. *J. Am. Anim. Hosp. Assoc.* 21 (2): 161–166.

114 Holtsinger, R.H., Beale, B.S., Bellah, J.R., and King, R.R. (1993). Spontaneous pneumothorax in the dog – a retrospective analysis of 21 cases. *J. Am. Anim. Hosp. Assoc.* 29 (3): 195–210.

115 Groblinger, K., Lorinson, D., and Wiskocil, L. (2001). Spontaneous pneumothorax caused by bullae pulmonales in four hiskies. *Vet. Surg.* 30: 304.

116 Lipscomb, V.J., Hardie, R.J., and Dubielzig, R.R. (2003). Spontaneous pneumothorax caused by pulmonary blebs and bullae in 12 dogs. *J. Am. Anim. Hosp. Assoc.* 39 (5): 435–445.

117 Kramek, B.A., Caywood, D.D., and Obrien, T.D. (1985). Bullous emphysema and recurrent pneumothorax in the dog. *J. Am. Vet. Med. Assoc.* 186 (9): 971–974.

118 Nelson, A.W. and Monnet, E. (2003). Lungs. In: *Textbook of Small Animal Surgery* (ed. D.H. Slatter), 880. Philadelphia: Saunders.

119 Dallman, M.J., Martin, R.A., and Roth, L. (1988). Pneumothorax as the primary problem in 2 cases of Bronchioloalveolar carcinoma in the dog. *J. Am. Anim. Hosp. Assoc.* 24 (6): 710–714.

120 Saheki, Y., Ishitani, R., and Miyamoto, Y. (1981). Acute fatal pneumothorax in canine dirofilariasis. *Nippon Juigaku Zasshi.* 43 (3): 315–328.

121 Smith, J.W., Scott-Moncrieff, J.C., and Rivers, B.J. (1998). Pneumothorax secondary to Dirofilaria immitis infection in two cats. *J. Am. Vet. Med. Assoc.* 213 (1): 91–93.

122 Berson, J.L., Rendano, V.T., and Hoffer, R.E. (1979). Recurrent pneumothorax secondary to ruptured pulmonary blebs: a case report. *JAAHA* 15: 707–711.

123 Busch, D.S. and Noxon, J.O. (1992). Pneumothorax in a dog infected with Dirofilaria immitis. *J. Am. Vet. Med. Assoc.* 201 (12): 1893.

124 Hopper, B.J., Lester, N.V., Irwin, P.J. et al. (2004). Imaging diagnosis: pneumothorax and focal peritonitis in a dog due to migration of an inhaled grass awn. *Vet. Radiol. Ultrasound* 45 (2): 136–138.

125 Rochat, M.C., Cowell, R.L., Tyler, R.D., and Johnson, E.M. (1990). Paragonimiasis in dogs and cats. *Compend. Contin. Educ. Pract.* 12 (8): 1093.

126 Stogdale, L., O'Connor, C.D., Williams, M.C., and Smuts, M.M. (1982). Recurrent pneumothorax associated with a pulmonary emphysematous bulla in a dog: surgical correction and proposed pathogenesis. *Can. Vet. J.* 23 (10): 281–287.

127 Bhandal, J. and Kuzma, A. (2008). Tracheal rupture in a cat: diagnosis by computed tomography. *Can. Vet. J.* 49 (6): 595–597.

128 Quandt JE. (2017). Postintubation Tracheal Tears in Cats. NAVC Clinician's Brief [Interner]. (June). https://www.cliniciansbrief.com/article/postintubation-tracheal-tears-cats.

129 Strickland, K.N. (2008). Congenital heart disease. In: *Manual of Canine and Feline Cardiology*, 4e (ed. L.P. Tilley, F.W.K. Smith, M.A. Oyama and M.M. Sleeper), 215–239. Philadelphia: W.B. Saunders.

130 Voges, A.K., Bertrand, S., Hill, R.C. et al. (1997). True diaphragmatic hernia in a cat. *Vet. Radiol. Ultrasound* 38 (2): 116–119.

131 Worth, A.J. and Machon, R.G. (2005). Traumatic diaphragmatic herniation: pathophysiology and management. *Compend. Contin. Educ. Pract.* 27 (3): 178–191.

132 Schmiedt, C.W., Tobias, K.M., and Stevenson, M.A. (2003). Traumatic diaphragmatic hernia in cats: 34 cases (1991–2001). *J. Am. Vet. Med. Assoc.* 222 (9): 1237–1240.

133 Fossum, T.W. (2000). Pleural and extrapleural diseases. In: *Textbook of Veterinary Internal Medicine* (ed. S.J. Ettinger and E.C. Feldman), 1098. Philadelphia: Saunders.

134 Lee, J.A. (2004). Respiratory distress and cyanosis in dogs. In: *Textbook of Respiratory Disease in Dogs and Cats* (ed. L. King), 12–17. Philadelphia: WB Saunders.

135 Mandell, D.C. (2004). Respiratory distress in cats. In: *Textbook of Respiratory Disease in Dogs and Cats* (ed. L. King), 12–17. Philadeophia: WB Saunders.

136 Macintire, D.K. and Drobatz, K. (2005). *Manual of Small Animal Emergency and Critical Care Medicine*. Philadelphia: Lippencott, Williams, & Wilkins.

137 Suave, V. (2009). Pleural space disease. In: *Small Animal Critical Care Medicine* (ed. D.C. Silverstein and K. Hopper), 49–52. Philadelphia: WB Saunders.

138 Silverstein, D.C. (2004). Pleural space disease. In: *Textbook of Respiratory Disease in Dogs and Cats* (ed. L. King), 49–52. Philadelphia: WB Saunders.

139 Evans, S.M. and Biery, D.N. (1980). Congenital peritoneopericardial diaphragmatic-hernia in the dog and cat – a literature-review and 17 additional case-histories. *Vet. Radiol.* 21 (3): 108–116.

140 Hay, W.H., Woodfield, J.A., and Moon, M.A. (1989). Clinical, echocardiographic, and radiographic findings of peritoneopericardial diaphragmatic-hernia in 2 dogs and a cat. *J. Am. Vet. Med. Assoc.* 195 (9): 1245–1248.

141 Reimer, S.B., Kyles, A.E., Filipowicz, D.E., and Gregory, C.R. (2004). Long-term outcome of cats treated conservatively or surgically for peritoneopericardial diaphragmatic hernia: 66 cases (1987–2002). *Javma -J. Am. Vet. Med. Assoc.* 224 (5): 728–732.

142 Reed, C.A. (1951). Pericardio-peritoneal Herniae in mammals, with description of a case in the domestic cat. *Anat. Rec.* 110 (1): 113–119.

143 Kittleson MD. Case 25: Peritoneopericardial Diaphragmatic Hernia. Case Studies in Small Animal Cardiovascular Medicine [Internet]. http://www.vetmed.ucdavis.edu/vmth/small_animal/cardio_kittleson/cases/case25/text.htm.

144 Baral, R.M. (2012). The thoracic cavity. In: *The Cat: Clinical Medicine and Management* (ed. S.E. Little), 892–913. St. Louis: Saunders Elsevier.

145 Day, M.J. (1997). Review of thymic pathology in 30 cats and 36 dogs. *J. Small Anim. Pract.* 38 (9): 393–403.

146 Vilafranca, M. and Font, A. (2005). Thymolipoma in a cat. *J. Feline Med. Surg.* 7 (2): 125–127.

147 Larsen MM. (2008). Radiographic interpretation of the mediastinum and pleural space (Proceedings). DVM 360 [Internet]. http://veterinarycalendar.dvm360.com/radiographic-interpretation-mediastinum-and-pleural-space-proceedings?id=&sk=&date=&%0A%09%09%09&pageID=2.

148 Risetto KC, Fan TM, Lucas P. (2008). An update on diagnosing and treating primary lung tumors. DVM 360 [Internet]. http://veterinarymedicine.dvm360.com/update-diagnosing-and-treating-primary-lung-tumors.

149 Withrow, S.J. (2007). Tumors of the respiratory system: lung cancer. In: *Withrow and MacEwen's Small Animal Clinical Oncology* (ed. S.J. Withrow and D.M. Vail), 517–525. Philadelphia: WB Saunders Co.

150 Ogilvie, G.K., Haschek, W.M., Withrow, S.J. et al. (1989). Classification of primary lung tumors in dogs: 210 cases (1975–1985). *J. Am. Vet. Med. Assoc.* 195 (1): 106–108.

151 Brodey, R.S. and Craig, P.H. (1965). Primary pulmonary neoplasms in the dog: a review of 29 cases. *J. Am. Vet. Med. Assoc.* 147 (12): 1628–1643.

152 Paoloni, M.C., Adams, W.M., Dubielzig, R.R. et al. (2006). Comparison of results of computed tomography and radiography with histopathologic findings in tracheobronchial lymph nodes in dogs with primary lung tumors: 14 cases (1999–2002). *J. Am. Vet. Med. Assoc.* 228 (11): 1718–1722.

153 Nielsen, S.W. and Horava, A. (1960). Primary pulmonary tumors of the dog. A report of sixteen cases. *Am. J. Vet. Res.* 21: 813–830.

154 Koblik, P.D. (1986). Radiographic appearance of primary lung-tumors in cats – a review of 41 cases. *Vet. Radiol.* 27 (3): 66–73.

155 Barr, F., Gruffyddjones, T.J., Brown, P.J., and Gibbs, C. (1987). Primary lung-tumors in the cat. *J. Small Anim. Pract.* 28 (12): 1115–1125.

156 Hahn, K.A. and McEntee, M.F. (1997). Primary lung tumors in cats: 86 cases (1979–1994). *J. Am. Vet. Med. Assoc.* 211 (10): 1257–1260.

157 Moulton, J.E., von Tscharner, C., and Schneider, R. (1981). Classification of lung carcinomas in the dog and cat. *Vet. Pathol.* 18 (4): 513–528.

158 McNiel, E.A., Ogilvie, G.K., Powers, B.E. et al. (1997). Evaluation of prognostic factors for dogs with primary lung tumors: 67 cases (1985–1992). *J. Am. Vet. Med. Assoc.* 211 (11): 1422–1427.

159 Ogilvie, G.K., Weigel, R.M., Haschek, W.M. et al. (1989). Prognostic factors for tumor remission and survival in dogs after surgery for primary lung-tumor – 76 cases (1975–1985). *J. Am. Vet. Med. Assoc.* 195 (1): 109–112.

160 Mehlhaff, C.J., Leifer, C.E., Patnaik, A.K., and Schwarz, P.D. (1984). Surgical-treatment of primary pulmonary neoplasia in 15 dogs. *J. Am. Anim. Hosp. Assoc.* 20 (5): 799–803.

161 Mcmillan, M.C., Kleine, L.J., and Carpenter, J.L. (1988). Fluoroscopically guided percutaneous fine-needle aspiration biopsy of thoracic lesions in dogs and cats. *Vet. Radiol.* 29 (5): 194–197.

162 Teske, E., Stokhof, A.A., Vandeningh, T.S.G.A.M. et al. (1991). Transthoracic needle aspiration biopsy of the lung in dogs with pulmonic diseases. *J. Am. Anim. Hosp. Assoc.* 27 (3): 289–294.

163 Kuehn NF. Neoplasia of the Respiratory System in Small Animals. Merck Manual: Veterinary Medicine [Internet]. https://www.msdvetmanual.com/respiratory-system/respiratory-diseases-of-small-animals/neoplasia-of-the-respiratory-system-in-small-animals.

164 Golder, F.J., Hewitt, M.M., and McLeod, J.F. (2013). Respiratory stimulant drugs in the post-operative setting. *Respir. Physiol. Neurobiol.* 189 (2): 395–402.

165 Mazzaferro, E.M. (2007). Warming the patient. *NAVC Clinician's Brief* (August): 13–15.

166 Reuss-Lamky, H. (2015). Hypothermia overview. *NAVC Clinician's Brief* (November): 12–16.

167 Bigby, S.E., Beths, T., Bauquier, S., and Carter, J.E. (2017). Postinduction apnoea in dogs premedicated with acepromazine or dexmedetomidine and anaesthetized with alfaxalone or propofol. *Vet. Anaesth. Analg.* 44 (5): 1007–1015.

168 Wilson, D.V. and Shih, A.C. (2015). Anesthetic emergencies and resuscitation. In: *Veterinary Anesthesia and Analgesia* (ed. K.A. Grimm, L.A. Lamont and W.J. Tranquilli). Philadelphia: Wiley Blackwell.

169 Muir, W., Lerche, P., Wiese, A. et al. (2008). Cardiorespiratory and anesthetic effects of clinical and supraclinical doses of alfaxalone in dogs. *Vet. Anaesth. Analg.* 35 (6): 451–462.

170 Muir, W., Lerche, P., Wiese, A. et al. (2009). The cardiorespiratory and anesthetic effects of clinical and supraclinical doses of alfaxalone in cats. *Vet. Anaesth. Analg.* 36 (1): 42–54.

171 Smith, J.A., Gaynor, J.S., Bednarski, R.M., and Muir, W.W. (1993). Adverse-effects of administration of propofol with various Preanesthetic regimens in dogs. *J. Am. Vet. Med. Assoc.* 202 (7): 1111–1115.

172 Oncken, A.K., Kirby, R., and Rudloff, E. (2001). Hypothermia in critically ill dogs and cats. *Compend. Contin. Educ. Pract.* 23 (6): 506–520.

173 McKelvey, D. and Hollingshead, K. (1994). *Small Animal Anesthesia: Canine and Feline Practice*. St. Louis: Mosby-Year Book.

174 Harvey R, editor. Crisis management: what to worry about. *AAHA*; 2009.

175 Lukasik, V. (2006). Anesthesia of the pediatric patient. *NAVTA J.* (Fall): 52–57.

176 Lee, J.A. and Cohn, L. (2015). Pediatric critical care. *Clin. Brief* 13 (2): 41–42.

177 Blackmon, N. (2015). Anesthetic considerations for geriatric dogs. *Vet. Team Brief* 3 (3): 24.

37

Abnormal Lung Sounds

37.1 Introduction to Lung Sounds

Physicians recognized that lung sounds existed long before the stethoscope was invented, when the only means of thoracic auscultation was to place an ear directly against the patient's chest [1].

Sound quality improved after French physician Rene Laennec created a working prototype of the stethoscope that is used in clinical practice today [1]. The original model, built from a wooden cylinder, allowed for the auscultation of abnormal sounds, which he described as "rales" [1, 2]. At the time, "rales" was understood to mean those respiratory sounds made by the dying [1, 2]. The same death rattle was described by the word, "rhonchus," by Greek physicians [2, 3].

Although technology has advanced the way in which medicine is practiced, word choice remains descriptive, yet ambiguous, when it comes to describing breath sounds [1, 2, 4]. In 1989, a publication by Roudebush et al. addressed the nebulousness of breath sound terminology among the veterinary profession [5]. His survey of 310 veterinary case reports revealed that over 20 different terms exist throughout the veterinary medical literature to describe variations of similar sounds [5]. Twelve of these alone describe what we would refer to today as crackles [5].

Breath sound descriptors are also inherently subjective: dry versus moist seem obvious and distinct, yet two clinicians hearing the same sound may classify it differently [2].

Crepitation is a second example of a sound that means something different to each individual [2]. Crepitation is intended to refer to high-pitched noise, yet some understand it to imply the acoustic version of palpable crepitus, the textural crunching or grating that is produced when bone pathologically rubs against bone, as in the case of a fracture.

There is a pressing need to standardize breath sounds, particularly within medical reports, so as to work toward universal understanding [1, 5, 6]. Because this standardization has yet to occur, it is at times difficult to interpret

what clinicians mean unless someone were to hear the described sound for oneself.

What can be agreed upon is that the airways produce normal and abnormal sounds.

Airway sounds occur when airflow through a structured space creates vibrations. How quickly air flows through the space as well as the turbulence of the air current collectively influence which vibrations can be heard, their loudness, and their frequencies [1, 7].

Within the respiratory tract, the trachea and the larger airways generate turbulent airflow [1]. Normal airway sounds arise from these structures, as compared to the smaller airways, whose laminar flow generates no sound in times of health [1].

Auscultation over the trachea yields normal, so-called bronchial sounds [7]. Bronchial sounds are harsh because they are generated from turbulent airflow [8]. They may be likened to wind on a stormy day [8]. Bronchial sounds are relatively loud and range in pitch from 75 to 1000 Hz [1].

Patient-specific factors, such as age and the depth of each breath, alter the amplitude and frequency range of a normal patient [1, 9]. Healthy older patients tend to have louder bronchial sounds, as do patients that are maximizing airflow volume and velocity through panting [1, 8]. Neither of these factors is considered abnormal [1].

In the normal patient, most of the sound that is heard on expiration is generated by the trachea and large bronchi, whereas lobar and subsegmental airways produce most inspiratory sounds [1, 10]. The latter tend to be low-pitched sounds with frequencies that are typically lower than 400 Hz [1, 10].

The quietest airway sounds arise from the periphery of the thoracic cavity [7]. These so-called vesicular sounds have been likened to the gentle rustling of leaves on a crisp autumn day. Vesicular sounds confirm that there is indeed air-filled lung tissue seated between the chest wall and the more turbulent, larger airways [7].

So-called bronchovesicular sounds fall somewhere in between the spectrum in terms of location within the chest, tone, and loudness [8].

All three of these sounds – bronchial, bronchovesicular, and vesicular – are normal and may be appreciated through thoracic auscultation of a healthy patient [8]. Bronchial sounds are heard best over the trachea, whereas auscultation of the lower airway is best for appreciating vesicular and bronchovesicular sounds [7].

Lung sounds are appreciated more easily in some patients than in others.

Lung sounds may be increased or decreased; discontinuous or continuous; normal or abnormal [1]. Abnormal sounds are collectively described as being adventitious [8].

37.1.1 Increased Lung Sounds

Increased lung sounds may be present in healthy patients as well as in the diseased.

Consider, for example, the hyperactive, hyperexcitable, or extremely anxious patient. These patients are likely to present with tachypnea. Normal airway sounds are accentuated in tachypneic patients [8, 11–16].

On the other hand, increased lung sounds may result from underlying pathology. Recall from Chapter 36, Section 36.3 that the list of differential diagnoses for tachypnea and dyspnea is extensive [8, 16–36].

Some of these conditions, such as infectious tracheobronchitis (ITB), increase bronchial sounds due to exaggerated turbulence of air flowing over the inflamed trachea and larger bronchi.

37.1.2 Decreased Lung Sounds

Decreased lung sounds may be present in health as well as in disease [1, 8].

Unlike humans, most companion animals have a full coat of fur that creates an additional barrier between the stethoscope and chest wall. In particularly thick-coated patients, such as Chow Chows, Siberian Huskies, and Alaskan Malamutes, the clinician may have a difficult time appreciating normal sounds because the fur muffles what sounds are able to pass through the coat.

Fur may also create sound artifacts that do not actually exist. The clinician that is a novice must learn how to differentiate these sounds from those that are real.

Obese patients may also be challenging to auscult because in these situations fat, in addition to fur, becomes an obstruction to sound. Furthermore, these patients may be more likely to pant. Although panting intensifies bronchial sounds, it obscures the quieter, vesicular sounds.

Pathological conditions, such as pleural effusion, may also reduce lung sounds. Quieter-than-normal or absent lung sounds secondary to pathology typically indicate that abnormal tissue or fluid has accumulated between the chest wall and the airways [7].

37.1.3 Discontinuous Lung Sounds

Discontinuous lung sounds are intermittent [1]. They occur sporadically throughout the respiratory cycle.

The most common example of discontinuous lung sounds in clinical practice is the crackle. Crackles will be discussed in Section 37.2.

37.1.4 Continuous Lung Sounds

Continuous lung sounds are long-lived as compared to discontinuous sounds [1]. They may be present throughout the entire respiratory cycle or they may arise in a certain segment of the cycle.

The most common example of continuous lung sounds in clinical practice is the wheeze. Wheezes will be discussed in Section 37.3.

37.2 Crackles

Crackles are brief, discontinuous, adventitious lung sounds [1, 2, 8, 37]. They sound like "popping" [8].

The reader can simulate crackles by wetting the thumb and index finger, sticking them together, then separating them within hearing range of your ear [37].

Crackles may also be described as crisp or crunchy, like the sound that the reader would hear if hair by the ear were rolled between two fingers, or the sound that is associated with pulling two strips of Velcro apart [1, 37].

Crackles may be present during the inspiratory half of the respiratory cycle, the expiratory half, or both [37].

Crackles may be unilateral or bilateral. There may be partial or complete involvement or one or more lung lobes.

There are two main types of crackles [1]:

- Coarse crackles
- Fine crackles

Coarse crackles are audible without a stethoscope and suggest that large upper airways are experiencing excessive intraluminal secretions [1, 8]. The mobilization of these secretions creates the classic sound that is associated with coarse crackles [1].

Fine crackles occur when small airways that were obstructed finally open [1]. Airway obstruction, in these clinical cases, is not due to intraluminal secretions [1]. Instead, it is typically due to cellular infiltrate or fluid accumulation within the pulmonary interstitial spaces [1]. When lung volume is small, particularly during exhalation, the interstitial pressure forces smaller airways to close. As the lungs expand during inhalation, this pressure is overcome and the smaller airways reopen [1]. "Popping" sounds result as hundreds of such airways snap back open [1].

Crackles may be present in the following disease processes [1, 8, 38–40]:

- Bronchial disease
  - Chronic bronchitis (refer to Chapter 35, Section 35.4.2)
  - Feline asthma (refer to Chapter 35, Section 35.4.1)
- Cardiogenic pulmonary edema (refer to Chapter 36, Sections 36.3.3 and 36.3.4)
  - Left-sided congestive heart failure (CHF)
    - Chronic valvular heart disease (CVHD)
    - Mitral regurgitation (MR)
    - Dilated cardiomyopathy (DCM)
    - Hypertrophic cardiomyopathy (HCM)
- Feline heartworm-associated respiratory disease (HARD) (refer to Chapter 35, Section 35.4.3)
- Lungworms (refer to Chapter 35, Section 35.4.4)
- Non-cardiogenic pulmonary edema (refer to Chapter 36, Section 36.3.5)
  - Accidental electrocution secondary to chewing electrical cords
  - Acute respiratory distress syndrome (ARDS)
  - Near choking
  - Near drowning
  - Sepsis
  - Smoke inhalation
  - Snakebites
  - Upper airway obstruction
- Pneumonia and bronchopneumonia
  - Aspiration
  - Bacterial
  - Fungal
  - Viral

Inflammation of the lung parenchyma is called pneumonia [38, 41]. When pneumonia involves the terminal bronchioles, it is classified as bronchopneumonia [38].

37.2.1 Aspiration Pneumonia

Aspiration pneumonia is a condition in which substances other than air inappropriately enter the respiratory tract. These substances may include vomitus, food, water, and saliva. Instead of remaining in the digestive tract, these substances are breathed into the lungs.

Aspiration pneumonia may result from pathology that involves the [41]

- Esophagus
- Larynx
- Nervous system.

Megaesophagus is a common risk factor for the development of aspiration pneumonia (see Figures 37.1a, b).

The Irish Setter, Great Dane, German Shepherd, Labrador Retriever, and Newfoundland are predisposed to congenital megaesophagus [42–44]. Megaesophagus can also be acquired, secondary to myasthenia gravis [45–47], hypoadrenocorticism, lead poisoning, and potentially hypothyroidism [42].

Aspiration pneumonia may also develop as a direct result of anesthetic events, during which time the patient loses conscious control over the airway [41, 48, 49].

Radiographic evidence that is supportive of a diagnosis of aspiration pneumonia includes right middle lung lobe consolidation [38, 41, 48] (see Figures 37.2a–f).

(a)
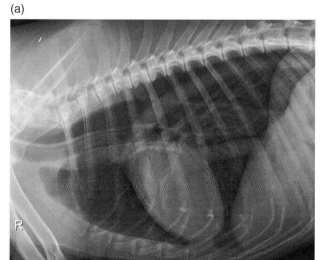
(b)
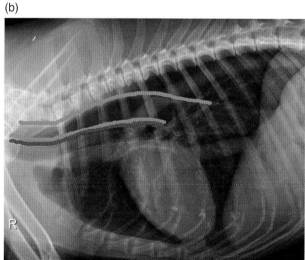

Figure 37.1 (a) This canine patient has radiographic evidence of megaesophagus. *Source:* Courtesy of Jason M. Eberhardt, DVM, MS, DACVIM. (b) This is the same patient that is depicted in Figure 37.1a. Note that the borders of the esophagus have been outlined in blue. The classic "tracheal stripe" sign that is confirmatory for megaesophagus has been outlined in red. The "tracheal stripe" sign is created by summation of the dorsal tracheal wall with the ventral wall of the esophagus. *Source:* Courtesy of Jason M. Eberhardt, DVM, MS, DACVIM.

(a)

(b)

(c)

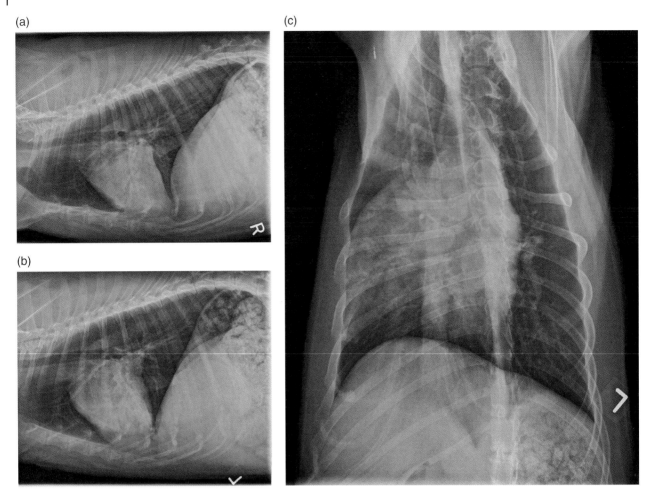

Figure 37.2 (a) Right lateral thoracic radiograph in a patient with aspiration pneumonia. *Source:* Courtesy of Daniel Foy, MS, DVM, DACVIM, DACVECC. (b) Left lateral thoracic radiograph in a patient with aspiration pneumonia. *Source:* Courtesy of Daniel Foy, MS, DVM, DACVIM, DACVECC. (c) Ventrodorsal (V/D) thoracic radiograph in a patient with aspiration pneumonia. Note the involvement of the right middle lung lobe. *Source:* Courtesy of Daniel Foy, MS, DVM, DACVIM, DACVECC. (d) Left lateral thoracic radiograph in a patient with aspiration pneumonia. *Source:* Courtesy of Daniel Foy, MS, DVM, DACVIM, DACVECC. (e) Right lateral thoracic radiograph in a patient with aspiration pneumonia. *Source:* Courtesy of Daniel Foy, MS, DVM, DACVIM, DACVECC. (f) V/D thoracic radiograph in a patient with aspiration pneumonia. Note the involvement of the right middle lung lobe. *Source:* Courtesy of Daniel Foy, MS, DVM, DACVIM, DACVECC.

Lung lobes other than the right middle may also be involved [48]. In other words, an unaffected right middle lung lobe does not effectively rule out aspiration pneumonia [48].

37.2.2 Bacterial Pneumonia

Bacterial pneumonia and bronchopneumonia occur with greater frequency in community-housed dogs, such as those populations that frequent kennels, grooming facilities, and shelters [41, 50]. Young dogs are at increased risk [41].

Commonly implicated bacteria include *Bordetella bronchiseptica* and *Mycoplasma* spp. [41].

Streptococcus zooepidemicus occurs less frequently in clinical practice [41]. However, when it does, the resultant pneumonia is typically hemorrhagic [51].

Patients with bacterial pneumonia typically present with a cough, fever, and clinical signs that are associated with general malaise: lethargy, apparent weakness, and inappetence [41]. As disease progresses, they are likely to become dyspneic [41].

Crackles are commonly heard [38]. Bronchial sounds may be increased, particularly if there is concurrent tracheobronchitis [38]. In addition, thoracic auscultation is likely to reveal muffled vesicular lung sounds, particularly when one or more lung lobes are consolidated [38].

Radiographic evidence that supports a diagnosis of bacterial pneumonia includes cranioventral involvement and an interstitial-to-alveolar pattern [41].

Air bronchograms are often present. Air bronchograms refer to the outlining of tubular airways. This occurs due to contrast that is created when radiolucent air, which appears black in radiographs, stands out

(d)

(f)

(e)

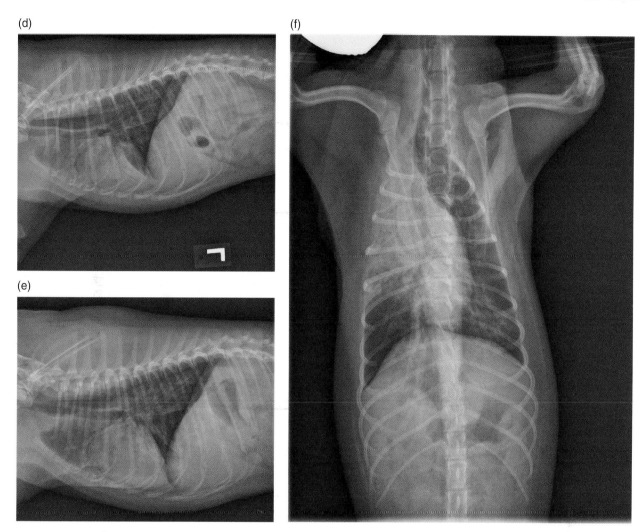

Figure 37.2 (Continued)

against the surrounding, fluid-filled radiopaque alveoli, which appear gray-white (see Figures 37.3a–c).

Note that distribution and patterns may be atypical [41, 52]. In other words, lack of cranioventral involvement and lack of an interstitial-to-alveolar pattern do not effectively rule out bacterial pneumonia [41, 52].

37.2.3 Fungal Pneumonia

Fungal infections may cause focal lesions. However, more often than not, their pathophysiology is multisystemic. The lungs are frequently involved.

The likelihood of contracting a fungal infection largely depends upon where a patient lives. Different regions of the globe are preferential habitats for particular species of fungi [41].

For example, recall that blastomycosis was first introduced in Chapter 9, Section 9.5.1 as a causative agent of nasal planum depigmentation. Blastomycosis is caused by *Blastomyces dermatitidis*. This organism is endemic

to North American soil [53, 54]. However, those who reside near the Mississippi, Missouri, and Ohio River valleys are most at risk for contracting disease [53].

Fungal pneumonia due to *B. dermatitidis* results in tachypnea, dyspnea, and cyanosis [53]. Many dogs present with concurrent lymphadenopathy and/or cutaneous signs, including nodules, papules, plaques, and depigmentation lesions of the nasal planum [53, 55]. Gastrointestinal, ocular, and/or neurological signs may also develop [53, 55].

In addition to blastomycosis, other causes of fungal pneumonia include the following [41, 56, 57]:

- Coccidioidomycosis
- Disseminated histoplasmosis

Young patients are at increased risk of contracting fungal pneumonia [41]. Coughing and respiratory distress are common clinical signs [41, 56, 57].

Perihilar lymphadenopathy is often appreciated on thoracic radiographs [41]. Radiography may also reveal a

(a)

(b)

(c)

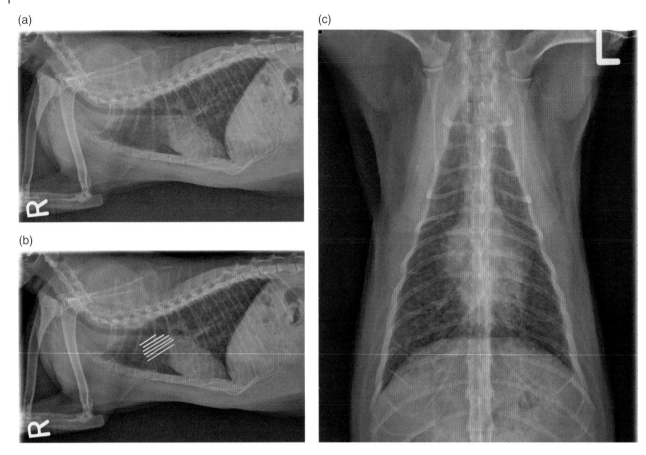

Figure 37.3 (a) Right lateral thoracic radiograph in a feline patient with air bronchograms in the cranioventral thorax. (b) Same radiograph as in Figure 37.3a. Three air bronchograms have been outlined in yellow, blue, and orange, respectively, for ease of observation. (c) Orthogonal view of the same feline patient depicted in Figure 37.3a.

miliary pattern [41]. A miliary pattern refers to the abundance of very small pulmonary nodules that are too numerous to count (see Figures 37.4a, b).

37.2.4 Viral Pneumonia

Viral pneumonia occurs less frequently than bacterial pneumonia among the companion animal population, and it occurs in dogs more often than in cats.

Canine distemper virus (CDV) and canine influenza virus (CIV) are the most common causes of viral pneumonia in dogs [41]. Refer to Chapter 35, Section 35.3.2 for more information on CIV. Refer to Part Eight of the textbook for more information on CDV.

It is rare, but possible, for canine herpesvirus (CHV) to cause pneumonia [58, 59].

37.2.5 Cardiogenic Pulmonary Edema and Left-Sided CHF

Recall from Chapter 36, Section 36.3.3 that pulmonary edema is the condition in which alveoli become fluid

filled [60]. This layer of fluid compromises gas exchange. Ineffective ventilation causes inadequate oxygenation over time.

Cardiac disease is a common cause of pulmonary edema, particularly in the canine patient. Specifically, left-sided CHF leads to cardiogenic pulmonary edema [61, 62].

The left ventricle of the heart pumps blood through the aorta, into systemic circulation [61, 62]. When the left ventricle fails as a pump, there is backflow of blood into the left atrium and, ultimately, the pulmonary vasculature [61, 62].

The lungs are said to be congested [60]. This congestion is audible as crackles upon thoracic auscultation [38].

This congestion is also visible on thoracic radiographs as pulmonary infiltrates [60]. Thoracic imaging may also reveal pulmonary venous distension and cardiomegaly [31, 60, 63]. The left atrium is particularly prominent and may appear, particularly on lateral films, as an atrial bulge (see Figures 37.5a–d).

Medical management of left-sided CHF is lifelong. Treatment is aimed at reducing pulmonary congestion

(a)

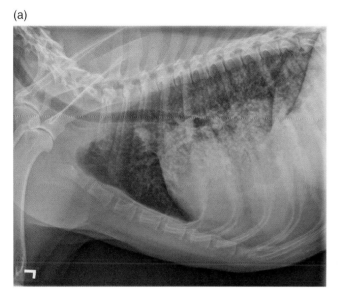

(b)

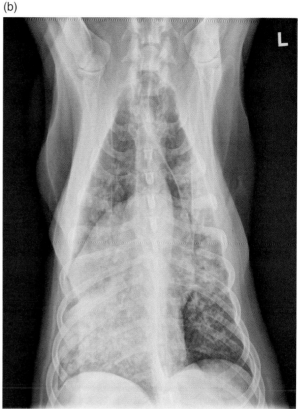

Figure 37.4 (a) Left lateral thoracic radiograph of a canine patient with blastomycosis. Note the miliary pattern that is associated with the lung fields. *Source:* Courtesy of Daniel Foy, MS, DVM, DACVIM, DACVECC. (b) Orthogonal view of the same patient depicted in Figure 37.4a. Note the miliary pattern that is associated with the lung fields. *Source:* Courtesy of Daniel Foy, MS, DVM, DACVIM, DACVECC.

through diuresis [60, 62–65]. Furosemide is routinely prescribed as a diuretic [60, 62].

Response to injectable furosemide is rapid, and it is evident when imaging studies are repeated (see Figures 37.6a–c).

37.3 Wheezes

Wheezes are another adventitious lung sound. Unlike crackles, wheezes are said to be continuous because their sound is prolonged. At more than 80 ms in duration, wheezes last, on average, four times longer than crackles [1].

Wheezes are "musical" sounds that result from vibrations of airway walls [8].

A patient that is wheezing likely has an airspace with increased resistance to airflow [1, 8]. This commonly occurs in cats or dogs that have reactive, or thickened airways [1, 8].

Wheezes may also occur in patients with partially collapsed or obstructed airways due to neighboring pulmonary disease [8].

Patients with asthma routinely wheeze during an acute attack [1, 8, 37].

Refer to Chapter 35, Section 35.4.1 for a review of feline asthma. Recall that asthma is a condition involving chronic inflammation of the bronchi and bronchioles [40, 66, 67]. Inflammation of the airway mucosa causes increased airway secretions [40, 66–68]. These narrow the airway lumen [40, 66–68].

During an asthma attack, the patient experiences bronchoconstriction [40, 66, 67]. This further reduces an already pathologically narrowed space [40, 66, 67].

Asthmatic cats typically present for recurrent coughing episodes and expiratory wheezing [40, 66, 67].

Asthmatic wheezes are more high-pitched than wheezes that are associated with bronchitis [37]. Historically, asthmatic wheezes were referred to as sibilant rhonchi to differentiate them from the sonorous rhonchi of bronchitis [37].

Bronchitis-induced wheezes sound less musical and more like a combination of snoring and moaning. These result from excessive secretions within the larger airways [37].

Refer to Chapter 35, Section 35.4.2 for a review of chronic bronchitis.

(a)

(b)

(c)

(d)

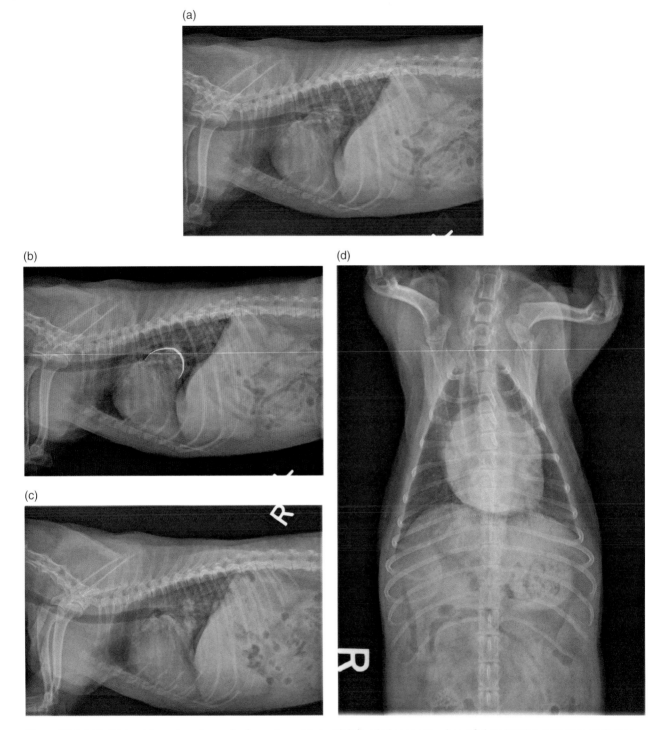

Figure 37.5 (a) Left lateral thoracic radiograph of a canine patient with left-sided congestive heart failure (CHF), pre-treatment. *Source:* Courtesy of Daniel Foy, MS, DVM, DACVIM, DACVECC. (b) Same radiograph as in Figure 37.5a. Left atrial enlargement is highlighted in light orange as a prominent atrial bulge from the cardiac silhouette. *Source:* Courtesy of Daniel Foy, MS, DVM, DACVIM, DACVECC. (c) Right lateral thoracic radiograph of a canine patient with left-sided CHF, pre-treatment. *Source:* Courtesy of Daniel Foy, MS, DVM, DACVIM, DACVECC. (d) Ventrodorsal (V/D) thoracic radiograph of a canine patient with left-sided CHF, pre-treatment. *Source:* Courtesy of Daniel Foy, MS, DVM, DACVIM, DACVECC.

(a)

(b)

(c)

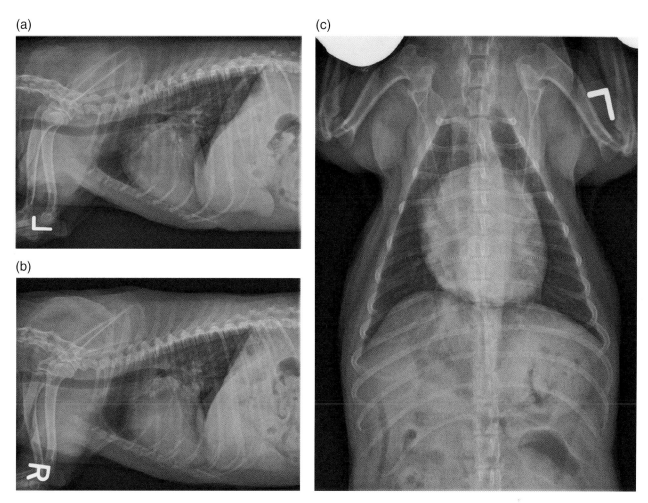

Figure 37.6 (a) Left lateral thoracic radiograph of a canine patient with left-sided congestive heart failure (CHF), after the administration of injectable furosemide. *Source:* Courtesy of Daniel Foy, MS, DVM, DACVIM, DACVECC. (b) Right lateral thoracic radiograph of a canine patient with left-sided CHF, after the administration of injectable furosemide. *Source:* Courtesy of Daniel Foy, MS, DVM, DACVIM, DACVECC. (c) Ventrodorsal (V/D) thoracic radiograph of a canine patient with left-sided CHF, after the administration of injectable furosemide. *Source:* Courtesy of Daniel Foy, MS, DVM, DACVIM, DACVECC.

Note that one does not require a stethoscope to hear all wheezes: some are audible through the mouth [1]. However, subtle wheezes may only be appreciated on auscultation [1].

Imaging studies are an essential component of the diagnostic work-up.

Thoracic radiographs suggest bronchial disease, such as asthma and chronic bronchitis, when they demonstrate thickened bronchial walls [67]. Each bronchus is outlined by a thicker-than-normal black circle [8]. This creates the so-called "donut" pattern [8, 68] (see Figures 37.7a–c).

Thoracic radiographs of canine patients with chronic bronchitis may also demonstrate bronchiectasis or atelectasis [67, 69].

Computed tomography (CT) or bronchoscopy may provide additional clues that bronchial disease is present.

Samples may be taken for cytologic or histopathologic evaluation at the time of bronchoscopy. Alternatively, the patient may endure transtracheal or endotracheal washes to obtain samples that guide decision making concerning the patient's treatment plan [69–71].

(a)

(b)

(c)

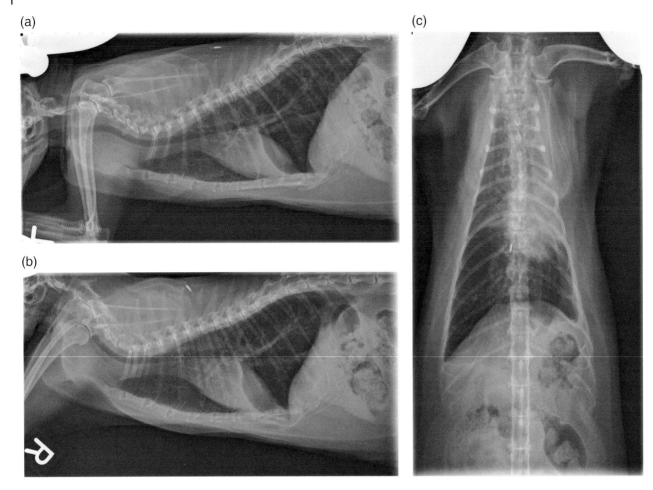

Figure 37.7 (a) Left lateral thoracic radiograph of a cat with feline asthma. *Source:* Courtesy of Daniel Foy, MS, DVM, DACVIM, DACVECC. (b) Right lateral thoracic radiograph of a cat with feline asthma. *Source:* Courtesy of Daniel Foy, MS, DVM, DACVIM, DACVECC. (c) Ventrodorsal (V/D) thoracic radiograph of a cat with feline asthma. *Source:* Courtesy of Daniel Foy, MS, DVM, DACVIM, DACVECC.

References

1 Hansen B. (2009). What's that noise? Interpreting lung sounds. DVM 360 [Internet]. http://veterinarycalendar.dvm360.com/whats-noise-interpreting-lung-sounds-proceedings.

2 Forgacs, P. (1978). The functional basis of pulmonary sounds. *Chest* 73 (3): 399–405.

3 Forgacs, P. (1978). *Lung Sounds*. London: Bailiere Tindall (MacMillan).

4 Melbye, H., Garcia-Marcos, L., Brand, P. et al. (2016). Wheezes, crackles and rhonchi: simplifying description of lung sounds increases the agreement on their classification: a study of 12 physicians' classification of lung sounds from video recordings. *BMJ Open Respir. Res.* 3 (1): e000136.

5 Roudebush, P. and Ryan, J. (1989). Breath sound terminology in the veterinary literature. *J. Am. Vet. Med. Assoc.* 194 (10): 1415–1417.

6 Robertson, A.J. and Coope, R. (1957). Rales, rhonchi, and Laennec. *Lancet* 273 (6992): 417–423.

7 Rijnberk, A. and van Sluijs, F.S. (2009). *Medical History and Physical Examination in Companion Animals*, 333 p. The Netherlands: Elsevier Limited.

8 Englar, R.E. (2017). *Performing the Small Animal Physical Examination*. Hoboken, NJ: Wiley.

9 Gross, V., Dittmar, A., Penzel, T. et al. (2000). The relationship between normal lung sounds, age, and gender. *Am. J. Respir. Crit. Care Med.* 162 (3 Pt 1): 905–909.

10 Kraman, S.S. and Wang, P.M. (1990). Airflow-generated sound in a hollow canine airway cast. *Chest* 97 (2): 461–466.

11 King, L. and Clarke, D. (2010). Emergency care of the patient with acute respiratory distress. *Vet. Focus* 20 (2): 36–43.

12 Horwitz, D.F. (2010). Hyperactivity in dogs. *NAVC Clinician's Brief* (April): 25–27.

13 Curtis TM. (2013). How to recognize and treat anxious dogs and cats. Veterinary Team Brief [Internet]. https://www.veterinaryteambrief.com/article/how-recognize-and-treat-anxious-dogs-and-cats.

14 Levine, E.D. (2008). Feline fear and anxiety. *Vet. Clin. North Am. Small Anim. Pract.* 38 (5): 1065–1079, vii.

15 Mazzaferro EM. (2012). The case: breathing difficulty in a "well" cat. NAVC Clinician's Brief [Internet]. https://www.cliniciansbrief.com/article/case-breathing-difficulty-well-cat.

16 Gough, A. and Murphy, K. (2015). *Differential Diagnosis in Small Animal Medicine*. Ames, IA: Wiley.

17 Miller, M.W. (2004). Diagnostic tree: dyspnea. *NAVC Clinician's Brief* (May): 54.

18 Dowers K. (2011). Working up pleural effusions in cats. DVM 360 [Internet]. http://veterinarycalendar.dvm360.com/working-pleural-effusions-cats-proceedings.

19 Rozanski E. (2011). Pulmonary contusions and other thoracic trauma (Proceedings). DVM 360 [Internet]. http://veterinarycalendar.dvm360.com/pulmonary-contusions-and-other-thoracic-trauma-proceedings.

20 Rishniw M. (2006). Dyspnea in a cat. NAVC Clinician's Brief [Internet]. Available from: https://www.cliniciansbrief.com/article/dyspnea-cat.

21 Statz G. (2014). The case: acute respiratory distress. NAVC Clinician's Brief [Internet]. https://www.cliniciansbrief.com/article/case-acute-respiratory-distress.

22 Hawkins, E.C. (2015). Bacterial pneumonia. *NAVC Clinician's Brief* (August): 69–75.

23 Lee, J.A. (2015). Top 5 clinical situations that can't wait. *NAVC Clinician's Brief* (June): 27–29.

24 Davis, A., Khorzad, R., and Whelan, M. (2013). Dynamic upper airway obstruction secondary to severe feline asthma. *J. Am. Anim. Hosp. Assoc.* 49 (2): 142–147.

25 Pachtinger, G.E. (2015). Septic shock. *NAVC Clinician's Brief* (March): 13–16.

26 Richardson, J.A. and Gwaltney-Brant, S.M. (2003). Consultant on call: ethylene glycol toxicosis in dogs and cats. *NAVC Clinician's Brief* (January): 13–19.

27 Sueda, K.L.C. (2016). Cho J. Trazodone. *Plumb's Therapeutics Briefs* (July): 55–57.

28 Pachtinger, G.E. and King, L. (2010). Fever of unknown origin. *NAVC Clinician's Brief* (March): 29–32.

29 Powell, L.L. (2008). Canine heatstroke. *NAVC Clinician's Brief* (August): 13–16.

30 Gorris F, Faut S, S. Daminet, de Rooster H, Saunders JH, Paepe D. (2017). Pyothorax in cats and dogs. Vlaams Diergeneeskundig Tijdschrift [Internet]. http://vdt.ugent.be/sites/default/files/Dutchart07.pdf.

31 Hogan, D.F. (2004). Congestive heart failure in the dog. *NAVC Clinician's Brief* (September): 16–19.

32 Boswood, A. (2010). Chronic valvular disease in the dog. *NAVC Clinician's Brief* (December): 17–21.

33 Bright, R.M. (2005). Diaphragmatic hernia. *NAVC Clinician's Brief* (April): 59–60.

34 Byers CG. (2011). Obesity in dogs, Part 1: Exploring the causes and consequences of canine obesity. DVM 360 [Internet]. http://veterinarymedicine.dvm360.com/obesity-dogs-part-1-exploring-causes-and-consequences-canine-obesity.

35 Riviere, J.E. and Papich, M.G. (2017). *Veterinary Pharmacology and Therapeutics*, 10e. Hoboken, NJ: Wiley.

36 Muir, W.W. 3rd and Gadawski, J.E. (1998). Respiratory depression and apnea induced by propofol in dogs. *Am. J. Vet. Res.* 59 (2): 157–161.

37 RnCeus Interactive™. (1996). Abnormal breath sounds. http://www.rnceus.com/resp/respabn.html].

38 Hackett T. (2009). Pulmonary parenchymal disease. DVM 360 [Internet]. http://veterinarycalendar.dvm360.com/pulmonary-parenchymal-disease-proceedings.

39 Dye, J.A., McKiernan, B.C., Rozanski, E.A. et al. (1996). Bronchopulmonary disease in the cat: historical, physical, radiographic, clinicopathologic, and pulmonary functional evaluation of 24 affected and 15 healthy cats. *J. Vet. Intern. Med.* 10 (6): 385–400.

40 Mason, R.A. and Rand, J. (2006). The coughing cat. In: *Problem-Based Feline Medicine* (ed. J. Rand), 90–108. Philadelphia: Elsevier Limited.

41 Palma, D. (2016). Common pulmonary diseases in dogs. *NAVC Clinician's Brief* (October): 77–109.

42 Washabau, R.J. (2003). Gastrointestinal motility disorders and gastrointestinal prokinetic therapy. *Vet. Clin. North Am. Small Anim. Pract.* 33 (5): 1007–1028, vi.

43 Holland, C.T., Satchell, P.M., and Farrow, B.R. (1996). Vagal esophagomotor nerve function and esophageal motor performance in dogs with congenital idiopathic megaesophagus. *Am. J. Vet. Res.* 57 (6): 906–913.

44 Holland, C.T., Satchell, P.M., and Farrow, B.R. (2002). Selective vagal afferent dysfunction in dogs with congenital idiopathic megaoesophagus. *Auton. Neurosci.* 99 (1): 18–23.

45 Gaynor, A.R., Shofer, F.S., and Washabau, R.J. (1997). Risk factors for acquired megaesophagus in dogs. *J. Am. Vet. Med. Assoc.* 211 (11): 1406–1412.

46 Shelton, G.D., Willard, M.D., Cardinet, G.H. 3rd, and Lindstrom, J. (1990). Acquired myasthenia gravis. Selective involvement of esophageal, pharyngeal, and facial muscles. *J. Vet. Intern. Med.* 4 (6): 281–284.

47 Shelton, G.D., Schule, A., and Kass, P.H. (1997). Risk factors for acquired myasthenia gravis in dogs: 1,154 cases (1991–1995). *J. Am. Vet. Med. Assoc.* 211 (11): 1428–1431.

48 Kogan, D.A., Johnson, L.R., Jandrey, K.F., and Pollard, R.E. (2008). Clinical, clinicopathologic, and radiographic findings in dogs with aspiration pneumonia: 88 cases (2004–2006). *J. Am. Vet. Med. Assoc.* 233 (11): 1742–1747.

49 Kogan, D.A., Johnson, L.R., Sturges, B.K. et al. (2008). Etiology and clinical outcome in dogs with aspiration pneumonia: 88 cases (2004–2006). *J. Am. Vet. Med. Assoc.* 233 (11): 1748–1755.

50 Radhakrishnan, A., Drobatz, K.J., Culp, W.T., and King, L.G. (2007). Community-acquired infectious pneumonia in puppies: 65 cases (1993–2002). *J. Am. Vet. Med. Assoc.* 230 (10): 1493–1497.

51 Priestnall, S. and Erles, K. (2011). Streptococcus zooepidemicus: an emerging canine pathogen. *Vet. J.* 188 (2): 142–148.

52 Jameson, P.H., King, L.A., Lappin, M.R., and Jones, R.L. (1995). Comparison of clinical signs, diagnostic findings, organisms isolated, and clinical outcome in dogs with bacterial pneumonia: 93 cases (1986-1991). *J. Am. Vet. Med. Assoc.* 206 (2): 206–209.

53 Kerl, M.E. (2003). Update on canine and feline fungal diseases. *Vet. Clin. North Am. Small Anim. Pract.* 33 (4): 721–747.

54 Werner, A. and Norton, F. (2011). Blastomycosis. *Compend. Contin. Educ. Vet.* 33 (8): E1–E4; quiz E5.

55 Roudebush, P. (1985). Mycotic pneumonias. *Vet. Clin. North Am. Small Anim. Pract.* 15 (5): 949–969.

56 Johnson, L.R., Herrgesell, E.J., Davidson, A.P., and Pappagianis, D. (2003). Clinical, clinicopathologic, and radiographic findings in dogs with coccidioidomycosis: 24 cases (1995–2000). *J. Am. Vet. Med. Assoc.* 222 (4): 461–466.

57 Clinkenbeard, K.D., Cowell, R.L., and Tyler, R.D. (1988). Disseminated Histoplasmosis in Dogs – 12 Cases (1981–1986). *J. Am. Vet. Med. Assoc.* 193 (11): 1443–1447.

58 Kumar, S., Driskell, E.A., Cooley, A.J. et al. (2015). Fatal Canid Herpesvirus 1 Respiratory Infections in 4 Clinically Healthy Adult Dogs. *Vet. Pathol.* 52 (4): 681–687.

59 Larsen MM. (2008). Radiographic evaluation of pulmonary patterns and disease. DVM 360 [Internet]. http://veterinarycalendar.dvm360.com/radiographic-evaluation-pulmonary-patterns-and-disease-proceedings.

60 Rozanski E. (2009). Pulmonary edema. DVM 360 [Internet]. http://veterinarycalendar.dvm360.com/print/328751?page=full.

61 Reece, W.O., Erickson, H.H., Goff, J.P., and Uemura, E.E. (2015). *Dukes' Physiology of Domestic Animals*, 13e, xii, 748 p. Ames, Iowa, USA: Wiley Blackwell.

62 Estrada, A. (2014). Heart disease: diagnosis & treatment. *NAVC Clinician's Brief* (March): 91–95.

63 Hoskins JD. (2008). Keys to managing end-stage heart failure. DVM 360 [Internet]. http://veterinarynews.dvm360.com/print/316908?page=full.

64 Spier A. (2007). Congestive heart failure: approaches to care. NAVC Clinician's Brief [Internet]. https://www.cliniciansbrief.com/article/congestive-heart-failure-approaches-care.

65 DeFrancesco, T. (2015). Mitral valve disease in a dog. *Plumb's Therapeutics Briefs* (May): 13–16.

66 Padrid P. (2011). Diagnosing and treating feline asthma (including the use of inhalants). DVM 360 [Internet]. http://veterinarycalendar.dvm360.com/diagnosing-and-treating-feline-asthma-including-use-inhalants-proceedings.

67 Tilley, L.P. and Smith, F.W.K. (2016). *Blackwell's Five-Minute Veterinary Consult. Canine and Feline*, 6e, lxix, 1622 p. Ames, Iowa, USA: Wiley.

68 Padrid, P. (2005). Feline asthma and bronchitis. *NAVC Clinician's Brief* (October): 37–40.

69 Kumrow, K.J. (2012). Canine chronic bronchitis: a review and update. *Today's Veterinary Practice* (November/December): 12–17.

70 Padrid, P.A., Hornof, W.J., Kurpershoek, C.J., and Cross, C.E. (1990). Canine chronic bronchitis. A pathophysiologic evaluation of 18 cases. *J. Vet. Intern. Med.* 4 (3): 172–180.

71 Carey SA, editor. (2018). Current therapy for canine chronic bronchitis. Michigan Veterinary Medical Association [Internet]. https://www.michvma.org/resources/Documents/MVC/2018%20Proceedings/carey_04.pdf.

Part Five

The Cardiovascular System

38

Abnormal Mucous Membranes and Capillary Refill Time (CRT)

38.1 Introduction to Mucous Membranes

Mucous membranes are normal epithelial linings of body cavities and organ surfaces [1, 2]. Sometimes these tissues are referred to collectively as mucosa [1, 2]. At body openings, such as the mouth, nostrils, urethra, and anus, the mucosa is continuous with skin [1, 2].

Mucous membranes are largely protective. Consider, for example, the stomach. The mucosa of the stomach functions to prevent gastric acid from eroding the stomach wall as ingesta is digested.

Likewise, the mucosa of the urinary bladder protects the bladder wall from irritants contained within urine, and the mucosa of the gall bladder exists to protect the gall bladder from bile.

Mucous membranes also secrete mucus. This secretion helps certain tissues trap particles before they gain deeper entry into the body. Consider, for example, the respiratory tract. Mucous secretions of the upper respiratory tract prevent particulate matter from inadvertently entering the lungs.

Secretions from mucous membranes also help to keep tissues moist.

Some, but not all of, mucous membranes are visible to the naked eye [3, 4]. These tissues can be evaluated during a physical examination to help the clinician gather additional information about the patient's hydration and vascular health [3, 4].

The most commonly examined mucous membranes in the dog and cat are located within the oral cavity as the gingiva, or gums [3–5]. In health, the gingiva should appear pinkish in color and moist [4–8] (see Figures 38.1a, b).

Note that you can appreciate glistening in both Figures 38.1a and b. You can imagine that if you were to touch either patient's gums, they would be moist, as opposed to tacky or dry [4–8] (see Figures 38.2a, b).

Certain patients will not allow you to examine their oral cavities thoroughly while awake. It may not be safe for the clinician to lift the patient's lip with his fingers in an attempt to evaluate or feel the gingiva. These patients may benefit from using a tongue depressor to safely raise the lip to note the gross appearance of the gums [4] (see Figures 38.3a, b).

If the clinician's safety or the handler's safety remains a concern, then an altered site may be evaluated, such as the conjunctiva [3–5] (see Figures 38.4a, b).

Alternatively, clinicians may attempt to examine those mucous membranes that are associated with the external genitalia, namely, the vulva or the prepuce [3–5, 9].

38.2 Tacky or Dry Mucous Membranes

Healthy gums should be moist. However, be aware that hypersalivation can create the illusion of moist gums when in fact the patient is dehydrated (see Figure 38.5).

Mucous membranes that are not moist are either tacky or dry [3–8].

If you were to touch tacky mucous membranes, your finger would transiently stick to the gums, just as if you were touching Elmer's glue that had yet to dry. Your finger would not remain attached if you were to attempt to remove it, but you would feel momentarily tethered.

Tacky gums are, in a sense, sticky.

Extremely tacky gums are said to be dry [3–8]. In cases where mucous membranes are dry, the clinician's finger figuratively glues itself to the gums. Yes, the finger can ultimately detach from the gums, but it takes more effort.

There is also a certain sound associated with touching a finger to dry gums. The sound is similar to what you would hear if you moistened your thumb and index finger, touched them together, then forced separation between the two. It is subtle, but audible, whereas there is no sound as one peels a finger off moistened gingiva.

Tacky or dry mucous membranes can be normal in healthy, panting dogs [6]. However, they more commonly result from true dehydration [4, 6]. In fact, in a patient that is not panting, tacky mucous membranes are one of the first signs of dehydration.

(a)   (b)

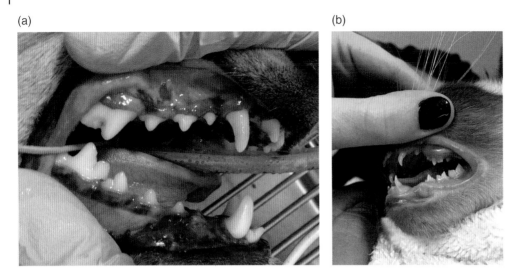

Figure 38.1 (a) Healthy pink mucous membranes in a canine patient. *Source:* Courtesy of Patricia Bennett, DVM. (b) Healthy pink mucous membranes in a feline patient. *Source:* Courtesy of Natalie J. Reeser.

(a)   (b)

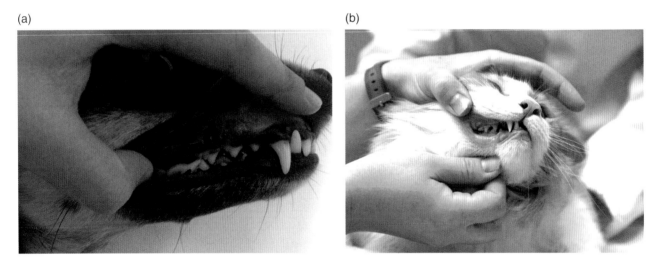

Figure 38.2 (a) Using one's fingertips to lift the lips of a canine patient to assess the patient's oral mucous membranes. *Source:* Courtesy of the Media Resources Department at Midwestern University. (b) Using one's fingertips to lift the lips of a feline patient to assess the patient's oral mucous membranes. *Source:* Courtesy of the Media Resources Department at Midwestern University.

A patient that is less than 5% dehydrated will have tacky mucous membranes [5, 6]. As dehydration intensifies to 6–8% of body weight, tacky gums transition to dry [5, 6].

Note that tacky mucous membranes are observable on physical examination before the skin tents [5, 6]. Skin tenting occurs when a patient is 6–8% dehydrated [5, 6] (see Figures 38.6).

The skin is checked for tenting by grasping a skin fold at the nape of the neck or between the shoulder blades [4]. This skin fold is lifted up and twisted to one side by the examiner's flick of the wrist [4]. This is called tenting the skin [4]. The skin fold is then released for observation by the clinician [4].

A hydrated patient has elastic skin [4]. There is, in other words, appreciable skin turgor [4]. This allows the fold of skin to snap back to its original position [4]. In other words, there is no "skin tent" [4].

A dehydrated patient experiences diminished skin elasticity [4]. The skin may not bounce back quickly to its starting position [4]. As dehydration progresses, the skin fold remains "tented" [4].

Skin tenting is an important test to perform in patients with tacky mucous membranes. It helps to clarify the level of dehydration.

Note, however, that the skin tent test is imperfect. Geriatric patients or patients that have excessive skin folds following extreme weight loss may have what

(a)

(b)

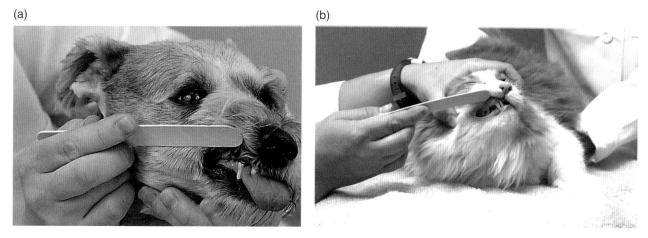

Figure 38.3 (a) Using a tongue depressor to lift the lips of a canine patient to assess the patient's oral mucous membranes. *Source:* Courtesy of the Media Resources Department at Midwestern University. (b) Using a tongue depressor to lift the lips of a feline patient to assess the patient's oral mucous membranes. *Source:* Courtesy of the Media Resources Department at Midwestern University.

(a)

(b)

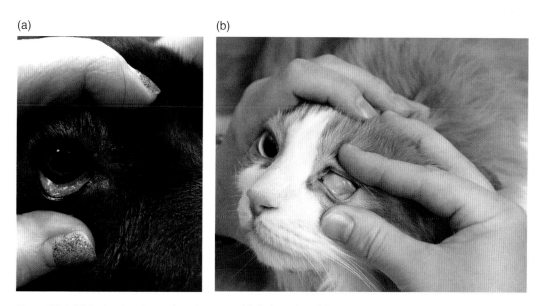

Figure 38.4 (a) Evaluating the conjunctiva to establish the color of this dog's mucous membranes. (b) Evaluating the conjunctiva of this cat. *Source:* Courtesy of the Media Resources Department at Midwestern University.

appears to be a skin tent in the absence of true dehydration [4].

Patients that are 8–10% dehydrated will have dry mucous membranes, skin tenting, and globes that have sunken into their respective orbits [5–8].

Dehydration may result from a number of causes, including hypovolemia. Hypovolemia occurs when there is a net loss of fluid from the intravascular space. This may be due to the following [5, 6, 10]:

- Insufficient intake of water
- Elevated core body temperature
- Elevated environmental temperature
- Vomiting
- Diarrhea
- Excessive volumes of urine being produced and excreted (polyuria)
- Excessive frequency of urination (pollakiuria)
- Excessive sweating, as from exercise or overexertion

Dehydration may also be due to loss of fluid from the skin, as through cutaneous burns, or loss of intravascular fluid because of hemorrhage [5, 6, 10].

Patients that are dehydrated benefit from a diagnostic work-up to identify the primary cause so that it can be resolved. Replacement fluid therapy is a mainstay of treatment to correct the dehydration; however, the problem will recur if the underlying issue is not addressed. There is also no "one-size-fits-all" approach to fluid therapy. Fluids must be tailored to each individual patient in terms of fluid type, fluid additives, volume to be infused, and rate of infusion [10].

Consult a fluid therapy or internal medicine resource for guidelines.

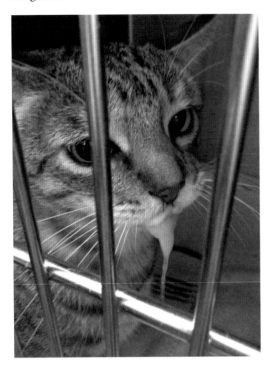

Figure 38.5 Ptyalism in a feline patient. Hypersalivation can make the gums seem moist, even when they are actually dry. This patient's ptyalism was triggered by the administration of oral buprenorphine. Nauseous patients may also hypersalivate. *Source:* Courtesy of Carolyn Deshaies, DVM.

38.3 Normal Mucous Membrane Colors

Most healthy mucous membranes are pink in color [3, 4]. The color is a direct reflection of vascular health. Mucosa has a healthy blood supply and its tissues are thin. This makes changes in oxygenation and perfusion visible. When mucosa is well-oxygenated and there is adequate blood flow through the vasculature, nonpigmented mucosa is pink [4].

Another measure of the health of the patient's circulatory system is the capillary refill time (CRT) [4, 11]. This can be assessed easily in patients with pink gums [4]. The clinician presses down on an area of the gumline firmly, with a finger [4]. The most common site for this in canine and feline patients is the gingiva that is associated with the lateral aspect of either maxillary canine tooth [4].

Pressure from a finger or tongue depressor forces blood out of the capillaries [4]. When the finger or tongue depressor is released, blood returns to capillaries [4]. Normal CRT ranges from one to two seconds [4, 11].

Some patients have naturally pigmented mucosa [4]. These pigments diminish what should be visible, making it more challenging to use mucous membranes as indicators of general well-being [4].

Pigmented gingiva may be mottled or solid black [4] (see Figures 38.7a–d).

(a)

(b)

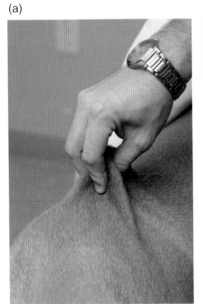
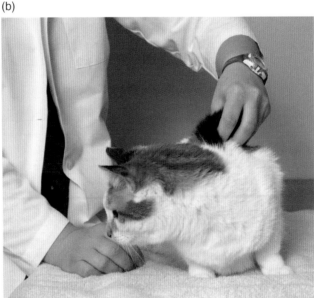

Figure 38.6 (a) Checking for a skin tent in a canine patient. *Source:* Courtesy of the Media Resources Department at Midwestern University. (b) Checking for a skin tent in a feline patient. *Source:* Courtesy of the Media Resources Department at Midwestern University.

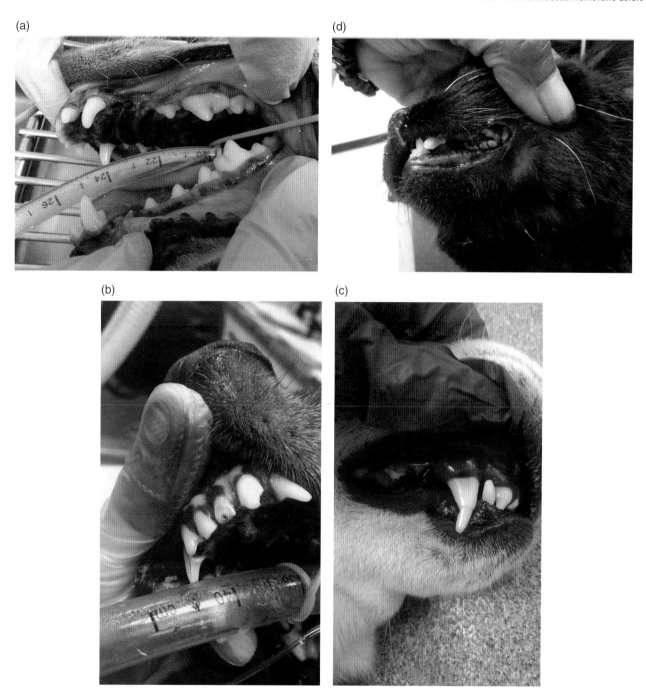

(a)

(d)

(b)

(c)

Figure 38.7 (a) Pigmented soft and hard palate, and mottled pink-black gingiva in a canine patient. (b) Pigmented soft palate, and mottled pink-black gingiva in a canine patient. This patient just so happens to have a fractured maxillary incisor. *Source:* Courtesy of Frank Isom, DVM. (c) Mostly black gingiva in a canine patient that had canine distemper virus (CDV) as a juvenile. Note the enamel damage that is associated with the right maxillary canine tooth. *Source:* Courtesy of Laura Polerecky, LVT. (d) Black gingiva in a feline patient that has extensive dental disease.

Recall from Chapter 9, Section 9.2 that hyperpigmentation results from increased melanin deposits within the skin [12]. Hereditary hyperpigmentation is most common in cream, red, and tricolor cats and is referred to as lentigo simplex [12, 13]. Lentigo simplex can be seen in dogs as well.

Patients with lentigo simplex develop macules of black-brown pigment that typically increase in number and enlarge with age [12, 13].

These patches develop anywhere on the skin; however, they concentrate on oral mucosa and the soft and hard palates [13–15]. This creates a mottled appearance.

38.4 Abnormal Mucous Membrane Colors

Mucous membrane color may change because of underlying pathology.

Abnormal mucous membrane colors include the following [4, 16–29]:

- Pale pink
- White
- Yellow or icteric
- Bluish-purple or cyanotic
- Chocolate brown
- Red, so-called hyperemic or "injected" (see Figures 38.8a–e)

38.4.1 Pale Pink or White Mucous Membranes

Pale pink or white mucous membranes are caused by either anemia or vasoconstriction [4, 29].

38.4.1.1 Anemia

Broadly, anemia may be due to [4, 17, 29]

- Decreased production of erythrocytes, as from bone marrow pathology
- Increased loss of erythrocytes, as from hemorrhage
- Increased destruction of erythrocytes, as in immune-mediated disease.

Patient presentation differs, depending upon whether anemia is acute or chronic [29].

Those with chronic anemia, such as cats that are infected by feline leukemia virus (FeLV), are usually more tolerant of decreased erythrocyte mass [29]. They are less burdened by anemia because they have had time to compensate.

Contrast these patients with those suffering from acute anemia. These patients have not had the opportunity to acclimate to a significantly decreased erythrocyte mass. Consider, for example, the hit-by-car patient with life-threatening hemoabdomen. This patient has experienced massive translocation of blood from the vasculature to the peritoneal cavity. The result is a significant drop in circulating blood volume [30]. Hypovolemic shock ensues [30].

In response to hypovolemic shock, canine patients typically present with tachycardia, tachypnea, and reduced blood pressure, whereas cats in shock tend to be bradycardic [11, 29, 30].

Additional signs of hypovolemic shock include the following [11, 30]:

- Prolonged CRT
- Weak femoral pulses
- Abnormal mentation
  - Dull
  - Depressed
  - Stuporous
  - Comatose
- Cold extremities or generalized hypothermia

Any patient that presents with pale pink or white mucous membranes should be evaluated for anemia. A complete blood count (CBC) and blood smear collectively are critical starting points for interpretation of decreased erythrocyte mass [17].

An elevated absolute reticulocyte count, for example, is suggestive of regenerative anemia. The presence of reticulocytosis tells the clinician that the bone marrow is capable of producing new erythrocytes and in fact is doing what it can to stimulate production of new red blood cells to make up for the body's deficit [17]. Erythrocytes are either being destroyed by the body's own defenses, as in cases of immune-mediated hemolytic anemia, or they are being lost from the circulation at one or more locations as hemorrhage [17].

Note that regeneration of erythrocytes is not instantaneous. A patient that presents within hours of acute hemorrhage into a body cavity will not yet have evidence of reticulocytosis. The body needs time to catch up and process the blood loss. It takes three to five days, on average, for reticulocytes to enter the bloodstream after blood loss, and five to seven days for reticulocytosis to peak [31].

Non-regenerative anemias typically result from bone marrow suppression, as occurs in cases of chronic kidney disease, or primary bone marrow disorders, such as FeLV-associated myelodysplasia [31].

Additional clues as to the source of the anemia may be provided by examining erythrocyte shape, mean corpuscular volume (MCV), and mean corpuscular hemoglobin concentration (MCHC). [17] For example, microcytosis, the condition of having a lower than normal MCV, is classically seen in cases of iron-deficiency anemia. For more information on erythrocyte shape and parameters, refer to a clinical pathology textbook or other related references [17, 31, 32].

38.4.1.2 Vasoconstriction

Vasoconstriction refers to the narrowing of the vasculature, particularly arteries and arterioles [30]. This occurs via muscular contraction of the vessel walls.

If vasoconstriction is generalized, then systemic blood pressure rises.

Focal vasoconstriction may also reduce blood flow to a particular tissue or region of the body.

When it occurs, vasoconstriction is typically due to either pharmacologic influences or shock.

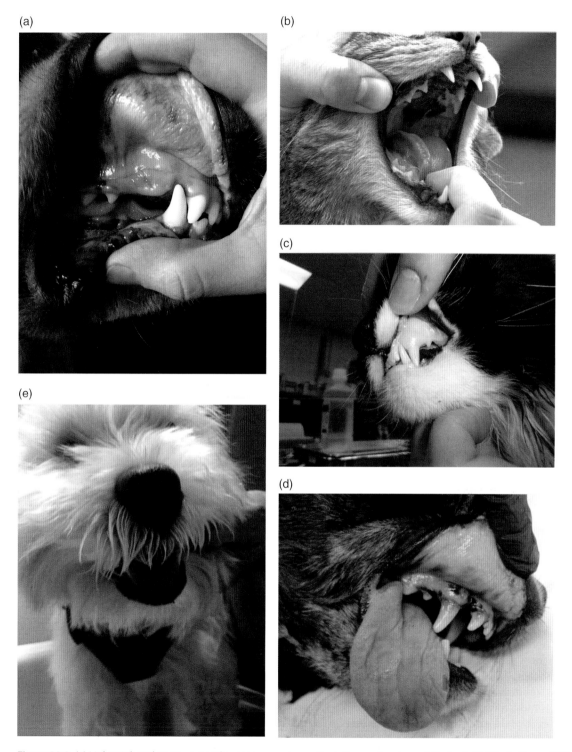

Figure 38.8 (a) Light pink oral mucous membranes in a canine patient. *Source:* Courtesy of Kimberly Wallitsch, Class of 2019, Midwestern University College of Veterinary Medicine. (b) Pale pink oral mucous membranes in a feline patient. *Source:* Courtesy of the Media Resources Department at Midwestern University. (c) White oral mucous membranes in a severely anemic feline patient. *Source:* Courtesy of Daniel Foy, MS, DVM, DACVIM, DACVECC. (d) Icteric oral mucous membranes in a canine patient. *Source:* Courtesy of Dr. Alexandra Brower. (e) Cyanotic tongue in a West Highland white terrier. *Source:* Courtesy of Rodolfo Oliveira Leal, DVM (Portugal), PhD, Dipl. ECVIM-CA (Internal Medicine).

The following medications are known to potentially cause vasoconstriction [33–35]:

- Decongestants
- Dopamine
- Epinephrine
- Stimulants
- Vasopressin, otherwise known as anti-diuretic hormone (ADH)

Other less common causes of vasoconstriction include histamine and hypothermia [36–38].

Histamine is released from mast cells within the body as a defense mechanism by the immune system. The binding of histamine to one of four receptor subtypes, H1 through H4, determines the course of action. When histamine binds to the H1 receptor, it promotes inflammation as well as allergic and anaphylactic reactions. Histamine causes site-specific vasoconstriction and site-specific vasodilation [37, 38].

Histamine tends to cause hyperemic or injected mucous membranes, whereas hypothermia results in pale pink to white gingiva.

When it occurs, hypothermia may be secondary to environmental conditions or, more commonly, anesthetic events, particularly if anesthesia is prolonged [36].

Hypothermic patients experience generalized vasoconstriction as the body attempts to reduce further loss of heat [36]. If vasoconstriction fails to maintain core body temperature, then the patient will start to shiver [36, 39]. Shivering may allow core body temperature to rise; however, it is energetically expensive to maintain [36]. The body's need for oxygen increases by as much as 200% in order to sustain shivering [36].

More often, vasoconstriction in veterinary medicine results from a specific type of shock [29, 30]. Hypovolemic and cardiogenic shock commonly result in vasoconstriction [29, 30, 40].

38.4.1.3 Hypovolemic Shock

Hypovolemic shock occurs when the body experiences a significant loss of circulating blood volume. Large amounts of blood volume, lost rapidly, are particularly detrimental to the body because tissues and organs are now acutely and inadequately perfused [30]. Poor perfusion implies inadequate delivery of oxygen to tissues [30, 41, 42].

Because tissues become starved for oxygen, they have to rely increasingly upon anaerobic metabolism [30]. Over time, this pathway results in a build-up of lactate [30]. As lactate levels rise, lactic acidosis becomes a concern [30].

In addition to poor oxygen delivery, tissues are not able to rid themselves of metabolic by-products, including cellular waste [41, 42].

Hemorrhage is the most obvious cause of a reduction in circulating blood volume [30]. Hemorrhage may result from the following [30]:

- Immune-mediated hemolytic anemia
- Immune-mediated thrombocytopenia
- Ingestion of anticoagulant rodenticide
- Neoplasia
- Surgery
  - Expected blood loss
  - Unexpected blood loss secondary to perioperative complications
- Trauma

In addition to hemorrhage, the following pathways can reduce circulating blood volume [30, 41, 42]:

- Dehydration
  - Net water loss from cutaneous burns
  - Net water loss from chronic diarrhea
  - Net water loss from persistent vomiting
  - Net water loss from polyuria
- Third space disease
  - Fluid build-up within the thoracic cavity
    - ○ Pleural effusion
    - ○ Pulmonary edema
  - Fluid build-up within the abdominal cavity
    - ○ Ascites

Patients in hypovolemic shock benefit from rapid administration of isotonic crystalloid fluids [30, 43–45]. Typically, patients receive one-fourth to one-third of their calculated shock dose. A full shock dose in dogs and cats is 90 ml/kg and 44–60 ml/kg respectively [30, 43–45]. Patients are then reassessed based upon the following parameters [30]:

- Blood pressure
- Core body temperature
- CRT
- Heart rate
- Mucous membrane color

Fluid therapy effectively restores circulating blood volume when hypovolemic shock is secondary to dehydration. Increasing circulating blood volume allows for improved tissue perfusion. As perfusion improves, mucous membranes pink up.

When hypovolemic shock is secondary to hemorrhage, fluid therapy plays an essential role in terms of patient stabilization. However, the inciting condition that caused the hemorrhage must still be addressed.

38.4.1.4 Cardiogenic Shock

Cardiogenic shock also results in vasoconstriction [29, 30, 40].

Cardiogenic shock occurs when cardiac function fails [46]. The heart is, at its core, a pump [47, 48]. It exists to pump blood through the vasculature as a vehicle for the delivery of oxygen and nutrients [47, 48].

When that pump fails, the amount of blood that the heart pumps per minute drops. In other words, the patient's cardiac output is reduced [46]. Cardiac output is a function of heart rate and stroke volume, the amount of blood that is pumped with each beat of the heart.

The heart may try to compensate for the reduction in cardiac output. For example, heart rate may increase to compensate for the decrease in stroke volume.

However, cardiomyopathy tends to be progressive and the heart becomes increasingly inefficient. As this occurs, blood may back up in vessels, waiting to be pumped out into systemic circulation. This excessive pre-load is common in cases of congestive heart failure (CHF).

The primary causes of left-sided CHF in companion animal practice include the following [49–53]:

- Chronic valvular heart disease (CVHD)/myxomatous valve degeneration/endocardiosis
  - Mitral regurgitation (MR)
- Dilated cardiomyopathy (DCM)
- Hypertrophic cardiomyopathy (HCM)

Recall from Chapter 36, Section 36.3.3 that left-sided CHF results in cardiogenic pulmonary edema [48, 49, 54]. Affected patients experience backflow of blood into the left atrium and, ultimately, the pulmonary vasculature [47–49] Pulmonary congestion develops and is visible on thoracic radiographs [49].

Clinically, pulmonary congestion may cause one or more of the following signs [46]:

- Adventitious lung sounds, including crackles (see Chapter 37, Section 37.2)
- Dyspnea (see Chapter 36, Section 36.2)
- Tachypnea (see Chapter 36, Section 36.2)

These clinical signs help the clinician to differentiate patients with cardiogenic shock from those with hypovolemic shock [46].

38.4.2 Icteric Mucous Membranes

Icterus is the accumulation of bile pigment within tissues [23]. Although this pigment can be deposited anywhere, it is most likely to gather in one or more of the following locations in dogs and cats [4]:

- Mucous membranes
- Sclera
- Skin

Recall from Chapter 28, Section 28.2 that icterus is the result of pre-hepatic, hepatic, or post-hepatic pathways [4, 23, 55–57].

38.4.2.1 Pre-Hepatic Icterus
Review Chapter 28, Section 28.2.1 for an overview of pre-hepatic icterus. Recall that pre-hepatic icterus is due to excessive hemolysis [55, 56, 58].

In the dog and cat, the most common causes of pre-hepatic icterus include the following [19, 55–72]:

- Adverse vaccine and/or drug reactions
  - Acetaminophen (refer to Chapter 28, Section 28.2.1.1)
  - New methylene blue
- Onion toxicity (refer to Chapter 28, Section 28.2.1.2)
- Infectious disease
  - Canine babesiosis
  - Cytauxzoonosis, as caused by *Cytauxzoon felis* (refer to Chapter 6, Section 6.5.8)
  - Feline hemobartonellosis, as caused by *Mycoplasma haemofelis* (refer to Chapter 6, Section 6.4.5)
  - Feline immunodeficiency virus (FIV)
  - FeLV
- Immune-mediated hemolytic anemia (IMHA) (refer to Chapter 28, Section 28.2.1.3)
- Transfusion reactions
- Neonatal isoerythrolysis

38.4.2.2 Hepatic Icterus
Review Chapter 28, Section 28.2.2 for an overview of hepatic icterus. Recall that hepatic icterus results from liver diseases.

The most common primary liver diseases that cause icterus include the following [55–57, 64, 73, 74]:

- Portosystemic shunts
  - Congenital
  - Acquired
- Infections
  - Toxoplasmosis, as caused by *Toxoplasma gondii*
  - Feline infectious peritonitis (FIP)
- Hepatic lipidosis (refer to Chapter 28, Section 28.2.2.1)
- Hepatitis
  - Copper-associated hepatitis, an inherited defect
- Cholangiohepatitis
  - Lymphocytic
  - Suppurative or neutrophilic
  - Fluke-associated
- Hepatic abscessation
- Neoplasia
  - Lymphoma
  - Biliary cystadenoma or cystadenocarcinoma
  - Hepatocellular or biliary carcinoma

The most common secondary liver diseases that cause icterus include the following [55–57, 64, 73]:

- Drugs and toxins
  - Acetaminophen
  - Diazepam
  - Ketoconazole

- Methimazole
- Phenols
- Aflatoxins
- Sepsis
- Metastatic neoplasia

38.4.2.3 Post-Hepatic Icterus

Review Chapter 28, Section 28.2.3 for an overview of post-hepatic icterus, which most often results from obstruction of the biliary tree [56]. Such obstruction may be due to the following [56, 75]:

- Choleliths
  - Gall bladder mucocoeles
- Neoplasia
  - Biliary
  - Duodenal
  - Pancreatic
- Pancreatitis

Bloodwork and abdominal imaging studies are an essential part of diagnosing the underlying cause of icterus in these patients.

Consult an internal medicine reference for additional information.

38.4.3 Cyanotic Mucous Membranes

Hypoxemia results in cyanosis [29].

Cyanotic mucous membranes appear to be bluish-purple due to an excess of desaturated hemoglobin in circulation [29, 76].

For mucous membranes to become cyanotic, oxygen saturation has to drop to 75%, which is significant [29]. If sustained, this level is incompatible with life. Therefore, patients with cyanotic mucous membranes have extremely guarded prognoses [29]. Supplemental oxygen therapy must be instituted immediately for the patient to survive in the short term [29].

Recall from Chapter 34, Section 34.1.5 that cyanotic mucous membranes are commonly identified in patients with obstructive airway disease [16]. These patients present in acute respiratory distress [24].

Note that obstructive airway disease may be associated with upper or lower airways [24]. In addition, the following causes may result in respiratory distress and cyanosis [24]:

- Abdominal distension
  - Ascites
  - Morbid obesity/Pickwickian Syndrome (see Chapter 36, Section 36.3.1)
- Pathology of the chest wall
  - So-called "flail chest"
- Pleural space disease
  - Neoplasia (see Chapter 36, Section 36.3.8)
  - Pleural effusion (see Chapter 36, Section 36.3.6)
  - Pneumothorax (see Chapter 36, Section 36.3.7)

- Pulmonary parenchymal disease
  - Cardiogenic edema (see Chapter 36, Sections 36.3.3 and 36.3.4)
  - Neoplasia (see Chapter 36, Section 36.3.9)
  - Non-cardiogenic edema (see Chapter 36, Section 36.3.5)
  - Pneumonia
    - Bacterial
    - Fungal
    - Viral
- Pulmonary vascular pathology
  - Heartworm disease (HWD)
  - Pulmonary thromboembolism (PTE)

Note that cyanosis may not be as readily apparent in a patient that is concurrently anemic [25, 29].

Bloodwork and imaging studies are an essential part of diagnosing the underlying cause of cyanosis in these patients.

Consult an internal medicine reference for additional information.

38.4.4 Chocolate Brown Mucous Membranes

Methemoglobinemia causes mucous membranes to take on a chocolate brown appearance [29].

Methemoglobin is a type of hemoglobin. Unlike hemoglobin, in which the iron in the heme group is in the Fe^{+2} (ferrous) state, methemoglobin carries iron in the Fe^{+3} (ferric) state. The result is that methemoglobin cannot bind oxygen effectively.

A common cause of methemoglobinemia in cats is acetaminophen toxicosis [26, 27, 77–81].

Recall from Chapter 28, Section 28.2.1.1 that cats are particularly sensitive to acetaminophen because they have great difficulty breaking it down into nontoxic metabolites within the liver [82–87]. Cats are largely unsuccessful at glucuronidation, due to a deficiency in the enzyme, glucuronyl transferase [82]. As a result, the toxic metabolite, N-acetyl-para-benzoquinone imine (NAPQI) accumulates [82, 83, 87–89].

NAPQI oxidizes ferrous iron, Fe^{+2}, to ferric iron, Fe^{+3} [82]. The resultant methemoglobin is inefficient at oxygen transport [82, 83, 88]. Patients typically present in respiratory distress [82, 84, 87–89]. For reasons that have yet to be discovered, facial and paw edema are also commonly seen in cases of acetaminophen toxicosis [77, 82, 84, 87, 88].

A second cause of methemoglobinemia is onion toxicosis. Review Chapter 28, Section 28.2.1.2 for additional information.

38.4.5 Hyperemic or "Injected" Mucous Membranes Secondary to Vasodilation

"Injected" mucous membranes are red [29].

Most commonly, this red color results from vasodilation [29]. Vasodilation causes blood to pool within capillary beds. Hence, blood flow is increased locally. The site of increased blood flow is said to be hyperemic. Hyperemia differs from hemorrhage. In the former example, blood is still contained within the vasculature.

Mucous membranes may be "injected." The skin may also take on a hyperemic appearance. When this happens at the level of skin, the skin may also appear to be warmer than usual.

Vasodilation may be physiologic or pathologic.

Physiologic causes of vasodilation include exercise. When the body has increased workload on account of exercising, nutrient and oxygen delivery are in demand. These demands are met through vasodilation, which increases the blood supply to regions of need.

Pathologic causes of vasodilation include early septic shock and heatstroke [16, 29].

38.4.5.1 Septic Shock

Septic shock is the result of sepsis, a condition that is characterized by an excessive inflammatory response to bacterial, viral, fungal, or parasitic infection [21, 46, 90, 91].

Sometimes sepsis is referred to as "blood poisoning."

Sepsis is, essentially, what results when the body's immune system goes into overdrive in an attempt to clear the bloodstream of infection. Inflammation triggers a cascade of events that, if uninterrupted, may cause organ failure [90].

Early septic shock, in dogs, is characterized by peripheral vasodilation [90]. The resultant hyperemia creates "brick red" mucous membranes [90]. In addition, canine patients that present in early septic shock often have one or more of the following abnormalities on physical examination [20, 90, 92, 93]:

- Abbreviated CRT (<1 s)
- Bounding pulses
- Elevated core body temperature
- Tachycardia
- Tachypnea

These changes reflect the hyperdynamic state that is associated with early sepsis and is attributed to the release of catecholamines and cortisol, among other hormones [90, 93].

As sepsis progresses, the body's compensatory mechanisms fail. Patients become extremely hypotensive [90]. In addition, those in late-stage septic shock typically present with one or more of the following abnormalities on physical examination [90, 92]:

- Pale mucous membranes
- Prolonged CRT
- Weak-to-poor peripheral pulses

Note that cats, unlike dogs, tend to skip the hyperdynamic phase of sepsis [90, 92]. Even in the early stages of sepsis, they present with clinical signs associated with late-stage sepsis. Also, unlike septic dogs, septic cats tend to be bradycardic and hypothermic [20, 21, 90, 92].

38.4.5.2 Heatstroke

Heatstroke is the condition by which the body is unable to effectively and efficiently dissipate heat [94].

The following conditions increase the risk of heatstroke either because they prevent proper dissipation of heat or because they generate heat [94]:

- Brachycephalic airway syndrome
- Central nervous system (CNS) disease
- Fever
- Hyperthyroidism
- Laryngeal paralysis
- Obesity
- Severe muscle fasciculation
- Status epilepticus
- Tracheal collapse
- Upper airway obstruction

Review the pathophysiology of heatstroke in Chapter 36, Section 36.3.2.

Peripheral vasodilation is common in patients with heatstroke. It is an attempt by the body to release heat to the environment.

As a result of peripheral vasodilation, mucous membranes appear "flushed" in the early stages of heatstroke [95].

Recall that as heatstroke progresses, circulating blood volume is reduced because of splanchnic blood pooling [95]. This causes hypotension [95].

Peripheral vasodilation and hypotension decrease cardiac output, and tissues are inadequately perfused [95]. "Injected" mucous membranes give way to generalized pallor in the late stages of heatstroke.

38.4.6 Hyperemic or "Injected" Mucous Membranes Secondary to Carbon Monoxide and Cyanide Poisoning

In addition to vasodilation, hyperemic membranes may result from carbon monoxide and/or cyanide poisoning [29]. The former interferes with the binding of oxygen to hemoglobin, and the latter decreases cells' ability to make use of oxygen. The result is a classic "cherry red" color to the skin and mucous membranes alike [29].

38.5 Petechiae and Ecchymoses

Broken capillaries cause minor bleeding that may be visible on the skin as 1 to 2 mm red-purple dots [96]. These lesions are called petechiae [29, 96]. Large petechiae are called ecchymoses [29, 96].

In addition to being associated with the skin, both petechiae and ecchymoses are visible along the surfaces of mucous membranes (see Figures 38.9a–f).

Patients with petechiae and/or ecchymoses may have evidence of systemic bleeding elsewhere.

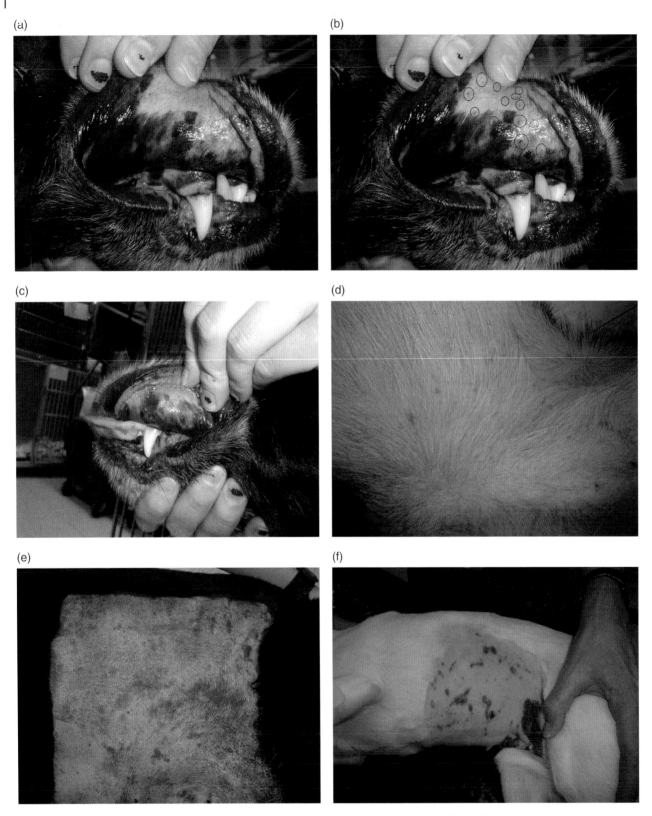

Figure 38.9 (a) Petechiae associated with the oral mucosa of a canine patient. *Source:* Courtesy of Daniel Foy, MS, DVM, DACVIM, DACVECC. (b) Same patient as in Figure 38.9a, with petechiae circled in purple. *Source:* Courtesy of Daniel Foy, MS, DVM, DACVIM, DACVECC. (c) Singular ecchymosis associated with the oral mucosa of a canine patient. *Source:* Courtesy of Daniel Foy, MS, DVM, DACVIM, DACVECC. (d) Petechiae associated with the ventrum of a canine patient. *Source:* Courtesy of Daniel Foy, MS, DVM, DACVIM, DACVECC. (e) Petechiae associated with the shaved abdomen of a canine patient. *Source:* Courtesy of Daniel Foy, MS, DVM, DACVIM, DACVECC. (f) Petechiae and ecchymoses associated with the shaved abdomen of a canine patient. *Source:* Courtesy of Daniel Foy, MS, DVM, DACVIM, DACVECC.

Hemorrhage may flow from body orifices, including the following [94]:

- The mouth, in the form of bloody sputum, hemoptysis, and hematemesis, bloody vomitus
- The nose, in the form of epistaxis
- The anus, in the form of hematochezia, blood in the stool
- The urogenital tract, in the form of hematuria, bloody urine

In addition to bleeding from orifices, hemorrhage may be housed within visible components of the body, such as the anterior chamber of the globe. Recall from Chapter 16, Section 16.1 that this clinical sign is called hyphema [96–101] (see Figure 38.10).

Hemorrhage may also be hidden internally, within the thoracic and abdominal cavities [94, 96].

Review the pathophysiology of bleeding disorders in Chapter 16, Section 16.2.2. Patients that present with petechiae and/or ecchymoses need to be screened for thrombocytopenia, hemolytic and non-hemolytic

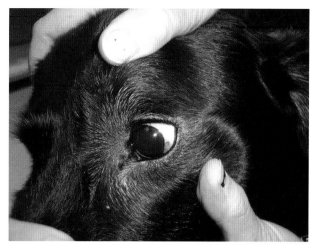

Figure 38.10 Hyphema in a canine patient. *Source:* Courtesy of Daniel Foy, MS, DVM, DACVIM, DACVECC.

anemia, and other coagulopathies, such as those caused by ingestion of anticoagulant rodenticide [96, 102–106].

References

1 Evans, H.E. and Miller, M.E. (2013). *Miller's Anatomy of the Dog*, 4e, xix, 850 p. St. Louis, Missouri: Elsevier.

2 Singh, B. and Dyce, K.M. (2018). *Dyce, Sack, and Wensing's Textbook of Veterinary Anatomy*, 5e. St. Louis, Missouri: Saunders.

3 Rozanski, E. (2017). Quiz: mucous membrane evaluation in dogs. *NAVC Clinician's Brief* (August).

4 Englar, R.E. (2017). *Performing the Small Animal Physical Examination*. Hoboken, NJ: Wiley.

5 Rudolph, L.W. (2016). Assessing patient hydration. *Veterinary Team Brief* (August): 18–22.

6 Rudloff, E. (2015). Assessment of hydration. In: *Small Animal Critical Care Medicine* (ed. D.C. Silverstein and K. Hopper), 307–310. St. Louis, MO: Elsevier.

7 Donohoe, C. (2016). Fluid therapy. In: *Small Animal Emergency and Critical Care for Veterinary Technicians* (ed. A. Battaglia and A. Steele), 61–77. St. Louis, MO: Elsevier.

8 Boag, A. and Hughes, D. (2007). Fluid therapy. In: *BSAVA Manual of Canine and Feline Emergency and Critical Care* (ed. L.G. King and A. Boag), 30–45. Gloucester, UK: BSAVA.

9 Cave, C. (2011). High dependency nursing. In: *The Complete Textbook of Veterinary Nursing* (ed. V. Aspinall), 421–438. St. Louis, MO: Elsevier.

10 Davis, H., Jensen, T., Johnson, A. et al. (2013). 2013 AAHA/AAFP fluid therapy guidelines for dogs and cats. *J. Am. Anim. Hosp. Assoc.* 49 (3): 149–159.

11 Nowers, T. (2015). Top 5 clinical differences between cats and dogs. *Veterinary Team Brief* (September): 20–21.

12 Patel, A. and Forsythe, P.J. (2008). *Saunders Solutions in Veterinary practice: Small Animal Dermatology*, 1e. China: Saunders, Ltd.

13 Little, S. (2012). *The Cat: Clinical Medicine and Management*, 1e. St. Louis, Missouri: Saunders Elsevier.

14 Hnilica, K. and Patterson, A.P. (2017). *Small Animal Dermatology: A Color Atlas and Therapeutic Guide*. St. Louis, Missouri: Elsevier, Inc.

15 Friberg, C. (2006). Feline facial dermatoses. *Vet. Clin. North Am. Small Anim. Pract.* 36 (1): 115–140, vi–vii.

16 Mandese, W.W. and Estrada, A.H. (2017). The basic cardiology examination. *NAVC Clinician's Brief* (May): 91–97.

17 Harvey, J.W. (2010). What type of anemia? *NAVC Clinician's Brief* (April): 34–38.

18 Caruso, K.J. (2003). The evidence at hand. *NAVC Clinician's Brief* (May): 9–10.

19 Cohn LA. (2012). What you should know about… Cytauxzoonosis. DVM 360 [Internet]. http://veterinarymedicine.dvm360.com/what-you-should-know-about-cytauxzoonosis.

20 Brady, C.A., Otto, C.M., Van Winkle, T.J., and King, L.G. (2000). Severe sepsis in cats: 29 cases (1986–1998). *J. Am. Vet. Med. Assoc.* 217 (4): 531–535.

21 Klainbart, S., Agi, L., Bdolah-Abram, T. et al. (2017). Clinical, laboratory, and hemostatic findings in cats

with naturally occurring sepsis. *J. Am. Vet. Med. Assoc.* 251 (9): 1025–1034.

22 Pachtinger, G.E. (2016). Distributive shock. *NAVC Clinician's Brief* (October).

23 Schaer, M. (2008). Icterus. *NAVC Clinician's Brief* (September): 8.

24 Leach, S. and Fine, D. (2011). Acute respiratory distress: the blue patient. *NAVC Clinician's Brief* (February): 69–74.

25 King, L.G. and Clarke, D. (2010). Emergency care of the patient with acute respiratory distress. *Vet. Focus.* 20 (2): 36–43.

26 Ilkiw, J.E. and Ratcliffe, R.C. (1987). Paracetamol toxicity in a cat. *Aust. Vet. J.* 64 (8): 245–247.

27 St. Omer, V.V. and Mcknight, E.D. (1980). Acetylcysteine for treatment of acetaminophen toxicosis in the cat. *J. Am. Vet. Med. Assoc.* 176 (9): 911–913.

28 Stewart, J.E., Haslam, A.K., and Puig, J. (2016). Pathology in practice. *J. Am. Vet. Med. Assoc.* 248 (9): 1009–1011.

29 Campbell VL. (2011). Critical care triage. DVM 360 [Internet]. http://veterinarycalendar.dvm360.com/critical-care-triage-proceedings.

30 Pachtinger, G.E. (2014). Hypovolemic shock. *NAVC Clinician's Brief* (October): 13–16.

31 Tasker S, editor. (2006). The differential diagnosis of feline anemia. World Congress: WSAVA/FECAVA/CSAVA.

32 Cohn, L.A. (2005). Severe anemia in a cat. *NAVC Clinician's Brief* (August): 37–38.

33 Java, M. and MacDonald, B. (2016). Cardiopulmonary resuscitation. *NAVC Clinician's Brief* (November).

34 MacIntire, D.K. and Tefend, M. (2004). Constant-rate infusions: practical use. *NAVC Clinician's Brief* (April): 25–28.

35 Plumb, D.C. (2011). *Plumb's Veterinary Drug Handbook*, 7e, 1187 p. Ames, Iowa: PharmaVet.

36 Reuss-Lamky, H. (2015). Hypothermia overview. *NAVC Clinician's Brief* (November): 12–16.

37 Levi, R., Rubin, L.E., and Gross, S.S. (1991). Histamine in cardiovascular function and dysfuction: recent developments. In: *Histamine and Histamine Antagonists* (ed. B. Uvnas), 347–382. Berlin: Springer.

38 Jin, H., Koyama, T., Hatanaka, Y. et al. (2006). Histamine-induced vasodilation and vasoconstriction in the mesenteric resistance artery of the rat. *Eur. J. Pharmacol.* 529 (1–3): 136–144.

39 Duffy, T. (ed.) (2007). *Thermoregulation of the Perioperative Patient.* Chicago, IL: Proc ACVS.

40 Rozanski, E. and Rondeau, M. (2002). Choosing fluids in traumatic hypovolemic shock: the role of crystalloids, colloids, and hypertonic saline. *J. Am. Anim. Hosp. Assoc.* 38 (6): 499–501.

41 Hopper, K., Silverstein, D., and Bateman, S. (2012). Shock syndromes. In: *Fluid Therapy in Small Animal Practice* (ed. S.P. DiBartola), 557–583. St. Louis, MO: Elsevier Saunders.

42 de Laforcade, A.M. (2009). Shock. In: *Small Animal Critical Care* (ed. D.C. Silverstein), 41–45. St. Louis, MO: Elsevier Saunders.

43 Boag, A.K. and Hughes, D. (2005). Assessment and treatment of perfusion abnormalities in the emergency patient. *Vet. Clin. North Am. Small Anim. Pract.* 35 (2): 319–342.

44 Chan, D.L. (2008). Colloids: current recommendations. *Vet. Clin. North Am. Small Anim. Pract.* 38 (3): 587–593, xi.

45 Choi, P.T., Yip, G., Quinonez, L.G., and Cook, D.J. (1999). Crystalloids vs. colloids in fluid resuscitation: a systematic review. *Crit. Care Med.* 27 (1): 200–210.

46 Pachtinger GE. (2013). The Many Types of Shock. NAVC Clinician's Brief [Internet]. https://www.cliniciansbrief.com/article/many-types-shock.

47 Reece, W.O., Erickson, H.H., Goff, J.P., and Uemura, E.E. (2015). *Dukes' Physiology of Domestic Animals*, 13e, xii, 748 p. Ames, Iowa, USA: Wiley Blackwell.

48 Estrada, A. (2014). Heart disease: diagnosis & treatment. *NAVC Clinician's Brief* (March): 91–95.

49 Rozanski E. (2009). Pulmonary edema. DVM 360 [Internet]. http://veterinarycalendar.dvm360.com/print/328751?page=full.

50 Atkins, A. (2011). Finding a consensus on canine CVHD. *NAVC Clinician's Brief* (July): 53–57.

51 Hogan, D.F. (2004). Congestive heart failure in the dog. *NAVC Clinician's Brief* (September): 16–19.

52 Saunders AB, Gordon SG. (2015). 6 Practical tips from cardiologists: heart failure in dogs. Today's Veterinary Practice [Internet]. (July/August). http://todaysveterinarypractice.navc.com/wp-content/uploads/2016/06/T1507F02.pdf.

53 Boswood, A. (2010). Chronic valvular disease in the dog. *NAVC Clinician's Brief* (December): 17–21.

54 Spier A. (2007). Congestive heart failure: approaches to care. NAVC Clinician's Brief [Internet]. https://www.cliniciansbrief.com/article/congestive-heart-failure-approaches-care.

55 Wray, J. (2017). *Canine Internal Medicine: What's Your Diagnosis?* Hoboken, NJ: Wiley.

56 Schaer M. The icteric dog and cat. http://www.delawarevalleyacademyvm.org/pdfs/may10/Icteric.pdf.

57 Lappin, M. (2001). *Feline Internal Medicine Secrets.* Philadelphia: Hanley & Belfus, Inc.

58 Schaer, M. (2010). Immune-mediated hemolytic anemia. *NAVC Clinician's Brief* (March): 78.

59 Caruso, K. (2004). Feline erythroparasites. *NAVC Clinician's Brief* (June): 36–38.

60 Fry, J.K. and Burney, D.P. (2012). Feline cytauxzoonosis. *NAVC Clinician's Brief* (July): 85 89.

61 Haber, M. (2005). Icterus & pancytopenia in a cat. *NAVC Clinician's Brief* (July): 21–23.

62 Bowles M. (2017). Identifying and treating 3 tick-borne diseases in dogs. DVM 360 [Internet]. http://veterinarymedicine.dvm360.com/identifying-and-treating-3-tick-borne-diseases-dogs.

63 Colleran E. (2017). Tick-borne disease in cats: two to watch for. DVM 360 [Internet]. http://veterinarynews.dvm360.com/tick-borne-disease-cats-two-watch.

64 Gordon J. (2011). Clinical approach to icterus in the cat (Proceedings). DVM 360 [Internet]. http://veterinarycalendar.dvm360.com/clinical-approach-icterus-cat-proceedings.

65 Meier, H.T. and Moore, L.E. (2000). Feline cytauxzoonosis: a case report and literature review. *J. Am. Anim. Hosp. Assoc.* 36 (6): 493–496.

66 Meinkoth, J.H. and Kocan, A.A. (2005). Feline cytauxzoonosis. *Vet. Clin. North Am. Small Anim. Pract.* 35 (1): 89–101, vi.

67 Holman, P.J. and Snowden, K.F. (2009). Canine hepatozoonosis and babesiosis, and feline cytauxzoonosis. *Vet. Clin. North Am. Small Anim. Pract.* 39 (6): 1035 1053, v.

68 Sherrill, M.K. and Cohn, L.A. (2015). Cytauxzoonosis: diagnosis and treatment of an emerging disease. *J. Feline Med. Surg.* 17 (11): 940–948.

69 Wang, J.L., Li, T.T., Liu, G.H. et al. (2017). Two tales of Cytauxzoon felis infections in domestic cats. *Clin. Microbiol. Rev.* 30 (4): 861–885.

70 Shaw N, Harrell K. (2008). IMHA. Diagnosing and treating a complex disease. DVM 360 [Internet]. http://veterinarymedicine.dvm360.com/imha-diagnosing-and-treating-complex-disease.

71 Day, M.J. (2012). Canine immune-mediated hemolytic anemia. *NAVC Clinician's Brief* (October): 53–57.

72 Archer, T. and Mackin, A. (2013). Diagnosis of immune-mediated hemolytic anemia. *Today's Veterinary Practice* (July/August): 32–36.

73 Norsworthy GD. (2011). The icteric cat: a case study. DVM 360 [Internet]. http://veterinarycalendar.dvm360.com/icteric-cat-case-study-proceedings.

74 Webb, C. (2013). Liver conditions in dogs. *NAVC Clinician's Brief* (May): 85–87.

75 eClin path2013. Cholestasis. Cornell University College of Veterinary Medicine [Internet]. http://www.eclinpath.com/chemistry/liver/cholestasis.

76 Tilley, L.P. and Smith, F.W.K. (2004). *The 5-Minute Veterinary Consult: Canine and Feline*, 3e. Baltimore, MD: Lippincott Williams & Wilkins.

77 Meadows, I. and Gwaltney-Brant, S. (2006). The 10 most common toxicoses in dogs. *Vet. Med.* 101 (3): 142–148.

78 Allen, A.L. (2003). The diagnosis of acetaminophen toxicosis in a cat. *Can. Vet. J.* 44 (6): 509–510.

79 Finco, D.C., Duncan, J.R., Schall, W.D., and Prasse, K.W. (1975). Acetaminophen toxicosis in the cat. *J. Am. Vet. Med. Assoc.* 166 (5): 469–472.

80 Nash, S.L., Savides, M.C., Oehme, F.W., and Johnson, D.E. (1984). The effect of acetaminophen on methemoglobin and blood glutathione parameters in the cat. *Toxicology* 31 (3–4): 329–334.

81 Savides, M.C., Oehme, F.W., Nash, S.L., and Leipold, H.W. (1984). The toxicity and biotransformation of single doses of acetaminophen in dogs and cats. *Toxicol. Appl. Pharmacol.* 74 (1): 26–34.

82 Allen, A.L. (2003). The diagnosis of acetaminophen toxicosis in a cat. *Can. Vet. J.* 44 (6): 509–510.

83 Sellon, R.K. (2001). Acetaminophen. In: *Small Animal Toxicology* (ed. M.E. Peterson and P.A. Talcott), 388–395. Toronto: WB Saunders.

84 Aronson, L.R. (1996). Acetaminophen toxicosis in 17 cats. *J. Vet. Emerg. Crit. Care* 6: 65–69.

85 Jones, R.D., Baynes, R.E., and Nimitz, C.T. (1992). Nonsteroidal anti-inflammatory drug toxicosis in dogs and cats: 240 cases (1989-1990). *J. Am. Vet. Med. Assoc.* 201 (3): 475 477.

86 Court, M.H. (2001). Acetaminophen UDP-glucuronosyltransferase in ferrets: species and gender differences, and sequence analysis of ferret UGT1A6. *J. Vet. Pharmacol. Ther.* 24 (6): 415–422.

87 Steenbergen, V. (2003). Acetaminophen and cats – a dangerous combination. *Vet. Tech.* 24 (1): 43–45.

88 Richardson, J.A. (2000). Management of acetaminophen and ibuprofen toxicoses in dogs and cats. *J. Vet. Emerg. Crit. Care* 10: 285–291.

89 Rumbeiha, W.K., Lin, Y.S., and Oehme, F.W. (1995). Comparison of N-acetylcysteine and methylene blue, alone or in combination, for treatment of acetaminophen toxicosis in cats. *Am. J. Vet. Res.* 56 (11): 1529–1533.

90 Pachtinger, G.E. (2015). Septic shock. *NAVC Clinician's Brief* (March): 13–16.

91 Purvis, D. and Kirby, R. (1994). Systemic inflammatory response syndrome: septic shock. *Vet. Clin. North Am. Small Anim. Pract.* 24 (6): 1225–1247.

92 Boller, E.M. and Otto, C.M. (2009). Sepsis and septic shock. In: *Small Animal Critical Care Medicine* (ed. D. Silverstein and K. Hopper), 454–459. Philadelphia: WB Saunders.

93 Bone, R.C., Balk, R.A., and Cerra, F.B. (1992). American College of Chest Physicians/Society of Critical Care Medicine Consensus Conference: definitions for sepsis and organ failure and guidelines for the use of innovative therapies in sepsis. *Crit. Care Med.* 20 (6): 864–874.

94 Powell, L.L. (2008). Canine heatstroke. *NAVC Clinician's Brief* (August): 13–16.

95 Stanley SM. (1980). A study of heat stroke and heat exhaustion in the dog. Iowa State University Digital Repository [Internet]. 42(1). https://lib.dr.iastate.edu/cgi/viewcontent.cgi?article=2978&context=iowastate_veterinarian.

96 Telle, M.R. and Betbeze, C. (2015). Hyphema: considerations in the small animal patient. *Top. Companion Anim. Med.* 30 (3): 97–106.

97 Jinks, M.R., Olea-Popelka, F., and Freeman, K.S. (2017). Causes and outcomes of dogs presenting with hyphema to a referral hospital in Colorado: a retrospective analysis of 99 cases. *Vet. Ophthalmol.* 21 (2): 160–166.

98 Hendrix, D.V.H. (2013). Diseases and surgery of the canine anterior uvea. In: *Veterinary Ophthalmology* (ed. K.N. Gelatt, B.C. Gilger and T.J. Kern), 1146–1198. Oxford: Wiley-Blackwell.

99 Komaromy, A.M., Ramsey, D.T., Brooks, D.E. et al. (1999). Hyphema. Part I. Pathophysiologic considerations. *Compend. Contin. Educ. Pract.* 21 (11): 1064–1069.

100 Nelms, S.R., Nasisse, M.P., Davidson, M.G., and Kirschner, S.E. (1993). Hyphema associated with retinal disease in dogs: 17 cases (1986–1991). *J. Am. Vet. Med. Assoc.* 202 (8): 1289–1292.

101 Nelson, R.W. and Couto, C.G. (2009). Disorders of hemostasis. In: *Small Animal Internal Medicine* (ed. R.W. Nelson and C.G. Couto), 1242–1259. Missouri: Mosby Elsevier.

102 Boudreaux, M.K. (1996). Platelets and coagulation – An update. *Vet. Clin. North Am. Small* 26 (5): 1065–1087.

103 Peterson, J.L., Couto, C.G., and Wellman, M.L. (1995). Hemostatic disorders in cats – a retrospective study and review of the literature. *J. Vet. Intern. Med.* 9 (5): 298–303.

104 Fogh, J.M. and Fogh, I.T. (1988). Inherited coagulation disorders. *Vet. Clin. North Am. Small Anim. Pract.* 18 (1): 231–243.

105 Hart, S.W. and Nolte, I. (1994). Hemostatic disorders in feline immunodeficiency virus-seropositive cats. *J. Vet. Intern. Med.* 8 (5): 355–362.

106 Lisciandro, S.C., Hohenhaus, A., and Brooks, M. (1998). Coagulation abnormalities in 22 cats with naturally occurring liver disease. *J. Vet. Intern. Med.* 12 (2): 71–75.

39

Palpably Cool or Cyanotic Extremities

39.1 Introduction to Thermoregulation

Survival depends upon the body's ability to maintain homeostasis, that is, a stable internal state in which certain variables are maintained within an optimal range in spite of external conditions [1].

Core body temperature is one factor that is tightly regulated, centrally, by the hypothalamus [2–4]. The hypothalamus acts like a thermostat [4]. When the core body temperature exceeds its optimal range, cooling mechanisms are turned on [4]. When the core body temperature drops beyond the safe zone, measures are taken to heat the body [4].

Cooling and heating mechanisms represent coordinated efforts between the brain, spinal cord, thorax, abdomen, skin, subcutaneous fat, and fur coat to effect physiologic and behavioral changes that restore the body's thermal set point [4–8].

In health, communication between body parts is effective in maintaining the core body temperature to within 0.2 °C of the optional range [4, 6]. This process is called thermoregulation [2–4]. Thermoregulation requires afferent thermal sensing by cells in most tissues within the body [4].

39.2 Measuring Body Temperature: Core versus Peripheral

Body temperature is measured via the thermometer, which can be placed in a number of body orifices to capture a numerical reading. Although axillary and tympanic routes are possible in companion animal patients, rectal temperature is more commonly measured [3, 4].

In dogs, normal rectal temperature fluctuates between 100.9 and 102.7 °F [4, 9–11]. Feline rectal temperature falls within a similar range [10].

However, rectal temperature provides a peripheral measurement, as opposed to reporting core body temperature [4].

Core body temperature, in the dog, is typically 0.72–2.0 °F greater than rectal temperature [4, 12]. Core body temperature is also more tightly regulated than the temperature at the periphery [4].

39.3 Introduction to Hypothermia

Detection of cold over heat appears to be prioritized by the mammalian body [4, 13]. The skin has 10 times more cold-sensing than heat-sensing receptors [4, 13]. Cold-sensing cells also use myelinated fibers to transmit messages to the spinal cord, whereas heat-sensing cells do not [4, 14]. Because myelin increases the velocity of information transfer, the hypothalamus recognizes peripheral detection of cold long before peripheral detection of heat [4, 14].

When the body temperature drops below the expected range, the patient is said to be hypothermic [2].

As the peripheral temperature drops below the optimal range, cold-sensing receptors fire with increasing frequency [4]. These signals trigger efferent responses that raise the temperature to within normal limits [4].

One response to hypothermia is peripheral vasoconstriction to conserve body heat [3]. This may result in palpably cool limbs.

A secondary response to hypothermia is shivering [3, 15]. Shivering is energetically expensive to maintain [3].

In addition to vasoconstriction and shivering, the hypothermic patient is likely to initiate piloerection [2]. Piloerection effectively traps air against the skin, provided that the fur coat is dry [2, 13]. Dry fur acts as an insulator to hold in the heat [2, 13].

Patients that are at greater risk of developing hypothermia include dogs and cats that are [2, 3, 16–23]

- Anesthetized
- Geriatric
- Ill
- Immobile
- Immune-compromised
- Neonates
- Small in stature and body weight.

Common Clinical Presentations in Dogs and Cats, First Edition. Ryane E. Englar.
© 2019 John Wiley & Sons, Inc. Published 2019 by John Wiley & Sons, Inc.

Neonates are, in fact, hypothermic, as compared to adult dogs and cats, until four to seven weeks of life [3, 23]. This is in large part due to their high surface area-to-mass ratio [2, 3]. They are also relatively inefficient producers of heat [2, 19–21].

Hypothermia is also a common complication of anesthesia [2, 4, 21]. Most anesthetic and analgesic agents dull the ability of the hypothalamus to be a functional hemostat [4, 24–26]. General anesthesia eliminates the patient's ability to generate heat through shivering [4]. Both epidural and spinal anesthesia block signals from cold-sensing receptors [4]. The hypothalamus does not receive the message that the core body temperature has dropped below the normal reference range [4]. Therefore, the hypothalamus does not initiate vasoconstriction [4].

Inhalant agents also contribute to heat loss through vasodilation [4]. In addition, inhalants bypass the nasal passageways [3]. Inhalants therefore reach the lower airways without having been warmed first [3].

In addition, air temperature and the temperature of surrounding objects affect patient heat loss [3, 4, 27–30]. Surgical theaters tend to operate at appreciably cooler ambient temperatures, and stainless steel induction and surgical tables are routinely non-insulated [3, 4, 27–30].

The insulating layer of fur is also eliminated altogether, through clipping, and the skin is made wet with surgical prep solutions [3, 4, 27–30].

39.4 Local Hypothermia

Hypothermia can be generalized or local [3]. Local hypothermia is colloquially referred to as frostbite.

Frostbite seems likely to occur in dogs and cats because their paws lack insulation [3, 31]. Distal limbs are also more likely to lose heat because, like neonates, they, too, have a high surface area-to-volume ratio [31].

Yet frostbite is relatively uncommon in companion animal practice. Why this is the case has only recently been explored. However, the veterinary literature is rich with reports that document how other species make use of counter-current heat exchange to maintain temperatures at one or more extremities, including the following [31–40]:

- Ears of rabbits
- Fins, flukes, and tongues of dolphins, manatees, and whales
- Flippers of penguins
- Ophthalmic retes of birds, ocean fish, and sharks

Dogs are also adaptable [31]. Their footpad vasculature is arranged in vein–artery–vein triads, with anastomoses between arteries and veins, arterioles and venules [31]. This counter-current heat exchange conserves body heat by recirculating it back to the body's core when the patient is challenged with a cold environment [31]. Warm arterial blood that is flowing to the distal limb transfers heat to the cool venous blood that is returning to the heart [31]. This allows the patient's core to remain at its optimal set point despite the patient's paws being cold to the touch [31].

This same mechanism is suspected in cats; however, to the author's knowledge, this has not been proven.

Cold footpads are palpable in dogs and are therefore evident on physical examination. It is important to note that cold footpads, in this circumstance, represent a normal physiologic response to the external environment. A patient that lives outdoors, but comes inside for a veterinary visit, is likely to have cold feet.

39.5 Abnormal Causes of Palpably Cool or Cyanotic Extremities

Despite the fact that dogs have footpad vasculature that preserves the core body temperature at the expense of the peripheral body temperature, there are conditions in which palpably cool extremities are abnormal. These include

- Arterial or aortic thromboembolism (ATE)
- Reverse patent ductus arteriosus (PDA)
- Shock.

39.5.1 Arterial Thromboembolism

A thrombus is a blood clot that forms within the vascular system, as opposed to outside of the vasculature, at the site of a wound [41].

Three factors are thought to contribute to thrombosis [42]. They are collectively referred to as Virchow's triad and include the following [41–50]:

- Changes in hemodynamics
  - Blood stasis
  - Turbulent blood flow
- Hypercoagulability
- Vessel or tissue injury

Cardiomyopathy, in and of itself, has the potential to promote thrombosis [42, 51, 52].

Consider, for example, enlargement of the left atria. The stretching of this chamber exposes endocardial collagen, which may incite platelet aggregation [41, 42, 44, 46, 48, 49].

When platelets aggregate, they activate the coagulation cascade [41, 42, 44, 46, 48, 49]. The resultant fibrin combines with platelet clumps to form an intracardiac thrombus [42].

The thrombus can break off from its site of origin, within the heart, and enter the aorta, where at some point it will occlude the arterial vasculature [41, 42].

The distal aortic trifurcation is the most common site of obstruction in cats in that more than 90% of emboli lodge here [42]. When they do, affected patients are said to have a "saddle thrombus" [41, 42].

Note that thrombi may also form within the left ventricle or the right side of the heart, although the left atrium is most typical [41, 42, 44–46, 48, 49, 53].

Cats with primary cardiomyopathy are at increased risk for ATE [42, 51, 53, 54]. Unfortunately, many cats that present with ATE have hidden cardiomyopathy, meaning that it has not yet been diagnosed [42, 53, 55, 56].

Of all feline cardiomyopathies, hypertrophic cardiomyopathy (HCM) is most often associated with ATE [51]. Because males are more likely to develop HCM, male cats appear to be at greater risk for development of ATE [51, 57].

Certain breeds are predisposed to HCM, including, but not limited to Maine Coons, Persians, Burmese, Siamese, American Shorthairs, Ragdolls, and Norwegian Forest cats [58].

Cats with cardiomyopathy that is secondary to hyperthyroidism are also at risk, even if the endocrinopathy itself is well managed [41, 51, 54, 58].

Non-cardiac causes of ATE are possible [51]. The most common among these is pulmonary neoplasia [51, 54]. However, in this case, a piece of the tumor rather than a true thrombus causes the vascular obstruction [51, 54].

Patients with a "saddle thrombus" present acutely with pelvic limb paresis or paralysis that involves one or both legs [41, 51, 58]. Bilateral involvement is most common [41]. In these cases, one limb may appear to be clinically worse than the other [41, 51].

Patients with embolization of the brachial artery present acutely with forelimb paresis or paralysis [41, 51].

Other sites are possible for ATE; however, these cases are infrequent and present with much less classic signs [41, 51].

The cat with "saddle thrombus" is in acute pain and often vocal [41, 51, 58]. It may appear overstimulated or frenzied [41]. It may present to the clinic in a full-blown state of open-mouth breathing [41].

The client may come home to find the cat dragging one or both limbs [51]. The affected limb(s) often lack(s) a femoral pulse [51]. The absence of this pulse is indicative of a vascular occlusion. Alternatively, the pulse may be weak and thready [41].

Without blood flow, the affected limb(s) become(s) cold [51]. The distal limb is colder than the proximal [51]. A cold paw is palpable on physical examination [51]. The patient is thus said to exhibit poikilothermy, meaning that its internal temperature varies depending upon the location where it is measured. This is pathological.

Many cats with ATE also exhibit rectal hypothermia [41, 54, 57, 59]. This is the direct result of ATE. However, it may be compounded by shock [41].

Because the affected limb's blood supply has been reduced, if not terminated, tissues experience varying degrees of hypoxemia [51]. Over time, paw pads and nail beds become cyanotic [41, 51].

Patients may or may not present in a state of congestive heart failure (CHF) [51]. Thoracic auscultation of these patients may reveal the following [41, 54]:

- Adventitious lung sounds
  - Crackles
- Arrhythmia
  - Tachycardia
- Gallop rhythm
- Heart murmur

Note that ATE is not ruled out by the absence of abnormal findings on thoracic auscultation [41, 54]. Evidence of CHF is present on radiographs and/or necropsy of 40–66% of cats with ATE, including those without abnormal findings on auscultation [41, 51, 53–55, 57].

A serum chemistry profile of affected patients is likely to demonstrate the following [41, 51]:

- Azotemia, secondary to poor systemic perfusion
- Elevation of creatine kinase (CK) due to muscle ischemia
- Stress hyperglycemia

Hyperkalemia may develop if and when perfusion is restored [51].

Echocardiography of affected patients is not necessary to make the diagnosis. However, after the patient is stabilized, echocardiography is a valuable tool to evaluate the severity of underlying cardiomyopathy [41, 51, 54]. The presence of so-called "smoke," that is, spontaneous echo contrast, is common [51, 59]. Some clinicians believe that "smoke" confers increased risk to the patient [51, 59]. The patient with "smoke" may be more likely to succumb to additional episodes of ATE [51, 59].

Historically, the majority of cats with ATE were euthanized on initial presentation [51]. However, although the average patient's prognosis is guarded, some patients do better than others [51]. Survival is most likely among those with unilateral involvement: as many as 70–80% survive to discharge [51, 53, 57, 59].

Refer to an internal medicine and/or emergency textbook for additional guidelines on how to develop a patient-specific therapeutic plan.

39.5.2 Congenital Heart Disease

Congenital heart disease is relatively uncommon in companion animal patients. When it occurs in the dog, the diagnosis is usually one of three types [60–64]:

- Aortic stenosis
- PDA
- Pulmonic stenosis

Less common canine congenital heart defects include the following [60–62]:

- Atrial septal defect (ASD)
- Persistent right aortic arch
- Tetralogy of Fallot
- Ventricular septal defect (VSD)

Congenital heart defects are even less common in cats [60–62].

A PDA is a specific type of abnormality in which a fetal structure persists in the patient after birth [60–62, 65, 66].

In the fetus, the ductus arteriosus connects the descending aorta to the pulmonary artery. This allows fetal blood to bypass the lungs [60–62, 65]. There is no need for the fetus to pump blood through the pulmonary tree because oxygen is delivered to the fetus through the placenta. This allows the lungs sufficient opportunity to develop.

Upon birth, the patient takes its first breath [67]. This requires its lungs to work for the very first time. At that point, the lungs take over the role of oxygenation. In response to this, the ductus arteriosus will close [67]. This closure takes place shortly after birth, typically within two to three days [61, 65, 68, 69].

Within a month of life, all that remains of the ductus arteriosus is a collection of elastic fibers, the ligamentum arteriosum [10, 63, 70].

The ductus arteriosus is said to be patent when closure of this structure does not occur [10]. The resultant defect is called a PDA. There are two forms of PDAs [10, 60–62]:

- Left-to-right
- Right-to-left

39.5.2.1 Left-to-Right PDA

The most common form of PDA is left-to-right [10, 60–62, 65]. In patients with this defect, the pressurized aorta shunts blood inappropriately into the pulmonary circulation. This blood constitutes an additional volume that the pulmonary vasculature was not expecting: in health, the pulmonary vasculature only receives blood from the pulmonary artery [10, 60–62].

The pulmonary circulation is now overwhelmed [10, 60–62]. In turn, it overwhelms the left atrium by pushing forward the additional blood volume.

Over time, volume overload of the left atrium into the left ventricle causes both chambers of the heart to dilate and hypertrophy [10, 60–62].

Patients present with continuous murmurs that have been described as sounding like washing machines [10, 60–62]. Femoral pulses are hyperkinetic [61]. In other words, they are bounding, like jackhammers [61].

Without surgical correction for the left-to-right PDA, the patient succumbs to left-sided CHF with pulmonary congestion [10, 60–63, 70].

Breeds at increased risk of PDAs include the following [10, 63, 67, 70–73]:

- Bichon Frise
- Chihuahua
- Cocker Spaniel
- Collie
- English Springer Spaniel
- Keeshond
- Maltese
- Miniature Poodle
- Pomeranian
- Shetland Sheepdog
- Shih Tzu
- Toy Poodle
- Yorkshire Terrier
- Welsh Corgi

39.5.2.2 Right-to-Left PDA

A right-to-left PDA, otherwise known as a reversed PDA, occurs much less frequently [61, 65, 74–76]. It results from a large-diameter PDA [61, 75]. This causes pulmonary vascular injury that leads to increased pulmonary vascular resistance [10, 60, 61, 63, 70].

When pulmonary vascular resistance, in the face of pulmonary hypertension, exceeds systemic vascular resistance, oxygen-poor blood follows the same pathway as in the fetus. That is, oxygen-poor blood is inappropriately shunted from the pulmonary artery to the aorta, distal to the brachiocephalic and left subclavian arteries [10, 60, 61, 63, 65, 70].

Cranial to these arteries, aortic blood is oxygen rich and delivers its typical supply to the head and forelimbs [65]. These structures therefore receive the same quality of arterial blood that they would have, had the patient not been affected by a reversed PDA.

Distal to the brachiocephalic and left subclavian arteries, arterial blood is diluted in terms of oxygen content because oxygen-poor blood has been shunted into systemic circulation [10, 60, 61, 63, 65, 70]. The arterial blood that reaches the caudal half of the patient is therefore compromised in terms of oxygen content [65]. Thus, caudal tissues experience significant hypoxemia [10, 60, 61, 63, 70].

On presentation, the patient demonstrates caudal cyanosis or so-called differential cyanosis [10, 60, 61, 63, 70, 75].

The cranial half of the body has pink mucous membranes because they are adequately perfused [10, 60, 61, 63, 70, 75]. The caudal half of the body becomes cyanotic [10, 60, 61, 63, 70, 75].

The body attempts to compensate through polycythemia [61, 65, 66]. However, this can only increase perfusion to tissues so much [63, 70]. As reversed PDAs progress, oral mucous membranes may become equally dark and congested [65].

Dogs and cats are typically clinical for reversed PDA as pediatric patients [61]. Onset is frequently sudden in the former species, as compared to more gradual in the latter [61]. It is not uncommon for dogs to present for reversed PDA within the first four months of life [61].

Patients with reversed PDA also present with continuous murmurs and hyperkinetic femoral pulses [10, 60–62]. In addition, during history taking, clients often report the following changes [65, 66, 76–81]:

- Ataxia of the pelvic limbs
- Exercise intolerance
- Collapse, or syncope
- Fainting episodes
- Hind end incoordination
- Hind end weakness
- Hind limb "lameness"
- Seizures

When they occur, seizures are secondary to increased viscosity of blood that is attributed to polycythemia [65, 78].

Unlike those with PDAs, patients with reversed PDAs are not surgical candidates [65]. Ligation of a reversed PDA would result in life-threatening pulmonary hypertension [65]. In order for the heart to continue to pump blood, its right side would need to raise its pressure significantly to exceed that of the pulmonary vasculature. This is not sustainable. Without means to alleviate the building pressures within the right side of the heart, the patient will succumb to right-sided heart failure [65].

Patients with reversed PDAs can only be managed medically, by means of prophylactic phlebotomy to thin the blood to decrease neurological clinical signs [65, 74–76, 78, 79, 81–85].

In addition, exercise, excitement, and stress must be reduced [65, 75].

Ultimately, patients succumb to hypoxemia, fatal cardiac arrhythmias, or thrombus formation [65, 74].

It is unlikely that a patient with reversed PDA will live beyond middle age [65, 68, 74, 80].

39.5.3 Shock

Shock is a medical condition in which body tissues do not receive the blood flow, oxygen, and/or nutrients that they need to sustain life. Recall from Chapter 38 that there are many different types of shock. Refer to Chapter 38 to review the pathophysiology of hypovolemic, cardiogenic, and septic shock.

39.5.3.1 Hypovolemic Shock
Recall from Chapter 38, Section 38.4.1.3 that hypovolemic shock results from a significant loss of circulating blood volume, as from hemorrhage, dehydration, or third space disease [86–88].

Dogs typically respond to hypovolemic shock with tachycardia and cats, with bradycardia [86, 89, 90].

Both species may also present with [86, 90]

- Prolonged capillary refill time (CRT)
- Weak femoral pulses
- Abnormal mentation
- Cold extremities or generalized hypothermia.

Cold extremities result from compensatory vasoconstriction [86, 89, 91].

39.5.3.2 Cardiogenic Shock
Recall from Chapter 38, Section 38.4.1.4 that cardiogenic shock presents similarly. As cardiac function fails, cardiac output drops [92]. The heart may try to compensate for reduced cardiac output by increasing the following:

- Cardiac contractility
- Heart rate
- Stroke volume
- Systemic vascular resistance

Vasoconstriction is a means by which the body raises systemic vascular resistance. This is the body's attempt to maintain normal blood pressure in the face of reduced cardiac output.

Vasoconstriction is likely to result in cool extremities, particularly as cardiomyopathy progresses and cardiac function declines.

39.5.3.3 Septic Shock
Recall from Chapter 38, Section 38.4.5.1 that late-stage septic shock is characterized by the following [93, 94]:

- Hypotension
- Pale mucous membranes
- Prolonged CRT
- Weak-to-poor peripheral pulses

Septic cats are also likely to be hypothermic [93–96]. Patients attempt to maintain core body temperature at all costs, even at the expense of the periphery. Therefore, septic cats tend to have poor peripheral perfusion, as evidenced by low rectal temperatures and palpably cool distal extremities.

References

1 Currie, W.B. (1988). *Structure and Function of Domestic Animals*, xiii, 443 p. Boston: Butterworths.

2 Brodeur, A., Wright, A., and Cortes, Y. (2017). Hypothermia and targeted temperature management in cats and dogs. *J. Vet. Emerg. Crit. Care* 27 (2): 151–163.

3 Reuss-Lamky, H. (2015). Hypothermia overview. *NAVC Clinician's Brief* (November): 12–16.

4 Clark-Price, S. (2015). Inadvertent perianesthetic hypothermia in small animal patients. *Vet. Clin. North Am. Small Anim. Pract.* 45 (5): 983–994.

5 Henshaw, R.E. (1978). Peripheral thermoregulation – hematologic or vascular adaptations. *J. Therm. Biol.* 3 (1): 31–37.

6 Prestrud, P. (1991). Adaptations by the arctic fox (Alopex-lagopus) to the polar winter. *Arctic* 44 (2): 132–138.

7 Duffy, T. (ed.) (2007). *Thermoregulation of the Perioperative Patient.* Chicago, IL: ProcACVS.

8 Tabor, B. (2007). Heatstroke in dogs. *Vet. Tech.* 28 (4).

9 Rijnberk, A. and Stokhof, A.A. (2009). General examination. In: *Medical History and Physical Examination in Companion Animals* (ed. A. Rijnberk and F.J. van Sluijs), 47–62. St. Louis: Saunders Elsevier.

10 Englar, R.E. (2017). *Performing the Small Animal Physical Examination.* Hoboken, NJ: Wiley.

11 Refinetti, R. and Piccione, G. (2003). Daily rhythmicity of body temperature in the dog. *J. Vet. Med. Sci.* 65 (8): 935–937.

12 Osinchuk, S., Taylor, S.M., Shmon, C.L. et al. (2014). Comparison between core temperatures measured telemetrically using the CorTemp(R) ingestible temperature sensor and rectal temperature in healthy Labrador retrievers. *Can. Vet. J.* 55 (10): 939–945.

13 Hall, J.E. (2011). Body temperature regulation, and fever. In: *Guyton and Hall Textbook of Medical Physiology* (ed. J.E. Hall), 867–877. Philadelphia: Saunders Elsevier.

14 Kurz, A. (2009). Physiology of thermoregulation. *Best Pract. Res. Clin. Anaesthesiol.* 22 (4): 627–644.

15 Duffy T, editor. (2007). Thermoregulation of the perioperative patient. Proc ACVS; Chicago, IL.

16 Oncken, A.K., Kirby, R., and Rudloff, E. (2001). Hypothermia in critically ill dogs and cats. *Comp. Cont. Educ. Pract.* 23 (6): 506–521.

17 Mallet, M.L. (2002). Pathophysiology of accidental hypothermia. *Qjm-Int. J. Med.* 95 (12): 775–785.

18 Sugano, Y. (1981). Seasonal-changes in heat-balance of dogs acclimatized to outdoor climate. *Jpn. J. Physiol.* 31 (4): 465–475.

19 Dhupa, N. (1995). Hypothermia in dogs and cats. *Comp. Cont. Educ. Pract.* 17 (1): 61–69.

20 Danzl, D.F. and Pozos, R.S. (1994). Current concepts – accidental hypothermia. *New Engl. J. Med.* 331 (26): 1756–1760.

21 Armstrong, S.R., Roberts, B.K., and Aronsohn, M. (2005). Perioperative hypothermia. *J. Vet. Emerg. Crit. Care* 15 (1): 32–37.

22 Lee, J. and Cohn, L. (2015). Pediatric critical care. *Clin. Brief* 13 (2): 41–42.

23 Blackmon, N. (2015). Anesthetic considerations for geriatric dogs. *Vet. Team Brief* 3 (3): 24.

24 Sessler, D.I. (2015). Temperature regulation and monitoring. In: *Miller's Anesthesia* (ed. R.D. Miller, N.H. Cohen and L.I. Eriksson), 1622–1646. St. Louis: Saunders Elsevier.

25 Saritas, Z.K., Saritas, T.B., Pamuk, K. et al. (2014). Comparison of the effects of lidocaine and fentanyl in epidural anesthesia in dogs. *Bratisl. Lek. Listy* 115 (8): 508–513.

26 Vainionpaa, M., Salla, K., Restitutti, F. et al. (2013). Thermographic imaging of superficial temperature in dogs sedated with medetomidine and butorphanol with and without MK-467 (L-659′066). *Vet. Anaesth. Analg.* 40 (2): 142–148.

27 Kaiser-Klinger S, editor. Troubleshooting emergency anesthesia. *IVECC*; 2008; Phoenix, AZ.

28 McKelvey, D. and Hollingshead, K. (1994). *Small Animal Anesthesia: Canine and Feline Practice.* St. Louis: Mosby-Year Book.

29 Harvey R, editor. Crisis management: what to worry about. *AAHA*; 2009.

30 Zeltzman P, editor. Hypothermia in surgical patients. *ACVS*; 2009; Phoenix, AZ.

31 Ninomiya, H., Akiyama, E., Simazaki, K. et al. (2011). Functional anatomy of the footpad vasculature of dogs: scanning electron microscopy of vascular corrosion casts. *Vet. Dermatol.* 22 (6): 475–481.

32 Arad, Z. and Midtgard, U. (1990). Ontogenetic development of the ophthalmic rete in relation to brain cooling in chickens and pigeons. *Am. J. Anat.* 187 (1): 98–103.

33 Bernal, D., Sepulveda, C., and Graham, J.B. (2001). Water-tunnel studies of heat balance in swimming mako sharks. *J. Exp. Biol.* 204 (Pt 23): 4043–4054.

34 Block, B.A. (1986). Structure of the brain and eye heater tissue in marlins, sailfish, and spearfishes. *J. Morphol.* 190 (2): 169–189.

35 Fritsches, K.A., Brill, R.W., and Warrant, E.J. (2005). Warm eyes provide superior vision in swordfishes. *Curr. Biol.* 15 (1): 55–58.

36 Ninomiya, H. (2000). The vascular bed in the rabbit ear: microangiography and scanning electron

microscopy of vascular corrosion casts. *Anat. Histol. Embryol.* 29 (5): 301–305.

37 Ninomiya, H. and Yoshida, E. (2007). Functional anatomy of the ocular circulatory system: vascular corrosion casts of the cetacean eye. *Vet. Ophthalmol.* 10 (4): 231–238.

38 Schmidt-Nielsen, K. (1981). Countercurrent systems in animals. *Sci. Am.* 244 (5): 118–128.

39 Heath, M.E. (1998). Gray whales in cold water. *Science* 280 (5364): 658–659.

40 Rommel, S.A. and Caplan, H. (2003). Vascular adaptations for heat conservation in the tail of Florida manatees (Trichechus manatus latirostris). *J. Anat.* 202 (4): 343–353.

41 Smith, S.A. and Tobias, A.H. (2004). Feline arterial thromboembolism: an update. *Vet. Clin. North Am. Small Anim. Pract.* 34 (5): 1245–1271.

42 Falconer, L. and Atwell, R. (2003). Feline aortic thromboembolism. *Aust. Vet. Pract.* 33 (1): 20–32.

43 Pion, P.D. and Kittleson, M.D. (1989). *Kirk's Current Veterinary Therapy X*, 295. Philadelphia: Saunders.

44 Rush, J.E. (1998). Therapy of feline hypertrophic cardiomyopathy. *Vet. Clin. North Am. Small Anim. Pract.* 28 (6): 1459–1479, ix.

45 Rush, J.E., Freeman, L.M., Brown, D.J., and Smith, F.W. Jr. (1998). The use of enalapril in the treatment of feline hypertrophic cardiomyopathy. *J. Am. Anim. Hosp. Assoc.* 34 (1): 38–41.

46 Rodriguez, D.B. and Harpster, N. (2002). Aortic thromboembolism associated with feline hypertrophic cardiomyopathy. *Comp. Cont. Educ. Pract.* 24 (6): 478–482.

47 Helenski, C.A. and Ross, J.N. Jr. (1987). Platelet aggregation in feline cardiomyopathy. *J. Vet. Intern. Med.* 1 (1): 24–28.

48 Fox, P.R., Sisson, D., and Moise, S.N. (eds.) (1999). *Textbook of Canine and Feline Cardiology: Principles and Practice.* Philadelphia: Saunders.

49 Fox, P.R. (2000). Feline cardiomyopathies. In: *Textbook of Veterinary Internal Medicine* (ed. S.J. Ettinger and E.C. Feldman), 896–923. Philadelphia: Saunders.

50 Hogan, D.F. (2017). Feline cardiogenic arterial thromboembolism: prevention and therapy. *Vet. Clin. North Am. Small Anim. Pract.* 47 (5): 1065–1082.

51 Fuentes, V.L. (2012). Arterial thromboembolism: risks, realities and a rational first-line approach. *J. Feline Med. Surg.* 14 (7): 459–470.

52 Borgeat, K., Wright, J., Garrod, O. et al. (2014). Arterial thromboembolism in 250 cats in general practice: 2004–2012. *J. Vet. Intern. Med.* 28 (1): 102–108.

53 Laste, N.J. and Harpster, N.K. (1995). A retrospective study of 100 cases of feline distal aortic thromboembolism: 1977–1993. *J. Am. Anim. Hosp. Assoc.* 31 (6): 492–500.

54 Smith, S.A., Tobias, A.H., Jacob, K.A. et al. (2003). Arterial thromboembolism in cats: acute crisis in 127 cases (1992–2001) and long-term management with low-dose aspirin in 24 cases. *J. Vet. Intern. Med.* 17 (1): 73–83.

55 Schoeman, J.P. (1999). Feline distal aortic thromboembolism: a review of 44 cases (1990–1998). *J. Feline Med. Surg.* 1 (4): 221–231.

56 Killingsworth, C.R., Eyster, G.E., Adams, T. et al. (1986). Streptokinase treatment of cats with experimentally induced aortic thrombosis. *Am. J. Vet. Res.* 47 (6): 1351–1359.

57 Moore, K.E., Morris, N., Dhupa, N. et al. (2000). Retrospective study of streptokinase administration in 46 cats with arterial thromboembolism. *J. Vet. Emerg. Crit. Care* 10: 245–257.

58 Rishniw, M. (2006). Feline aortic thromboembolism. *NAVC Clinician's Brief* (November): 17–20.

59 Schober, K.E. and Marz, I. (2003). Doppler echocardiographic assessment of left atrial appendage flow in cats with cardiomyopathy. *J. Vet. Intern. Med.* 17 (5): 739.

60 Côté, E. (2015). *Clinical Veterinary Advisor. Dogs and Cats*, 3e, xxxvii, 1642 p. St. Louis, Missouri: Elsevier Mosby.

61 Tilley, L.P., Smith, F.W.K., and Tilley, L.P. (2007). *Blackwell's Five-Minute Veterinary Consult: Canine and Feline*, 4e, lx, 1578 p. Ames, Iowa: Blackwell.

62 Aiello, S.E. and Moses, M.A. (2016). *The Merck Veterinary Mannual*, 11e. Whitehouse Station, NJ: Merck & Co., Inc.

63 Bulmer, B.J. (2011). The cardiovascular system. In: *Small Animal Pediatrics: the First 12 Months of Life* (ed. M.E. Peterson and M.A. Kutzler), 289–304. St. Louis, MO: Saunders/Elsevier.

64 Schrope, D.P. (2015). Prevalence of congenital heart disease in 76,301 mixed-breed dogs and 57,025 mixed-breed cats. *J. Vet. Cardiol.* 17 (3): 192–202.

65 Arora, M. (2001). Reversed patent ductus arteriosus in a dog. *Can. Vet. J.* 42 (6): 471–472.

66 Scurtu, I., Pestean, C., Lacatus, R. et al. (2106). Reverse PDA – less common type of patent ductus arteriosus – case report. *Bull. UASVM Vet. Med.* 73 (2): 351–355.

67 Broaddus, K. and Tillson, M. (2010). Patent ductus arteriosus in dogs. *Compend Cont. Educ. Vet.* 32 (9): E3.

68 Oliver, N.B. (1988). Congenital heart disease in dogs. In: *Canine and Feline Cardiology* (ed. P.R. Fox), 360–365. New York: Churchill Livingstone.

69 Nelson, R.W. and Couto, C.G. (1998). *Small Animal Internal Medicine.* St. Louis: Mosby.

70 Strickland, K.N. (2008). Congenital heart disease. In: *Manual of Canine and Feline Cardiology*, 4e

(ed. L.P. Tilley, F.W.K. Smith, M.A. Oyama and M.M. Sleeper), 215–239. Philadelphia: W.B. Saunders.

71 Orton, E.C. (2003). Cardiac surgery. In: *Textbook of Small Animal Surgery* (ed. D. Slatter), 955–959. Philadelphia: WB Saunders.

72 Fossum, T.W. (2007). *Small Animal Surgery*. St. Louis: Mosby Elsevier.

73 Buchanan, J.W. and Patterson, D.F. (2003). Etiology of patent ductus arteriosus in dogs. *J. Vet. Intern. Med.* 17 (2): 167–171.

74 Bonagura, J.D. and Darke, P.G. (1989). Congenital heart disease. In: *Textbook of Veterinary Internal Medicine* (ed. S.J. Ettinger and E.C. Feldman), 892–943. Philadelphia: WB Saunders.

75 Houghton, H.E. and Ware, W.A. (1996). Patent ductus arteriosus in dogs. *Iowa State University Veterinarian* 58 (2).

76 Cote, E. and Ettinger, S.J. (2001). Long-term clinical management of right-to-left ("reversed") patent ductus arteriosus in 3 dogs. *J. Vet. Intern. Med.* 15 (1): 39–42.

77 Goodwin, J.K. and Holland, M. (1995). Contrast echoaortography as an aid in the diagnosis of right-to-left shunting patent ductus-arteriosus. *Vet. Radiol. Ultrasound* 36 (2): 157–159.

78 Jeang, D.D. (1988). Hypertensive patent ductus arteriosus in a miniature dachshund. *Mod. Vet. Pract.* 69: 25–29.

79 Legendre, A.M., Appleford, M.D., Eyster, G.E., and Dade, A.W. (1974). Secondary polycythemia and seizures due to right to left shunting patent ductus arteriosus in a dog. *J. Am. Vet. Med. Assoc.* 164 (12): 1198–1201.

80 Oswald, G.P. and Orton, E.C. (1993). Patent ductus arteriosus and pulmonary hypertension in related Pembroke Welsh corgis. *J. Am. Vet. Med. Assoc.* 202 (5): 761–764.

81 Pyle, R.L., Park, R.D., Alexander, A.F., and Hill, B.L. (1981). Patent ductus arteriosus with pulmonary hypertension in the dog. *J. Am. Vet. Med. Assoc.* 178 (6): 565–571.

82 Sisson, D., Thomas, W.P., and Bonagura, J.D. (2000). Congenital heart disease. In: *Textbook of Veterinary Internal Medicine* (ed. S.J. Ettinger and E.C. Feldman), 737–787. Philadelphia: Saunders.

83 Goodwin, J.K., Cooper, R.C., and Weber, W.J. (1992). The medical-management of pets with congenital heart-defects. *Vet. Med. US* 87 (7): 670–675.

84 Campbell, K.L. (1990). Diagnosis and management of polycythemia in dogs. *Comp. Cont. Educ. Pract.* 12 (4): 543–550.

85 Ware, W.A. and Bonagura, J.D. (1988). Multiple congenital cardiac anomalies and Eisenmengers syndrome in a dog. *Comp. Cont. Educ. Pract.* 10 (8): 932–949.

86 Pachtinger, G.E. (2014). Hypovolemic shock. *NAVC Clinician's Brief* (October): 13–16.

87 Hopper, K., Silverstein, D., and Bateman, S. (2012). Shock syndromes. In: *Fluid Therapy in Small Animal Practice* (ed. S.P. DiBartola), 557–583. St. Louis, MO: Elsevier Saunders.

88 de Laforcade, A.M. (2009). Shock. In: *Small Animal Critical Care* (ed. D.C. Silverstein), 41–45. St. Louis, MO: Elsevier Saunders.

89 Campbell VL. (2011). Critical care triage. DVM 360 [Internet]. http://veterinarycalendar.dvm360.com/ critical-care-triage-proceedings.

90 Nowers, T. (2015). Top 5 clinical differences between cats and dogs. *Veterinary Team Brief* (September): 20–21.

91 Rozanski, E. and Rondeau, M. (2002). Choosing fluids in traumatic hypovolemic shock: the role of crystalloids, colloids, and hypertonic saline. *J. Am. Anim. Hosp. Assoc.* 38 (6): 499–501.

92 Pachtinger GE. (2013). The Many Types of Shock. NAVC Clinician's Brief [Internet]. https://www. cliniciansbrief.com/article/many-types-shock.

93 Pachtinger, G.E. (2015). Septic shock. *NAVC Clinician's Brief* (March): 13–16.

94 Boller, E.M. and Otto, C.M. (2009). Sepsis. In: *Small Animal Critical Care Medicine* (ed. D. Silverstein and K. Hopper), 454–459. Philadelphia: WB Saunders.

95 Klainbart, S., Agi, L., Bdolah-Abram, T. et al. (2017). Clinical, laboratory, and hemostatic findings in cats with naturally occurring sepsis. *J. Am. Vet. Med. Assoc.* 251 (9): 1025–1034.

96 Brady, C.A., Otto, C.M., Van Winkle, T.J., and King, L.G. (2000). Severe sepsis in cats: 29 cases (1986–1998). *J. Am. Vet. Med. Assoc.* 217 (4): 531–535.

40

Collapse

40.1 Differentiating Syncopal Collapse from Seizures

Collapse is a medical term to describe the event that occurs when a patient loses postural tone [1–4]. The patient, in effect, becomes weak and falls to the ground. Without postural tone, the body is unable to maintain itself upright, coordinated, and balanced [5].

Episodes of collapse are either syncopal or seizure-related [1–3, 6, 7].

Syncope is akin to fainting [6]. The patient loses consciousness suddenly [6]. This results in collapse, followed by spontaneous recovery [6].

Syncope may be [6]:

- Cardiogenic
- Hypotensive
- Neurally mediated.

Cardiogenic syncope is most common among companion animal Patients. It results from insufficient cardiac output due to altered structure and/or function of the heart [6].

Hypotensive syncope is caused by the following [6]:

- Drug-induced vasodilation
- Significant hypovolemia
  - Diarrhea
  - Emesis
  - Excessive diuresis
  - Extreme blood loss

Neurally mediated syncope occurs when an adrenergic surge causes a poorly understood autonomic reflex. This is common in humans [6, 8]. Emotional shock, such as phobias, or the sight of blood, may trigger fainting [6, 8]. Although less commonly appreciated in companion animal patients, fainting can also occur in startled dogs, for example, those that are ramped in fight-or-flight scenarios [8].

Neurally mediated syncope is situational and may include precipitating events such as the following [6, 8]:

- Agitation
- Barking
- Bathing
- Coughing
- Defecation
- Grooming
- Pain
- Stair climbing
- Urination
- Vomiting

Syncope may also result from hypoglycemia [6]. In addition, hypoxemia secondary to chronic respiratory diseases and pulmonary hypertension may trigger syncopal episodes [6].

Note that syncope is distinct from a seizure [6]. Although seizures are also sudden, involuntary events that are characterized by loss of muscle control, they are associated with abnormal neuroelectrical discharges. Excessive or synchronous firing of abnormal cells within the brain trigger seizure activity. Although seizures vary by type, the most recognizable ones are convulsive.

Based upon the descriptions above, syncope and epilepsy are uniquely different in terms of their origin and as such require distinct diagnostic investigations. However, based upon historical description, they are often difficult to differentiate [4, 7, 9, 10].

Misdiagnosis is common in human and veterinary medicine [7, 9, 10]. This stems from the fact that much of presumptive diagnosis is based upon patient history rather than clinically abnormal findings [7, 9–18]. The physical examination is typically unremarkable by the time the patient presents for evaluation [7, 11–18].

In general, syncope is preceded by pelvic limb weakness and/or ataxia [6]. These occur when cerebral perfusion is reduced, but not yet to the point of losing consciousness [6]. When consciousness is lost, it is typically brief, on the order of one minute or less [6]. Patients are most often flaccid at time of collapse [6].

Seizures, on the other hand, have historically been described by their abnormal tonic–clonic motor signs, with or without autonomic activity [2, 6]. On average, seizures last longer than syncopal episodes, and patients are typically slower to recover [6]. The postictal phase that immediately follows a seizure is often characterized by confusion. This may last minutes to hours. Transient behavioral changes and compromised vision are common during this period.

Although these descriptions sound distinct, the reality is that it is challenging to differentiate syncope from seizures based upon observation or recounted history alone [3, 9].

Episode duration is difficult for clients to describe. Although seizures tend to be longer than syncopal episodes, both may seem "long" to the observer, for whom the event may be perceived as frightening [3].

It used to be thought that vocalization, micturition, and defecation were only associated with seizures and could be distinguishing features [3]. However, vocalization and micturition may also be associated with syncopal events [3].

Although flaccid paralysis is most common during syncope, syncopal episodes may also be characterized by stiffness, seizure-like rigidity, and/or opisthotonos, in which the head and cervical spine are arched backward [3, 19].

Although muscle twitches have historically been linked to seizures, recent case reports demonstrate that syncopal episodes may also be characterized by involuntary muscle activity [9]. For example, Penning describes a cat that underwent facial tics, lip chewing, and leg actions that simulated running in place during a syncopal episode [9]. The patient also demonstrated ptyalism, a feature that is often associated with seizure activity [9]. It was only after a continuous electrocardiogram (ECG) was placed in the form of a Holter monitor that the patient was diagnosed with syncope secondary to high-grade atrioventricular (AV) block [9].

Although reflex syncope has been described, reflex seizures also exist [10]. A case report by Motta and Dutton describes a canine patient that seized in response to intense physical exercise [10].

Therefore, seizures may look like syncope, and syncope may look like seizures [4, 9, 20].

A definitive diagnosis is difficult to reach in the majority of patients without access to additional diagnostic aids [4].

40.2 Diagnostic Confirmation of Syncope

Episodes of collapse are frustrating for the client and clinician alike because they are intermittent. In between episodes, the patient is typically described as "normal." This means that unless the patient presents to the clinic in the middle of an event, the physical examination is unlikely to provide insight as to the cause of collapse [7, 9, 11–18].

Urinalysis and baseline bloodwork, in the form of a complete blood count (CBC) and serum chemistry panel, provide a minimum database for ruling out hypoglycemia, anemia, electrolyte imbalances, and renal and hepatic dysfunction [2].

Depending upon the patient, signalment, and index of suspicion, additional labwork may be indicated [2]:

- Serologic screening
  - Feline immunodeficiency virus (FIV)
  - Feline leukemia virus (FeLV)
  - Heartworm disease (HWD)
  - Rickettsial exposure
- Thyroid testing

When laboratory findings are unremarkable, meaning that there are no electrolyte imbalances that could explain collapse in terms of metabolic dysfunction, the diagnostic work-up shifts gears to focus on either cardiovascular or neurological disease [21].

In the presence of abnormal or muffled heart sounds, including murmurs, thoracic imaging is indicated [2].

If an arrhythmia is present or there are pulse deficits on physical examination, then the patient should submit to an ECG to evaluate the heart rhythm [2]. Bradyarrhythmias often precipitate syncope.

However, it is not uncommon for a spot-check, in-house ECG to be normal [21]. On average, an in-clinic ECG records three minutes of cardiac activity. This represents a mere 0.2% of cardiac depolarizations within a 24-hour period [22].

The reality is that arrhythmias are often transient [22, 23]. Because of this, they often go undetected when patients are screened with routine ECG [21, 23]. The patient thus goes undiagnosed, and episodes are likely to persist. This diagnostic delay puts the patient at increased risk: there is an association between syncope and sudden death in dogs with some, but not all, cardiomyopathy [24]. This includes myxomatous mitral valve disease (MVD) and arrhythmogenic right ventricular cardiomyopathy (ARVC), otherwise known as Boxer dog cardiomyopathy [24–30].

Continuous ambulatory electrocardiography, so-called Holter monitoring, has revolutionized the clinician's ability to diagnose transient arrhythmias [23]. The diagnostic yield is superior to that obtained by routine echocardiography [31]. Cardiac arrhythmia is more likely to be identified or excluded as the cause for the patient's clinical signs [31].

Holter monitoring became a staple of human medicine in the 1960s [22]. Its use has since extended into veterinary practice [22]. Holter monitoring of both dogs and cats has been described [22, 23, 31–40] (see Figure 40.1).

An additional advantage of Holter monitoring is that it is more likely to capture the patient's normal resting heart rate as opposed to one elevated by stress in the clinic setting [22].

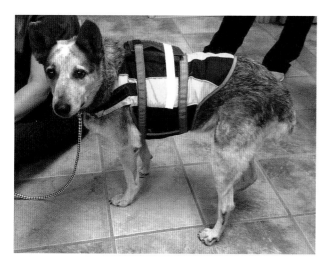

Figure 40.1 Canine patient outfitted with a continuous ambulatory electrocardiography device. This device is held in place via a wearable harness. *Source:* Courtesy of Grady Gray.

Even so, Holter monitors are an imperfect system. Some patients may feel hindered by the harness that is worn to secure the monitor to the body [21]. They may alter their physical activity accordingly [21].

Holter monitors may also still miss intermittent arrhythmias, given that storage is limited to a 24–48 h period [21].

More recently, implantable devices have been studied for use in dogs [21, 41, 42]. These devices are implanted over the left apex of the heart in subcutaneous tissue, where they continuously record data [21]. Patient caretakers also can make use of a remote activating device to flag data taken during a witnessed event [21]. This facilitates diagnosis by earmarking what went on at the level of the patient's heart immediately before, during, and after the event [21]. Devices can be programmed to autoactivate as well based upon preset parameters, such as heart rate [21]. Data is retrievable via computer for evaluation by a veterinary cardiologist [21].

Implantable loop recorders are battery operated and last up to 14 months [21].

Although few studies describe the use of these devices, they appear to be successful at capturing recurrent syncope and providing a definitive diagnosis [21, 41–44].

40.3 Brief Review of Cardiac Physiology

The heart functions as a mechanical pump [45]. The rate at which the heart pumps depends upon an intrinsic electrical conduction system [45]. This system generates impulses that spread through the heart and signal muscle tissue to contract in a coordinated fashion [45].

To facilitate conduction of these impulses, the heart has two nodes [45]:

- The sinoatrial (SA) node
- The AV node

Both nodes are collections of cells [45].

The SA node sits in the right atrium [45]. It is the originator of the impulse [45]. It has been called the heart's pacemaker.

The SA node sends impulses to the AV node, which is located at the base of the atrial septum [45]. The AV node then directs the impulse to the ventricles to initiate ventricular contraction [45].

The AV node also functions as an understudy [45]. In the event that the SA node fails as the heart's pacemaker, the AV node can take over [45].

40.4 Cardiogenic Syncope

Cardiogenic syncope is a common cause of collapse among companion animal patients [6]. It most often results from the following [6, 46–50]:

- ARVC
- Bradyarrhythmias
  - Atrial standstill
  - AV heart block
    o Second-degree
    o Third-degree
  - Sick sinus syndrome
- Cardiac disease
  - Acquired valvular disease
  - Aortic stenosis
  - Arterial or aortic thromboembolism (ATE) (refer to Chapter 39, Section 39.5.1)
  - Chemodectomas
  - Congestive heart failure (CHF) (refer to Chapter 36, Section 36.3.3 and Chapter 38, Section 38.4.1.4)
  - Dilated cardiomyopathy (DCM)
  - Hypertrophic cardiomyopathy (HCM)
  - Patent ductus arteriosus (PDA)
  - Pericardial effusion (refer to Chapter 42)
  - Pulmonary hypertension (refer to Chapter 39, Section 39.5.2.2)
  - Pulmonic stenosis (PS)
- Shock (refer to Chapter 38, Sections 38.4.1.3, 38.4.1.4, 38.4.5.1, and Chapter 39, Section 39.5.3)
- Ventricular tachycardia

40.4.1 Arrhythmogenic Right Ventricular Cardiomyopathy

ARVC was identified in the 1980s as a disease of Boxer dogs [28–30]. Affected dogs developed fatty infiltration of the heart secondary to cardiac muscle atrophy [28–30,

51, 52]. Because of its tendency to affect Boxers, this condition is sometimes referred to as, simply, Boxer dog cardiomyopathy [28, 51, 52].

The condition is genetic in Boxer dogs and is characterized as an autosomal dominant trait [28, 29, 53]. The trait codes for a mutation in the striatin gene, which results in structurally weak connections between desmosomes in affected dogs [29, 54].

Without the connectivity that is integral to the stability of the heart, myocytes become dysfunctional [29]. Inflammation of the heart and secondary fibrosis are associated sequelae [29, 55].

Diagnosis occurs in the adult dog, most typically at middle age [28, 29].

Affected dogs fit into one of three categories [28–30]:

- Asymptomatic
  - Occasional ventricular premature complexes (VPCs) appear as incidental findings on ECG
- Symptomatic
  - History of exercise intolerance
  - History of syncope
  - Evidence of tachyarrhythmias
    ○ Ventricular tachycardia
- Symptomatic, with CHF secondary to systolic dysfunction and ventricular dilation

Holter monitoring plays an important role in diagnosis because ECG abnormalities are rarely continuous [28, 29]. Arrhythmias are transient and sporadic [28, 29]. They are likely to be missed on routine, in-house ECG [28, 29].

Sudden death is a possibility among affected patients [28, 29].

Note that Boxer dogs are not the only ones to develop ARVC. Although occurrence is rare, ARVC has also been reported in a handful of case reports involving cats [56, 57].

40.4.2 Bradyarrhythmias

Bradyarrhythmias refer to those heart rhythms that collectively have a slower than expected heart rate [58]. In dogs, this is roughly defined as less than 60 beats/minute [58]. Cats are considered bradycardic at rates less than 140 [58].

The heart rate may be regularly slow, as in sinus bradycardia, or the patient may experience stretches of sinus arrest, that is, a pause in the heart rhythm [47, 58].

An ECG is required to differentiate between bradyarrhythmias as this is not feasible based upon cardiothoracic auscultation alone [58].

40.4.2.1 Sinus Bradycardia
Sinus bradycardia may result from the following [58]:

- High vagal tone
  - Central nervous system disease
  - Gastrointestinal disease
  - Respiratory disease

- Hyperkalemia (see Chapter 45, Section 45.3)
- Hypothermia, especially in cats
- Overzealous response to beta blockers, calcium channel blockers, or digoxin
- Particular anesthetic, analgesic, and other pharmaceutical agents
- Sepsis in cats

Sinus bradycardia in and of itself does not tend to cause syncope unless pauses between heartbeats last for several seconds [58]. In these situations, sick sinus syndrome is suspected [58].

40.4.2.2 Sick Sinus Syndrome
Sick sinus syndrome is named for a faulty SA node. In health, the SA node is responsible for initiating the heartbeat and establishing the resting heart rate. However, in dogs with sick sinus syndrome, the SA node fails to discharge as often as it ought to. This results in long pauses between heartbeats.

If the pause is long enough, another part of the heart may fire off an escape rhythm [59]. These ventricular escape beats are evident on ECG readings of affected patients, after which, a normal sinus rhythm resumes [59, 60].

Other patients fail to generate escape rhythms and experience true asystole [59]. These patients are likely to experience a syncopal episode [59]. Clients may also describe weakness and incoordination [59, 61, 62].

Miniature Schnauzers, Cocker Spaniels, and West Highland White Terriers are predisposed to this condition, the underlying cause of which remains unknown [46, 58, 59, 63–65].

Female dogs may be overrepresented [66].

Diagnosis is achieved by ECG [59]. Continuous ambulatory electrocardiography is often indicated, given the transient, intermittent nature of episodes [59].

Asymptomatic patients may simply be monitored with periodic ECGs [59].

Symptomatic patients may respond positively to positive chronotropic drugs [66]. However, most affected patients require treatment in the form of a pacemaker to alleviate clinical signs [58]. Pacemaker implantation carries a high success rate in the dog [59, 67].

Minor risks include seroma or hematoma formation at the site of implantation [59, 60, 67, 68].

Major risks include dislodgement of pacemaker leads [59, 67–69].

40.4.2.3 AV Block
AV block occurs when the electrical message from the atria to the ventricles is interrupted [45].

There are different types of AV block [58]:

- First-degree
- Second-degree
- Third-degree

In first-degree AV block, all impulses go through the atria to the ventricles as expected; however, there is an appreciable delay in message transmission. This delay can be observed as a prolonged PR interval on the ECG. First-degree AV block is not always pathological. Young, healthy dogs may have this as a result of high vagal tone.

Most patients with first-degree AV block are asymptomatic. That is, they do not present for syncopal episodes. Instead, first-degree AV block tends to be an incidental finding on ECG.

Second- and third-degree AV block are more likely to be associated with syncope [58].

In second-degree AV block, some, but not all, impulses are blocked from the atria to the ventricles. This is evident on ECG as a P wave that is not followed by a QRS complex. In other words, the signal was circumvented before ventricular contraction was initiated.

High vagal tone may cause second-degree AV block. Other common causes of second-degree AV block include

- AV node disease
- Hyperkalemia
- Opiates.

There are two versions of second-degree AV block:

- Mobitz type I
- Mobitz type II

In Mobitz type I second-degree AV block, the P-R interval is variable. This interval progressively lengthens until there is a skipped QRS. The pattern then restarts.

In Mobitz type II second-degree AV block, the P-R interval is consistent before and after the dropped beat.

All second-degree AV block can result in syncope [58].

Third-degree AV block, or complete AV block, is most likely to result in syncope because all SA-generated impulses are blocked at the AV node. This results in ventricular contractions that are spontaneous, meaning that they occur independently of what is going on at the level of the atria. This results in inefficient pumping of blood through the heart into systemic circulation.

Myocardial disease is likely in cats with complete AV block, much more so than in dogs [58, 67, 69, 70].

Sudden death is a valid concern for canine patients with complete AV block [58, 71]. Roughly one-quarter die within a month of diagnosis, although pacemaker implantation may extend the median survival time [58, 71].

Cats are less likely than dogs to spontaneously die as a result of complete AV block [58]. Their median survival is, on average, one year following diagnosis [70]. However, pacemakers do not appear to improve survival time in cats [58].

40.4.2.4 Atrial Standstill
Compared to sick sinus syndrome and AV block, atrial standstill is much less common in companion animal practice [47]. Atrial standstill occurs when there is faulty conduction by the atria themselves [47, 58]. When the atria fail to contract, the ventricles must take over the rhythm for the rest of the heart. This results in a junctional or ventricular escape rhythm [47, 58].

On ECG, atrial standstill is evident as a lack of P waves [58].

Although uncommon, atrial standstill is most likely to be seen in patients with severe hyperkalemia. Consider, for example, those patients with the following [58]:

- Acute renal failure (ARF)
- Addisonian crisis
- Urinary tract obstruction (UTO)

In addition, English Springer Spaniels appear to be predisposed [46, 72, 73].

40.4.3 Structural Dysfunction of the Heart and Cardiac Disease

Structural dysfunction within the heart itself, as from underlying cardiomyopathy, is a common cause of cardiogenic syncope [6]. For example, valvular insufficiency may precipitate CHF that in turn causes inadequate cardiac output [6]. If decline in cardiac output is sudden or significant in times of volume, then syncope may result.

Refer to Chapter 36, Section 36.3.3 and Chapter 38, Section 38.4.1.4 to recall the pathophysiology of CHF and its associated sequelae. Fainting is just one of many potential complications.

However, CHF is not the only example in which structural abnormalities result in cardiac dysfunction. The following pathologies represent additional causes of syncope that may be diagnosed in clinical practice.

40.4.3.1 Acquired Valvular Disease
Valvular disease is common in the dog [74–76].

In particular, MVD targets senior small-breed dogs, including the Miniature Poodle, Pomeranian, Yorkshire Terrier, Chihuahua, and King Charles Cavalier Spaniel [74, 77].

MVD is characterized by progressive degeneration of the mitral valve [50]. Valve leaflets develop nodules that, over time, prevent the valve from forming a tight seal every time it closes in the cardiac cycle [50]. The valve is said to be "leaky" [50]. Every time the heart beats, a fraction of blood flows backward, through the mitral valve and back into the left atrium [50].

Over time, left atrial pressure and volume increases [50]. The natural response of the left atrium is to dilate [50].

Eventually, backflow of blood causes pressure in the pulmonary vein to rise [50].

Left-sided CHF, characterized by congestion of the lungs, is common in advanced disease [74].

40.4.3.2 Aortic Stenosis

Aortic stenosis is a congenital heart defect that causes pressure overload on the left side of the heart. Congenital heart disease is rarer in kittens than in puppies [48, 78].

A specific type of aortic stenosis is subaortic stenosis (SAS). SAS is one of the most common congenital defects in dogs [48, 49, 79].

SAS is characterized by a fibrous band just below the aortic semilunar valves. This prevents the left ventricle from emptying completely. The band is, in a sense, a mechanical obstruction to blood flow [50].

In an attempt to overcome this obstruction and improve pumping efficiency, the left ventricle increases chamber pressure [50]. This requires the left ventricular wall to thicken [50].

Unfortunately, this thickening is counterproductive. Myocardial oxygen demand has now increased, yet the left ventricle is no more efficient [50]. There is still mechanical occlusion to blood flow [50].

The Boxer dog, English Bulldog, German Shepherd, Golden Retriever, Great Dane, Newfoundland, and Bull Terrier are overrepresented [50].

Syncope is common in cases of SAS and may be triggered by bouts of exercise or play. Sudden death is possible [48].

Reference a cardiology textbook for treatment options and recommendations. Balloon dilation of the outflow tract may be performed to improve clinical signs [80]. However, patient prognosis depends upon the severity of the obstruction and for that reason remains guarded.

40.4.3.3 Chemodectomas

Chemodectomas are uncommonly diagnosed in companion animal medicine [81]. These are rare tumors associated with either the carotid or aortic bodies [81]. Of the two sites, the latter are the most likely sites of tumor development [80]. These bodies represent collections of cells that are strategically placed to detect changes in arterial blood oxygen concentration [81]. When blood gas profiles stray from the norm; these cells coordinate changes in respiration, heart rate, and blood pressure to maintain homeostasis [81].

Chemodectomas are more likely to occur in brachycephalic breeds, including bulldogs [81–88]. It is thought perhaps that the chronic hypoxemia associated with brachycephalic dogs is a risk factor for development of this tumor [81]. This theory appears to carry weight in human medicine in that carotid body tumors are more likely to develop in humans with chronic obstructive pulmonary disease [89].

Middle-aged dogs and males are also overrepresented [81–88].

Patients with chemodectomas of the aortic bodies present for coughing and dyspnea [80]. Coughing may be secondary to CHF or heart enlargement that causes dorsal displacement of the trachea (see Figures 40.2a–c).

When chemodectomas involve the carotid bodies, patients may present for a cervical mass [80]. This may be grossly or palpably apparent. Because of location, it may also result in signs of dysphagia or regurgitation [80].

Either type of chemodectoma may result in syncope [80, 81].

Sudden death is possible if major arteries are invaded by the tumor, due to acute and life-threatening hemorrhage [80].

40.4.3.4 Dilated Cardiomyopathy

DCM is an acquired heart disease for which Doberman Pinschers and Irish Wolfhounds are overrepresented [90]. The etiology of DCM in dogs is unknown as compared to cats, in which DCM has been primarily linked to taurine deficiency [90, 91].

Affected dogs and cats develop dilation of the left ventricle.

As disease progresses, the left atrium dilates, too.

Although the heart is now enlarged, it is essentially ineffectual. Its contractility is appreciably reduced. The heart is somewhat flaccid, with incomplete contractions.

Blood is pumped out into systemic circulation via the aorta at significantly decreased velocity.

Ultimately, blood backs up from the left ventricle into the left atrium, and from the left atrium into the pulmonary tree. Lung congestion ensues.

Atrial fibrillation and ventricular arrhythmias are common in affected dogs, which often present for exercise intolerance or syncope [90, 92].

Sudden death occurs in approximately one-third to one-half of dogs that acquire this disease [90].

Reference a cardiology textbook for treatment options and recommendations. Medical management is lifelong and aims to stabilize the patient, improve cardiac function, and slow ventricular response rate in patients that develop atrial fibrillation [80].

40.4.3.5 Hypertrophic Cardiomyopathy

HCM is the most common form of inherited cardiomyopathy in the cat [93, 94].

Maine Coon cats inherit HCM as an autosomal dominant trait [95, 96]. This trait codes for a mutation in myosin-binding protein C (MYBPC3) [95, 97, 98]. This same mutation has been identified in Ragdoll cats with HCM as well as in Maine Coons [95].

Other predisposed breeds may include the Persian, Burmese, Siamese, American Shorthair, and Norwegian Forest cats [99].

Males are more likely than females to develop HCM [100–102].

(a)

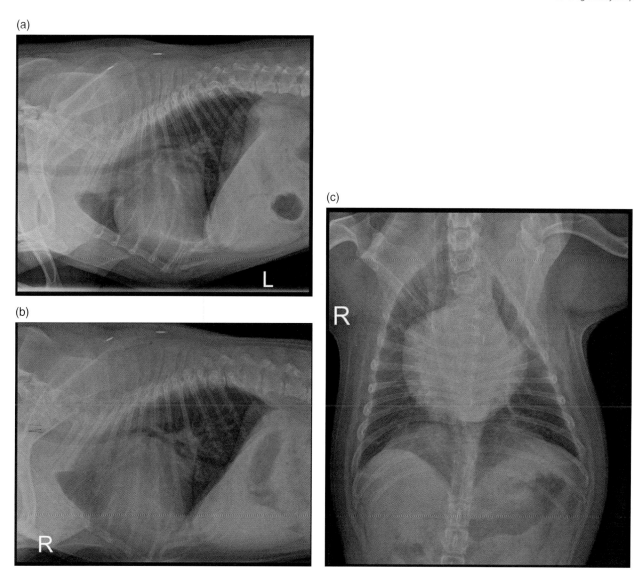

(b)

(c)

Figure 40.2 (a) Left lateral thoracic radiograph of a seven-year-old, castrated male French bulldog with an enlarged heart and congestive heart failure (CHF) secondary to chemodectoma. *Source:* Courtesy of Kelly C. Money. (b) Right lateral thoracic radiograph of the dog shown in (a). *Source:* Courtesy of Kelly C. Money. (c) Ventrodorsal (V-D) thoracic radiograph of the dog shown in (a). *Source:* Courtesy of Kelly C. Money.

Many cats with HCM are asymptomatic [103, 104]. Syncope is, in other words, possible, but rare [103, 105–107].

A heart murmur may be the only evidence of an underlying structural issue on physical examination [93].

HCM may also be associated with ATE [100]. Recall from Chapter 39, Section 39.5.1 that a "saddle thrombus" is the most typical presentation of ATE, and that bilateral involvement of the pelvic limbs is likely [108].

Patients affected by HCM are in acute pain [99, 100, 108]. They drag the affected limb(s) [100]. On physical examination, the affected limb(s) often lack(s) a femoral pulse [100].

Compromised blood flow causes the affected limb(s) to become cold [100]. Associated paw pads and nail beds are likely to become cyanotic [108, 109].

Sudden death associated with HCM is possible [80, 110].

Reference a cardiology textbook for treatment options for HCM and recommendations for medical management of HCM-associated ATE [80].

40.4.3.6 Pulmonic Stenosis
PS is similar to SAS in terms of pathophysiology, only the location of the mechanical obstruction is different [48, 49, 79].

Instead of affecting the aortic semilunar valves. PS creates an outflow obstruction at the level of the pulmonic valve.

This prevents the right ventricle from emptying completely.

In an attempt to overcome this obstruction and improve pumping efficiency, the right ventricle increases chamber pressure [50]. This requires the right ventricular wall to thicken [50].

Predisposed breeds include the Beagle dog, Cocker Spaniel, English Bulldog, Bull Mastiff, Samoyed, Schnauzer, and West Highland White Terrier [50].

If patients are mildly affected, they may not require treatment. However, severe cases may require surgical intervention. Insertion of a balloon catheter into the outflow tract to reduce the mechanical obstruction is both feasible and successful in many patients.

Reference a cardiology textbook for treatment guidelines and recommendations [80].

40.4.4   Ventricular Tachycardia

Ventricular tachycardia is common in cases of ARVC and DCM [28–30, 111]. Ventricular tachycardia refers an abnormally rapid heart rate that originates within the ventricles. Ventricular contractions occur independently of atrial contractions. These result in wide, so-called bizarre QRS complexes that are not tied to P waves on ECG [111].

Tissue perfusion is suboptimal during bouts of ventricular tachycardia. Syncope results from diminished perfusion of the brain [51–53, 112].

Sudden death is common

40.4.5   Chronic Respiratory Disease and Syncope

Note that syncope does not always stem exclusively from cardiac disease [113]. Pulmonary hypertension may also induce this clinical sign. Causes of pulmonary hypertension include the following [113]:

- Chronic bronchitis (see Chapter 35, Section 35.4.2)
- HWD and heartworm associated respiratory disease (HARD)
- Laryngeal paralysis (see Chapter 34, Section 34.4)
- Pulmonary fibrosis
- Pulmonary thromboembolism

Refer to Chapter 35, Section 35.4.3 for a review of HWD and HARD. Recall that dogs with HWD are more likely than cats to present for coughing, exercise intolerance, labored breathing, and syncope [114, 115].

Cats with HWD and HARD are frequently misdiagnosed with asthma [114, 115]. However, syncope in cats can occur secondary to HWD [19]. A case report by Malik et al. in 1998 describes a heartworm-positive cat that presented for evaluation of "fainting" spells and heavy breathing [19].

Pulmonary hypertension causes exercise intolerance and syncope because the associated ventilation-perfusion mismatch ultimately leads to hypoxemia [113, 116–119]. The hypoxic patient does not have adequate perfusion. There is insufficient cardiac output to sustain functions that require additional input, such as exercise or excitement [113]. Affected patients are likely to experience syncopal episodes with exertion [113].

References

1 Kraus MS, editor. (2004). Syncope in small breed dogs. Clinician's Brief [Internet]. https://www.cliniciansbrief.com/column/what039s-take-home/syncope-small-breed-dogs.

2 Thawley, V. and Silverstein, D. (2012). Collapse. *NAVC Clinician's Brief* (November): 14–15.

3 Estrada, A. (2017). Differentiating syncope from seizure. *NAVC Clinician's Brief* (July): 50–55.

4 Barnett, L., Martin, M.W., Todd, J. et al. (2011). A retrospective study of 153 cases of undiagnosed collapse, syncope or exercise intolerance: the outcomes. *J. Small Anim. Pract.* 52 (1): 26–31.

5 Gurfinkel, V., Cacciatore, T.W., Cordo, P. et al. (2006). Postural muscle tone in the body axis of healthy humans. *J. Neurophysiol.* 96 (5): 2678–2687.

6 Schwartz DS, editor. (2009). The Syncopal Dog. World Small Animal Veterinary Association World Congress Proceedings; Sao Paulo, Brazil.

7 Dutton, E., Dukes-McEwan, J., and Cripps, P.J. (2017). Serum cardiac troponin I in canine syncope and seizures. *J. Vet. Cardiol.* 19 (1): 1–13.

8 Kraus MS. (2017). Syncope: diagnosis and treatment. https://d12geb6i3t2qxg.cloudfront.net/webinar_resources/uploads/2017/01/Syncope_Diagnosis_and_Treatment_Marc_Kraus.pdf.

9 Penning, V.A., Connolly, D.J., Gajanayake, I. et al. (2009). Seizure-like episodes in 3 cats with intermittent high-grade atrioventricular dysfunction. *J. Vet. Intern. Med.* 23 (1): 200–205.

10 Motta, L. and Dutton, E. (2013). Suspected exercise-induced seizures in a young dog. *J. Small Anim. Pract.* 54 (4): 213–218.

11 Grubb, B.P., Gerard, G., Roush, K. et al. (1991). Differentiation of convulsive syncope and epilepsy with head-up tilt testing. *Ann. Intern. Med.* 115 (11): 871–876.

12 Linzer, M., Grubb, B.P., Ho, S. et al. (1994). Cardiovascular causes of loss of consciousness in patients with presumed epilepsy: a cause of the increased sudden death rate in people with epilepsy? *Am. J. Med.* 96 (2): 146–154.

13 Scheepers, B., Clough, P., and Pickles, C. (1998). The misdiagnosis of epilepsy: findings of a population study. *Seizure* 7 (5): 403–406.

14 Sheldon, R., Rose, S., Ritchie, D. et al. (2002). Historical criteria that distinguish syncope from seizures. *J. Am. Coll. Cardiol.* 40 (1): 142–148.

15 Smith, D., Defalla, B.A., and Chadwick, D.W. (1999). The misdiagnosis of epilepsy and the management of refractory epilepsy in a specialist clinic. *QJM* 92 (1): 15–23.

16 Zaidi, A., Clough, P., Cooper, P. et al. (2000). Misdiagnosis of epilepsy: many seizure-like attacks have a cardiovascular cause. *J. Am. Coll. Cardiol.* 36 (1): 181–184.

17 Chadwick, D. and Smith, D. (2002). The misdiagnosis of epilepsy. *BMJ* 324 (7336): 495–496.

18 Werz, M.A. (2005). Idiopathic generalized tonic-clonic seizures limited to exercise in a young adult. *Epilepsy Behav.* 6 (1): 98–101.

19 Malik, R., Church, D.B., and Eade, I.G. (1998). Syncope in a cat. *Aust. Vet. J.* 76 (7): 465, 70-1.

20 Bailey, K.S. and Dewey, C.W. (2009). The Seizuring Cat. Diagnostic work-up and therapy. *J. Feline Med. Surg.* 11 (5): 385–394.

21 MacKie, B.A., Stepien, R.L., and Kellihan, H.B. (2010). Retrospective analysis of an implantable loop recorder for evaluation of syncope, collapse, or intermittent weakness in 23 dogs (2004–2008). *J. Vet. Cardiol.* 12 (1): 25–33.

22 Miller, R.H., Lehmkuhl, L.B., Bonagura, J.D., and Beall, M.J. (1999). Retrospective analysis of the clinical utility of ambulatory electrocardiographic (Holter) recordings in syncopal dogs: 44 cases (1991–1995). *J. Vet. Intern. Med.* 13 (2): 111–122.

23 Goodwin, J.K. (1998). Holter monitoring and cardiac event recording. *Vet. Clin. North Am. Small Anim. Pract.* 28 (6): 1391–1407, viii.

24 Rasmussen, C.E., Falk, T., Domanjko Petric, A. et al. (2014). Holter monitoring of small breed dogs with advanced myxomatous mitral valve disease with and without a history of syncope. *J. Vet. Intern. Med.* 28 (2): 363–370.

25 Borgarelli, M., Savarino, P., Crosara, S. et al. (2008). Survival characteristics and prognostic variables of dogs with mitral regurgitation attributable to myxomatous valve disease. *J. Vet. Intern. Med.* 22 (1): 120–128.

26 Buchanan, J.W. (1977). Chronic valvular disease (endocardiosis) in dogs. *Adv. Vet. Sci. Comp. Med.* 21: 75–106.

27 Detweiler, D.K., Patterson, D.F., Hubben, K., and Botts, R.P. (1961). The prevalence of spontaneously occurring cardiovascular disease in dogs. *Am. J. Public Health Nations Health* 51: 228–241.

28 Meurs, K.M. (2004). Boxer dog cardiomyopathy: an update. *Vet. Clin. North Am. Small Anim. Pract.* 34 (5): 1235–1244, viii.

29 Meurs, K.M. (2017). Arrhythmogenic right ventricular cardiomyopathy in the boxer dog: an update. *Vet. Clin. North Am. Small Anim. Pract.* 47 (5): 1103–1111.

30 Palermo, V., Stafford Johnson, M.J., Sala, E. et al. (2011). Cardiomyopathy in Boxer dogs: a retrospective study of the clinical presentation, diagnostic findings and survival. *J. Vet. Cardiol.* 13 (1): 45–55.

31 Bright, J.M. and Cali, J.V. (2000). Clinical usefulness of cardiac event recording in dogs and cats examined because of syncope, episodic collapse, or intermittent weakness: 60 cases (1997–1999). *J. Am. Vet. Med. Assoc.* 216 (7): 1110–1114.

32 Ware WA, editor. (1997). Holter monitoring in cats. 15th Annual Forum, American College of Veterinary Internal Medicine.

33 Goodwin, J.K., Lombard, C.W., and Ginez, D.D. (1992). Results of continuous ambulatory electrocardiography in a cat with hypertrophic cardiomyopathy. *J. Am. Vet. Med. Assoc.* 200 (9): 1352–1354.

34 Vannoort, R., Vanhemel, N.M., Voorhout, G., and Stokhof, A.A. (1993). Ambulatory electrocardiographic (Holter) monitoring in the dog. *Tijdschr. Diergeneeskd.* 118: S66–S67.

35 Hall, L.W., Dunn, J.K., Delaney, M., and Shapiro, L.M. (1991). Ambulatory electrocardiography in dogs. *Vet. Rec.* 129 (10): 213–216.

36 Ulloa, H.M., Houston, B.J., and Altrogge, D.M. (1995). Arrhythmia prevalence during ambulatory electrocardiographic monitoring of beagles. *Am. J. Vet. Res.* 56 (3): 275–281.

37 Calvert, C.A., Jacobs, G.J., and Pickus, C.W. (1996). Bradycardia-associated episodic weakness, syncope, and aborted sudden death in cardiomyopathic Doberman pinschers. *J. Vet. Intern. Med.* 10 (2): 88–93.

38 Marino, D.J., Matthiesen, D.T., Fox, P.R. et al. (1994). Ventricular arrhythmias in dogs undergoing Splenectomy – a prospective-study. *Vet. Surg.* 23 (2): 101–106.

39 Moise, N. and DeFrancesco, T.C. (1995). Twenty-four hour ambulatory electrocardiography (Holter monitoring). In: *Kirk's Current Veterinary Therapy XII* (ed. J.D. Bonagura), 792–799. Philadelphia: WB Saunders.

40 Moise, N.S., Gilmour, R.F. Jr., Riccio, M.L., and Flahive, W.F. Jr. (1997). Diagnosis of inherited ventricular tachycardia in German shepherd dogs. *J. Am. Vet. Med. Assoc.* 210 (3): 403–410.

41 Santilli, R.A., Ferasin, L., Voghera, S.G., and Perego, M. (2010). Evaluation of the diagnostic value of an implantable loop recorder in dogs with unexplained syncope. *J. Am. Vet. Med. Assoc.* 236 (1): 78–82.

42 James, R., Summerfield, N., Loureiro, J. et al. (2008). Implantable loop recorders: a viable diagnostic tool in veterinary medicine. *J. Small Anim. Pract.* 49 (11): 564–570.

43 Ferasin, L. (2009). Recurrent syncope associated with paroxysmal supraventricular tachycardia in a Devon Rex cat diagnosed by implantable loop recorder. *J. Feline Med. Surg.* 11 (2): 149–152.

44 Willis, R., McLeod, K., Cusack, J., and Wotton, P. (2003). Use of an implantable loop recorder to investigate syncope in a cat. *J. Small Anim. Pract.* 44 (4): 181–183.

45 Reece, W.O., Erickson, H.H., Goff, J.P., and Uemura, E.E. (2015). *Dukes' Physiology of Domestic Animals*, 13e, xii, 748 p. Ames, Iowa, USA: Wiley Blackwell.

46 Scansen, B.A. (2011). Interventional cardiology for the criticalist. *J. Vet. Emerg. Crit. Care* 21 (2): 123–136.

47 Bulmer, B. (2012). Interpreting ECGs with confidence: Part 2. *NAVC Clinician's Brief* (June): 102–105.

48 Strickland, K.N. (2008). Congenital heart disease. In: *Manual of Canine and Feline Cardiology*, 4e (ed. L.P. Tilley, F.W.K. Smith, M.A. Oyama and M.M. Sleeper), 215–239. Philadelphia: W.B. Saunders.

49 Bulmer, B.J. (2011). The cardiovascular system. In: *Small Animal Pediatrics: The First 12 Months of Life* (ed. M.E. Peterson and M.A. Kutzler), 289–304. St. Louis, MO: Saunders/Elsevier.

50 Englar, R.E. (2017). *Performing the Small Animal Physical Examination*. Hoboken, NJ: Wiley.

51 Harpster, N. (1983). Boxer cardiomyopathy. In: *Current Veterinary Therapy VIII* (ed. R. Kirk), 329–337. Philadelphia: WB Saunders.

52 Harpster, N.K. (1991). Boxer cardiomyopathy. A review of the long-term benefits of antiarrhythmic therapy. *Vet. Clin. North Am. Small Anim. Pract.* 21 (5): 989–1004.

53 Meurs, K.M., Spier, A.W., Miller, M.W. et al. (1999). Familial ventricular arrhythmias in boxers. *J. Vet. Intern. Med.* 13 (5): 437–439.

54 Meurs, K.M., Mauceli, E., Lahmers, S. et al. (2010). Genome-wide association identifies a deletion in the 3′ untranslated region of Striatin in a canine model of arrhythmogenic right ventricular cardiomyopathy. *Hum. Genet.* 128 (3): 315–324.

55 Al-Jassar, C., Bikker, H., Overduin, M., and Chidgey, M. (2013). Mechanistic basis of desmosome-targeted diseases. *J. Mol. Biol.* 425 (21): 4006–4022.

56 Harvey, A.M., Battersby, I.A., Faena, M. et al. (2005). Arrhythmogenic right ventricular cardiomyopathy in two cats. *J. Small Anim. Pract.* 46 (3): 151–156.

57 Fox, P.R., Maron, B.J., Basso, C. et al. (2000). Spontaneously occurring arrhythmogenic right ventricular cardiomyopathy in the domestic cat: a new animal model similar to the human disease. *Circulation* 102 (15): 1863–1870.

58 DeFrancesco, T.C. (2013). Management of cardiac emergencies in small animals. *Vet. Clin. North Am. Small Anim. Pract.* 43 (4): 817–842.

59 Burrage, H. (2012). Sick sinus syndrome in a dog: treatment with dual-chambered pacemaker implantation. *Can. Vet. J.-Revue Veterinaire Canadienne* 53 (5): 565–568.

60 James, R. (2007). Use of pacemakers in dogs. *In Pract.* 29 (9): 503–511.

61 Kavanagh, K. (2002). Sick sinus syndrome in a bull terrier. *Can. Vet. J.* 43 (1): 46–48.

62 Vailati, M.C., Schwartz, D.S., Galli, N.M. et al. (2011). ECG of the month. Sick sinus syndrome in a dog. *J. Am. Vet. Med. Assoc.* 238 (7): 850–852.

63 Bulmer, B. (2011). Sick sinus syndrome. In: *Clinical Veterinary Advisor: Dogs and Cats* (ed. E. Cote), 1022–1024. St. Louis: Elsevier.

64 Hamlin, R.L., Smetzer, D.L., and Breznock, E.M. (1972). Sinoatrial syncope in Miniature Schnauzers. *J. Am. Vet. Med. Assoc.* 161 (9): 1022–1028.

65 Moneva-Jordan, A., Corcoran, B.M., French, A. et al. (2001). Sick sinus syndrome in nine West Highland white terriers. *Vet. Rec.* 148 (5): 142–147.

66 Ward, J.L., DeFrancesco, T.C., Tou, S.P. et al. (2016). Outcome and survival in canine sick sinus syndrome and sinus node dysfunction: 93 cases (2002–2014). *J. Vet. Cardiol.* 18 (3): 199–212.

67 Johnson, M.S., Martin, M.W., and Henley, W. (2007). Results of pacemaker implantation in 104 dogs. *J. Small Anim. Pract.* 48 (1): 4–11.

68 Oyama, M.A., Sisson, D.D., and Lehmkuhl, L.B. (2001). Practices and outcome of artificial cardiac pacing in 154 dogs. *J. Vet. Intern. Med.* 15 (3): 229–239.

69 Wess, G., Thomas, W.P., Berger, D.M., and Kittleson, M.D. (2006). Applications, complications, and outcomes of transvenous pacemaker implantation in 105 dogs (1997–2002). *J. Vet. Intern. Med.* 20 (4): 877–884.

70 Kellum, H.B. and Stepien, R.L. (2006). Third-degree atrioventricular block in 21 cats (1997–2004). *J. Vet. Intern. Med.* 20 (1): 97–103.

71 Schrope, D.P. and Kelch, W.J. (2006). Signalment, clinical signs, and prognostic indicators associated with high-grade second- or third-degree atrioventricular block in dogs: 124 cases (January 1, 1997–December 31, 1997). *J. Am. Vet. Med. Assoc.* 228 (11): 1710–1717.

72 Lai, S.R. (2009). Atrioventricular muscular dystrophy in a 5-month-old English springer spaniel. *Can. Vet. J.* 50 (12): 1286–1287.

73 MacAulay, K. (2002). Permanent transvenous pacemaker implantation in an Ibizan hound cross with persistent atrial standstill. *Can. Vet. J.* 43 (10): 789–791.

74 Abbott, J.A. (2008). Acquired valvular disease. In: *Manual of Canine and Feline Cardiology*, 4e (ed. L.P. Tilley, F.W.K. Smith, M.A. Oyama and M.M. Sleeper), 110–138. Philadelphia: W.B. Saunders.

75 Chandler, M.L. (2016). Impact of obesity on cardiopulmonary disease. *Vet. Clin. North Am. Small Anim. Pract.* 817–830.

76 Olson, L.H., Haggstrom, J., and Henrik, D.P. (2010). Acquired valvular heart disease. In: *Textbook of Veterinary Internal Medicine* (ed. S.J. Ettinger and E.C. Feldman), 1299–1319. St. Louis: Saunders Elsevier.

77 Oyama, M.A. (2011). Canine heart failure – early diagnosis, prompt treatment. *NAVC Clinician's Brief* 9 (5).

78 Kittleson, M.D. (1998). The approach to the patient with cardiac disease. In: *Small Animal Cardiovascular Medicine* (ed. M.D. Kittleson and R.D. Kienle), 195–217. St. Louis: Mosby.

79 Schrope, D.P. (2015). Prevalence of congenital heart disease in 76,301 mixed-breed dogs and 57,025 mixed-breed cats. *J. Vet. Cardiol.* 17 (3): 192–202.

80 Tilley, L.P., Smith, F.W.K., and Tilley, L.P. (2007). *Blackwell's Five-Minute Veterinary Consult: Canine and Feline*, 4e, lx, 1578 p. Ames, Iowa: Blackwell.

81 Phan, A., Yates, G.D., Nimmo, J., and Holloway, S.A. (2013). Syncope associated with swallowing in two British Bulldogs with unilateral carotid body tumours. *Aust. Vet. J.* 91 (1–2). 47–51.

82 Hayes, H.M. (1975). An hypothesis for the aetiology of canine chemoreceptor system neoplasms, based upon an epidemiological study of 73 cases among hospital patients. *J. Small Anim. Pract.* 16 (5): 337–343.

83 Hayes, H.M. and Sass, B. (1988). Chemoreceptor neoplasia: a study of the epidemiological features of 357 canine cases. *Zentralbl. Veterinarmed. A* 35 (6): 401–408.

84 Dean, M.J. and Strafuss, A.C. (1975). Carotid body tumors in the dog: a review and report of four cases. *J. Am. Vet. Med. Assoc.* 166 (10): 1003–1006.

85 Obradovich, J.E., Withrow, S.J., Powers, B.E., and Walshaw, R. (1992). Carotid body tumors in the dog. Eleven cases (1978–1988). *J. Vet. Intern. Med.* 6 (2): 96–101.

86 Owen, T.J., Bruyette, D.S., and Layton, C.E. (1996). Chemodectoma in dogs. *Compend. Contin. Educ. Pract.* 18 (3): 253–264.

87 Patnaik, A.K., Liu, S.K., Hurvitz, A.I., and McClelland, A.J. (1975). Canine chemodectoma (extra-adrenal paragangliomas)–a comparative study. *J. Small Anim. Pract.* 16 (12): 785–801.

88 Yates, W.D., Lester, S.J., and Mills, J.H. (1980). Chemoreceptor tumors diagnosed at the Western College of Veterinary Medicine 1967–1979. *Can. Vet. J.* 21 (4): 124–129.

89 Chedid, A. and Jao, W. (1974). Hereditary tumors of the carotid bodies and chronic obstructive pulmonary disease. *Cancer* 33 (6): 1635–1641.

90 Oyama, M.A. and Cardiomyopathy, C. (2008). *Manual of Canine and Feline Cardiology*, 4e (ed. L.P. Tilley, F.W.K. Smith, M.A. Oyama and M.M. Sleeper), 139–150. Philadelphia: W.B. Saunders.

91 Kienle, R.D. (2008). Feline cardiomyopathy. In: *Manual of Canine and Feline Cardiology*, 4e (ed. L.P. Tilley, F.W.K. Smith, M.A. Oyama and M.M. Sleeper), 151–175. Philadelphia: W.B. Saunders.

92 Mazzaferro, E.M. (2006). Acute collapse. *NAVC Clinician's Brief* (December): 15–16.

93 Fuentes, V.L. (2006). Cardiomyopathy: establishing a diagnosis. In: *Consultations in Feline Internal Medicine*, 5e (ed. J.R. August), 301–310. St. Louis: Saunders Elsevier.

94 Ferasin, L., Sturgess, C.P., Cannon, M.J. et al. (2003). Feline idiopathic cardiomyopathy: a retrospective study of 106 cats (1994–2001). *J. Feline Med. Surg.* 5 (3): 151–159.

95 Haggstrom, J., Fuentes, V.L., and Wess, G. (2015). Screening for hypertrophic cardiomyopathy in cats. *J. Vet. Cardiol.* 17: S134–S149.

96 Kittleson, M.D., Meurs, K.M., Munro, M.J. et al. (1999). Familial hypertrophic cardiomyopathy in Maine coon cats: an animal model of human disease. *Circulation* 99 (24): 3172–3180.

97 Meurs, K.M., Norgard, M.M., Ederer, M.M. et al. (2007). A substitution mutation in the myosin binding protein C gene in ragdoll hypertrophic cardiomyopathy. *Genomics* 90 (2): 261–264.

98 Meurs, K.M., Sanchez, X., David, R.M. et al. (2005). A cardiac myosin binding protein C mutation in the Maine coon cat with familial hypertrophic cardiomyopathy. *Hum. Mol. Genet.* 14 (23): 3587–3593.

99 Rishniw, M. (2006). Feline aortic thromboembolism. *NAVC Clinician's Brief* (November): 17–20.

100 Fuentes, V.L. (2012). Arterial thromboembolism. Risks, realities and a rational first-line approach. *J. Feline Med. Surg.* 14 (7): 459–470.

101 Moore, K.E., Morris, N., Dhupa, N. et al. (2000). Retrospective study of streptokinase administration in 46 cats with arterial thromboembolism. *J. Vet. Emerg. Crit. Care* 10: 245–257.

102 Ferasin, L. (2012). Feline cardiomyopathy. *In Pract.* 34 (4): 204–213.

103 Cote, E. and Harpster, N.K. (2009). Feline cardiac arrhythmias. In: *Kirk's Current Veterinary Therapy*

XIV (ed. R.W. Kirk), 731–739. St. Louis, MO: Elsevier Saunders.

104 Dirven, M.J., Cornelissen, J.M., Barendse, M.A. et al. (2010). Cause of heart murmurs in 57 apparently healthy cats. *Tijdschr. Diergeneeskd.* 135 (22): 840–847.

105 Laste, N.J. and Harpster, N.K. (1995). A retrospective study of 100 cases of feline distal aortic thromboembolism: 1977–1993. *J. Am. Anim. Hosp. Assoc.* 31 (6): 492–500.

106 Smith, S.A., Tobias, A.H., Jacob, K.A. et al. (2003). Arterial thromboembolism in cats: acute crisis in 127 cases (1992–2001) and long-term management with low-dose aspirin in 24 cases. *J. Vet. Intern. Med.* 17 (1): 73–83.

107 Gordon, S.G. (2006). Cardiomyopathy – therapeutic decisions. In: *Consultations in Feline Internal Medicine*, 5e (ed. J.R. August), 311–317. St. Louis: Saunders Elsevier.

108 Smith, S.A. and Tobias, A.H. (2004). Feline arterial thromboembolism: an update. *Vet. Clin. North Am. Small Anim. Pract.* 34 (5): 1245–1271.

109 Gompf, R.E. (2008). The history and physical examination. In: *Manual of Canine and Feline Cardiology* (ed. L.P. Tilley, F.W.K. Smith, M.A. Oyama and M.M. Sleeper), 2–23. St. Louis: Elsevier Saunders.

110 Fox, P.R. and Schober, K.E. (2015). Management of asymptomatic (occult) feline cardiomyopathy: challenges and realities. *J. Vet. Cardiol.* 17: S150–S158.

111 Jones, A. and Estrada, A. (2014). Top 5 arrhythmias in dogs and cats. *NAVC Clinician's Brief* (January): 94–100.

112 Thomason, J.D., Kraus, M.S., Surdyk, K.K. et al. (2008). Bradycardia-associated syncope in 7 Boxers with ventricular tachycardia (2002–2005). *J. Vet. Intern. Med.* 22 (4): 931–936.

113 Campbell, F.E. (2007). Cardiac effects of pulmonary disease. *Vet. Clin. North Am. Small Anim. Pract.* 37 (5): 949–962, vii.

114 Litster, A.L. and Atwell, R.B. (2008). Feline heartworm disease: a clinical review. *J. Feline Med. Surg.* 10 (2): 137–144.

115 Tilley, L.P. and Smith, F.W.K. (2016). *Blackwell's Five-Minute Veterinary Consult. Canine and Feline*, 6e, lxix, 1622 p. Ames, Iowa, USA: Wiley.

116 Hoeper, M.M., Oudiz, R.J., Peacock, A. et al. (2004). End points and clinical trial designs in pulmonary arterial hypertension: clinical and regulatory perspectives. *J. Am. Coll. Cardiol.* 43 (12 Suppl S): 48S–55S.

117 Barst, R.J., McGoon, M., Torbicki, A. et al. (2004). Diagnosis and differential assessment of pulmonary arterial hypertension. *J. Am. Coll. Cardiol.* 43 (12 Suppl S): 40S–47S.

118 Johnson, L. (1999). Diagnosis of pulmonary hypertension. *Clin. Tech. Small Anim. Pract.* 14 (4): 231–236.

119 Johnson, L., Boon, J., and Orton, E.C. (1999). Clinical characteristics of 53 dogs with Doppler-derived evidence of pulmonary hypertension: 1992–1996. *J. Vet. Intern. Med.* 13 (5): 440–447.

41

Jugular Vein Distension and Jugular Pulses

41.1 An Anatomical Review of the Jugular Vein

Recall from studying anatomy that veins represent vascular channels through which blood returns to the heart [1, 2].

As compared to arteries, veins tend to be low pressure, thin-walled conduits [1, 3]. Because their walls lack a high percentage of collagen and elastin, veins expand readily [1]. They can contain large volumes of blood under relatively low pressure [1].

Unlike arteries, healthy veins are pulseless [1]. Blood flow through veins depends largely upon muscular contractions, which compress the vessels to encourage venous return to the heart [1].

Venous blood continues to flow forward, in large part because intravascular valves prevent backflow [1]. These valves are greatest in number in vessels furthest from the heart [1].

In addition, the inspiratory half of the respiratory cycle causes the thoracic cavity to carry a net negative pressure. This contributes to forward, rather than backward, flow [1].

Blood is ultimately returned to the heart by means of the cranial vena cava and the caudal vena cava [1, 2]. The cranial vena cava drains the head, neck, and forelimbs [1, 2].

The external jugular veins are paired vessels, one on each side of the neck, that empty into the cranial vena cava [1, 2].

The external jugular veins are superficial and accessible for venipuncture in both the dog and cat [1, 4].

In health, neither is grossly apparent without a restrainer manually holding off the vessel [4, 5].

41.2 Venous Return

If venous return is reduced, then the external jugular veins may become visibly distended [4].

Venous return refers to blood flow back to the heart from peripheral vessels [6]. How much blood returns to the heart determines how much blood can be pumped out during the next phase of the cardiac cycle, ventricular contraction [6].

The movement of any fluid from point A to point B depends upon pressure gradients. Blood is no different. Pressure gradients within the vasculature dictate the direction in which blood flows as well as the speed by which it gets there [6, 7].

If right atrial pressure decreases, then venous return increases [6, 7]. If right atrial pressure increases, then venous return decreases [6, 7].

In addition to pressure, vascular resistance affects venous return [7]. Vascular resistance refers to the impediment(s) that must be overcome to move blood forward through the system. Vascular resistance can be affected by the following:

- Blood viscosity
- Vessel length
- Vessel diameter

Blood that is more viscous is more resistant to flow than blood that is thinner in consistency [6]. Blood develops high viscosity when the patient is hemoconcentrated. Elevations in erythrocyte concentration thicken the blood, making blood flow through the system sluggish.

Vessels that have smaller diameters have increased resistance to flow as compared to those with larger diameters [6]. Very small changes in vessel radius create dynamic changes in blood flow because resistance is inversely proportional to the fourth power of the vessel's radius [6].

Smooth muscle lines the walls of the vasculature [6]. Smooth muscle will respond to circulating hormones and local mediators by adjusting vessel diameter. Vasoconstriction increases systemic vascular resistance and may be triggered by smooth muscle agonists, including circulating catecholamines and locally produced endothelin [6, 8].

The catecholamines, epinephrine and norepinephrine, increase venous return by inducing vasoconstriction of most systemic arteries and veins. In addition, catecholamines increase heart rate and cardiac contractility to pump out more blood with each heartbeat.

Endothelin causes venoconstriction, which increases blood flow back to the heart [6, 8, 9].

Collectively, endothelin and the catecholamines improve cardiac output.

By contrast, the presence of vascular smooth muscle antagonists, such as nitric oxide, prostacyclin, and prostaglandins, dilates arterioles. This reduces venous return [6, 8, 9].

Venous return may also be compromised by [6, 8, 9]

- A true obstruction to blood flow through the vasculature
- Compression of the vasculature by surrounding tissue, causing an apparent obstruction to blood flow.

41.3 Clinically Apparent Signs of Poor Venous Return

In a normal patient, the external jugular veins are neither palpable nor visible without the restrainer applying direct pressure at the thoracic inlet [10].

When pressure is applied to the neck of a normal patient at the level of the thoracic inlet, then the external jugular vein on that same side will fill. The vessel will stay distended until the pressure is released, at which point the external jugular vein will rapidly disappear from view [10].

In a patient that has compromised venous return, the external jugular vein will stay distended, whether or not manual pressure is applied to the thoracic inlet [4, 10–12].

Jugular vein distension is best assessed with the patient in either a standing or a seated position [12]. Holding the head and neck in extension improves visualization [10].

Jugular vein distension will be difficult to appreciate in patients with long fur coats because the fur obstructs the view of the neck. The clinician may need to wet the fur over the cervical region with alcohol to facilitate inspection [10]. Shaving the neck may also be necessary [10].

In addition to jugular vein distension, both external jugular veins may develop a visible pulse with each heartbeat [4, 5, 11].

If a pulse is present that extends more than one-third of the way up the neckline from the thoracic inlet, then it is a jugular pulse, and it is considered abnormal [11].

Atrial contraction and filling are responsible for the jugular pulse wave that is visible.

Other physical examination findings that are suggestive of poor venous return include "stocking up" of the ventral thorax and abdomen [4]. This refers to the development of edema, that is, abnormal water retention in gravity-dependent regions of the body. When "stocking up" involves the abdominal cavity, it is referred to as abdominal effusion or ascites [4, 13].

Edema secondary to poor venous return may also be present at the level of the tarsal joints or, in males, at and around the prepuce [4].

41.4 The Pathophysiology of Jugular Vein Distension and Jugular Pulses

Section 41.2 provided a brief outline of the physiology that causes jugular vein distension and/or jugular pulses. This section will introduce specific diseases that cause one or both clinical signs.

Several pathological conditions impair venous return in companion animal patients.

The most common etiology is right-sided heart failure [4, 12].

Recall from Chapter 38, Section 38.4.1.4 that the heart is a pump [14, 15]. Its purpose is to push blood through the vasculature as a vehicle for the delivery of oxygen and nutrients to tissues [14, 15].

Whereas the left ventricle of the heart receives oxygenated blood from the lungs and pumps it into systemic circulation, the right ventricle of the heart receives deoxygenated blood from the periphery and delivers it to the lungs to refuel.

Right-sided heart failure is often associated with increased filling pressure within the right ventricle [12, 13]. When the right side of the heart fails, it becomes ineffective as a pump. This causes a backlog of blood waiting to progress through the vasculature. Blood backs up from the right ventricle into the right atrium, and from the right atrium into the cranial and caudal vena cava.

Blood backing up into the caudal vena cava causes distension of abdominal vessels, including those that are connected to the liver. Hepatomegaly is likely to result.

Blood backing up into the cranial vena cava causes both external jugular veins to become distended [4].

Note that not all patients with right-sided heart failure develop jugular vein distension and/or jugular pulses [11]. These clinical features are far more likely to occur in dogs than cats [11]. Even so, only about 7 out of every 10 dogs with right-sided heart failure will present with jugular distension [11]; cats rarely do [11].

Right-sided heart failure may result from structural and/or functional cardiac dysfunction, including the following [4, 11, 12, 16–18]:
- Failure of the heart to pump
  - Dilated cardiomyopathy (DCM) (see Chapter 40, Section 40.4.3.4)
  - Doxorubicin-associated cardiac toxicity
  - Hyperthyroidism
- Volume overload of the right ventricle
  - Tricuspid valve dysplasia
- Pressure overload of the right ventricle
  - Heartworm disease (see Chapter 35, Section 35.4.3 and Chapter 40, Section 40.4.5)
  - Pulmonary hypertension
  - Pulmonary thromboembolism (see Chapter 38, Section 38.4.3)
  - Pulmonic stenosis (see Chapter 40, Section 40.4.3.6)
- Inability to fill the right ventricle
  - Neoplasia
    ○ Cranial vena cava
    ○ Caudal vena cava
    ○ Right atrium
  - Pericardial effusion and cardiac tamponade (see Chapter 42)
  - Restrictive pericarditis
  - Tricuspid valve stenosis

Severe arrhythmias may also cause jugular distension [11]. For example, when electrical impulses are not coordinated between the atria and ventricles, the atria may contract prematurely, against a closed tricuspid valve [11]. In this clinical scenario, blood cannot move forward into the ventricles [11]. Instead, blood must follow the path of least resistance, which is backward movement, directly into the venous system [11].

41.5 Diagnostic Work-Up for Patients with Jugular Vein Distension and/or Jugular Pulses

Patients that present with external jugular vein distension and/or jugular pulses should undergo a diagnostic work-up for right-sided heart failure.

As with all clinical presentations, history taking and physical examination should be prioritized over diagnostic testing in the initial phases of the work-up, provided that the patient is stable.

During history taking, clients may report changes in attitude or activity level. They may describe that the patient appears weak, lethargic, or exercise intolerant.

Dogs with right-sided heart failure tend to develop hepatomegaly and ascites, without concurrent pleural effusion.

Cats with right-sided heart failure frequently present with both.

Both pleural effusion and ascites can adversely affect the respiratory cycle. Breaths may become rapid and shallow.

If pleural effusion is present and/or if there is pericardial effusion, then the patient is likely to have muffled heart sounds. This is evident on cardiopulmonary auscultation.

Another physical examination tool to test the heart's ability to circulate blood properly is the hepatojugular reflex [10–12]. To assess this reflex, the clinician compresses the patient's abdomen for 10–30 s [10–12]. Compression of the abdomen increases venous return [10–12].

A normal patient can handle this increase in blood volume flowing back to the heart [10–12]. However, a patient with right-sided heart failure is intolerant of volume overload [10–12]. This patient experiences a back-up of blood into the cranial vena cava and, ultimately, the external jugular veins [10–12]. The external jugular veins respond to the added volume by distending [10–12].

After taking a history and performing a physical examination, imaging studies are essential to evaluate the patient for cardiac disease [18].

Thoracic radiographs may depict an enlarged cardiac silhouette [17] (see Figures 41.1a, b).

Thoracic radiographs may depict right-sided cardiomegaly. When the right side of the heart enlarges, it may take on the shape of a "reverse D" on dorsoventral (D/V) thoracic radiographs [13] (see Figures 41.2a, b).

When the right side of the heart enlarges, it may have increased sternal contact on lateral thoracic radiographs [13] (see Figure 41.3).

Cardiac imaging in the form of an echocardiogram and Doppler echocardiography is likely to provide a definitive diagnosis [18]. These tools can confirm structural issues with heart valves, including the tricuspid, such as valvular insufficiency and valvular stenosis [18].

In addition, electrocardiography is an important diagnostic for cardiac arrhythmias [18].

(a)

(b)

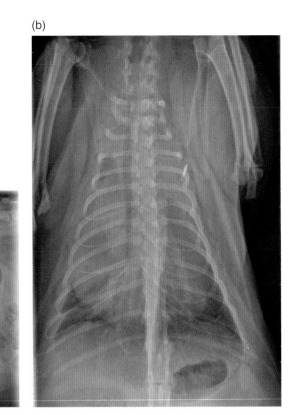

Figure 41.1 (a) Right lateral thoracic radiograph of a feline patient with an enlarged cardiac silhouette. This patient was subsequently diagnosed with pericardial effusion. *Source:* Courtesy of Daniel Foy, MS, DVM, DACVIM, DACVECC. (b) Ventrodorsal (V/D) thoracic radiograph of the same patient that was depicted in Figure 41.1a. Note the enlarged cardiac silhouette. *Source:* Courtesy of Daniel Foy, MS, DVM, DACVIM, DACVECC.

(a)   (b)

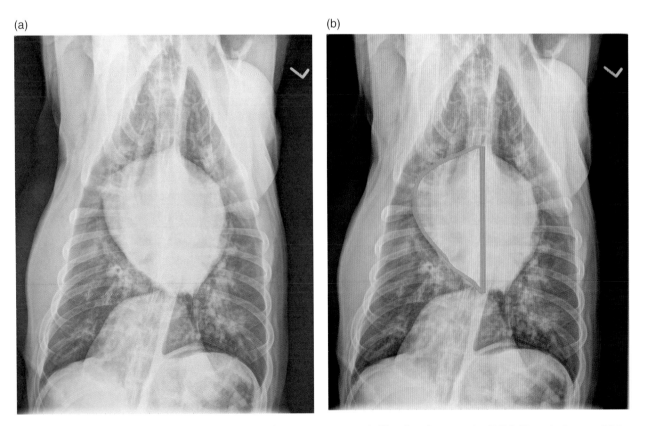

Figure 41.2 (a) Dorsoventral (D/V) thoracic radiograph of a canine patient with dilated cardiomyopathy (DCM). Note the "reverse D" shape that implies right-sided cardiomegaly. *Source:* Courtesy of Daniel Foy, MS, DVM, DACVIM, DACVECC. (b) Same radiograph as seen in Figure 41.2a, with the "reverse D" shape outlined in orange. *Source:* Courtesy of Daniel Foy, MS, DVM, DACVIM, DACVECC.

Figure 41.3 Right lateral thoracic radiograph of a canine patient with DCM. Note the increased sternal contact that is suggestive of right-sided heart enlargement. *Source:* Courtesy of Daniel Foy, MS, DVM, DACVIM, DACVECC.

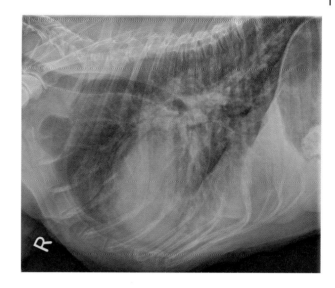

References

1 Evans, H.E. and Miller, M.E. (2013). *Miller's Anatomy of the Dog*, 4e, xix, 850 p. St. Louis, Missouri: Elsevier.

2 Singh, B. and Dyce, K.M. (2018). *Dyce, Sack, and Wensing's Textbook of Veterinary Anatomy*, 5e. St. Louis, Missouri: Saunders.

3 Engen, R.L. (2004). Dynamics of the cardiovascular system. In: *Dukes' Physiology of Domestic Animals*, 12e (ed. W.O. Reece), 181–191. Ithaca: Cornell University Press.

4 Englar, R.E. (2017). *Performing the Small Animal Physical Examination*. Hoboken, NJ: Wiley.

5 Gompf, R.E. (2008). The history and physical examination. In: *Manual of Canine and Feline Cardiology* (ed. L.P. Tilley, S. FWK, M. Oyama and M.M. Sleeper), 2–23. St. Louis, Missouri: Saunders, an imprint of Elsevier Inc.

6 Hall, J.E. and Guyton, A.C. (2011). *Guyton and Hall Textbook of Medical Physiology*, 12e, xix, 1091 p. Philadelphia, PA: Saunders/Elsevier.

7 Young, D.B. (2010). *Control of Cardiac Output*. San Rafael, CA: Morgan & Claypool Life Sciences.

8 Sandoo, A., van Zanten, J.J., Metsios, G.S. et al. (2010). The endothelium and its role in regulating vascular tone. *Open Cardiovasc. Med. J.* 4: 302–312.

9 Miller, V.M., Komori, K., Burnett, J.C. Jr., and Vanhoutte, P.M. (1989). Differential sensitivity to endothelin in canine arteries and veins. *Am. J. Phys.* 257 (4 Pt 2): H1127–H1131.

10 Estrada, A. (2017). Cardiac physical examination. NAVC Clinician's Brief [Internet]. https://www.cliniciansbrief.com/article/basic-cardiology-examination.

11 Cole, S.G. and Drobatz, K.J. (2008). Emergency management and critical care. In: *Manual of Canine and Feline Cardiology* (ed. L.P. Tilley, F.W.K. Smith, M. Oyama and M.M. Sleeper), 2–23. Philadelphia: Saunders.

12 Hogan, D.F. (2008). Cardiac examination & history. *NAVC Clinician's Brief* (July): 49–53.

13 MacDonald, K. (2011). Back to basics: clinical cardiovascular exam and diagnostic testing. DVM 360 [Internet]. http://veterinarycalendar.dvm360.com/back-basics-clinical-cardiovascular-exam-and-diagnostic-testing-proceedings.

14 Reece, W.O., Erickson, H.H., Goff, J.P., and Uemura, E.E. (2015). *Dukes' Physiology of Domestic Animals*, 13e, xii, 748 p. Ames, Iowa, USA: Wiley Blackwell.

15 Estrada, A. (2014). Heart disease: diagnosis & treatment. *NAVC Clinician's Brief* (March): 91–95.

16 Oyama, M.A. (2011). Clinical notes: Canine heart failure – early diagnosis, prompt treatment. NAVC Clinician's Brief [Internet]. 9(5). https://repository.upenn.edu/cgi/viewcontent.cgi?article=1002&context=vet_papers.

17 Wey, A.C. (2005). Cardiomegaly. *NAVC Clinician's Brief* (March): 7–8.

18 Boswood, A. (2010). Chronic valvular disease in the dog. *NAVC Clinician's Brief* (December): 17–21.

42

Muffled Heart Sounds

42.1 The Cardiac Cycle and Origin of Heart Sounds

Recall that the heart is a pump [1, 2]. It functions to push blood through a network of vessels to deliver oxygen and nutrients to tissues of the body [1, 2]. In order to achieve forward flow, the system has to work harmoniously through a coordinated cycle of contraction (systole) and relaxation (diastole). This cycle is referred to as the cardiac cycle [3, 4].

The cardiac cycle coordinates movement of blood through the system [3, 4]. To understand this system, let us trace the path of oxygenated blood that has a starting point within the left ventricle.

During systole, this blood is pumped from the left ventricle out of the heart, through the aorta. The aorta connects to a series of arteries, arterioles, and capillary beds that perfuse tissues with oxygen [3, 4].

Deoxygenated blood is gathered up by venules. These pool into veins that track blood back to the right atrium. Blood fills the right atrium and right ventricle during diastole [3, 4].

When systole recurs, blood is forced out from the right ventricle, through the pulmonary artery, and into the lungs. Within the lungs at the level of the alveoli, blood is re-oxygenated. Re-oxygenated blood returns to the heart through the pulmonary vein to fill the left atrium and left ventricle during diastole [3, 4].

The cycle repeats [3–5].

Note that this simplification only focuses on one side of the heart at any given point in time. In reality, both sides of the heart are working simultaneously to pump blood through both the pulmonary and systemic circulations [3, 4].

In order for this system to effectively move blood in a net forward direction, the heart relies upon valves [3, 4]. Valves minimize backflow [3, 4]. There are two primary sets of valves within the heart [3, 4]:

- The atrioventricular (AV) valves
  - The right AV, or tricuspid, valve, which sits between the right atrium and right ventricle

- The left AV, or mitral, valve, which sits between the left atrium and left ventricle
- The semilunar valves
  - The aortic valve, which separates the left ventricle and the aorta
  - The pulmonic valve, which separates the right ventricle and the pulmonary artery

During systole, the AV valves close. This prevents blood from flowing backward, that is, from the ventricles to the atria [3–5].

At the beginning of diastole, the aortic and pulmonic valves close to allow blood to fill the heart. Blood from the lungs fills the left side of the heart via the pulmonary vein; blood from systemic circulation fills the right side of the heart via the cranial and caudal vena cava [3–5].

The closing of heart valves results in normal heart sounds [3–5].

At their most basic, normal heart sounds consist of "lub-dub."

The first heart sound, the "lub," is called S1. S1 is created by closure of the AV valves to facilitate ventricular contraction [3–6].

The second heart sound, the "dub," is called S2. S2 is created by closure of the pulmonic and aortic valves to allow the heart to fill [3–6].

In the normal patient, these sounds should be crisp and easy to differentiate during auscultation of the heart with a stethoscope [3, 6].

Additional heart sounds, such as S3 and S4, are unlikely to be heard in the normal patient [3, 6]; however, these may be heard during pathology [3, 6]:

- Conditions that involve ventricular dilation, such as dilated cardiomyopathy (DCM), may promote the heart sound, S3. S3 occurs on the coat tails of S2 as blood flows from the atria into the ventricles.
- Conditions that involve atrial dilation, such as hypertrophic cardiomyopathy (HCM), may promote the heart sound, S4. S4 occurs with atrial contraction, just prior to S1.

Common Clinical Presentations in Dogs and Cats, First Edition. Ryane E. Englar.
© 2019 John Wiley & Sons, Inc. Published 2019 by John Wiley & Sons, Inc.

The presence of S3 or S4 creates so-called gallop rhythms [3]. These are beyond the scope of this chapter.

42.2 Indistinct Heart Sounds

S1 and S2 should be audible and clear in all canine and feline patients [3, 6]. When they are not, heart sounds are said to be muffled. This means that the heart sounds very far away.

Muffled heart sounds typically result from abnormal tissue or fluid getting in between the heart and the stethoscope, which is firmly placed against the body wall. This creates an extra layer or obstacle through which sound has to travel to be heard.

Morbidly obese patients may have indistinct heart sounds because the insulating layer of fat represents a sound barrier.

Muffled heart sounds may also result from cardiac or respiratory pathology, including pericardial and pleural effusions [7–14].

42.3 Structure and Function of the Pericardium

The pericardium is a two-layered sac that surrounds the heart [7, 15–17]. The innermost layer is the visceral pericardium, otherwise known as the epicardium. This layer directly contacts the myocardium. The outermost layer, the parietal pericardium, attaches to the diaphragm, via the phrenopericardial ligament, as well as to the exterior of the following vessels [7, 15–17]:

- Ascending aorta
- Cranial vena cava
- Caudal vena cava
- Main pulmonary artery
- Pulmonary veins

Between the two layers of the pericardium is a scant amount of serous fluid [7, 15, 16]. In health, this fluid approximates 0.25 ml/kg of body weight [7, 17].

A patient can live without the pericardium [7]. The pericardium is not essential for survival.

Its presence is largely protective [7, 17]. It lessens the risk of cardiac infections and adhesions to the heart because it serves as a barrier [17]. The pericardium is also believed to support the heart in a central position [7, 17].

42.4 The Pathophysiology of Pericardial Effusion

Unlike veins, the pericardium is not elastic [7]. Its compliance is poor, and it will not stretch to support acute accumulations of intrapericardial fluid [7].

When fluid increases in volume within the pericardial sac, the patient is said to have pericardial effusion [9].

Pericardial effusion compresses the heart [7]. This phenomenon is referred to as cardiac tamponade [7, 9, 17]. Specifically, cardiac tamponade refers to the collapse of the right atrium during diastole [9].

In health, intrapericardial pressure is less than both right ventricular and left ventricular diastolic pressures [7, 18, 19].

Pericardial effusion increases intrapericardial pressure [7, 17, 18]. When intrapericardial pressure becomes equal to ventricular diastolic pressure, the heart's ability to fill with blood is impaired [7, 18]. The walls of the various chambers of the heart begin to collapse in systole [7]. When this occurs, the heart becomes an inefficient pump. Forward flow of blood decreases. The patient attempts to compensate via tachycardia and peripheral vasoconstriction [7].

When the intrapericardial pressure exceeds the right atrial pressure, the patient experiences cardiogenic shock. Death is imminent without medical intervention [7, 9].

Another unique feature of cardiac tamponade is that the phase of the respiratory cycle influences the ventricular stroke volume [7]. The intrapleural pressure becomes negative every time a patient inhales [7]. At the same time, the intrapericardial pressure decreases [7]. This drop in the intrapericardial pressure allows the right ventricle to fill better [7].

Because the pericardium is not a compliant tissue, a stretch in one compartment of the heart occurs at the expense of another [7]. As the right ventricle expands, the left ventricular volume is reduced, which in turn decreases the left ventricular stroke volume [7]. There is a corresponding drop in the systolic systemic arterial pressure [7].

When the patient exhales, the reverse is true [7]. The intrapericardial pressure increases. This impairs filling of the right ventricle. Because the right ventricle is not expanded to its maximum capacity, the left ventricular volume is able to increase [7]. This results in a greater left ventricular stroke volume [7]. There is a corresponding increase in the systolic systemic arterial pressure [7].

This cycle repeats with each breath: inspiration depresses the systolic systemic arterial pressure as compared to expiration, which causes an increase [7].

Respiration always influences the arterial pulse amplitude. However, this effect is exaggerated in cases of pericardial effusion. When it occurs, it is called pulsus paradoxus [7].

Femoral pulses may vary in intensity in patients that are clinical for pericardial effusion. These fluctuations may be palpable on physical examination as pulses that alternate between weak and strong [20]. When this occurs, the patient is said to exhibit pulsus alternans [9].

42.5 Etlologles of Pericardial Effusion

Pericardial effusion is relatively rare in companion animal patients [7, 9, 10, 21].

In the dog, pericardial effusion is most often either idiopathic or neoplastic [7, 9, 17, 18, 22–25]. The most common neoplastic causes of pericardial effusion in dogs are the following [7, 9, 17, 18, 22–25]:

- Chemodectoma
- Ectopic thyroid carcinoma
- Hemangiosarcoma (HSA)
- Lymphosarcoma (LSA)
- Mesothelioma
- Metastatic adenocarcinoma

Idiopathic pericardial effusion is common in dogs [17]. Large-breed, middle-aged dogs seem to be predisposed [17]. Males appear in the veterinary medical literature more so than females [17].

Less commonly, dogs may develop pericardial effusion secondary to the following [9, 17]:

- Coagulopathy
  - Disseminated intravascular coagulation (DIC)
  - Anticoagulant rodenticide toxicity
- Congestive heart failure (CHF)
- Infectious pericarditis
- Left atrial rupture, secondary to advanced valvular endocardiosis
- Penetrating trauma
- Uremia

Infectious pericarditis is typically due to coccidioidomycosis or Valley Fever, which is more likely to occur in dogs in the southwestern United States [9, 26].

In the cat, the most common cause of pericardial effusion is cardiomyopathy [7, 10, 27–29]. In particular, the following heart-associated conditions have been linked to pericardial effusion in cats [7, 10, 27–29]:

- CHF
- DCM
- HCM
- Hyperthyroidism
- Mitral valve dysplasia
- Restrictive cardiomyopathy (RCM)

Infectious disease is also a cause of pericardial effusion in cats, particularly feline infectious peritonitis (FIP) [17].

Less common causes of pericardial effusion in cats include the following [7, 8, 10, 18, 21]:

- Coagulopathy
- Neoplasia
  - LSA
  - Metastatic neoplasia
- Uremia

42.6 Patient Presentations Relative to Pericardial Effusion

Patients with pericardial effusion often present for general malaise [9]. Clients may report lethargy or inappetence [9]. Patients may be intolerant of exercise [9]. In severe cases, they may present for collapse [9, 13]. Refer to Chapter 40 to explore other causes of collapse in the companion animal patient. Collapse is more likely to occur when canine patients develop pericardial effusion secondary to cardiac disease as opposed to idiopathic pericardial effusion [17].

Physical examination of patients with pericardial effusion varies, depending upon the stage in which they present [9].

Muffled heart and/or lung sounds are consistent with pericardial effusion [7–14]. Patients may also demonstrate compensatory tachycardia [7, 9].

Weak femoral pulses are typical; however, patients may exhibit pulsus alternans [11, 17].

In addition, because signs of right-sided congestion predominate, patients with pericardial effusion may present with the following clinical signs [17, 23, 25, 30–32]:

- Ascites
- Hepatomegaly
- Jugular vein distension +/– jugular pulses (see Chapter 41)
- Labored respiration
- Positive hepatojugular reflex (see Chapter 41)

42.7 Diagnostic Work-Up for Muffled Heart Sounds

Imaging is the primary means by which muffled heart sounds are evaluated [9].

Thoracic radiographs may be unremarkable in cases involving acute hemorrhage [9]. Acute hemopericardium is most often associated with HSA [9].

By contrast, chronic effusions are typically associated with an enlarged cardiac silhouette, in which the heart takes on a characteristically globoid or basketball shape [8, 17, 33] (see Figure 42.1).

Chronic effusions are typically slowly progressive, with gradual accumulation of pericardial fluid [9]. This process is typical of patients with primary pericardial disease, such as idiopathic pericarditis, mesothelioma, or a heart-base tumor [9].

Note that an enlarged cardiac silhouette is not pathognomonic for pericardial effusion [17]. Enlarged cardiac silhouettes may also result from an enlargement of one or more cardiac chambers, generalized cardiomyopathy, and peritoneopericardial hernias [34] (see Figures 42.2a–d).

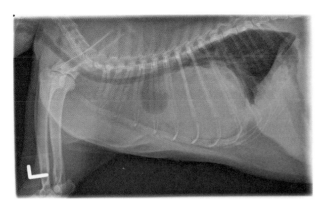

Figure 42.1 Left lateral thoracic radiograph of a feline patient with an enlarged cardiac silhouette. This patient was subsequently diagnosed with pericardial effusion. *Source:* Courtesy of Daniel Foy, MS, DVM, DACVIM, DACVECC.

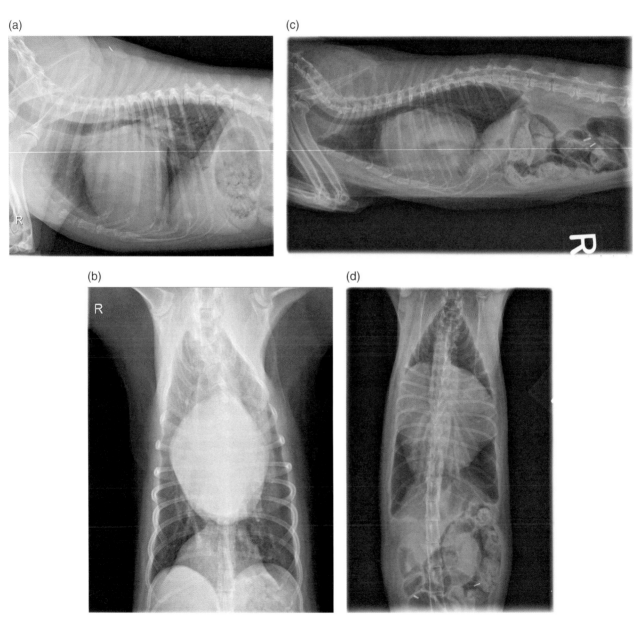

(a)

(c)

(b)

(d)

Figure 42.2 (a) Right lateral thoracic radiograph of a canine patient with generalized cardiomegaly. This patient did not have pericardial effusion. *Source:* Courtesy of Daniel Foy, MS, DVM, DACVIM, DACVECC. (b) Orthogonal view of the same patient that was depicted in Figure 42.2a. *Source:* Courtesy of Daniel Foy, MS, DVM, DACVIM, DACVECC. (c) Right lateral thoracic radiograph of a patient with a peritoneopericardial hernia. *Source:* Courtesy of Daniel Foy, MS, DVM, DACVIM, DACVECC. (d) Orthogonal view of the same patient that was depicted in Figure 42.2c. *Source:* Courtesy of Daniel Foy, MS, DVM, DACVIM, DACVECC.

(a)

(b)

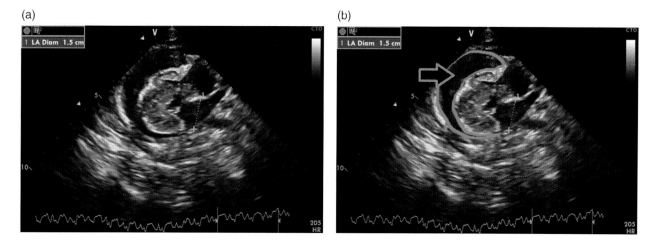

Figure 42.3 (a) Long-axis view echocardiogram showing pericardial effusion. *Source:* Courtesy of Justin Thomason, DACVIM (cardiology; SAIM), Wildcat Cardiology and Christy Zimmer Coyle, RVT. (b) Same figure as above with the region of pericardial effusion outlined in orange. *Source:* Courtesy of Justin Thomason, DACVIM (cardiology; SAIM), Wildcat Cardiology and Christy Zimmer Coyle, RVT.

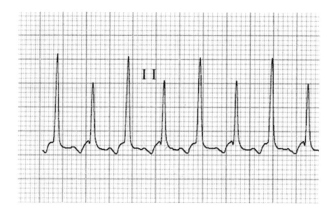

Figure 42.4 Electrical alternans as depicted on Lead 2 of an electrocardiogram (ECG) of a canine patient with pericardial effusion.

Cases of pericardial effusion may also exhibit the following radiographic changes [17]:

- Ascites
- Distension of the caudal vena cava
- Hepatomegaly
- Pleural effusion

When patients have HSA, pulmonary metastases are common [17].

If a heart-base tumor is present, the trachea may deviate dorsally [17].

As an imaging modality, echocardiography is more sensitive than thoracic radiography in the detection of pericardial effusion, particularly when it consists of only a small volume of fluid [7, 9, 11, 12, 17, 30, 31, 35].

In health, the two-layered pericardium is visualized through echocardiography as a single echogenic structure [7].

When there is pericardial effusion, a hypoechoic space arises between the heart and the pericardium [7, 9, 17] (see Figures 42.3a, b).

Echocardiography may also confirm cardiac tamponade [9].

In addition to diagnosing pericardial effusion, echocardiography is a valuable tool to scan the heart and heart base for tumors [9, 17]. HSA is most frequently implicated in canine cases involving right atrial or right auricular masses [9, 17, 36]. However, HSA may also involve the heart base [36]. HSA is rare in cats [17].

By the time HSA has been diagnosed within the heart, metastasis is likely [17].

Other heart-base tumors include chemodectomas, otherwise known as aortic body tumors [17]. These are consistently well-circumscribed, locally invasive, 2–3 cm masses [36].

Note that tumors may be hidden from view if they are associated with the right auricle [9].

In addition to echocardiography, electrocardiography (ECG) may support a diagnosis of large-volume pericardial effusion by demonstrating electrical alternans [17]. Electrical alternans refers to a change in the QRS complex amplitude that varies from beat to beat [17]. Classically, every other "R" is of high amplitude as compared to those in between, which are of consistently lower amplitude (see Figure 42.4).

Electrical alternans is the result of the heart freely swinging within a distended pericardial sac [17].

42.8 Pericardiocentesis

Pericardiocentesis is the medical procedure by which the fluid is removed from the pericardial space [9, 17, 33].

In a dog, an over-the-needle or through-the-needle a catheter is introduced at the aseptically prepared site, the right fifth intercostal space, just below the costochondral junction [9]. The needle is advanced into the pericardial sac [9]. Upon flashback of blood, the catheter is threaded into position, and the needle is removed.

In a cat, a 23- or 25-gauge butterfly set is an appropriate choice [9].

ECG monitoring is considered standard of care during pericardiocentesis [9, 33]. Ventricular premature contractions (VPCs) are likely to occur during this procedure [9, 33]. These worsen if the catheter makes contact with the heart [9].

Refer to a cardiology or emergency medicine reference for clarification concerning the proper technique.

As with any procedure, complications may arise. These include the following [17, 33]:

- Cardiac arrest
- Death
- Ectopy
- Laceration of a major coronary artery
- Laceration of the heart

As fluid is removed from the pericardial sac, the intra-pericardial pressure decreases [9]. This resolves cardiac tamponade [9].

A positive response to pericardiocentesis is a reduction in heart rate [9]. Recall that tachycardia is a compensatory reaction to pericardial effusion in an attempt to improve cardiac output.

Samples are collected for fluid analysis [9]. Most of the time, these samples are hemorrhagic and of limited diagnostic value [9, 17]. However, culturing of pericardial fluid is important to rule out septic peritonitis in cases where cytology or fluid pH suggests an infectious or inflammatory etiology [17, 33].

It is important to observe the fluid for clots. When pericardial effusions are hemorrhagic, the blood does not clot. The presence of clotted blood indicates that a vessel – or the heart itself – was perforated as a complication of the procedure [9].

Following pericardiocentesis, pericardial effusion may recur.

Medical therapy alone is rarely effective [9]. Chemotherapy can be used as a palliative agent in the management of heart-associated tumors [9]. Refer to an oncology textbook to explore chemotherapeutic drugs that are appropriate for the management of heart-base masses and HSA.

Pericardiectomy is more effective than medical management of restrictive pericardial disease [9]. Seek direction from a surgery textbook to explore the surgical approach and to review potential complications.

42.9 Pleural Effusion

Pleural effusion may also result in muffled heart sounds. Pleural effusion is the buildup of fluid within the chest cavity itself, between the lungs and the body wall. This fluid creates a barrier between the stethoscope and the heart.

In addition to muffling heart sounds, this fluid restricts the ability of the lungs to expand [37]. Patients struggle to breathe during the inspiratory part of the respiratory cycle. They present with inspiratory dyspnea, tachypnea, and/or open mouth breathing [37].

When they do breathe, breaths tend to be rapid and shallow [38].

Lung sounds of affected patients are also muffled, especially ventrally [37].

Patients are critical and may decline rapidly. Refer to Chapter 36, Section 36.3.6 for additional details on medical management.

References

1 Reece, W.O., Erickson, H.H., Goff, J.P., and Uemura, E.E. (2015). *Dukes' Physiology of Domestic Animals*, 13e, xii, 748 p. Ames, Iowa, USA: Wiley Blackwell.

2 Estrada, A. (2014). Heart disease: diagnosis & treatment. *NAVC Clinician's Brief* (March): 91–95.

3 Englar, R.E. (2017). *Performing the Small Animal Physical Examination*. Hoboken, NJ: Wiley.

4 Hall, J.E. and Guyton, A.C. (2011). *Guyton and Hall Textbook of Medical Physiology*, 12e, xix, 1091 p. Philadelphia, PA: Saunders/Elsevier.

5 Dyce, K.M., Sack, W.O., and Wensing, C.J.G. (2010). *Textbook of Veterinary Anatomy*, 4e, xii, 834 p. St. Louis, MO: Saunders/Elsevier.

6 Stokhof, A.A. and De Rick, A. (2009). Circulatory system. In: *Medical History and Physical Examination in Companion Animals* (ed. A. Rijnberk and F.J. van Sluijs), 75–85. St. Louis: Saunders.

7 De Madron, E. (2015). Pericardial diseases. In: *Clinical Echocardiography of the Dog and Cat* (ed. E. De Madron, V. Chetboul and C. Bussadori), 259–270. St. Louis: Elsevier.

8 Wey, A.C. (2005). Cardiomegaly. *NAVC Clinician's Brief* (March): 7–8.

9 Laste, N.J. (2016). Pericardial canine effusion. *NAVC Clinician's Brief* (January): 65–72.

10 Hall, D.J., Shofer, F., Meier, C.K., and Sleeper, M.M. (2007). Pericardial effusion in cats: a retrospective study of clinical findings and outcome in 146 cats. *J. Vet. Intern. Med.* 21 (5): 1002–1007.

11 DeFrancesco, T.C. (2013). Management of cardiac emergencies in small animals. *Vet. Clin. North Am. Small Anim. Pract.* 43 (4): 817–842.

12 Scansen, B.A. (2011). Interventional cardiology for the criticalist. *J. Vet. Emerg. Crit. Care (San Antonio)* 21 (2): 123–136.

13 MacDonald, K. (2009). Pericardial effusion: causes and clinical outcomes in dogs. DVM 360 [Internet]. http://veterinarycalendar.dvm360.com/pericardial-effusion-causes-and-clinical-outcomes-dogs-proceedings-0.

14 Bille, C., Bomassi, E., and Libermann, S. (2010). Muffled heart sounds in a dog. *Compend. Contin. Educ. Vet.* 32 (6): E1–E3.

15 Evans, H.E. and Miller, M.E. (2013). *Miller's Anatomy of the Dog*, 4e, xix, 850 p. St. Louis, Missouri: Elsevier.

16 Singh, B. and Dyce, K.M. (2018). *Dyce, Sack, and Wensing's Textbook of Veterinary Anatomy*, 5e. St. Louis, Missouri: Saunders.

17 Ware, W.A. (2015). Pericardial diseases. In: *Small Animal Critical Care Medicine*, 2e (ed. D. Silverstein and K. Hopper), 239–246. St. Louis: Saunders.

18 Sisson, D. and Thomas, W.P. (1999). Pericardial disease and cardiac tumors. In: *Textbook of Canine and Feline Cardiology* (ed. P.R. Fox, D. Sisson and N.S. Moise), 679–701. Philadelphia: WB Saunders.

19 Lorell, B.H. and Braunwald, E. (1992). Pericardial diseases. In: *Heart Diseases: A Textbook of Cardiovascular Medicine* (ed. E. Braunwald), 1465–1516. Philadelphia: WB Saunders.

20 Rijnberk, A. and Stokhof, A.A. (2009). General examination. In: *Medical History and Physical Examination in Companion Animals* (ed. A. Rijnberk and F.J. van Sluijs), 47–62. St. Louis: Saunders.

21 Reed, J.R. (1988). Pericardial diseases. In: *Canine and Feline Cardiology* (ed. P.R. Fox), 495–518. New York: Churchill Livingstone.

22 Berg, R.J., Wingfield, W.E., and Hoopes, P.J. (1984). Idiopathic hemorrhagic pericardial effusion in eight dogs. *J. Am. Vet. Med. Assoc.* 185 (9): 988–992.

23 Berg, R.J. and Wingfield, W. (1984). Pericardial-effusion in the dog – a review of 42 cases. *J. Am. Anim. Hosp. Assoc.* 20 (5): 721–730.

24 Johnson, M.S., Martin, M., Binns, S., and Day, M.J. (2004). A retrospective study of clinical findings, treatment and outcome in 143 dogs with pericardial effusion. *J. Small Anim. Pract.* 45 (11): 546–552.

25 Gibbs, C., Gaskell, C.J., Darke, P.G.G., and Wotton, P.R. (1982). Idiopathic pericardial hemorrhage in dogs – a review of 14 cases. *J. Small Anim. Pract.* 23 (9): 483–500.

26 Heinritz, C.K., Gilson, S.D., Soderstrom, M.J. et al. (2005). Subtotal pericardectomy and epicardial excision for treatment of coccidioidomycosis-induced effusive-constrictive pericarditis in dogs: 17 cases (1999–2003). *J. Am. Vet. Med. Assoc.* 227 (3): 435–440.

27 Harpster, N.K. (1987). The cardiovascular system. In: *Diseases of the Cat: Medicine and Surgery* (ed. J. Holzworth), 820–887. Philadelphia, PA: WB Saunders.

28 Rush, J.E., Keene, B.W., and Fox, P.R. (1990). Pericardial disease in the cat – a retrospective evaluation of 66 cases. *J. Am. Anim. Hosp. Assoc.* 26 (1): 39–46.

29 Owens, J.M. (1977). Pericardial-effusion in cat. *Vet. Clin. N. Am.* 7 (2): 373–383.

30 Ware, W.A. (2011). Pericardial diseases. In: *Cardiovascular Disease in Small Animal Medicine* (ed. W.A. Ware), 320–339. London: Manson Publishing.

31 Tobias, A.H. (2010). Pericardial diseases. In: *Textbook of Veterinary Internal Medicine* (ed. S.J. Ettinger and E.C. Feldman), 1342–1352. Philadelphia: WB Saunders.

32 Vogtli, T., Gaschen, F., Vogtli-Burger, R., and Lombard, C. (1997). Hemorrhagic pericardial effusion in dogs. A retrospective study of 10 cases (1989–1994) with a review of the literature. *Schweiz. Arch. Tierheilkd.* 139 (5): 217–224.

33 Paul, A.L. (2016). Pericardiocentesis. *NAVC Clinician's Brief* (July): 97–103.

34 Oura, T.J., Young, A.N., Keene, B.W. et al. (2015). A valentine-shaped cardiac silhouette in feline thoracic radiographs is primarily due to left atrial enlargement. *Vet. Radiol. Ultrasound* 56 (3): 245–250.

35 Thomas, W.P., Sisson, D., Bauer, T.G., and Reed, J.R. (1984). Detection of cardiac masses in dogs by two-dimensional echocardiography. *Vet. Radiol.* 25 (2): 65–72.

36 MacDonald, K.A., Cagney, O., and Magne, M.L. (2009). Echocardiographic and clinicopathologic characterization of pericardial effusion in dogs: 107 cases (1985–2006). *J. Am. Vet. Med. Assoc.* 235 (12): 1456–1461.

36 Dowers, K. (2011). Working up pleural effusions in cats. DVM 360 [Internet]. http://veterinarycalendar.dvm360.com/working-pleural-effusions-cats-proceedings.

38 Mitchell, S.L., McCarthy, R., Rudloff, E., and Pernell, R.T. (2000). Tracheal rupture associated with intubation in cats: 20 cases (1996–1998). *J. Am. Vet. Med. Assoc.* 216 (10): 1592–1595.

43

Abnormal Heart Sounds
Murmurs

43.1 Reviewing Heart Sounds

Recall from Chapter 42, Section 42.1 that there are two primary sets of valves within the heart [1, 2]:

- The right and left atrioventricular (AV) valves, the tricuspid and mitral valve, respectively
- The aortic and pulmonic semilunar valves

These valves are coordinated in order to effectively move blood forward through pulmonic and systemic circulations [1, 2].

As these valves close, they create heart sounds in the normal patient [1–4]. S1 and S2 are the basic heart sounds that form the characteristic "lub-dub" of each normal heartbeat [1–4].

Closure of the AV valves to facilitate ventricular contraction creates S1 [1–3, 5]. Closure of the pulmonic and aortic valves to allow the heart to fill creates S2 [1–3, 5].

Auscultation of the normal patient with a stethoscope yields these sounds [1, 5]. S1 is typically louder and lower in pitch than S2 [6, 7]. S1 is also longer in duration [7].

Both sounds should be crisp and discrete [1, 6, 7].

43.2 Laminar Versus Turbulent Blood Flow and the Development of Murmurs

As blood moves through pulmonic and systemic circulation, laminar flow keeps it streamlined [2]. Concentric layers of blood move through vessels in parallel [2]. At the center of each vessel, blood is moving at its fastest [2].

Laminar flow creates efficiency of movement [2]. Interactions between the blood and vessel walls are reduced and a net forward flow of blood results with minimal energy loss [2].

Turbulence is the opposite of laminar blood flow [2]. When blood flow is turbulent, blood does not flow linearly [2]. Its path is chaotic and illogical [2].

When laminar flow is disrupted, platelets are brought in close proximity to vessel walls. This may predispose the patient to form blood clots if coagulation factors are activated.

Turbulent blood flow is more likely than laminar blood flow to damage the endothelium. More energy is also required to push turbulent blood forward [2].

Turbulence may be created by [2]

- Blood flowing at higher-than-expected velocities
- Blood that is thinner than expected, for example, anemic blood
- Increased cardiac output.

Turbulence creates a characteristic whooshing sound that can be heard with a stethoscope. This sound is a heart murmur [1, 2, 7]. A heart murmur signifies that laminar blood flow has been disrupted [1, 2, 7].

When murmurs are auscultated, they should be described by their [7–9]

- Character:
  - Crescendo murmurs increase in intensity toward completion.
  - Diamond-shaped or crescendo-decrescendo murmurs first increase and then decrease toward completion. These are typically associated with turbulence across the right or left ventricular outflow tracts, as occurs with aortic or pulmonic stenosis (PS).
  - Decrescendo murmurs decrease in intensity toward completion.
  - Regurgitant murmurs sound harsh because they are caused by blood leaking backward through circulation, as in a left-to-right shunt in a patient with a ventricular septal defect (VSD).
  - Systolic clicks are typically heard over the left apex and are high-frequency sounds that are most often associated with mitral valve disease.
- Intensity or grade (see Section 43.3)
- Location in the cardiac cycle
  - Systolic
  - Holosystolic

– Diastolic
– Continuous
• Point of maximal intensity (PMI):
  – The location at which the murmur is the loudest:
    ○ Apical murmurs are loudest at the apex of the heart.
    ○ Basilar murmurs are loudest at the heart base.
    ○ Parasternal murmurs are common in cats [4].
  – The valve that the loudest part of the murmur is nearest:
    ○ Pulmonic
    ○ Aortic
    ○ Mitral
    ○ Tricuspid

To expand upon murmur location, systolic murmurs are whooshing sounds that occur between S1 and S2 [1, 8]:

S1	WHOOSH	S2		S1	WHOOSH	S2
"Lub"	*WHOOSH*	*"Dub"*		*"Lub"*	*WHOOSH*	*"Dub"*

Diastolic murmurs are whooshing sounds that occur between S2 and S1 [1, 8]:

S1	S2	WHOOSH	S1	S2	WHOOSH	S1	S2	WHOOSH
"Lub"	*"Dub"*	*WHOOSH*	*"Lub"*	*"Dub"*	*WHOOSH*	*"Lub"*	*"Dub"*	*WHOOSH*

Continuous murmurs occur throughout the entire cardiac cycle [1, 7]. Because the whooshing sound is constant, these are sometimes referred to as machinery or "washing machine" murmurs [7].

Note that systolic murmurs are more common in companion animal practice [4, 7, 10].

43.3 Grading Heart Murmurs

Murmurs are graded by their intensity on a scale of 1 to 6 [1, 6–8].

Grade 1 murmurs are the softest of all murmurs [7]. They are difficult to auscultate and may be present intermittently [7]. Sometimes, the only indication of their presence is an apparently prolonged S1, which occurs when the murmur blends into the first heart sound [1].

Grade 2 murmurs are more distinct than Grade 1 murmurs, although they are not much louder [1, 7]. They tend to concentrate over one valve [7]. Because of this, Grade 2 murmurs are said to be focal [7].

Grade 3 murmurs are obvious murmurs of moderate intensity [1, 7]. These may be focal or they may radiate to other areas of the chest [7].

Grade 4 murmurs are louder than Grade 3 and more extensive in terms of their distribution patterns [7].

Grade 5 murmurs are loud and they radiate widely [7]. In addition, they are associated with a palpable thrill [7].

A palpable thrill is a vibration that can be felt across the chest wall [1, 7].

Grade 6 murmurs are the loudest type, and are routinely audible without a stethoscope, or with a stethoscope that is barely touching the body wall [1, 7].

43.4 Innocent Heart Murmurs

Innocent heart murmurs are benign findings in some, but not all, puppies and kittens [7, 10–16]. They are more common than was once thought [14, 15, 17, 18]. Twenty-eight percent of puppies in a 2015 study by Sazatmàri et al. had an innocent murmur [13].

Neonates and pediatric patients have physiologic anemia; that is, they have lower hematocrits than adults [13, 19]. This means that their blood is thinner and is therefore more likely to become turbulent in flow rather than laminar. Turbulent blood flow is associated with murmurs [1, 2, 7].

Innocent heart murmurs may also result from the elevated heart rate that is typical of pediatric patients as compared to adults [11].

Finally, innocent murmurs are thought to be associated with turbulence within the heart and vessels as the heart is still developing [1].

When innocent heart murmurs occur, they tend to be soft in intensity, left-sided, and systolic [1, 11].

As affected patients age, these murmurs become quieter until they ultimately resolve [7, 11]. On average, innocent heart murmurs disappear by five or six months of age [11].

If, on the other hand, the murmur persists and/or worsens with each visit, then referral to a veterinary cardiologist is ideal to rule out congenital heart disease [13–15]. Echocardiography is indicated as part of the work-up for a persistent and/or progressing murmur [11, 20]. It is superior to survey radiography for the detection of congenital heart disease [10, 21].

43.5 Physiologic Heart Murmurs

Physiologic, or functional, murmurs result from conditions outside of the heart, rather than structural issues with the heart itself. These conditions include the following [10]:

• Anemia
• Fever
• High sympathetic tone
• Hypertension
• Hyperviscosity syndrome
• Hypoproteinemia
• Pain, particularly in cats
• Pregnancy

Once the aforementioned condition resolves, so, too, does the murmur [10]. For example, stress and excitement in cats causes high sympathetic tone. This may be sufficient to produce a physiologic murmur in an otherwise healthy cat [7, 22].

The following patients are also more likely to have physiologic murmurs that persist in spite of being healthy [7, 23, 24]:

- Athletic dogs
- Deep-chested, large-breed dogs, such as Boxers
- Thin-chested cats and dogs, such as Greyhounds

Like innocent murmurs, physiologic murmurs are benign [10]. Physiologic murmurs tend to be soft in intensity and high in frequency [7, 10]. They also tend to be systolic [10]. Many are loudest near the aortic or pulmonic valve [16, 25, 26]. Physiologic murmurs tend to be focal, rather than radiating throughout the chest [16, 25, 26].

43.6 Congenital Heart Disease

It is difficult to differentiate innocent or physiologic murmurs from pathology based upon solely the physical examination and cardiothoracic auscultation [10, 13–15, 27–29]. Although innocent murmurs tend to quieten, if not resolve, by six months of age, they may persist [7, 11].

An evaluation by a veterinary cardiologist, paired with echocardiography, is the best approach to rule out congenital heart disease [11, 13–15, 20].

Congenital heart disease is more likely to be present in patients with the following physical examination findings [10]:

- Arrhythmia
- Continuous murmur
- Cyanosis
- Diastolic murmur
- Femoral pulse abnormalities
  - Bounding pulses
  - Hypokinetic pulses
- Jugular vein distension and/or pulsation (see Chapter 41)
- Murmurs that radiate to the carotid arteries
- Right-sided murmurs

Congenital heart disease is more likely to occur in the dog than in the cat: its incidence is 4 to 8.5 dogs out of every 1000 compared to 0.2–1.0 cats out of 1000 that present to university clinics annually [10, 30, 31].

The incidence in dogs translates to 1 affected patient out of every 151 [31].

Congenital defects may be associated with volume and/or pressure overload of the heart, including the following [1, 20, 31–40]:

- Atrial septal defect (ASD)
- Mitral valve dysplasia (MVD)
- Patent ductus arteriosus (PDA)*
  - Left-to-right
  - Right-to-left
- PS*
- Subaortic stenosis (SAS)*
- Tetralogy of Fallot
  - Dextroposition or overriding of the aorta
  - PS
  - Right ventricular hypertrophy
  - VSD
- Tricuspid valve dysplasia (TVD)
- VSD***

Those conditions that are starred (*) above reflect the most common congenital defects in dogs within the United States [10, 35–37, 39].

The condition that is starred (***) above, VSD, reflects a congenital defect that is more commonly seen in cats than dogs [20].

Auscultation is an important starting point when evaluating murmurs. However, auscultation alone cannot discern which murmurs are innocent versus which are reflective of cardiac disease [28, 29, 41–43].

Young patients that present for lethargy, stunted growth, or cyanosis are more likely to have true heart disease as opposed to just an innocent murmur [12].

Refer to Chapter 39, Section 39.5.2 for more information about some of the aforementioned congenital heart conditions.

43.6.1 Atrial Septal Defect

An ASD is an abnormal connection between the right and left atria [44]. Because the left side of the heart is under higher pressure than the right, oxygenated blood from the left atrium is shunted into the right atrium [44]. This added volume overloads the right atrium [44]. Cats are more likely to be affected than dogs; however, this defect is relatively uncommon among types of congenital cardiac disease [20, 44].

ASD may not cause an audible murmur [7]. However, when it does, it is a soft, left-sided murmur with a PMI at the base of the heart, over the pulmonic valve [20]. This location is because volume overload of the right side of the heart leads to functional PS [44].

The murmur that results from ASD is holosystolic [20].

43.6.2 Patent Ductus Arteriosus

PDA is a congenital defect in which the fetal vascular structure, the ductus arteriosus, persists after birth [1, 31, 32, 45–49]. Rather than closing over to form the ligamentum arteriosum, the ductus arteriosus remains patent [1, 31, 32].

Review Chapter 39, Section 39.5.2 to explore the pathophysiology associated with PDAs [1, 45–47]. Recall that left-to-right PDAs are more common than right-to-left PDAs [1, 45–48].

Patients with left-to-right PDAs experience shunting of blood from the pressurized aorta into the pulmonary circulation. This additional volume overwhelms the pulmonary vasculature, which drains into the left atrium [1, 45–47]. Over time, the left atrium becomes overwhelmed [1, 45–47]. Congestive heart failure (CHF) with pulmonary congestion secondary to left-sided volume overload is likely [1, 31, 32, 45–47].

The classic PDA murmur is continuous [1, 45–47]. Some have described it as the "washing machine" murmur. Others have said that it mimics wind blowing through a tunnel [7]. In addition to this characteristic murmur, patients with PDA most often have bounding pulses on physical examination [46].

Breeds at increased risk of PDAs include the following [1, 31, 32, 50–53]:

- Bichon Frise
- Chihuahua
- Cocker Spaniel
- Collie
- English Springer Spaniel
- Keeshond
- Maltese
- Miniature Poodle
- Pomeranian
- Shetland Sheepdog
- Shih Tzu
- Toy Poodle
- Yorkshire Terrier
- Welsh Corgi

43.6.3 Pulmonic Stenosis

PS is a congenital defect in which there is an outflow obstruction at the level of the pulmonic valve. This obstruction prevents the right ventricle from emptying completely (see Figures 43.1a, b).

To overcome this obstruction, the right ventricle has to pump harder to force blood out through the right ventricular outflow tract [1]. Over time, this increase in pressure causes the right ventricular wall to thicken [1].

Predisposed breeds include the following [1, 34]:

- Beagle
- Cocker Spaniel
- English Bulldog
- Bull Mastiff
- Samoyed

- Schnauzer
- West Highland White Terrier

PS is characterized by a left-sided, holosystolic murmur with a PMI at the base of the heart [20].

Syncope and common death are possible sequelae of PS [20].

Refer to Chapter 40 for a review of the differential diagnoses for collapse as well as a brief discussion of treatment options for management of PS.

43.6.4 Subaortic Stenosis

SAS is a congenital defect in which there is an outflow obstruction just below the aortic semilunar valves. This prevents the left ventricle from emptying completely. The band is, in a sense, a mechanical obstruction to blood flow [1] (see Figure 43.2).

To overcome this obstruction, the left ventricle has to pump harder to force blood out through the left ventricular outflow tract [1]. Over time, this increase in pressure causes the left ventricular wall to thicken [1].

Predisposed breeds include the following [1, 34]:

- Boxer
- English Bulldog
- German Shepherd
- Golden Retriever
- Great Dane
- Newfoundland
- Bull Terrier

SAS is characterized by a left-sided, holosystolic murmur with a PMI at the base of the heart. The murmur is likely to radiate to the right side of the chest and to the carotid arteries [20].

Syncope and common death are common sequelae of SAS [20]. Refer to Chapter 40 for a review of the differential diagnoses for collapse as well as a brief discussion of treatment options for management of SAS.

43.6.5 Ventricular Septal Defect

VSD is an abnormal connection between the right and left ventricle [44] (see Figures 43.3a, b).

Because most defects are small, the left ventricular pressure is maintained as it should be, at a level higher than right ventricular pressure [44].

However, moderate-to-large defects will volume-overload the right side of the heart [44]. The blood that is shunted from left to right ultimately ends up in the pulmonary circulation [44]. This means that more blood returns from the lungs to the left side of the heart [44]. In time, the left side of the heart becomes volume overloaded as well. The cycle perpetuates until CHF ensues [44].

Figure 43.1 (a) Echocardiography (right parasternal long axis view): Severe right ventricular concentric hypertrophy in a young animal consistent with pulmonic stenosis (PS). In addition, note the lead II ECG. The ECG is consistent with normal sinus rhythm with right axis deviation due to the RVH. *Source:* Courtesy of Justin Thomason, DACVIM (cardiology; SAIM), Wildcat Cardiology and Christy Zimmer Coyle, RVT. (b) Echocardiography (left basilar view): This Spectral Doppler tracing is consistent with severe PS. From the Bernoulli equation, the pressure gradient is equal to 92 mmHg. *Source:* Courtesy of Justin Thomason, DACVIM (cardiology; SAIM), Wildcat Cardiology and Christy Zimmer Coyle, RVT.

(a)

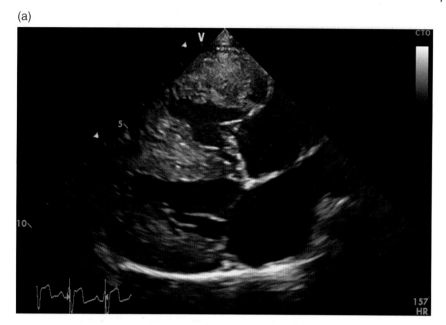

(b)

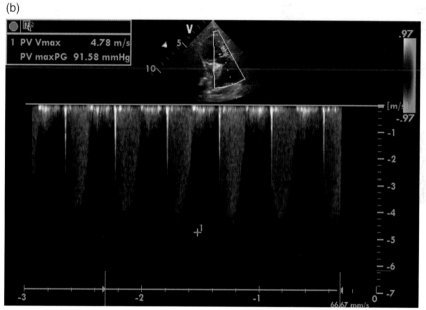

The English Springer Spaniel is predisposed to VSD [34]. VSD may not cause an audible murmur [7]. However, when it does, it is a right-sided, holosystolic murmur with a PMI at the base of the heart [20].

43.7 Acquired Heart Disease and Murmurs

Murmurs are not unique to pediatric patients. Murmurs may be acquired. These are most commonly systolic and benefit from a diagnostic work-up by a board-certified veterinary cardiologist to obtain a definitive diagnosis [10]. Pairing history taking and the physical examination with echocardiography provides a thorough approach to case management.

Without cardiac imaging, provisional diagnoses can be made based upon murmur characteristics, such as intensity, character, and PMI [10]. However, auscultation alone is prone to error [10]. For example, a study of murmurs in Whippet dogs demonstrated low specificity concerning auscultation: 89% of dogs with murmurs were incorrectly diagnosed based upon the acoustics of their murmurs [10].

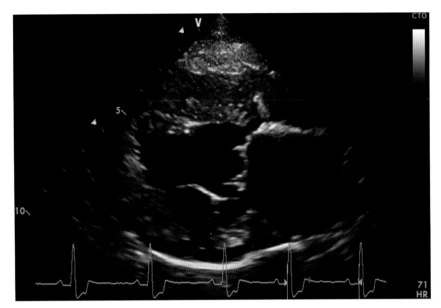

Figure 43.2 Echocardiography (right parasternal long axis view): There is evidence of left ventricular concentric hypertrophy. Concentric hypertrophy is secondary to pressure overload. In a young dog, consider subaortic stenosis (SAS). In a geriatric dog, consider systemic hypertension. *Source:* Courtesy of Justin Thomason, DACVIM (cardiology; SAIM), Wildcat Cardiology and Christy Zimmer Coyle, RVT.

(a)

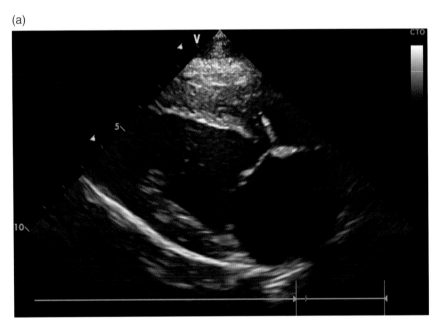

(b)

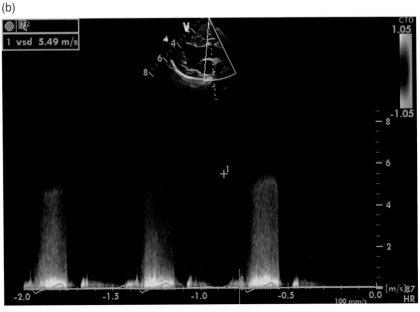

Figure 43.3 (a) Echocardiography (right parasternal long axis view): Echocardiogram is consistent with a ventricular septal defect (VSD). *Source:* Courtesy of Justin Thomason, DACVIM (cardiology; SAIM), Wildcat Cardiology and Christy Zimmer Coyle, RVT. (b) Echocardiography (right parasternal long axis view): This Spectral Doppler tracing is consistent with a velocity across the VSD of 5.49 m/s. From the Bernoulli equation, the pressure gradient is equal to approximately 121 mmHg. This elevated gradient is consistent with resistive VSD (small). This is one of the heart conditions in which the louder the heart murmur, the better the prognosis. *Source:* Courtesy of Justin Thomason, DACVIM (cardiology; SAIM), Wildcat Cardiology and Christy Zimmer Coyle, RVT.

43.7.1 Acquired Murmurs in the Adult and Geriatric Dog

Acquired murmurs may be pathological or nonpathological [10]. Nonpathological implies that the murmur could be physiologic, for example, secondary to anemia [10]. The nonpathological murmur could also be due to individual variation or "normal" for a particular breed [10].

This section will emphasize pathological murmurs.

Acquired, pathological left-sided, systolic, apical murmurs in the adult or geriatric dog are most commonly due to mitral regurgitation (MR) [10, 34]. MR may result from [10]

- Degenerative or myxomatous atrioventricular valve disease
- Dilated cardiomyopathy (DCM) (see Chapter 40, Section 40.4.3.4)
- Infectious endocarditis.

Of the aforementioned conditions, degenerative mitral valve disease (DMVD) is the most common to occur in adult dogs, especially small breeds, such as the Dachshund and the Cavalier King Charles Spaniel [4, 10, 34, 54–58]. Synonyms for DMVD have historically included endocardiosis and chronic valvular disease [55, 56]. Contrary to popular thought, large-breed dogs may also develop DMVD [54, 59].

DMVD is characterized by progressive changes in mitral valve morphology [56]. Valve leaflets enlarge and become thickened [56]. As these changes in tissue thickness progress, valve leaflets begin to bulge [56]. They ultimately prolapse into the associated atrium [56, 60–62]. This change is evident on echocardiography [56] (see Figures 43.4a, b).

In addition, chordae tendineae often elongate and may even rupture [56].

The net result is MR [56]. Mild MR does not have any significant impact on the cardiac chamber, wall thickness, heart function as a pump, or systemic circulation [56]. However, as MR worsens, the heart compensates for the diminished stroke volume by increasing the heart rate and the force of contraction [56]. Over time, there is pathologic remodeling of the heart [56]. Left atrial and left ventricular wall hypertrophy ensues [56]. If MR is severe enough, CHF may develop [56].

Physical examination findings that are supportive of early DMVD include a low-grade murmur with a PMI over the mitral valve, with or without a systolic click [56]. Murmurs may be intermittent [56]. Murmur intensity may worsen with exercise or stress [56, 63].

Even low-grade murmurs should be evaluated by echocardiography to evaluate patients for valve morphology and for the presence or absence of MR [56]. The use of spectral or color-flow Doppler can detect and quantify MR [56, 63–67].

Note that the presence of DMVD does not necessarily mean that all affected dogs will become symptomatic [54, 68, 69].

Although involvement of the mitral valve is most common and has been highlighted here, myxomatous degeneration may include other valves [56]. For example, degenerative tricuspid valve disease is more likely when adult dogs present with acquired, right-sided murmurs [10] (see Figure 43.5).

These patients may develop concurrent pulmonary hypertension [10].

43.7.2 Acquired Murmurs in the Adult and Geriatric Cat

Systolic murmurs are more common in apparently healthy cats than was once thought. Depending upon which study is consulted, anywhere from 16 to 44% of cats in shelters and clinics have murmurs [10, 22, 70–72]. Because feline murmurs can be caused by stress, fear, and pain, they are more easily detected in cats, the more that they are handled and/or examined [10, 22, 71, 72].

As is true of canine patients, acquired murmurs in cats may be pathological or nonpathological [10]. Nonpathological implies that the murmur could be physiologic, for example, secondary to anemia [10]. The nonpathological murmur could also be due to high sympathetic tone in the cat, as caused by stress, fear, or pain [10].

If a feline patient with a murmur also has a clinical finding of pallor on physical examination, then it should be evaluated for anemia [10]. Hematocrits less than 20% may cause a physiologic murmur [10]. Diagnostic confirmation and treatment of the anemia should resolve the murmur [10].

If a feline patient with a murmur also presents with clinical signs that are suggestive of systemic hypertension, such as retinopathy, then a diagnostic work-up to evaluate systolic arterial blood pressure should be launched [10]. If systolic arterial blood pressures exceed 180 mmHg, then the primary cause of hypertension should be explored and addressed [10]. This may in turn improve the murmur [10].

Murmurs may also develop secondary to hyperthyroidism in senior cats [10]. Senior feline patients with a murmur should be screened for hyperthyroidism if they exhibit signs that are suggestive of endocrinopathy [10]. These signs include weight loss in spite of a normal-to-increased appetite [1]. If patients are hyperthyroid, then case management should be aimed at addressing the endocrinopathy [10]. Once the patient becomes euthyroid, the murmur is then reassessed [10].

(a)

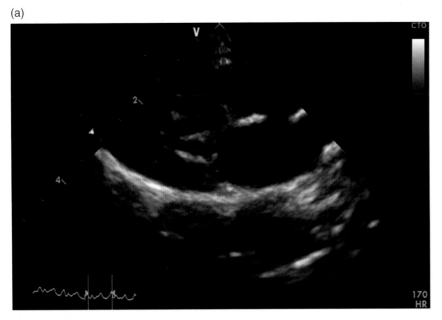

Figure 43.4 (a) Echocardiography (left caudal view). Echocardiogram is consistent with thickened mitral valves with prolapse evident into the left atrium. *Source:* Courtesy of Justin Thomason, DACVIM (cardiology; SAIM), Wildcat Cardiology and Christy Zimmer Coyle, RVT. (b) Echocardiography (right parasternal short axis view): Echocardiogram is consistent with thickened mitral valves secondary to myxomatous valvular disease. Color-flow Doppler reveals moderate mitral regurgitation (blue-green color). *Source:* Courtesy of Justin Thomason, DACVIM (cardiology; SAIM), Wildcat Cardiology and Christy Zimmer Coyle, RVT.

(b)

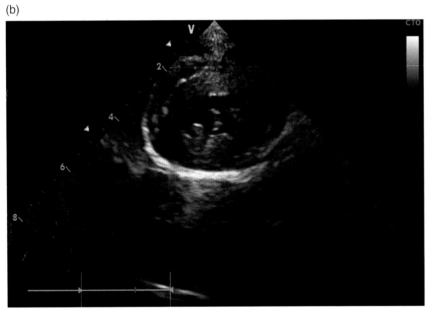

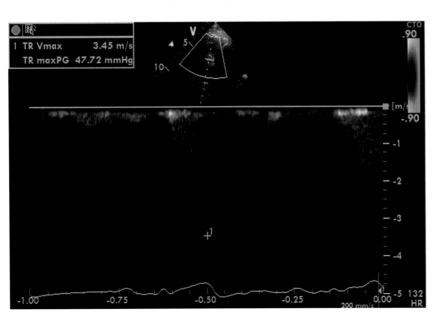

Figure 43.5 Echocardiography (left caudal view): Echocardiogram images consistent with tricuspid regurgitation (blue-green color flow). *Source:* Courtesy of Justin Thomason, DACVIM (cardiology; SAIM), Wildcat Cardiology and Christy Zimmer Coyle, RVT.

Figure 43.6 Echocardiography (right parasternal long axis view): Echocardiogram in a cat with concentric hypertrophy of the left ventricle. In a geriatric cat without systemic hypertension and/or hyperthyroidism, genetic HCM is likely. *Source:* Courtesy of Justin Thomason, DACVIM (cardiology; SAIM), Wildcat Cardiology and Christy Zimmer Coyle, RVT.

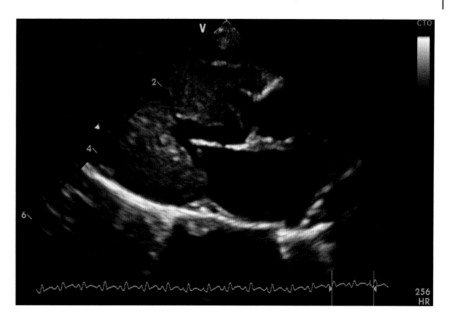

One concern in cats with murmurs is that as many as 55% may seem outwardly healthy, but have echocardiographic evidence of cardiac disease [72].

Among heart diseases in adult and senior cats, hypertrophic cardiomyopathy (HCM) is the most common [10, 22, 70–79].

Maine Coon cats, Persians, Burmese, Siamese, American Shorthairs, Ragdolls, and Norwegian Forest cats are predisposed to HCM [80].

HCM is a condition that involves thickening of the left ventricle (see Figure 43.6).

This hypertrophy is often associated with left atrial dilation [81]. Left ventricular hypertrophy compromises the compliance of this chamber [81]. In order to fill the left ventricle, the left atrium has to raise its pressure [81]. This in turn increases the pressure of the pulmonary vein, which is tasked with the filling of the left atrium [81].

The pathophysiology of HCM is a vicious cycle [81]. The body attempts to compensate for reduced filling and cardiac output by increasing heart rate [81]. Tachycardia requires the myocardium to work harder, such that the heart's need for oxygen increases [81]. However, the heart remains inefficient [81]. Coronary perfusion time decreases [81]. This perpetuates ischemia [81].

In addition, the stiffness of the left ventricle impairs its ability to relax during diastole. This further hinders filling [81].

Additional structural changes are often present with HCM, including MR and dynamic left ventricular outflow obstruction [81]. The latter results from the mitral valve becoming displaced against the inner wall of the left ventricle. This causes a mechanical obstruction for blood that is attempting to pass from the left ventricle

through the aortic valve and into systemic circulation. These structural changes are evident on Doppler studies via echocardiography [81].

Cats with HCM tend to be young to middle-aged at time of diagnosis [81]. Males are overrepresented in many studies [81].

Physical examination findings that are supportive of a diagnosis of HCM include a heart murmur, with or without a gallop rhythm [81]. Gallop rhythms will be discussed in Chapter 44.

Cardiothoracic auscultation alone may prompt an investigation that leads to diagnosis. In other words, many cats with HCM are asymptomatic. The murmur associated with the disease process is an incidental finding on examination [78]. Some of these patients remain asymptomatic and do not die from HCM [82–84].

Other cats become symptomatic for HCM.

If patients have developed left-sided CHF secondary to HCM, then the following abnormalities may be present on physical examination [81]:

- Crackles
- Dyspnea
- Tachypnea

Recall from Chapter 37, Section 37.2 that crackles are brief, discontinuous, adventitious lung sounds that sound like "popping" [1, 85–87].

In left-sided CHF, pulmonary interstitial spaces become saturated with fluid. This fluid obstructs small airways.

Fine crackles occur when intrathoracic pressure increases sufficiently to force obstructed airways to open [85].

Recall from Chapter 39, Section 39.5.1 that HCM is often associated with thrombi formation (see Figure 43.7).

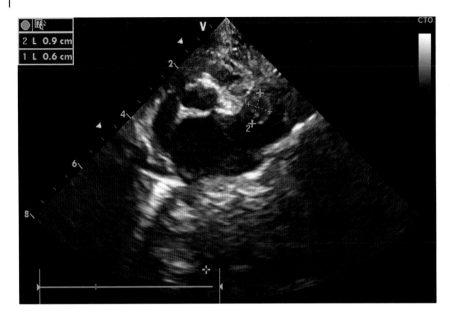

Figure 43.7 Echocardiography (right parasternal short axis basilar view): Echocardiogram is consistent with left atrial dilation with a thrombus noted in the left atrium. *Source:* Courtesy of Justin Thomason, DACVIM (cardiology; SAIM), Wildcat Cardiology and Christy Zimmer Coyle, RVT.

In particular, aortic thromboembolism (ATE), also known as "saddle thrombus" is of significant concern in cats with HCM [88].

Patients with ATE present acutely with pelvic limb paresis or paralysis that involves one or both legs [80, 88, 89]. Bilateral involvement is most common [89].

These cats are in acute pain [80, 88, 89].

Patients with HCM may also experience sudden death [77, 82]. This may occur before or after diagnosis.

Echocardiography is an essential part of the diagnostic work-up for cats with murmurs, particularly because there is a high prevalence of occult heart disease in this species [72, 90].

As an imaging modality, the echocardiogram allows for measurement of chamber size. Measurements are not foolproof [90, 91]. For example, the left atrium can be altered by dehydration and/or iatrogenic fluid overload secondary to rehydration therapy [90, 91]. However, measurements do provide contextual data that may help the clinician to discern the pathophysiology underlying each patient's presentation.

Note that HCM is not the only cause of murmurs in the adult or geriatric cat. Other causes of systolic murmurs in cats include the following [92]:

- Degenerative myxomatous atrioventricular valve disease
  - MR
  - Tricuspid regurgitation
- Dynamic left ventricular outflow obstruction
  - SAS (see Section 43.6.4)
- Dynamic right ventricular outflow obstruction
  - PS (see Section 43.6.3)

In addition, adult cats with murmurs may also have been overlooked as pediatric patients with tricuspid dysplasia or VSD [10].

It is also essential that adult or geriatric cats be screened for other systemic conditions that could be responsible for causing their murmurs. Murmurs in cats are often secondary to noncardiac disease, such as hyperthyroidism, the sequelae of which lead to cardiac changes.

43.8 Challenges Associated with Cardiothoracic Auscultation

Cardiothoracic auscultation is a clinical skill. It takes time and experience to learn appropriate stethoscope placement against the chest, classify heart sounds as normal and abnormal, and describe these abnormalities with reference to the cardiac cycle, character of the sound, and the murmur's PMI. These are challenges for any novice.

Novices must learn how to screen out the following sounds to zero in on the heart [11]:

- Respiratory sounds
- Shivering
- Rubbing of fur against the bell or diaphragm of the stethoscope

If the aforementioned sounds are confused with the heart, the novice may erroneously believe that an abnormality exists.

In addition, the novice must learn how to use each part of the stethoscope for its intended purpose [11]. The stethoscope consists of ear pieces, tubing, the bell, and the diaphragm.

The fit of the stethoscope's ear pieces is essential to the success of the auscultation [11].

The flat-side of the stethoscope, the diaphragm, preferentially transmits high-frequency sounds to the listener. Both S1 and S2 are heard well with the diaphragm. The diaphragm is designed for firm placement against the chest wall.

By contrast, the bell preferentially transmits low-frequency sounds. This facilitates the hearing of gallop sounds, S3 and S4. The bell is designed for a soft touch, that is, gentle placement against the chest wall.

Using too much force against the chest with the bell can create sound artifacts that are suggestive of a murmur, when in fact the murmur is not there.

Additional challenges to auscultation are species- and patient-specific [11].

Cats, for example, have very small hearts. This may make it challenging to differentiate apical from basilar murmurs based upon auscultation alone. Similarly, it can be a challenge to appreciate the PMI [10].

Auscultation is performed best with the cat or dog standing, but veterinary patients do not always cooperate [11].

Auscultation is also more accurate when the cat or dog is quiet [11]. Unfortunately, panting in dogs and purring in cats complicate the ability to hear heart sounds crisply and to make clinical judgments [11].

Panting may be discouraged by closing a dog's mouth and keeping it closed during auscultation. This forces the dog to breathe through its nose, which should allow the clinician to hear the heart better.

Purring is a bit more challenging; however, it may be deterred by one of the following means [1, 11]:

- Asking the client to refrain from petting the cat during auscultation.
- Turning on the faucet in the examination room. The sound of water running is often a deterrent.
- Encouraging the cat to sniff a cotton ball that has been moistened with alcohol. Alcohol has an odor that is aversive to cats. Citrus scents may also be deterrents. This is my least preferred method.

Excited patients are likely to be tachycardic. Murmurs are inducible in cats more so than dogs. Their intensity is likely to change with excitement or heart rate [10, 22, 71]. Allowing the patient to have a "time out" may be of benefit. Auscultating the patient once it is more relaxed may allow for more accurate results [11].

References

1 Englar, R.E. (2017). *Performing the Small Animal Physical Examination*. Hoboken, NJ: Wiley.

2 Hall, J.E. and Guyton, A.C. (2011). *Guyton and Hall Textbook of Medical Physiology*, 12e, xix, 1091 p. Philadelphia, Pa: Saunders/Elsevier.

3 Dyce, K.M., Sack, W.O., and Wensing, C.J.G. (2010). *Textbook of Veterinary Anatomy*, 4e, xii, 834 p. St. Louis, Mo: Saunders/Elsevier.

4 Hogan, D.F. (2008). Cardiac examination & history. *NAVC Clinician's Brief* (July): 49–53.

5 Stokhof, A.A. and De Rick, A. (2009). Circulatory System. In: *Medical History and Physical Examination in Companion Animals* (ed. A. Rijnberk and F.J. van Sluijs), 75–85. St. Louis: Saunders.

6 Estrada, A. Cardiac physical examination. NAVC Clinician's Brief [Internet]. https://www.cliniciansbrief.com/article/cardiac-physical-examination

7 Mandese, W.W. and Estrada, A.H. (2017). The basic cardiology examination. *NAVC Clinician's Brief* (May): 91–97.

8 Gompf, R.E. (2008). The history and physical examination. In: *Manual of Canine and Feline Cardiology* (ed. L.P. Tilley, F.W.K. Smith, M. Oyama and M.M. Sleeper), 2–23. St. Louis, Missouri: Saunders, an imprint of Elsevier Inc.

9 Kittleson, M.D. and Kienle, R.D. (2005). Physical exam. In: *Small Animal Cardiovascular Medicine* (ed. M.D. Kittleson and R.D. Kienle). Maryland Heights, MO: Mosby Elsevier.

10 Cote, E., Edwards, N.J., Ettinger, S.J. et al. (1998). Management of incidentally detected heart murmurs in dogs and cats. *J. Vet. Cardiol.* 17 (4): 245–261.

11 DeFrancesco, T. (2012). Cardiac auscultation 101. *NC State College of Veterinary Medicine [Internet]*. https://cvm.ncsu.edu/wp-content/uploads/2015/06/DeFrancesco2012_CardiacAusculation.pdf.

12 Stepien, R.L. (ed.) (2005). *How Worried Should I Be about this Heart Murmur?* Orlando, Florida: North American Veterinary Conference (NAVC).

13 Szatmari, V., van Leeuwen, M.W., and Teske, E. (2015). Innocent cardiac murmur in puppies: prevalence, correlation with hematocrit, and auscultation characteristics. *J. Vet. Intern. Med.* 29 (6): 1524–1528.

14 Dennis, S. (2013). Sound advice for heart murmurs. *J. Small Anim. Pract.* 54 (9): 443–444.

15 Fonfara, S. (2015). Listen to the sound: what is normal? *J. Small Anim. Pract.* 56 (2): 75–76.

16 Bavegems, V.C., Duchateau, L., Polis, I.E. et al. (2011). Detection of innocent systolic murmurs by

auscultation and their relation to hematologic and echocardiographic findings in clinically normal whippets. *J. Am. Vet. Med. Assoc.* 238 (4): 468–471.

17 Tavel, M.E. (2006). Cardiac auscultation: a glorious past – and it does have a future. *Circulation* 113 (9): 1255–1259.

18 Bavegems, V.C., Duchateau, L., Polis, I.E. et al. (2011). Detection of innocent systolic murmurs by auscultation and their relation to hematologic and echocardiographic findings in clinically normal Whippets. *J. Am. Vet. Med. Assoc.* 238 (4): 468–471.

19 Peterson, M.E. and Kutzler, M.A. (2011). *Small Animal Pediatrics: The First 12 Months of Life*, xvi, 526 p. St. Louis, Mo: Saunders/Elsevier.

20 MacDonald, K. (2011). Murmurs in puppies and kittens. DVM 360 [Internet]. http://veterinarycalendar.dvm360.com/murmurs-puppies-and-kittens-proceedings

21 Tse, Y.C., Rush, J.E., Cunningham, S.M. et al. (2013). Evaluation of a training course in focused echocardiography for noncardiology house officers. *J. Vet. Emerg. Crit. Care* 23 (3): 268–273.

22 Wagner, T., Fuentes, V.L., Payne, J.R. et al. (2010). Comparison of auscultatory and echocardiographic findings in healthy adult cats. *J. Vet. Cardiol.* 12 (3): 171–182.

23 Garcia, J.L. (2015). Journal Scan: Physiological heart murmurs are more common in our veterinary patients than we may think. DVM 360 [Internet]. http://veterinarymedicine.dvm360.com/journal-scan-physiological-heart-murmurs-are-more-common-our-veterinary-patients-we-may-think

24 Drut, A., Ribas, T., Floch, F. et al. (2015). Prevalence of physiological heart murmurs in a population of 95 healthy young adult dogs. *J. Small Anim. Pract.* 56 (2): 112–118.

25 Sisson, D.D. and Ettinger, S.J. (1999). The physical examination. In: *Textbook of Canine and Feline Cardiology: Principles and Clinical Practice* (ed. P.R. Fox, D.D. Sisson and N.S. Moise), 46–64. Philadelphia: WB Saunders.

26 Kvart, C. and Haggstrom, J. (2002). Heart sounds and murmurs in dogs and cats. In: *Cardiac Auscultation and Phonocardiography in Dogs, Horses, and Cats* (ed. C. Kvart), 21–71. Uppsala, Sweden: Selbstverlag.

27 Marinus, S.M., van Engelen, H., and Szatmari, V. (2017). N-terminal pro-B-type natriuretic peptide and phonocardiography in differentiating innocent cardiac murmurs from congenital cardiac anomalies in asymptomatic puppies. *J. Vet. Intern. Med.* 31 (3): 661–667.

28 Abbott, J. (2001). Auscultation: what type of practice makes perfect? *J. Vet. Intern. Med.* 15 (6): 505–506.

29 Naylor, J.M., Yadernuk, L.M., Pharr, J.W., and Ashburner, J.S. (2001). An assessment of the ability of diplomates, practitioners, and students to describe and interpret recordings of heart murmurs and arrhythmia. *J. Vet. Intern. Med.* 15 (6): 507–515.

30 Patterson, D.F. (1968). Epidemiologic and genetic studies of congenital heart disease in the dog. *Circ. Res.* 23 (2): 171–202.

31 Strickland, K.N. (2008). Congenital heart disease. In: *Manual of Canine and Feline Cardiology*, 4e (ed. L.P. Tilley, F.W.K. Smith, M.A. Oyama and M.M. Sleeper), 215–239. Philadelphia: W.B. Saunders.

32 Bulmer, B.J. (2011). The cardiovascular system. In: *Small Animal Pediatrics: The First 12 Months of Life* (ed. M.E. Peterson and M.A. Kutzler), 289–304. St. Louis, Mo: Saunders/Elsevier.

33 Schrope, D.P. (2015). Prevalence of congenital heart disease in 76,301 mixed-breed dogs and 57,025 mixed-breed cats. *J. Vet. Cardiol.* 17 (3): 192–202.

34 Rishniw, M. (2011). Canine heart murmur. *NAVC Clinician's Brief* (May): 49–52.

35 Oliveira, P., Domenech, O., Silva, J. et al. (2011). Retrospective review of congenital heart disease in 976 dogs. *J. Vet. Intern. Med.* 25 (3): 477–483.

36 Buchanan, J.W. (1998). Prevalence of cardiovascular disorders. In: *Textbook of Canine and Feline Cardiology* (ed. P.R. Fox, D.D. Sisson and N.S. Moise), 457–470. Philadelphia: W.B. Saunders.

37 Baumgartner, C. and Glaus, T.M. (2003). Congenital cardiac diseases in dogs: a retrospective analysis. *Schweiz. Arch. Tierheilkd.* 145 (11): 527–533, 35-6.

38 Hunt, G.B., Church, D.B., Malik, R., and Bellenger, C.R. (1990). A retrospective analysis of congenital cardiac anomalies (1977–1989). *Aust. Vet. Pract.* 20 (2): 70–75.

39 Tidholm, A. (1997). Retrospective study of congenital heart defects in 151 dogs. *J. Small Anim. Pract.* 38 (3): 94–98.

40 MacDonald, K.A. (2006). Congenital heart diseases of puppies and kittens. *Vet. Clin. North Am. Small Anim. Pract.* 36 (3): 503–531. vi.

41 Mackie, A.S., Jutras, L.C., Dancea, A.B. et al. (2009). Can cardiologists distinguish innocent from pathologic murmurs in neonates? *J. Pediatr.* 154 (1): 50–54. e1.

42 Pyle, R.L. (2000). Interpreting low-intensity cardiac murmurs in dogs predisposed to subaortic stenosis. *J. Am. Anim. Hosp. Assoc.* 36 (5): 379–382.

43 Shub, C. (2003). Echocardiography or auscultation? How to evaluate systolic murmurs. *Can. Fam. Physician* 49: 163–167.

44 Tilley, L.P. and Smith, F.W.K. (2004). *The 5-Minute Veterinary Consult: Canine and Feline*, 3e. Baltimore, MD: Lippincott Williams & Wilkins.

45 Côté, E. (2015). *Clinical Veterinary Advisor. Dogs and Cats*, 3e, xxxvii, 1642 p. St. Louis, Missouri: Elsevier Mosby.

46 Tilley, L.P., Smith, F.W.K., and Tilley, L.P. (2007). *Blackwell's Five-Minute Veterinary Consult: Canine and Feline*, 4e, lx, 1578 p. Ames, Iowa: Blackwell.

47 Aiello, S.E. and Moses, M.A. (2016). *The Merck Veterinary Manual*. Whitehouse Station, NJ: Merck & Co., Inc.

48 Arora, M. (2001). Reversed patent ductus arteriosus in a dog. *Can. Vet. J.* 42 (6): 471–472.

49 Scurtu, I., Pestean, C., Lacatus, R. et al. (2106). Reverse PDA – less common type of patent Ductus Arteriosus – case report. *Bull. Univ. Agric. Sci. Vet. Med. Cluj Napoca* 73 (2): 351–355.

50 Broaddus, K. and Tillson, M. (2010). Patent ductus arteriosus in dogs. *Compend. Contin. Educ. Vet.* 32 (9): E3.

51 Orton, E.C. (2003). Cardiac Surgery. In: *Textbook of Small Animal Surgery* (ed. D. Slatter), 955–959. Philadelphia: WB Saunders.

52 Fossum, T.W. (2007). *Small Animal Surgery*. St. Louis: Mosby Elsevier.

53 Buchanan, J.W. and Patterson, D.F. (2003). Etiology of patent ductus arteriosus in dogs. *J. Vet. Intern. Med.* 17 (2): 167–171.

54 Borgarelli, M. and Haggstrom, J. (2010). Canine degenerative Myxomatous mitral valve disease: natural history, clinical presentation and therapy. *Vet. Clin. N. Am. Small.* 40 (4): 651–663.

55 Fox, P.R. (2012). Pathology of myxomatous mitral valve disease in the dog. *J. Vet. Cardiol.* 14 (1): 103–126.

56 Haggstrom, J., Pedersen, H.D., and Kvart, C. (2004). New insights into degenerative mitral valve disease in dogs. *Vet. Clin. N. Am. Small.* 34 (5): 1209–1226.

57 Sisson, D.D., Kvart, C., and Darke, P. (1999). Acquired valvular heart disease. In: *Textbook of Canine and Feline Cardiology* (ed. P.R. Fox, D.D. Sisson and N.S. Moise), 536–565. Philadelphia: WB Saunders Company.

58 Haggstrom, J., Hoglund, K., and Borgarelli, M. (2009). An update on treatment and prognostic indicators in canine myxomatous mitral valve disease. *J. Small Anim. Pract.* 50 (Suppl 1): 25–33.

59 Borgarelli, M., Zini, E., D'Agnolo, G. et al. (2004). Comparison of primary mitral valve disease in German Shepherd dogs and in small breeds. *J. Vet. Cardiol.* 6 (2): 27–34.

60 Buchanan, J.W. (1977). Chronic valvular disease (endocardiosis) in dogs. *Adv. Vet. Sci. Comp. Med.* 21: 75–106.

61 Kogure, K. (1980). Pathology of chronic mitral valvular disease in the dog. *Nippon Juigaku Zasshi* 42 (3): 323–335.

62 Whitney, J.C. (1974). Observations on the effect of age on the severity of heart valve lesions in the dog. *J. Small Anim. Pract.* 15 (8): 511–522.

63 Pedersen, H.D., Haggstrom, J., Falk, T. et al. (1999). Auscultation in mild mitral regurgitation in dogs: observer variation, effects of physical maneuvers, and agreement with color Doppler echocardiography and phonocardiography. *J. Vet. Intern. Med.* 13 (1): 56–64.

64 Kittleson, M.D. (1998). Myxomatous atrioventricular valvular degeneration. In: *Small Animal Cardiovascular Medicine* (ed. M.D. Kittleson and R.D. Kienle), 297–318. St. Louis: Mosby.

65 Muzzi, R.A., de Araujo, R.B., Muzzi, L.A. et al. (2003). Regurgitant jet area by Doppler color flow mapping: quantitative assessment of mitral regurgitation severity in dogs. *J. Vet. Cardiol.* 5 (2): 33–38.

66 Kittleson, M.D. and Brown, W.A. (2003). Regurgitant fraction measured by using the proximal isovelocity surface area method in dogs with chronic myxomatous mitral valve disease. *J. Vet. Intern. Med.* 17 (1): 84–88.

67 Doiguchi, O. and Takahashi, T. (2000). Examination of quantitative analysis and measurement of the regurgitation rate in mitral valve regurgitation by the "proximal isovelocity surface area" method. *J. Vet. Med. Sci.* 62 (1): 109–112.

68 Chetboul, V., Serres, F., Tissier, R. et al. (2009). Association of plasma N-terminal pro-B-type natriuretic peptide concentration with mitral regurgitation severity and outcome in dogs with asymptomatic degenerative mitral valve disease. *J. Vet. Intern. Med.* 23 (5): 984–994.

69 Borgarelli, M., Savarino, P., Crosara, S. et al. (2008). Survival characteristics and prognostic variables of dogs with mitral regurgitation attributable to myxomatous valve disease. *J. Vet. Intern. Med.* 22 (1): 120–128.

70 Cote, E., Manning, A.M., Emerson, D. et al. (2004). Assessment of the prevalence of heart murmurs in overtly healthy cats. *J. Am. Vet. Med. Assoc.* 225 (3): 384–388.

71 Paige, C.F., Abbott, J.A., Elvinger, F., and Pyle, R.L. (2009). Prevalence of cardiomyopathy in apparently healthy cats. *J. Am. Vet. Med. Assoc.* 234 (11): 1398–1403.

72 Nakamura, R.K., Rishniw, M., King, M.K., and Sammarco, C.D. (2011). Prevalence of echocardiographic evidence of cardiac disease in apparently healthy cats with murmurs. *J. Feline Med. Surg.* 13 (4): 266–271.

73 Bonagura, J.D. (2000). Feline echocardiography. *J. Feline Med. Surg.* 2 (3): 147–151.

74 Dirven, M.J., Cornelissen, J.M., Barendse, M.A. et al. (2010). Cause of heart murmurs in 57 apparently healthy cats. *Tijdschr. Diergeneeskd.* 135 (22): 840–847.

75 Cardiomyopathy, F.V.L. (2006). Establishing a diagnosis. In: *Consultations in Feline Internal Medicine*, vol. 5 (ed. J.R. August), 301–310. St. Louis: Saunders Elsevier.

76 Ferasin, L., Sturgess, C.P., Cannon, M.J. et al. (2003). Feline idiopathic cardiomyopathy: a retrospective study of 106 cats (1994–2001). *J. Feline Med. Surg.* 5 (3): 151–159.

77 Rishniw, M. and Pion, P.D. (2011). Is treatment of feline hypertrophic cardiomyopathy based in science or faith? A survey of cardiologists and a literature search. *J. Feline Med. Surg.* 13 (7): 487–497.

78 Freeman, L.M., Rush, J.E., Stern, J.A. et al. (2017). Feline hypertrophic Cardiomyopathy: a spontaneous large animal model of human HCM. *Cardiol. Res.* 8 (4): 139–142.

79 Payne, J.R., Brodbelt, D.C., and Luis Fuentes, V. (2015). Cardiomyopathy prevalence in 780 apparently healthy cats in rehoming centres (the CatScan study). *J. Vet. Cardiol.* 17 (Suppl 1): S244–S257.

80 Rishniw, M. (2006). Feline aortic thromboembolism. *NAVC Clinician's Brief* (November): 17–20.

81 Bonagura, J.D. (1997). Feline hypertrophic cardiomyopathy. *Vet. Q.* 19: S5–S6.

82 Payne, J.R., Borgeat, K., Connolly, D.J. et al. (2013). Prognostic indicators in cats with hypertrophic cardiomyopathy. *J. Vet. Intern. Med.* 27 (6): 1427–1436.

83 Atkins, C.E., Gallo, A.M., Kurzman, I.D., and Cowen, P. (1992). Risk factors, clinical signs, and survival in cats with a clinical diagnosis of idiopathic hypertrophic cardiomyopathy: 74 cases (1985–1989). *J. Am. Vet. Med. Assoc.* 201 (4): 613–618.

84 Liu, S.K., Maron, B.J., and Tilley, L.P. (1981). Feline hypertrophic cardiomyopathy: gross anatomic and quantitative histologic features. *Am. J. Pathol.* 102 (3): 388–395.

85 Hansen, B. (2009). What's that noise? Interpreting lung sounds. DVM 360 [Internet]. http://veterinarycalendar. dvm360.com/whats-noise-interpreting-lung-sounds-proceedings.

86 RnCeus. (1996). *Abnormal breath sounds: RnCeus Interactive™, LLC;* [Available from: http://www.rnceus. com/resp/respabn.html].

87 Forgacs, P. (1978). The functional basis of pulmonary sounds. *Chest* 73 (3): 399–405.

88 Fuentes, V.L. (2012). ARTERIAL THROMBOEMBOLISM risks, realities and a rational first-line approach. *J. Feline Med. Surg.* 14 (7): 459–470.

89 Smith, S.A. and Tobias, A.H. (2004). Feline arterial thromboembolism: an update. *Vet. Clin. North Am. Small Anim. Pract.* 34 (5): 1245–1271.

90 Ferasin, L. (2009). Feline myocardial disease 2: diagnosis, prognosis and clinical management. *J. Feline Med. Surg.* 11 (3): 183–194.

91 Campbell, F.E. and Kittleson, M.D. (2007). The effect of hydration status on the echocardiographic measurements of normal cats. *J. Vet. Intern. Med.* 21 (5): 1008–1015.

92 Rishniw, M. and Thomas, W.P. (2002). Dynamic right ventricular outflow obstruction: a new cause of systolic murmurs in cats. *J. Vet. Intern. Med.* 16 (5): 547–552.

44

Gallop Rhythms

44.1 Brief Review of Normal Heart Sounds, S1 and S2

Recall from Chapter 42, Section 42.1 and Chapter 43, Section 43.1 that the heart is a pump that coordinates forward flow of blood through the vasculature through atrial and ventricular contractions, and a series of valves that guard against backflow [1, 2]. It is the closure of particular sets of valves that creates the normal heart sounds, S1 and S2 [1, 2]. S1 and S2 create the characteristic "lub-dub" sound that is associated with each heartbeat [1–4]:

S1	S2	S1	S2
"Lub"	"Dub"	"Lub"	"Dub"

S1 is the result of atrioventricular (AV) valve closure: the left-sided mitral and the right-sided tricuspid valves close to facilitate ventricular contraction [1–3, 5].

S2 is the result of semilunar valve closure: the left-sided aortic and the right-sided pulmonic valves close during diastole to allow filling of the heart with blood in anticipation of the next phase of the cardiac cycle [1–3, 5].

S1 and S2 should both be audible on cardiothoracic auscultation of the normal patient [1].

44.2 Introduction to Abnormal Heart Sounds, S3 and S4

It is abnormal to hear additional heart sounds on cardiothoracic auscultation [5]. Two heart sounds, in particular, are associated with a decrease in ventricular compliance: S3 and S4 [6].

S3 is sometimes referred to as the ventricular gallop sound [7]. It occurs in early diastole, when the ventricles are filling with blood [6, 7]. Ordinarily, this event does not translate into a heart sound [7]. However, certain cardiac pathologies result in diastolic dysfunction [7].

Affected patients require greater investment of pressure to encourage filling of the ventricles [7]. This creates a third heart sound, S3 [5, 7]. The result is a so-called gallop rhythm [1, 5]:

1	2–3	1	2–3	1	2–3	1	2–3

S4 is sometimes referred to as the atrial gallop sound [7]. It occurs during the "atrial kick," that is, when the atria contract just before ventricular systole [6]. The purpose of the "atrial kick" is to increase preload by providing one last push of blood into the ventricles before it is pumped into systemic circulation. S4 develops in patients that have impaired ventricular relaxation [7]. Because their ventricles are inadequately relaxed, they have greater filling pressures [7]. The atria must exert more energy than is normal to force additional blood volume into the ventricles to maintain cardiac output [7]. This creates a fourth heart sound, S4 [5, 7]. The result is a different type of gallop rhythm [1, 5]:

4–1	2	4–1	2	4–1	2	4–1	2

S3 and S4 usually occur in isolation from one another; that is, a patient is more likely to have just one of the two abnormal heart sounds. However, there are rare occasions when a patient has both. When this occurs, the patient is said to have a summation gallop [7]:

4–1	2–3	4–1	2–3	4–1	2–3	4–1	2–3

Both S3 and S4 are detected best by the bell of the stethoscope because they are of low frequency [8, 9].

Gallop rhythms are so named because they sound like the bounding gait of a horse [6]. However, it may be more appropriate to consider gallop rhythms as gallop sounds. Gallop sounds are not arrhythmias, but they are sometimes confused with them when referred to as gallop rhythms. Arrhythmias are irregular heartbeats [1]. These can be detected via electrocardiography, whereas gallop rhythms cannot. Gallop rhythms simply refer to the addition of one or more heart sounds. Neither S3 nor S4 is apparent on electrocardiograms (ECGs).

44.3 The Ventricular Gallop, S3

The most common causes of the ventricular gallop are [1, 7]

- Congestive heart failure (CHF) secondary to dilated cardiomyopathy (DCM)
- Patent ductus arteriosus (PDA)
- Severe mitral regurgitation (MR).

44.3.1 Dilated Cardiomyopathy

Recall from Chapter 40, Section 40.4.3.4 that DCM is an acquired heart disease that has increased prevalence in Doberman Pinschers and Irish Wolfhounds [10]. Cats tend to develop DCM because of taurine deficiency, as compared to dogs, in which the etiology of DCM remains unknown [10, 11].

DCM results in a dilated, flaccid left ventricle that is inefficient at best. Cardiac contractility is greatly reduced, and systole is incomplete. Blood that is pumped into systemic circulation is at reduced velocity. Ultimately, blood backs up from the left ventricle into the left atrium, and from the left atrium into the pulmonary tree. Left-sided CHF is common.

Affected dogs often present for exercise intolerance or syncope [10, 12]. S3 may be present on cardiothoracic auscultation. Patients may also demonstrate atrial fibrillation and ventricular arrhythmias on ECG.

Taurine deficiency is rare in cats. When it occurs, it is most typically because of an inappropriate diet. Cats cannot synthesize taurine; they must ingest it in their food.

When feline taurine levels drop 50% below normal, retinal degeneration is likely [13–17].

Review Chapter 15, Section 15.4.5 for a discussion of at-risk cats and taurine-deficient diets.

In addition to blindness, taurine deficiency causes DCM in cats [18–22].

44.3.2 Patent Ductus Arteriosus

Review the pathophysiology of PDA as outlined in Chapter 39, Section 39.5.2 and Chapter 43, Section 43.6.2. Recall that left-to-right PDAs are more common than right-to-left PDAs [1, 23–26].

Patients with left-to-right PDAs have abnormal circulation in that blood from the pressurized aorta is directed into the pulmonary circulation. This volume overloads the pulmonary vasculature and, by extension, the left atrium [1, 23–25]. CHF secondary to left-sided volume overload is likely [1, 23–25, 27, 28].

On physical examination, affected patients have a continuous, "washing machine" murmur [1, 23–25]. Although it is often impossible to hear over this murmur, S3 may be audible.

Refer to the aforementioned sections for more information regarding breed predispositions and clinical presentations.

44.3.3 Severe Mitral Regurgitation

Recall from Chapter 40, Section 40.4.3.1 and Chapter 43, Section 43.7.1 that degenerative mitral valve disease (DMVD) is common in adult dogs, especially in small breeds [4, 29–35].

Affected dogs develop morphological changes in the mitral valve, including valve thickening, bulging, and eventual prolapse [33, 36–38]. This results in MR [33]. When MR is mild, cardiac function is relatively unchanged [33]. However, severe MR leads to pathologic remodeling of the heart [33]. To compensate for diminished stroke volume, the heart increases the heart rate and force of contraction [33]. Over time, the left atrium and left ventricle undergo hypertrophy [33]. CHF secondary to left-sided volume overload is likely [33].

On physical examination, affected patients have a systolic murmur that varies in intensity depending upon the stage of disease. In addition, cardiothoracic auscultation may reveal a ventricular gallop [1, 7].

44.4 The Atrial Gallop, S4

Common causes of the atrial gallop are [1, 7, 39–43]

- Hypertrophic cardiomyopathy (HCM)
- Systemic hypertension.

Third-degree AV block is also a cause of the atrial gallop; however, its frequency of occurrence is low as compared to the pathologies outlined above [7].

44.4.1 Hypertrophic Cardiomyopathy

Review the pathophysiology of HCM as outlined in Chapter 39, Section 39.5.1 and Chapter 43, Section 43.7.2. Recall that HCM is the most common heart disease among adult cats [29, 44–54].

Affected cats develop left ventricular hypertrophy. Less blood volume is able to fill the left ventricle at any given point in time, so it backs up into the left atrium, which dilates [55]. The left atrium struggles to fill the noncompliant left ventricle. Filling the left ventricle requires the left atrium to increase chamber pressure [55]. In turn, the pressure of the pulmonary vein has to increase in order to fill the left atrium [55].

As HCM progresses, CHF secondary to left-sided volume overload is likely [55]. Patients in CHF will often present with tachypnea and/or open-mouth breathing [55]. In addition, cardiothoracic auscultation is likely to reveal adventitious lung sounds, crackles.

Concerning the heart, a systolic murmur is often present, with or without a gallop rhythm [55–57].

Note that the murmur and/or gallop rhythm may also be present in otherwise asymptomatic cats [53, 58–61].

Refer to the aforementioned sections for more information regarding breed predispositions and classic clinical presentations, including aortic thromboembolism (ATE), the so-called "saddle thrombus."

44.4.2 Systemic Hypertension

Recall from Chapter 15, Section 15.4.2.2 that feline hypertension is defined as having persistently elevated, systolic blood pressure at greater than 160–170 mmHg and/or elevated diastolic pressures greater than 100 mmHg [62–67].

Recall from Chapter 15, Section 15.4.2 that canine hypertension is defined as having persistently elevated, systolic pressures of 180–200 mmHg and/or elevated diastolic pressures greater than 100 mmHg [64, 68, 69].

Hypertension may be primary or secondary [62, 64, 65, 70–72]. Both cause ventricular hypertrophy that results in the development of an atrial gallop.

Primary systemic hypertension is more common in dogs than cats, although it may be more common in cats than was once believed [64, 73–77].

Secondary systemic hypertension results from the following [62, 64–67, 70, 72, 78–85]:

- Acromegaly
- Chronic anemia
- Diabetes mellitus
- Erythropoietin
- High-salt diets (cats)
- Hyperadrenocorticism
- Hyperthyroidism***
- Pheochromocytomas
- Primary hyperaldosteronism
- Renal disease***

Those conditions that are starred (***) above reflect those causes of secondary systemic hypertension that most often result in the atrial gallop.

Refer to Chapter 15, Section 15.4.2 for more information regarding target organ damage secondary to systemic hypertension, particularly retinopathy.

Recall from Chapter 43, Section 43.7.2, that feline hyperthyroidism can also cause systolic murmurs.

Refer to Part Seven of the text to explore renal disease in greater depth, including its link to hypertension.

44.5 The Diagnostic Work-Up for Gallop Rhythms

Because gallop rhythms are abnormal findings on cardiothoracic auscultation, the presence of S3 and/or S4 in a companion animal patient warrants a diagnostic investigation into the source of the gallop [5].

As outlined in Sections 44.3 and 44.4, gallop rhythms may stem from primary cardiac pathology or systemic disease [1, 7, 39–43, 62, 64–67, 70, 72, 78–85]. Both avenues should be explored as potential causes of the gallop.

Bloodwork and urinalysis are a critical first step in exploring overall patient health.

The following blood tests provide an important baseline:

- Complete blood count (CBC)
- Chemistry profile
- Total thyroxine (TT4)

The aforementioned tests, in combination with urinalysis, establish organ function and screen for hyperthyroidism. In particular, the clinician is looking for evidence of renal and/or thyroid dysfunction. Both are commonly linked to systemic hypertension. For that reason, the patient's blood pressure (BP) should be evaluated.

Note that hypertension may also be primary. BP should therefore be a part of every patient's baseline when evaluating the dog or cat for a gallop rhythm.

In addition to diagnostic testing of body fluids, thoracic imaging is an important part of case management. Radiographs of the chest may confirm CHF or other thoracic disease. Radiographic evidence of cardiomegaly is suggestive of cardiomyopathy.

Echocardiography is preferred over thoracic radiography for the detection of congenital heart disease [29, 86]. Echocardiograms also provide greater detail concerning the internal structure of the heart, and they are capable of confirming structural changes that may be the source of the gallop.

ECGs are also important add-on tests that evaluate the patient for the presence of arrhythmias. Although the gallop itself will not be visible on ECGs, affected patients may have an underlying arrhythmogenic cardiomyopathy.

References

1 Englar, R.E. (2017). *Performing the Small Animal Physical Examination*. Hoboken, NJ: Wiley.

2 Hall, J.E. and Guyton, A.C. (2011). *Guyton and Hall Textbook of Medical Physiology*, 12e, xix, 1091 p. Philadelphia, PA: Saunders/Elsevier.

3 Dyce, K.M., Sack, W.O., and Wensing, C.J.G. (2010). *Textbook of Veterinary Anatomy*, 4e, xii, 834 p. St. Louis, MO: Saunders/Elsevier.

4 Hogan, D.F. (2008). Cardiac examination & history. *NAVC Clinician's Brief* (July): 49–53.

5 Stokhof, A.A. and De Rick, A. (2009). Circulatory system. In: *Medical History and Physical Examination in Companion Animals* (ed. A. Rijnberk and F.J. van Sluijs), 75–85. St. Louis: Elsevier Limited.

6 Estrada, A. Cardiac physical examination. NAVC Clinician's Brief [Internet]. https://www.cliniciansbrief.com/article/cardiac-physical-examinatio

7 Lorenz, M.C., Neer, T.M., and DeMars, P. (2009). *Small Animal Medical Diagnosis*, 3e. Ames, Iowa: Blackwell Publishing.

8 DeFrancesco, T. (2012). Cardiac auscultation 101. *NC State College of Veterinary Medicine [Internet]*. https://cvm.ncsu.edu/wp-content/uploads/2015/06/DeFrancesco2012_CardiacAusculation.pdf.

9 Garcia, J.L. (2014). Lecture Link: Feline cardiology review. DVM 360 [Internet]. http://veterinarymedicine.dvm360.com/lecture-link-feline-cardiology-review.

10 Oyama, M.A. (2008). Canine cardiomyopathy. In: *Manual of Canine and Feline Cardiology*, 4e (ed. L.P. Tilley, S. FWK, M.A. Oyama and M.M. Sleeper), 139–150. Philadelphia: W.B. Saunders.

11 Kienle, R.D. (2008). Feline cardiomyopathy. In: *Manual of Canine and Feline Cardiology*, 4e (ed. L.P. Tilley, F.W.K. Smith, M.A. Oyama and M.M. Sleeper), 151–175. Philadelphia: W.B. Saunders.

12 Mazzaferro, E.M. (2006). Acute collapse. *NAVC Clinician's Brief* (December): 15–16.

13 Aguirre, G.D. (1978). Retinal degeneration associated with the feeding of dog foods to cats. *J. Am. Vet. Med. Assoc.* 172 (7): 791–796.

14 Schmidt, S.Y., Berson, E.L., and Hayes, K.C. (1976). Retinal degeneration in cats fed casein. I. Taurine deficiency. *Invest. Ophthalmol.* 15 (1): 47–52.

15 Schmidt, S.Y., Berson, E.L., Watson, G., and Huang, C. (1977). Retinal degeneration in cats fed casein. III. Taurine deficiency and ERG amplitudes. *Invest. Ophthalmol. Vis. Sci.* 16 (7): 673–678.

16 Berson, E.L., Hayes, K.C., Rabin, A.R. et al. (1976). Retinal degeneration in cats fed casein. II. Supplementation with methionine, cysteine, or taurine. *Invest. Ophthalmol.* 15 (1): 52–58.

17 Hayes, K.C. (1976). A review on the biological function of taurine. *Nutr. Rev.* 34 (6): 161–165.

18 Novotny, M.J., Hogan, P.M., and Flannigan, G. (1994). Echocardiographic evidence for myocardial failure induced by taurine deficiency in domestic cats. *Can. J. Vet. Res.* 58 (1): 6–12.

19 Sisson, D.D., Knight, D.H., Helinski, C. et al. (1991). Plasma taurine concentrations and M-mode echocardiographic measures in healthy cats and in cats with dilated cardiomyopathy. *J. Vet. Intern. Med.* 5 (4): 232–238.

20 Pion, P.D., Kittleson, M.D., Rogers, Q.R., and Morris, J.G. (1987). Myocardial failure in cats associated with low plasma taurine: a reversible cardiomyopathy. *Science* 237 (4816): 764–768.

21 Pion, P.D., Kittleson, M.D., Rogers, Q.R., and Morris, J.G. (1990). Taurine deficiency myocardial failure in the domestic cat. *Prog. Clin. Biol. Res.* 351: 423–430.

22 Pion, P.D., Kittleson, M.D., Thomas, W.P. et al. (1992). Clinical findings in cats with dilated cardiomyopathy and relationship of findings to taurine deficiency. *J. Am. Vet. Med. Assoc.* 201 (2): 267–274.

23 Côté, E. (2015). *Clinical Veterinary Advisor. Dogs and Cats*, 3e, xxxvii, 1642 p. St. Louis, Missouri: Elsevier Mosby.

24 Tilley, L.P., Smith, F.W.K., and Tilley, L.P. (2007). *Blackwell's Five-minute Veterinary Consult: Canine and Feline*, 4e, Ix, 1578 p. Ames, Iowa: Blackwell.

25 Aiello, S.E., Moses, M.A., and Allen, D.G. (2016). *The Merck Veterinary Manual*. Whitehouse Station, NJ: Merck & Co., Inc.

26 Arora, M. (2001). Reversed patent ductus arteriosus in a dog. *Can. Vet. J.* 42 (6): 471–472.

27 Strickland, K.N. (2008). Congenital heart disease. In: *Manual of Canine and Feline Cardiology*, 4e (ed. L.P. Tilley, F.W.K. Smith, M.A. Oyama and M.M. Sleeper), 215–239. Philadelphia: W.B. Saunders.

28 Bulmer, B.J. (2011). The cardiovascular system. In: *Small Animal Pediatrics: The First 12 Months of Life* (ed. M.E. Peterson and M.A. Kutzler), 289–304. St. Louis, MO: Saunders/Elsevier.

29 Cote, E., Edwards, N.J., Ettinger, S.J. et al. (2015). Management of incidentally detected heart murmurs in dogs and cats. *J. Vet. Cardiol.* 17 (4): 245–261.

30 Rishniw, M. (2011). Canine heart murmur. *NAVC Clinician's Brief* (May): 49–52.

31 Borgarelli, M. and Haggstrom, J. (2010). Canine degenerative Myxomatous mitral valve disease: natural history, clinical presentation and therapy. *Vet. Clin. North Am. Small* 40 (4): 651–663.

32 Fox, P.R. (2012). Pathology of myxomatous mitral valve disease in the dog. *J. Vet. Cardiol.* 14 (1): 103–126.

33 Haggstrom, J., Pedersen, H.D., and Kvart, C. (2004). New insights into degenerative mitral valve disease in dogs. *Vet. Clin. North Am. Small.* 34 (5): 1209–1226.

34 Sisson, D.D., Kvart, C., and Darke, P. (1999). Acquired valvular heart disease. In: *Textbook of Canine and Feline Cardiology* (ed. P.R. Fox, D.D. Sisson and N.S. Moise), 536–565. Philadelphia: WB Saunders Company.

35 Haggstrom, J., Hoglund, K., and Borgarelli, M. (2009). An update on treatment and prognostic indicators in canine myxomatous mitral valve disease. *J. Small Anim. Pract.* 50 (Suppl 1): 25–33.

36 Buchanan, J.W. (1977). Chronic valvular disease (endocardiosis) in dogs. *Adv. Vet. Sci. Comp. Med.* 21: 75–106.

37 Kogure, K. (1980). Pathology of chronic mitral valvular disease in the dog. *Nippon Juigaku Zasshi* 42 (3): 323–335.

38 Whitney, J.C. (1974). Observations on the effect of age on the severity of heart valve lesions in the dog. *J. Small Anim. Pract.* 15 (8): 511–522.

39 Stepien, R.L. (2011). Feline systemic hypertension: diagnosis and management. *J. Feline Med. Surg.* 13 (1): 35–43.

40 Syme, H.M., Barber, P.J., Markwell, P.J., and Elliott, J. (2002). Prevalence of systolic hypertension in cats with chronic renal failure at initial evaluation. *J. Am. Vet. Med. Assoc.* 220 (12): 1799–1804.

41 Elliott, J., Barber, P.J., Syme, H.M. et al. (2001). Feline hypertension: clinical findings and response to antihypertensive treatment in 30 cases. *J. Small Anim. Pract.* 42 (3): 122–129.

42 Chetboul, V., Lefebvre, H.P., Pinhas, C. et al. (2003). Spontaneous feline hypertension: clinical and echocardiographic abnormalities, and survival rate. *J. Vet. Intern. Med.* 17 (1): 89–95.

43 Jacobs, G., Hutson, C., Dougherty, J., and Kirmayer, A. (1986). Congestive heart failure associated with hyperthyroidism in cats. *J. Am. Vet. Med. Assoc.* 188 (1): 52–56.

44 Cote, E., Manning, A.M., Emerson, D. et al. (2004). Assessment of the prevalence of heart murmurs in overtly healthy cats. *J. Am. Vet. Med. Assoc.* 225 (3): 384–388.

45 Paige, C.F., Abbott, J.A., Elvinger, F., and Pyle, R.L. (2009). Prevalence of cardiomyopathy in apparently healthy cats. *J. Am. Vet. Med. Assoc.* 234 (11): 1398–1403.

46 Wagner, T., Fuentes, V.L., Payne, J.R. et al. (2010). Comparison of auscultatory and echocardiographic findings in healthy adult cats. *J. Vet. Cardiol.* 12 (3): 171–182.

47 Bonagura, J.D. (2000). Feline echocardiography. *J. Feline Med. Surg.* 2 (3): 147–151.

48 Dirven, M.J., Cornelissen, J.M., Barendse, M.A. et al. (2010). Cause of heart murmurs in 57 apparently healthy cats. *Tijdschr. Diergeneeskd.* 135 (22): 840–847.

49 Nakamura, R.K., Rishniw, M., King, M.K., and Sammarco, C.D. (2011). Prevalence of echocardiographic evidence of cardiac disease in apparently healthy cats with murmurs. *J. Feline Med. Surg.* 13 (4): 266–271.

50 Fuentes, V.L. (2006). Cardiomyopathy: establishing a diagnosis. In: *Consultations in Feline Internal Medicine*, 5e (ed. J.R. August), 301–310. St. Louis: Saunders Elsevier.

51 Ferasin, L., Sturgess, C.P., Cannon, M.J. et al. (2003). Feline idiopathic cardiomyopathy: a retrospective study of 106 cats (1994–2001). *J. Feline Med. Surg.* 5 (3): 151–159.

52 Rishniw, M. and Pion, P.D. (2011). Is treatment of feline hypertrophic cardiomyopathy based in science or faith? A survey of cardiologists and a literature search. *J. Feline Med. Surg.* 13 (7): 487–497.

53 Freeman, L.M., Rush, J.E., Stern, J.A. et al. (2017). Feline hypertrophic cardiomyopathy: a spontaneous large animal model of human HCM. *Cardiol. Res.* 8 (4): 139–142.

54 Payne, J.R., Brodbelt, D.C., and Luis Fuentes, V. (2015). Cardiomyopathy prevalence in 780 apparently healthy cats in rehoming centres (the CatScan study). *J. Vet. Cardiol.* 17 (Suppl 1): S244–S257.

55 Bonagura, J.D. (1997). Feline hypertrophic cardiomyopathy. *Vet. Q.* 19: S5–S6.

56 Rush, J.E., Freeman, L.M., Fenollosa, N.K., and Brown, D.J. (2002). Population and survival characteristics of cats with hypertrophic cardiomyopathy: 260 cases (1990–1999). *J. Am. Vet. Med. Assoc.* 220 (2): 202–207.

57 Tilley, L.P., Liu, S.K., Gilbertson, S.R. et al. (1977). Primary myocardial disease in the cat. A model for human cardiomyopathy. *Am. J. Pathol.* 86 (3): 493–522.

58 Payne, J.R., Borgeat, K., Connolly, D.J. et al. (2013). Prognostic indicators in cats with hypertrophic cardiomyopathy. *J. Vet. Intern. Med.* 27 (6): 1427–1436.

59 Atkins, C.E., Gallo, A.M., Kurzman, I.D., and Cowen, P. (1992). Risk factors, clinical signs, and survival in cats with a clinical diagnosis of idiopathic hypertrophic cardiomyopathy: 74 cases (1985–1989). *J. Am. Vet. Med. Assoc.* 201 (4): 613–618.

60 Liu, S.K., Maron, B.J., and Tilley, L.P. (1981). Feline hypertrophic cardiomyopathy: gross anatomic and quantitative histologic features. *Am. J. Pathol.* 102 (3): 388–395.

61 Trehiou-Sechi, E., Tissier, R., Gouni, V. et al. (2012). Comparative echocardiographic and clinical features of hypertrophic cardiomyopathy in 5 breeds of cats: a retrospective analysis of 344 cases (2001–2011). *J. Vet. Intern. Med.* 26 (3): 532–541.

62 Maggio, F., DeFrancesco, T.C., Atkins, C.E. et al. (2000). Ocular lesions associated with systemic hypertension in cats: 69 cases (1985–1998). *J. Am. Vet. Med. Assoc.* 217 (5): 695–702.

63 Samsom, J., Rogers, K., and Wood, J.L. (2004). Blood pressure assessment in healthy cats and cats with hypertensive retinopathy. *Am. J. Vet. Res.* 65 (2): 245–252.

64 Henik, R.A. (1997). Systemic hypertension and its management. *Vet. Clin. North Am. Small Anim. Pract.* 27 (6): 1355–1372.

65 Littman, M.P. (1994). Spontaneous systemic hypertension in 24 cats. *J. Vet. Intern. Med.* 8 (2): 79–86.

66 Morgan, R.V. (1986). Systemic hypertension in four cats: ocular and medical findings. *J. Am. Anim. Hosp. Assoc.* 22: 615–621.

67 Stiles, J., Polzin, D.J., and Bistner, S.I. (1994). The prevalence of retinopathy in cats with systemic hypertension and chronic-renal-failure or hyperthyroidism. *J. Am. Anim. Hosp. Assoc.* 30 (6): 564–572.

68 Remillard, R.L., Ross, J.N., and Eddy, J.B. (1991). Variance of indirect blood pressure measurements and prevalence of hypertension in clinically normal dogs. *Am. J. Vet. Res.* 52 (4): 561–565.

69 Ritchie, C.M., Sheridan, B., Fraser, R. et al. (1990). Studies on the pathogenesis of hypertension in Cushing's disease and acromegaly. *Q. J. Med.* 76 (280): 855–867.

70 Henik, R.A., Snyder, P.S., and Volk, L.M. (1997). Treatment of systemic hypertension in cats with amlodipine besylate. *J. Am. Anim. Hosp. Assoc.* 33 (3): 226–234.

71 Komaromy, A.M., Andrew, S.E., Denis, H.M. et al. (2004). Hypertensive retinopathy and choroidopathy in a cat. *Vet. Ophthalmol.* 7 (1): 3–9.

72 Turner, J.L., Brogdon, J.D., Lees, G.E., and Greco, D.S. (1990). Idiopathic hypertension in a cat with secondary hypertensive retinopathy associated with a high-salt diet. *J. Am. Anim. Hosp. Assoc.* 26 (6): 647–651.

73 Brown, S.A. and Henik, R.A. (1998). Diagnosis and treatment of systemic hypertension. *Vet. Clin. North Am. Small Anim. Pract.* 28 (6): 1481–1494. ix.

74 Sansom, J., Barnett, K.C., Dunn, K.A. et al. (1994). Ocular-disease associated with hypertension in 16 cats. *J. Small Anim. Pract.* 35 (12): 604–611.

75 Bovee, K.C., Littman, M.P., Saleh, F. et al. (1986). Essential hereditary hypertension in dogs: a new animal model. *J. Hypertens. Suppl.* 4 (5): S172–S171.

76 Tippett, F.E., Padgett, G.A., Eyster, G. et al. (1987). Primary hypertension in a colony of dogs. *Hypertension* 9 (1): 49–58.

77 Littman, M.P., Robertson, J.L., and Bovee, K.C. (1988). Spontaneous systemic hypertension in dogs: five cases (1981–1983). *J. Am. Vet. Med. Assoc.* 193 (4): 486–494.

78 Ross, L.A. (1992). Hypertension and chronic renal failure. *Semin. Vet. Med. Surg. (Small Anim.)* 7 (3): 221–226.

79 Kobayashi, D.L., Peterson, M.E., Graves, T.K. et al. (1990). Hypertension in cats with chronic renal failure or hyperthyroidism. *J. Vet. Intern. Med.* 4 (2): 58–62.

80 Jensen, J., Henik, R.A., Brownfield, M., and Armstrong, J. (1997). Plasma renin activity and angiotensin I and aldosterone concentrations in cats with hypertension associated with chronic renal disease. *Am. J. Vet. Res.* 58 (5): 535–540.

81 Snyder, P.S. (1998). Amlodipine: a randomized, blinded clinical trial in 9 cats with systemic hypertension. *J. Vet. Intern. Med.* 12 (3): 157–162.

82 Peterson, M.E., Taylor, R.S., Greco, D.S. et al. (1990). Acromegaly in 14 cats. *J. Vet. Intern. Med.* 4 (4): 192–201.

83 Cowgill, L.D., James, K.M., Levy, J.K. et al. (1998). Use of recombinant human erythropoietin for management of anemia in dogs and cats with renal failure. *J. Am. Vet. Med. Assoc.* 212 (4): 521–528.

84 Chun, R., Jakovljevic, S., Morrison, W.B. et al. (1997). Apocrine gland adenocarcinoma and pheochromocytoma in a cat. *J. Am. Anim. Hosp. Assoc.* 33 (1): 33–36.

85 Flood, S.M., Randolph, J.F., Gelzer, A.R., and Refsal, K. (1999). Primary hyperaldosteronism in two cats. *J. Am. Anim. Hosp. Assoc.* 35 (5): 411–416.

86 Tse, Y.C., Rush, J.E., Cunningham, S.M. et al. (2013). Evaluation of a training course in focused echocardiography for noncardiology house officers. *J. Vet. Emerg. Crit. Care* 23 (3): 268–273.

45

Bradycardia

45.1 Introduction to Bradyarrhythmias

Bradyarrhythmias were first introduced in Chapter 40, Section 40.4. Recall that these heart rhythms are characterized by bradycardia, that is, a low heart rate [1]. Note that the heart rate may be consistently slow or the patient may experience bouts of sinus arrest, that is, pauses in the normal heart rhythm [1, 2].

When bradyarrhythmias cause one or more pauses that last for several seconds, then cardiogenic syncope is possible. Recall that these bradyarrhythmias include [2–7]

- Atrial standstill
- Atrioventricular (AV) heart block
- Sick sinus syndrome.

Review the pathophysiology of each in Chapter 40, Section 40.4.2.1. Recognize that it is not possible to differentiate between bradyarrhythmias based upon cardiothoracic auscultation alone [1]; electrocardiography is indicated.

45.2 Introduction to Sinus Bradycardia

This chapter will focus on sinus bradycardia, a heart rhythm in which there is a regular heartbeat. The heart rate is simply slower than normal.

Bradycardic dogs have a heart rate that is less than 60 beats per minute [1]. Cats are considered bradycardic at rates less than 140 [1].

Recall from Chapter 40 that sinus bradycardia may result from the following [1, 8–26]:

- Electrolyte imbalances
  - Hyperkalemia***
- High vagal tone***
- Hypothermia***

- Overzealous response to β-blockers, calcium channel blockers, or digoxin
- Administration of certain pharmaceutical agents
  - α-2-adrenergic agonists
    - Dexmedetomidine
    - Medetomidine
    - Xylazine
- Opioids
- Phenothiazines
  - Acepromazine
  - Prostaglandin (PG) F2α
  - Sodium nitroprusside
- Sepsis in cats

Those that are starred (***) will be explored in greater detail here.

45.3 Hyperkalemia and Sinus Bradycardia

Potassium is one of the most important electrolytes in the body [27]. As the body's primary intracellular cation, potassium contributes to the function of nerves and muscle, specifically cardiac and skeletal, by generating the normal resting cell membrane potential [27, 28]. For this reason, its serum concentrations are tightly regulated between 3.5 and 5.5 mEq/l, depending upon which laboratory is referenced [27].

When serum potassium exceeds the normal reference range, cardiac and neuromuscular cells are adversely impaired due to alterations in the transmembrane resting potential [27–29].

The following cardiac changes are evident on electrocardiograms (ECGs) of hyperkalemic patients [27, 28, 30–38]:

- Bradycardia
- Lengthened P–R intervals
- Small-to-nonexistent P waves
- So-called tented T-waves, meaning that they are tall and spiked, with a base that is narrow
- Widened QRS complexes

Common Clinical Presentations in Dogs and Cats, First Edition. Ryane E. Englar.
© 2019 John Wiley & Sons, Inc. Published 2019 by John Wiley & Sons, Inc.

Bradycardia results from prolonged depolarization and repolarization of the myocardium [28, 29].

Note that the progression of ECG changes is proportional to the degree to which serum potassium climbs [27, 28]. If serum potassium exceeds 7.5 mEq/l and medical management is not instituted, then patient fatality is likely [28, 34].

Patients that are hyperkalemic to the point of having cardiac changes on ECG are typically ill on initial presentation [29, 30, 39].

Owners may relay historical findings of weakness and collapse [30].

A common presenting complaint in male cats with hyperkalemia is related to the urinary tract [29, 39, 40]. Owners may report dysuria, stranguria, hematuria, or anuria, secondary to urinary tract obstruction (UTO) or rupture [29, 30].

Other causes of hyperkalemia in companion animal patients include the following [27, 28, 30]:

- Acute renal failure (ARF) or acute kidney injury (AKI)
- Extensive muscle trauma
- Hypoadrenocorticism, an endocrinopathy that is otherwise known as Addison's disease
- Metabolic acidosis
- Pharmaceutical drugs
  - Angiotensin-converting enzyme (ACE) inhibitors
  - Potassium-sparing diuretics
- Reperfusion syndrome
- Trichuriasis, also known as whipworm infestation

History taking and the physical examination are essential diagnostic tools in cases that involve bradycardic patients, because certain findings may make the clinician suspicious of hyperkalemia.

A thorough patient profile involving current pharmaceutical history – which medications the patient is taking, at which dose, and with what frequency – may lead the clinician to suspect that bradycardia is secondary to hyperkalemia.

Patients with a history of weight loss and intermittent, large-bowel diarrhea that may or may not contain frank blood benefit from screening for whipworms.

In some cases, physical examination findings are nearly pathognomonic for pathology that could explain the patient's bradycardia. Consider, for example, the case of a "blocked" cat. A blocked cat has a urethral obstruction that results in decreased urinary excretion of potassium [27, 28, 30]. Because of underlying hyperkalemia, these patients tend to be bradycardic on presentation. In addition, palpation of the abdomen on physical examination will reveal a firm, turgid, painful urinary bladder. This finding is sufficient to formulate a presumptive diagnosis of UTO.

All patients that are bradycardic and ill should undergo, at minimum, baseline bloodwork testing, including a serum chemistry profile, to evaluate them for hyperkalemia.

45.4 Hypothermia and Sinus Bradycardia

Hypothermia is defined as a drop in core body temperature below the established reference range [41–43]. Companion animal patients are said to be hypothermic when their core body temperature drop below 99 °F [43].

Recall from Chapter 39, Section 39.3 that the body is primed to detect changes in core temperature, and that body temperature is regulated at the level of the hypothalamus [44–46]. Review how the body responds to hypothermia in an attempt to maintain homeostasis [41, 45, 47, 48].

Any patient may become hypothermic. However, patients are most at risk for developing hypothermia if they are [41, 43, 47, 49–55]

- Anesthetized
- Geriatric
- Immobile
- Immune-compromised
- Neonates
- Small in size and/or body weight
- Severely ill.

Recall that it is normal for neonatal cats and dogs to be hypothermic until four to seven weeks of life [47, 55].

Hypothermia depresses the baroreceptor reflex [42, 56, 57].

Remember that baroreceptors are collections of nerve endings within the vasculature and heart that respond to changes in arterial pressure [58]. They are particularly concentrated within the aortic arch and internal carotid arteries [58].

Baroreceptors work by sensing intraluminal stretch within vessels [58]. Stretch results from changes in intraluminal pressure. Increased stretch, as detected by baroreceptors, is interpreted as elevated blood pressure (BP), whereas decreased stretch translates into reduced BP.

At low pressures, baroreceptors are relatively inactive. Although they are constantly reporting back to higher centers about BP, they do not increase their firing rate until they perceive increased vascular wall stretch [58].

As stretch increases, so, too, does the rate at which baroreceptors fire [58]. This increased rate inhibits sympathetic outflow, resulting in less norepinephrine that is available to bind to cardiovascular targets. Because norepinephrine causes vasoconstriction, less of it in the circulation causes vasodilation. At the same time, less sympathetic activity shifts the balance in favor of the parasympathetic pathway. Activation of the parasympathetic nervous system results in reflex bradycardia. The net result is a reduction in BP.

On the other hand, if BP drops too low, then baroreceptors will reduce their rate of firing [58]. This activates the sympathetic nervous system to increase heart rate and cause vasoconstriction. Both actions in turn remedy hypotension by restoring BP to a more appropriate range.

So how does this system of checks and balances relate to hypothermia?

Hypothermia reduces BP. Ordinarily, the baroreceptor reflex would become activated to counter hypotension. However, hypothermia dampens this reflex. As a result, the body is at a loss to respond to hypotension through activation of the sympathetic nervous system, and hypotension persists. The patient's heart rate does not elevate, as it should, to combat hypotension. Instead, heart rate continues to drop as core body temperature moves further and further from the normal reference range [58].

Hypothermia is commonly seen in ill cats, particularly those that are hypotensive [59]. Whereas dogs tend to respond to shock initially with a hyperdynamic phase, cats are so sensitive that they decompensate rapidly [59]. Shocky cats become hypothermic because they are bradycardic and have poor cardiac output [59]. However, the resultant hypotension exacerbates the bradycardia [59]. It becomes a vicious cycle. Cats are difficult to resuscitate from hypotensive shock [59]. Warming their core body temperature is an important aspect of case management to restore the baroreceptor reflex and reverse bradycardia.

Hypothermia is also a common complication of anesthesia [41, 44, 53, 60]. Most anesthetic and analgesic agents dull the ability of the hypothalamus to serve as a functional thermostat [44, 53, 61–63].

In addition, general anesthesia eliminates the patient's ability to shiver to produce heat [44, 64].

Inhalant agents also contribute to heat loss because they bypass the nasal passageways [47]. They reach the lower airways without having been warmed first [47]. This chills the respiratory tract, which reduces core body temperature.

In addition, patients are chilled because of air temperature and the temperature of surrounding objects while under anesthesia and undergoing medical or surgical procedures [44, 47, 65–68]. Operating rooms are typically set at cooler ambient temperatures, and stainless steel induction and surgical tables are infrequently insulated [44, 47, 53, 65–68].

Surgical prep, in particular clipping or shaving the fur, effectively removes the patient's insulating layer. Fur at the periphery of the surgical field is often wet with surgical prep solutions [44, 47, 65–69]. This exacerbates heat loss.

Open-chest and abdominal procedures also contribute to hypothermia [53].

All of these factors contribute to hypothermia during the perioperative, operative, and immediate postoperative periods. Hypothermia promotes bradycardia [43, 53, 70, 71].

In addition, hypothermia prolongs recovery from general anesthesia [42]. This is particularly concerning because postoperative hypothermia is associated with increased morbidity and mortality in humans [53, 72].

Monitoring core body temperature is critical throughout anesthesia to minimize changes that could be detrimental to the patient. When core body temperature drops, active measures must be taken to guard against further loss and to remedy the current situation.

45.5 High Vagal Tone and Sinus Bradycardia

Vagal tone describes the activity of the tenth cranial nerve, the vagus. The vagus nerve is located in the medulla oblongata and contributes to the autonomic nervous system. In particular, the vagus nerve promotes parasympathetic activity. The parasympathetic nervous system is sometimes referred to as the "rest and digest" or "feed and breed" system [73]: It is not, in other words, associated with "fight or flight."

When the vagus nerve fires, it is supportive of those activities that support the patient that is at rest, including the following [58, 73]:

- Bradycardia
- Defecation
- Digestion
- Lacrimation
- Pupil constriction
- Salivation
- Urination

Vagal tone is a measure of how well the parasympathetic nervous system is activated at any given point in time. When there is high vagal tone, parasympathetic activity is maximized [58, 73].

Therefore, physiologic and pathologic conditions that promote high vagal tone will result in bradycardia [58, 73]. These include the following [1]:

- Central nervous system disease
  - Increased intracranial pressure (ICP)
  - Increased intraocular pressure (IOP)
- Gastrointestinal disease

- Respiratory disease
- Severe pain

For example, compression of the eye or traction applied to extraocular muscles, as may occur during enucleation, induces the oculocardiac reflex [74, 75]. This reflex is characterized by a drop in heart rate that is mediated via the vagus and trigeminal nerves [76]. Brachycephalic and pediatric patients are most at risk for developing this response. If it occurs, manipulation of the eye or surrounding tissues should be discontinued [76]. Intravenous administration of glycopyrrolate may be required to resolve the bradycardia [76]. Note, however, that bradycardia is not the only potential sequelae of the oculocardiac reflex [76]. Patients may also develop life-threatening arrhythmias and even cardiopulmonary arrest [76].

A second example is the Cushing reflex or the vasopressor response. Increased ICP results in Cushing's triad [77, 78]:

- Bradycardia
- Increased BP
- Slow and often irregular respiration.

Cerebral arterioles are compressed when ICP exceeds mean arterial blood pressure [79–81]. This compression reduces blood flow to the brain [79–81]. The body's initial response to cerebral ischemia is to activate the sympathetic nervous system [79–81]. This stimulates adrenergic receptors to cause vasoconstriction, which increases BP in an attempt to restore blood flow to the brain [79–81]. In addition, epinephrine raises the heart rate and contractility to increase cardiac output [79–81]. This tachycardia is not long-lasting [79–81].

When baroreceptors detect elevations in BP, they fire with increasing frequency to inhibit sympathetic outflow and trigger a parasympathetic response [58]. Activation of the parasympathetic nervous system results in reflex bradycardia. The net result is a reduction in BP.

References

1 DeFrancesco, T.C. (2013). Management of cardiac emergencies in small animals. *Vet. Clin. North Am. Small Anim. Pract.* 43 (4): 817–842.

2 Bulmer, B. (2012). Interpreting ECGs with confidence: Part 2. *NAVC Clinician's Brief* (June): 102–105.

3 Schwartz, D.S. (ed.) (2009). The syncopal dog. *World Small Animal Veterinary Association World Congress Proceedings*; Sao Paulo, Brazil.

4 Scansen, B.A. (2011). Interventional cardiology for the criticalist. *J. Vet. Emerg. Crit. Care (San Antonio)* 21 (2): 123–136.

5 Strickland, K.N. (2008). Congenital heart disease. In: *Manual of Canine and Feline Cardiology*, 4e (ed. L.P. Tilley, F.W.K. Smith, M.A. Oyama and M.M. Sleeper), 215–239. Philadelphia: W.B. Saunders.

6 Bulmer, B.J. (2011). The cardiovascular system. In: *Small Animal Pediatrics: The First 12 Months of Life* (ed. M.E. Peterson and M.A. Kutzler), 289–304. St. Louis, Mo: Saunders/Elsevier.

7 Englar, R.E. (2017). *Performing the Small Animal Physical Examination*. Hoboken, NJ: Wiley.

8 Ko, J.C.H., Fox, S.M., and Mandsager, R.E. (2001). Effects of preemptive atropine administration on incidence of medetomidine-induced bradycardia in dogs. *J. Am. Vet. Med. Assoc.* 218 (1): 52–58.

9 Bartram, D.H., Diamond, M.J., Tute, A.S. et al. (1994). Use of medetomidine and butorphanol for sedation in dogs. *J. Small Anim. Pract.* 35 (10): 495–498.

10 Ko, J.C., Thurmon, J.C., Benson, G.J. et al. (1994). Hemodynamic and anesthetic effects of etomidate infusion in medetomidine-premedicated dogs. *Am. J. Vet. Res.* 55 (6): 842–846.

11 Thurmon, J.C., Ko, J.C., Benson, G.J. et al. (1994). Hemodynamic and analgesic effects of propofol infusion in medetomidine-premedicated dogs. *Am. J. Vet. Res.* 55 (3): 363–367.

12 Vainio, O. (1989). Introduction to the clinical pharmacology of medetomidine. *Acta Vet. Scand. Suppl.* 85: 85–88.

13 Young, L.E., Brearley, J.C., Richards, D.L.S. et al. (1990). Medetomidine as a premedicant in dogs and its reversal by atipamezole. *J. Small Anim. Pract.* 31 (11): 554–559.

14 Forsyth, S. (ed.) (2001). Perioperative use of opioids in dogs and cats. World Small Animal Veterinary Association World Congress; Vancouver, Canada.

15 Dohoo, S.E. and Dohoo, I.R. (1996). Postoperative use of analgesics in dogs and cats by Canadian veterinarians. *Can. Vet. J.* 37 (9): 546–551.

16 Dohoo, S.E. and Dohoo, I.R. (1998). Attitudes and concerns of Canadian animal health technologists toward postoperative pain management in dogs and cats. *Can. Vet. J.* 39 (8): 491–496.

17 Carroll, G.L. (1999). Analgesics and pain. *Vet. Clin. North Am. Small* 29 (3): 701.

18 Mazzaferro, E. and Wagner, A.E. (2001). Hypotension during anesthesia in dogs and cats: recognition, causes, and treatment. *Comp. Cont. Educ. Pract.* 23 (8): 728.

19 Bergstrom, K. (1988). Cardiovascular and pulmonary effects of a new sedative/analgesic (medetomidine) as a preanaesthetic drug in the dog. *Acta Vet. Scand.* 29 (1): 109–116.

20 Clarke, K.W. and England, G.C.W. (1989). Medetomidine, a new sedative-analgesic for use in the

dog and its reversal with atipamezole. *J. Small Anim. Pract.* 30 (6): 343–348.

21 Lemke, K.A. and Tranquilli, W.J. (1994). Anesthetics, arrhythmias, and myocardial sensitization to epinephrine. *J. Am. Vet. Med. Assoc.* 205 (12): 1679–1684.

22 Short, C.E. (1991). Effects of anticholinergic treatment on the cardiac and respiratory systems in dogs sedated with medetomidine. *Vet. Rec.* 129 (14): 310–313.

23 Pypendop, B.H. and Verstegen, J.P. (1998). Hemodynamic effects of medetomidine in the dog: a dose titration study. *Vet. Surg.* 27 (6): 612–622.

24 Paddleford, R.R. and Harvey, R.C. (1999). Alpha(2) agonists and antagonists. *Vet. Clin. North Am. Small* 29 (3): 737.

25 Hintze, T.H., Martin, E.G., Messina, E.J., and Kaley, G. (1979). Prostacyclin (PGI2) elicits reflex bradycardia in dogs: evidence for vagal mediation. *Proc. Soc. Exp. Biol. Med.* 162 (1): 96–100.

26 Hintze, T.H., Panzenbeck, M.J., Messina, E.J., and Kaley, G. (1981). Prostacyclin (PGI2) lowers heart rate in the conscious dog. *Cardiovasc. Res.* 15 (9): 538–546.

27 DiBartola, S.P. (2012). *Fluid, Electrolyte, and Acid-Base Disorders in Small Animal Practice*, 4e, xiv, 744 p. St. Louis, Mo: Saunders/Elsevier.

28 Odunyano, A. (2014). Management of potassium disorders. *NAVC Clinician's Brief* (March): 69–72.

29 Lee, J.A. and Drobatz, K.J. (2006). Historical and physical parameters as predictors of severe hyperkalemia in male cats with urethral obstruction. *J. Vet. Emerg. Crit. Care* 16 (2): 104–111.

30 Tilley, L.P., Smith, F.W.K., and Tilley, L.P. (2007). *Blackwell's Five-Minute Veterinary Consult: Canine and Feline*, 4e, lx, 1578 p. Ames, Iowa: Blackwell.

31 Schaer, M. (1977). Hyperkalemia in cats with urethral obstruction. Electrocardiographic abnormalities and treatment. *Vet. Clin. North Am.* 7 (2): 407–414.

32 Parks, J. (1975). Electrocardiographic abnormalities from serum electrolyte imbalance due to feline urethral obstruction. *J. Am. Anim. Hosp. Assoc.* 11: 101–109.

33 Surawicz, B. (1967). Relationship between electrocardiogram and electrolytes. *Am. Heart J.* 73 (6): 814–834.

34 Tag, T.L. and Day, T.K. (2008). Electrocardiographic assessment of hyperkalemia in dogs and cats. *J. Vet. Emerg. Crit. Care* 18 (1): 61–67.

35 Dreifus, L.S. and Pick, A. (1956). A clinical correlative study of the electrocardiogram in electrolyte imbalance. *Circulation* 14 (5): 815–825.

36 Ettinger, P.O., Regan, T.J., and Oldewurtel, H.A. (1974). Hyperkalemia, cardiac conduction, and the electrocardiogram: a review. *Am. Heart J.* 88 (3): 360–371.

37 Cote, E. (2010). Feline arrhythmias: an update. *Vet. Clin. North Am. Small* 40 (4): 643.

38 Tilley, L.P. (1993). *Essentials of Canine and Feline Electrocardiography*. Philadelphia: Lea & Febiger.

39 Lee, J.A. and Drobatz, K.J. (2003). Characterization of the clinical characteristics, electrolytes, acid-base, and renal parameters in male cats with urethral obstruction. *J. Vet. Emerg. Crit. Care* 13 (4): 227–233.

40 Lawler, D.F., Sjolin, D.W., and Collins, J.E. (1985). Incidence rates of feline lower urinary-tract disease in the United-States. *Feline Pract.* 15 (5): 13–16.

41 Brodeur, A., Wright, A., and Cortes, Y. (2017). Hypothermia and targeted temperature management in cats and dogs. *J. Vet. Emerg. Crit. Care (San Antonio)* 27 (2): 151–163.

42 Pottie, R.G., Dart, C.M., Perkins, N.R., and Hodgson, D.R. (2007). Effect of hypothermia on recovery from general anaesthesia in the dog. *Aust. Vet. J.* 85 (4): 158–162.

43 Oncken, A.K., Kirby, R., and Rudloff, E. (2001). Hypothermia in critically ill dogs and cats. *Comp. Cont. Educ. Pract.* 23 (6): 506.

44 Clark-Price, S. (2015). Inadvertent perianesthetic hypothermia in small animal patients. *Vet. Clin. North Am. Small Anim. Pract.* 45 (5): 983–994.

45 Hall, J.E. (2011). Body temperature regulation, and fever. In: *Guyton and Hall Textbook of Medical Physiology* (ed. J.E. Hall), 867–877. Philadelphia: Saunders Elsevier.

46 Kurz, A. (2009). Physiology of thermoregulation. *Best Pract. Res. Clin. Anaesthesiol.* 22 (4): 627–644.

47 Reuss-Lamky, H. (2015). Hypothermia overview. *NAVC Clinician's Brief* (November): 12–16.

48 Duffy, T. (ed.) (2007). *Thermoregulation of the Perioperative Patient*. Proc ACVS. Chicago, IL: ACVS.

49 Mallet, M.L. (2002). Pathophysiology of accidental hypothermia. *Qjm-Int. J. Med.* 95 (12): 775–785.

50 Sugano, Y. (1981). Seasonal-changes in heat-balance of dogs acclimatized to outdoor climate. *Jpn. J. Physiol.* 31 (4): 465–475.

51 Dhupa, N. (1995). Hypothermia in dogs and cats. *Comp. Cont. Educ. Pract.* 17 (1): 61–68.

52 Danzl, D.F. and Pozos, R.S. (1994). Current concepts - accidental hypothermia. *N. Engl. J. Med.* 331 (26): 1756–1760.

53 Armstrong, S.R., Roberts, B.K., and Aronsohn, M. (2005). Perioperative hypothermia. *J. Vet. Emerg. Crit. Care* 15 (1): 32–37.

54 Lee, J. and Cohn, L. (2015). Pediatric critical care. *Clin. Brief* 13 (2): 41–42.

55 Blackmon, N. (2015). Anesthetic considerations for geriatric dogs. *Vet. Team Brief* 3 (3): 24.

56 Frank, S.M., Fleisher, L.A., Breslow, M.J. et al. (1997). Perioperative maintenance of normothermia reduces the incidence of morbid cardiac events. A randomized clinical trial. *JAMA* 277 (14): 1127–1134.

57 Tanaka, M., Nagasaki, G., and Nishikawa, T. (2001). Moderate hypothermia depresses arterial baroreflex

control of heart rate during, and delays its recovery after, general anesthesia in humans. *Anesthesiology* 95 (1): 51–55.

58 Reece, W.O., Erickson, H.H., Goff, J.P., and Uemura, E.E. (2015). *Dukes' Physiology of Domestic Animals*, 13e, xii, 748 p. Ames, Iowa, USA: Wiley Blackwell.

59 Tello, L.H. (ed.) (2009). *Feline as Emergency Patient: Trauma*. Sao Paulo, Brazil: WSAVA.

60 Hosgood, G. and Scholl, D.T. (2002). Evaluation of age and American Society of Anesthesiologists (ASA) physical status as risk factors for perianesthetic morbidity and mortality in the cat. *J. Vet. Emerg. Crit. Care* 12 (1): 9–15.

61 Sessler, D.I. (2015). Temperature regulation and monitoring. In: *Miller's Anesthesia* (ed. R.D. Miller, N.H. Cohen and L.I. Eriksson), 1622–1646. St. Louis: Saunders Elsevier.

62 Saritas, Z.K., Saritas, T.B., Pamuk, K. et al. (2014). Comparison of the effects of lidocaine and fentanyl in epidural anesthesia in dogs. *Bratisl. Lek. Listy* 115 (8): 508–513.

63 Vainionpaa, M., Salla, K., Restitutti, F. et al. (2013). Thermographic imaging of superficial temperature in dogs sedated with medetomidine and butorphanol with and without MK-467 (L-659′066). *Vet. Anaesth. Analg.* 40 (2): 142–148.

64 Matsukawa, T., Kurz, A., Sessler, D.I. et al. (1995). Propofol linearly reduces the vasoconstriction and shivering thresholds. *Anesthesiology* 82 (5): 1169–1180.

65 Kaiser-Klinger, S. (ed.) (2008). *Troubleshooting Emergency Anesthesia*. Phoenix, AZ: IVECC.

66 McKelvey, D. and Hollingshead, K. (1994). *Small Animal Anesthesia: Canine and Feline Practice*. St. Louis: Mosby-Year Book.

67 Harvey, R. (ed.) (2009). *Crisis Management: What to Worry About*. AAHA.

68 Zeltzman, P. (2009). *Hypothermia in Surgical Patients*. Phoenix, AZ: ACVS.

69 Sessler, D.I. (1997). Perioperative thermoregulation and heat balance. *Ann. N. Y. Acad. Sci.* 813: 757–777.

70 Orts, A., Alcaraz, C., Delaney, K.A. et al. (1992). Bretylium tosylate and electrically induced cardiac arrhythmias during hypothermia in dogs. *Am. J. Emerg. Med.* 10 (4): 311–316.

71 Yoshida, M., Shibata, K., Itoh, H., and Yamamoto, K. (2001). Cardiovascular responses to the induction of mild hypothermia in the presence of epidural anesthesia. *Anesthesiology* 94 (4): 678–682.

72 Slotman, G.J., Jed, E.H., and Burchard, K.W. (1985). Adverse effects of hypothermia in postoperative patients. *Am. J. Surg.* 149 (4): 495–501.

73 McCorry, L.K. (2007). Physiology of the autonomic nervous system. *Am. J. Pharm. Educ.* 71 (4): 78.

74 Kim, H.S., Kim, S.D., Kim, C.S., and Yum, M.K. (2000). Prediction of the oculocardiac reflex from pre-operative linear and nonlinear heart rate dynamics in children. *Anaesthesia* 55 (9): 847–852.

75 Paton, J.F., Boscan, P., Pickering, A.E., and Nalivaiko, E. (2005). The yin and yang of cardiac autonomic control: vago-sympathetic interactions revisited. *Brain Res. Brain Res. Rev.* 49 (3): 555–565.

76 Bryant, S. (ed.) (2010). *Anesthesia for Veterinary Technicians*. Ames, Iowa: Blackwell Publishing.

77 Ayling, J. (2002). Managing head injuries. *Emerg. Med. Serv.* 31 (8): 42.

78 Fodstad, H., Kelly, P.J., and Buchfelder, M. (2006). History of the Cushing reflex. *Neurosurgery* 59 (5): 1132–1137; discussion 7.

79 Beiner, J.M., Olgivy, C.S., and DuBois, A.B. (1997). Cerebral blood flow changes in response to elevated intracranial pressure in rabbits and bluefish: a comparative study. *Comp. Biochem. Physiol. A Physiol.* 116 (3): 245–252.

80 Hackett, J.G., Abboud, F.M., Mark, A.L. et al. (1972). Coronary vascular responses to stimulation of chemoreceptors and baroreceptors: evidence for reflex activation of vagal cholinergic innervation. *Circ. Res.* 31 (1): 8–17.

81 Woodman, O.L. and Vatner, S.F. (1987). Coronary vasoconstriction mediated by alpha 1- and alpha 2-adrenoceptors in conscious dogs. *Am. J. Physiol.* 253 (2 Pt 2): H388–H393.

46

Tachycardia

46.1 Introduction to Tachyarrhythmias

Tachyarrhythmias are heart rhythms that are characterized by tachycardia, that is, a rapid heart rate [1]. Note that the heart rate may be consistently fast or the patient may experience bursts of tachycardia interposed between periods of normal heart rhythm [1, 2].

Tachyarrhythmias were first touched upon in Chapter 40, Sections 40.4.1 and 40.4.4 in reference to the cardiac pathology, arrhythmogenic right ventricular cardiomyopathy (ARVC). Recall that ARVC commonly causes ventricular tachycardia, an abnormally rapid heart rate that originates within the ventricles ([3–6]). Ventricular contractions occur independently of atrial contractions, resulting in wide, so-called bizarre QRS complexes that are not tied to P waves on the electrocardiogram (ECG) ([6–8]).

Note that ventricular tachycardia is not the only form of tachyarrhythmias [1, 2]. Other forms include [1, 2, 6, 8–12] the following:

- Atrial fibrillation
- Atrial flutter
- Supraventricular tachycardia
- Ventricular fibrillation

Most tachyarrhythmias are associated with clinical emergencies [11, 13]. The heart may be driven to pump so fast that there is inadequate filling of the heart with each beat. This leads to a decrease in blood flow to the body [14–17].

If blood flow to the brain is sufficiently reduced, then cardiogenic syncope is likely [14–17]. Patients often present for weakness and/or collapse. Sudden death is possible [11, 13].

Refer to Chapter 40 for a review of collapse.

Recognize that it is not possible to differentiate between tachyarrhythmias based upon cardiothoracic auscultation alone [1, 11, 13, 18]. Electrocardiography is indicated [19].

46.2 Introduction to Sinus Tachycardia

This chapter will focus on sinus tachycardia, a heart rhythm in which there is a regular heartbeat [20–22]. The heart rate is simply faster than normal [22].

Recognition of tachycardia on physical examination requires one to know the normal heart rate for both cats and dogs. Note that the normal reference range varies for both species depending upon which references are consulted. In general, the following ranges of heart rate constitutes normal [23–26]:

- Cat:
  - 140–210 beats per minute (bpm)
- Dog:
  - Small-breed: 90–120 bpm
  - Medium-breed: 70–110 bpm
  - Large-breed: 60–90 bpm

In large part, this variation between numerical values in reference material is due to the fact that most data concerning heart rate is gathered on clinical examinations, and most veterinary patients are physiologically stressed in the examination room. The so-called "white coat syndrome" complicates our understanding of our patients' "normal" heart rate [27–30]. What is "normal" for us to auscultate during a physical examination is likely higher than the patient's resting heart rate when in a more familiar setting, such as the home environment.

In general, dogs are considered to be tachycardic when their heart rate is greater than 140–180 bpm [20, 21]. Note that this is not a hard-fast rule. Reference ranges for heart rate require some degree of flexibility based upon the size of the dog. For example, a large-breed dog with a heart rate of 115 is likely to be considered tachycardic, whereas a small-breed dog with the same heart rate is considered normal.

Cats may be considered tachycardic at rates greater than 180–210 bpm [19, 31]. Cats are definitively tachycardic at rates greater than 240 bpm [20].

Common Clinical Presentations in Dogs and Cats, First Edition. Ryane E. Englar.
© 2019 John Wiley & Sons, Inc. Published 2019 by John Wiley & Sons, Inc.

Because cats are so often tachycardic in the veterinary clinic, some consider this to be a normal physical examination finding in the feline patient [19, 31, 32].

46.3 Causes of Sinus Tachycardia

Sinus tachycardia may be physiologic or pathologic [13].

Causes of physiologic sinus tachycardia include the following [8, 11, 13, 20, 22, 33]:

- Anxiety
- Excitement
- Exercise
- Fear
- Hyperthermia
- Pain
- Restraint
- Stress

Causes of pathologic sinus tachycardia include the following [8, 11, 13, 20, 22, 33, 34]:

- Anemia
- Aortic thromboembolism (ATE)
- Congestive heart failure (CHF)
- Fever
- Hyperthyroidism
- Hypotension
- Hypovolemia
  - Dehydration
  - Hemorrhage
- Hypoxia
- Infectious disease
- Low cardiac output
- Pheochromocytoma
- Pulmonary thromboembolism (PTE)

Sinus tachycardia may also result from the administration of certain pharmaceutical agents, including the following [13]:

- Atropine
- β-agonists
- Epinephrine
- Glycopyrrolate
- Ketamine

Finally, sinus tachycardia may result from inappropriate depth of anesthesia, meaning that the patient's maintenance anesthesia is too light [13].

46.4 Sinus Tachycardia due to Increased Sympathetic Tone

Sinus tachycardia is often the result of high sympathetic tone [13, 31].

Sympathetic tone describes the body's response to impulses from the sympathetic nervous system. Recall that the sympathetic nervous system is one arm of the autonomic nervous system [24].

The sympathetic nervous system opposes the parasympathetic nervous system [24]. The former facilitates "fight or flight," whereas the latter has been described as the "feed and breed" or "rest and digest" pathway [24, 35].

High sympathetic tone occurs when messages from the sympathetic nervous system exceed those from the parasympathetic nervous system. These messages involve the activation of certain receptors by and unable neurotransmitters [24].

Messages from the sympathetic nervous system typically involve the activation of adrenergic receptors by catecholamines, such as norepinephrine (noradrenaline) or epinephrine (adrenaline) [24].

When catecholamines bind to adrenergic receptors, the following cardiovascular actions result [24, 36–41]:

- Chronotropy, or increased heart rate
- Dromotropy, or increased cardiac conduction velocities
- Increased blood pressure (BP)
- Inotropy, or increased force of contraction
- Preferential vasoconstriction to shunt blood away from the skin, mucosa, and viscera via
  - Cutaneous arteries
  - Mucosal arteries
  - Splanchnic arteries
  - Renal arteries
- Preferential vasodilation to shunt blood to the heart and skeletal muscle via
  - Coronary vessels
  - Skeletal vessels

In addition to these cardiovascular actions, sympathetic stimulation results in [24]

- Activation of sweat glands
  - Paw pads
- Bronchodilation
- Mydriasis
- Urine retention
  - Detrusor muscle relaxation
  - Contraction of the trigone

High sympathetic tone has many effects on the body, and impacts multiple body systems [24]. Increased heart rate is just one result of high sympathetic tone [13, 31].

The clinic setting is a stressful environment for most of our patients. It is therefore not surprising that many present with tachycardia because of high sympathetic tone.

In such cases of physiologic sinus tachycardia, there is no indication to treat the arrhythmia itself [19]. When the cause of the sinus tachycardia is removed, normal sinus rhythm is restored [13, 22].

Therefore, if anything, treat the cause. For example, address stress in cats by taking measures to support a feline-friendly practice. This may mean incorporating any number of the following measures into the clinic [23, 42–65]:

- Creating cat-only waiting rooms, offering shelving to keep carriers off the ground, and/or using barriers such as walls or screens to create the illusion of hideaways in the waiting room so that cats feel securely hidden from view
- Minimizing waiting times
- Directing cats immediately into examination rooms
- Creating cat-only boarding and hospital wards
- Stacking cages or "kitty condos" so that cats do not have to face each other
- Hanging clean towels over cage doors of stable patients to allow patients to hide
- Dimming bright overhead lights
- Removing white coats to lessen "white coat syndrome"
- Reducing sound
- Using a relaxed tone
- Avoiding shushing at cats: shushing sounds remarkably similar to hissing
- Avoiding direct stares
- Using easy-to-clean, non-slip mats, soft foam, or towels on examination room tables so that patients feel secure in their footing
- Limiting initial physical touch to the head and neck/ avoiding the back and abdomen
- Avoiding aversive scents, such as alcohol, citrus, aloe, pine, or eucalyptus
- Using synthetic feline facial pheromone
- Taking your time with the exam: you must "go slow to go fast" [42]
- Working around the cat: Allow the cat to stay in its carrier rather than dumping the cat out

Many of these same concepts may be applied to canine patients. Practices that handle dogs should develop techniques that foster low-stress handling, a concept that was pioneered by Dr. Sophia Yin [66]. The coined phrase implies the need for gentle restraint. However, its philosophy expands far beyond handling skills. At its core, low-stress handling is about understanding patient behavior, that is, what motivates the patient to act or react [23].

Additional measures that may be taken to reduce stress in dogs include the following [23, 67–82]:

- Avoiding human-centered social behaviors that may be perceived as threatening by dogs
  - Direct eye contact
  - Hugs or other forms of embrace
  - Reaching out suddenly

- Using easy-to-clean, non-slip mats on low-profile, electronic floor scales
- Placing scales away from corners, where patients may feel trapped, without the ability to escape
- Cleaning examination rooms thoroughly in between use, given that scent recognition is strong in the dog. Dogs may pick up messages from a number of sources, including
  - Anal sac secretions
  - Feces
  - Paw pad secretions
  - Sebaceous gland secretions
  - Urine
  - Vaginal secretions
- Using dog-appeasing pheromone (DAP)
  - DAP is naturally produced by intermammary sebaceous glands shortly after parturition
  - It is thought to convey a sense of security to the pups before and after nursing
  - Synthetic analogs of DAP have been commercialized to target a variety of behavioral concerns, particularly those that are fear-based

Physiologic sinus tachycardia due to high sympathetic tone may be unavoidable. In these situations, it may be helpful to stage veterinary appointments and/or prescribe anxiolytic medications that are administered to the patient prior to the clinic visit. In-clinic sedation may also be necessary to facilitate patient procedures while minimizing patient stress.

46.5 Pathologic Sinus Tachycardia

When sinus tachycardia is caused by pathologic mechanisms, it is important to recognize that it is often a compensatory reflex [19]. Consider, for example, a patient with CHF. This patient is likely to be tachycardic in an attempt to improve cardiac output. Sinus tachycardia, in other words, is the body's attempt to compensate for its need for increased blood flow [21, 31]. In this case, treating the sinus tachycardia alone, for example, with propranolol, to slow the heart rate is ill-advised [19]. Sinus tachycardia is present for a reason. It would better serve the patient to diagnose its underlying disease, that is, the source of the CHF. Management is most successful when it attempts to remedy the underlying pathology as opposed to treating the surface issue, sinus tachycardia.

Similarly, if sinus tachycardia in a dehydrated patient is secondary to hypovolemia, then manage the hypovolemia by administering intravenous fluids.

If the patient is exhibiting sinus tachycardia because it is too light under general anesthesia, then deepen the plane of anesthesia.

The bottom line is to dig beneath the surface. A diagnostic investigation is essential to the success of therapy and patient outcomes. Identify what is causing the pathologic sinus tachycardia and address it. Sinus tachycardia is likely to improve when the cause of it has been addressed, if not resolved.

46.6 Sinus Arrhythmia

Sinus arrhythmia is common in companion animal patients, particularly those dogs with high vagal tone.

Recall from Chapter 45, Section 45.5 that vagal tone describes the activity of the tenth cranial nerve, the vagus. The vagus nerve is a messenger of the parasympathetic nervous system.

As compared to the sympathetic activity, parasympathetic activity promotes the following [24, 35]:

- Bradycardia
- Defecation
- Digestion
- Lacrimation
- Pupil constriction
- Salivation
- Urination

High vagal tone maximizes parasympathetic activity [24, 35]. In the process of doing so, high vagal tone may result in or contribute to sinus arrhythmia.

Sinus arrhythmia is a heart rhythm that is tied to the respiratory cycle [6, 13, 23]. Inspiration increases heart rate; exhalation lowers it [6, 13, 23].

Dogs are more likely than cats to exhibit sinus arrhythmia, in large part because cats are largely driven by sympathetic tone in a clinic setting [6]. The sympathetic-driven elevation in feline heart rate causes sufficient tachycardia that is not conducive to the development of sinus arrhythmia [6].

Sinus arrhythmias vary in frequency, duration, and severity [18]. On cardiothoracic auscultation, sinus arrhythmias sound like an irregular heart rhythm. It is sometimes difficult for novices to differentiate sinus arrhythmia from abnormal rhythms based upon sound alone [18].

An ECG is an important diagnostic tool for confirming the presence or absence of sinus arrhythmia [18].

References

1 DeFrancesco, T.C. (2013). Management of cardiac emergencies in small animals. *Vet. Clin. North Am. Small Anim. Pract.* 43 (4): 817–842.

2 Bulmer, B. (2012). Interpreting ECGs with confidence: part 2. *NAVC Clinician's Brief* (June): 102–105.

3 Meurs, K.M. (2004). Boxer dog cardiomyopathy: an update. *Vet. Clin. North Am. Small Anim. Pract.* 34 (5): 1235–1244, viii.

4 Meurs, K.M. (2017). Arrhythmogenic right ventricular cardiomyopathy in the boxer dog: an update. *Vet. Clin. North Am. Small Anim. Pract.* 47 (5): 1103–1111.

5 Palermo, V., Stafford Johnson, M.J., Sala, E. et al. (2011). Cardiomyopathy in boxer dogs: a retrospective study of the clinical presentation, diagnostic findings and survival. *J. Vet. Cardiol.* 13 (1): 45–55.

6 Jones, A. and Estrada, A. (2014). Top 5 arrhythmias in dogs and cats. *NAVC Clinician's Brief* (January): 94–100.

7 Leach, S. (2016). Ventricular tachycardia. *Veterinary Team Brief* (May): 23–27.

8 French, A. (ed.) (2008). Arrhythmias: recognition and treatment. World Small Animal Veterinary Congress, Dublin, Ireland.

9 Bulmer, B. (2012). Management tree: tachyarrhythmia. *NAVC Clinician's Brief* (June): 107.

10 MacDonald, K. (2009). Get with the beat! Analysis and treatment of cardiac arrhythmias. DVM 360 [Internet]. http://veterinarycalendar.dvm360.com/get-with-beat-analysis-and-treatment-cardiac-arrhythmias-proceedings.

11 Stepien, R.L. (ed.) (2008). *Emergency Arrhythmias.* British Small Animal Veterinary Congress.

12 Ettinger, S.J., Feldman, E.C., and Côté, E. (2017). *Textbook of Veterinary Internal Medicine: Diseases of the Dog and the Cat,* 8e, 2 volumes (lviii, 2181, 1–90 p.). St. Louis, Missouri: Elsevier.

13 Tilley, L.P., Smith, F.W.K., and Tilley, L.P. (2007). *Blackwell's Five-Minute Veterinary Consult: Canine and Feline,* 4e, lx, 1578 p. Ames, Iowa: Blackwell.

14 Thomason, J.D., Kraus, M.S., Surdyk, K.K. et al. (2008). Bradycardia-associated syncope in 7 boxers with ventricular tachycardia (2002–2005). *J. Vet. Intern. Med.* 22 (4): 931–936.

15 Harpster, N. (1983). Boxer cardiomyopathy. In: *Current Veterinary Therapy VIII* (ed. R. Kirk), 329–337. Philadelphia: WB Saunders.

16 Harpster, N.K. (1991). Boxer cardiomyopathy. A review of the long-term benefits of antiarrhythmic therapy. *Vet. Clin. North Am. Small Anim. Pract.* 21 (5): 989–1004.

17 Meurs, K.M., Spier, A.W., Miller, M.W. et al. (1999). Familial ventricular arrhythmias in boxers. *J. Vet. Intern. Med.* 13 (5): 437–439.

18 Ware, W. (2013). *Cardiovascular Disease in Small Animal Medicine*. Boca Raton, FL: Taylor & Francis Group, LLC.

19 Cote, E., MacDonald, K.A., Meurs, K.M., and Sleeper, M.M. (2011). *Feline Cardiology*. Ames, Iowa: Wiley.

20 Rozanski, E.A. and Rush, J.E. (2012). *Small Animal Emergency and Critical Care Medicine: A Color Handbook*. London: Manson Publishing.

21 Sawyer, D. (2008). *The Practice of Veterinary Anesthesia: Small Animals, Birds, Fish and Reptiles*. Jackson, WY: Trenton NewMedia.

22 Constable, P.D., Blood, D.C., and Radostits, O.M. (2017). *Veterinary Medicine: A Textbook of the Diseases of Cattle, Horses, Sheep, Pigs, and Goats*, 11e, 2 volumes. St. Louis, Missouri: Elsevier.

23 Englar, R.E. (2017). *Performing the Small Animal Physical Examination*. Hoboken, NJ: Wiley.

24 Reece, W.O., Erickson, H.H., Goff, J.P., and Uemura, E.E. (2015). *Dukes' Physiology of Domestic Animals*, 13e, xii, 748 p. Ames, Iowa, USA: Wiley Blackwell.

25 Nowers, T. (2015). Top 5 clinical differences between cats & dogs. *Veterinary Team* Brief [Internet]. (September). https://www.veterinaryteambrief.com/article/top-5-clinical-differences-between-cats-dogs.

26 Bulmer, B. (2012). Common cardiac arrhythmias. *NAVC Clinician's Brief* [Internet]. https://www.cliniciansbrief.com/article/common-cardiac-arrhythmias

27 Verdecchia, P., Schillaci, G., Borgioni, C. et al. (1995). White coat hypertension and white coat effect - similarities and differences. *Am. J. Hypertens.* 8 (8): 790–798.

28 Ogedegbe, G. (2008). White-coat effect: unraveling its mechanisms. *Am. J. Hypertens.* 21 (2): 135.

29 Cardillo, C., Defelice, F., Campia, U., and Folli, G. (1993). Psychophysiological reactivity and cardiac end-organ changes in white coat hypertension. *Hypertension* 21 (6): 836–844.

30 Palmer, B.M., Lynch, J.M., Snyder, S.M., and Moore, R.L. (2001). Renal hypertension prevents run training modification of cardiomyocyte diastolic Ca2+ regulation in male rats. *J. Appl. Physiol.* 90 (6): 2063–2069.

31 August, J.R. (2010). *Consultations in Feline Internal Medicine*. St. Louis, MO: Saunders.

32 Yamaki, F.L., Soares, E.C., Pereira, G.G. et al. (2014). Twenty-four hour ambulatory electrocardiography (Holter monitoring) in normal unsedated cats. *Acta Sci. Vet.* 42.

33 Rand, J. (2006). *Problem-Based Feline Medicine*, xiv, 1479 p. Edinburgh; New York: Saunders.

34 Saunders, A.B. and Gordon, S.G. (2015). 6 Practical tips from cardiologists: heart failure in dogs. *Today's Veterinary Practice* (July/August).

35 McCorry, L.K. (2007). Physiology of the autonomic nervous system. *Am. J. Pharm. Educ.* 71 (4): 78.

36 Lake, C.R. (1979). Relationship of sympathetic nervous system tone and blood pressure. *Nephron* 23 (2–3): 84–90.

37 Narkiewicz, K. and Somers, V.K. (1999). Interactive effect of heart rate and muscle sympathetic nerve activity on blood pressure. *Circulation* 100 (25): 2514–2518.

38 Corcoran Lecture, J.S. (1993). Sympathetic hyperactivity and coronary risk in hypertension. *Hypertension* 21 (6 Pt 2): 886–893.

39 Mark, A.L. (1996). The sympathetic nervous system in hypertension: a potential long-term regulator of arterial pressure. *J. Hypertens. Suppl.* 14 (5): S159–S165.

40 Mancia, G., Grassi, G., Parati, G., and Zanchetti, A. (1997). The sympathetic nervous system in human hypertension. *Acta Physiol. Scand. Suppl.* 640: 117–121.

41 Somers, V.K., Anderson, E.A., and Mark, A.L. (1993). Sympathetic neural mechanisms in human hypertension. *Curr. Opin. Nephrol. Hypertens.* 2 (1): 96–105.

42 Rodan, I., Sundahl, E., Carney, H. et al. (2011). AAFP and ISFM feline-friendly handling guidelines. *J. Feline Med. Surg.* 13 (5): 364–375.

43 Rodan, I., Sundahl, E., Carney, H. et al. (2011). Feline focus: AAFP and ISFM feline-friendly handling guidelines. *Compendium* 33 (12): E3.

44 Bowen, J. and Heath, S. (2005). *An Overview of Feline Social Behaviour and Communication: Behaviour Problems in Small Animals: Practice Advice for the Veterinary Team*. Philadelphia: Saunders.

45 Levine, E.D. (2008). Feline fear and anxiety. *Vet. Clin. North Am. Small Anim. Pract.* 38 (5): 1065–1079, vii.

46 Scherk, M. (2013). The cat-friendly practice. In: *BSAVA Manual of Feline Practice: A Foundation Manual* (ed. A. Harvey and S. Tasker). Gloucester, England: British Small Animal Veterinary Association.

47 Brunt, J. (2012). The cat-friendly practice. In: *The Cat* (ed. S. Little), 20–25. St. Louis: Elsevier Saunders.

48 Rubert, R., Long, L.D., and Hutchinson, M.L. (2007). Creating a healing environment in the ICU. In: *Critical Care Nursing: Synergy for Optimal Outcomes* (ed. R. Kaplow and S.R. Hardin), 27–39. Jones and Bartlett Publishers.

49 Fontaine, D.K., Briggs, L.P., and Pope-Smith, B. (2001). Designing humanistic critical care environments. *Crit. Care Nurs. Q.* 24 (3): 21–34.

50 Morgan, K.N. and Tromborg, C.T. (2007). Sources of stress in captivity. *Appl. Anim. Behav. Sci.* 102 (3–4): 262–302.

51 Veranic, P. and Jezernik, K. (2001). Succession of events in desquamation of superficial urothelial cells as a

response to stress induced by prolonged constant illumination. *Tissue Cell* 33 (3): 280–285.

52 Pollard, J.C. and Littlejohn, R.P. (1994). Behavioral-effects of light conditions on Red Deer in a holding pen. *Appl. Anim. Behav. Sci.* 41 (1–2): 127–134.

53 Gunter, R. (1951). The absolute threshold for vision in the cat. *J. Physiol. Lond.* 114 (1–2): 8–15.

54 Miller, P.E. and Murphy, C.J. (1995). Vision in dogs. *J. Am. Vet. Med. Assoc.* 207 (12): 1623–1634.

55 Marino, C.L., Cober, R.E., Iazbik, M.C., and Couto, C.G. (2011). White-coat effect on systemic blood pressure in retired racing greyhounds. *J. Vet. Intern. Med.* 25 (4): 861–865.

56 Belew, A.M., Barlett, T., and Brown, S.A. (1999). Evaluation of the white-coat effect in cats. *J. Vet. Intern. Med.* 13 (2): 134–142.

57 Herron, M.E. and Shreyer, T. (2014). The pet-friendly veterinary practice: a guide for practitioners. *Vet. Clin. North Am. Small* 44 (3): 451.

58 Crowell-Davis, S.L. (2007). White coat syndrome: prevention and treatment. *Comp. Cont. Educ. Pract.* 29 (3): 163–165.

59 Rodan, I. (2010). Understanding feline behavior and application for appropriate handling and management. *Top. Companion Anim. Med.* 25 (4): 178–188.

60 Heath, S. (2009). Aggression in cats. In: *BSAVA Manual of Canine and Feline Behavioural Medicine*, 2e (ed. D. Horwitz and D. Mills), 233. Gloucester: British Small Animal Veterinary Association.

61 Pereira, J.S., Fragoso, S., Beck, A. et al. (2015). Improving the feline veterinary consultation: the usefulness of Feliway spray in reducing cats' stress. *J. Feline Med. Surg.*.

62 Gunn-Moore, D.A. and Cameron, M.E. (2004). A pilot study using synthetic feline facial pheromone for the management of feline idiopathic cystitis. *J. Feline Med. Surg.* 6 (3): 133–138.

63 Griffith, C.A., Steigerwald, E.S., and Buffington, C.A. (2000). Effects of a synthetic facial pheromone on behavior of cats. *J. Am. Vet. Med. Assoc.* 217 (8): 1154–1156.

64. Frank, D., Beauchamp, G., and Palestrini, C. (2010). Systematic review of the use of pheromones for treatment of undesirable behavior in cats and dogs. *JAVMA J. Am. Vet. Med. A* 236 (12): 1308–1316.

65 Kronen, P.W., Ludders, J.W., Erb, H.N. et al. (2006). A synthetic fraction of feline facial pheromones calms but does not reduce struggling in cats before venous catheterization. *Vet. Anaesth. Analg.* 33 (4): 258–265.

66 Yin, S. (2016). Low stress handling® – from the veterinary technicians' perspective. *CattleDog Publishing* [Internet]. https://drsophiayin.com/low-stress-handling.

67 Overall, K.L. (1997). Normal canine behavior. In: *Clinical Behavioral Medicine for Small Animals* (ed. K.L. Overall), 10–44. St. Louis: Mosby.

68 Bradshaw, J.W.S. and Brown, S.L. (1990). Behavioral adaptations of dogs to domestication. In: *Pets, Benefits, and Practice* (ed. I.H. Berger), 18–24. London: British Veterinary Association Publications.

69 Pageat, P. and Gaultier, E. (2003). Current research in canine and feline pheromones. *Vet. Clin. North Am. Small Anim. Pract.* 33 (2): 187–211.

70 Landsberg, G.M., Beck, A., Lopez, A. et al. (2015). Dog-appeasing pheromone collars reduce sound-induced fear and anxiety in beagle dogs: a placebo-controlled study. *Vet. Rec.* 177 (10): 260.

71 Tod, E., Brander, D., and Waran, N. (2005). Efficacy of dog appeasing pheromone in reducing stress and fear related behaviour in shelter dogs. *Appl. Anim. Behav. Sci.* 93 (3–4): 295–308.

72 Grigg, E.K. and Piehler, M. (2015). Influence of dog appeasing pheromone (DAP) on dogs housed in a long-term kennelling facility. *Vet. Rec. Open* 2 (1): e000098.

73 Mills, D.S., Ramos, D., Estelles, M.G., and Hargrave, C. (2006). A triple blind placebo-controlled investigation into the assessment of the effect of dog appeasing pheromone (DAP) on anxiety related behaviour of problem dogs in the veterinary clinic. *Appl. Anim. Behav. Sci.* 98 (1–2): 114–126.

74 Denenberg, S. and Landsberg, G.M. (2008). Effects of dog-appeasing pheromones on anxiety and fear in puppies during training and on long-term socialization. *JAVMA J. Am. Vet. Med. A.* 233 (12): 1874–1882.

75 Estelles, M.G. and Mills, D.S. (2006). Signs of travel-related problems in dogs and their response to treatment with dog-appeasing pheromone. *Vet. Rec.* 159 (5): 143.

76 Gaultier, E., Bonnafous, L., Vienet-Legue, D. et al. (2008). Efficacy of dog-appeasing pheromone in reducing stress associated with social isolation in newly adopted puppies. *Vet. Rec.* 163 (3): 73–80.

77 Gaultier, E., Bonnafous, L., Vienet-Lague, D. et al. (2009). Efficacy of dog-appeasing pheromone in reducing behaviours associated with fear of unfamiliar people and new surroundings in newly adopted puppies. *Vet. Rec.* 164 (23): 708–714.

78 Sheppard, G. and Mills, D.S. (2003). Evaluation of dog-appeasing pheromone as a potential treatment for dogs fearful of fireworks. *Vet. Rec.* 152 (14): 432–436.

79 Mills, D.S., Estelles, M.G., Coleshaw, P.H., and Shorthouse, C. (2003). Retrospective analysis of

the treatment of firework fears in dogs. *Vet. Rec.* 153 (18): 561–562.

80 Levine, E.D. and Mills, D.S. (2008). Long-term follow-up of the efficacy of a behavioural treatment programme for dogs with firework fears. *Vet. Rec.* 162 (20): 657–659.

81 Levine, E.D., Ramos, D., and Mills, D.S. (2007). A prospective study of two self-help CD based desensitization and counter-conditioning programmes

with the use of dog appeasing pheromone for the treatment of firework fears in dogs (*Canis familiaris*). *Appl. Anim. Behav. Sci.* 105 (4): 311–329.

82 Taylor, K. and Mills, D.S. (2007). A placebo-controlled study to investigate the effect of dog appeasing pheromone and other environmental and management factors on the reports of disturbance and house soiling during the night in recently adopted puppies (*Canis familiaris*). *Appl. Anim. Behav. Sci.* 105 (4): 358–368.

Part Six

The Digestive System

47

Abnormal Gut Sounds

47.1 Introduction to Normal Gut Sounds

It has been known for hundreds of years that the normal gut makes sounds [1–3]. Hippocrates referred to sound emanating from the gut as borborygmus [2]. Borborygmus remains in common use among medical terminology today, although gut noise is sometimes referred to in the plural as borborygmi [4, 5].

Borborygmi are sounds that are intestinal in origin and resonate as loud gurgles that result from peristaltic contractions [2, 6, 7].

It has been suggested that the frequency and intensity of these sounds may be characteristic of bowel pathology [2]. For this reason, the human medical profession spent a good portion of the 1800s trying to classify these sounds into the following categories: "splashings, rattling, or rustling noises" [2].

Unfortunately, differentiating between these sounds is easier said than done, and no one sound is pathognomonic for a particular disease. Moreover, many of the same sounds that exist in pathological conditions exist in health [2].

47.2 The Role of Abdominal Auscultation

Gut sounds are nonspecific [8]. In addition, their auscultation is somewhat subjective – what one person may consider hypoactive, another may consider normoactive [6, 8–11]. For this reason, the usefulness of abdominal auscultation has been called into question by the human medical profession [11–14]. Although human medical students continue to be trained in abdominal auscultation, many clinicians no longer attempt it in practice. A 2014 study by Felder et al. found that 44% of clinicians self-reported that they "rarely listened to bowel sounds" [11].

Despite the potential for subjectivity, abdominal auscultation remains a vital part of the veterinary physical examination, particularly in large animal medicine. In cattle, the presence or absence of rumen contractions is associated with certain pathology. In horses, lack of movement in the gut, so-called ileus, is a significant concern. Large animal practitioners are used to abdominal auscultation because they have trained themselves to tune in to subtleties and trends in sound quality and frequency.

In the author's experience, small animal practitioners vary in their approach to the abdominal examination of dogs and cats. Some auscultate the abdomen and some do not. Those that do tend to auscultate prior to abdominal palpation. It is thought that abdominal palpation may shift intestinal loops within the abdominal cavity and alter gut sounds [5, 15, 16].

The purpose of auscultating for gut sounds is to obtain information regarding the motility and gut content of the digestive tract [5]. For borborygmi to be audible, the motile bowel must contain some fluid and gas [5]. If borborygmi are not heard, then the bowel is either empty or not moving, or both [5, 7].

47.3 The Technique of Abdominal Auscultation

To auscultate the abdomen, the diaphragm of the stethoscope is placed along the ventral and ventrolateral abdominal walls [5, 7, 10].

When gut sounds are heard, they may be

- Hyperactive
- Normoactive
- Hypoactive
- Absent.

In human medicine, auscultation time varies from 30 s to 7 min before it is concluded that the patient lacks gut sounds [10, 17, 18]. The veterinary medical literature is sparse in terms of such documentation. What we do know is that auscultation of the abdomen requires patience [7]. It may take 2 to 3 minutes to appreciate borborygmi in patients with delayed gut motility [5].

47.4 Hyperactive Gut Sounds

Borborygmi may be exaggerated in the following conditions [4, 19–21]:

- Aerophagia
  - Brachycephalic canine breeds
  - Working and/or sporting dog breeds
    o Extreme bouts of exercise
- Enteritis
- Excessive fermentation of ingesta by bacteria
  - Nonabsorbable oligosaccharides
    o Soybeans
    o Legumes
  - Fermentable fibers
    o Pectin
- Functional bowel disorders
  - Inflammatory bowel disease (IBD)
- Gastritis
- Gastrointestinal parasites
- Hepatitis
- Malabsorption
- Maldigestion
- Exocrine pancreatic insufficiency (EPI)
- Small intestinal bacterial overgrowth (SIBO)

Patients with hyperactive gut sounds may or may not have concurrent flatulence [19]. They may also exhibit intermittent inappetence, particularly if they develop abdominal discomfort secondary to increased intestinal gas [19]. These patients may stand with an arched back in an attempt to lessen gut pain [19].

History plays an important role in establishing if there is a temporal association between increased gut sounds, flatulence, and other events [21]. For example, it is important to expand upon the following topics during history taking [21]:

- Have there been any changes to the diet?
- Has the patient been guilty of dietary indiscretion?
- What is the patient's activity level or exercise and when does exercise occur relative to eating?
- When did the patient last eat?
- Has the patient experienced stress?
- Is the patient taking any medications, prescribed or over-the-counter, including supplements?
- Has bowel activity been irregular?
- Is the patient vomiting?
- Is the patient having diarrhea?

- If yes, describe the following relative to the diarrhea:
  o Color
  o Consistency or Quality
  o Frequency
  o With or without tenesmus, that is, straining
  o With or without hematochezia, that is, blood
  o With or without steatorrhea, that is, the presence of abnormal amounts of fecal fat

Physical examination of affected patients may also reveal [21]

- Flatulence during abdominal palpation
- Palpable gas distension within the intestinal tract
- Gastric tympany.

As an isolated finding in an otherwise asymptomatic dog or cat, increased borborygmi is not a concern.

Increased borborygmi becomes a concern when it is paired with additional findings, such as diarrhea or weight loss [21]. In these clinical scenarios, the patient benefits from a diagnostic work-up that explores potential causes of maldigestion and/or malabsorption. In particular, two digestive tract pathologies, EPI and IBD, come to mind. Refer to Chapter 51 for additional information about these two topics.

47.5 Hypoactive-to-Absent Gut Sounds

As an isolated finding in an otherwise asymptomatic dog or cat, decreased borborygmi is not a concern.

However, borborygmi may be reduced to absent in the following concerning conditions [5, 16, 22–25]:

- Anorexia
- Ascites
- Gastrointestinal obstruction
  - Complete
  - Partial
  - Strangulating
- Peritonitis
- Post-laparotomy

History plays an important role in establishing if there is a temporal association between decreased or absent gut sounds and other events [21]. For example, it is important to expand upon the following topics during history taking as were outlined in Section 47.4 [21]:

- Have there been any changes to the diet?
- Has the patient had a decreased appetite?
- Has the patient become anorexic?
- When did the patient last eat?
- Has the patient experienced stress?
- Is the patient taking any medications, prescribed or over the counter, including supplements?

- Has bowel activity been irregular?
- Is the patient regurgitating?
- Is the patient vomiting?
  - If yes, describe the following related to emesis:
    ○ Amount
    ○ Color
    ○ Consistency
    ○ Frequency
    ○ Relationship to drinking
      ▪ Does vomiting occur after drinking water?
      ▪ How soon after drinking water does vomiting occur?
    ○ Relationship to eating
      ▪ Does vomiting occur after eating?
      ▪ How soon after eating does vomiting occur?
    ○ Presence or absence of hematemesis, that is, blood in the vomit
- Does the patient have a history of eating non-food items, so-called "foreign bodies"?
- Has the patient ever had a gastrointestinal obstruction before?
- Has the patient recently had surgery on the gastrointestinal tract?

History alone should confirm or refute anorexia as a cause of diminished or nonexistent gut sounds [21].

If ascites is responsible for diminished gut sounds, it should be detectable on physical examination either grossly, or upon palpation, as a fluid wave [5, 7].

To assess for a fluid wave, the clinician typically stands behind the patient, with patient and clinician facing the same direction [5]. The palm of the clinician's left hand is placed flush against the left side of the patient's abdomen [5]. The clinician then performs ballottement with his right hand, that is, he taps the right abdominal wall with his right fingertips to bounce internal structures off the opposite wall [5].

The process is repeated by balloting the left abdominal wall to feel for any abnormal response against the right [5]. If there is appreciable fluid within the peritoneal cavity, the clinician will feel a wave of fluid against the wall opposite to the one that was tapped [5]. This is not appreciated in a healthy patient; only in a patient with abdominal effusion [5, 7].

Abdominal effusion may also be evident on radiographs as:

- Increased density throughout the abdomen
- Poor definition of soft tissue structures.

See Figure 47.1.

If there is a palpable fluid wave, then fluid should be sampled via abdominocentesis to determine its source [5, 26, 27]. It could be reflective of underlying peritonitis [5].

In vomiting dogs with painful abdomens and reduced-to-absent gut sounds, clinicians should suspect gastroin-

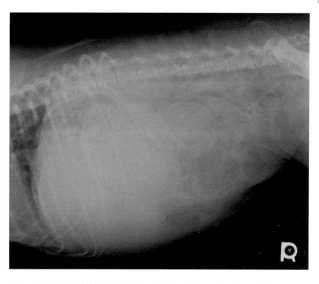

Figure 47.1 Right lateral abdominal radiograph of a canine patient with a hemoabdomen. Note the increased density throughout the abdominal cavity. There is also poor definition of soft tissue structures.

testinal obstruction, particularly in those patients that are young or are repeat offenders [22, 24, 28, 29]. Dogs most often ingest nonlinear foreign bodies [22, 24, 28, 29]. These include, but are not limited to the following [22, 24, 28, 29]:

- Balls
- Bones
- Bottle caps
- Coins
- Cords
- Corn cobs
- Fabric
- Fish hooks
- Fruit seeds
- Plastic
- Rubber
- Stones
- Tampons
- Toys
- Wrappers

Cats are less likely to ingest nonlinear foreign bodies [22, 30]. Cats are more likely to develop an obstructive trichobezoars, that is, hairballs [22, 30].

Survey radiographs will outline radiopaque foreign bodies, such as stones [22] (see Figure 47.2).

Not all foreign bodies are radiopaque. In these clinical scenarios, radiographs support the diagnosis when they demonstrate the following signs of intestinal obstruction [22, 31–33]:

- Focal intestinal distension
- Focal soft tissue opacity within stomach or intestines

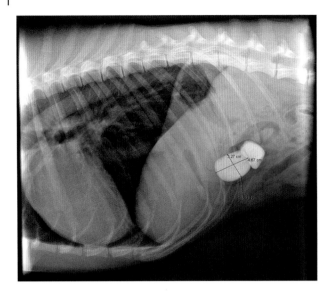

Figure 47.2 Abdominal radiograph of a canine patient that ingested river rocks. These were removed surgically. *Source:* Courtesy of Ashley Benson.

- Parallel, distended intestinal loops
- Sharp hairpin turns between intestinal loops (see Figures 47.3a, b).

Abdominal radiographs are often equivocal [22]. These cases may benefit from the use of contrast medium to enhance visualization of the gastrointestinal tract [22].

Cats are more likely to ingest linear foreign bodies, in particular, string and thread, with or without the needle attached [22, 34–37] (see Figures 47.4a–c.)

Although it is less commonly seen in clinical practice, dogs may also ingest linear foreign bodies [22, 35, 37]. These may also consist of string and thread, but are more likely to include tape, nylon hosiery, cord, carpet, and fabric [22, 35, 37].

Plication of intestinal loops is typically palpable on physical examination of patients with linear foreign bodies [22, 34–37]. These patients may also have a string looped around the base of their tongue or teeth [22, 34–37]. Sedation may be required to allow for intraoral inspection. [22]

On occasion, a string foreign body will be evident protruding from the patient's anus [22, 34–37].

Survey radiographs are often confirmatory for linear foreign bodies. Abdominal radiographic findings that support a diagnosis of linear foreign body include the following [22, 36, 37]:

- Comma-shaped gas bubbles
- Peritonitis
- Plication of intestines
- Radiopaque foreign body, such as a needle

Ultrasonography is also able to detect intestinal plication and in this way may be used to confirm the diagnosis of linear foreign body [22].

47.6 Concluding Remarks About Abdominal Auscultation

Subjectivity of gut sounds remains a concern for both human and veterinary medicine. Agreement between

(a)

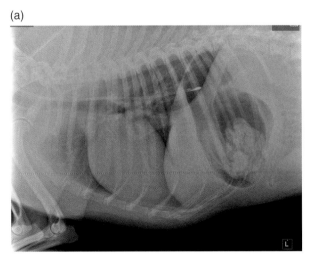

(b)

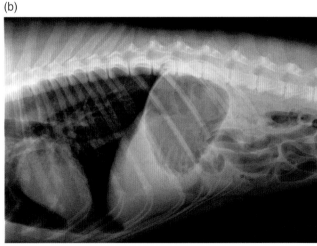

Figure 47.3 (a) Abdominal radiograph of a canine patient that has a soft tissue "mass effect" within the body of the stomach. This was a nonlinear foreign body that had to be removed surgically. *Source:* Courtesy of Kara Thomas, DVM, CVMA. (b) Abdominal radiograph of a canine patient, in which a foreign body was suspected. Note that there is appreciable gas distension of the stomach and gas distension of several loops of bowel. *Source:* Courtesy of Kara Thomas, DVM, CVMA.

(a)

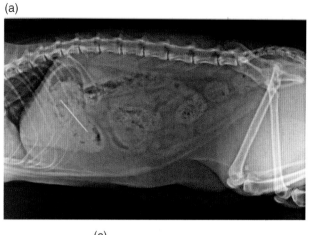

(b) (c)

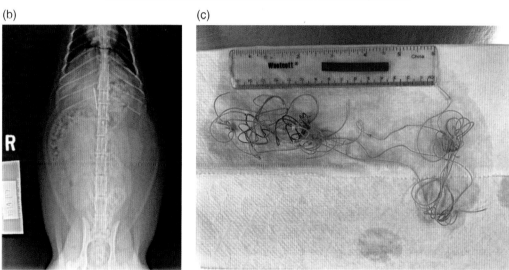

Figure 47.4 (a) Left lateral abdominal radiograph of a feline patient that swallowed a needle. The needle is lodged within the body of the cat's stomach. *Source:* Courtesy of Jennifer Lang. (b). Orthogonal radiographic view of the same patient depicted in (a). Note the radiopaque needle. *Source:* Courtesy of Jennifer Lang. (c) Linear foreign body that was removed rectally, via enema, in a feline patient. *Source:* Courtesy of Pamela Mueller, DVM.

clinicians as to what constitutes normal versus abnormal is not always consistent, and it is difficult to know based upon a single snapshot in time whether what is heard is normal for the patient.

The most important takeaway is that changes in gut sounds are not concerning when they are isolated findings in otherwise asymptomatic patients.

Increased gut sounds raise concern when paired with evidence of maldigestion or malabsorption, such as weight loss and diarrhea.

Decreased to absent gut sounds raise concern when paired with evidence of anorexia and/or vomiting.

When increased or decreased gut sounds are appreciated in sick patients, diagnostic work-ups are indicated.

References

1 Cannon, W.B. (1902). The movements of the intestines studied by means of the Rontgen rays. *J. Med. Res.* 7 (1): 72–75.

2 Cannon, W.B. (1905). Auscultation of the rhythmic sounds produced by the stomach and intestines. APS [Internet]. https://www.physiology.org/doi/pdf/10.1152/ajplegacy.1905.14.4.339.

3 Cannon, W.B. and Murphy, F.T.I.V. (1906). The movements of the stomach and intestines in some surgical conditions. *Ann. Surg.* 43 (4): 512–536.

4 Côté, E. (2015). *Clinical Veterinary Advisor. Dogs and Cats*, 3e, xxxvii, 1642 p. St. Louis, Missouri: Elsevier Mosby.

5 Englar, R.E. (2017). *Performing the Small Animal Physical Examination*. Hoboken, NJ: Wiley.

6 Gu, Y., Lim, H.J., and Moser, M.A. (2010). How useful are bowel sounds in assessing the abdomen? *Dig. Surg.* 27 (5): 422–426.

7 Rothuizen, J., Schrauwen, E., Theyse, L.F.H., and Verhaert, L. (2009). Digestive tract. In: *Medical History and Physical Examination in Companion Animals* (ed. A. Rijnberk and F.J. van Sluijs), 86–100. St. Louis, MO: Elsevier Limited.

8 Ching, S.S. and Tan, Y.K. (2012). Spectral analysis of bowel sounds in intestinal obstruction using an electronic stethoscope. *World J. Gastroenterol.* 18 (33): 4585–4592.

9 Gade, J., Kruse, P., Andersen, O.T. et al. (1998). Physicians' abdominal auscultation. A multi-rater agreement study. *Scand. J. Gastroenterol.* 33 (7): 773–777.

10 Baid, H. (2009). A critical review of auscultating bowel sounds. *Br. J. Nurs.* 18 (18): 1125–1129.

11 Felder, S., Margel, D., Murrell, Z., and Fleshner, P. (2014). Usefulness of bowel sound auscultation: a prospective evaluation. *J. Surg. Educ.* 71 (5): 768–773.

12 Fletcher, R.H. and Fletcher, S.W. (1992). Has medicine outgrown physical diagnosis? *Ann. Intern. Med.* 117 (9): 786–787.

13 West, M. and Klein, M.D. (1982). Is abdominal auscultation important? *Lancet* 2 (8310): 1279.

14 Zuin, M., Rigatelli, G., Andreotti, A.N. et al. (2017). Is abdominal auscultation a still relevant part of the physical examination? *Eur. J. Intern. Med.* 43: e24–e25.

15 Dye, T. (2003). The acute abdomen: a surgeon's approach to diagnosis and treatment. *Clin. Tech. Small Anim. Pract.* 18 (1): 53–65.

16 Saxon, W.D. (1994). The acute abdomen. *Vet. Clin. North Am. Small Anim. Pract.* 24 (6): 1207–1224.

17 Epstein, O. (2008). The abdomen. In: *Clinical Examination* (ed. O. Epstein, G.D. Perkin and J. Cookson), 186–225. Edinburgh: Mosby Elsevier.

18 Cox, C. and Steggall, M. (2009). A step-by-step buide to performing a complete abdominal examination. *Gastrointestinal Nursing* 7 (1): 17–19.

19 Tams, T.R. (2003). *Handbook of Small Animal Gastroenterology*, 2e, xiv, 486 p. St. Louis, Mo: Saunders.

20 Ettinger, S.J., Feldman, E.C., and Côté, E. (2017). *Textbook of Veterinary Internal Medicine: Diseases of the Dog and the Cat*, 8e, 2 volumes (lviii, 2181, 1–90 p.). St. Louis, Missouri: Elsevier.

21 Cave, N. (2013). Gastrointestinal gas: eructation, Borborygmus, and flatulence. In: *Canine and Feline Gastroenterology* (ed. R. Washabau and M.J. Day), 124–128. St. Louis, MO: Saunders.

22 Papazoglou, L.G., Patsikas, M.N., and Rallis, T. (2003). Intestinal foreign bodies in dogs and cats. *Comp. Cont. Educ. Pract.* 25 (11): 830.

23 Rijnberk, A. and van Sluijs, F.S. (2009). *Medical History and Physical Examination in Companion Animals*, vol. 333. The Netherlands: Elsevier Limited.

24 Guilford, W.G. and Strombeck, D.R. (1996). Intestinal obstruction, pseudo-obstruction, and foreign bodies. In: *Strombeck's Small Animal Gastroenterology* (ed. W.B. Guilford, S.A. Center and D.R. Strombeck), 487–502. Philadelphia: WB Saunders.

25 Morris, I.R., Darby, C.F., Hammond, P., and Taylor, I. (1983). Changes in small bowel myoelectrical activity following laparotomy. *Br. J. Surg.* 70 (9): 547–548.

26 Walters, P.C. (2000). Approach to the acute abdomen. *Clin. Tech. Small Anim. Pract.* 15 (2): 63–69.

27 Walters, J.M. (2003). Abdominal paracentesis and diagnostic peritoneal lavage. *Clin. Tech. Small Anim. Pract.* 18 (1): 32–38.

28 Capak, D., Simpraga, M., Maticic, D. et al. (2001). Incidence of foreign-body-induced ileus in dogs. *Berl. Munch. Tierarztl. Wochenschr.* 114 (7–8): 290–296.

29 Clark, W.T. (1968). Foreign bodies in small intestine of dog. *Vet. Rec.* 83 (5): 115.

30 Barrs, V.R., Beatty, J.A., Tisdall, P.L. et al. (1999). Intestinal obstruction by trichobezoars in five cats. *J. Feline Med. Surg.* 1 (4): 199–207.

31 O'Brien, T.R. (1978). Small intestine. In: *Radiographic Diagnosis of Abdominal Disorders in the Dog and Cat: Radiographic Interpretation, Clinical Signs, Pathophysiology* (ed. T.R. O'Brien), 259–351. Philadelphia: WB Saunders.

32 McNeel, S.V. (1994). The small bowel. In: *Textbook of Veterinary Diagnostic Radiology* (ed. D.E. Thrall), 524–543. Philadelphia: WB Saunders.

33 Lamb, C.R. and Hansson, K. (1994). Radiological identification of non-opaque intestinal foreign-bodies. *Vet. Radiol. Ultrasound* 35 (2): 87–88.

34 Basher, A.W.P. and Fowler, J.D. (1987). Conservative versus surgical-management of gastrointestinal linear foreign-bodies in the cat. *Vet. Surg.* 16 (2): 135–138.

35 Evans, K.L., Smeak, D.D., and Biller, D.S. (1994). Gastrointestinal linear foreign-bodies in 32 dogs - a retrospective evaluation and feline comparison. *J. Am. Anim. Hosp. Assoc.* 30 (5): 445–450.

36 Felts, J.F., Fox, P.R., and Burk, R.L. (1984). Thread and sewing needles as gastrointestinal foreign-bodies in the cat - a review of 64 cases. *J. Am. Vet. Med. Assoc.* 184 (1): 56–59.

37 Root, C.R. and Lord, P.F. (1971). Linear radiolucent gastrointestinal foreign-bodies in cats and dogs - their radiographic appearance. *J. Am. Vet. Radiol. Soc.* 12: 45.

48

Abnormal Ingestive Behaviors

48.1 Introduction to Ingestive Behaviors

Ingestive behaviors are those pertaining to eating and drinking. The purpose of ingestive behaviors is to maintain a steady state, homeostasis [1–4]. From a physiological standpoint, this requires eating and drinking to maintain caloric intake and hydration. Nonphysiological factors, such as the social aspects of eating, also play a role in establishing hunger and satiety [3]. However, unlike humans, companion animal patients are heavily dependent upon owners, who determine which food is fed, how much, and how often.

48.2 Introduction to Abnormal Ingestive Behaviors

A common abnormal ingestive behavior that is observed among companion animal patients is pica [5–7]. Pica refers to the intentional consumption of non-food items [8–10]. Which non-food items are preferred depends upon the patient; however, the assortment of non-food items that can be ingested is quite varied.

Pica includes, but is not limited to, the consumption of the following [9–13]:

- Adhesive tape
- Articles of clothing, including hair bands, shoelaces, and threads
- Fabric softener sheets
- Grass and other plant material
- Grout
- Hardware
- Jewelry
- Litter
- Paper or cardboard
- Plastic
- Rocks
- Rubber
- Sand and soil
- Sponges
- Toiletries and cosmetics
- Toys
- Wood (see Figures 48.1a, b.)

Cats that are affected by pica are typically young – less than one year of age – at onset [14]. Studies vary concerning whether or not there is a sex predilection [10]. Males were overrepresented in one study [6]. Indoor-only cats are affected more than indoor-outdoor or outdoor-only cats [9].

Wool sucking by cats is another form of pica, even though the fabric is heavily mouthed, rather than ingested [9]. Siamese cats and other Oriental breeds appear predisposed to wool sucking [8, 9, 14, 15]. These same breeds may be more likely than others to develop additional behavioral anomalies, including psychogenic alopecia [16].

Pica is a concern because it jeopardizes the human–animal bond [10]. Clients may be more likely to relinquish cats to shelters when cats destroy human belongings; clients may be more likely to pursue euthanasia if exploratory surgery is indicated to manage gastrointestinal obstructions [10].

When non-food items include feces, the term, coprophagia, is used instead of pica [8, 17, 18]. A dog or cat is said to be coprophagic when it ingests its own feces and/or the feces of others [5, 17]. This includes the feces of other species [5, 17]. Dogs seem more likely to exhibit coprophagic behavior than cats [5, 17]. This behavior is particularly problematic for clients [17, 19, 20]. Clients who witness this behavior tend to view it as both detrimental to the health of the dog and distasteful [17].

Be careful not to confuse pica with destructive chewing [21] (see Figures 48.2a–c).

(a) (b)

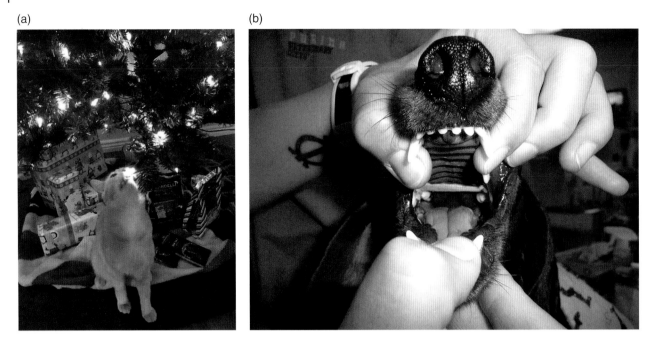

Figure 48.1 (a) Cat exhibiting pica by ingesting needles off a Christmas tree. *Source:* Courtesy of Denise V. Sorbet. (b) This canine patient developed a stick foreign body because of ingesting wood.

48.3 Causes of Abnormal Ingestive Behaviors

Pica or its variations, coprophagia and wool sucking, may stem from medical or behavioral issues [8].

Medical causes of pica include, but are not limited to the following [8, 11, 12, 17, 22–24]:

- Anemia
  - Iron-deficiency anemia
- Dietary or nutrient deficiency
- Drug-induced
  - Glucocorticoids
  - Phenobarbital
- Gastrointestinal parasites
  - Giardiasis
  - Roundworms
  - Hookworms
  - Tapeworms
  - Whipworms
- Malabsorptive and/or maldigestion syndromes
  - Exocrine pancreatic insufficiency (EPI)
  - Inflammatory bowel disease (IBD)
- Metabolic disease
  - Diabetes mellitus
  - Hyperadrenocorticism
  - Hyperthyroidism

- Neuropathy
  - Abnormal hunger and satiety signals within the central nervous system
- Poor plane of nutrition
  - Starvation, as from neglect
- Portosystemic shunt (PSS)
- Structural disease
  - Esophageal stricture
  - Megaesophagus

Behavioral causes of pica include, but are not limited to the following [7–10, 15, 16, 18, 21, 22, 25–31]:

- Age-related
  - Teething
- Anxiety
- Attention seeking
- Early weaning
- Lack of enrichment
- Maternal nesting behavior
- Obsessive–compulsive disorder (OCD)
- Play solicitation
- Removing the source of the punishment, that is, consuming feces to remove evidence of house soiling
- Response to stress
- Taste preference
  - Feces from animals that eat meat-rich diets may be savory to certain dogs

(a)
(b)

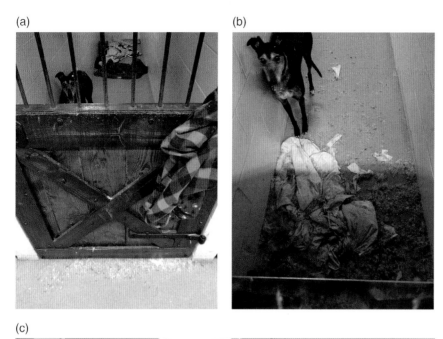

(c)

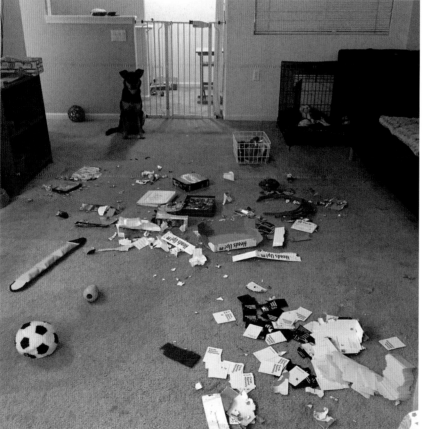

Figure 48.2 (a) Canine patient with separation anxiety, prior to destructive behavior. *Source:* Courtesy of Tradel Harris, DVM. (b) Canine patient with separation anxiety, demonstrating destructive behavior. *Source:* Courtesy of Tradel Harris, DVM. (c) Canine patient with destructive chewing. *Source:* Courtesy of Nikalette Gros, Student Veterinarian 2019.

48.4 The Diagnostic Work-Up for Abnormal Ingestive Behaviors

The patient history plays an integral role in distinguishing medical from behavioral ingestive anomalies [8]. In particular, the following topics should be stressed during history taking when evaluating a patient for pica [8]:

- Appetite
  - What is typical for the patient?
  - Has the patient's appetite changed, and if so, for how long?
- Behavioral history
- Body weight
  - What is the patient's "normal" body weight?
  - Has the patient's body weight changed? If so:
    o Over how long of a period did it change?
    o Was the change intentional (owner-driven)?
    o What, if anything else, may have precipitated this change?
- Current medications
- Description of bowel movements
  - Fecal score to establish consistency, shape, and firmness
  - Frequency of defecation
- Deworming history, including prophylactic endoparasite control
- Diet
  - Quantity
  - Quality
- Lifestyle
  - Activity level
  - Environment
  - Sources of environmental enrichment

The history alone may be beneficial in establishing a medical cause of pica, for example, an inadequate or inappropriate plane of nutrition.

A pharmaceutical history is beneficial because it may reveal that the patient is taking medications that induce polyphagia, for instance, glucocorticoids.

If the patient has a history of unusual licking – licking of the air or licking of surfaces – then an underlying gastrointestinal disorder is a more likely culprit [8, 12, 32].

The owner may report finding "worms" in the patient's stool. Follow-up fecal flotation is essential to confirm endoparasitism.

If the client reports weight loss in a dog despite increased appetite, and loose yellow-to-gray, malodorous feces, then EPI will be prioritized as a differential diagnosis [31]. Based upon this history, the clinician is more likely to pursue pancreatic function tests, such as serum trypsin-like immunoreactivity (TLI) [31].

EPI is a condition in which the pancreatic acinar cells produce insufficient amounts of digestive enzymes [31]. This results in inadequate breakdown of ingesta into absorbable nutrients [31]. When undigested food reaches the small intestine, much of it is unfit for absorption across the gut wall [31]. Small intestinal bacterial overgrowth (SIBO) is likely [31]. German Shepherds and rough-coated Collies are at greater risk than other breeds for development of EPI secondary to pancreatic acinar atrophy. [31] Chronic pancreatitis and pancreatic neoplasia may also lead to EPI [31].

In addition to history taking, the physical examination is an important diagnostic tool in establishing patient body condition score (BCS) and overall health. Anemic, underweight, malnourished, and/or endoparasite-infested patients tend to be unthrifty. Coat quality may also be poor.

A plantigrade stance, paired with a history of polydipsia (PD) and polyuria (PU), is supportive of diabetes mellitus [8].

A palpable thyroid nodule in a cat is suggestive of hyperthyroidism [33].

Baseline bloodwork in the form of a complete blood count (CBC) and chemistry profile provides additional details that are of value. The CBC may confirm anemia and/or hypoproteinemia, which is supportive of maldigestion or malabsorption [8].

The presence of microcytosis and target cells raises the index of suspicion that the patient may have a portosystemic shunt (PSS) [8]. Concurrent hypoalbuminemia and low blood urea nitrogen (BUN) support this suspicion [8].

Patients with gastrointestinal parasitism or eosinophilic IBD may have peripheral eosinophilia [8].

Other laboratory findings may be suggestive of endocrinopathy [8]. For example, elevations in feline aspartate aminotransferase (AST), alanine aminotransferase (ALT), and alkaline phosphatase (ALP or ALK PHOS) support additional testing for hyperthyroidism. Serum total thyroxine (TT4) testing is indicated for any cat with weight loss despite increased appetite, particularly those cats with liver enzyme elevations on baseline chemistry profiles.

If hyperadrenocorticism (HAC) is suspected, then an ACTH stimulation test or low-dose dexamethasone suppression test may be pursued. HAC is driven either by the pituitary or adrenal glands and is characterized by an excess of circulating cortisol. Dogs with HAC often present for PU/PD and polyphagia. They tend to be potbellied and may have a history of poor wound healing. They often have concurrent dermatopathy. Bloodwork that is supportive of HAC includes elevations in ALT and ALP as well as hyperglycemia and hypercholesterolemia secondary to lipolysis, which is stimulated by increased endogenous cortisol.

If a PSS is suspected, then bile acids testing is indicated. A PSS is a congenital or an acquired condition in which blood bypasses the liver, allowing toxins, such as ammonia, to enter systemic circulation. Congenital, extrahepatic PSSs occur more often in small breeds, such as Maltese dogs and Yorkshire Terriers [8].

Imaging studies are indicated in patients that are suspected to have esophageal disease [8]. A history of regurgitation raises the index of suspicion for megaesophagus or esophageal stricture [8].

When a medical cause for pica is established, treatment targets the pathology with the hope that pica will cease once the medical problem has resolved [8].

If a medical cause for ingestive anomalies cannot be determined, then abnormal behavior is likely [8]. In this circumstance, treatment is aimed at removing opportunities for pica [8]. In the ideal world, items that patients target for ingestion would be relocated out of their reach [8].

Alternatively, items can be coated with aversive flavors, such as bitter apple or bitter orange, to deter ingestion. Basket muzzles can be useful, particularly for repeat canine offenders [8].

Leash-walking is particularly effective against coprophagia, although it may not necessarily be convenient for clients.

Some clients may find it easier to lace their dog's feces with bitter or hot substances, such as cayenne pepper, as a deterrent [8]. The hope is that dogs that ingest these substances will develop taste aversion to fecal matter.

Others may prefer to sprinkle commercial products, such as FOR-BID, onto meals [8]. When these products are digested and incorporated into feces, they reportedly create an unsavory taste that may deter the dog from future fecal ingestion. Success is variable.

References

1 Currie, W.B. (1988). *Structure and Function of Domestic Animals*, xiii, 443 p. Boston: Butterworths.

2 Hall, J.E. (2016). *Guyton and Hall Textbook of Medical Physiology*, 13e, xix, 1145 p. Philadelphia, PA: Elsevier.

3 Bellisle, F. (2009). How and why should we study ingestive behaviors in humans? *Food Qual. Prefer.* 20 (8): 539–544.

4 Carlson, N. (2017). *Physiology of Behavior*. England: Pearson Education Limited.

5 Nijsse, R., Mughini-Gras, L., Wagenaar, J.A., and Ploeger, H.W. (2014). Coprophagy in dogs interferes in the diagnosis of parasitic infections by faecal examination. *Vet. Parasitol.* 204 (3–4): 304–309.

6 Bamberger, M. and Houpt, K.A. (2006). Signalment factors, comorbidity, and trends in behavior diagnoses in cats: 736 cases (1991–2001). *J. Am. Vet. Med. Assoc.* 229 (10): 1602–1606.

7 Houpt, K. (1982). Ingestive behavior problems of dogs and cats. *Vet. Clin. North Am. Small Anim. Pract.* 12 (4): 683–692.

8 Tilley, L.P. and Smith, F.W.K. (2004). *The 5-Minute Veterinary Consult: Canine and Feline*, 3e. Baltimore, MD: Lippincott Williams & Wilkins.

9 Stepita, M.E. (2016). Feline anxiety and fear-related disorders. In: *August's Consultations in Feline Internal Medicine*, vol. 7 (ed. S. Little), 900–910. St. Louis, MO: Elsevier, Inc.

10 Demontigny-Bedard, I., Beauchamp, G., Belanger, M.C., and Frank, D. (2016). Characterization of pica and chewing behaviors in privately owned cats: a case-control study. *J. Feline Med. Surg.* 18 (8): 652–657.

11 Kvitko-White, H.L., Cook, A.K. (2014). Managing iron deficiency anemia. DVM360 [Internet] http://veterinarymedicine.dvm360.com/managing-iron-deficiency-anemia.

12 Becuwe-Bonnet, V., Belanger, M.C., Frank, D. et al. (2012). Gastrointestinal disorders in dogs with excessive licking of surfaces. *J. Vet. Behav.* 7 (4): 194–204.

13 Knight, R.W. (1967). Predisposition of Siamese cats to cat woollen articles. *Vet. Rec.* 81 (24): 641–642.

14 Bradshaw, J.W.S., Neville, P.F., and Sawyer, D. (1997). Factors affecting pica in the domestic cat. *Appl. Anim. Behav. Sci.* 52 (3–4): 373–379.

15 Overall, K.L. and Dunham, A.E. (2002). Clinical features and outcome in dogs and cats with obsessive-compulsive disorder: 126 cases (1989–2000). *J. Am. Vet. Med. Assoc.* 221 (10): 1445–1452.

16 Sawyer, L.S., Moon-Fanelli, A.A., and Dodman, N.H. (1999). Psychogenic alopecia in cats: 11 cases (1993–1996). *J. Am. Vet. Med. Assoc.* 214 (1): 71–74.

17 Wells, D.L. (2003). Comparison of two treatments for preventing dogs eating their own faeces. *Vet. Rec.* 153 (2): 51–53.

18 Houpt, K.A. (1991). Feeding and drinking behavior problems. *Vet. Clin. North Am. Small Anim. Pract.* 21 (2): 281–298.

19 Beaver, B.V. (1994). Owner complaints about canine behavior. *J. Am. Vet. Med. Assoc.* 204 (12): 1953–1955.

20 Wells, D.L. and Hepper, P.G. (2000). Prevalence of behaviour problems reported by owners of dogs purchased from an animal rescue shelter. *Appl. Anim. Behav. Sci.* 69 (1): 55–65.

21 Beaver, B.V.G. (2009). *Canine Behavior: Insights and Answers*, 2e. St. Louis, Mo: Saunders/Elsevier.

22 Hart, B.L. and Hart, L.A. (1985). *Canine and Feline Behavioral Therapy*, 123–124. Philadelphia: Lea & Febiger.

23 Overall, K.L. (1997). *Clinical Behavioral Medicine for Small Animals*. London: Mosby Year Book.

24 McKeown, D., Luescher, A., and Machum, M. (1988). Coprophagia: food for thought. *Can. Vet. J.* 29 (10): 849–850.

25 Neville, P.F. (1991). Treatment of behaviour problems in cats. *In Practice* 13: 43–47.

26 Neville, P.F. (ed.) (1996). *Treatment of Fabric-Eating Disorder in Cats*. North American Veterinary Conference (NAVC). Orlando, FL: Eastern States Veterinary Association.

27 Horwitz, D.F. (2007). Chewing in dogs. *NAVC Clinician's Brief* (November): 15–16.

28 Crowell-Davis, S.L. (2007). Stereotypic behavior and compulsive disorder. *Comp. Cont. Educ. Pract.* 29 (10): 625–628.

29 Landsberg, G., Hunthausen, W., and Ackerman, L. (2003). Stereotypic and compulsive disorders. In: *Handbook of Behavior Problems of the Dog and the Cat* (ed. G. Landsberg and W. Hunthausen), 195–225. Edinburgh: Saunders.

30 Frank, D. (2013). Repetitive behaviors in cats and dogs: are they really a sign of obsessive-compulsive disorders (OCD)? *Can. Vet. J.* 54 (2): 129–131.

31 Morgan, J.A., Moore, L.E. (2009). A quick review of canine exocrine pancreatic insufficiency. DVM360 [Internet]. http://veterinarymedicine.dvm360. com/quick-review-canine-exocrine-pancreatic-insufficiency.

32 Pike AL. Medical causes of behavior problems in dogs and cats. https://michvma.org/resources/Documents/ MVC/2017%20Proceedings/pike%2005.pdf.

33 Pike, A.L. Medical causes of behavior problems in dogs and cats. Michigan Veterinary Medical Association [Internet]. https://michvma.org/resources/Documents/ MVC/2017%20Proceedings/pike%2005.pdf.

49

Abnormal Numbers of Teeth and Enamel Defects

49.1 Introduction to Dentition

Cats and dogs have diphyodont dentition, meaning that they have two sets of teeth in a lifetime. The first set consists of deciduous teeth. Deciduous teeth are sometimes referred to as "baby teeth" or "milk teeth." These develop during embryonic life and erupt in pediatric patients. They are smaller than the permanent set of incisors (I), canines (C), premolars (P), and molars (M) that ultimately replace them [1, 2] (see Figures 49.1a, b).

There are fewer deciduous teeth in both the pediatric dog and cat than in the adult [1–6].

49.1.1 Normal Canine Dentition

Puppies have 28 deciduous teeth as compared to a permanent set of 42 [1–6].

The dental formula of an immature dog is [1–6]

- $2 \times (I3/3, C1/1, P3/3)$

The dental formula of an adult dog is [1–6]

- $2 \times (I3/3, C1/1, P4/4, M2/3)$

Eruption of deciduous incisors and canines occurs between three and four weeks old; eruption of deciduous premolars occurs between four and twelve weeks old [1, 2, 7, 8] (see Figure 49.2).

Permanent incisors and canine teeth erupt between three and four months old [1, 7, 8]. Permanent premolars erupt between four and six months, and permanent molars, between five and seven months [1, 7, 8].

Given the timeline above, it is not uncommon for certain age groups of puppies to have both deciduous and permanent teeth present in the mouth at the same time [8]. This is considered age-appropriate mixed dentition [1, 2, 8] (see Figures 49.3a–c).

49.1.2 Normal Feline Dentition

Cats have 26 deciduous teeth as compared to a permanent set of 30 [1, 4–6].

The dental formula of an immature cat is [1, 4–6]

- $2 \times (I3/3, C1/1, P3/2)$

The dental formula of an adult cat is [1, 4–6]

- $2 \times (I3/3, C1/1, P3/2, M1/1)$

Deciduous incisors erupt between two and three weeks of age, followed by the deciduous canines [1, 8]. Deciduous premolars may erupt as late as six weeks of age [1, 8].

Eruption of permanent teeth begins with the permanent incisors between three and four months of age [1, 8] and is complete by five to six months of age [1, 8, 9]. Typically, the molars are the last to erupt [5, 8, 10].

Given the timeline above, it is not uncommon for certain age groups of kittens to have both deciduous and permanent teeth present in the mouth at the same time. This is considered age-appropriate mixed dentition [1, 8] (see Figures 49.4a, b).

49.1.3 Modified Triadan System of Nomenclature for Dentition

During a sedated intraoral examination, each tooth is inspected, and pertinent findings must be documented in the medical record. Forty-two teeth in a dog and thirty teeth in a cat can be challenging to keep track of, without a standard system of nomenclature [1].

The Modified Triadan System of nomenclature was developed to facilitate the identification of individual teeth in veterinary medicine [4, 6, 10, 11].

Each tooth is assigned a three-digit identification number.

The dental arcade determines the first digit in this number [1, 4, 6, 10, 11]:

- Every tooth in the right maxillary arcade has an identification number that starts with one.
- Every tooth in the left maxillary arcade has an identification number that starts with two.
- Every tooth in the left mandibular arcade has an identification number that starts with three.
- Every tooth in the right mandibular arcade has an identification number that starts with four.

Common Clinical Presentations in Dogs and Cats, First Edition. Ryane E. Englar.
© 2019 John Wiley & Sons, Inc. Published 2019 by John Wiley & Sons, Inc.

(a)

(b)

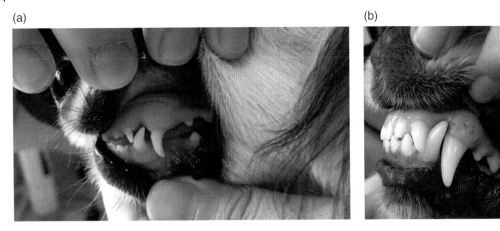

Figure 49.1 (a) Deciduous teeth in a puppy. *Source:* Courtesy of Shirley Yang, DVM. (b) Permanent teeth in an adult dog. *Source:* Courtesy of Christiana and Kaylee Otterson.

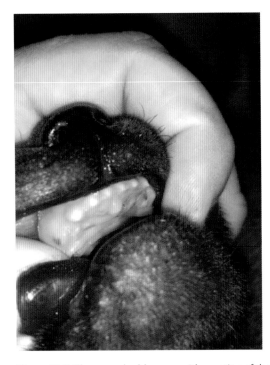

Figure 49.2 Three-week-old puppy with eruption of the maxillary deciduous incisors. *Source:* Courtesy of Lauren Bessert.

The teeth are then numbered beginning from midline. For instance, each arcade has three incisors. So in the right maxillary arcade, the incisor nearest the midline is given the identification number 101; the middle incisor is 102; and the third incisor from the midline is 103 [11].

Canine teeth are always numbered four [1, 4, 6, 10, 11]:

- The canine tooth of the right maxillary arcade is thereby numbered 104, 1 signifying the arcade and 4 signifying the tooth number.

- The canine tooth of the left maxillary arcade is thereby numbered 204, 2 signifying the arcade and 4 signifying the tooth number.
- The canine tooth of the left mandibular arcade is thereby numbered 304, 3 signifying the arcade and 4 signifying the tooth number.
- The canine tooth of the right mandibular arcade is thereby numbered 404, 4 signifying the arcade and 4 signifying the tooth number.

49.1.3.1 The Dog

The last tooth in the maxillary arcade for the dog is assigned the number 10 [1, 4, 6, 10, 11]:

- The second of two molars that are associated with the dog's right maxillary arcade is thereby numbered 110, the first "1" signifying the arcade and 10 signifying the tooth number.
- The second of two molars that are associated with the dog's left maxillary arcade is thereby numbered 210, the 2 signifying the arcade and 10 signifying the tooth number.

The last tooth in the mandibular arcade for the dog is given the number 11 [1, 4, 6, 10, 11]:

- The third of three molars that are associated with the dog's left mandibular arcade is thereby numbered 311, the 3 signifying the arcade and 11 signifying the tooth number.
- The third of three molars that are associated with the dog's right mandibular arcade is thereby numbered 411, the 4 signifying the arcade and 11 signifying the tooth number.

The remaining teeth (the premolars) are filled in numerically, counting down from the last molar [1, 11] (see Figures 49.5a, b).

(a)　　　　　　　　　　(b)　　　　　　　　　　(c)

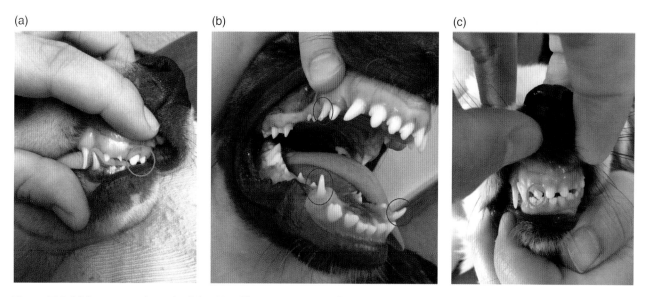

Figure 49.3 (a) Age-appropriate mixed dentition. The permanent maxillary incisors are circled in blue. *Source:* Courtesy of Lauren Beren, student veterinarian. (b) Age-appropriate mixed dentition. The deciduous canine teeth are circled in dark blue. *Source:* Courtesy of Jule Schweighoefer. (c) Age-appropriate mixed dentition. The deciduous maxillary incisor that is circled in blue is loose and is about to become dislodged. *Source:* Courtesy of Shirley Yang, DVM.

(a)　　　　　　　　　　(b)

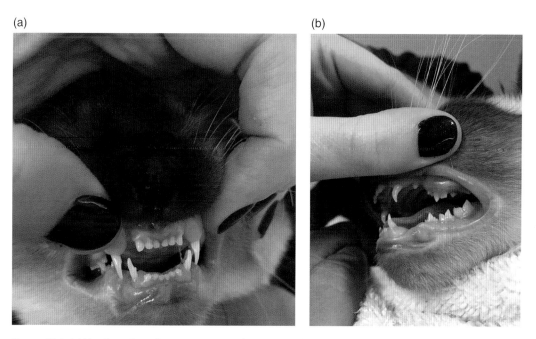

Figure 49.4 (a) Head-on view of age-appropriate dentition in a kitten. Note that all four canine teeth are deciduous. *Source:* Courtesy of Natalie J. Reeser. (b) Lateral view of age-appropriate dentition in a kitten. Note that the canine teeth are deciduous. *Source:* Courtesy of Natalie J. Reeser.

49.1.3.2 The Cat

The last tooth in the maxillary arcade for the cat is assigned the number 9 [1, 4, 6, 10, 11]:

- The one and only molar that is associated with the cat's right maxillary arcade is thereby numbered 109, the first "1" signifying the arcade and 9 signifying the tooth number.

- The one and only molar that is associated with the cat's left maxillary arcade is thereby numbered 209, the first "2" signifying the arcade and 9 signifying the tooth number.
- The one and only molar that is associated with the cat's left mandibular arcade is thereby numbered 309, the first "1" signifying the arcade and 9 signifying the tooth number.

(a)

(b)

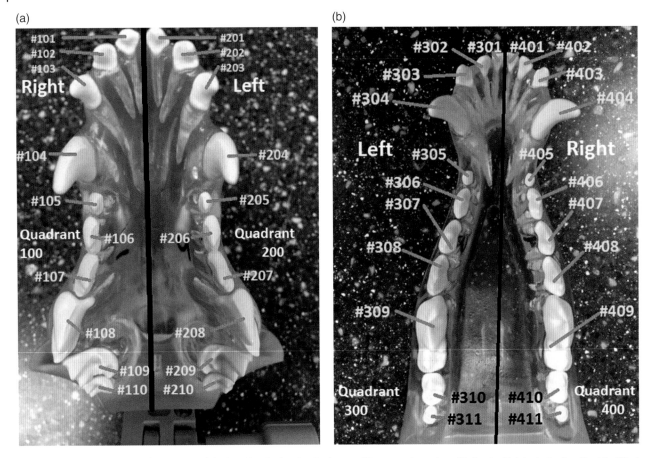

Figure 49.5 (a) Dental model showing adult dentition in the dog in the maxillary arcades only, with the teeth labeled using the Modified Triadan System. (b). Dental model showing adult dentition in the dog in the mandibular arcades only, with the teeth labeled using the Modified Triadan System.

- The one and only molar that is associated with the cat's right mandibular arcade is thereby numbered 409, the first "1" signifying the arcade and 9 signifying the tooth number.

The remaining teeth (the premolars) are filled in numerically, counting down from nine, when moving caudal to the midline (see Figures 49.6a, b).

Because cats have fewer teeth than dogs, cats are missing teeth #105, 205, 305, 306, 405, and 406 as compared to dogs.

49.2   Supernumerary Teeth

When a patient has one or more extra teeth, the extras are referred to as supernumerary teeth [2, 12–15]. Sometimes this condition is called hyperdontia or polyodontia [12].

Any type of tooth – incisor, canine, premolar, or molar – can be present as an extra. However, incisors and premolars are most commonly implicated [2]. Boxer dogs and Mastiffs are more likely to present with extra incisors [13]. In cats, supernumerary teeth are most often the fourth mandibular premolars [14].

One concern is that supernumerary teeth may cause crowding. In dolichocephalic breeds, this is less of an issue because there is sufficient space to accommodate most extras. When crowding is not of concern, supernumerary teeth can remain [15].

However, brachycephalic breeds already have foreshortened skulls [2, 16–19]. Supernumerary teeth in these breeds are likely to create spatial issues within the oral cavity [14, 15]. Misalignment of teeth predisposes the patient to premature periodontal disease [14, 15]. Surgical extraction of supernumerary teeth is advisable when crowding becomes clinically relevant [12, 13, 15].

Like brachycephalic breeds, cats often lack sufficient space to accommodate extra teeth, and extraction of supernumerary teeth is often indicated [12, 13].

49.3   Persistent or Retained Deciduous Teeth

Dogs are more likely than cats to have one or more deciduous teeth fail to fall out [8, 14]. These persistent or retained deciduous teeth linger as their

(a)

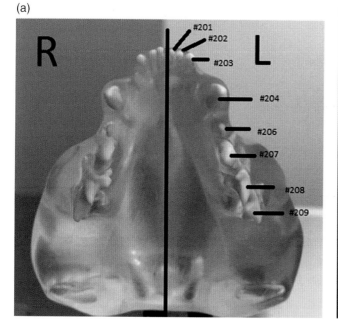

(b)

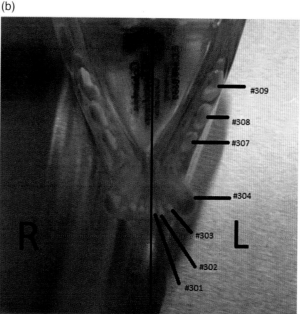

Figure 49.6 (a) Dental model showing adult dentition in the cat in the maxillary arcades only, with the teeth labeled using the Modified Triadan System. (b) Dental model showing adult dentition in the cat in the mandibular arcades only, with the teeth labeled using the Modified Triadan System.

permanent replacements erupt. In this clinical scenario, both the deciduous and permanent teeth share the same gingival collar [8]. This forces the permanent tooth to be malpositioned [8, 20].

Retained deciduous canines are commonplace is clinical practice. When the maxillary canine is involved, the permanent tooth tends to erupt rostral to the deciduous one [8]. When the mandibular canine is involved, the deciduous tooth is often labial to the permanent one [8] (see Figures 49.7a–d).

Most other permanent teeth will be deviated lingually if their deciduous counterparts are retained [14].

Retained deciduous teeth should be extracted when possible [8, 14]. Note that retained canine teeth have long, thin roots that are easily fractured in the process of removing them (see Figure 49.8).

Surgical excision is a delicate process, and care should be taken to avoid inadvertently damaging the erupting permanent canine tooth [8].

49.4 Hypodontia

Absence of teeth altogether, anodontia, is rare in the canine and feline patient [21]. However, one or more teeth may be congenitally absent [12]. This condition, hypodontia, is more likely to be seen in clinical practice [12, 21]. Kelly Blue Terriers and hairless breeds are over-represented [15, 22, 23].

Hypodontia may involve deciduous teeth, permanent teeth, or both [15].

Incisors and premolars are more likely to be missing than molars and canine teeth [15].

Note that hypodontia may also be acquired [15]. For example, teeth may be missing secondary to trauma [15].

Dental radiographs are necessary to confirm hypodontia [15]. A differential diagnosis for hypodontia is an impacted tooth, that is, one that fails to erupt because of a physical barrier in its path [15].

Hypodontia is not a medical concern; it is an aesthetic issue [12].

49.5 Resorptive Lesions

Tooth resorption (TR) is common in feline patients and is sometimes referred to as feline odontoclastic resorptive lesion (FORL) [12, 24–27]. Other synonyms that appear in the veterinary medical literature include neck lesions, cervical line erosions, and external odontoclastic resorptions [24].

Studies vary widely in terms of prevalence: 20–75% of cats are affected by one or more lesion [15, 26–33]. Young Burmese and Siamese cats (<12 months of age) appear to be at increased risk [30, 34]. Other breeds tend to be predisposed when over six years of age [30, 34].

TR involves one or more teeth, the dentin of which becomes eroded [24]. Note that this is a process [24, 27]. Over time, the following outcomes are possible [25, 27]:

- The entire tooth may be consumed.
- The root(s) undergo(es) complete resorption.

(a)

(c)

(b)

(d)

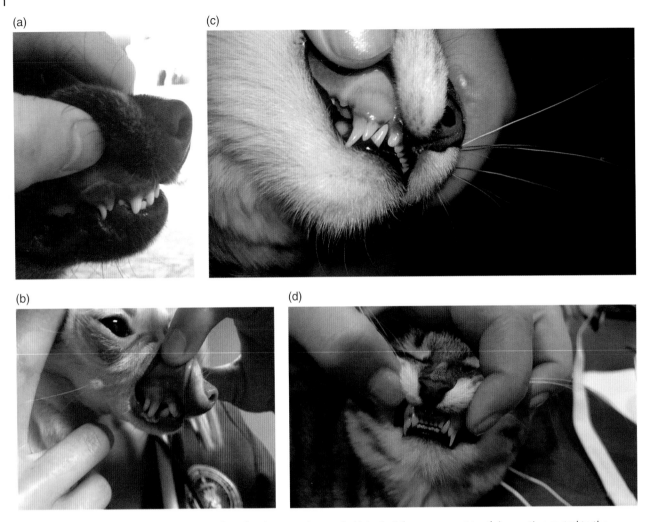

Figure 49.7 (a) Dog with retained right maxillary deciduous canine tooth. Note that the permanent tooth is erupting rostral to the deciduous one, which is typical. (b) Chihuahua with retained right maxillary deciduous canine tooth. *Source:* Courtesy of John A. Schwartz. (c) Cat with bilaterally retained maxillary canine teeth. Because this photograph is a profile view, only the retained right maxillary deciduous canine tooth is evident. *Source:* Courtesy of Hannah Butler. (d) Head-on view of the same cat depicted in Figure 49.7c. Note that both maxillary canine deciduous teeth have been retained. *Source:* Courtesy of Hannah Butler.

- – With nothing to anchor the crown to the jaw, the crown falls out.
- – The patient is now said to have hypodontia.
- The crown breaks off, leaving root remnants behind in alveolar bone.
  - – Root remnants act as a foreign body.
  - – The periodontium becomes irritated and inflamed.
  - – The patient's mouth becomes painful to manipulate.

Classification of TR is complex [14]. Five stages of TR have been described in the cat [14]. The details of these stages are beyond the scope of this text; however, in general, they progress in terms of intensity [14]:

- Stage 1 is least invasive: lesions are limited to the enamel or cementum.
- Stage 2 lesions involve the dentin.
- Stage 3 involves exposure of the pulp.

- Stage 4 lesions destabilize the structure of affected teeth.
- Stage 5 is most extensive: only tooth roots of affected teeth remain.

A thorough intraoral exam under anesthesia and radiographic evaluation of all dental arcades are both necessary for staging to be accurate [14, 33] (see Figure 49.9).

Early and mid-stage FORLs are likely to be underreported if the clinician is reliant upon gross observation skills alone [25, 33].

Note that FORLs are not the same as dental caries or cavities [24]. Caries develop when the acid by-products of bacterial fermentation of carbohydrates damage the surface of one or more teeth [24]. Over time, a cavity forms because acid-induced demineralization of the enamel and dentin allows bacteria to gain entry to and

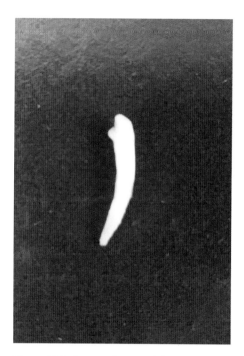

Figure 49.8 Extracted retained deciduous canine tooth from a Yorkshire terrier dog. Note the long root. *Source:* Courtesy of Kelli L. Crisfulli, RVT.

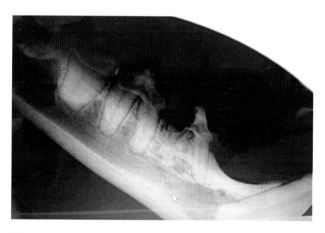

Figure 49.9 Radiographic evidence of FORL. Note how the crown appears to be dissolving. *Source:* Courtesy of Genevieve LaFerriere, DVM.

subsequently cause infection within the pulp [24, 35]. The pulp is the innermost layer of the tooth that houses blood vessels and nerve endings.

TR is a separate process by which dentin erodes. Depending upon the stage, treatment for TR may involve the following [33, 36, 37]:

- Conservative management
- Tooth extraction
- Coronal amputation

Conservation management may be appropriate for lesions that are only evident radiographically in a patient that has no overt pain or discomfort [33]. This is rarely the case by the time the patient presents to the clinic for evaluation [33].

Many patients with FORLs present with one or more of the following clinical signs [24]:

- Blood-tinged saliva
- Decreased appetite
- Difficulty with prehension of food
- Ptyalism

These clinical signs are suggestive of underlying oral discomfort that is often secondary to TR [24].

Because most patients with TR are clinical at time of presentation, extraction of affected teeth is performed more often than conservative management [33, 36, 37].

When resorption is so extensive that it is impossible to remove all tooth substance, coronal amputation is indicated [33]. This technique requires specialty training and is beyond the scope of this text.

49.6 Enamel Defects

Odontogenesis is the process by which teeth form from embryonic cells [38–41]. Tooth structure will be impacted by any disruption in this process [38].

In dogs, enamel forms between two weeks of age and three months [42]. Traumatic or systemic disturbances that take place during this time frame can also alter the anatomy of one or more teeth [38].

Severe fever and exposure to epitheliotropic viruses, such as canine distemper virus (CDV), have been associated with enamel defects [38, 43–45]. Specifically, these have been linked to one particular type of defect, diffuse enamel hypoplasia [38].

Diffuse enamel hypoplasia is a condition in which a patient's enamel is thinner than it ought to be [38]. Defects may be linear or pit-like, as is common for human patients [38, 46] (see Figure 49.10).

In dogs, however, defects are more often circumferential, meaning that they stretch around the entire crown [38] (see Figure 49.11).

Dentin is exposed when patches of enamel are quite thin [38]. This leads to dental staining [38].

Dental staining may also occur if tetracycline antibiotics are prescribed during pregnancy or to pediatric patients <6 months of age [38, 43, 47–51]. Teeth will stain yellow-brown [38]. This permanent stain is because tetracycline irreversibly binds to a certain mineral in teeth, calcium orthophosphate [38, 48, 52]. This

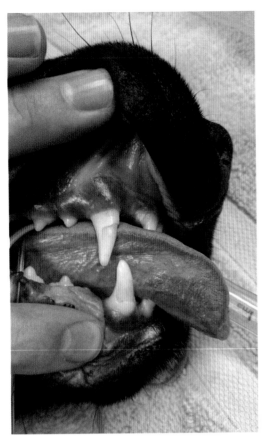

Figure 49.10 Pit-like enamel defects in a canine patient. *Source:* Courtesy of Adam Riley.

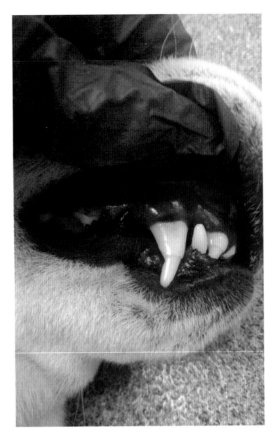

Figure 49.11 Circumferential enamel defects in a canine patient. These defects occurred secondary to CDV. *Source:* Courtesy of Laura Polerecky, LVT.

creates a color change that darkens with exposure to light.

Doxycycline and minocycline will also stain teeth, although staining is less pronounced [51, 52].

Staining is aesthetically displeasing to the eye [38]. Dentin exposure may also lead to dentin sensitivity or pulpitis [42].

Pulpitis is inflammation of the pulp. When pulp becomes inflamed, it may experience minor hemorrhage. Just as hemorrhage under the skin causes a visible bruise, pulpitis causes the affected tooth to discolor. The discoloration occurs from within the tooth, which may appear pink-purple to gray (see Figure 49.12).

Note that pulpitis is not solely the result of dentin exposure. It more commonly results from focal trauma.

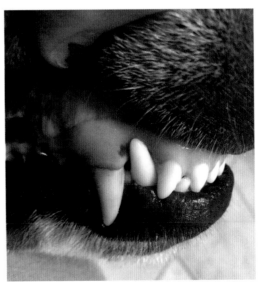

Figure 49.12 Pulpitis at the tip of the right maxillary canine tooth. *Source:* Courtesy of Kimberly Wallitsch.

References

1 Englar, R.E. (2017). *Performing the Small Animal Physical Examination*. Hoboken, NJ: Wiley.

2 Evans, H.E. (2013). The digestive apparatus and abdomen. In: *Miller's Anatomy of the Dog, 4e, xix, 850 p* (ed. H.E. Evans and M.E. Miller). St. Louis, Missouri: Elsevier

3 Evans, H.E. (1993). The digestive apparatus and abdomen. In: *Miller's Anatomy of the Dog*, 3e (ed. H.E. Evans and M.E. Miller), 385–462. Philadelphia: W.B. Saunders.

4 Holmstrom, S.E. and Holmstrom, S.E. (2013). *Veterinary Dentistry: A Team Approach*, 2e, viii, 434 p. St. Louis, Mo: Elsevier/Mosby.

5 Lobprise, H.B. and Wiggs, R.B. (2000). *The Veterinarian's Companion for Common Dental Procedures*. Lakewood, Colorado: AAHA Press.

6 Shipp, A.D. and Fahrenkrug, P. (1992). *Practitioners' Guide to Veterinary Dentistry*, 237. Glendale, CA: Griffin Printing, Inc.

7 Fulton, A.J., Fiani, N., and Verstraete, F.J. (2014). Canine pediatric dentistry. *Vet. Clin. North Am. Small Anim. Pract.* 44 (2): 303–324.

8 Bellows, J. (2011). Tooth eruption and exfoliation in dogs and cats. DVM 360 [Internet]. http://veterinarynews.dvm360.com/tooth-eruption-and-exfoliation-dogs-and-cats.

9 Rijnberk, A. and van Sluijs, F.S. (2009). *Medical History and Physical Examination in Companion Animals*, 333. The Netherlands: Elsevier Limited.

10 Reiter, A.M. and Soltero-Rivera, M.M. (2014). Applied feline oral anatomy and tooth extraction techniques: an illustrated guide. *J. Feline Med. Surg.* 16 (11): 900–913.

11 Floyd, M.R. (1991). The modified Triadan system: nomenclature for veterinary dentistry. *J. Vet. Dent.* 8 (4): 18–19.

12 DuPont, G. (2010). Dental and oral examination: A visual atlas of dental and oral pathology. DVM 360 [Internet]. http://veterinarycalendar.dvm360.com/dental-and-oral-examination-visual-atlas-dental-and-oral-pathology-proceedings.

13 Peterson, M.E. and Kutzler, M.A. (2011). *Small Animal Pediatrics: The First 12 Months of Life*, xvi, 526 p. St. Louis, Mo.: Saunders/Elsevier.

14 Marretta, S.M. (ed.) (2001). Feline dentistry. Atlantic Coast Veterinary Conference.

15 Verhaert, L. (ed.) (2001). Developmental disturbances of teeth. World Small Animal Veterinary Association World Congress; Vancouver, Canada.

16 Haworth, K.E., Islam, I., Breen, M. et al. (2001). Canine TCOF1; cloning, chromosome assignment and genetic analysis in dogs with different head types. *Mamm. Genome* 12 (8): 622–629.

17 Wayne, R.K. (1986). Cranial morphology of domestic and wild canids – the influence of development on morphological change. *Evolution* 40 (2): 243–261.

18 Young, A. and Bannasch, D. (2006). Morphological variation in the dog. In: *The Dog and its Genome* (ed. E.A. Ostrander, U. Giger and Lindblad-Toh), 47–65. Cold Spring Harbor, NY: Cold Spring Harbor Laboratory Press.

19 Schoenebeck, J.J. and Ostrander, E.A. (2013). The genetics of canine skull shape variation. *Genetics* 193 (2): 317–325.

20 Schaer, M. and Gaschen, F. (2016). *Clinical Medicine of the Dog and Cat*, 3e. Boca Raton, FL: Taylor & Francis Group.

21 Slatter, D.H. (1985). *Textbook of Small Animal Surgery*. Philadelphia: W.B. Saunders.

22 Pearson, L.K. (2018). Congenital and inherited anomalies of the teeth. Merck Veterinary Manual [Internet]. https://www.merckvetmanual.com/digestive-system/congenital-and-inherited-anomalies-of-the-digestive-system/congenital-and-inherited-anomalies-of-the-teeth.

23 Foil, C. (1993). *Veterinary Pediatrics* (ed. J.D. Hoskins), 366. Philadelphia: WB Saunders.

24 Bellows, J. (2016). External tooth resorption in cats: part 1: pathogenesis, classification, & diagnosis. *Today's Vet. Pract.* (January/February): 20–25.

25 Johnston, N. (2000). Acquired feline oral cavity disease part 2: feline odontoclastic resorptive lesions. *In Pract.* 22 (4): 188–197.

26 Reiter, A.M., Lewis, J.R., and Okuda, A. (2005). Update on the etiology of tooth resorption in domestic cats. *Vet. Clin. North Am. Small Anim. Pract.* 35 (4): 913–942, vii.

27 Reiter, A.M., Lyon, K.F., Nachreiner, R.F., and Shofer, F.S. (2005). Evaluation of calciotropic hormones in cats with odontoclastic resorptive lesions. *Am. J. Vet. Res.* 66 (8): 1446–1452.

28 Reiter, A.M. and Mendoza, K.A. (2002). Feline odontoclastic resorptive lesions an unsolved enigma in veterinary dentistry. *Vet. Clin. North Am. Small Anim. Pract.* 32 (4): 791–837, v.

29 Gorrel, C. and Larsson, A. (2002). Feline odontoclastic resorptive lesions: unveiling the early lesion. *J. Small Anim. Pract.* 43 (11): 482–488.

30 Lommer, M.J. and Verstraete, F.J. (2000). Prevalence of odontoclastic resorption lesions and periapical radiographic lucencies in cats: 265 cases (1995–1998). *J. Am. Vet. Med. Assoc.* 217 (12): 1866–1869.

31 Lund, E.M., Bohacek, L.K., Dahlke, J.L. et al. (1998). Prevalence and risk factors for odontoclastic resorptive lesions in cats. *J. Am. Vet. Med. Assoc.* 212 (3): 392–395.

32 Verstraete, F.J., van Aarde, R.J., Nieuwoudt, B.A. et al. (1996). The dental pathology of feral cats on Marion Island, part II: periodontitis, external odontoclastic resorption lesions and mandibular thickening. *J. Comp. Pathol.* 115 (3): 283–297.

33 Gorrel, C. (ed.) (2003). Feline odontoclastic resorptive lesions. World Small Animal Veterinary Association World Congress; Hamshire, UK.

34 Clarke, D.E. and Caiafa, A. (2014). Oral examination in the cat: a systematic approach. *J. feline Med. Surg.* 16 (11): 873–886.

35 von Arx, T., Schawalder, P., Ackermann, M., and Bosshardt, D.D. (2009). Human and feline invasive cervical resorptions: the missing link?–Presentation of four cases. *J. Endod.* 35 (6): 904–913.

36 DuPont, G. (1995). Crown amputation with intentional root retention for advanced feline resorptive lesions–a clinical study. *J. Vet. Dent.* 12 (1): 9–13.

37 Carmichael, D.T. (2005). Dental corner: how to detect and treat feline odontoclastic resorptive lesions. DVM 360 [Internet]. http://veterinarymedicine.dvm360.com/dental-corner-how-detect-and-treat-feline-odontoclastic-resorptive-lesions?id=&sk=&date=&pageID=2.

38 Boy, S., Crossley, D., and Steenkamp, G. (2016). Developmental structural tooth defects in dogs – experience from veterinary dental referral practice and review of the literature. *Front Vet. Sci.* 3: 9.

39 Cobourne, M.T. and Sharpe, P.T. (2003). Tooth and jaw: molecular mechanisms of patterning in the first branchial arch. *Arch. Oral Biol.* 48 (1): 1–14.

40 Seppala, M., Zoupa, M., Onyekwelu, O., and Cobourne, M.T. (2006). Tooth development: 1. Generating teeth in the embryo. *Dent. Update.* 33 (10): 582–584, 6–8, 90–1.

41 Sharpe, P.T. (2001). Neural crest and tooth morphogenesis. *Adv. Dent. Res.* 15: 4–7.

42 Beckman, B. (2012). Dental enamel defects in dogs. DVM 360 [Internet]. http://veterinarynews.dvm360.com/dental-enamel-defects-dogs.

43 Miles, A.E.W., Grigson, C., and Colyer, F. (1990). *Colyer's Variations and Diseases of the Teeth of Animals.* xvi, 672 p. Cambridge England; New York: Cambridge University Press.

44 Bittegeko, S.B., Arnbjerg, J., Nkya, R., and Tevik, A. (1995). Multiple dental developmental abnormalities following canine distemper infection. *J. Am. Anim. Hosp. Assoc.* 31 (1): 42–45.

45 Dubielzig, R.R. (1979). The effect of canine distemper virus on the ameloblastic layer of the developing tooth. *Vet. Pathol.* 16 (2): 268–270.

46 Hillson, S. and Bond, S. (1997). Relationship of enamel hypoplasia to the pattern of tooth crown growth: a discussion. *Am. J. Phys. Anthropol.* 104 (1): 89–103.

47 Schuster, A. and Shwachman, H. (1956). The tetracyclines; applied pharmacology. *Pediatr. Clin. N. Am.* 295–303.

48 Wallman, I.S. and Hilton, H.B. (1962). Teeth pigmented by tetracycline. *Lancet* 1 (7234): 827–829.

49 van der Bijl, P. and Pitigoi-Aron, G. (1995). Tetracyclines and calcified tissues. *Ann. Dent.* 54 (1–2): 69–72.

50 Sanchez, A.R., Rogers, R.S. 3rd, and Sheridan, P.J. (2004). Tetracycline and other tetracycline-derivative staining of the teeth and oral cavity. *Int. J. Dermatol.* 43 (10): 709–715.

51 Grossman, E.R. (1986). Tetracycline and staining of the teeth. *J. Am. Med. Assoc.* 255 (18): 2442–2443.

52 Good, M.L. and Hussey, D.L. (2003). Minocycline: stain devil? *Br. J. Dermatol.* 149 (2): 237–239.

50

Acute Abdomen

50.1 The Clinical Presentation of Acute Abdomen

Acute abdomen is a catchall phrase for sudden, intense abdominal pain [1–9]. It is not pathognomonic for any one particular disease. Instead, it represents a spectrum of conditions that constitute medical emergencies, some of which are life-threatening [1–9].

Because any number of body systems may be involved, the clinical presentation of acute abdomen varies. Common presentations include the following [1–3, 7–21]:

- Abnormal posturing
  - Dogs often present hunched, with either an arched back or the so-called "prayer posture."
  - This posture mirrors that of a "play bow" except the patient is not playing; it is sick (see Figure 50.1).
    - Forelimbs are extended.
    - Chest is lowered to the floor.
    - Rump is elevated.
- Abdominal distension
  - Secondary to fluid: ascites
  - Secondary to food: so-called "food bloat" (see Figure 50.2).
  - Secondary to gas: "bloat"
  - Secondary to "mass effect"
    - Displaced organ
    - Torsion of organ
    - Abdominal mass
- Changes in attitude
  - Depression
- Changes in mobility
  - Inability to settle
    - Pacing
    - Restlessness
  - Alternatively, unwilling or unable to move
    - Trembling
    - Stiff stance as if frozen in place

- Changes in perfusion parameters
  - Delayed capillary refill time (CRT)
  - Pale mucous membranes (see Chapter 38, Section 38.4.1)
  - Poor pulse quality
- Collapse (review Chapter 40)
- Dehydration
- Elevated heart rate and respiratory rate, with or without an elevation in core body temperature
- History of altered appetite
  History of vomiting, with or without diarrhea
  - Hypersalivation
  - Productive or unproductive retching
- Tenseness on abdominal palpation
  - Abdominal splinting

50.2 Potential Causes of Acute Abdomen

Acute abdomen may truly originate from the gastrointestinal tract. For example, one or more of the following digestive or hepatobiliary organs may be involved [1–3, 5, 7, 22–24]:

- Stomach
  - Gastric dilatation
  - Gastric dilatation-volvulus (GDV) ***
  - Gastric foreign body ***
  - Gastric perforation
  - Gastritis ***
  - Gastrointestinal ulceration
  - Neoplasia
  - Pyloric stenosis
- Small intestine
  - Bowel perforation
  - Bowel stricture (see Figure 50.3a)
  - Endoparasitism ***

- Enteritis ***
  - Infectious ***
    - Canine parvovirus (CPV) ***
    - Feline panleukopenia virus
- Gastroenteritis ***
- Ileus ***
- Intestinal obstruction ***
- Intestinal torsion
- Intussusception ***
- Neoplasia ***

- Large intestine
  - Colitis ***
  - Colonic perforation
  - Constipation ***
  - Neoplasia
- Pancreas
  - Pancreatic abscess
  - Pancreatic ischemia
  - Pancreatic duct obstruction
  - Pancreatitis ***
  - Neoplasia
- Liver
  - Cholangiohepatitis ***
  - Hepatic abscess
  - Hepatitis
    - Infectious
    - Toxic
  - Liver lobe torsion
  - Neoplasia *** (see Figure 50.3b)
- Gall bladder
  - Bile peritonitis
  - Biliary mucocele
  - Cholecystitis ***
  - Gall bladder obstruction
  - Gall bladder rupture
  - Gall stones
  - Neoplasia
- Other
  - Duodenocolic ligament entrapment
  - Mesenteric thromboembolism
  - Mesenteric lymph node disease
  - Mesenteric torsion

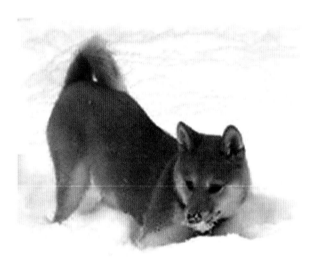

Figure 50.1 Shiba Inu demonstrating a "play bow." This dog is playful. Note that this same play posture is displayed by patients that present for acute abdomen. Sometimes, this display is referred to as the "prayer posture." *Source:* Courtesy of Alan Fink Fine Art.

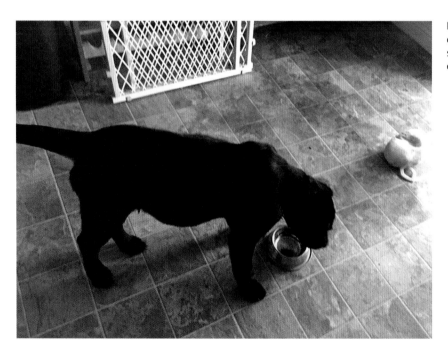

Figure 50.2 Labrador Retriever puppy demonstrating abdominal distension secondary to food bloat. *Source:* Courtesy of Kat Blincoe.

- Mesenteric volvulus
- Post-laparotomy dehiscence or traumatic evisceration
  (see Figures 50.3c, d)
    o Body wall
    o Hollow organ

Items that are starred above (***) represent relatively common clinical presentations in a primary care setting.

Although it may be tempting to view acute abdomen as strictly a gastrointestinal problem, it is important to recognize that many other organs or organ systems may be involved [1–5, 7, 10, 18, 25]:

- Body wall defect ***
  - Hernia with strangulated viscera
    o Inguinal (see Figure 50.4)
    o Perineal
    o Scrotal
    o Umbilical (see Figure 50.5)

- Metabolic disturbances
  - Hypoadrenocorticism (Addison's disease) ***
- Musculoskeletal system
  - Discospondylitis
  - Intervertebral disc disease (IVDD) ***
- Spleen
  - Neoplasia ***
  - Splenic hematoma (see Figure 50.6)
  - Splenic torsion
- Urogenital system
  - Acute renal failure (ARF) or acute kidney injury (AKI) ***
  - Cystitis ***
  - Intra-abdominal testicular torsion in a cryptorchid patient
  - Metritis
  - Neoplasia
  - Prostatic abscess
  - Prostatitis ***

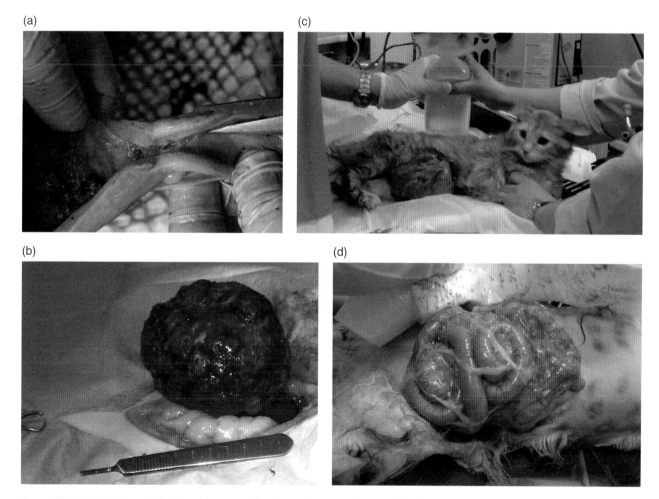

(a)

(c)

(b)

(d)

Figure 50.3 (a) Small intestinal stricture in a crocodile. *Source:* Courtesy of Laura Polerecky, LVT. (b) Intraoperative photograph of hepatobiliary neoplasia in a cat. (c) Evisceration in a cat. *Source:* Courtesy of Daniel Foy, MS, DVM, DACVIM, DACVECC. (d) Close-up of same cat in (c). *Source:* Courtesy of Daniel Foy, MS, DVM, DACVIM, DACVECC.

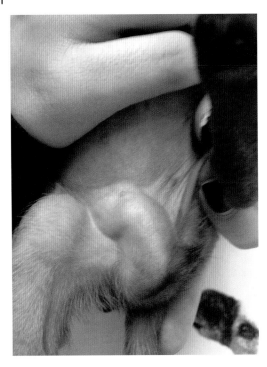

Figure 50.4 Inguinal hernia. *Source:* Courtesy of Pamela Mueller, DVM.

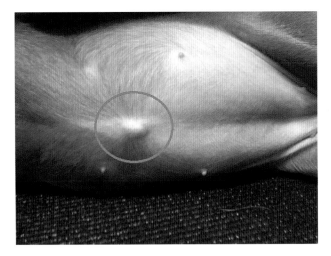

Figure 50.5 Umbilical hernia evident on visual inspection of a canine patient in lateral recumbency.

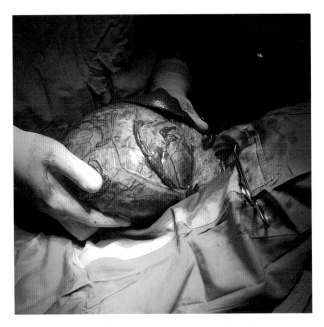

Figure 50.6 Splenic hematoma in a canine patient. *Source:* Courtesy of Frank Isom, DVM.

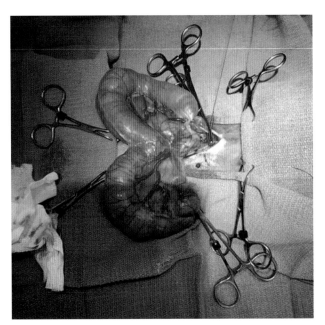

Figure 50.7 Pyometra. *Source:* Courtesy of Samantha B. Thurman, DVM.

- Pyelonephritis ***
- Pyometra *** (see Figure 50.7)
- Torsion
  - Testicular (see Figure 50.8) (refer to Chapter 55)
  - Uterine
- Ureteral rupture
- Urethral tears

- Urinary bladder rupture
- Urinary calculi or urolithiasis ***
  - Bladder stones *** (see Figures 50.9a, b)
  - Nephroliths
  - Ureteroliths
- Urinary tract obstruction (UTO) ***
  - Especially male cats
- Other
  - Peritonitis ***
  - Steatitis

Items that are starred above (***) represent relatively common clinical presentations in a primary care setting.

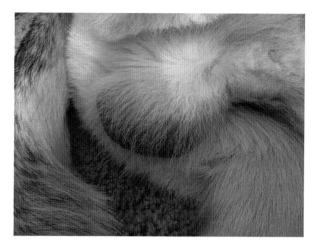

Figure 50.8 Swollen and bruised scrotum secondary to suspected testicular torsion in a canine patient. *Source:* Courtesy of Jule Schweighoefer.

50.3 Signalment, History Taking, and Acute Abdomen Presentations

It can be overwhelming to consider all of these differential diagnoses at once. For the student clinician, it can be especially difficult to know where to begin. There is just so much to consider.

The student clinician faces the additional challenge of having to discern which conditions are surgical versus medical emergencies when time is of the essence. In cases of acute abdomen, patient instability often requires rapid decision making. Unlike wellness examinations, acute abdomen cases are time-sensitive: the clinician does not have the luxury of unlimited time with which to make case management decisions.

Furthermore, these cases are often emotionally charged or distressing to the client: clinicians have to not only stabilize the patient, but also encourage the owner to make quick decisions about diagnostic and therapeutic interventions.

An advisable approach would be to take a step back from the lists of differential diagnoses.

Begin with signalment and history taking to gather patient-specific data. With time, these lead to pattern recognition. As students have more opportunities to experience clinical cases, they learn what is most, versus least, likely and manage cases accordingly.

For example, consider the patient's age when the clinical presentation is acute abdomen [3, 4]:

- Puppies are more likely than adult dogs to develop CPV.
- Kittens are more likely to develop viral gastroenteritis secondary to feline panleukopenia.

(a)

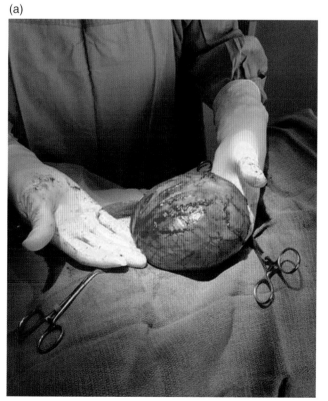

(b)

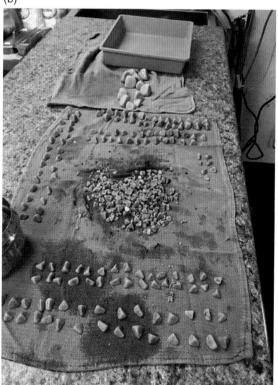

Figure 50.9 (a) Intraoperative photograph depicting a canine patient undergoing cystotomy. *Source:* Courtesy of Samantha Thurman, DVM. (b) Postoperative photograph depicting all cystic calculi that were removed from the canine patient that was depicted in (a). *Source:* Courtesy of Samantha Thurman, DVM.

- Young adult patients are most at risk of developing Addison's disease.
- A six-month-old puppy is more likely to present for acute abdomen secondary to foreign body ingestion than a twelve-year-old dog.
- Intra-abdominal masses secondary to neoplastic disease are more likely to occur in middle-aged to older patients. It would be rare, for instance, to diagnose splenic hemangiosarcoma in a six-month old puppy.

In addition, consider the patient's breed when the clinical presentation is acute abdomen [1, 3, 4, 7, 26–30]:

- Dachshunds are prone to developing IVDD.
- Dalmatians and English Bulldogs are more likely to develop a specific type of urinary calculi, urates.
- Large-breed and deep-chested dogs are most at risk for developing GDV.
  - Alaskan Malamutes
  - German Shepherds
  - Great Danes
  - Irish Wolfhounds
  - Labrador Retrievers
  - Saint Bernards
- Deep-chested dogs may also be more likely to experience splenic torsion.
- Miniature Schnauzers are predisposed to pancreatitis, in addition to calcium oxalate and struvite urolithiasis.
- Standard Poodles are at increased risk of developing Addison's disease.

Consider also the patient's sex, sexual status, and species when the clinical presentation is acute abdomen [1, 3, 4, 7, 31–33]:

- An intact female is at risk for pyometra.
- Male cats are more likely than females to develop UTO.
- Prostatitis and prostatic abscesses are more common occurrences in the intact, as opposed to castrated, male.

Signalment alone can narrow down the list of differential diagnoses.

History taking further refines the list of differentials by providing additional insight. In particular, the following topics should be stressed during history taking when evaluating a patient with acute abdomen [1, 4, 34]:

- Abdominal distension
  - Has the owner noticed a bloated appearance?
    ○ How distended is the abdomen?
    ○ Did the abdomen become distended acutely?
    ○ Is the abdomen continuing to expand?
- Abnormal ingestive behaviors
  - Does the patient have a history of pica?

- Activity level
  - What is the patient's activity level?
  - Has the patient's actively level acutely changed?
- Appetite
  - What is the patient's appetite typically?
  - Has the patient's appetite acutely changed?
- Back pain
  - Does the patient have a history of back pain and/or IVDD?
- Current medications
  - Is the patient currently taking a non-steroidal anti-inflammatory drug (NSAID) such as carprofen?
    ○ Dose
    ○ Dosing frequency
    ○ Duration of treatment
  - Was the patient inadvertently given the NSAID, ibuprofen?
    ○ When?
    ○ How much?
    ○ How often?
- Dietary history
  - What is the patient fed on a regular basis?
  - Is the patient fed meals or is the patient free-fed?
    ○ How much food is offered during a 24-h period?
    ○ How much food is ingested during a 24-h period?
  - Is the patient's diet commercial dog or cat food?
    ○ Brand
    ○ Formulation (dry, canned, semi-moist)
    ○ Has the client changed brands recently?
  - Is the patient's diet home-prepared?
    ○ What are the ingredients?
    ○ How was it designed or formulated?
    ○ Is it missing any essential nutrients?
  - Is the patient eating a raw diet?
    ○ This heightens the risk of Salmonellosis.
- Diarrhea
  - Is the patient having diarrhea?
    ○ Is the patient having small bowel diarrhea?
      ▪ Normal to mild increase in the frequency of defecation
      ▪ Normal to increased fecal volume
      ▪ May contain melena (see Figure 50.10)
      ▪ Negative for mucus
      ▪ Negative for tenesmus
      ▪ Negative for urgency
      ▪ Commonly associated with weight loss if chronic issue
      ▪ Commonly associated with emesis
    ○ Is the patient having large bowel diarrhea?
      ▪ Increased frequency of defecation
      ▪ Increased water content/decreased fecal volume
      ▪ May contain fresh blood (hematochezia) (see Figure 50.11)
      ▪ Frequently contains mucus

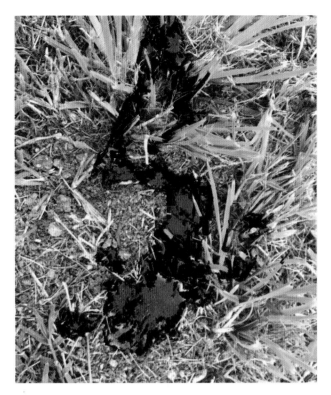

Figure 50.10 Melena from a canine patient. The black color indicates the presence of digested blood. This means that the blood originated from the upper gastrointestinal tract. *Source:* Courtesy of Beki Cohen Regan, DVM, DACVIM (Oncology).

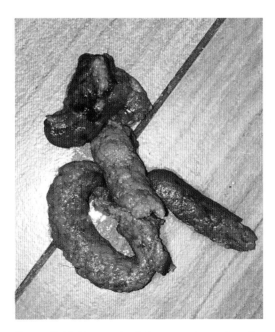

Figure 50.11 Hematochezia from a canine patient. Note the presence of fresh red blood coating the soft stool. This color of blood means that it originated from the lower gastrointestinal tract. *Source:* Courtesy of Frank Isom, DVM.

- Associated with tenesmus
- Associated with urgency
- Not associated with weight loss
- May be associated with vomiting
- Emesis
  - Is the patient regurgitating or vomiting?
  - Is the patient coughing so violently that it is triggering emesis?
    - Is emesis productive?
      - Contents of vomitus
      - Description of vomitus (color, consistency)
      - When did the patient vomit?
      - How often has the patient vomited?
      - Is the patient vomiting food?
        - How soon after ingesting food does the patient vomit?
      - Can the patient keep water down?
        - How soon after ingesting water down the patient vomit?
    - Does the vomitus contain blood? (see Figure 50.12)
      - This occurrence is called hematemesis.
    - Does the vomitus contain bile?
- Exposure to conspecifics
  - Does the patient live with conspecifics?
    - If yes, are they exhibiting similar, if not the same, clinical signs
  - Does the patient interact with and/or come into close contact with conspecifics?
    - Doggie day care
    - Grooming
    - Kenneling
- Exposure to toxins
  - Antifreeze
  - Lily toxicosis (cats)

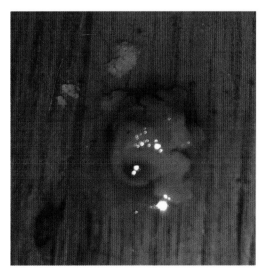

Figure 50.12 Hematemesis from a canine patient. *Source:* Courtesy of Ballroom Dance School Manhattan.

– Anticoagulant rodenticide
  ○ Internal hemorrhage, including potential for hemoabdomen
● Reproductive history
  – Intact female
    ○ When was the patient last in heat, that is, in estrus?
● Urinary history: does the patient have a history of:
  – Urinary tract infections (UTI)
  – Urolithiasis
  – UTO
● Vaccination history:
  – Is the patient up to date (UTD) on vaccines?
  – Against which diseases has the patient been vaccinated?

Although these topics should be addressed in every consultation for acute abdomen, not all can be incorporated into history taking immediately [3]. The patient must first be triaged [3]. Triage emphasizes the following [3]:

● Signalment
  – Age
  – Sex
  – Sexual status
  – Breed
  – Species
● Abbreviated history
  – Chief complaint (cc)
  – Onset of cc
  – Progression of cc
● Assessment of major body systems
  – Cardiopulmonary
    ○ Airway status
      ■ Oxygenation
      ■ Patency of airway
    ○ Circulation
      ■ Heart rate
      ■ Pulse quality
  – Neurologic status
    ○ Alert
    ○ Depressed
    ○ Dull
    ○ Obtunded
    ○ Comatose
  – Urogenital
    ○ Urinary bladder palpation

The purpose of triage is to establish the stability of the patient. Patient stability dictates how much time the clinician has to intervene. Patients that are not stable must be tended to urgently, which means that history-taking topics frequently need to be tabled [3].

Critical patients include dogs with GDV or patients with uncontrolled hemorrhage [3]. Identification of

these cases is relatively straightforward: a deep-chested dog that presents for acute onset of nonproductive retching and taut abdominal distension has GDV until proven otherwise [3].

Similarly, a "rock hard," turgid urinary bladder in a male cat is most likely UTO.

Other cases are not so clear-cut. These cases benefit from exhaustive history taking, which may resume after triage determines that the patient is stable [3].

50.4 The Physical Examination and Acute Abdomen Presentations

The triage examination is intentionally an abbreviated patient assessment to establish patient stability [3]. Patients still require a full physical examination to gain additional insight into the most likely differential diagnoses. This includes a rectal examination in adult dogs. Cats typically do not submit to rectal examinations without sedation, and even then, one can only typically advance a pinkie finger.

In particular, the following physical exam-based findings may help to refine the clinician's understanding of acute abdomen as it presents in specific patients [2, 3, 10, 21, 35–49]:

● Abdominal auscultation
  – Hyperactive gut sounds are supportive of gastritis, enteritis, malabsorption, and maldigestion (refer to Chapter 47, Section 47.4).
  – Hypoactive gut sounds are supportive of ascites, gastrointestinal obstruction, and peritonitis (refer to Chapter 47, Section 47.5).
● Abdominal palpation
  – A palpable fluid wave is suggestive of ascites, that is, abdominal effusion.
    ○ Abdominal effusions could be hemorrhagic, as from trauma.
    ○ Effusions also result from uroabdomen and septic peritonitis, as from leakage of gastrointestinal contents from a bowel perforation.
  – Focal thickening of the small bowel may be the result of foreign body ingestion.
  – Palpable plication, or bunching of the intestine, is abnormal and occurs typically in cases involving a linear (string) foreign body.
● Integumentary system
  – Hemorrhage at the umbilicus is suggestive of hemoabdomen.
  – Petechiae and/or ecchymoses may indicate coagulopathy (see Figures 50.13a, b).
  – Icterus may be secondary to hepatitis or coagulopathy (see Figures 50.14a–c).

(a)

(b)

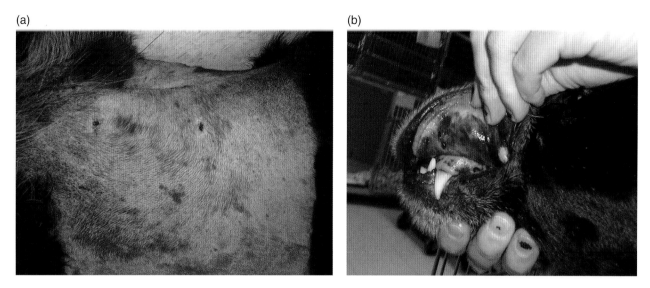

Figure 50.13 (a) Petechiae along the ventrum of a canine patient. *Source:* Courtesy of Daniel Foy, MS, DVM, DACVIM, DACVECC. (b) Ecchymoses within the oral cavity of a canine patient. *Source:* Courtesy of Daniel Foy, MS, DVM, DACVIM, DACVECC.

(a)

(b)

(c)

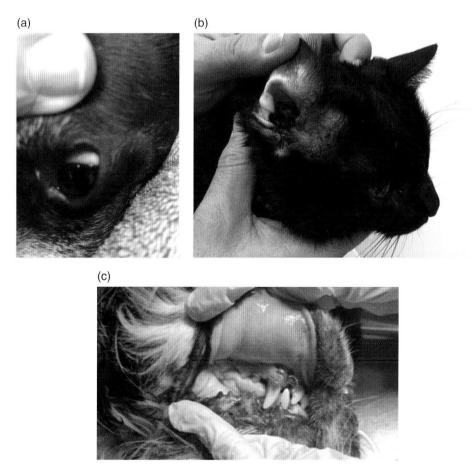

Figure 50.14 (a) Subtle icterus within the sclera of a dog. *Source:* Courtesy of Pamela Mueller, DVM. (b) Markedly icteric skin of a cat. (c) Markedly icteric mucous membranes in a Cocker Spaniel. *Source:* Courtesy of Rodolfo Oliveira Leal, DVM (Portugal), PhD, Dipl. ECVIM-CA (Internal Medicine) and Maria Joana Dias, DVM (Portugal).

- Musculoskeletal
  - Guarding against certain movements is suggestive of musculoskeletal pain
    - For example, cervical ventroflexion may be protective, guarding against neck pain secondary to neck-associated IVDD.
- Not resisting pressure applied to one or more regions of the spine
  - For example, a normal response for a dog that has pressure applied to its lumbar spine is to push back to counter the pressure.
  - A dog with lower back-associated IVDD is likely to drop its back in the direction in which pressure is applied.
- Oral examination
  - A string foreign body may be discovered at the base of the tongue.
- Rectal examination
  - Evidence of hematochezia on the exam glove is suggestive of a lower digestive tract bleed, as from colitis.
  - Evidence of melena on the exam glove is suggestive of an upper digestive tract bleed, as from the stomach or small bowel.
  - Pain on palpation of the prostate is suggestive of prostatic pathology, such as prostatitis.
  - Sublumbar lymphadenopathy is suggestive of regional inflammation, infection, or neoplastic disease.

Note that abdominal palpation in a patient with acute abdomen should be firm, yet gentle [11, 18, 21, 42]. Given that the patient is already tender, start with superficial palpation of the abdomen before applying deep pressure [10, 11, 18, 21]. Applying too much pressure to an acute abdomen patient could potentially lead to damage. For example, it is possible to rupture intra-abdominal masses, such as splenic hemangiosarcoma, via palpation that is heavy-handed.

50.5 The Diagnostic Approach to Acute Abdomen

The diagnostic approach to acute abdomen typically consists of baseline bloodwork and imaging [3].

Even in those patients for whom the diagnosis is fairly obvious based upon clinical presentation – for example, the dog with presumptive GDV – baseline bloodwork is of value in assessing whole body health and the patient's preparedness for surgery. How the rest of the body is responding to the primary problem may factor into whether or not the client is willing to proceed with treatment. It is equally important for the surgeon and anesthetist to be able to predict anticipated complications before they arise so that s/he is able to respond in a time-sensitive manner.

Bloodwork typically involves a complete blood count (CBC) and chemistry profile [3]. A CBC will provide baseline data concerning the erythrogram and leukogram, as well as platelet counts, whereas the chemistry profile will provide an overview of the patient's electrolytes, blood glucose, and renal and hepatic health [3].

Dehydration may be evident on the CBC as elevations in both packed cell volume (PCV) and total protein (TP) [18].

If PCV is lower than anticipated, then the patient may be experiencing blood loss [18]. This is more likely to be true of chronic blood loss [18]. It takes time for acute blood loss to result in a diminished PCV mostly because the loss is initially compensated for by splenic contraction [18].

If albumin is low, it can be difficult to pinpoint the source. Hypoalbuminemia may result from the following [18]:

- Blood loss
- Protein-losing enteropathy (PLE)
  - These patients typically have a history of marked weight loss (see Figure 50.15)
- Protein-losing nephropathy (PLN)
- Poor albumin production

In addition, the following diagnostic tests may be indicated [3]:

- Coagulation panel
- Fecal float and cytology

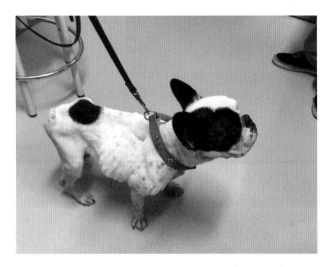

Figure 50.15 Emaciation in a canine patient with protein-losing enteropathy (PLE). *Source:* Courtesy of Rodolfo Oliveira Leal, DVM (Portugal), PhD, Dipl. ECVIM-CA (Internal Medicine).

- Pancreatic lipase immunoreactivity (PLI) test or other assessment of pancreatic function
- Urinalysis and urine sediment

Whether or not to proceed with these tests depends in large part upon the clinician's index of suspicion concerning each potential diagnosis. Signalment and history taking are important contributing factors.

Abdominal imaging is also an important part of the secondary survey [3].

Abdominal radiographs are a common starting point for survey imaging [5]. Although they lack the detail that can be obtained by ultrasound and computed tomography (CT), digital radiographs offer rapid turnaround time in terms of diagnostic results [2]. This is valuable when critical patients present for acute abdomen; they require immediate intervention.

Abdominal radiographs can readily highlight the following [2, 3, 5, 18, 25, 50]:

- Ascites
  - Ground glass appearance to images
  - Image quality will demonstrate poor contrast or will be fuzzy despite appropriate radiographic technique
- Body wall defects (see Figures 50.16a, b)

(a)

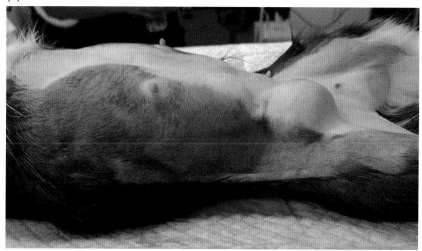

(b)

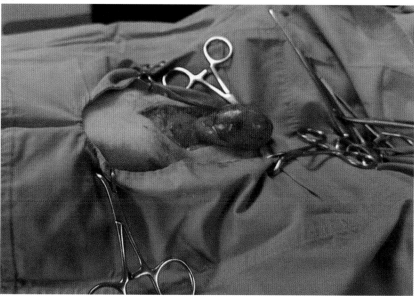

Figure 50.16 (a) Body wall defect in a feline patient. The prominent bulge represents the urinary bladder, which has herniated through the abdominal wall. *Source:* Courtesy of Pet Pantry of Lancaster County. (b) Same patient as depicted in (a), at surgery. *Source:* Courtesy of Pet Pantry of Lancaster County.

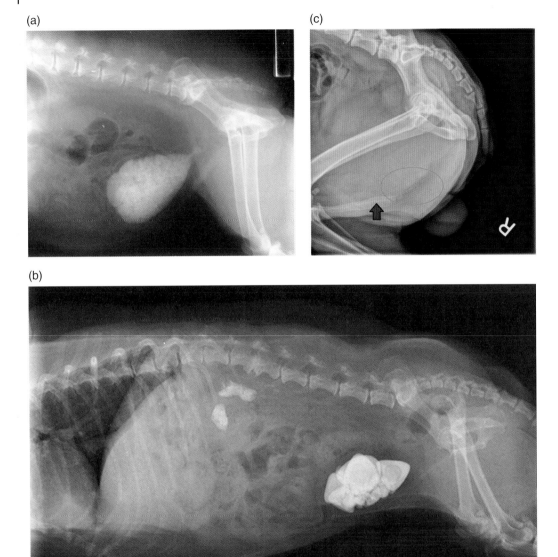

Figure 50.17 (a) Cystic calculi, as evident on a lateral radiograph. *Source:* Courtesy of Daniel Foy, MS, DVM, DACVIM, DACVECC. (b) Cystic calculi and nephroliths, as evident on a lateral radiograph. *Source:* Courtesy of Joseph Onello, DVM, of Central Mesa Veterinary Hospital. (c) Urethral calculi, circled in orange. Note their location proximal to the os penis (solid blue arrow). *Source:* Courtesy of Daniel Foy, MS, DVM, DACVIM, DACVECC.

- Calculi (see Figures 50.17a–c)
  - Cystic, meaning originating from the urinary bladder
  - Renal
  - Ureteral
  - Urethral
- Evidence of IVDD or diskospondylitis
- Gastric dilatation without volvulus (see Figures 50.18a, b)
- GDV (see Figures 50.19a, b)
- Hemoabdomen (see Figure 50.20)
  - Ground glass appearance to images
    - Image quality will demonstrate poor contrast or will be fuzzy despite appropriate radiographic technique
- "Mass effect"
- Gas-distended colon
- Gas-distended small bowel
- Diaphragmatic hernia
  - Herniation of abdominal contents into thoracic cavity
- Obstipation (see Figure 50.21)
- Organomegaly
  - The stomach axis will be deviated caudally in cases of hepatomegaly

(a)

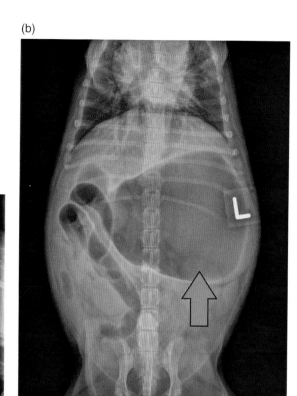
(b)

Figure 50.18 (a) Gastric dilatation without volvulus secondary to foreign body ingestion in a canine patent. Left lateral radiograph. Stomach has been identified (orange arrow). *Source:* Courtesy of Daniel Foy, MS, DVM, DACVIM, DACVECC. (b) Orthogonal radiographic view of the same patient depicted in (a). *Source:* Courtesy of Daniel Foy, MS, DVM, DACVIM, DACVECC.

(b)

(a)

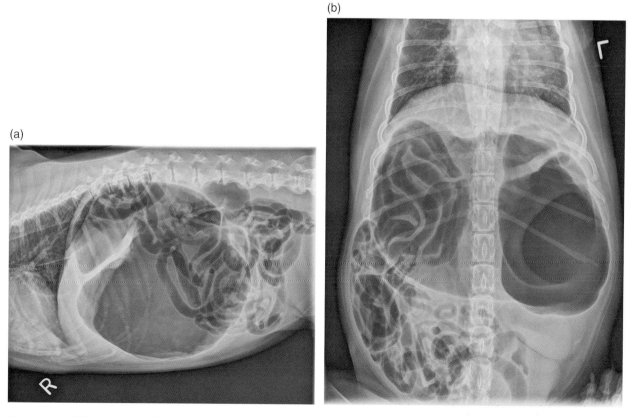

Figure 50.19 (a) Right lateral radiograph, diagnostic for GDV. Note also the gas-filled loops of bowel. *Source:* Courtesy of Daniel Foy, MS, DVM, DACVIM, DACVECC. (b) Orthogonal radiographic view of the same patient depicted in (a). *Source:* Courtesy of Daniel Foy, MS, DVM, DACVIM, DACVECC.

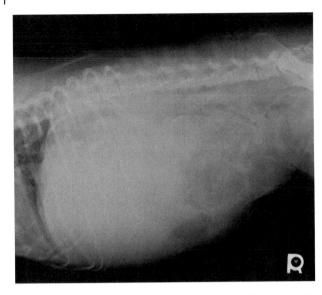

Figure 50.20 Right lateral abdominal radiograph of a patient with hemoabdomen. Note the hazy or "ground glass" appearance of abdominal cavity contents that makes it difficult to appreciate details surrounding abdominal architecture.

- The urinary bladder will be displaced cranially by prostatic enlargement, which may also displace the colon dorsally
- Renomegaly
- Splenomegaly
    ○ May be secondary to drug administration, for example, thiobarbiturates
    ○ May be pathological
- Pneumoperitoneum, that is, free gas within the peritoneal space, or retroperitoneal gas
    - Emphysematous cystitis
    - Ruptured hepatobiliary abscess or urinary bladder

- Pyometra will be evident as a tubular structure of soft tissue opacity between the urinary bladder and the descending colon on either lateral view
- Skeletal fractures
    - Ribs
    - Vertebrae

Recall from Chapter 47, Section 47.5 that abdominal radiographs may also support a presumptive diagnosis of foreign body obstruction. The following radiographic findings are supportive of this pathology [2, 47, 50–53]:

- Focal intestinal distension
- Focal soft tissue opacity within stomach or intestines
- Parallel, distended intestinal loops
- Sharp hairpin turns between intestinal loops (see Figures 50.22a–e)

Foreign bodies may also be linear. These create their own characteristic patterns on radiographs [47, 54, 55]:

- Comma-shaped gas bubbles
- Peritonitis
- Plication of intestines
- Radiopaque foreign body, such as a needle

Survey abdominal radiographs should consist of at least two orthogonal views [2, 5, 25]. A ventrodorsal (V/D) view and either right or left lateral view are considered standard, except in the case of GDV, in which the right lateral view is diagnostic [2, 11, 18, 21, 56].

The use of contrast medium may be indicated in survey abdominal radiographs that are inconclusive, for example, to provide more detail in cases of presumptive gastrointestinal obstruction [2, 5, 18].

Contrast medium is not limited to use in the gastrointestinal tract [2, 11, 18, 21, 50]. Contrast also plays a role in

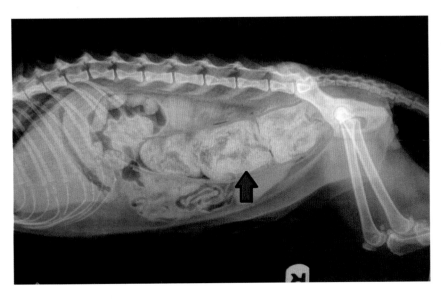

Figure 50.21 Right lateral abdominal radiograph of an obstipated feline patient. The descending colon (blue arrow) has been appreciably distended by fecal balls. The walls of the colon have been outlined in orange. *Source:* Courtesy of Daniel Foy, MS, DVM, DACVIM, DACVECC.

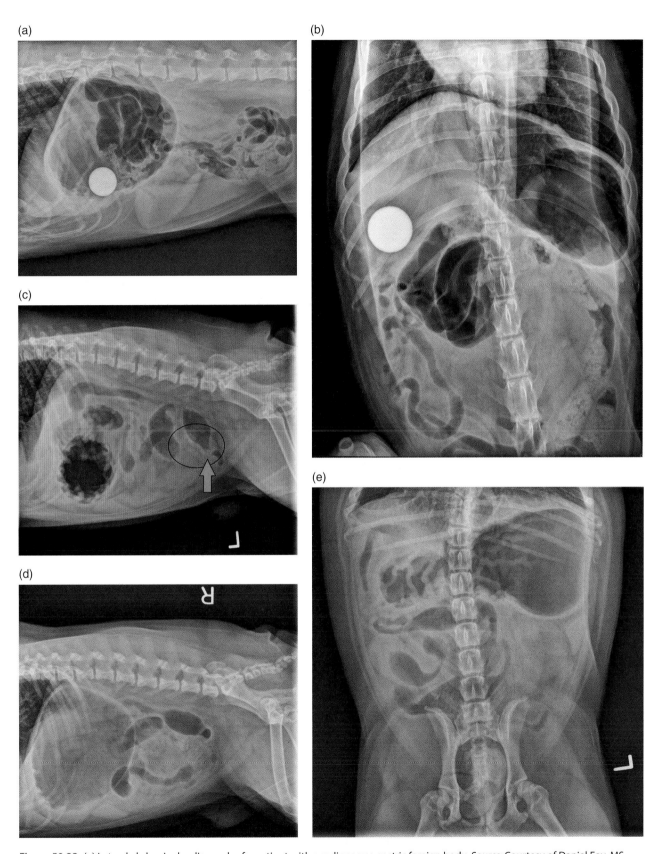

Figure 50.22 (a) Lateral abdominal radiograph of a patient with a radiopaque gastric foreign body. *Source:* Courtesy of Daniel Foy, MS, DVM, DACVIM, DACVECC. (b) Orthogonal radiographic view of the same patient depicted in (a). *Source:* Courtesy of Daniel Foy, MS, DVM, DACVIM, DACVECC. (c) Left lateral abdominal radiograph of a canine patient that developed a foreign body obstruction secondary to corn cob ingestion. The corn cob is visible (circled in black, orange arrow). *Source:* Courtesy of Daniel Foy, MS, DVM, DACVIM, DACVECC. (d) Right lateral abdominal radiograph of the same patient depicted in (c). *Source:* Courtesy of Daniel Foy, MS, DVM, DACVIM, DACVECC. (e) Ventrodorsal (V/D) radiograph of the same patient depicted in (c). *Source:* Courtesy of Daniel Foy, MS, DVM, DACVIM, DACVECC.

highlighting tears within the urinary tract [2, 50]. For example, positive contrast cystography can facilitate detection of a urinary bladder rupture [2, 50].

Abdominal ultrasound is an alternative means of imaging the abdominal cavity. Like radiography, ultrasonography is noninvasive. However, ultrasonography is particularly advantageous when finer details are required, or when ultrasound-guided fine needle aspirates (FNAs) are anticipated.

As a diagnostic tool, abdominal ultrasonography can support the following diagnoses [2, 3, 5, 50, 57–67]:

- Biliary tract obstruction
- Bowel obstruction
- Organomegaly
- Pancreatitis
- Peritoneal effusion
  - When only a small amount of free-floating fluid is present, it is most visible between the liver lobes or near the apex of the urinary bladder
- Prostatitis
- Pyometra
- Urolithiasis

In cases of abdominal effusion, sampling should occur via abdominocentesis to determine the source of the fluid [5, 6, 10, 42, 68]:

- In cases where urinary bladder rupture is a concern, potassium and/or blood urea nitrogen (BUN) and creatinine levels can be compared between the serum and the effusion [6].
  - If potassium is greater in the abdominal fluid than in serum, then urinary tract rupture is likely [6].
  - If BUN or creatinine is greater in abdominal fluid than in serum, then urinary tract rupture is likely [6].

Abdominal effusions are also present in cases of peritonitis [42].

Septic peritonitis is likely if analysis of the abdominal effusion reveals the following [6]:

- Elevated protein
- Increased neutrophil count
- Intracellular bacteria

Cultures are indicated when bacteria is present in abdominal effusions [6].

Septic peritonitis is likely if the glucose concentration of abdominal fluid is lower than the blood glucose concentration [6]. A blood-to-fluid glucose (BFG) difference of 20 mg/dL supports a diagnosis of septic peritoneal effusion.

50.6 Common Clinical Scenarios Involving Acute Abdomen

This chapter introduced the concept of acute abdomen and intended to provide an overview of underlying causes.

Those conditions that occur commonly in clinical practice will be reviewed in subsequent chapters; however, a handful of the most common clinical scenarios will be mentioned in brief here.

50.6.1 Gastric Dilatation-Volvulus

GDV, otherwise called "bloat" or "gastric torsion," is a condition in which the stomach distends significantly with gas and then rotates [42, 69].

When volvulus occurs, the stomach migrates from its normal anatomical position [42]. The right-sided pylorus becomes cranioventral relative to the body of the stomach [42]. The pylorus then moves to the left of the midline [42]. Eventually, the pylorus is positioned dorsal to the esophagus and the fundus, still to the left of midline [42, 69].

GDV is a life-threatening condition. As the stomach expands, it exerts pressure against the diaphragm [1]. This restricts the patient's ability to expand the lungs [1]. Respiration is impaired [1].

Stomach expansion also compromises venous return from the abdomen, and torsion of the stomach occludes its own blood supply [1]. Splenic infarction is common [1]. Progressive hypoxia and hypovolemic shock are inevitable [1, 69–73].

On physical examination of the healthy patient, the stomach is not palpable unless the patient has significantly overindulged in food, causing gastric distension [1, 42]. In this case, the patient's stomach would feel doughy upon palpation.

In a patient with GDV, the stomach is not only palpable beyond the costal margins of the cranial abdomen, it is visibly distended [1, 42, 69]. When viewed from behind, the patient develops an abdominal silhouette that billows out like a rounded cow.

On palpation, the stomach of a patient with GDV is very taut and painful [69].

In addition to being bloated, patients with GDV often present with ptyalism and nonproductive retching [69, 74].

Deep-chested dogs are most at risk for GDV [27, 75, 76].

50.6.2 Pancreatitis

Pancreatitis is an inflammatory process involving the pancreas [1]. It may be acute or chronic [1]. When the pancreas becomes inflamed, its digestive enzymes activate within acinar cells [1]. This results in autodigestion [1].

The etiology of pancreatitis is often unknown. However, the following factors may incite pancreatitis [1]:

- Duodenal reflux
- High fat diet

- Hyperlipoproteinemia
- Pancreatic duct obstruction

Concurrent hepatobiliary or intestinal inflammation in cats may also trigger pancreatitis in cats because they have unique hepatobiliary and gastrointestinal anatomy [77, 78].

Recall from Chapter 28, Section 28.2.3 that the common bile duct extends from the liver to the duodenum. It represents a shared route for both the cystic and hepatic ducts [77, 78].

In dogs, the major duodenal papilla is where the common bile duct enters the duodenum. As it does, it is adjacent to, but not conjoined with the pancreatic duct. The pancreatic duct empties its contents into the duodenum at a separate location, the minor duodenal papilla [77, 78].

Cats are unique in that the common bile duct and pancreatic ducts both empty into the major duodenal papilla [77, 78]. For this reason, pancreatitis in cats often reflects an extension of other disease, that is, focal enteritis, hepatitis, or cholecystitis [1]. Any pathology that affects the major duodenal papilla has the potential to create ascending inflammation or infection through the pancreas [77, 78].

Breed also appears to influence the likelihood of the patient developing pancreatitis. Miniature schnauzers are predisposed [1].

Siamese cats may also be at increased risk [1].

Patients with pancreatitis are in pain. Pain may be localized to the right, ventromedial cranial abdomen on abdominal palpation; however, the pancreas itself is not typically palpable unless there is a significant-sized pancreatic tumor [41, 79, 80].

50.6.3 Pyometra

Pyometra is a uterine infection: the uterus is distended with purulent material [81]. Pyometras may be further defined as being open or closed [1]. In an open pyometra, the cervix is open [1]. This allows uterine contents to drain freely [1]. Drainage will be evident grossly on visual inspection. The uterus of an open pyometra is often palpable, although it will not be as distended as that of a closed pyometra. In a closed pyometra, the cervix is closed. This prevents drainage of uterine discharge. The uterus continues to expand, and patients are systemically ill.

Common systemic signs of illness in patients with pyometra include the following [1]:

- Anorexia
- Depression
- Lethargy
- Vomiting
- Polydipsia
- Polyuria

Most dogs with pyometra have cycled previously, and present between 2.4 and 7.25 years of age [81–87].

Pyometra is less common in cats, occurring in 2.2% of intact queens by the time they reach 13 years of age [42, 88]. Oriental and exotic purebreds such as the Siamese, Korat, Ocicat, and Bengal are predisposed, with pyometra occurring younger in life than it does within the general population [88].

Risk factors for the development of pyometra include the following [81, 85, 87, 89, 90]:

- Being nulliparous
- Having been in estrus within 12 weeks prior to presentation
- Prior hormonal therapy with estrogens or progestins
- Past pregnancy termination

The uterus of a patient with pyometra palpates as a tubular structure on abdominal palpation.

Pyometras are confirmed via imaging: either radiography or abdominal ultrasound are viable options for obtaining a definitive diagnosis.

50.6.4 Urinary Tract Obstruction

A UTO is the condition by which urine cannot flow through the urinary tract [1, 42]. The obstruction to flow may be within the lumen of the urinary tract itself. Consider, for example, urethral plugs, protein-rich conglomerations of inflammatory cells and urinary crystals [91, 92]. These commonly lead to UTO, particularly in male cats because the male urethra is narrower than the female's [93].

Obstruction to the flow of urine can also be intramural. Consider, for example, an enlarged prostate, prostatitis, or prostatic neoplasia in male dogs [1].

Patients with UTO often present for the following [1, 42]:

- Anorexia
- Abdominal distension
- Depressed or dull mentation
- Dysuria, difficulty with urination
- Hematuria, blood in the urine
- Pollakiuria, increased frequency of attempts to urinate
- Recumbency
- Stranguria, straining to urinate
- Vocalization
- Vomiting

In cases of UTO, the urinary bladder becomes progressively distended and painful [1, 42]. It will palpate as "rock hard" [1, 42]. Care should be taken to palpate gently: iatrogenic urinary bladder rupture is possible [93].

UTO represents one extreme of feline lower urinary tract disease (FLUTD). It is a medical emergency. Refer to Chapter 65 for additional information.

References

1 Tilley, L.P. and Smith, F.W.K. (2004). *The 5-Minute Veterinary Consult: Canine and Feline*, 3e, lviii, 1487 p. Baltimore, MD: Lippincott Williams & Wilkins.

2 Heeren, V., Edwards, L., and Mazzaferro, E.M. (2004). Acute abdomen: diagnosis. *Compend. Contin. Educ. Pract.* 26 (5): 350–363.

3 Pachtinger, G. (2013). Acute abdomen in dogs & cats: step-by-step approach to patient care. *Today's Veterinary Practice* (September/October): 14–19.

4 Durkan, S. (2008). Approach to the acute abdomen. DVM 360 [Internet]. http://veterinarycalendar.dvm360.com/approach-acute-abdomen-proceedings?id=&sk=&date=&pageID=2.

5 Boag, A. and Hughes, D. (2004). Emergency management of the acute abdomen in dogs and cats: 1. Investigation and initial stabilisation. *In Pract.* 26 (9): 476–483.

6 Swinney, G. (2011). The acute abdomen and septic peritonitis. Australian Veterinary Association [Internet]. www.ava.com.au/sites/default/files/AVA_website/pdfs/NSW_Division/THE%20ACUTE%20ABDOMEN%20AND%20SEPTIC%20PERITONITIS_GSwinney.pdf.

7 Mazzaferro, E.M. (2003). Triage and approach to the acute abdomen. *Clin. Tech. Small Anim. Pract.* 18 (1): 1–6.

8 Tello, L.H. (2011). *Editor Dealing with the Acute Abdomen Patient*. World Small Animal Veterinary Association World Congress.

9 Burrows, C.F. (ed.) (2002). *The Acute Abdomen*. World Small Animal Veterinary Association World Congress.

10 Walters, P.C. (2000). Approach to the acute abdomen. *Clin. Tech. Small Anim. Pract.* 15 (2): 63–69.

11 Franks, J.N. and Howe, L.M. (2000). Evaluating and managing acute abdomen. *Vet. Med.* 95 (1): 56–69.

12 Kleine, L.J. (1997). *Radiology and Acute Abdominal Disorders in Teh Dog and Cat: Part 1. The Compendium Collection*, 336–341. Yardley, PA: Veterinary Learning Systems.

13 Davenport, D.J. and Martin, R.A. (1992). Acute abdomen. In: *Veterinary Emergency and Critical Care Medicine* (ed. R.J. Murtaugh and P.M. Kaplan), 153–162. St. Louis: Mosby.

14 Leveille, C.R. (1992). The acute abdomen. In: *Current Veterinary Therapy XI.* (ed. J.D. Bonagura and R.W. Kirk), 125–131. Philadelphia: WB Saunders.

15 Mann, F.A. (2002). Acute abdomen: evaluation and emergency treatment. In: *Kirk's Current Veterinary Therapy XIII* (ed. J.D. Bonagura), 160–164. Philadelphia: WB Saunders.

16 Brady, C.A., Otto, C.M., Van Winkle, T.J., and King, L.G. (2000). Severe sepsis in cats: 29 cases (1986–1998). *J. Am. Vet. Med. Assoc.* 217 (4): 531–535.

17 Macintire, D.K. (1988). The acute abdomen – differential diagnosis and management. *Semin. Vet. Med. Surg.* 3 (4): 302–310.

18 Dye, T. (2003). The acute abdomen: a surgeon's approach to diagnosis and treatment. *Clin. Tech. Small Anim. Pract.* 18 (1): 53–65.

19 Crowe, D. (1988). Symposium on the acute abdomen – introduction – responding to a life-threatening condition. *Vet. Med.* 83 (7): 651–709.

20 Crowe, D.T. (1988). The 1st steps in handling the acute abdomen patient. *Vet. Med.* 83 (7): 654–674.

21 Saxon, W.D. (1994). The acute abdomen. *Vet. Clin. North Am. Small Anim. Pract.* 24 (6): 1207–1224.

22 Spevakow, A.B., Nibblett, B.M., Carr, A.P., and Linn, K.A. (2010). Chronic mesenteric volvulus in a dog. *Can. Vet. J.* 51 (1): 85–88.

23 Junius, G., Appeldoorn, A.M., and Schrauwen, E. (2004). Mesenteric volvulus in the dog: a retrospective study of 12 cases. *J. Small Anim. Pract.* 45 (2): 104–107.

24 Matushek, K.J. and Cockshutt, J.R. (1987). Mesenteric and gastric volvulus in a dog. *J. Am. Vet. Med. Assoc.* 191 (3): 327–328.

25 Bischoff, M.G. (2003). Radiographic techniques and interpretation of the acute abdomen. *Clin. Tech. Small Anim. Pract.* 18 (1): 7–19.

26 Brockman, D.J., Washabau, R.J., and Drobatz, K.J. (1995). Canine gastric dilatation/volvulus syndrome in a veterinary critical care unit: 295 cases (1986–1992). *J. Am. Vet. Med. Assoc.* 207 (4): 460–464.

27 Glickman, L.T., Glickman, N.W., Perez, C.M. et al. (1994). Analysis of risk factors for gastric dilatation and dilatation-volvulus in dogs. *J. Am. Vet. Med. Assoc.* 204 (9): 1465–1471.

28 Glickman, L.T., Glickman, N.W., Schellenberg, D.B. et al. (2000). Non-dietary risk factors for gastric dilatation-volvulus in large and giant breed dogs. *J. Am. Vet. Med. Assoc.* 217 (10): 1492–1499.

29 Glickman, L.T., Glickman, N.W., Schellenberg, D.B. et al. (2000). Incidence of and breed-related risk factors for gastric dilatation-volvulus in dogs. *J. Am. Vet. Med. Assoc.* 216 (1): 40–45.

30 Hosgood, G. (1994). Gastric dilatation-volvulus in dogs. *J. Am. Vet. Med. Assoc.* 204 (11): 1742–1747.

31 Hogg, A.H. (1947). Prostatic disease in the dog; clinical manifestations and treatment. *Vet. Rec.* 59 (5): 47–53.

32 Hornbuckle, W.E., MacCoy, D.M., Allan, G.S., and Gunther, R. (1978). Prostatic disease in the dog. *Cornell Vet.* 68 (Suppl 7): 284–305.

33 Biddle, D. and Macintire, D.K. (2000). Obstetrical emergencies. *Clin. Tech. Small Anim. Pract.* 15 (2): 88–93.

34 Gaschen, F. (ed.) (2006). Large intestinal diarrhea – causes and treatment. WSAVA World Congress.

35 Rusbridge, C. (2005). Neurological diseases of the Cavalier King Charles spaniel. *J. Small Anim. Pract.* 46 (6): 265–272.

36 Ryan, T.M., Platt, S.R., Llabres-Diaz, F.J. et al. (2008). Detection of spinal cord compression in dogs with cervical intervertebral disc disease by magnetic resonance imaging. *Vet. Rec.* 163 (1): 11–15.

37 Brisson, B.A. (2010). Intervertebral disc disease in dogs. *Vet. Clin. North Am. Small Anim. Pract.* 40 (5): 829–858.

38 Denny, H.R. (1978). The surgical treatment of cervical disc protrusions in the dog: a review of 40 cases. *J. Small Anim. Pract.* 19 (5): 251–257.

39 Morgan, P.W., Parent, J., and Holmberg, D.L. (1993). Cervical pain secondary to intervertebral disc disease in dogs – radiographic findings and surgical implications. *Prog. Vet. Neurol.* 4 (3): 76–80.

40 Rothuizen, J., Schrauwen, E., Theyse, L.F.H., and Verhaert, L. (2009). Digestive tract. In: *Medical History and Physical Examination in Companion Animals*, 2e (ed. A. Rijnberk and F.J. Sluijs), 86–100. Edinburgh, New York: Saunders/Elsevier.

41 Rijnberk, A. and van Sluijs, F.S. (2009). *Medical History and Physical Examination in Companion Animals*, 333. The Netherlands: Elsevier Limited.

42 Englar, R.E. (2017). *Performing the Small Animal Physical Examination*. Hoboken, NJ: Wiley.

43 Tams, T.R. (2003). *Handbook of Small Animal Gastroenterology*, 2e, xiv, 486 p. St. Louis, MO: Saunders.

44 Ettinger, S.J., Feldman, E.C., and Côté, E. (2017). *Textbook of Veterinary Internal Medicine: Diseases of the Dog and the Cat*, 8e, 2 volumes (lviii, 2181, I-90 p.). St. Louis, Missouri: Elsevier.

45 Côté, E. (2015). Clinical veterinary advisor. In: *Dogs and cats*, 3e, vol. xxxvii, 1642. St. Louis, Missouri: Elsevier Mosby.

46 Cave, N. (2013). Gastrointestinal gas: eructation, borborygmus, and flatulence. In: *Canine and Feline Gastroenterology* (ed. R. Washabau and M.J. Day), 124–128. St. Louis, MO: Saunders.

47 Papazoglou, L.G., Patsikas, M.N., and Rallis, T. (2003). Intestinal foreign bodies in dogs and cats. *Compend. Contin. Educ. Pract.* 25 (11): 830–844.

48 Guilford, W.G. and Strombeck, D.R. (1996). Intestinal obstruction, pseudo-obstruction, and foreign bodies. In: *Strombeck's Small Animal Gastroenterology* (ed. W.B. Guilford, S.A. Center and D.R. Strombeck), 487–502. Philadelphia: WB Saunders.

49 Morris, I.R., Darby, C.F., Hammond, P., and Taylor, I. (1983). Changes in small bowel myoelectrical activity following laparotomy. *Br. J. Surg.* 70 (9): 547–548.

50 Thrall, D.E. (1998). *Textbook of Veterinary Diagnostic Radiology*. Philadelphia: WB Saunders.

51 O'Brien, T.R. (1978). Small intestine. In: *Radiographic Diagnosis of Abdominal Disorders in the Dog and Cat: Radiographic Interpretation, Clinical Signs, Pathophysiology* (ed. T.R. O'Brien), 259–351. Philadelphia: WB Saunders.

52 McNeel, S.V. (1994). The small bowel. In: *Textbook of Veterinary Diagnostic Radiology* (ed. D.E. Thrall), 524–543. Philadelphia: WB Saunders.

53 Lamb, C.R. and Hansson, K. (1994). Radiological identification of non-opaque intestinal foreign-bodies. *Vet. Radiol. Ultrasound* 35 (2): 87–88.

54 Root, C.R. and Lord, P.F. (1971). Linear radiolucent Gastrointestinal foreign-bodies in cats and dogs – their radiographic appearance. *J. Am. Vet. Radiol. Soc.* 12: 45–53.

55 Felts, J.F., Fox, P.R., and Burk, R.L. (1984). Thread and sewing needles as Gastrointestinal foreign-bodies in the cat – a review of 64 cases. *J. Am. Vet. Med. Assoc.* 184 (1): 56–59.

56 Aronson, L.R., Brockman, D.J., and Brown, D.C. (2000). Gastrointestinal emergencies. *Vet. Clin. North Am. Small Anim. Pract.* 30 (3): 555–579, vi.

57 Cruz-Arambulo, R. and Wrigley, R. (2003). Ultrasonography of the acute abdomen. *Clin. Tech. Small Anim. Pract.* 18 (1): 20–31.

58 Nyland, T.G., Matoon, J.S., and Herrgesel, E.J. (2002). Liver. In: *Small Animal Diagnostic Ultrasound* (ed. T.G. Nyland and J.S. Matoon), 144–157. Philadelphia: WB Saunders.

59 Hess, R.S., Saunders, H.M., Van Winkle, T.J. et al. (1998). Clinical, clinicopathologic, radiographic, and ultrasonographic abnormalities in dogs with fatal acute pancreatitis: 70 cases (1986–1995). *J. Am. Vet. Med. Assoc.* 213 (5): 665–670.

60 Nyland, T.G., Matoon, J.S., Herrgesel, E.J., and Tract, U. (2002). *Small Animal Diagnostic Ultrasound* (ed. T.G. Nyland and J.S. Matoon), 158–195. Philadelphia: WB Saunders.

61 Grooters, A.M. and Biller, D.S. (1995). Ultrasonographic findings in renal disease. In: *Current Veterinary Therapy XII: Small Animal Practice* (ed. J.D. Bonagura and R.W. Kirk), 933–937. Philadelphia: WB Saunders.

62 Finn, S.T. and Wrigley, R. (1989). Ultrasonography and ultrasound-guided biopsy of the canine prostate. In: *Current Veterinary Therapy X: Small Animal Practice* (ed. R.W. Kirk and J.D. Bonagura), 1227–1239. Philadelphia: WB Saunders.

63 Matton, J.S. and Nyland, T.G. (2002). Ovaries and uterus. In: *Small Animal Diagnostic Ultrasound* (ed. T.G. Nyland and J.S. Matoon), 231–249. Philadelphia: WB Saunders.

64 Peter, A.T. and Jakovljevic, S. (1992). Real-time ultrasonography of the small animal reproductive-organs. *Compend. Contin. Educ. Pract. Vet.* 14 (6): 739–744.

65 Poffenbarger, E.M. and Feeney, D.A. (1986). Use of gray-scale ultrasonography in the diagnosis of reproductive disease in the bitch: 18 cases (1981–1984). *J. Am. Vet. Med. Assoc.* 189 (1): 90–95.

66 Lamb, C.R. (1990). Abdominal ultrasonography in small animals – intestinal-Tract and mesentery, kidneys, adrenal-glands, uterus and prostate. *J. Small Anim. Pract.* 31 (6): 295–304.

67 Felkai, C., Voros, K., and Fenyves, B. (1995). Lesions of the renal pelvis and proximal ureter in various nephro-urological conditions – an ultrasonographic study. *Vet. Radiol. Ultrasound* 36 (5): 397–401.

68 Walters, J.M. (2003). Abdominal paracentesis and diagnostic peritoneal lavage. *Clin. Tech. Small Anim. Pract.* 18 (1): 32–38.

69 Monnet, E. (2003). Gastric dilatation volvulus syndrome in dogs. *Vet. Clin. North Am. Small Anim. Pract.* 33 (5): 987–1005, vi.

70 Hall, J.A. (1989). Canine gastric dilatation – volvulus update. *Sem. Vet. Med. Surg.* 4 (3): 188–193.

71 Wingfield, W.E., Cornelius, L.M., and Deyoung, D.W. (1974). Pathophysiology of the gastric dilation-torsion complex in the dog. *J. Small Anim. Pract.* 15 (12): 735–739.

72 Orton, E.C. and Muir, W.W. 3rd (1983). Hemodynamics during experimental gastric dilatation-volvulus in dogs. *Am. J. Vet. Res.* 44 (8): 1512–1515.

73 Muir, W.W. (1982). Gastric dilatation-volvulus in the dog, with emphasis on cardiac arrhythmias. *J. Am. Vet. Med. Assoc.* 180 (7): 739–742.

74 Brourman, J.D., Schertel, E.R., Allen, D.A. et al. (1996). Factors associated with perioperative mortality in dogs with surgically managed gastric dilatation-volvulus: 137 cases (1988–1993). *J. Am. Vet. Med. Assoc.* 208 (11): 1855–1858.

75 Sullivan, M. and Yool, D.A. (1998). Gastric disease in the dog and cat. *Vet. J.* 156 (2): 91–106.

76 Schaible, R.H., Ziech, J., Glickman, N.W. et al. (1997). Predisposition to gastric dilatation volvulus in relation to genetics of thoracic conformation in Irish setters. *J. Am. Anim. Hosp. Assoc.* 33 (5): 379–383.

77 Evans, H.E. and Miller, M.E. (2013). *Miller's Anatomy of the Dog*, 4e, xix, 850 p. St. Louis, Missouri: Elsevier.

78 Singh, B. and Dyce, K.M. (2018). *Dyce, Sack, and Wensing's Textbook of Veterinary Anatomy*, 5e. St. Louis, Missouri: Saunders.

79 Defarges, A. (2015). The physical examination. *Clinician's Brief* September: 73–80.

80 Ettinger, S.J. (2010). The physical examination of the dog and cat. In: *Textbook of Veterinary Internal Medicine* (ed. S.J. Ettinger and E.C. Feldman), 1–9. St. Louis: Saunders Elsevier.

81 Pretzer, S.D. (2008). Clinical presentation of canine pyometra and mucometra: a review. *Theriogenology* 70 (3): 359–363.

82 Johnston, S.D., Root Kustritz, M.V., and Olson, P.S. (2001). Disorders of the canine uterus and uterine tubes (oviducts). In: *Canine and Feline Theriogenology*, 1e (ed. S.D. Johnston, M.V. Root Kustritz and P.S. Olson), 206–224. Philadelphia, PA: Saunders.

83 Feldman, E.C. and Nelson, R.W. (2004). Cystic endometrial hyperplasia/pyometra complex. In: *Canine and Feline Endocrinology and Reproduction*, 3e (ed. E.C. Feldman and R.W. Nelson), 852–867. St. Louis, Mo: Saunders.

84 Hardy, R.M. and Osborne, C.A. (1974). Canine pyometra: pathogenesis, physiology, diagnosis and treatment of uterine and extra-uterine lesions. *J. Am. Anim. Hosp. Assoc.* 10: 245–268.

85 Dow, C. (1957). The cystic hyperplasia–pyometra complex in the bitch. *Vet. Rec.* 69: 1409–1415.

86 Ewald, B.H. (1961). A survey of the cystic hyperplasia–pyometra complex in the bitch. *Small Anim. Clin.* 1: 383–386.

87 Wheaton, L.G., Johnson, A.L., Parker, A.J., and Kneller, S.K. (1989). Results and complications of surgical-treatment of pyometra – a review of 80 cases. *J. Am. Anim. Hosp. Assoc.* 25 (5): 563–568.

88 Hagman, R., Strom Holst, B., Moller, L., and Egenvall, A. (2014). Incidence of pyometra in Swedish insured cats. *Theriogenology* 82 (1): 114–120.

89 Bowen, R.A., Behrendt, M.D., Wheeler, S.L. et al. (1985). Efficacy and toxicity of estrogens commonly used to terminate canine pregnancy. *J. Am. Vet. Med. Assoc.* 186 (8): 783–788.

90 Sutton, D.J., Geary, M.R., and Bergman, J.G.H.E. (1997). Prevention of pregnancy in bitches following unwanted mating: a clinical trial using low dose oestradiol benzoate. *J. Reprod. Fertil.* 239–243.

91 Gerber, B., Boretti, F.S., Kley, S. et al. (2005). Evaluation of clinical signs and causes of lower urinary tract disease in European cats. *J. Small Anim. Pract.* 46 (12): 571–577.

92 Kruger, J.M., Osborne, C.A., Goyal, S.M. et al. (1991). Clinical-evaluation of cats with lower urinary-tract disease. *J. Am. Vet. Med. Assoc.* 199 (2): 211–216.

93 Little, S.E. (2012). The lower urinary tract. In: *The Cat: Clinical Medicine and Management* (ed. S.E. Little), 980–1013. St. Louis: St. Louis.

51

Changes in Fecal Appearance

51.1 Introduction to Fecal Formation, Appearance, and Score

Digestion is the process by which ingesta is metabolized into usable bits of fuel that can be absorbed into the bloodstream, transported to various tissues, and used for energy [1]. Within the small intestine, the digestion of carbohydrates, fats, and proteins is facilitated by pancreatic enzymes [1].

The digestion of carbohydrates and proteins continues into the large intestine [1]. Here, both types of organic compounds are converted into short-chain fatty acids (SCFAs) and ammonia [1]. These by-products of digestion are then absorbed across the bowel wall [1].

The bowel as a whole is also responsible for recovering and recycling digestive gland secretions [1]. These secretions, including saliva, constitute a large amount of fluid [1]. Approximately 60% of this fluid is recovered by the proximal small intestine, the duodenum and jejunum [1]. In health, the remainder of fluid is reabsorbed by the ileum and large intestine [1].

What remains in the descending colon is fecal matter, the remnant by-products of digestion that are slated for elimination from the body [1]. Feces contain undigested material as well as bacteria and metabolic waste, including bilirubin and sloughed epithelial cells that line the lumen of the gut. [1]

Defecation is the process by which this material is excreted from the body in bulk [1].

Fecal amount, shape, and consistency are in large part determined by the patient's overall health and diet [1]. In health, canine and feline feces should be formed, yet compressible [2–4]. Stool is routinely palpable within the descending colon during routine physical examination [4].

Even when the descending colon lacks fecal material, it is palpable and distinguishable from small intestine because the colonic wall is stiffer. [3]

Note that the colon is dynamic [1]. It can stretch up to several times its normal diameter due to retained fecal matter [1].

As stool is retained, it becomes drier, firmer, and less compressible [5].

If, on the other hand, gastrointestinal transit time is abbreviated, stool becomes looser, that is, more liquid in consistency and therefore, devoid of shape [5].

Fecal scoring has recently been developed as a more objective way to describe direct fecal examination [5]. So-called fecal scores facilitate conversations about stool shape and consistency within members of the veterinary team, including clients [5] (see Figure 51.1).

There is no universal fecal scoring system. Many nutritional companies, including Nestlé-Purina, have devised their own to encourage dialogue [5]. Scores provide definition and allow veterinary clients and clinicians to be on the same page. What one person considers diarrhea, another may not [5]. However, using a fecal score chart, it is easier to define one's gross observations relative to the patient's bowel habits.

Using the Nestlé-Purina system, dogs and cats with a fecal score of two or three are considered normal.

Note that it is also important to consider what is normal for the patient. For example, a patient may always have a fecal score of four on diet "x," but a fecal score of two on diet "y." Diet contributes significantly to fecal amount, shape, and consistency; so, too, do overall gastrointestinal health and individual patient factors.

51.2 Stool with Low Fecal Scores

A fecal score of 1 using the Nestlé-Purina system indicates that feces are drier than normal. This stool is not pliable and tends to be expelled as pellets rather than logs.

Stool typically becomes hardened when it is retained in the colon [6]. This increase in gut transit time enhances

Common Clinical Presentations in Dogs and Cats, First Edition. Ryane E. Englar.
© 2019 John Wiley & Sons, Inc. Published 2019 by John Wiley & Sons, Inc.

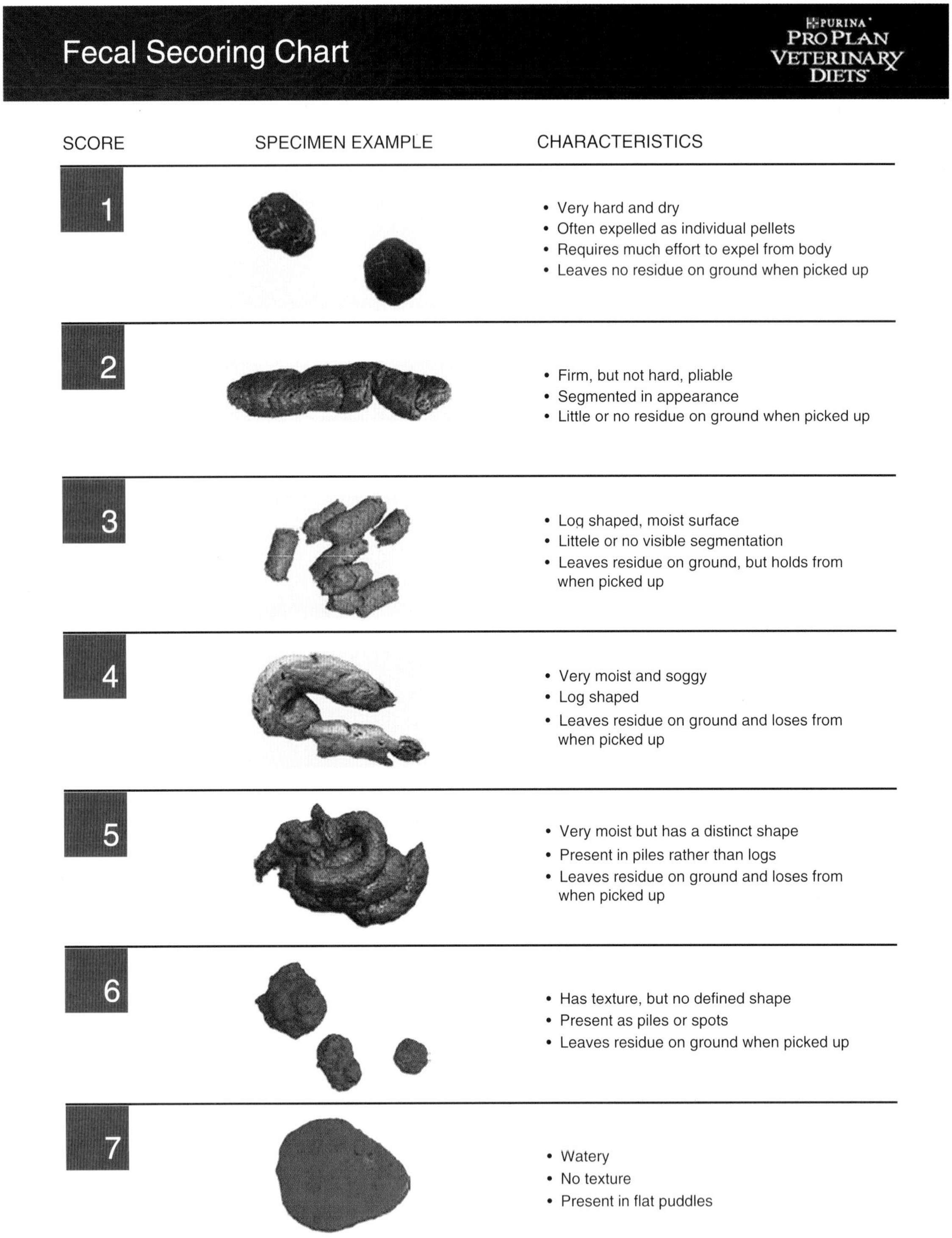
Fecal Secoring Chart
PURINA
PRO PLAN
VETERINARY
DIETS
SCORE
SPECIMEN EXAMPLE
CHARACTERISTICS
1
• Very hard and dry
• Often expelled as individual pellets
• Requires much effort to expel from body
• Leaves no residue on ground when picked up
2
• Firm, but not hard, pliable
• Segmented in appearance
• Little or no residue on ground when picked up
3
• Loq shaped, moist surface
• Littele or no visible segmentation
• Leaves residue on ground, but holds from when picked up
4
• Very moist and soggy
• Log shaped
• Leaves residue on ground and loses from when picked up
5
• Very moist but has a distinct shape
• Present in piles rather than logs
• Leaves residue on ground and loses from when picked up
6
• Has texture, but no defined shape
• Present as piles or spots
• Leaves residue on ground when picked up
7
• Watery
• No texture
• Present in flat puddles

Figure 51.1 Fecal scoring system. *Source:* Courtesy of Nestlé-Purina.

water resorption across the bowel wall [6]. The more water that is reabsorbed, the drier the feces [6].

Gut transit time may be increased for a variety of reasons, including the following [6–16]:

- Decreased exercise
- Dietary factors
  - Decreased water intake
  - Excess fiber

- Foreign body ingestion (see Chapter 48)
- Ingestion of bones
- Ingestion of hair, causing a trichobezoar (hairball)
- Drugs
  - Anticholinergic agents
  - Kaolin pectin or Kaopectate®
  - Opioids
- Environmental factors
  - Dirty litter box, causing the patient to hold its bowels
  - Hospitalization
  - Increased ambient temperatures, causing increased water resorption
- Mechanical obstruction
  - Atresia ani
  - Atresia coli
  - Manx cat deformities
  - Neoplasia
    ○ Colon
    ○ Prostate
      - Benign prostatic hypertrophy
      - Prostatic neoplasia
    ○ Rectum (see Figures 51.2a, b)
  - Pelvic fracture(s) or other cause(s) of narrowed pelvic canal
  - Perineal hernia
  - Polyp
  - Prostatic hypertrophy
  - Rectal prolapse (see Figures 51.3a, b)
  - Sublumbar lymphadenopathy
- Metabolic disease
  - Hypercalcemia
  - Hyperparathyroidism

- Hypokalemia secondary to chronic renal failure (CRF) or chronic kidney disease (CKD)
- Hypothyroidism
- Neuromuscular disease
  - Intervertebral disc disease (IVDD)
  - Paraplegia
  - Smooth muscle dysfunction
    ○ Idiopathic megacolon in cats
  - Spinal cord disease
  - Tail pull injury, causing sacral nerve damage
- Pain during defecation
  - Painful posturing
    ○ Dislocated limb(s)
    ○ Fractured limb(s) or pelvis
    ○ Osteoarthritis
  - Painful evacuation of stool (see Figures 51.4a–c)
    ○ Anal sacculitis
    ○ Anal stricture
    ○ Perianal fistula
- Supplements
  - Iron
- Toxicosis
  - Lead

Increased gut transit time leads to constipation [6]. Constipation is characterized as the condition by which stools are passed infrequently, incompletely, or with difficulty [6, 8–10, 15–19]. If and when stools cannot be passed at all, the patient is said to be obstipated [6, 8, 18–20]. Obstipation implies that the patient is refractory to standard treatment for constipation and colonic function may be permanently compromised [8, 19, 20].

Obstipation with resultant megacolon, that is, a permanently distended colon, is more common in cats than

(a)

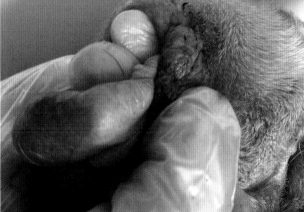

(b)

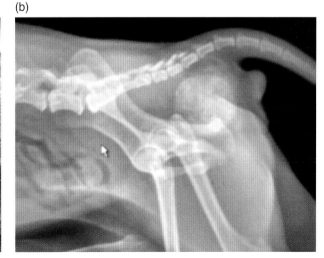

Figure 51.2 (a) Grossly visible rectal tumors in a canine patient. *Source:* Courtesy of Pamela Mueller, DVM. (b) Lateral abdominal radiograph demonstrating soft tissue opacity ("mass effect") in the rectal canal of a seven-year-old Yorkshire terrier that presented with tenesmus, that is, straining to defecate. *Source:* Courtesy of Pamela Mueller, DVM.

(a) (b)

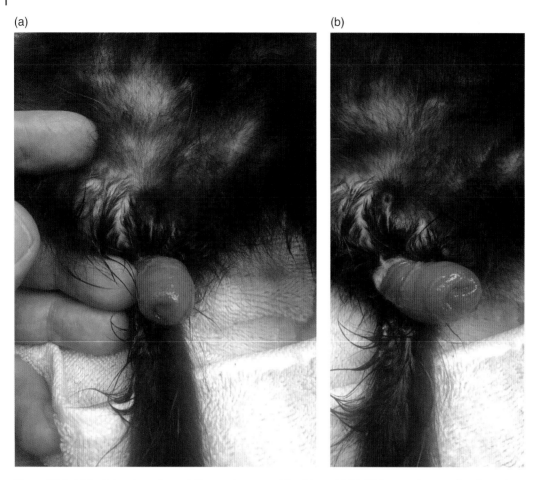

Figure 51.3 (a) Rectal prolapse in a cat. *Source:* Courtesy of Frank Isom, DVM. (b) Progressive rectal prolapse in a cat. *Source:* Courtesy of Frank Isom, DVM.

(a) (b) (c)

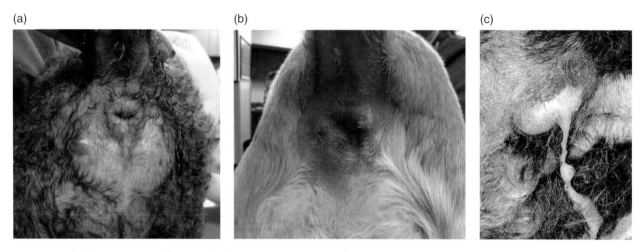

Figure 51.4 (a) Canine patient with perianal irritation. *Source:* Courtesy of Patricia Bennett, DVM. (b) Second example of a canine patient with perianal irritation. *Source:* Courtesy of Patricia Bennett, DVM. (c) Ruptured anal sac. *Source:* Courtesy of Shannon Carey, DVM.

dogs, and is the result of chronic obstipation [8, 18, 20, 21] (see Figures 51.5a–d).

In human medicine, megacolon is defined as having a colonic diameter greater than 6.5 cm at the pelvic brim [22]. Although there is no exact guideline in veterinary medicine by which to define megacolon, it has been theorized that the colonic diameter of a cat should be less than the length of the body of vertebra L7 [18, 23].

(a)

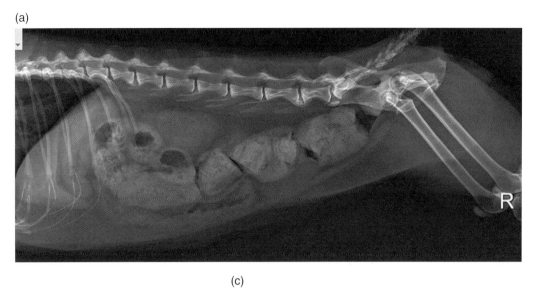

(b)   (c)

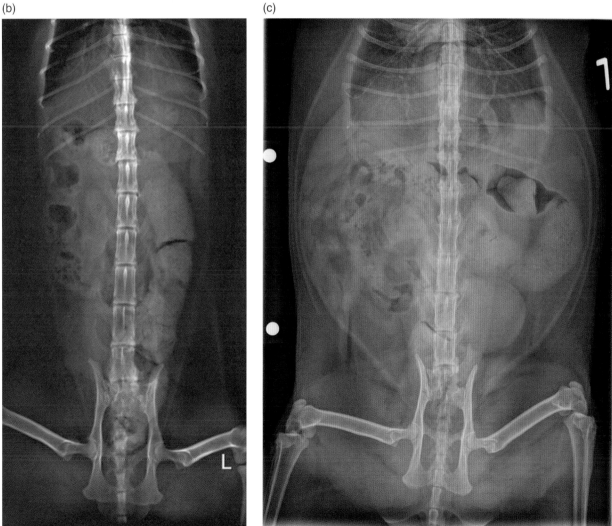

Figure 51.5 (a) Right lateral abdominal radiograph of an obstipated feline patient. *Source:* Courtesy of AMM. (b) Orthogonal radiographic view of the same patient that was depicted in (a). *Source:* Courtesy of AMM. (c) Right lateral abdominal radiograph of an obstipated feline patient. *Source:* Courtesy of Daniel Foy, MS, DVM, DACVIM, DACVECC. (d) Orthogonal radiographic view of the same patient depicted in (c). *Source:* Courtesy of Daniel Foy, MS, DVM, DACVIM, DACVECC.

(d)

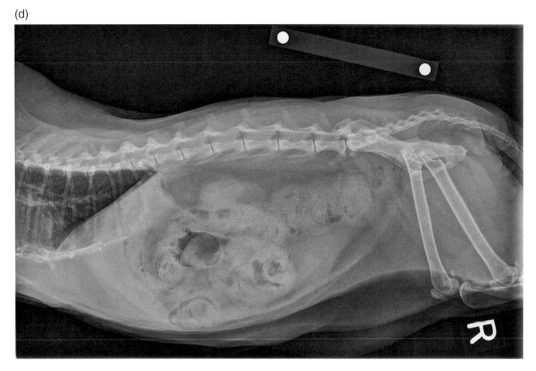

Figure 51.5 (Continued)

(a)   (b)

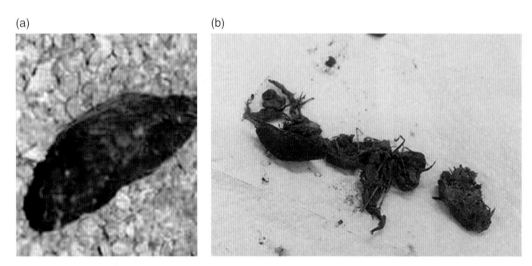

Figure 51.6 (a) Feline feces with fecal score of 1, using the Nestlé-Purina scale. This fecal matter is hard and likely to crumble with manipulation, as opposed to being pliable. (b) Canine feces with fecal score of 1, using the Nestlé-Purina scale. This fecal matter is also hard and likely to crumble with manipulation, as opposed to being pliable. *Source:* Courtesy of Liz Glicksman, DVM.

When the diameter of the colon increases beyond this point, colonic propulsion of the feces is hindered [4]. This encourages fecal retention [4]. Retained feces become harder and more difficult to expel from the lower digestive tract [4] (see Figures 51.6a, b).

Fecal balls back up, further stretching out the colon [4]. It is a vicious cycle.

Patients often present for dyschezia and tenesmus, that is, straining to defecate [4, 18]. Straining may be so great that liquid matter may shoot around the retained fecal balls, causing breakthrough diarrhea [4].

Nausea secondary to colonic distention, vomiting, and/or anorexia are likely sequelae [4, 24].

The passage of frank blood, hematochezia, may be present [9]. When this occurs, it signifies mucosal irritation secondary to the retention of hardened feces [9] (see Figure 51.7).

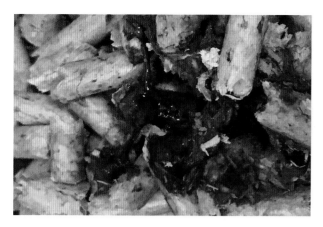

Figure 51.7 Hematochezia in a feline patient. The fresh red color indicates colonic or rectal bleeding as opposed to small intestinal bleeding. *Source:* Courtesy of Jule Schweighoefer.

If cats strain excessively for long periods, they are at increased risk of developing rectal prolapse [24] (see Figures 50.3a, b).

Minor prolapses of the rectum involve only the mucous membrane; however, as the condition increases in severity, the entire mesorectum may be exteriorized [25].

Two-thirds of cases of megacolon in cats are idiopathic [8–10, 18, 20]. Pelvic canal narrowing represents the second most common cause of megacolon in cats, followed by pelvic nerve injury [8, 10].

51.3 Stool with High Fecal Scores

A fecal score of 4 through 7 using the Nestlé-Purina system indicates that feces are increasingly wetter than normal. This stool is progressively loose. By the time fecal matter scores a 7 out of 7, it is shapeless and forms flat puddles.

Stool typically becomes wet and diarrheic when transit time through the gut is reduced [6]. The quicker stool moves through the digestive tract, the less time the body has to reabsorb water across the bowel wall. As more water is lost in the feces, the stool becomes soupier and resembles what one classically imagines as diarrhea.

Diarrhea often results from a hypermotile gut.

In addition, diarrhea may also result from one or more of the following pathways [6, 26, 27]:

- Increased gut wall permeability as caused by intestinal inflammation, which leads to a leaky gut and excess fluid loss via the digestive tract
- Osmotic diarrhea
  - Ingestion of food that is osmotically active, but poorly digested
    - High-fiber diets

- Administration of medications that are osmotically active, but poorly digested
  - Lactulose
  - Magnesium sulfate
  - Sugar alcohols
    - Mannitol
    - Sorbitol
    - Xylitol
- Secretory diarrhea
  - Bacterial toxins
  - Impaired electrolyte absorption
  - Luminal secretagogues
    - Bile acids
    - Non-osmotic laxatives
  - Overstimulation of the parasympathetic nervous system
  - Reduced absorptive surface, for instance, due to gut resection

Diarrhea can also be classified based upon where it originates within the gut, for instance, whether it is associated with the small or large bowel.

Small bowel diarrhea tends to be voluminous and associated with weight loss [4, 5, 28]. It typically does not involve fecal mucus, increased frequency of defecation, tenesmus, or dyschezia [4, 28, 29].

When it occurs, small bowel diarrhea may be due to the following [4, 5, 28–36]:

- Dietary indiscretion***
- Enteritis
  - Bacterial
  - Fungal
    - Histoplasmosis
    - Phycomycosis
    - Pythiosis
  - Parasitic***
    - Hookworms
    - Protozoa
    - Roundworms
    - Tapeworms
  - Viral***
    - Canine parvovirus type 1 (CPV-1, minute virus)
    - Canine parvovirus type 2 (CPV-2)***
    - Coronavirus
    - Feline immunodeficiency virus (FIV)
    - Feline leukemia virus (FeLV)
    - Feline panleukopenia virus, otherwise referred to as feline parvovirus***
- Exocrine pancreatic insufficiency (EPI)
- Food allergy
- Food intolerance
- Hypoadrenocorticism
- Hyperthyroidism
- Pancreatitis

- Portosystemic shunt
- Protein-losing enteropathy (PLE)
  - Inflammatory bowel disease (IBD)
    o Eosinophilic
    o Granulomatous enteritis
    o Lymphocytic-plasmacytic
  - Intestinal lymphangiectasia
  - Intestinal neoplasia
    o Lymphoma
- Small intestinal bacterial overgrowth (SIBO) as from malabsorptive small bowel disease
- Toxicosis

Those conditions that are starred above (***) represent the most common causes of small bowel diarrhea in pediatric companion animal patients [34].

Chronic enteropathies, such as PLE, IBD, intestinal lymphangiectasia, and intestinal lymphoma, are beyond the scope of this chapter.

Small bowel diarrhea tends to be liquid, with a fecal score of 6 or 7, using the Nestlé-Purina system.

If there is blood in small bowel diarrhea, it tends to be passed in the form of digested blood or melena. Melena has the appearance of black tar (see Figure 51.8).

On the other hand, large bowel diarrhea tends to be smaller in terms of volume and semi-formed or gelatinous, with a fecal score of 4 or 5.

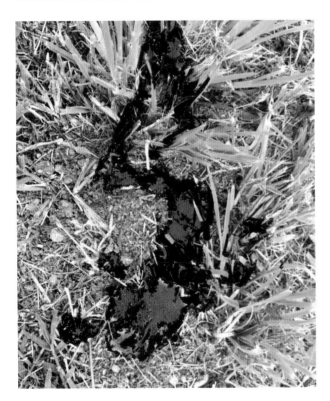

Figure 51.8 Melena from a canine patient. Note the appearance: melena looks like black tar. The black color indicates digested blood, meaning that fecal blood originated from the proximal digestive tract.

Large bowel diarrhea does not tend to be associated with weight loss.

Large bowel diarrhea contains an excess of mucus. The patient also typically exhibits increased frequency and urgency of defecation, with tenesmus.

Large bowel diarrhea may or may not be associated with hematochezia (see Figures 51.9a, b).

When it occurs, large bowel diarrhea may be due to the following [5, 6, 34, 37–39]:

- Dietary indiscretion***
- Infectious colitis
  - *Campylobacter* spp.
  - *Clostridium* spp.
  - *Cryptosporidium* spp.
  - *Entamoeba histolytica*
  - *Escherichia coli*
  - *Giardia* spp.
  - *Histoplasma capsulatum*
  - *Salmonella* spp.
  - *Prototheca*
- Endoparasitism
  - Hookworms
  - *Tritrichomonas foetus*
  - Whipworms***
- Food allergy
- Food intolerance
- Histiocytic ulcerative colitis
- IBD
- Neoplasia

Those conditions that are starred above (***) represent the most common causes of acute colitis in companion animal patients [39–41].

Causes of chronic colitis, such as food allergy, food intolerance, histiocytic ulcerative colitis, IBD, and neoplasia, are beyond the scope of this chapter.

51.4 Bacterial Diarrhea

Neonates are more susceptible than adults to bacterial diarrhea, particularly that which is caused by the following agents [34, 42, 43]:

- *Campylobacter* spp.
- *Clostridium* spp.
- *E. coli*
- *Salmonella* spp.
- *Yersinia enterocolitica*

Fecal culture will confirm the presence of *Salmonella* and *Campylobacter* spp. [34] Toxin assays can confirm the presence of *Clostridium* spp. [34]

The primary challenge associated with isolating bacteria in cases involving acute or chronic diarrhea is determining

(a)

(b)

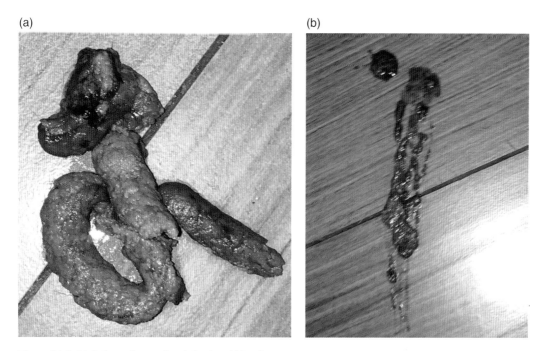

Figure 51.9 (a) Soft stool coated with fresh red blood in a canine patient. *Source:* Courtesy of Frank Isom, DVM. (b) Liquid diarrhea with evidence of fresh hemorrhage. *Source:* Courtesy of Frank Isom, DVM.

whether the bacteria are in fact causing pathology or are simply present within the gastrointestinal tract [34].

As an added complication, many bacteria are opportunistic: they will not cause disease in and of themselves, but they may cause disease if the gastrointestinal environment is disrupted [34, 42].

51.4.1 Campylobacter

Both healthy and diarrheic patients may have fecal matter that contains *Campylobacter* spp. [44–49]. It is particularly abundant in stool of young patients, and those that are stressed [44]. *Campylobacter* spp. are gram-negative, curved bacteria. When viewed under light microscopy, *Campylobacter* spp. take on a seagull wing S-shape (see Figure 51.10).

Note that this shape is not pathognomonic for *Campylobacter* spp. [44]. Other bacteria with this characteristic shape include *Helicobacter, Arcobacter,* and *Anaerobiospirillum* [44].

Furthermore, just because *Campylobacter*-like organisms (CLOs) are present on fecal examination does not mean that they are necessarily pathogenic [44]. Colonization of the gut with *Campylobacter* spp. can be normal [44].

However, *Campylobacter* spp. are zoonotic [44, 50–55]. It is the responsibility of the veterinary team to bring this to the attention of the client.

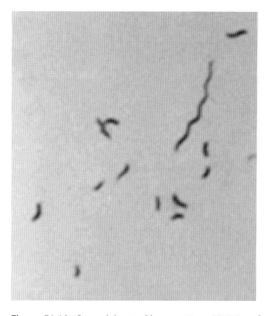

Figure 51.10 *Campylobacter*-like organisms (CLOs) on fecal examination. Note the characteristic gull wing or S-shape.

51.4.2 Clostridium difficile

The gram-positive, anaerobic, spore-forming bacteria, *Clostridium difficile*, is more commonly referenced in the human medical literature; however, it can also cause enteritis in dogs [32, 44, 56–58]. Prevalence is greater in shelters, kennels, and veterinary hospitals [44, 59–63].

Unlike the disease in humans, *C. difficile*-associated diarrhea in dogs does not appear to be linked to antibiotic use [44].

Clinical signs are quite variable, ranging from mild and self-limiting to hemorrhagic and fatal [44].

Diagnosis is typically via fecal culture [44].

51.4.3 Clostridium perfringens

Like C. difficile, Clostridium perfringens is a gram-positive, anaerobic, spore-forming bacterium [44]. There are five major types, A through E, depending upon which toxic gene(s) is/are present [44]. Type A most commonly occurs in dogs and cats [44]. Because it can be found in the fecal matter of both healthy and diarrheic animals, it is difficult to equate its presence with pathology [44, 57, 64–66].

When viewed under light microscopy, *Clostridium* spp. take on a characteristic safety pin shape (see Figure 51.11).

Clinically, *Clostridium* spp. tend to induce large bowel diarrhea [44]. However, diarrhea may also be mixed, meaning that it is of small and large bowel origin [44].

51.4.4 Salmonella

Unlike *Clostridium* spp., *Salmonella* spp. are rarely present in the stool of healthy dogs and cats [44]. *Salmonella* is a gram-negative bacterium that is more prevalent among the following populations [44, 67–70]:

- Cats that ingest songbirds
- Dogs that are fed raw meat
- Geriatric dogs
- Pediatric patients
- Stray dogs

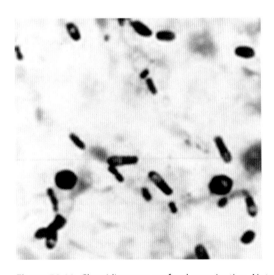

Figure 51.11 *Clostridium* spp. on fecal examination. Note the characteristic safety pin shape of the purple-staining organisms.

Diarrhea may be mild and self-limiting or severe and hemorrhagic [44, 71].

Diagnosis is typically via fecal culture [44].

Like *Campylobacter*, *Salmonella* is zoonotic [44, 72–79]. The handling of contaminated animal-based treats, such as pig ears, as well as raw food diets remains of concern to the human population [44].

51.5 Viral Diarrhea

As compared to bacterial diarrhea, viral diarrhea is relatively common among pediatric companion animal patients [34]. In particular, dogs less than six months of age are most susceptible to viral enteritis [80].

51.5.1 CPV-1 or Minute Virus

CPV-1 is a nonenveloped DNA virus that replicates only among rapidly dividing cells, such as the gut [80].

CPV-1 targets puppies less than six weeks of age, including fetal pups, by virtue of its ability to cross the placenta [34, 80]. Fetal death is one potential outcome of exposure to this virus [34]. When neonates are infected, they are more likely to present for diarrhea and/or vomiting [34]. In addition, they may exhibit respiratory distress or sudden death [34].

Diagnostic tests are not available clinically, as they are for CPV-2 [34]. In academic settings, CPV-1 may be confirmed through fecal electron microscopy, but this diagnostic tool is not routinely available to private practitioners and as such is impractical [34].

Disease progresses rapidly, and treatment is relatively unsuccessful [34].

CPV-1 is not currently a disease against which one can be vaccinated [34, 43].

51.5.2 CPV-2

CPV-2 is also a nonenveloped DNA virus that requires rapidly dividing cells, such as the gut, to replicate [80].

CPV-2 causes canine parvoviral enteritis [80]. In its original form, it only affected dogs [80]. However, newer strains 2a and 2b are capable of infecting felids [80].

Unvaccinated dogs and pups that have not yet developed protective antibody titers are most are risk [34, 80]. There also appears to be a breed predisposition for CPV-2 among Rottweilers, Doberman Pinschers, Labrador Retrievers, German Shepherds, and Staffordshire Terriers [34, 80, 81].

At the microscopic level, CPV-2 causes lymphocytolysis. This results in leukopenia, secondary to neutropenia and lymphopenia [34]. Blood loss in stool causes anemia, and malabsorptive syndrome secondary to small intestinal villi destruction leads to hypoproteinemia [34].

Clinically, patients present for fever, bloody diarrhea, and vomiting [34, 80]. Rapid loss of fluid through the gastrointestinal tract leads to life-threatening dehydration [34, 80].

Sepsis, intestinal intussusception, and disseminated intravascular coagulation (DIC) may also result [34, 80].

Diagnosis is possible via in-house fecal ELISA antigen testing [34, 80]. This test offers rapid turn-around time and is practical in the clinic setting [34, 80]. However, false positives may occur 5–15 days after vaccination with a modified live virus (MLV) [34, 80, 82].

Treatment is largely supportive and emphasizes rehydration, to combat fluid loss and electrolyte imbalance [34, 80]. Because the mucosal barrier of the gastrointestinal tract is disrupted and will pave the way for sepsis, prophylactic parenteral broad-spectrum antibiotic therapy is indicated [34, 80]. Anti-nausea therapy and prokinetic agents, such as metoclopramide, are also mainstays of treatment [34, 80].

Survival is common in cases that are diagnosed early if aggressive therapy is instituted [34, 80].

Vaccinations are protective if they are administered in accordance with the manufacturer's recommendations [34, 80].

51.5.3 Feline Panleukopenia

Feline panleukopenia is caused by a DNA virus that targets unvaccinated cats, particularly those that are less than one year of age [83]. Feline panleukopenia is extraordinarily stable in the environment and is therefore spread most often by indirect contact [83].

Queens may also transmit the virus in utero [83]. When infection occurs early in gestation, fetal resorption may occur [83]. Queens may also develop subsequent infertility [83]. If infection occurs late in gestation, then live kittens will be birthed that have varying neurological damage, secondary to cerebellar hypoplasia [83]. Because the cerebellum is responsible for coordinated, fluid movement, hypoplasia results in variable ataxia and hypermetria, that is, a high-stepping gait [83]. Movement is disjointed and jerky [83]. Affected kittens typically have a wide-based stance, as if trying to improve their balance [83]. They are also likely to develop intention tremors [83].

Most neonatal or pediatric infections with feline panleukopenia are subclinical [83].

When infections are clinical, they target the central nervous system (CNS) and/or the gut [83]. The CNS can be affected up until nine days old [83]. Three-to-five month old kittens are more likely to be afflicted with gastrointestinal disease [83]. These kittens present for anorexia,

depression, and fever [83]. Vomiting is more likely to be seen than diarrhea; however, either is possible [83].

Physical examination typically reveals marked dehydration, and intestinal loops are thickened on abdominal palpation [83].

Diagnosis is possible via in-house fecal testing using the ELISA for CPV antigen [34, 80]. This test offers rapid turn-around time and is practical in the clinic setting [34, 80].

Diagnosis is also supported by significant leukopenia [83]. Neutropenia precedes lymphopenia [83]. Concurrent anemia is more likely indicative of FeLV [83].

Fecal culture may be necessary to rule out feline salmonellosis, which can mimic feline panleukopenia [83].

51.6 Parasitic Diarrhea

Endoparasitism is most common among pediatric patients; however, dogs and cats of any age may be affected [34].

51.6.1 Roundworms

Roundworms, otherwise known as ascarids, are a type of zoonotic helminth that can cause infection of pets and humans alike [84–86].

Roundworms are considered ubiquitous. They are present in the soil and can cause infection when dogs and cats ingest roundworm eggs. Pups may become infected through the placenta and via nursing. Kittens also acquire roundworms by ingesting infected milk [84–86]. Because of vertical transmission, puppies and kittens are assumed to have roundworm infections, and prophylactic deworming is considered routine [42, 84–86].

Clinically important roundworms in dogs and cats include the following [84–86]:

- *Toxocara canis*
- *Toxocara cati*
- *Toxocara leonina*

Patients typically present with a rounded or so-called "buddha belly". Diarrhea and/or vomiting may also be present, in combination with poor weight gain and stunted growth. Patients may be described as unthrifty. They also may also present with dull coats.

Diagnosis is via observation of roundworm eggs via fecal flotation or gross observation of roundworms in the feces (see Figures 51.12a–c).

The zoonotic potential associated with ascarids, visceral and ocular larval migrans, is a significant concern [84–89]. Liver damage secondary to visceral larval migrans occurs less often than ocular larval migrans. At least 750 cases of uveitis, vision loss, and blindness are

(a)   (b)

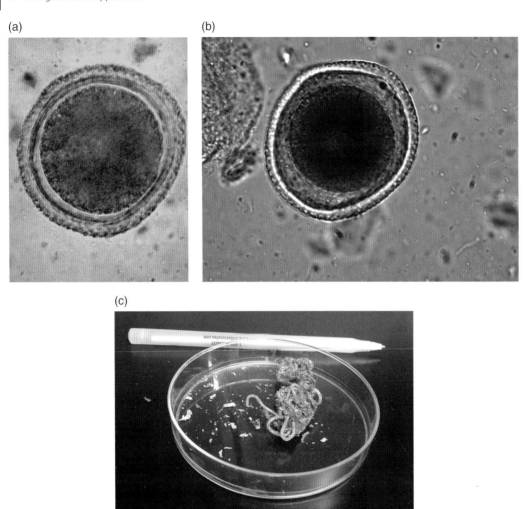

(c)

Figure 51.12 (a) *Toxocara canis* egg on fecal examination, using light microscopy. (b) *Toxocara cati* egg on fecal examination, using light microscopy. *Source:* Courtesy of Dr. Araceli Lucio-Forster, Cornell University College of Veterinary Medicine. (c) Adult *Toxocara cati* in a stool sample. *Source:* Courtesy of Dr. Araceli Lucio-Forster, Cornell University College of Veterinary Medicine.

diagnosed every year in humans in the United States (U.S.) alone, secondary to toxocariasis [85, 87, 89].

Children are particularly at risk of developing larval migrans because they are more likely to play in and therefore ingest dirt [85].

To lessen the risk for zoonotic transmission, the Centers for Disease Control (CDC) recommends monthly deworming of companion animal patients.

51.6.2 Hookworms

Hookworms are another type of zoonotic helminth that can cause infection of pets and humans alike [84–86].

Hookworms are most prevalent in the southern United States, especially the coastal regions [85].

Hookworms are acquired by dogs and cats through nursing [84, 85, 90]. Infective larvae may also penetrate the skin [84, 85].

Clinically important hookworms in dogs and cats include the following [34]:

– *Ancylostoma caninum*
– *Ancylostoma tubaeforme*
– *Uncinaria stenocephala*

Patients typically present with pallor due to rapidly progressing anemia: hookworms ingest a large amount of blood from their hosts [84]. Dark, tarry stool and diarrhea are also possible.

Diagnosis is via observation of hookworm eggs via fecal flotation or gross observation of hookworms in the feces (see Figures 51.13a, b).

The zoonotic potential associated with hookworms, cutaneous and visceral larval migrans, is a significant concern [84, 85]. Larvae penetrate the skin of humans, particularly those who come into contact with moist or wet sand or soil [85]. Sandboxes and beaches are

(a)

(b)

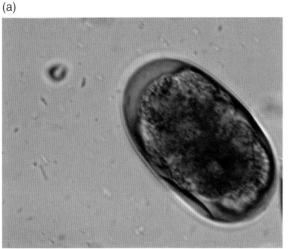
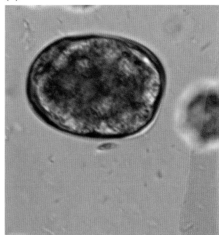

Figure 51.13 (a) *Uncinaria* egg on fecal examination, using light microscopy. *Source:* Courtesy of Dr. Araceli Lucio-Forster, Cornell University College of Veterinary Medicine. (b) *Ancylostoma* egg on fecal examination, using light microscopy. *Source:* Courtesy of Dr. Araceli Lucio-Forster, Cornell University College of Veterinary Medicine.

additional risk factors [85]. Infected humans develop pruritic papules that transition into visible tunnels as larvae migrate through the skin. Migration can be long-lasting, on the order of weeks to months. If larvae migrate beneath the skin to deeper tissues, then the human host can succumb to visceral larval migrans, which is characterized most often by an eosinophilic enteritis [84, 85].

51.6.3 Tapeworms

Tapeworms are zoonotic, parasitic flatworms or cestodes [86].

Clinically important tapeworms in dogs and cats include [34]

– *Dipylidium caninum*
– *Echinococcus granulosus*
– *Taenia* spp.

Recall from Chapter 6, Section 6.4.3 that fleas are vectors of *D. caninum*, which is present worldwide, but especially prevalent in North American cats [91–104].

Adult tapeworms attach themselves to the small intestinal wall of their host. As these hermaphrodites mature, eggs are produced and stored within terminal segments called proglottids. Each proglottid contains egg capsules or packets, each containing 5–30 hexacanth ova [86] (see Figure 51.14).

Once a proglottid is full of eggs, it detaches and is shed in the host's feces. Proglottids are visible to the naked eye and may resemble grains of white rice or cucumber seeds [86, 105] (see Figures 51.15a–e).

D. caninum eggs are released from terminal segments into the environment when each proglottid breaks open.

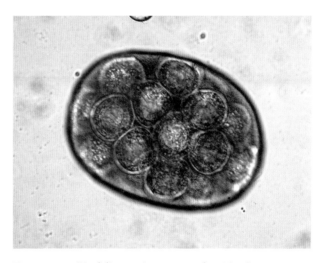

Figure 51.14 *Dipylidium caninum* egg packet, 20×. *Source:* Courtesy of Dr. Araceli Lucio-Forster, Cornell University College of Veterinary Medicine.

In the adult cat or dog, *D. caninum* may cause perianal pruritus, but is otherwise merely an inconvenience for the patient and an eyesore for the client.

If the cestode burden is great enough, a young or debilitated patient may present for an unthrifty coat and a pot-bellied appearance, with abdominal distension. Diarrhea or constipation may result from heavy infestation.

Humans, particularly children, become infected when they unknowingly ingest whole fleas that contain *D. caninum* [94, 106, 107]. Children may develop pruritus, diarrhea, and tapeworm segments [85].

Taenia spp. are another kind of cestode. *Taenia taeniaeformis* is found in both the cat and the dog, whereas *Taenia pisiformis* is found primarily in domestic and

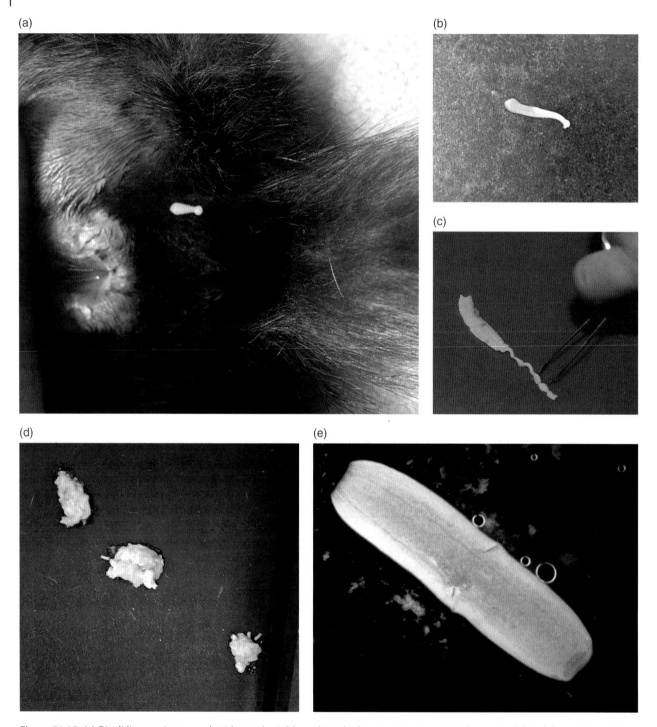

Figure 51.15 (a) *Dipylidium caninum* proglottid, grossly visible to the naked eye as it scoots across the perineal fur of this canine patient. *Source:* Courtesy of Frank Isom, DVM. (b) *Dipylidium caninum* proglottid. *Source:* Courtesy of Sarah Bashaw, DVM. (c) *Dipylidium caninum* proglottids. *Source:* Courtesy of Daria Turchenkova. (d) Masses of *Dipylidium caninum* proglottids from a canine patient that presented for elective sterilization surgery as part of a veterinary nonprofit rural outreach program. *Source:* Courtesy of Hannah Butler. (e) Magnified *Dipylidium* segment. *Source:* Courtesy of Dr. Araceli Lucio-Forster, Cornell University College of Veterinary Medicine.

wild canids. These species cause disease when hosts ingest infected rodents or hares [86].

Diagnosis is via observation of eggs via fecal flotation (see Figures 51.16a, b).

Humans become infected with *Taenia* when their hands are contaminated with canine feces that contain tapeworm eggs [85]. Accidental ingestion of these eggs leads to infection [85]. Infections are rare, but can lead to

(a)
(b)

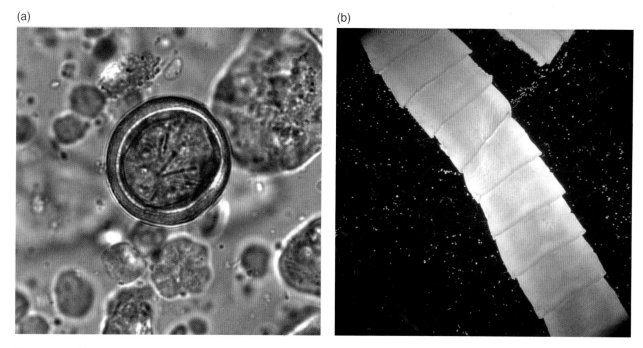

Figure 51.16 (a) *Taenia* egg, 40×. *Source:* Courtesy of Dr. Araceli Lucio-Forster, Cornell University College of Veterinary Medicine. (b) Magnified *Taenia* segment. *Source:* Courtesy of Dr. Araceli Lucio-Forster, Cornell University College of Veterinary Medicine.

cyst formation within the CNS, eye, muscle, or subcutaneous tissues [85].

Infection of humans with *E. granulosus* is of greater concern because it causes hydatid disease, that is, the development of cystic growths in the liver and other viscera [85]. This is more prevalent in the northern United States, Canada, and Alaska [85]. Dogs become infected when they are fed viscera of moose and caribou [85]. These dogs then become a source of exposure for the humans with whom they interact [85].

51.6.4 Whipworms

Whipworms are large intestinal parasites that are most commonly passed by vertical transmission [37]. However, adult dogs may also acquire whipworms by ingesting infected wildlife or infected feces, soil, or water.

They are named for their whip-like appearance: they have a wider head that tapers to a narrow tail [86].

Trichuris vulpis is a clinically important canine whipworm [34]. Dogs that are infected with *T. vulpis* typically present for diarrhea, weight loss, anemia, and/or hematochezia [37].

Diagnosis is via observation of eggs via fecal flotation [37]. Eggs are football-shaped with polar plugs at both ends [37] (see Figure 51.17).

Note that this shape is not pathognomonic for whipworms [37]. Respiratory parasites, such as the capillarids *Eucoleus (Capillaria) aerophila* and *Eucoleus (Capillaria)*

boehmi, are shaped similarly [37]. These can be distinguished from *T. vulpis* because the capillarid eggs tend to be smaller in size [37].

51.6.5 Protozoa

Protozoal diarrhea is common in pediatric companion animal patients [34].

Clinically important protozoa in dogs and cats include the following [34]:

– Coccidia
– *Cryptosporidium* spp.
– *Giardia* spp.
– *Tritrichomonas foetus*

51.6.5.1 Coccidiosis

Coccidiosis is caused by any number of coccidia species, including *Hammondia*, *Isospora*, and *Sarcocystis* spp. [86]. In addition, cats may become infected with *Besnoitia* spp. [86]. Of these, *Isospora* spp. are most commonly implicated in clinical infections among dogs and cats.

Coccidia tend to be host-specific.

Feline coccidiosis is most often caused by *Isospora felis* and *Isospora rivolta*; canine coccidiosis is most often caused by *Isospora canis*, *Isospora ohioensis*, *Isospora burrowsi*, and *Isospora neorivolta*.

When coccidiosis occurs in companion animal patients, it most often develops during times of stress,

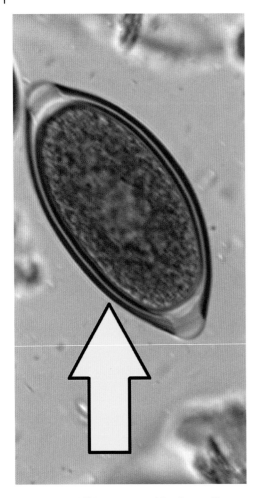

Figure 51.17 Whipworm egg, 20×. *Source:* Courtesy of Dr. Araceli Lucio-Forster, Cornell University College of Veterinary Medicine.

such as weaning. Diarrhea is frequent, and may be accompanied by weight loss and dehydration. Diarrhea may or may not be bloody.

Diagnosis is via observation of eggs via fecal flotation (see Figures 51.18a–d).

Most infections with *Coccidia* spp. are self-limiting; however, they can be effectively managed with sulfa-containing drugs [34].

51.6.5.2 Cryptosporidiosis

Cryptosporidiosis is another cause of protozoal, pediatric diarrhea in dogs and cats [34, 108].

Cryptosporidium canis and *Cryptosporidium felis* infect dogs and cats, respectively [108]. Both of these are zoonotic, and are likely to spread to immunocompromised people, including children [108].

Small bowel diarrhea is the most common clinical sign in companion animal patients. It may range in severity from mild and self-limiting to chronic and associated with weight loss and anorexia [109].

Oocysts are detected on fecal examination [108]. False negatives are common due to intermittent shedding [109]. Detection also requires attention to detail because oocysts are very small and easy to miss [109].

51.6.5.3 Giardiasis

Giardiasis causes small bowel diarrhea and potentially weight loss, stunted growth, and unthriftiness [34, 108–110]. Pediatric patients are more likely to be symptomatic [34, 109–111]. Adult infections may be clinical or subclinical [108–110]. Diarrhea may become chronic if the patient remains untreated [108].

Patients typically become infected through ingestion of cysts found in contaminated food or water [85, 110, 112]. Cysts are resistant to cold temperatures and damp environments [110, 112]. Cysts release trophozoites within the small bowel [112]. Trophozoites can be free-floating throughout the lumen, or they may attach to intestinal mucosa via a ventral sucking disc [112]. As these parasites move toward the colon, they undergo encystation [112].

Prevalence is relatively low: 5% in healthy cats and dogs, as compared to 15% in sick patients [110, 113].

Diagnosis is achieved by one or more of the following [108, 110, 114]:

- Identification of fecal cysts via zinc sulfate fecal flotation or a direct saline smear
- Identification of trophozoites in fresh fecal smears
- Fecal antigen detection test (see Figures 51.19a, b)

Sensitivity of microscopic identification is low [85, 109, 115, 116].

Trophozoites may be recognized by their classic pattern of activity: their movement takes on a typical "falling leaf motion" under 100× magnification [110].

Although zoonotic transmission is possible in human patients that are immunocompromised, for instance, those with human immunodeficiency virus (HIV), genotypes of *Giardia* that commonly infect dogs and cats are not the same as those that commonly infect people [85, 117, 118].

51.6.5.4 T. Foetus

Trichomoniasis causes waxing and waning large bowel diarrhea in cats [5, 119, 120]. Diarrheic samples from affected cats may contain fresh blood and/or mucus [119]. Stool is characteristic of cow-pie consistency and malodorous [119]. Severe cases may exhibit perineal inflammation, fecal incontinence, and/or rectal prolapse [109, 119]. However, other than focal disease, affected cats appear to be systemically healthy [119].

Diagnosis is via light microscopy. Trophozoites may be observed on fecal smears with saline, at 20× to 40× magnification [119].

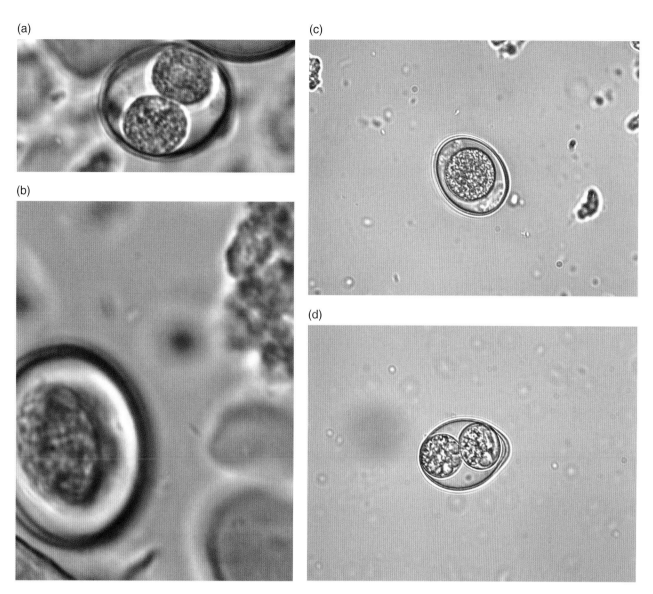

Figure 51.18 (a) *Isospora felis*. *Source:* Courtesy of Dr. Araceli Lucio-Forster, Cornell University College of Veterinary Medicine. (b) *Isospora rivolta*. *Source:* Courtesy of Dr. Araceli Lucio-Forster, Cornell University College of Veterinary Medicine. (c) *Isospora canis*. *Source:* Courtesy of Dr. Araceli Lucio-Forster, Cornell University College of Veterinary Medicine. (d) *Isospora ohioensis*. *Source:* Courtesy of Dr. Araceli Lucio-Forster, Cornell University College of Veterinary Medicine.

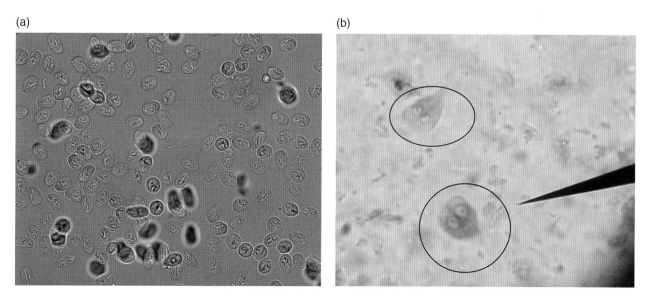

Figure 51.19 (a) *Giardia* cysts in a feline patient, 40×. Concentrated from feces by zinc sulfate centrifugal flotation. *Source:* Courtesy of Araceli Lucio-Forster, PhD. (b) *Giardia* trophozoite in a fecal smear. *Source:* Courtesy of Robert Eisemann.

T. foetus is often mistaken for *Giardia* [119]. Like *Giardia*, *T. foetus* is a highly motile flagellate [119]. However, compared to the "falling leaf" action of *Giardia*, *T. foetus* is characterized by a jerky, forward-rolling motion [119]. *T. foetus* is also distinct based upon morphology: it has a single nucleus, as compared to the classic "owl eyes" appearance that is associated with *Giardia* [109]. In addition, *T. foetus* has an undulating membrane [109, 119, 121] (see Figure 51.20).

Co-infection with *Giardia* is common [119].

Prevalence is higher among young cats, particularly those in shelters or catteries [109, 122].

It is difficult to diagnose *T. foetus* because trichomonads are shed intermittently [119]. They are also less hardy than *Giardia* because they do not form cysts [109]. They therefore do not survive refrigeration or fecal flotation [109, 119]. Fecal culture using In Pouch™ TF Feline may increase yield [109, 119]. Pouches are inoculated with a fecal sample that approximates the size of a peppercorn [119]. Stool must be freshly collected, either from a voided sample or via rectal loop collection [119]. Pouch contents are examined every other day for 12 days [119].

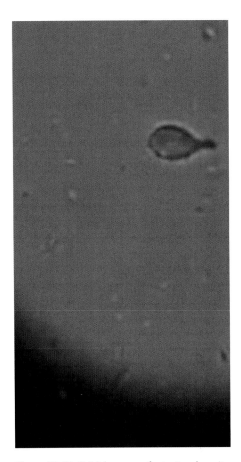

Figure 51.20 *Tritrichomonas foetus* trophozoite, as seen on light microscopy.

T. foetus can also be diagnosed via polymerase chain reaction (PCR) [109, 121, 122]. This diagnostic test is expensive; however, it is also the most sensitive diagnostic tool of those discussed here [109].

51.7 Abnormal Fecal Color

In addition to fecal score, fecal color provides important information regarding gastrointestinal health.

Abnormal fecal colors include the following [5]:

- Black tar
- Fresh red streaks
- Pale or colorless, yellow or gray

When stool takes on the appearance of black tar, it signifies an upper bowel bleed. When blood from the small bowel is digested, it mixes with stool to form melena. Refer to Figure 51.8.

When stool takes on the appearance of fresh red streaks, it signifies a lower bowel bleed. When blood from the lower bowel is present, it mixes with stool to form hematochezia. Refer to Figure 51.7.

When stool appears pale or colorless, it is referred to as acholic feces [5]. Acholic feces result from either EPI or a bile duct obstruction. Recall from Chapter 48, Section 48.4 that EPI is characterized by insufficient production of digestive enzymes by pancreatic acinar cells [123]. Ingesta is not properly broken down into absorbable nutrients [123]. The resultant stool may also be greasy, because it contains an excessive amount of undigested fat [5]. This kind of feces is called steatorrhea (see Figures 51.21a–c).

51.8 Diagnostic Work-Up

As is evident by this chapter, which is not by any means exhaustive, abnormal fecal scores can be caused by a number of structural, metabolic, and infectious disease processes. Consider, for example, diarrhea in the canine or feline patient. It may be overwhelming for the student clinician to consider all possible causes of diarrheic stool.

So where should one begin?

Signalment facilitates the clinician's prioritization of differential diagnoses [5]. For instance, a young, unvaccinated dog that presents for blood diarrhea is more likely to have parvovirus than a 12-year-old, fully vaccinated, Labrador Retriever. Likewise, a young, unvaccinated kitten that presents for diarrhea is more likely to have gastrointestinal parasites than a fully vaccinated, indoor-only, senior cat in a single-pet household. On the other hand, an elderly cat with a history of diarrhea and

Figure 51.21 (a) Soft yellow feces in a canine patient with EPI. (b) Cow-pie stool with excessive mucus in a canine patient with EPI. (c) Steatorrhea in a canine patient with EPI.

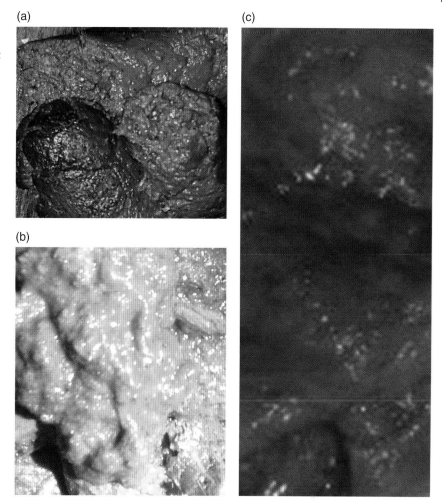

weight loss, despite polyphagia, is more likely to have hyperthyroidism.

History taking also plays an essential role in diagnosis, particularly when it comes to diarrheic stool [5]. By tracking how disease has progressed and concurrent clinical signs, history can piece together a story of small or large bowel diarrhea, or primary versus secondary gastrointestinal disease [5].

Open-ended questions, such as "Describe your patient's bowel habits," provide additional clues as to the source of the patient's issue [5]. This phraseology allows the client to expand upon gross observations at home [5].

Additionally, fecal scoring provides additional detail as to the consistency of bowel movements: what they are now versus what they were previously [5].

The physical examination also provides important clues in terms of the following patient parameters [4, 5]:

- Abdominal auscultation (refer to Chapter 47)
  - Hypermotile gut sounds
  - Hypomotile gut sounds
- Abdominal distension (refer to Chapter 50, Section 50.1)
  - Distension may be due to fluid, gas, or "mass effect."
- Abdominal splinting (refer to Chapter 50, Section 50.1)
  - The presence of this is suggestive of abdominal pain.
- Body condition score (BCS)
- Core body temperature
  - An elevated temperature may indicate infectious disease.
  - A truly low body temperature may indicate sepsis or shock.
  - An obstipated patient may have an apparently low body temperature due to the inadvertent insertion of the thermometer into a fecal ball.
- Hydration
  - Capillary refill time (CRT)
  - Cornea
  - Mucous membranes
  - Skin turgor
- Mentation
- Posture

Diagnostic tests can be thought of as additional tools that round out the patient's database [5].

Gross fecal examination is an important part of any work-up for abnormal fecal appearance. Start by evaluating fecal amount, color, and consistency. Reference the Nestlé-Purina fecal scoring system or a comparable scale to assess fecal moisture [5].

Prepare a direct fecal smear with saline to evaluate for *Giardia* trophozoites, *T. foetus*, or *Coccidia* spp. [5]

Fecal flotation can effectively diagnose roundworms, hookworms, tapeworms, and coccidia [5]. Zinc sulfate centrifugation may also be used to identify *Giardia* cysts, although its utility is dependent upon the examiner's level of experience [5].

Fecal cytology with staining, such as Diff-Quik or gram staining, may highlight gull-like CLOs or the characteristic safety pin shape of *Clostridium* spp. [5] *Cryptosporidium* spp. are more likely to be seen with acid-fast stains [5].

Fecal antigen tests increase the likelihood of detection for *Giardia* spp. [5]

Fecal culture may be helpful, although it is important to recognize that many bacterial populations are present in health as well as in disease [5].

In addition to fecal testing, many patients with signs of systemic illness benefit from baseline bloodwork, such as a complete blood count (CBC) and chemistry panel [5].

Those patients that raise the index of suspicion for EPI would benefit from undergoing serum trypsin-like immunoreactivity (TLI) testing [5].

Patients with ileal disease may benefit from serum cobalamin (vitamin B12) testing because deficiencies are common [5].

Survey radiographs are valuable in cases of nonproductive tenesmus to evaluate patients for obstipation and associated megacolon [5].

Ultrasonography is beneficial to assess for localized disease, such as intestinal tumors and enlarged mesenteric lymph nodes [5]. Liver and pancreatic architecture can also be appreciated [5].

Diagnostic investigations for gastrointestinal disease are inherently complex, and often require a multistep approach to work toward finding a solution.

References

1 Argenzio, R.B. (2004). Digestive and absorptive functions of the intestines. In: *Dukes' Physiology of Domestic Animals*, 12e (ed. H.H. Dukes and W.O. Reece), xiv, 999 p. Ithaca: Comstock Pub. Associates.

2 Evans, H.E. (1993). The digestive apparatus and abdomen. In: *Miller's Anatomy of the Dog*, 3e, 385–461. Philadelphia: Saunders Elsevier.

3 Dyce, K.M., Sack, W.O., and Wensing, C.J.G. (1996). *Textbook of Veterinary Anatomy*, 2e, xiii, 856 p. Philadelphia: Saunders.

4 Englar, R.E. (2017). *Performing the Small Animal Physical Examination*. Hoboken, NJ: Wiley.

5 Greco, D.S. Diagnosis and dietary management of gastrointestinal disease: purina veterinary diets. https://www.purinaproplanvets.com/media/1202/gi_quick_reference_guide.pdf (accessed 2 May 2019).

6 Tilley, L.P. and Smith, F.W.K. (2004). *The 5-Minute Veterinary Consult: Canine and Feline*, 3e, lviii, 1487 p. Baltimore, MD: Lippincott Williams & Wilkins.

7 Rothuizen, J., Schrauwen, E., Theyse, L.F.H., and Verhaert, L. (2009). Digestive tract. In: *Medical History and Physical Examination in Companion Animals* (ed. A. Rijnberk and F.J. van Sluijs), 86–100. Philadelphia: Elsevier, Ltd.

8 Trevail, T., Gunn-Moore, D., Carrera, I. et al. (2011). Radiographic diameter of the colon in normal and constipated cats and in cats with megacolon. *Vet. Radiol. Ultrasound* 52 (5): 516–520.

9 Washabau, R. (2001). Feline constipation, obstipation, and megacolon: prevention, diagnosis, and treatment. World Small Animal Veterinary Association World Congress [Internet]. https://www.vin.com/VINDBPub/SearchPB/Proceedings/PR05000/PR00118.htm.

10 Washabau, R. (1997). Constipation, obstipation, and megacolon. In: *Consultations in Feline Internal Medicine*, 3e (ed. J.R. August), 104–112. Philadelphia: Saunders.

11 Bredal, W.P., Thoresen, S.I., and Kvellestad, A. (1994). Atresia-coli in a 9-week-old kitten. *J. Small Anim. Pract.* 35 (12): 643–645.

12 Vandenbroek, A.H.M., Else, R.W., and Hunter, M.S. (1988). Atresia Ani and Urethrorectal fistula in a kitten. *J. Small Anim. Pract.* 29 (2): 91–94.

13 Yam, P. (1997). Decision making in the management of constipation in the cat. *In Pract.* 19 (8): 434–440.

14 Hudson, E.B., Farrow, C.S., and Smith, S.L. (1979). Acquired Megacolon in a cat. *Mod. Vet. Pract.* 60 (8): 625–627.

15 Washabau, R. and Holt, D. (2000). Feline constipation and idiopathic megacolon. In: *Kirk's Current Veterinary Therapy*, 13e (ed. J.D. Bonagura), 648–652. Philadelphia: WB Saunders.

16 Freiche, V., Houston, D., Weese, H. et al. (2011). Uncontrolled study assessing the impact of a psyllium-enriched extruded dry diet on faecal consistency in cats with constipation. *J. Feline Med. Surg.* 13 (12): 903–911.

17 Jones, B.D. (2000). Constipation, tenesmus, dyschezia, and faecal incontinence. In: *Textbook of Veterinary Internal Medicine* (ed. S.J. Ettinger and E.C. Feldman), 129–135. Philadelphia: Saunders.

18 White, R.N. (2002). Surgical management of constipation. *J. Feline Med. Surg.* 4 (3): 129–138.

19 Scherk, M. (2003). Feline megacolon. World Small Animal Veterinary Association World Congress [Internet]. https://www.vin.com/apputil/content/defaultadv1.aspx?pId=8768&meta=generic&id=3850188&print=1.

20 Rosin, E., Walshaw, R., Mehlhaff, C. et al. (1988). Subtotal colectomy for treatment of chronic constipation associated with idiopathic megacolon in cats: 38 cases (1979–1985). *J. Am. Vet. Med. Assoc.* 193 (7): 850–853.

21 Kudisch, M. and Pavletic, M.M. (1993). Subtotal colectomy with surgical stapling instruments via a trans-cecal approach for treatment of acquired megacolon in cats. *Vet. Surg.* 22 (6): 457–463.

22 Preston, D.M., Lennard-Jones, J.E., and Thomas, B.M. (1985). Towards a radiologic definition of idiopathic megacolon. *Gastrointest. Radiol.* 10 (2): 167–169.

23 O'Brien, T.R. (1978). *Radiographic Diagnosis of Abdominal Disorders in the Dog and Cat: Radiographic Interpretation, Clinical Signs, Pathophysiology*, xi, 682 p. Philadelphia: Saunders.

24 Baral, R.M. (2012). Diseases of the intestines. In: *The Cat: Clinical Medicine and Management* (ed. S.E. Little), 466–477. St. Louis: Saunders Elsevier.

25 Holt, P. (1985). Anal and perianal surgery in dogs and cats. *In Pract.* 7 (3): 82–89.

26 Schiller, L.R. (1999). Secretory diarrhea. *Curr. Gastroenterol. Rep.* 1 (5): 389–397.

27 Thiagarajah, J.R., Donowitz, M., and Verkman, A.S. (2015). Secretory diarrhoea: mechanisms and emerging therapies. *Nat. Rev. Gastroenterol. Hepatol.* 12 (8): 446–457.

28 Gaschen, F. (ed.) (2006). Small intestinal diarrhea – causes and treatment. WSAVA World Congress.

29 Allenspach, K. (2013). Diagnosis of small intestinal disorders in dogs and cats. *Vet. Clin. North Am. Small Anim. Pract.* 43 (6): 1227–1240, v.

30 Marks, S.L. and Kather, E.J. (2003). Bacterial-associated diarrhea in the dog: a critical appraisal. *Vet. Clin. North Am. Small Anim. Pract.* 33 (5): 1029–1060.

31 Greene, C.E. (1998). Enteric bacterial infections. In: *Infectious Diseases of the Dog and Cat* (ed. C.E. Greene), 243–245. St. Louis, Mo: Saunders/Elsevier.

32 Cave, N.J., Marks, S.L., Kass, P.H. et al. (2002). Evaluation of a routine diagnostic fecal panel for dogs with diarrhea. *J. Am. Vet. Med. Assoc.* 221 (1): 52–59.

33 Guilford, W.G. and Strombeck, D.R. (1996). Gastrointestinal tract infections, parasites, and

toxicosis. In: *Stromback's Small Animal Gastroenterology*, 3e (ed. W.G. Guilford and S.A. Center), 411–432. Philadelphia: W.B. Saunders.

34 Magne, M.L. (2006). Selected topics in pediatric gastroenterology. *Vet. Clin. North Am. Small Anim. Pract.* 36 (3): 533–548, vi.

35 Matz, M.E. (2006). Chronic diarrhea in a dog. *NAVC Clinician's Brief* (April): 75–77.

36 Sokolow, S.H., Rand, C., Marks, S.L. et al. (2005). Epidemiologic evaluation of diarrhea in dogs in an animal shelter. *Am. J. Vet. Res.* 66 (6): 1018–1024.

37 Zajac, A.M. (2003). A case of canine diarrhea. *NAVC Clinician's Brief* (April): 13–14.

38 German, A.J. (2006). Large bowel diarrhea. *NAVC Clinician's Brief* (February): 54–55.

39 Lecoindre, P. and Gaschen, F.P. (2011). Chronic idiopathic large bowel diarrhea in the dog. *Vet. Clin. North Am. Small Anim. Pract.* 41 (2): 447–456.

40 Leib, M.S. (2008). Large intestine. In: *Small animal gastroenterology* (ed. J.M. Steiner), 217–230. Hannover, Germany: Schluetersche.

41 Allenspach, K. (2010). Diseases of the large intestine. In: *Textbook of Veterinary Internal Medicine*, 7e (ed. S.J. Ettinger and E.C. Feldman), 1573–1594. St. Louis: Saunders Elsevier.

42 Hall, E.J. and German, A.J. (2005). Diseases of the small intestine. In: *Textbook of Veterinary Internal Medicine*, 6e (ed. S.J. Ettinger and E.C. Feldman), 1332–1378. Philadelphia: WB Saunders.

43 Hoskins, J.D. and Dimski, D. (1990). The digestive system. In: *Veterinary Pediatrics* (ed. J.D. Hoskins), 133–187. Philadelphia: WB Saunders.

44 Weese, J.S. (2011). Bacterial enteritis in dogs and cats: diagnosis, therapy, and zoonotic potential. *Vet. Clin. North Am. Small Anim. Pract.* 41 (2): 287–309.

45 Burnens, A.P., Angeloz-Wick, B., and Nicolet, J. (1992). Comparison of *campylobacter* carriage rates in diarrheic and healthy pet animals. *Zentralbl. Veterinarmed. B* 39 (3): 175–180.

46 Fox, J.G., Hering, A.M., Ackerman, J.I., and Taylor, N.S. (1983). The pet hamster as a potential reservoir of human campylobacteriosis. *J. Infect. Dis.* 147 (4): 784.

47 Acke, E., Whyte, P., Jones, B.R. et al. (2006). Prevalence of thermophilic *campylobacter* species in cats and dogs in two animal shelters in Ireland. *Vet. Rec.* 158 (2): 51–54.

48 Rossi, M., Hanninen, M.L., Revez, J. et al. (2008). Occurrence and species level diagnostics of *Campylobacter* spp., enteric *Helicobacter* spp. and *Anaerobiospirillum* spp. in healthy and diarrheic dogs and cats. *Vet. Microbiol.* 129 (3–4): 304–314.

49 Sandberg, M., Bergsjo, B., Hofshagen, M. et al. (2002). Risk factors for *campylobacter* infection in Norwegian cats and dogs. *Prev. Vet. Med.* 55 (4): 241–253.

50 Adak, G.K., Cowden, J.M., Nicholas, S., and Evans, H.S. (1995). The public health laboratory service national case-control study of primary indigenous sporadic cases of *campylobacter* infection. *Epidemiol. Infect.* 115 (1): 15–22.

51 Damborg, P., Olsen, K.E., Moller Nielsen, E., and Guardabassi, L. (2004). Occurrence of *Campylobacter jejuni* in pets living with human patients infected with *C. jejuni*. *J. Clin. Microbiol.* 42 (3): 1363–1364.

52 Fullerton, K.E., Ingram, L.A., Jones, T.F. et al. (2007). Sporadic *campylobacter* infection in infants: a population-based surveillance case-control study. *Pediatr. Infect. Dis. J.* 26 (1): 19–24.

53 Gillespie, I.A., O'Brien, S.J., Adak, G.K. et al. (2003). Point source outbreaks of *campylobacter* jejuni infection–are they more common than we think and what might cause them? *Epidemiol. Infect.* 130 (3): 367–375.

54 Tam, C.C., Higgins, C.D., Neal, K.R. et al. (2009). Chicken consumption and use of acid-suppressing medications as risk factors for *Campylobacter* enteritis, England. *Emerg. Infect. Dis.* 15 (9): 1402–1408.

55 Tenkate, T.D. and Stafford, R.J. (2001). Risk factors for *campylobacter* infection in infants and young children: a matched case-control study. *Epidemiol. Infect.* 127 (3): 399–404.

56 Weese, J.S. and Armstrong, J. (2003). Outbreak of *Clostridium difficile*-associated disease in a small animal veterinary teaching hospital. *J. Vet. Intern. Med.* 17 (6): 813–816.

57 Weese, J.S., Staempfli, H.R., Prescott, J.F. et al. (2001). The roles of *Clostridium difficile* and enterotoxigenic *Clostridium perfringens* in diarrhea in dogs. *J. Vet. Intern. Med.* 15 (4): 374–378.

58 Weese, J.S., Weese, H.E., Bourdeau, T.L., and Staempfli, H.R. (2001). Suspected *Clostridium difficile*-associated diarrhea in two cats. *J. Am. Vet. Med. Assoc.* 218 (9): 1436–1439, 21.

59 al Saif, N. and Brazier, J.S. (1996). The distribution of *Clostridium difficile* in the environment of South Wales. *J. Med. Microbiol.* 45 (2): 133–137.

60 Borriello, S.P., Honour, P., Turner, T., and Barclay, F. (1983). Household pets as a potential reservoir for *Clostridium difficile* infection. *J. Clin. Pathol.* 36 (1): 84–87.

61 Clooten, J., Kruth, S., Arroyo, L., and Weese, J.S. (2008). Prevalence and risk factors for *Clostridium difficile* colonization in dogs and cats hospitalized in an intensive care unit. *Vet. Microbiol.* 129 (1–2): 209–214.

62 Madewell, B.R., Bea, J.K., Kraegel, S.A. et al. (1999). *Clostridium difficile*: a survey of fecal carriage in cats in a veterinary medical teaching hospital. *J. Vet. Diagn. Investig.* 11 (1): 50–54.

63 Riley, T.V., Adams, J.E., O'Neill, G.L., and Bowman, R.A. (1991). Gastrointestinal carriage of *Clostridium difficile* in cats and dogs attending veterinary clinics. *Epidemiol. Infect.* 107 (3): 659–665.

64 Marks, S.L., Kather, E.J., Kass, P.H., and Melli, A.C. (2002). Genotypic and phenotypic characterization of *Clostridium perfringens* and *Clostridium difficile* in diarrheic and healthy dogs. *J. Vet. Intern. Med.* 16 (5): 533–540.

65 Cassutto, B.H. and Cook, L.C. (2002). An epidemiological survey of *Clostridium perfringens*-associated enterotoxemia at an army veterinary treatment facility. *Mil. Med.* 167 (3): 219–222.

66 McKenzie, E., Riehl, J., Banse, H. et al. (2010). Prevalence of diarrhea and enteropathogens in racing sled dogs. *J. Vet. Intern. Med.* 24 (1): 97–103.

67 Tsai, H.J., Huang, H.C., Lin, C.M. et al. (2007). *Salmonellae* and *campylobacters* in household and stray dogs in northern Taiwan. *Vet. Res. Commun.* 31 (8): 931–939.

68 Joffe, D.J. and Schlesinger, D.P. (2002). Preliminary assessment of the risk of *Salmonella* infection in dogs fed raw chicken diets. *Can. Vet. J.* 43 (6): 441–442.

69 Morley, P.S., Strohmeyer, R.A., Tankson, J.D. et al. (2006). Evaluation of the association between feeding raw meat and *Salmonella enterica* infections at a greyhound breeding facility. *J. Am. Vet. Med. Assoc.* 228 (10): 1524–1532.

70 Lefebvre, S.L., Reid-Smith, R., Boerlin, P., and Weese, J.S. (2008). Evaluation of the risks of shedding *Salmonellae* and other potential pathogens by therapy dogs fed raw diets in Ontario and Alberta. *Zoonoses Public Health* 55 (8–10): 470–480.

71 Choudhary, S.P., Kalimuddin, M., Prasad, G. et al. (1985). Observations on natural and experimental salmonellosis in dogs. *J. Diarrhoeal Dis. Res.* 3 (3): 149–153.

72 Wright, J.G., Tengelsen, L.A., Smith, K.E. et al. (2005). Multidrug-resistant *Salmonella Typhimurium* in four animal facilities. *Emerg. Infect. Dis.* 11 (8): 1235–1241.

73 Wall, P.G., Threllfall, E.J., Ward, L.R., and Rowe, B. (1996). Multiresistant *Salmonella typhimurium* DT104 in cats: a public health risk. *Lancet* 348 (9025): 471.

74 Tauni, M.A. and Osterlund, A. (2000). Outbreak of *Salmonella typhimurium* in cats and humans associated with infection in wild birds. *J. Small Anim. Pract.* 41 (8): 339–341.

75 Schotte, U., Borchers, D., Wulff, C., and Geue, L. (2007). Salmonella Montevideo outbreak in military kennel dogs caused by contaminated commercial feed, which was only recognized through monitoring. *Vet. Microbiol.* 119 (2–4): 316–323.

76 Pitout, J.D., Reisbig, M.D., Mulvey, M. et al. (2003). Association between handling of pet treats and infection with *Salmonella enterica* serotype Newport expressing the AmpC beta-lactamase, CMY-2. *J. Clin. Microbiol.* 41 (10): 4578–4582.

77 Centers for Disease C, Prevention (2001). Outbreaks of multidrug-resistant *Salmonella typhimurium* associated with veterinary facilities–Idaho, Minnesota, and Washington, 1999. *MMWR Morb. Mortal. Wkly Rep.* 50 (33): 701–704.

78 Centers for Disease C, Prevention (2008). Multistate outbreak of human salmonella infections caused by contaminated dry dog food–United States, 2006–2007. *MMWR Morb. Mortal. Wkly Rep.* 57 (19): 521–524.

79 Centers for Disease C, Prevention (2008). Update: recall of dry dog and cat food products associated with human salmonella Schwarzengrund infections–United States, 2008. *MMWR Morb. Mortal. Wkly Rep.* 57 (44): 1200–1202.

80 McCaw, D.L. and Hoskins, J.D. (2006). Canine viral enteritis. In: *Infectious Diseases of the Dog and Cat*, 3e (ed. C.E. Greene), 63–73. St. Louis, Mo.: Saunders/Elsevier.

81 Glickman, L.T., Domanski, L.M., Patronek, G.J., and Visintainer, F. (1985). Breed-related risk factors for canine parvovirus enteritis. *J. Am. Vet. Med. Assoc.* 187 (6): 589–594.

82 Rewerts, J.M. and Cohn, L.A. (2000). CVT update: diagnosis and treatment of parvovirus. In: *Kirk's Current Veterinary Therapy XIII* (ed. J.D. Bonagura), 629–632. Philadelphia: WB Saunders.

83 Greene, C.E. and Addie, D.D. (2006). Feline parvovirus infections. In: *Infectious Diseases of the Dog and Cat*, 3e (ed. C.E. Greene), 78–88. St. Louis, Mo.: Saunders/Elsevier.

84 CDC. Guidelines for Veterinarians: Prevention of Zoonotic Transmission of Ascarids and Hookworms. CDC [Internet]. https://www.cdc.gov/parasites/zoonotichookworm/resources/prevention.pdf (accessed 2 May 2019).

85 Schantz, P.M. (2007). Zoonotic parasitic infections contracted from dogs and cats: How frequent are they? DVM 360 [Internet]. http://veterinarymedicine.dvm360.com/zoonotic-parasitic-infections-contracted-dogs-and-cats-how-frequent-are-they.

86 Bowman, D.D. and Georgi, J.R. (2009). *Georgis' Parasitology for Veterinarians*, 9e ix, 451 p.p. St. Louis, MO: Saunders/Elsevier.

87 Schantz, P.M. (2004). Larva migrans syndromes caused by Toxocara species and other helminths. In: *Infectious Diseases* (ed. S.L. Gorbach, J.G. Bartlett and N.R. Blacklow), 1529–1535. Philadelphia: WB Saunders.

88 Glickman, L.T. and Schantz, P.M. (1982). Epidemiology and pathogenesis of zoonotic toxocariasis. *Epidemiol. Rev.* 3: 230–250.

89 Schantz, P.M. (1989). Toxocara larva migrans now. *Am. J. Trop. Med. Hyg.* 41: 21–34.

90 Burke, T.M. and Roberson, E.L. (1985). Prenatal and lactational transmission of *Toxocara canis* and *Ancylostoma caninum*: experimental infection of the bitch at midpregnancy and at parturition. *Int. J. Parasitol.* 15 (5): 485–490.

91 Blagburn, B.L. and Dryden, M.W. (2009). Biology, treatment, and control of flea and tick infestations. *Vet. Clin. N. Am. Small Anim. Pract.* 39 (6): 1173–1200.

92 Dryden, M.W. and Rust, M.K. (1994). The cat flea – biology, ecology and control. *Vet. Parasitol.* 52 (1–2): 1–19.

93 Rust, M.K. and Dryden, M.W. (1997). The biology, ecology, and management of the cat flea. *Annu. Rev. Entomol.* 42: 451–473.

94 Traversa, D. (2013). Fleas infesting pets in the era of emerging extra-intestinal nematodes. *Parasit. Vectors* 6: 59.

95 Flick, S.C. (1973). Endoparasites in cats: current practice and opinions. *Feline Pract.* 4: 21–34.

96 Hitchcock, D.J. (1953). Incidence of gastro-intestinal parasites in some Michigan kittens. *North Am. Vet.* 34: 428–429.

97 Arundel, J.H. (1970). Control of helminth parasites of dogs and cats. *Aust. Vet. J.* 46 (4): 164–168.

98 Baker, M.K., Lange, L., Verster, A., and van der Plaat, S. (1989). A survey of helminths in domestic cats in the Pretoria area of Transvaal, Republic of South Africa. Part 1: the prevalence and comparison of burdens of helminths in adult and juvenile cats. *J. S. Afr. Vet. Assoc.* 60 (3): 139–142.

99 Boreham, R.E. and Boreham, P.F.L. (1990). *Dipylidium-Caninum* – life-cycle, Epizootiology, and control. *Compend. Contin. Educ. Pract. Vet.* 12 (5): 667–675.

100 Collins, G.H. (1973). A limited survey of gastro-intestinal helminths of dogs and cats. *N. Z. Vet. J.* 21 (8): 175–176.

101 Coman, B.J. (1972). A survey of the gastro-intestinal parasites of the feral cat in Victoria. *Aust. Vet. J.* 48 (4): 133–136.

102 Coman, B.J. (1972). Helminth parasites of the dingo and feral dog in Victoria with some notes on the diet of the host. *Aust. Vet. J.* 48 (8): 456–461.

103 Coman, B.J., Jones, E.H., and Driesen, M.A. (1981). Helminth parasites and arthropods of feral cats. *Aust. Vet. J.* 57 (7): 324–327.

104 Engbaek, K., Madsen, H., and Larsen, S.O. (1984). A survey of helminths in stray cats from Copenhagen with ecological aspects. *Z. Parasitenkd.* 70 (1): 87–94.

105 Griffiths, H.J. (1978). *Handbook of Veterinary Parasitology*. Minnesota: University of Minnesota.

106 Dobler, G. and Pfeffer, M. (2011). Fleas as parasites of the family Canidae. *Parasit. Vectors* 4: 139.

107 Kramer, F. and Mencke, N. (2001). *Flea Biology and Control*. Berlin, Germany: Springer-Verlag Berlin and Heidelberg GmbH & Co.

108 Bowman, D. (2009). Canine and feline cryptosporidiosis and giardiasis. DVM 360 [Internet]. http://veterinarycalendar.dvm360.com/canine-and-feline-cryptosporidiosis-and-giardiasis-proceedings.

109 Little S. (2011). Diarrhea in kittens and young cats. WSAVA World Congress; Jeju, Korea.

110 Scorza, V. (2013). Giardiasis. *NAVC Clinician's Brief* (February): 71–86.

111 Tangtrongsup, S. and Scorza, V. (2010). Update on the diagnosis and management of giardia spp infections in dogs and cats. *Top. Companion Anim. Med.* 25 (3): 155–162.

112 Barr, S.C. (2006). Enteric protozoal infections. In: *Infectious Diseases of the Dog and Cat* (ed. C.E. Greene), 736–742. St. Louis, MO: Elsevier, Inc.

113 Ballweber, L.R., Xiao, L., Bowman, D.D. et al. (2010). Giardiasis in dogs and cats: update on epidemiology and public health significance. *Trends Parasitol.* 26 (4): 180–189.

114 Steiner, J.M. (2010). Workup of dogs with chronic diarrhea. DVM 360 [Internet]. http://veterinarycalendar.dvm360.com/workup-dogs-with-chronic-diarrhea-basics-proceedings.

115 Dryden, M.W., Payne, P.A., and Smith, V. (2006). Accurate diagnosis of *Giardia* spp and proper fecal examination procedures. *Vet. Ther.* 7 (1): 4–14.

116 Hackett, T. and Lappin, M.R. (2003). Prevalence of enteric pathogens in dogs of north-Central Colorado. *J. Am. Anim. Hosp. Assoc.* 39 (1): 52–56.

117 Slifko, T.R., Smith, H.V., and Rose, J.B. (2000). Emerging parasite zoonoses associated with water and food. *Int. J. Parasitol.* 30 (12–13): 1379–1393.

118 Thompson, R.C. (2004). The zoonotic significance and molecular epidemiology of giardia and giardiasis. *Vet. Parasitol.* 126 (1–2): 15–35.

119 Gookin, J.L. (2006). Trichomoniasis. In: *Infectious Diseases of the Dog and Cat* (ed. C.E. Greene), 745–750. St. Louis, MO: Elsevier, Inc.

120 Levy, M.G., Gookin, J.L., Poore, M. et al. (2003). *Tritrichomonas foetus* and not *Pentatrichomonas hominis* is the etiologic agent of feline trichomonal diarrhea. *J. Parasitol.* 89 (1): 99–104.

121 Steiner, J.M. (2012). Chronic diarrhea in a Himalayan cat. *NAVC Clinician's Brief* (July): 79–82.

122 Steiner, J.M. (2007). Chronic diarrhea in cats. *NAVC Clinician's Brief* (March): 12–13.

123 Morgan, J.A. and Moore, L.E. (2009). A quick review of canine exocrine pancreatic insufficiency. DVM360 [Internet]. http://veterinarymedicine.dvm360.com/quick-review-canine-exocrine-pancreatic-insufficiency.

52

Dysphagia and Regurgitation

52.1 Introduction to Deglutition

Deglutition is the process by which a patient swallows. For swallowing to be effective, meaning that a bolus of food is successfully passed onward from the mouth to the stomach, the patient must coordinate a number of actions [1, 2]. These include, but are not limited to the following [1, 3, 4]:

- Prehension, the physical handling of food to get it into the mouth
- Mastication, the act of chewing the food to break it into bite-sized pieces
  - Requires functional masticatory muscles
  - Requires the ability to open and close the jaw
  - Requires functional dentition
- Lubrication of food with saliva
  - Requires functional salivary glands
  - Requires patent salivary ducts
- Manipulation of the bolus of food by the tongue to press it backward into the pharynx
  - Requires functional cranial nerves
    ○ Cranial nerve IX, the glossopharyngeal nerve
    ○ Cranial nerve XII, the hypoglossal nerve
- Reflex movement of the bolus into the esophagus via peristaltic contractions
  - Simultaneous closure of the larynx by the epiglottis to inhibit respiration
  - Relaxation of the upper esophageal sphincter, that is, the paired cricopharyngeus and thyropharyngeus muscles, to accept the bolus of food into the proximal esophagus
  - Closure of the paired cricopharyngeus and thyropharyngeus muscles to prevent retrograde movement of the bolus
- Restoration of the epiglottis to its relaxed position
- Continuation of normal respiration

The esophagus is a tubular structure that is responsible for transporting the bolus of food from the oropharynx to the stomach [1].

As is true of all other regions of the gastrointestinal tract, the esophagus is multilayered [1, 5]. Mucosa forms the innermost lining [1, 5]. From the inside out, the remaining layers are the submucosa, muscularis, and the fibrous coat, or adventitia [1, 5, 6].

Striated muscle makes up the muscularis layer of the canine esophagus [1, 5]. By comparison, the caudal third of the esophageal muscularis layer is composed of smooth muscle in the cat [1]. A bolus of food travels faster via striated muscle than via smooth muscle [4].

Peristaltic waves move the bolus of food from the proximal to the distal esophagus [1, 7]. The bolus must then pass through the lower esophageal sphincter to enter the stomach [1].

Pathology may occur at any step along the process, leading to an assortment of clinical signs, including the following [1–3, 8–11]:

- Dysphagia, or difficulty swallowing
- Pseudoptyalism, or inability to swallow normal saliva
- Ptyalism, or increased production of saliva
- Regurgitation
- Trismus, or lockjaw, that is, inability to fully open the jaw

52.2 Introduction to Dysphagia

Dysphagia is a broad clinical sign that encompasses difficulty swallowing at any point in the pathway. Because deglutition is such a complex process, dysphagia can be further divided into several clinical presentations, based upon where in the pathway the process breaks down [1, 2, 8–10]:

- Oral dysphagia
- Pharyngeal dysphagia
- Cricopharyngeal dysphagia
- Esophageal dysphagia

52.2.1 Oral Dysphagia

Oral dysphagia refers to difficulty with either the prehension of food or its transport to the base of the tongue [1, 2, 8–10].

These patients may have an anatomical defect, such as a cleft palate, which alters the flow of food to the back of the throat in anticipation of swallowing [10]. Recall from Chapter 33, Section 33.8 that a cleft of the secondary palate is a split in the roof of the mouth [12]. This leads to abnormal communication between the oral and nasal cavities [12] (see Figures 52.1a, b).

Clefts of the secondary palate are present at birth [12].

Clients may report that milk drips out of the nose during nursing [12]. After weaning, solid foods will emerge from the nasal cavity during feeding [12].

An oral examination is confirmatory of the diagnosis: clefts are apparent when the patient's mouth is opened [12–14].

Cleft palates can be surgically repaired [12].

Note that clefts are not the only cause of oral dysphagia. Patients may instead have abnormal dentition and/or periodontal disease that requires them to modify their eating behavior to facilitate bolus transfer to the base of the tongue [10] (see Figures 52.2a, b).

An oral examination will confirm dental disease, although patients that are in pain may require sedation.

Patients with oral dysphagia could also have a pain unrelated to the teeth, as from stomatitis or an oral mass [10]. If sufficiently painful, this could cause the patient to modify its eating habits (see Figures 52.3a–e).

One can imagine how the patients that are depicted in Figures 52.3a–e would have a difficult time with prehension.

Likewise, patients who chew on electrical cords may experience traumatic burns that make eating painful [10].

In all cases, the patient is likely to have trouble with passage of food through the mouth.

Owners of these patients are likely to report changes in eating behavior [8]. For example, patients with oral masses on the right side of the mouth may learn to eat on the left side of the mouth to minimize pain associated with inadvertent chewing of the mass, rather than the food.

It is also relatively common for owners to report a head tilt while eating, or tossing the head back while eating as if to facilitate passage of the food bolus to the base of the tongue [8].

Patients that present for dysphagia of any sort benefit from a thorough oral examination to assess the following structures [13]:

- Buccal cavity
- Dentition
- Gingiva

(a)

(b)

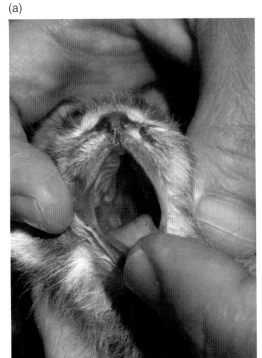 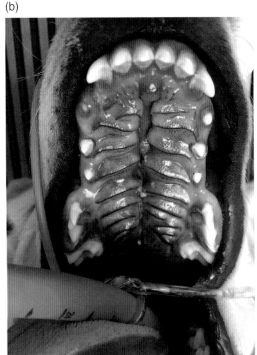

Figure 52.1 (a) Cleft palate in a kitten. *Source:* Courtesy of Kate Anderson, DVM. (b) Cleft palate in a five-month-old, spayed female, Labrador retriever dog. *Source:* Courtesy of Jackie Kucskar, DVM.

(a)

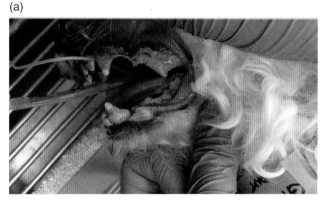

(b)

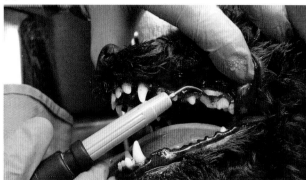

Figure 52.2 (a) Severe, diffuse dental disease in a canine patient. *Source:* Courtesy of Dr. Lauren Griggs. (b) Slab fracture of the left maxillary carnassial tooth in a canine patient. *Source:* Courtesy of Dr. Lauren Griggs.

- Mucosa
- Oropharynx
- Palate
- Sublingual space
- Tongue

Extraoral structures may also contribute to dysphagia and therefore should be evaluated as part of a thorough patient evaluation [13]. Items of particular interest include the following [13]:

- Assessment of facial symmetry
- Palpation
  - Angular processes of the mandible
  - Intermandibular space
  - Maxilla
  - Right and left bodies of the mandible
  - Temporomandibular joint (TMJ)
  - Zygomatic arches

Palpation of these structures is important because it may reveal underlying pain or discomfort that could be associated with the musculoskeletal or neurological systems.

Consider, for example, masticatory muscle myositis [8–10], which is characterized as an immune-mediated condition [3]. Affected patients may present for unusual carriage of the jaw and ptyalism [3]. When the clinician attempts to open the jaw, s/he is unsuccessful and/or the patient resists [3]. There is pain on palpation over the TMJ bilaterally, and swelling of the masseter and temporalis muscles may be grossly apparent [3].

Patients with masticatory muscle myositis typically have elevations in creatine kinase [3].

Diagnosis of masticatory muscle myositis is typically via 2 M antibody titer test [3]. 2 M fibers are exclusively in masticatory muscles [3, 15, 16]. When this titer is greater than 1:100, it implies autoantibody formation against the muscles of mastication [3].

Masticatory muscle myositis is medically managed with immunosuppressive doses of steroids [3].

Dysphagia may also occur in patients with masticatory muscle atrophy [8, 9]. These patients tend to develop a sunken-in appearance over the masseter and/or temporalis muscles [13] (see Figures 52.4a–c).

This, too, may affect patients' ability to manipulate and break down food into manageable boluses.

52.2.2 Pharyngeal Dysphagia

Pharyngeal dysphagia refers to those patients that can prehend food normally, but fail to get it to the back of the throat via tongue action or cannot swallow it when they do [1, 8–10]. These patients have an abnormal gag reflex [9]. They may exaggerate chewing actions and attempt to facilitate swallowing by flexing and extending the neck, but tongue and/or pharyngeal weakness prevents the bolus from getting into proper position [9].

Myopathies and/or neuromuscular disease are typically responsible for pharyngeal weakness, for example, muscular dystrophy and myasthenia gravis [1, 17–22].

52.2.2.1 Muscular Dystrophy

Muscular dystrophy is a relatively rare, inherited, noninflammatory, and progressive disease that is characterized by a deficiency of the muscle membrane protein, dystrophin [9]. Because dystrophin is globally deficient, affected patients exhibit whole body weakness, as opposed to focal weakness involving the tongue and esophagus [9].

In addition to difficulty swallowing, patients with muscular dystrophy also exhibit a stiff, stilted gait [9]. Patients may appear to bunny-hop in the pelvic limbs, and may develop a plantigrade stance [9]. Patients are intolerant of exercise [9]. They may develop limb tremors secondary to muscular weakness [9]. They may also

(a)

(b)

(c)

(d)

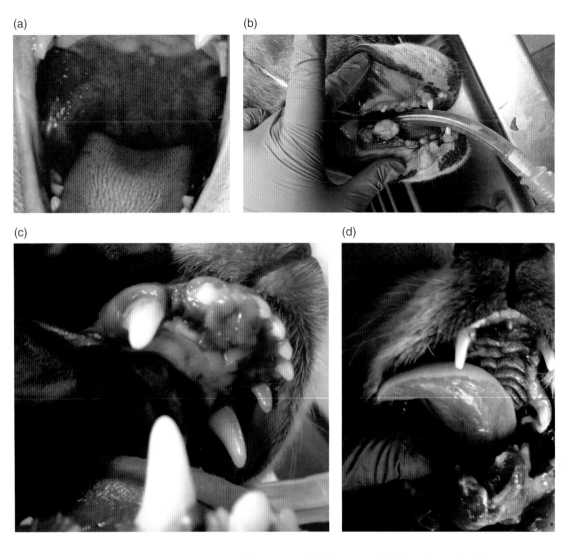

(e)

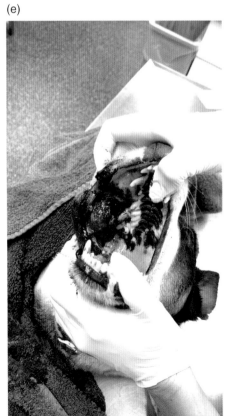

Figure 52.3 (a) Feline stomatitis. Note the raw hamburger appearance at the back of the throat. (b) Extensive canine gingival hyperplasia. *Source:* Courtesy of Dr. Lauren Griggs. (c) Canine oral mass, in close association with the maxillary incisors. (d) Canine oral mass, in close association with the mandibular arcades. *Source:* Courtesy of Dr. Stephanie Harris. (e) Canine oral mass, in close association with the right buccal cavity. *Source:* Courtesy of Kelli L. Crisfulli, RVT.

(a)

(c)

(b)

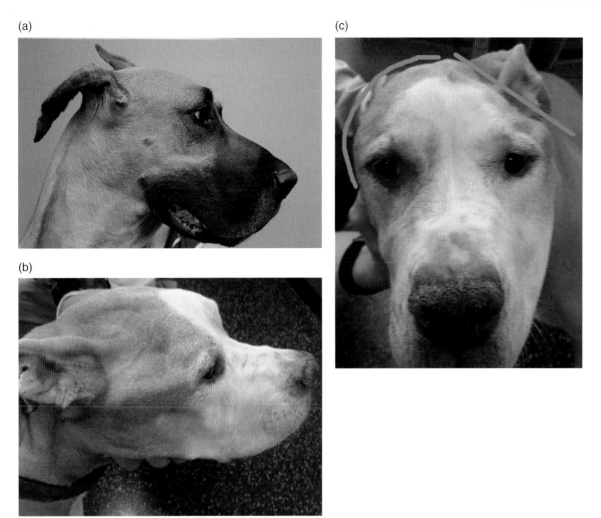

Figure 52.4 (a) This Great Dane appears to have normal muscles of mastication based upon gross visual examination. *Source:* Courtesy of the Media Resources Department at Midwestern University. (b) This patient has marked temporalis muscle atrophy, when viewed in profile. *Source:* Courtesy of Daniel Foy, MS, DVM, DACVIM, DACVECC. (c) This patient has marked asymmetry of the temporalis muscles when comparing the left to the right. *Source:* Courtesy of Daniel Foy, MS, DVM, DACVIM, DACVECC.

develop difficulties with respiration because the diaphragm, as a muscle, is compromised [9].

Because the condition is sex-linked, males are more likely to be affected than females [9]. Golden Retrievers, Irish Terriers, Labrador Retrievers, Samoyeds, Belgian Shepherds, and Bouvier des Flandres are predisposed [9].

52.2.2.2 Myasthenia Gravis

Myasthenia gravis is a relatively rare condition among companion animal patients [9].

In the congenital form, patients have abnormal acetylcholine receptors [9]. These result in faulty communication of messages across the neuromuscular junction [9]. Jack Russell Terriers, Springer Spaniels, and Smooth Fox Terriers are at increased risk [9].

When myasthenia gravis is acquired, patients develop autoantibodies against acetylcholine receptors [9]. This form of myasthenia gravis is more likely to occur in German Shepherds and Labrador Retrievers [9].

Patients that have either the congenital or acquired form of myasthenia gravis typically appear normal at rest [9]. With mild exertion, they rapidly become fatigued [9]. Exercise intolerance is progressive [9]. In addition, the development of megaesophagus in affected patients is common [9].

Presumptive diagnosis is made by administering edrophonium chloride intravenously and noticing restoration of muscle strength [9]. Definitive diagnosis of acquired myasthenia gravis is via serum acetylcholine receptor antibody titer [9].

Patients with myasthenia gravis are medically managed with anticholinesterase drugs so that acetylcholine persists at the neuromuscular junction [9].

52.2.2.3 Rabies

Note that rabies must also be considered in all cases that involve apparent pharyngeal weakness [23].

52.2.3 Cricopharyngeal Dysphagia

Recall the role of the paired cricopharyngeus and thyropharyngeus muscles in deglutition. These muscles comprise the upper esophageal sphincter, and must relax to accept the bolus of food into the proximal esophagus [1, 3, 4]. Note that, as these muscles relax, the pharyngeal muscles must constrict in order to hand over the bolus of food [2].

Patients with cricopharyngeal dysphagia have normal prehension and a normal gag reflex; however, they are unable to successfully swallow [1, 8–10].

This may result from cricopharyngeal achalasia, the inability to relax the upper esophageal sphincter, or dyssynchrony, meaning that relaxation occurs, but is delayed [1, 2, 24–29].

Diagnosis of both forms of cricopharyngeal dysphagia is made via contrast videofluoroscopy [1, 24, 29–32].

Surgical correction via myotomy or myectomy of the cricopharyngeal muscles is effective at reducing, if not resolving, dysphagia [6, 28].

52.2.4 Esophageal Dysphagia

Esophageal dysphagia refers to difficulty transporting the bolus of food from the esophagus to the stomach [1, 2].

Causes of esophageal dysphagia include the following [1, 2, 33]:

- Esophageal "mass"
  - Esophageal stricture
  - Foreign body
  - Extraluminal compression of the esophagus
    ○ Cardiomegaly
    ○ Hilar lymphadenopathy
    ○ Mediastinal mass
    ○ Vascular ring abnormalities
      ● Persistent right aortic arch (PRAA)
  - Intraluminal mass that occludes the lumen of the esophagus
- Esophagitis
- Megaesophagus
  - Primary
  - Secondary

52.2.4.1 Esophageal Masses: Real and Apparent

Foreign body ingestion of any sort can lead to a complete or partial esophageal obstruction. In particular, bones, plastic, and trichobezoars can become lodged within the esophagus and/or lead to the development of an esophageal stricture [33].

Foreign bodies may or may not be apparent on survey radiographs of the neck and thorax [1, 34]. Radiodense objects, such as needles and fishhooks, are easily identified; however, wood foreign bodies may present a greater challenge [1, 34–39]. In such cases, the stick itself is not evident, but the resultant subcutaneous emphysema between muscle planes may be visible [1, 38].

Sometimes only esophageal narrowing, at the level of the obstruction, or esophageal dilation, after the point of obstruction, is present on survey radiographs (see Figures 52.5a–d).

Esophageal foreign bodies frequently incite inflammation of the mucosa [34]. Esophageal strictures are common sequelae [34].

Contrast survey radiography may facilitate visualization of an esophageal foreign body, esophageal stricture, vascular ring anomaly, or esophageal masses [1].

Esophageal strictures are best highlighted by feeding barium-soaked kibble: liquid will easily pass through the stricture, but kibble will not [1].

Vascular ring anomalies are beyond the scope of this text, but typically result from a PRAA [1, 24, 40]. Weanlings present for regurgitation because the esophagus becomes strangled by an encircling branch of the aorta that has failed to regress [40].

Contrast-enhanced videofluoroscopy is another modality by which deglutition can be evaluated [1]. Liquid barium is administered to the patient, who then swallows [1]. The clinician is able to track boluses all the way to the stomach, in real time [1]. Afterward, s/he can review the still shots of the recording, frame by frame, to evaluate oropharyngeal and esophageal function [1]. Digitally captured fluoroscopic images facilitate diagnosis of structural and functional abnormalities [1] (see Figures 52.6a–e).

52.2.4.2 Esophagitis

When the esophageal mucosa becomes inflamed, the patient is said to have esophagitis [33, 34]. Esophagitis is thought to occur more frequently than is currently recognized in companion animal patients [33].

Risk factors for developing esophagitis include the following [33]:

- Abnormal ingestive behaviors
  - Sharp foreign bodies are more likely to penetrate the esophagus, causing injury
  - Abrasive foreign bodies are more likely to scuff the esophagus, causing erosions
  - Chemical ingestion, as from the ingestion of cleaning products, may cause esophageal burns
- Brachycephalic breeds and Shar Pei dogs
  - These breeds are more likely to have abnormal lower esophageal sphincters

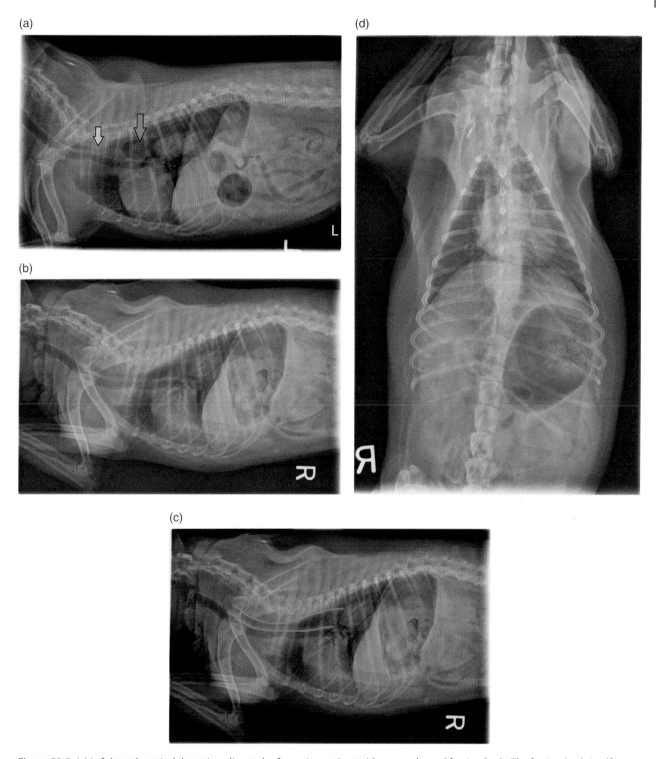

Figure 52.5 (a) Left lateral cervical thoracic radiograph of a canine patient with an esophageal foreign body. The foreign body itself is not apparent. However, note the point of esophageal constriction (blue arrow), followed by the point of esophageal dilation (orange arrow) that raises the index of suspicion that there is an esophageal obstruction. *Source:* Courtesy of Daniel Foy, MS, DVM, DACVIM, DACVECC. (b) Right lateral cervical thoracic radiograph of the same canine patient depicted in Figure 52.5a. *Source:* Courtesy of Daniel Foy, MS, DVM, DACVIM, DACVECC. (c) Right lateral cervical thoracic radiograph of the same canine patient depicted in Figure 52.5a. The esophagus is visible and has been outlined in orange. *Source:* Courtesy of Daniel Foy, MS, DVM, DACVIM, DACVECC. (d) Ventrodorsal (V/D) thoracic radiograph of the same canine patient depicted in Figure 52.5a. *Source:* Courtesy of Daniel Foy, MS, DVM, DACVIM, DACVECC.

(a)

(b)

(c)

(d)

(e)

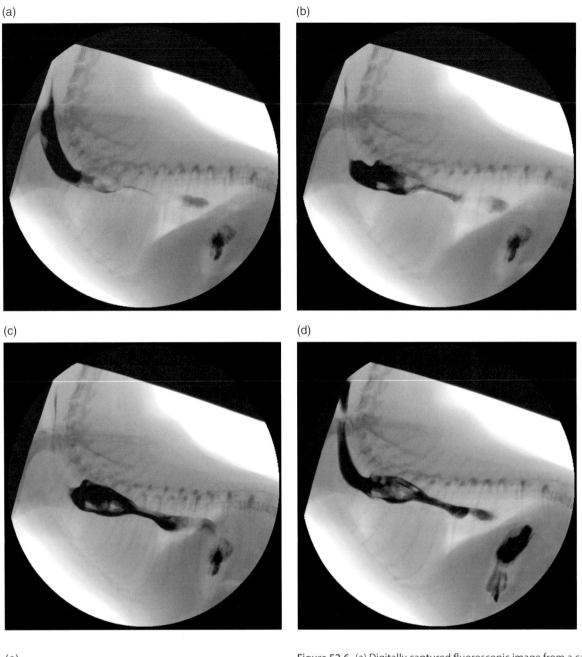
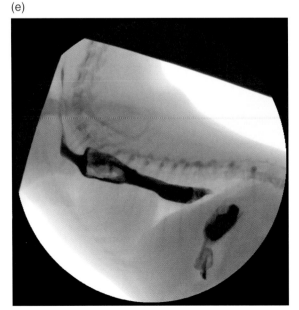

Figure 52.6 (a) Digitally captured fluoroscopic image from a canine patient with an esophageal foreign body. *Source:* Courtesy of Daniel Foy, MS, DVM, DACVIM, DACVECC. (b) Digitally captured fluoroscopic image from a canine patient with an esophageal foreign body. Same patient as depicted in Figure 52.6a. *Source:* Courtesy of Daniel Foy, MS, DVM, DACVIM, DACVECC. (c) Digitally captured fluoroscopic image from a canine patient with an esophageal foreign body. Same patient as depicted in Figure 52.6a. *Source:* Courtesy of Daniel Foy, MS, DVM, DACVIM, DACVECC. (d) Digitally captured fluoroscopic image from a canine patient with an esophageal foreign body. Same patient as depicted in Figure 52.6a. *Source:* Courtesy of Daniel Foy, MS, DVM, DACVIM, DACVECC. (e) Digitally captured fluoroscopic image from a canine patient with an esophageal foreign body. Same patient as depicted in Figure 52.6a. *Source:* Courtesy of Daniel Foy, MS, DVM, DACVIM, DACVECC.

– Abnormal lower esophageal sphincters increase the risk for gastroesophageal reflux
– Reflux burns the esophagus as a result of low gastric pH

- Delayed gastric emptying
- "Dry pilling" may lead to esophageal ulceration and/or stricture
  – Bisphosphonates
  – Clindamycin (cats) [34]
  – Doxycycline (cats) [34, 41, 42]
- Esophageal infection
  – *Pythium insidiosum*
  – *Spirocerca lupi*
- Frequent vomiting
- General anesthesia
- Hiatal hernia
- Hypergastrinemia, for example, as caused by a gastrinoma [34]
- Radiation therapy
- Trichobezoars, or hairballs

When esophagitis is secondary to general anesthesia, clinical signs tend to develop one to three days post-procedure [34]. Patients may present for the following [34]:

- Anorexia or reduced appetite
- Dysphagia
  – Gagging
  – Hypersalivation
  – Repeated swallowing or attempts to swallow
  – Retching
- General malaise
- Odynophagia, or painful swallowing
- Regurgitation

If esophagitis leads to stricture formation, then regurgitation is likely to develop one to four weeks after the inciting event [34].

In most strictures, regurgitation occurs within a short time frame after eating [34]. However, if the stricture is distal, regurgitation may be delayed: food sits in the esophagus cranial to site of obstruction [34].

Regurgitation is the hallmark sign of esophageal disease [34, 43].

Regurgitation is characterized as the passive evacuation of ingesta from the esophagus [43, 44]. Unlike vomiting, in which there is centrally mediated, active expulsion of stomach and/or duodenal contents, regurgitation is a passive, locally mediated process [43, 44]. Nausea is not typically associated with regurgitation, whereas it quite commonly precedes vomiting [44].

Material that is regurgitated is typically tubular in structure, as a result of being housed within the esophagus [43]. Food is undigested and may be mixed with water [43]. Frothy saliva may be present as foam, but not bile [43].

Regurgitation may result in aspiration pneumonia [34, 43]. Signs of aspiration pneumonia include the following [33, 34, 43]:

- Adventitious lung sounds
  – Crackles
- Anorexia or reduced appetite
- Cough
- Depression
- Dyspnea
- Fever
- Increased respiratory effort
- Increased respiratory rate
- Lethargy
- Mucopurulent nasal discharge
- Respiratory distress

52.2.4.3 Megaesophagus

Megaesophagus is the condition of having a dilated, hypomotile esophagus [8, 9]. This results in regurgitation of both food and water [8, 9]. Patients with megaesophagus are likely to experience stunted growth or weight loss because what is ingested does not always make it into the lower digestive tract for processing [8, 9].

Regurgitation is an inciting factor for aspiration pneumonia in affected patients [33, 34, 43].

On physical examination, patients with megaesophagus may have a palpable esophagus that bulges outward at the thoracic inlet [8, 9, 24]. Pain may be associated with esophageal palpation [8, 9].

Megaesophagus may be [8, 9]

- Congenital [45–47]
- Acquired [22, 45, 48, 49].

Congenital megaesophagus is more likely to occur in the following [2, 43, 45–47]:

- Fox Terriers
- German Shepherd
- Great Dane
- Irish Setter
- Labrador Retriever
- Newfoundland
- Shar Pei

Among cats, the Siamese breed is predisposed [9, 43].

Most patients that are afflicted with congenital megaesophagus develop clinical signs at weaning [8, 9, 43].

Megaesophagus can also be acquired [8, 9]. Idiopathic acquired megaesophagus is common [2, 8, 9].

Other causes of acquired megaesophagus include the following [2, 22, 45, 48, 49]:

- Botulism
- Dysautonomia

(a)

(b)

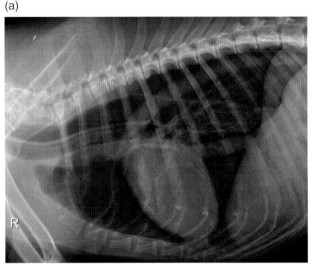 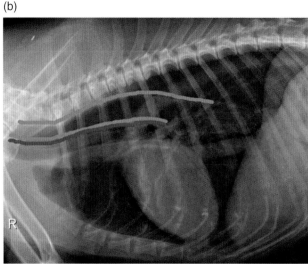

Figure 52.7 (a) This canine patient has radiographic evidence of megaesophagus. *Source:* Courtesy of Jason M Eberhardt, DVM, MS, DACVIM. (b) This is the same patient that is depicted in Figure 52.7a. Note that the borders of the esophagus have been outlined in blue. The classic "tracheal stripe" sign that is confirmatory for megaesophagus has been outlined in red. The "tracheal stripe" sign is created by summation of the dorsal tracheal wall with the ventral wall of the esophagus. *Source:* Courtesy of Jason M. Eberhardt, DVM, MS, DACVIM.

- Esophageal obstruction
- Hypoadrenocorticism
- Hypothyroidism
- Lead poisoning
- Myasthenia gravis
- Polymyositis
- Polyneuritis
- Systemic lupus erythematosus (SLE)
- Thallium toxicosis

The patient's history and clinical signs facilitate diagnosis making [2]. Survey thoracic radiographs are often diagnostic for megaesophagus [8, 9, 24] (see Figures 52.7a, b).

Caution must be taken not to over-interpret radiographs of anesthetized patients or patients that are hyperexcitable [2]. In both cases, it is not atypical to see air within the esophagus [2]. This air may be misconstrued as megaesophagus [2].

In all cases of megaesophagus, the clinician should attempt to establish the underlying etiology [2].

References

1 Pollard, R.E. (2012). Imaging evaluation of dogs and cats with Dysphagia. *ISRN Vet. Sci.* 2012: 238505.

2 Marks, S.L. (ed.) (2008). Dysphagia and regurgitation in dogs - more common than you think!. Canine Medicine Symposium.

3 Specht, A. (2017). Trismus & ptyalism. *NAVC Clinician's Brief* (March): 40–42.

4 Argenzio, R.A. (2004). Gastrointestinal motility. In: *Dukes' Physiology of Domestic Animals*, 12e (ed. H.H. Dukes and W.O. Reece), 391–404. Ithaca: Comstock Pub. Associates.

5 Evans, H.E. (1993). The digestive apparatus and abdomen. In: *Miller's Anatomy of the Dog*, 3e, xvi, 1113 p (ed. H.E. Evans and M.E. Miller). Philadelphia: W.B. Saunders.

6 Watrous, B.J. (2007). The esophagus. In: *Veterinary Diagnostic Radiology* (ed. D.E. Thrall), 494–511. St. Louis, MO: Saunders Elsevier.

7 Jergens, A.E. (2010). Diseases of esophagus. In: *Textbook of Veterinary Internal Medicine* (ed. S.J. Ettinger and E.C. Feldman), 1487–1499. St. Louis, MO: Saunders Elsevier.

8 Côté, E. (2015). *Clinical Veterinary Advisor. Dogs and Cats*, 3e, xxxvii, 1642 p. St. Louis, Missouri: Elsevier Mosby.

9 Tilley, L.P. and Smith, F.W.K. (2004). *The 5-Minute Veterinary Consult : Canine and Feline*, 3e, lviii, 1487 p. Baltimore, MD: Lippincott Williams & Wilkins.

10 Ettinger, S.J., Feldman, E.C., and Côté, E. (2017). *Textbook of Veterinary Internal Medicine : Diseases of the Dog and the Cat*, 8e, 2 volumes (lviii, 2181, I-90 p.). St. Louis, Missouri: Elsevier.

11 Allen, J. (2014). Ptyalism & pseudoptyalism. *NAVC Clinician's Brief* (June): 12–13.

12 Fiani, N., Verstraete, F.J., and Arzi, B. (2016). Reconstruction of congenital nose, cleft primary palate,

and lip disorders. *Vet. Clin. North Am. Small Anim. Pract.* 46 (4): 663–675.

13 Englar, R.E. (2017). *Performing the Small Animal Physical Examination*. Hoboken, NJ: Wiley.

14 Stokhof, A.A. and Venker-van Haagen, A.J. (2009). Respiratory system. In: *Medical History and Physical Examination in Companion Animals* (ed. A. Rijnberk and F.J. van Sluijs), 63–74. Philadephia: Saunders Elsevier.

15 Evans, J., Levesque, D., and Shelton, G.D. (2004). Canine inflammatory myopathies: a clinicopathologic review of 200 cases. *J. Vet. Intern. Med.* 18 (5): 679–691.

16 Shelton, G.D., Cardinet, G.H. 3rd, and Bandman, E. (1987). Canine masticatory muscle disorders: a study of 29 cases. *Muscle Nerve* 10 (8): 753–766.

17 Toyoda, K., Uchida, K., Matsuki, N. et al. (2010). Inflammatory myopathy with severe tongue atrophy in Pembroke Welsh Corgi dogs. *J. Vet. Diagn. Investig.* 22 (6): 876–885.

18 Ryckman, L.R., Krahwinkel, D.J., Sims, M.H. et al. (2005). Dysphagia as the primary clinical abnormality in two dogs with inflammatory myopathy. *J. Am. Vet. Med. Assoc.* 226 (9): 1519–1523. 01.

19 Peeters, M.E. and Ubbink, G.J. (1994). Dysphagia-associated muscular dystrophy: a familial trait in the bouvier des Flandres. *Vet. Rec.* 134 (17): 444–446.

20 Peeters, M.E., Venker-van Haagen, A.J., Goedegebuure, S.A., and Wolvekamp, W.T. (1991). Dysphagia in Bouviers associated with muscular dystrophy; evaluation of 24 cases. *Vet. Q.* 13 (2): 65–73.

21 Hutt, F.B. and De Lahunta, A. (1971). A lethal glossopharyngeal defect in the dog. *J. Hered.* 62 (5): 291–293.

22 Shelton, G.D., Willard, M.D., Cardinet, G.H. 3rd, and Lindstrom, J. (1990). Acquired myasthenia gravis. Selective involvement of esophageal, pharyngeal, and facial muscles. *J. Vet. Intern. Med.* 4 (6): 281–284.

23 Braund, K.G. (1980). Encephalitis and meningitis. *Vet. Clin. North Am. Small Anim. Pract.* 10 (1): 31–56.

24 Carlisle, W.T. and Egger, E.L. (1980). Differential diagnosis of persistent dysphagia and regurgitation in the young. *Iowa State Univ. Vet.* [Internet] 42 (1): 14–18. Available from: https://lib.dr.iastate.edu/cgi/viewcontent.cgi?article=2975&context=iowastate_veterinarian.

25 Kyles, A.E. (2002). Esophagus. In: *Textbook of Small Animal Surgery* (ed. D.H. Slatter), 573–592. Philadelphia: WB Saunders.

26 Ladlow, J. and Hardie, R.J. (2000). Cricopharyngeal achalasia in dogs. *Compend. Contin. Educ. Pract.* 22 (8): 750–755.

27 Davidson, A.P., Pollard, R.E., Bannasch, D.L. et al. (2004). Inheritance of cricopharyngeal dysfunction in golden retrievers. *Am. J. Vet. Res.* 65 (3): 344–349.

28 Papazoglou, L.G., Mann, F.A., Warnock, J.J., and Song, K.J.E. (2006). Cricopharyngeal dysphagia in dogs: the lateral approach for surgical management. *Compend. Contin. Educ. Pract.* 28 (10): 696–704.

29 Warnock, J.J., Marks, S.L., Pollard, R. et al. (2003). Surgical management of cricopharyngeal dysphagia in dogs: 14 cases (1989–2001). *J. Am. Vet. Med. Assoc.* 223 (10): 1462–1468.

30 Pollard, R.E., Marks, S.L., Davidson, A., and Hornof, W.J. (2000). Quantitative videofluoroscopic evaluation of pharyngeal function in the dog. *Vet. Radiol. Ultrasound* 41 (5): 409–412.

31 Pollard, R.E., Marks, S.L., Leonard, R., and Belafsky, P.C. (2007). Preliminary evaluation of the pharyngeal constriction ratio (PCR) for fluoroscopic determination of pharyngeal constriction in dysphagic dogs. *Vet. Radiol. Ultrasound* 48 (3): 221–226.

32 Watrous, B.J. (1983). Clinical presentation and diagnosis of dysphagia. *Vet. Clin. North. Am. Small Anim. Pract.* 13 (3): 437–459.

33 Bissett, S. (2012). Esophagitis. *NAVC Clinician's Brief* (June): 23–26.

34 Sherding, R.G. (2011). Esophagitis and esophageal stricture. DVM 360 [Internet]. http://veterinarycalendar.dvm360.com/esophagitis-and-esophageal-stricture-proceedings.

35 Bright, S.R., Mellanby, R.J., and Williams, J.M. (2002). Oropharyngeal stick injury in a Bengal cat. *J. Feline Med. Surg.* 4 (3): 153–155.

36 Doran, I.P., Wright, C.A., and Moore, A.H. (2008). Acute oropharyngeal and esophageal stick injury in forty-one dogs. *Vet. Surg.* 37 (8): 781–785.

37 Billen, F., Day, M.J., and Clercx, C. (2006). Diagnosis of pharyngeal disorders in dogs: a retrospective study of 67 cases. *J. Small Anim. Pract.* 47 (3): 122–129.

38 Griffiths, L.G., Tiruneh, R., Sullivan, M., and Reid, S.W. (2000). Oropharyngeal penetrating injuries in 50 dogs: a retrospective study. *Vet. Surg.* 29 (5): 383–388.

39 Kang, M.H., Lim, C.Y., and Park, H.M. (2011). Nasopharyngeal tooth foreign body in a dog. *J. Vet. Dent.* 28 (1): 26–29.

40 Buchanan, J.W. (2004). Tracheal signs and associated vascular anomalies in dogs with persistent right aortic arch. *J. Vet. Intern. Med.* 18 (4): 510–514.

41 Leib, M.S. (ed.) (2005). *Doxcyline Esophagitis / Stricture in Cats*. Orlando, Floria: NAVC.

42 McGrotty, Y.L. and Knottenbelt, C.M. (2002). Oesophageal stricture in a cat due to oral administration of tetracyclines. *J. Small Anim. Pract.* 43 (5): 221–223.

43 Sherding, R.G. (2011). Regurgitation, dysphagia, and esophageal dysmotility. DVM 360 [Internet]. http://veterinarycalendar.dvm360.com/regurgitation-dysphagia-and-esophageal-dysmotility-proceedings.

44 Gallagher, A. (2012). Regurgitation or vomiting? *NAVC Clinician's Brief* (June): 33–35.

45 Washabau, R.J. (2003). Gastrointestinal motility disorders and gastrointestinal prokinetic therapy. *Vet. Clin. North Am. Small Anim. Pract.* 33 (5): 1007–1028, vi.

46 Holland, C.T., Satchell, P.M., and Farrow, B.R. (1996). Vagal esophagomotor nerve function and esophageal motor performance in dogs with congenital idiopathic megaesophagus. *Am. J. Vet. Res.* 57 (6): 906–913.

47 Holland, C.T., Satchell, P.M., and Farrow, B.R. (2002). Selective vagal afferent dysfunction in dogs with congenital idiopathic megaoesophagus. *Auton. Neurosci.* 99 (1): 18–23.

48 Gaynor, A.R., Shofer, F.S., and Washabau, R.J. (1997). Risk factors for acquired megaesophagus in dogs. *J. Am. Vet. Med. Assoc.* 211 (11): 1406–1412.

49 Shelton, G.D., Schule, A., and Kass, P.H. (1997). Risk factors for acquired myasthenia gravis in dogs: 1,154 cases (1991–1995). *J. Am. Vet. Med. Assoc.* 211 (11): 1428–1431.

53

Halitosis

53.1 Halitosis, Defined

Halitosis is the appropriate medical terminology for bad breath [1, 2]. Simply put, halitosis is a displeasing odor that arises from the oral cavity. It may be apparent on physical examination during intraoral evaluation. It may also be detected when the clinician stands within breathing room of a panting canine patient. More frequently, clients complain of halitosis during the veterinary consultation [3–6]. They often ask what can be done to remedy the situation with the hope that there is an easy fix [6].

53.2 Causes of Halitosis

The most common cause of halitosis is periodontal disease [1, 2].

Other causes of halitosis include the following [1–3, 5, 7–18]:

- Abnormal ingestive behavior or pica (see Chapter 48)
  - Chemical burns secondary to the ingestion of caustic substances
  - Coprophagy, the ingestion of fecal matter
  - Electrical burns secondary to chewing on electric cords
- Extraoral factors
  - Dermatitis, including lip fold pyoderma (see Chapter 12, Section 12.3.1) [13]
  - Dirty or wet "beards" of dogs with abundant facial fur, such as Schnauzers
  - Gastrointestinal obstruction
    - Foreign body
    - Neoplasia
    - Stricture
  - Hepatopathy
  - Inflammatory bowel disease (IBD)
  - Megaesophagus (see Chapter 52, Section 52.2.4)
  - Metabolic dysfunction
    - Ketones secondary to diabetic ketoacidosis (DKA)
    - Uremia secondary to renal disease

- Rhinitis (see Chapter 33)
  - Sinusitis
  - Small intestinal bacterial overgrowth (SIBO)
- Oral factors
  - Abscess
    - Soft tissue
    - Tooth root (see Figure 53.1a)
  - Cleft palate (see Chapter 33, Section 33.8 and Chapter 52, Section 52.2.1) (refer to Figures 52.1a and b)
  - Eosinophilic granuloma complex (see Chapter 12, Section 12.3.2)
  - Fracture
    - Jaw
    - One or more teeth (see Figure 53.1b)
  - Malocclusion (see Figure 53.1c)
  - Neoplasia and associated tissue necrosis
  - Oronasal fistula (see Figure 53.1d)
  - Pathologic bleeding, hemorrhage, as is associated with
    - Coagulopathy
    - Oral tumors
  - Physiologic bleeding associated with teething
  - Retained teeth (see Chapter 49, Section 49.3) (see Figure 53.1e)
  - Stomatitis
  - Supernumerary teeth (see Chapter 49, Section 49.2)
  - Tooth resorption (see Chapter 49, Section 49.5)

53.3 Periodontal Disease and Halitosis

The most common cause of halitosis is periodontal disease, a condition that affects the periodontium [1, 2, 19]. The periodontium refers to the supporting structures that surround the teeth [19–21]:

- Alveolar bone
- Gingiva
- Periodontal ligament

Common Clinical Presentations in Dogs and Cats, First Edition. Ryane E. Englar.
© 2019 John Wiley & Sons, Inc. Published 2019 by John Wiley & Sons, Inc.

(a)

(b)

(d)

(c)

(e)

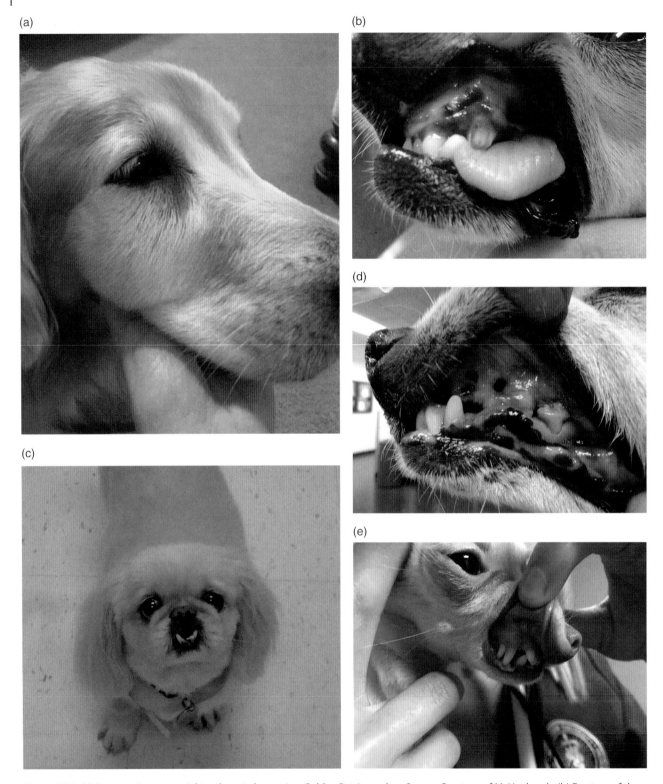

Figure 53.1 (a) Presumptive carnassial tooth root abscess in a Golden Retriever dog. *Source:* Courtesy of M. Upchurch. (b) Fracture of the left maxillary canine tooth in a dog. *Source:* Courtesy of Patricia Bennett, DVM. (c) Significant underbite in a canine patient. (d) Oronasal fistula in a canine patient. *Source:* Courtesy of Patricia Bennett, DVM. (e) Retained right maxillary deciduous canine tooth. *Source:* Courtesy of John A. Schwartz.

(a)

(b)

(c)

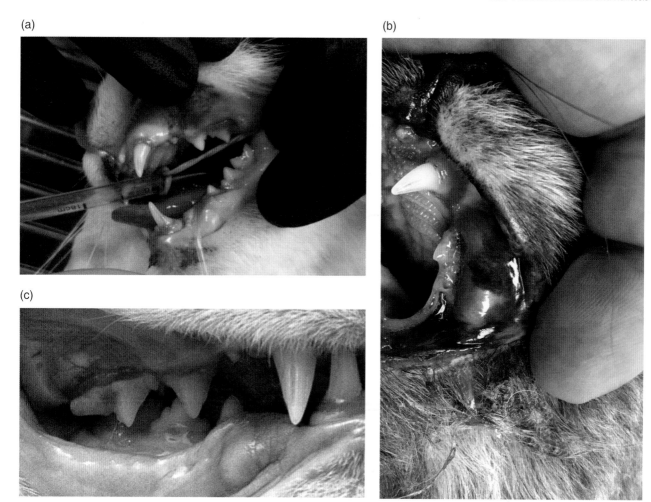

Figure 53.2 (a) Focal gingivitis associated with this cat's left maxillary and mandibular canine tooth. *Source:* Courtesy of Dr. Elizabeth Robbins. (b) Marked gingivitis associated with this feline patient's left maxillary dental arcade. *Source:* Courtesy of Frank Isom, DVM. (c) Marked gingivitis associated with this feline patient's right maxillary dental arcade. *Source:* Courtesy of the Media Resources Department at Midwestern University.

A patient is said to have periodontal disease when one or more of the aforementioned structures is inflamed [19, 22].

Gingivitis, inflammation of the gum line, represents the earliest stage of periodontal disease [19]. It may be focal or diffuse (see Figures 53.2a–c).

Intraoral bacterial populations contribute to gingival irritation as well as subgingival disease [1, 2, 19, 22].

The glycoproteins that are in saliva cover the surfaces of teeth in a slick film [1, 2, 19]. This film is disrupted during professional teeth cleaning; however, it reestablishes itself within hours after dental prophylaxis [1, 2, 19]. Bacteria take up residence within this film to form plaque [1, 2, 19].

Plaque mineralizes within a few days to form dental calculus [1, 2, 19] (see Figures 53.3a, b).

The immune system initiates an inflammatory response against plaque and calculus [1, 2, 19, 22]. This response

has the potential to damage the supporting structures of the teeth [1, 2, 19]. For example, gingival recession is common [1, 2, 19]. The gingival sulci deepen into pockets [1, 2, 19]. These pockets allow food to accumulate. Because of this abundant food source, bacteria thrive. However, bacterial metabolism produces volatile compounds that damage the integrity of intraoral tissues [1, 2, 19, 22].

Over time, the following sequelae may result [1, 2, 19, 23–26]:

- Exposure of tooth roots
- Focal infection
- Loss of alveolar bone and/or the periodontal ligament
- Increased mobility of affected teeth
  Loss of affected teeth
  - Affected teeth may fall out
  - Affected teeth may require surgical extraction (see Figures 53.4a, b)

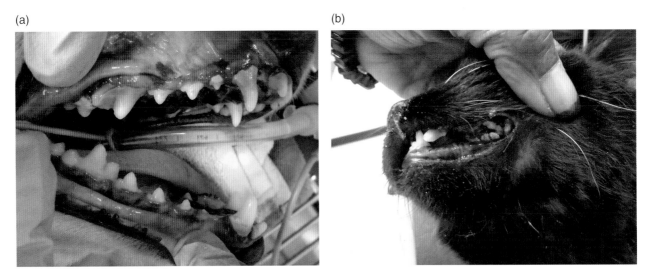

Figure 53.3 (a) Diffuse dental calculus in a canine patient that presented for dental prophylaxis. (b) Dental calculus in a feline patient that presented for dental prophylaxis. *Source:* Courtesy of Patricia Bennett, DVM.

(a)

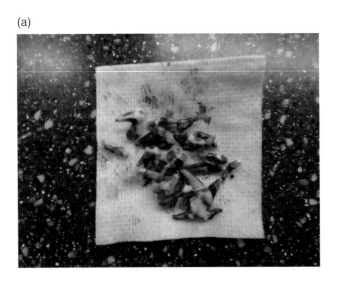

(b)

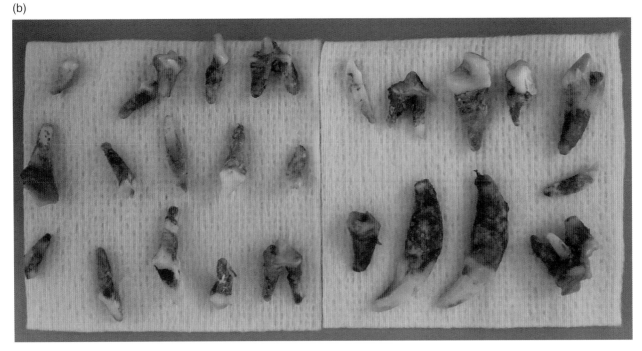

Figure 53.4 (a) These teeth had to be surgically extracted due to periodontal disease. (b) These teeth had to be surgically extracted due to periodontal disease. *Source:* Courtesy of Joseph Onello, DVM.

Assessing cats and dogs for periodontal disease requires an extensive oral examination under general anesthesia. This evaluation should take care to assess the following [19, 23, 24, 27]:

- Each and every tooth in the oral cavity
- Each gingival sulcus, looking for evidence of pocketing
- Root exposure
- The integrity of the surrounding alveolar bone

When periodontal disease is diagnosed, it may involve one or more teeth [19]. Each tooth is assigned a score based upon staging nomenclature that was developed by the American Veterinary Dental College [20–24, 28, 29].

- PD 0: Negative for gingivitis, with radiographically normal periodontium.
- PD 1: Gingivitis is present as the only indication of periodontal disease. The periodontium is radiographically normal.

- PD 2: Gingivitis is present, and radiographic signs of periodontal disease are present: at most there is 25% loss of periodontal attachment.
- PD 3: Gingivitis is present, and radiographic signs are progressive: there is between 25 and 50% loss of periodontal attachment.
- PD 4: Periodontal disease is advanced, with >50% loss of periodontal attachment.

Note that whole mouth radiographs are required to stage any patient for periodontal disease [1, 2, 19] (see Figures 53.5a–d).

Periodontal disease is an important consideration for oral health in every veterinary patient. Any patient may develop periodontal disease; however, the following patients are at an increased risk [21]:

- Small-breed dogs and brachycephalic patients
  - More likely to have malocclusions
  - More likely to have overcrowding of teeth
  - More likely to have retained deciduous teeth

(a) (b)

(c) (d)

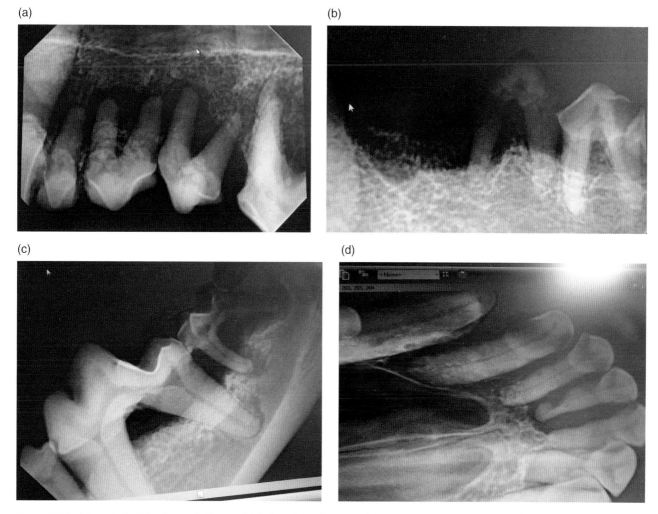

Figure 53.5 (a) Sample dental radiograph. Note multiple furcations, that is, tooth root exposure. *Source:* Courtesy of Patricia Bennett, DVM. (b) Sample dental radiograph. *Source:* Courtesy of Patricia Bennett, DVM. (c) Sample dental radiograph. Note multiple furcations, that is, tooth root exposure. *Source:* Courtesy of Patricia Bennett, DVM. (d) Sample dental radiograph. *Source:* Courtesy of Patricia Bennett, DVM.

- Those with abnormal ingestive behaviors
  - Chewing on rocks increases the likelihood of gingival trauma and/or fractured teeth
- Those that consume only soft or semi-moist foods
  - Less mechanical abrasion
- Those with a history of systemic illness that adversely impacted enamel development (see Chapter 49, Section 49.6)
  - Canine distemper virus (CDV)
- Those with a history of chronic disease that may reduce immune health or impair wound healing
  - Feline immunodeficiency virus (FIV)
  - Feline leukemia virus (FeLV)
  - Hyperadrenocorticism
  - Hypothyroidism

Periodontal disease contributes substantially to halitosis [1, 2, 19]. Oral malodor results from a combination of decomposing food and by-products of bacterial metabolism [1, 2]. These noxious substances include the following [2]:

- Dimethyl sulfide
- Hydrogen sulfide
- Methyl mercaptan
- Volatile fatty acids

These compounds contain sulfur [2]. Sulfur is produced primarily by gram-negative anaerobic bacteria, such as *Actinomyces, Bacteroides,* and *Fusobacterium* spp. [2, 3, 5].

Sulfur confers an unpleasant odor to the mouth [2].

The best way to manage halitosis from periodontal disease is to treat the patient's periodontal disease [2].

Clients may also be directed to use oral care products that contain zinc [2]. Zinc, among other metal ions, has a high affinity for sulfur [2]. Zinc–sulfur complexes inhibit microbial proliferation [2].

Chlorhexidine rinses and pastes may also reduce odor and control plaque [2].

53.4 Malocclusions and Halitosis

A malocclusion occurs when there is misalignment of the teeth [2]. Misalignment may result from a primary dental issue or a primary skeletal issue [2, 19].

Class 1 malocclusions are the result of the former clinical scenario: the jaw is the correct length, but one or more teeth are malpositioned [2, 19].

Overcrowding is a type of Class 1 malocclusion that is commonly seen in toy breeds, small-breed dogs, and brachycephalic patients (see Figures 53.6a, b).

Class 2 and Class 3 malocclusions are skeletal issues involving jaw length [23, 28].

A Class II malocclusion occurs when the mandible is shorter than expected [2, 19]. This results in so-called "parrot mouth," that is, an overbite [2, 19]. The maxillary dental arcades protrude beyond the mandibular arcades [2, 19] (see Figure 53.7).

(a)

(b)

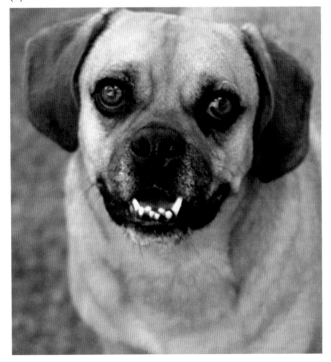
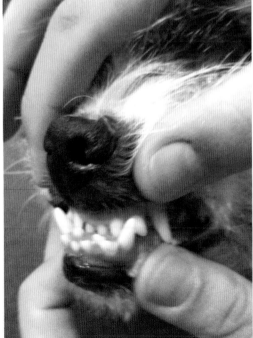

Figure 53.6 (a) Crowding of the teeth in this brachycephalic patient has led to irregularly spaced mandibular incisors. *Source:* Courtesy of Shelby Newton. (b) Note the irregular spacing between #301–303. *Source:* Courtesy of David A. May.

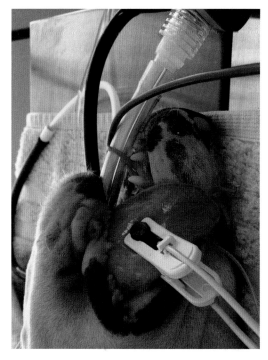

Figure 53.7 This patient has a prominent overbite. *Source:* Courtesy of Jeana E. Barrow, MS.

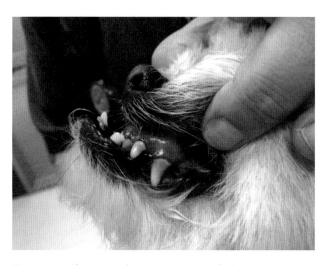

Figure 53.8 This patient has a prominent underbite.

If this is severe, the mandibular canine teeth may contact the hard palate, causing mechanical irritation or ulceration. It is possible for an oronasal fistula to develop if the mandibular canine teeth penetrate through the hard palate [23, 28, 30].

A Class III malocclusion is characterized by either mandibular prognathism, a longer than normal mandible, or maxillary brachygnathism, a shorter than normal maxilla [2, 19]. This results in so-called "monkey mouth," that is, an underbite [2, 19]. The mandibular dental arcades protrude beyond the maxillary dental arcades [28, 30] (see Figure 53.8).

Malocclusions of any class may contribute to halitosis because they create abnormal surfaces that support plaque formation. For example, the overcrowding of the teeth creates additional nooks and crannies in which food particles can hide. This adds to the amount of particulate matter that is decomposing within the oral cavity at any given point in time [3, 5, 31–33]. Putrefaction causes a distinct odor.

53.5 Oral Tumors and Halitosis

Oral cavity tumors are relatively common clinical presentations in companion animal practice. They come in a variety of shapes and sizes, and may progress rapidly (see Figures 53.9a, b).

As these masses grow, they may ulcerate and/or become necrotic. Those that do contribute to halitosis. As tissues decompose and/or become secondarily infected, a rancid or rotting odor is quite common.

Indirectly, oral tumors that hemorrhage also have a distinct odor that comes from the smell of blood (see Figures 53.10a, b).

The majority of oral cavity tumors in the cat are malignant [15, 34–36]. The most common type of oral malignancy in the cat is squamous cell carcinoma (SCC) [12, 14, 16, 34, 35].

SCC is most likely to target the following locations in the cat [15, 34]:

- Beneath the tongue
- Buccal mucosa
- Caudal pharynx
- Lip
- Mandible
- Maxilla
- Tongue

Metastasis from SCC was once thought to be relatively uncommon; however, recent research suggests that spread to the mandibular lymph nodes occurs in slightly more than one-third of all cases [15, 37–40].

Complete surgical excision offers the best prognosis in theory; however, rarely is the lesion in a location that is amenable to complete resection [15].

The following are considered risk factors for the development of SCC in cats [15, 41–43]:

- Eating canned food
- Eating tuna
- Ingesting environmental tobacco smoke and soot
- Wearing flea collars

Note that SCC is not the only type of oral malignancy in cats, nor is it restricted to this one particular species [15]. SCC may also affect dogs [15].

(a)   (b)

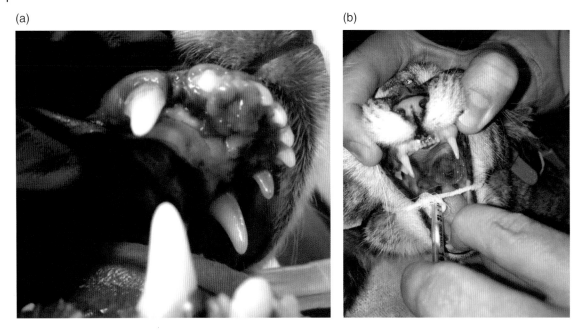

Figure 53.9 (a) Oral mass associated with the maxillary arcades of teeth in this canine patient. (b) Squamous cell carcinoma (SCC) associated with the caudal pharynx of this feline patient. *Source:* Courtesy of Beki Cohen Regan, DVM, DACVIM (Oncology).

(a)   (b)

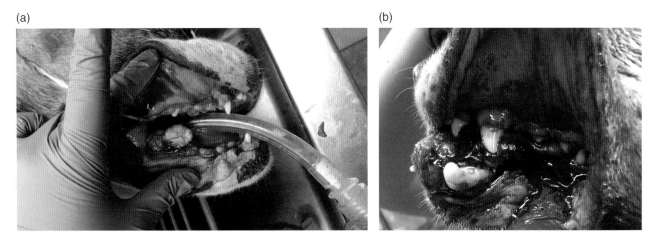

Figure 53.10 (a) Extensive gingival hyperplasia in a canine patient. The tissue is friable and irritated, causing it to hemorrhage with minimal manipulation. *Source:* Courtesy of Dr. Lauren Griggs. (b) Aggressive, extensive, hemorrhagic oral mass. *Source:* Courtesy of Dr. Stephanie Harris.

In addition to SCC, the following tumor types are possible [2, 11, 15, 34, 42]:

- Chondrosarcoma
- Fibrosarcoma
- Lymphoma
- Mast cell tumor
- Melanoma
- Osteosarcoma
- Plasma cell tumor
- Salivary adenocarcinoma

Fibrosarcoma is the second most common oral malignancy in the cat [2].

In the dog, malignant melanoma is the most common oral malignancy, followed by SCC and then fibrosarcoma [2].

Concerning malignant melanoma in dogs, the following breeds may be predisposed [2]:

- Chow Chows
- Cocker Spaniels
- German Shepherds

The incidence of malignant melanoma is also more likely in dogs with pigmented mucous membranes [2].

Male dogs also appear in the medical literature concerning malignant melanoma more so than females [2].

Note that not all growths in the oral cavity are malignant [2]. Benign growths within the oral cavity are also possible, and may resemble neoplasia [15]. Consider, for example, bacterial and fungal abscesses, granulomas, and osteomyelitis [15].

Patients with oral tumors tend to present with one or more of the following clinical signs [15]:

- Blood-tinged saliva
- Decreased appetite
- Discolored coat from salivary staining
- Dysphagia
- Inability to close the mouth
- Increased mobility of neighboring teeth
- Oral swelling
- Pain upon opening the mouth
- Ptyalism
- Reduction in grooming behaviors
- Thick, ropy saliva
- Weight loss (see Figures 53.11a, b)

Oral examination will confirm the presence of a neoplastic growth [15]. However, additional diagnostic testing to evaluate cellular morphology is essential to diagnose mass type [15].

Fine-needle aspiration is unrealistic in an awake patient. It is unlikely to obtain a representative sample in a safe manner – safe for the handler, clinician, and patient alike [15]. An incisional biopsy is the preferred sampling technique because it will provide information about cellular architecture [15].

Imaging of tumors is an important secondary step to establish the invasiveness of the growth relative to vital structures [15]. Radiographs can provide important information in terms of how much bone is involved, and to what extent [15]. For example, radiographs may demonstrate osteolysis and tooth resorption [15].

However, radiographs are not ideal as a stand-alone imaging modality for surgical planning [15]. Thirty to fifty percent of bone mineral content must be lost in order to be detected on radiographic film [15]. Therefore, computed tomography (CT) and/or magnetic resonance imaging (MRI) are considered superior [15].

(a)　　　　　　　　(b)

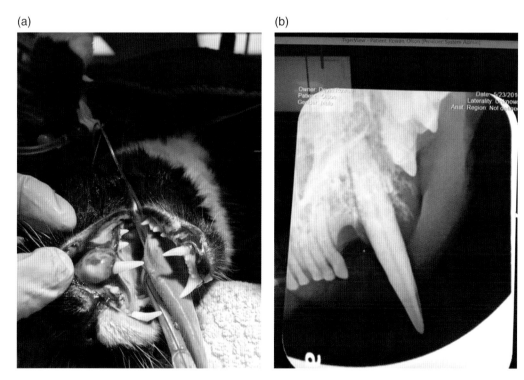

Figure 53.11 (a) Pronounced, firm gingival swelling associated with the left maxillary canine tooth in this feline patient. This was later diagnosed as squamous cell carcinoma (SCC). (b) Dental radiograph taken from the same patient depicted in Figure 53.11a. Note the destruction of the supportive tissue surrounding the root of the affected canine tooth. On physical examination, the affected tooth exhibited mobility.

References

1 Côté, E. (2015). *Clinical Veterinary Advisor. Dogs and Cats*, 3e, xxxvii, 1642 p. St. Louis, Missouri: Elsevier Mosby.

2 Tilley, L.P. and Smith, F.W.K. (2004). *The 5-Minute Veterinary Consult: Canine and Feline*, 3e, lviii, 1487 p. Baltimore, MD: Lippincott Williams & Wilkins.

3 Eubanks, D.L. (2009). "Doggy breath": what causes it, how do I evaluate it, and what can I do about it? *J. Vet. Dent.* 26 (3): 192–193.

4 Simone, A., Jensen, L., Setser, C. et al. (1994). Assessment of oral malodor in dogs. *J. Vet. Dent.* 11 (2): 71–74.

5 Eubanks, D.L. (2006). Canine oral malodor. *J. Am. Anim. Hosp. Assoc.* 42 (1): 77–79.

6 Low, S.B., Peak, R.M., Smithson, C.W. et al. (2014). Evaluation of a topical gel containing a novel combination of essential oils and antioxidants for reducing oral malodor in dogs. *Am. J. Vet. Res.* 75 (7): 653–657.

7 Bellows, J. (2012). Halitosis. *NAVC Clinician's Brief* (April): 24–25.

8 Tabor, B. (2008). Understanding and treating diabetic ketoacidosis. *Vet. Tech.* [Internet] 29 (4). Available from: http://www.vetfolio.com/internal-medicine/understanding-and-treating-diabetic-ketoacidosis.

9 Sherding, R.G. (2011). Regurgitation, dysphagia, and esophageal dysmotility. DVM 360 [Internet]. http://veterinarycalendar.dvm360.com/regurgitation-dysphagia-and-esophageal-dysmotility-proceedings.

10 Mace, S., Shelton, G.D., and Eddlestone, S. (2012). Megaesophagus. *Compend Contin. Educ. Vet.* 34 (2): E1.

11 Ehrhart, N. (2013). Common oral tumors in dogs and cats. *NAVC Clinician's Brief* (January).

12 Perrone, J.R. (2016). Top 5 feline oral health concerns. Veterinary Team Brief. (January/February).

13 Reiter, A. Oral inflammatory and ulcerative disease in small animals. Merck Veterinary Manual [Internet]. https://www.merckvetmanual.com/digestive-system/diseases-of-the-mouth-in-small-animals/oral-inflammatory-and-ulcerative-disease-in-small-animals.

14 Pellin, M. and Turek, M. (2016). A review of feline oral squamous cell carcinoma. *Today's Veterinary Practice* (November/December): 24–33.

15 Bilgic, O., Duda, L., Sanchez, M.D., and Lewis, J.R. (2015). Feline oral squamous cell carcinoma: clinical manifestations and literature review. *J. Vet. Dent.* 32 (1): 30–40.

16 Garrett, L.D. and Marretta, S.M. (2007). Feline oral squamous cell carcinoma: an overview. DVM 360 [Internet]. http://veterinarymedicine.dvm360.com/feline-oral-squamous-cell-carcinoma-overview.

17 Soltero-Rivera, M.M., Krick, E.L., Reiter, A.M. et al. (2014). Prevalence of regional and distant metastasis in cats with advanced oral squamous cell carcinoma: 49 cases (2005–2011). *J. Feline Med. Surg.* 16 (2): 164–169.

18 Cornell Feline Health Center. Oral Cavity tumors. Cornell University College of Veterinary Medicine [Internet]. https://www2.vet.cornell.edu/departments-centers-and-institutes/cornell-feline-health-center/health-information/feline-health-topics/oral-cavity-tumors.

19 Englar, R.E. (2017). *Performing the Small Animal Physical Examination*. Hoboken, NJ: Wiley.

20 American Veterinary Dental College. (1988). Periodontal disease: information for pet owners. AVDC [Internet]. https://www.avdc.org/periodontaldisease.html.

21 Royal Veterinary College. (2002). Veterinary periodontal disease. RVC [Internet]. www.rvc.ac.uk/review/dentistry/Shared_Media/pdfs/perio_print.pdf.

22 Reiter, A.M. Periodontal disease in small animals. Merck Veterinary Manual [Internet]. https://www.merckvetmanual.com/digestive-system/dentistry/periodontal-disease-in-small-animals.

23 Holmstrom, S.E. and Holmstrom, S.E. (2013). *Veterinary Dentistry: A Team Approach*, 2e, viii, 434 p. St. Louis, Mo: Elsevier/Mosby.

24 Lobprise, H.B. and Wiggs, R.B. (2000). *The Veterinarian's Companion for Common Dental Procedures*. Lakewood, Colorado: AAHA Press.

25 Clarke, D.E. and Caiafa, A. (2014). Oral examination in the cat: a systematic approach. *J. Feline Med. Surg.* 16 (11): 873–886.

26 Reiter, A.M. and Soltero-Rivera, M.M. (2014). Applied feline oral anatomy and tooth extraction techniques: an illustrated guide. *J. Feline Med. Surg.* 16 (11): 900–913.

27 Lemmons, M. (2013). Clinical feline dental radiography. *Vet. Clin. North Am. Small Anim. Pract.* 43 (3): 533–554.

28 American Veterinary Dental College (AVDC), AVDC Nomenclature. [Internet]. https://www.avdc.org/Nomenclature/Nomen-Intro.html (accessed 6 May 2019).

29 Holmstrom, S.E. (2012). Veterinary dentistry in senior canines and felines. *Vet. Clin. North Am. Small Anim. Pract.* 42 (4): 793–808, viii.

30 Shipp, A.D. and Fahrenkrug, P. (1992). *Practitioners' Guide to Veterinary Dentistry*, 237. Glendale, CA: Griffin Printing, Inc.

31 Culham, N. and Rawlings, J.M. (1998). Oral malodor and its relevance to periodontal disease in the dog. *J. Vet. Dent.* 15 (4): 165–168.

32 Hennet, P., Delille, B., and Davot, J.L. (1995). Oral malodor in dogs: measurement using a sulfide monitor. *J. Vet. Dent.* 12 (3): 101–103.

33 Rawlings, J.M. and Culham, N. (1998). Studies of oral malodor in the dog. *J. Vet. Dent.* 15 (4): 169–173.

34 Liptak, J.M. and Withrow, S.J. (2007). Oral tumors. In: *Small Animal Clinical Oncology* (ed. S.J. Withrow and D.M. Vail), 455–478. St. Louis, MO: Saunders Elsevier.

35 Stebbins, K.E., Morse, C.C., and Goldschmidt, M.H. (1989). Feline oral neoplasia: a ten-year survey. *Vet. Pathol.* 26 (2): 121–128.

36 Harvey, C.E. and Emily, P. (1993). Oral neoplasms. In: *Small Animal Dentistry* (ed. C.E. Harvey and P. Emily), 306. St. Louis: Mosby.

37 Hayes, A.M., Adams, V.J., Scase, T.J., and Murphy, S. (2007). Survival of 54 cats with oral squamous cell carcinoma in United Kingdom general practice. *J. Small Anim. Pract.* 48 (7): 394–399.

38 Hutson, C.A., Willauer, C.C., Walder, E.J. et al. (1992). Treatment of mandibular squamous-cell carcinoma in cats by use of mandibulectomy and radiotherapy – 7 cases (1987–1989). *J. Am. Vet. Med. Assoc.* 201 (5): 777–781.

39 Gendler, A., Lewis, J.R., Reetz, J.A., and Schwarz, T. (2010). Computed tomographic features of oral squamous cell carcinoma in cats: 18 cases (2002–2008). *J. Am. Vet. Med. A.* 236 (3): 319–325.

40 Reeves, N.C.P., Turrel, J.M., and Withrow, S.J. (1993). Oral squamous-cell carcinoma in the cat. *J. Am. Anim. Hosp. Assoc.* 29 (5): 438–441.

41 Bertone, E.R., Snyder, L.A., and Moore, A.S. (2003). Environmental and lifestyle risk factors for oral squamous cell carcinoma in domestic cats. *J. Vet. Intern. Med.* 17 (4): 557–562.

42 Marretta, J.J., Garrett, L.D., and Marretta, S.M. (2007). Feline oral squamous cell carcinoma: an overview. *Vet. Med.-Us.* 102 (6): 392–406.

43 Snyder, L.A., Bertone, E.R., Jakowski, R.M. et al. (2004). p53 expression and environmental tobacco smoke exposure in feline oral squamous cell carcinoma. *Vet. Pathol.* 41 (3): 209–214.

54

Emesis

54.1 Introduction to Emesis

Emesis is the appropriate medical term for the act of vomiting, that is, the forceful expulsion of ingesta from the stomach and out of the body, through the oral cavity [1–10].

Vomiting is a reflex that requires neural integration at the level of the lateral reticular formation of the medulla oblongata [1, 2, 7, 8, 11]. This so-called vomiting center receives input from four primary sources that collectively communicate the body's need for gastric evacuation [1–3, 5, 7, 9, 11–13]:

- Cerebral cortex
- Chemoreceptor trigger zone (CRTZ)
- Peripheral sensory receptors
- Vestibular apparatus

These four regions may be thought of as relay stations that pass the message on to the vomiting center so that it can initiate vomiting when emesis is warranted [3, 11].

The cerebral cortex plays a significant role in prompting emesis in humans [1]. Consider, for example, how stress, anxiety, and excitement can trigger the vomiting reflex [2]. It is thought that animals may also experience psychogenic vomiting, although the mechanisms associated with this have not yet been established [1, 2].

The CRTZ, which is positioned within the floor of the fourth ventricle of the medulla, screens the blood for chemical red flags [1, 2, 11]. This is possible because the blood–brain barrier is incomplete at this location, allowing the CRTZ to function as a chemical sensor [1, 2, 11, 12]. The presence of certain substances in the bloodstream raises alarm and will trigger communication between the CRTZ and the vomiting center. These include the following [1, 2, 13]:

- Drugs
  - Antibiotics
  - Apomorphine
  - Cardiac glycosides
  - Chemotherapeutic agents
  - Morphine
  - Non-steroidal anti-inflammatory drugs (NSAIDs)
  - Salicylates
- Toxins
  - Bacterial
  - Uremic

Peripheral sensory receptors are widely distributed throughout the body; however, their greatest concentration is within abdominal viscera [1, 2]. If one or more visceral organs become distended, the degree of stretch is registered and translated into an electrical impulse that is received by the vomiting center [1, 2]. Inflammation without significant distension can also trigger the vomiting reflex, particularly within the following organs and tissues [1]:

- Antrum of stomach
- Bowel
  - Small intestine
    - Especially the duodenum
  - Large intestine
- Pancreas
- Peritoneum

This explains why, for example, constipated cats often vomit: large bowel distension provides feedback to the vomiting center to initiate emesis.

Although organs of the digestive tract are most frequently implicated in vomiting, non-digestive organs can also trigger emesis. For instance, the heart and genitourinary tract also report to the emetic center via the vagus and sympathetic nerve trunk [1, 12].

Finally, the vestibular system provides inputs to the vomiting center. Recall from Chapter 23, Section 23.4.4 that the vestibular system is tasked with maintaining the body's sense of balance [14–18]. A body that is balanced is able to coordinate posture and eye position relative to where the head is positioned and how it moves through space [14, 19].

To be functional, the vestibular system requires both central and peripheral components [14].

Common Clinical Presentations in Dogs and Cats, First Edition. Ryane E. Englar.

The central vestibular system is composed of the brainstem, the cerebellum, and two caudal cerebellar peduncles [20, 21]. Within the brainstem, there are eight vestibular nuclei [20, 21]. These communicate via the medial longitudinal fasciculus and the third, fourth, and sixth cranial nerves, with the spinal cord, the cerebrum, and the extraocular muscles [20–22].

The peripheral vestibular system is composed of the middle ear and inner ear, including the semicircular canals, the utricle and saccule, and the eighth cranial nerve, CN VIII, the vestibulocochlear nerve [20–22].

It is the peripheral vestibular system that provides inputs to the vomiting center via CN VIII [2]. This explains why patients with vestibular disease or other disorders of balance, including motion sickness, vomit [1, 2, 11].

54.2 The Act of Vomiting and the Vomitus

The vomiting center integrates messages that it receives from all sources [11]. Once the decision to initiate vomiting is made, the vomiting center launches a coordinated series of actions to evacuate the stomach [1, 2, 11].

Nausea precedes vomiting [1, 2]. Cats and dogs that are nauseous exhibit one or more of the following clinical signs [2, 5, 11]:

- Lip licking
- Pronounced, frequent swallowing
- Ptyalism

As the patient prepares to vomit, stomach tone decreases and proximal small bowel contractions increase [2]. These peristaltic waves cause bile and pancreatic juices to flow retrograde into the stomach [2, 5].

Retching is initiated when the patient reflexively closes the glottis while moving the chest wall and diaphragm in the same manner as they would during inspiration [2, 11]. Simultaneously, the antral and pyloric parts of the stomach contract [2]. This leads to emesis [2].

During the act of vomiting, stomach contents are forcibly brought into the esophagus and out through the mouth [2, 11]. For this to occur, the cardia of the stomach has to relax [2].

Vomiting is an active process [2, 4]. Expelling ingesta in this matter requires force. The patient has to work to bring material up and out of the digestive tract.

Those observing the vomiting patient should notice abdominal contractions and heaving. These create a very different clinical picture than regurgitation [23]. It is critical that these two processes are differentiated based upon clinical appearance because they are not the same [4].

Each has its own differential list, and there is not much overlap between the two.

Recall that regurgitation was first introduced in Chapter 52, Section 52.2.4.2 as the hallmark sign of esophageal disease [24, 25].

Regurgitation is characterized as the passive evacuation of ingesta from the esophagus [4, 23, 24]. Food falls out of the upper digestive tract without abdominal contractions. There is no effort with regurgitation, whereas vomiting consumes energy. Nausea also does not typically precede regurgitation, unlike vomiting [23, 24].

Regurgitated material is typically tubular because it was housed within the esophagus [24]. It is often undigested and may be mixed with water and frothy saliva, but not bile [24]. Vomiting, on the other hand, is often rich in bile. Bile is green to yellow-brown fluid that is made by the liver and stored by the gall bladder.

Bile is typically released to assist with digestion; however, it is typically seen with vomiting, particularly when emesis occurs on an empty stomach (see Figures 54.1a–d).

Vomitus may also contain blood, semi-digested food, and/or non-food items (see Figures 54.2a–e).

54.3 Consequences of Vomiting

As an isolated event, vomiting is unlikely to cause harm other than general malaise: it is not uncommon for patients to appear "off" immediately following the episode.

However, vomiting that is protracted is likely to cause dehydration [1, 2].

Dehydration is determined by a number of physical examination and clinicopathologic parameters that include the following [1, 26, 27]:

- Capillary refill time (CRT)
- Complete blood count (CBC)
  - Hemoconcentration, with increased total solids, points to dehydration
- Mucous membrane moisture
  - Tacky mucous membranes are suggestive of dehydration in a non-panting patient
- Pulse quality
- Serum chemistry panel
  - Pre-renal azotemia is supportive of dehydration
- Skin turgor
- Urine specific gravity (USG)
  - Concentrated urine is supportive of dehydration

Skin turgor is an assessment of the skin's elasticity [26]. It can be evaluated by grasping a generous fold of skin at the nape of the neck or between the shoulder blades, and lifting it up gently, but firmly [26]. Some refer to this process as checking for a skin tent (see Figures 54.3a, b).

(a)

(b)

(c)

(d)

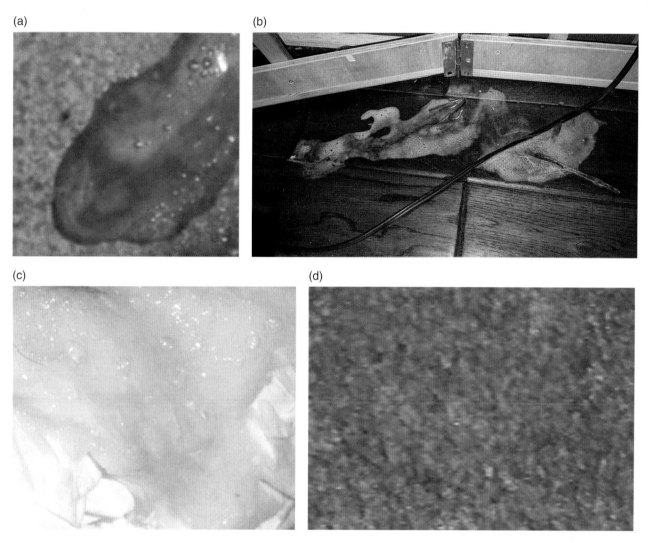

Figure 54.1 (a) The typical appearance of bile in vomitus. (b) The typical appearance of bile in vomitus, which also contains isolated bits of vegetation. *Source:* Courtesy of Tara Beugel. (c) Bile on a sheet. (d) Bile-stained carpet.

The skin fold is released [26]. One of two outcomes is possible [26]:

- In a euhydrated patient, skin elasticity causes the fold to return to its normal position almost instantaneously. In other words, there is not a persistent skin tent.
- As the patient dehydrates, the skin loses elasticity. It is slow to bounce back. In cases of severe dehydration, it does not return to its normal position at all. Rather, it stays tented.

The smallest percentage at which dehydration is clinically detectable is 5% [26].

Moderate to severe dehydration may cause hypovolemic shock [11].

Dehydration may also lead to imbalances in electrolytes [2, 11]. Water, sodium, chloride, hydrogen, and potassium are lost in vomitus [2]. Of these, potassium deficiency is most common in patients with protracted vomiting [2].

Vomiting may also cause disturbances in the patient's whole body acid–base status [2, 11]. Metabolic acidosis and metabolic alkalosis are possible [2]. Either change in acid–base status may be fatal [11].

In addition to causing dehydration, vomiting may also cause abdominal discomfort [1, 2]. This may be apparent on physical examination as a patient that guards its abdomen.

Vomiting may also lead to aspiration pneumonia [11, 24, 25]. Recall from Chapter 52, Section 52.2.4.2 that signs of aspiration pneumonia include the following [24, 25, 28]:

- Adventitious lung sounds
  - Crackles
- Anorexia or reduced appetite
- Cough

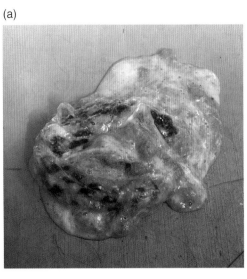

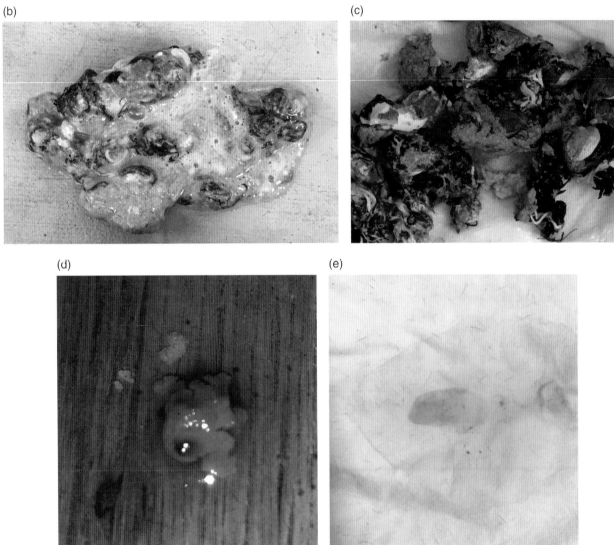

Figure 54.2 (a) Canine vomitus. *Source:* Courtesy of Kimberly Wallitsch. (b) Canine vomitus containing multiple foreign bodies. *Source:* Courtesy of Kimberly Wallitsch. (c). Same foreign bodies as depicted in Figure 54.2b, rinsed off so that they are easier to visualize. *Source:* Courtesy of Kimberly Wallitsch. (d) Hematemesis, blood in the vomitus, from a canine patient. *Source:* Courtesy of Ballroom Dance School Manhattan. (e) Blood-tinged vomitus from a cat that soaked into a sheet.

(a)

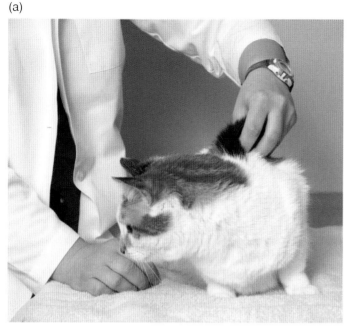

(b)

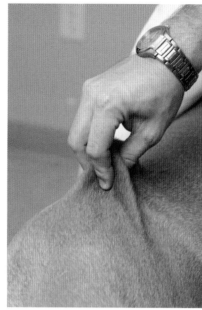

Figure 54.3 (a) Assessing a cat's hydration status by checking for a skin tent at the nape of the neck. *Source:* Courtesy of the Media Resources Department at Midwestern University. (b) Assessing a dog's hydration status by checking for a skin tent between the shoulder blades. *Source:* Courtesy of the Media Resources Department at Midwestern University.

- Depression
- Dyspnea
- Fever
- Increased respiratory effort
- Increased respiratory rate
- Lethargy
- Mucopurulent nasal discharge
- Respiratory distress

54.4 Gastrointestinal Causes of Vomiting

Emesis is a common clinical presentation in companion animal practice [1, 4–9, 11, 29–34].

The list of differential diagnoses for emesis is remarkably diverse and extensive. This assortment of pathologies can overwhelm even a seasoned practitioner.

It may be helpful to consider causes of emesis as falling into one of two categories: gastrointestinal or "other." Here, "other" is a catch-all phrase for any cause that originates from outside of the gut, including systemic maladies.

Gastrointestinal causes of vomiting are perhaps the easiest to consider. Because emesis is a gastrointestinal reflex, it is logical to consider how pathology within the digestive tract itself can lead to vomiting.

Gastrointestinal causes of vomiting include, but are not limited to the following [30–34]:

- Bilious vomiting syndrome***
- Delayed gastric emptying, prolonged gut transit time, and/or obstruction [35–37]
  - Bile duct obstruction
  - Cholelithiasis
  - Cholestasis***
  - Constipation***
  - Dysautonomia
  - Foreign body obstruction*** (see Chapter 50, Section 50.5)
    - Gastric
    - Intestinal
      - Small bowel
      - Large bowel
  - Gastric dilatation-volvulus (GDV) *** (see Chapter 50, Section 50.6.1)
  - Ileus***
  - Intestinal volvulus
  - Intussusception***
  - Polyps
  - Pyloric stenosis
- Dietary indiscretion***
- Hypergastrinemia
- Infection***
  - Bacterial***
    - *Campylobacter* spp. (see Chapter 51, Section 51.4.1)
    - Salmonellosis (see Chapter 51, Section 51.4.4)
  - Fungal
  - Parasitic***

- ○ Ascarids, or roundworms (see Chapter 51, Section 51.6.1) [38–40]
  - Toxocara canis
  - Toxocara cati
  - Toxocara leonina
- – *Giardia* (see Chapter 51, Section 51.6.5.3)
- – Hookworms (see Chapter 51, Section 51.6.2) [41]
  - Ancylostoma caninum
  - Ancylostoma tubaeforme
  - Uncinaria stenocephala
- ○ *Physaloptera* (dogs)
- ○ Whipworms (see Chapter 51, Section 51.6.4)
- – Viral***
  - ○ Canine coronavirus
  - ○ Canine distemper virus (CDV)
  - ○ Canine parvovirus (see Chapter 51, Section 51.5.2)
  - ○ Feline infectious peritonitis
  - ○ Feline panleukopenia virus, otherwise referred to as feline parvovirus (see Chapter 51, Section 51.5.3)
- Gastrointestinal inflammation
  - – Adverse food reaction***
    - ○ Food allergy
    - ○ Food intolerance
  - – Cholangitis-cholangiohepatitis***
  - – Colitis***
  - – Enteritis***
  - – Gastritis***
    - ○ With or without *Helicobacter*
    - ○ Often caused by ingestion of household plants [34]
      - Azalea
      - Daffodil
      - Holly
      - Honeysuckle
      - Jasmine
      - Mistletoe
      - Poinsettia
      - Rhododendron
  - – Gastroenteritis***
  - – Gastric or gastroduodenal ulceration
  - – Hepatitis***
  - – Inflammatory bowel disease (IBD)***
  - – Lymphangiectasia
  - – Pancreatitis***
- Hepatic lipidosis***
- Mastocytosis
- Neoplasia
  - – Gastric
    - ○ Malignant
      - Adenocarcinoma***
      - Lymphosarcoma***
    - – Benign
      - Adenomatous polyps
      - Leiomyoma

- – Hepatobiliary
  - ○ Malignant
    - Canine hepatocellular carcinoma***
    - Lymphosarcoma in cats***
  - ○ Benign
    - Biliary cystadenoma in cats
    - Canine hepatocellular adenomas
- – Intestinal
  - ○ Malignant
    - Adenocarcinoma***
    - Lymphosarcoma***
    - Leiomyosarcoma
- – Benign
  - Adenomatous polyps
  - Leiomyoma

Items that are starred above (***) represent relatively common clinical presentations in a primary care setting.

54.5 Non-gastrointestinal Causes of Vomiting

Other factors that are systemic or unrelated to the gastrointestinal tract itself may trigger emesis. These processes include, but are not limited to the following [2, 4, 11, 32, 34, 42–52]:

- Anaphylaxis***
- Diaphragmatic hernia
- Drugs***
- Fear
- Heat stroke***
- Neurologic disease***
  - – Cerebellar disturbances
  - – Increased intracranial pressure (ICP)
    - ○ Central nervous system (CNS) tumors
    - ○ Cerebral edema, for example, secondary to head trauma
    - ○ Hydrocephalus
  - – Inflammatory disease
    - ○ Encephalitis
    - ○ Meningitis
  - – Vestibular disturbances
- Pain***
- Postoperative***/Anesthetic related***
- Splenic pathology
  - – Abscess
  - – Infarction
  - – Neoplasia***
  - – Torsion
- Steatitis
- Stress
- Systemic disease and/or metabolic dysfunction

- Diabetic ketoacidosis (DKA) ***
- Heartworm disease (HWD) ***
  o Vomiting is a common sign of HWD in cats, but not dogs
- Hepatopathy
  o Cirrhosis
  o Hepatic encephalopathy***
  o Hepatitis
  o Liver failure***
- Hyperthyroidism***
- Hypoadrenocorticism (Addison's disease) ***
- Peritonitis
- Pyometra***
- Uremia secondary to renal failure, acute or chronic***
- Urinary tract disease***
  o Cystitis
  o Pyelonephritis
  o Urinary tract infection (UTI)
  o Urinary tract obstruction (UTO)
    ▪ Stricture
    ▪ Urolithiasis
- Toxins
  - Chocolate and cocoa bean shell mulch
    o Methylxanthine toxicity
    o Theobromine toxicity
  - Ethylene glycol***
  - Heavy metals
    o Lead
    o Zinc
  - Lilies***
  - Mycotoxins
  - Sago palm
  - Xylitol

Items that are starred above (***) represent relatively common clinical presentations in a primary care setting.

54.6 The Role of Signalment and History Taking in Presentations of Acute Vomiting

As demonstrated above, by Sections 54.4 and 54.5, lists of gastrointestinal and extra-gastrointestinal causes of vomiting are extensive. Sometimes it is difficult to know where to begin in the diagnostic process.

The student clinician faces the additional challenge of having to discern which conditions are surgical emergencies. These cases mirror many of those that were introduced in Chapter 50 ("Acute Abdomen") – for example, GDV. The instability of these surgical candidates often requires rapid decision making. The clinician does not have the luxury of unlimited time with which to make case management decisions.

Many presentations of acute vomiting are also emotionally charged and/or distressing to the client. Clinicians have to not only stabilize the patient, but also convince the owner to make quick decisions about diagnostic and therapeutic interventions.

An advisable approach would be to take a step back from the lists of differential diagnoses.

Begin with signalment and history taking to gather patient-specific data that over time leads to pattern recognition. As students have more opportunities to experience clinical cases, they learn what is most, versus least, likely and how to manage cases accordingly.

For example, consider the patient's age when the clinical presentation is acute vomiting [1, 11]:

- Puppies are more likely than adult dogs to develop CPV.
- Kittens are more likely than adult cats to develop feline panleukopenia virus.
- Young patients are most at risk of developing hypoadrenocorticism.
- A six-month-old puppy is more likely to present for acute abdomen secondary to foreign body ingestion than a 12-year-old dog.
- Younger dogs are also more likely to present for vomiting secondary to foreign-body-induced ileus, intussusception, and dietary indiscretion [11]. By contrast, older dogs are more likely to develop intra-abdominal neoplastic disease.
- Similarly, young cats are at increased risk of foreign body ingestion, gastrointestinal viruses, and parasites, whereas older cats are more likely to develop hyperthyroidism and/or renal disease.

In addition, consider the patient's breed when the clinical presentation is acute vomiting [8, 11, 32, 53–60]:

- Belgian Shepherd dogs are more likely to develop gastric carcinoma.
- Large-breed, deep-chested dogs are most at risk for developing GDV [57, 61, 62].
- Miniature Schnauzers are predisposed to pancreatitis.
- Purebred cats are predisposed to lymphoplasmacytic gastroenteritis.
- Rottweilers, Doberman Pinschers, Labrador Retrievers, German Shepherds, and Staffordshire Terriers are predisposed to CPV [41, 63, 64].
- Siamese cats are more likely to develop pyloric stenosis and gastrointestinal adenocarcinoma.
- Standard poodles are at increased risk of developing Addison's disease.
- Toy breeds are more likely to develop hypertrophic pyloric gastropathy.

- Certain small-breed dogs are also more likely to develop extrahepatic portosystemic shunts, resulting in hepatic encephalopathy. One of the many sequelae associated with hepatic encephalopathy is vomiting.

Consider also the patient's sex, sexual status, and species when the clinical presentation is acute abdomen [8, 11, 32, 53–55, 65–67]:

- An intact female is at risk for pyometra.
- Female dogs are more likely than males to develop Addison's disease.
- Male cats are more likely than females to develop UTO and duodenal adenomatous polyps.

Signalment alone can appreciably narrow down the list of differential diagnoses to those that are more likely.

History taking further refines the list of differentials.

In particular, history taking should clarify whether the patient is truly vomiting or is in fact regurgitating. In addition, the client should be questioned as to the following [10]:

- Is emesis productive?
  - Contents of vomitus
  - Description of vomitus (color, consistency)
  - Is the vomiting projectile? [2]
    ○ This may be suggestive of pyloric obstruction
- Is the vomiting cyclical?
- Does the patient appear nauseous before vomiting?
  ○ Lip licking
  ○ Ptyalism
  - When does the patient vomit?
    ○ Only in the morning or after fasting?
    ○ Sporadically?
    ○ Only after meals?
  - How often has the patient vomited?
  - Is the patient vomiting food?
    ○ How soon after ingesting food does the patient vomit?
  - Can the patient keep water down?
    ○ How soon after ingesting water down the patient vomit?
  - Does the vomitus contain blood? (see Chapter 50, Figure 50.12)
    ○ This occurrence is called hematemesis.
      ■ Fresh blood, as from recent large bowel mucosal bleeds, will appear red [2].
      ■ Older bleeds may result in a brown "coffee-ground" appearance because the blood is partially digested [2].
  - Does the vomitus contain bile?
  - Does the vomitus smell like feces?
    ○ If so, this is suggestive of an intestinal obstruction or bowel-associated bacterial overgrowth [2].

In addition to questions concerning emesis, history taking should lean on many of the same questions as pertained to case presentations of acute abdomen.

Recall from Chapter 50, Section 50.3 the importance of inquiring about the following topics [4, 6, 10, 32, 53, 68]:

- Abdominal distension
  - Has the owner noticed a bloated appearance?
    ○ How distended is the abdomen?
    ○ Did the abdomen become distended acutely?
    ○ Is the abdomen continuing to expand?
- Abnormal ingestive behaviors
  - Does the patient have a history of pica?
- Activity level
  - What is the patient's activity level?
  - Has the patient's actively level acutely changed?
- Appetite
  - What is the patient's normal appetite?
  - Has the patient's appetite acutely changed?
- Current medications
  - Is the patient currently taking an NSAID such as carprofen?
    ○ Dose
    ○ Dosing frequency
    ○ Duration of treatment
- Was the patient inadvertently given the NSAID, ibuprofen?
    ○ When?
    ○ How much?
    ○ How often?
- Dietary history
  - What is the patient fed on a regular basis?
  - Is the patient fed meals or is the patient free-fed?
    ○ How much food is offered during a 24-hour period?
    ○ How much food is ingested during a 24-hour period?
  - Is the patient's diet commercial dog or cat food?
    ○ Brand
    ○ Formulation (dry, canned, semi-moist)
    ○ Has the client changed brands recently?
  - Is the patient's diet home-prepared?
    ○ What are the ingredients?
    ○ How was it designed or formulated?
    ○ Is it missing any essential nutrients?
  - Is the patient eating a raw diet?
    ○ This heightens the risk of Salmonellosis
- Diarrhea
  - Is the patient having diarrhea?
    ○ Is the patient having small bowel diarrhea?
      ■ Normal to mild increase in the frequency of defecation
      ■ Normal to increased fecal volume
      ■ May contain melena (see Chapter 50, Figure 50.10)

- Negative for mucus
- Negative for tenesmus
- Negative for urgency
- Commonly associated with weight loss if chronic issue
- Commonly associated with emesis
  ○ Is the patient having large bowel diarrhea?
    - Increased frequency of defecation
    - Increased water content/decreased fecal volume
    - May contain fresh blood (hematochezia) (see Chapter 50, Figure 50.11)
    - Frequently contains mucus
    - Associated with tenesmus
    - Associated with urgency
    - Not associated with weight loss
    - May be associated with vomiting
- Exposure to conspecifics
  - Does the patient live with conspecifics?
    ○ If yes, are the conspecifics exhibiting the same clinical signs as the patient?
  - Does the patient interact with and/or come into close contact with conspecifics?
    ○ Doggie day care
    ○ Grooming
    ○ Kenneling
- Exposure to toxins
  - Anticoagulant rodenticide
    ○ Internal hemorrhage, including potential for hemoabdomen
  - Antifreeze
  - Chocolate
  - Cocoa beans or cocoa mulch
  - Lily toxicosis (cats)
  - Sago palm
  - Xylitol
- Reproductive history
  - Intact female
    ○ When was the patient last in heat, that is, in estrus?
    ○ Does the patient have vaginal bleeding at today's visit?
    ○ Is there vulvar discharge of any kind?
- Urinary history: does the patient have a history of:
  - Dysuria
  - Hematuria
  - Stranguria
  - UTIs
  - Urolithiasis
  - UTO?
- Vaccination history
  - Is the patient up-to-date (UTD) on vaccines?
  - Against which diseases has the patient been vaccinated?

The client should also be asked about any other signs that may not outwardly seem related. These clinical signs may provide clues as to what other body systems may be involved and contributing, if not causing, the presenting complaint, emesis.

Consider, for example, the following clinical signs [1, 42, 69, 70]:

- Neurologic signs, including seizures, increase the likelihood of CNS disease, such as cerebral swelling, hepatic encephalopathy, lead toxicosis and/or systemic disease.
- Polyuria (PU) and polydipsia (PD) in an intact female, adult, cat or dog increases the likelihood of pyometra.
- PU and PD also raise the index of suspicion of endocrinopathies, such as diabetes mellitus, or renal disease.
- Respiratory distress or coughing may suggest asthma or HWD, particularly in cats.
- Weight loss in spite of a ravenous appetite in a middle-aged to older cat is suggestive of hyperthyroidism.

As was true of patients that present for acute abdomen, patients that present for acute vomiting should be triaged [54]. Review this portion of patient evaluation in Chapter 50, Section 50.4 [54].

Recall that the purpose of triage is to establish the stability of the patient. Patients that are critical must be tended to urgently, which means that history-taking topics frequently need to be tabled until the patient is stable [54].

54.7 The Physical Examination and Presentations of Acute Vomiting

The triage examination is intentionally an abbreviated patient assessment [54]. The patient still requires a complete physical examination.

The following physical examination findings were taken directly from Chapter 50, Section 50.4. They highlight important areas of concern for a patient that presents for acute vomiting [1, 26, 31, 54, 71–86]:

- Abdominal auscultation
  - Hyperactive gut sounds are supportive of gastritis, enteritis, malabsorption, and maldigestion (refer also to Chapter 47, Section 47.4)
  - Hypoactive gut sounds are supportive of ascites, gastrointestinal obstruction, and peritonitis (refer also to Chapter 47, Section 47.5)
- Abdominal pain
  - A patient that is displaying a so-called "prayer posture" is likely to be experiencing cranial abdominal pain.

- This position is akin to a play bow, only the patient is not attempting to play. Its head and forelimbs are lowered to the ground as its rump remains held high in the air.
- Abdominal palpation
  - A palpable fluid wave is suggestive of abdominal effusion
    - Abdominal effusions could be hemorrhagic, as from trauma.
    - Effusions also result from uroabdomen and septic peritonitis.
  - Focal thickening of the small bowel may be the result of foreign body ingestion.
  - Focal pain assists with localization of disease:
    - A dog with cranial abdominal pain is more likely to have pancreatitis than colitis.
    - A dog with caudal abdominal pain is more likely to have a prostatic abscess than gastritis.
  - Plication of the intestines is palpably abnormal and is suggestive of a linear (string) foreign body.
  - The stomach is not normally palpable in health in either dogs or cats [2, 26]. Ordinarily, the stomach is seated beneath the rib cage [2].
    - A palpable stomach suggests that it is either distended with food or air, or displaced caudally in the abdomen by an enlarged liver [2].
- Cardiovascular assessment
  - Patients with hypovolemic shock secondary to fluid loss in the vomitus are likely to have poor skin turgor, dry mucous membranes, and changes in heart rate and pulse quality.
    - Dogs tend to become tachycardic [87].
    - Cats tend to become bradycardic [87].
  - Patients with diffusely red or muddy gums may be septic. Such patients are also likely to develop fever and evidence of coagulopathy.
- Integumentary system
  - Icteric skin signifies that bile is accumulating in the body [88].
    - This pigment can be detected throughout the skin
    - It may also involve the sclera and/or the mucous membranes [26].
  - Skin tenting is indicative of dehydration
- Lymphadenopathy
  - One or more swollen peripheral lymph nodes may be associated with inflammation or neoplasia.
- Oral examination
  - A linear (string) foreign body may be discovered at the base of the tongue.
  - Oral erosions may be secondary to uremia, the ingestion of caustic chemicals, and/or electrical burns.
- Rectal examination
  - A rectal examination should be performed in all vomiting adult dogs.

- Cats do not typically tolerate rectal examinations without sedation.
- Evidence of hematochezia on the exam glove is suggestive of a lower digestive tract bleed, as from colitis.
- Evidence of melena on the exam glove is suggestive of an upper digestive tract bleed, as from the stomach or small bowel.
- Pain on palpation of the prostate is suggestive of prostatic pathology, such as prostatitis.
- Sublumbar lymphadenopathy is suggestive of regional inflammation, infection, or neoplastic disease.
- Respiratory system
  - Patients with increased respiratory rate and effort may be dyspneic.
  - Pain, stress, and fear can also elevate both of these vital parameters.

54.8 The Diagnostic Approach to Acute Vomiting

Triage, history taking, and physical examination should collectively reveal enough data to allow patients to be sorted into one of the following categories [8]:

- Stable and systemically "well"; that is, no further intervention is indicated.
- Stable, but conservative intervention is indicated.
- Stable, but aggressive intervention is indicated.
- Unstable.

Patients that are stable and do not require further intervention at this time may have an abbreviated history of vomiting as a single isolated event. Perhaps a feline patient vomited a hairball, or maybe a canine patient vomited once after being fed a novel treat. Examination of these "well" patients is unremarkable, and unless emesis recurs, no additional testing or treatment is warranted.

Many cases of vomiting in companion animal patients are self-limiting [9, 11, 89]. Many canine patients that vomit once do not even present to the veterinarian for evaluation [89].

Of those patients that do present to the clinic, most require only conservative intervention [9, 11, 89]. They may be slightly dehydrated. These patients may benefit from subcutaneous or intravenous fluid therapy to restore fluid and electrolyte balance [5, 90].

Conservative treatment may also involve a brief period of rest for the digestive tract [5, 9]. For example, it is not uncommon for veterinarians to advise withholding food for 12 to 48 h, depending upon the patient's response to treatment [5]. When vomiting ceases, a bland diet may be introduced in small portions, frequently, to provide substrate that is easier to digest [5, 10].

Stable patients with acute vomiting may also benefit from antiemetic drugs to break the cycle of vomiting [5, 7, 10]. These drugs may include the following [5, 7, 9, 90]:

- Neurokinin-1 receptor antagonists, such as maropitant citrate
- Serotonin antagonists, such as ondansetron or mirtazapine

Depending upon the case, gastric protectants and prokinetic drugs such as the following may also be of use [5, 7, 9, 90]:

- Cisapride, to stimulate esophageal peristalsis in cats
  - Cisapride works in cats by targeting the smooth muscle of the distal esophagus.
  - Because the canine esophagus is strictly composed of striated muscle, cisapride has no effect on esophageal motility in dogs.
- H2 receptor antagonists, such as famotidine (Pepcid), cimetidine (Tagamet), and ranitidine (Zantac)
- Antidopaminergics, such as metoclopramide
- Proton pump inhibitors, such as omeprazole
- Sucralfate

Many times, these mild cases resolve without ever identifying the underlying cause [11]. Dietary indiscretions are often blamed [11]. Infectious agents and toxins also rank high on the list of considered differentials [11].

When patients do not spontaneously resolve, with or without conservative treatment, a diagnostic work-up is indicated.

Note that a diagnostic work-up is never wrong, and in fact it may be advisable to be more aggressive than less so when considering the potential for complications to arise.

To treat or not to treat, and how forceful to be in terms of launching a diagnostic investigation, truly depends upon the individual patient, the client's comfort, and the clinician's confidence level [11]. The benefits and risks of diagnostic and treatment options must be discussed with transparency, and shared decision making must result in a plan to which all parties can agree.

Clients must also be informed that there is no guarantee of patient response and that diagnostic interventions, if not deemed necessary now, may become necessary later [11].

Some cases could go either way in terms of patient stability, and it is challenging at times for the inexperienced clinician to feel settled about moving forward with a plan that does not include a full work-up.

It is far easier to recognize that a patient is unstable and to devise a plan accordingly. Patients with one or more of the following clinical signs may be unstable at time of presentation or they may become unstable [8, 10, 90]:

- Abdominal distension
- Abnormal mentation
  - Depressed
  - Obtunded
  - Comatose
- Arrhythmias
  - Bradyarrhythmias (see Chapter 45)
  - Tachyarrhythmias (see Chapter 46)
- Ascites
- Breakthrough bouts of emesis despite withholding food and water to rest the stomach
- Hematemesis
- Hypothermia
- Icterus
- Malaise
- Marked abdominal pain
- Melena
- Moderate to severe dehydration
- Pallor
- PU and PD
- Pyrexia
- Rapid weight loss
- UTO
- Vaginal discharge

Patients that fail to respond to supportive care and those patients for which vomiting has become a chronic concern also require intervention [8].

Intervention for presentations of acute vomiting in dogs and cats typically consists of baseline bloodwork, urinalysis, and imaging [1, 2, 4, 91].

Bloodwork typically involves a CBC and chemistry profile [54].

As was reviewed in Chapter 50, a CBC evaluates the erythrogram and leukogram, as well as platelet counts, whereas the chemistry profile measures the patient's electrolytes, blood glucose, renal and hepatic health [54].

Patients with gastric disease most often demonstrate the following changes on their leukogram [2]:

- Eosinopenia
- Lymphopenia
- Neutrophilia
- ± Monocytosis

This pattern is called a stress leukogram [2].

If a stress leukogram is absent in a vomiting patient, then a baseline cortisol or ACTH stimulation test should be considered to rule out hypoadrenocorticism [2].

Dehydration may be evident on the CBC as elevations in both packed cell volume (PCV) and total protein (TP) [92].

If PCV is lower than anticipated, then the patient may be experiencing blood loss [92]. This is more likely to be true of chronic blood loss [92]. It takes time for acute blood loss to result in a diminished PCV mostly because the loss is initially compensated for by splenic contraction [92].

If albumin is low, it can be difficult to pinpoint the source. Hypoalbuminemia may result from the following [92]:

- Blood loss
  Protein-losing enteropathy (PLE)
  – These patients typically have a history of marked weight loss (see Chapter 50, Figure 50.15)
- Protein-losing nephropathy (PLN)
- Poor albumin production

The chemistry profile may flag regions of concern in terms of renal or hepatic health. Amylase and lipase elevations may support a preliminary diagnosis of pancreatitis in dogs, if the test value is three or more times greater than the normal reference range [4, 6]. However, amylase and lipase are of limited value, particularly in cats, and a normal test in a dog does not rule out pancreatitis [4, 6].

The chemistry profile may also confirm electrolyte imbalances that need to be corrected through inpatient care with intravenous fluid therapy.

Urinalysis and urine sediment are essential prior to the initiation of fluid therapy to establish a baseline specific gravity and to evaluate renal function [1, 2]. A dehydrated patient is expected to have a higher-than-normal USG. A low USG in the face of clinical dehydration is supportive of renal dysfunction: the kidneys should concentrate the urine in the face of hypovolemia.

Urinalysis may also confirm glucosuria and ketonuria, which are the hallmark of DKA.

In addition, fecal examination is critical to screen for gastrointestinal parasites and their ova. Fecal tests are imperfect in that some parasites shed intermittently. They also depend upon the examiner's experience.

Cats that are vomiting also benefit from being screened for hyperthyroidism and HWD disease via total thyroxine (T4) and a heartworm antibody test, respectively [4, 6]. Vomiting in cats can be caused by either disease.

Cats that are vomiting may also benefit from folate and cobalamin testing [10].

Patients with cranial abdominal pain may have pancreatitis. The serum pancreatic lipase immunoreactivity (PLI) test is highly sensitive, much more so than amylase and lipase [4, 6].

Abdominal imaging is also an important part of the diagnostic work-up for vomiting [54].

As was true for patients with "acute abdomen," abdominal radiographs are a common starting point for survey imaging of patients with acute vomiting [2, 93]. Although they lack the detail that can be obtained by ultrasound and computed tomography (CT), they offer rapid turnaround time in terms of diagnostic results [79]. This is valuable when critical patients present for acute abdomen: they require immediate intervention.

Recall from Chapter 50, Section 50.5 that abdominal radiographs can detect the following [54, 79, 92–95]:

- Ascites
- Body wall defects (see Chapter 50, Figures 50.16a, b)
- Calculi (see Chapter 50, Figures 50.17a–c)
- Foreign body
- Gastric dilatation without volvulus (see Chapter 50, Figures 50.18a, b)
- GDV (see Chapter 50, Figures 50.19a, b)
- Hemoabdomen (see Chapter 50, Figure 50.20)
- "Mass effect"
- Gas-distended colon
- Gas-distended small bowel
- Gastric axis displacement
- Diaphragmatic hernia
- Obstipation (see Chapter 50, Figure 50.21)
- Obstructive pattern that is suggestive of a foreign body ingestion (refer to Chapter 50, Section 50.5)
- Organomegaly
  – Hepatomegaly
  – Prostatomegaly
  – Renomegaly
  – Splenomegaly
- Pneumoperitoneum
- Pyometra

Recall from Chapter 50, Section 50.5 that survey abdominal radiographs should consist of at least two orthogonal views, and that they may be taken with or without contrast [79, 92, 93, 95]. Contrast medium may facilitate the detection of gastric motility disorders and/or digestive tract obstructions [2].

Other means of abdominal imaging that are appropriate for clinical presentations involving acute vomiting include abdominal ultrasonography, endoscopy, and fluoroscopy [2, 4, 6, 10].

As was outlined in Chapter 50, Section 50.5, abdominal ultrasonography can support the following diagnoses [54, 79, 93, 94, 96–106]:

- Biliary tract obstruction
- Bowel obstruction
- Organomegaly
- Pancreatitis
- Peritoneal effusion
- Prostatitis
- Pyometra
- Urolithiasis

Endoscopy and fluoroscopy are beyond the scope of this chapter.

Abdominal exploratory may be indicated in cases with unknown etiologies that are not responding well to treatment [4, 6, 35, 36]. One advantage of this approach is that it facilitates tissue collection for histopathologic examination. Biopsies are most likely to provide a definitive diagnosis.

54.9 Common Clinical Scenarios Involving Acute Vomiting

This chapter introduced the concept of emesis, with an emphasis on acute vomiting, with the objective of providing an overview of the underlying causes. A handful of the most common clinical scenarios will be introduced in brief here.

54.9.1 Bilious Vomiting Syndrome

Bilious vomiting syndrome is a poorly understood condition that describes a subset of canine patients that appear healthy with the exception of vomiting bile shortly after rising in the morning [107]. Young, mixed-breed, castrated males with chronic vomiting of bile in the morning hours are overrepresented [107].

The pathophysiology underlying bilious vomiting syndrome is unclear [107]. Some have attributed it to poor gastric motility [107, 108]. Others assume that duodenal reflux into the stomach is due to pressure differentials in which duodenal pressure exceeds that of an empty stomach [107].

Regardless of the mechanism, bile enters the stomach routinely in affected patients after an overnight fast [107]. This creates a sour stomach and may perpetuate a cycle of vomiting by damaging the stomach lining [107, 109–111].

Bilious vomiting syndrome is intended to be a diagnosis of exclusion [107]. However, many patients are labeled with this condition without having the benefit of a full work-up, particularly if they present with the stereotypical signs [107].

Treatment is typically aimed at reducing the length of time between meals and feeding the last meal of the night late [107]. Increasing meal frequency is thought to reduce the amount of time that the stomach is empty and therefore lessen the chance for a sour stomach [107].

The use of gastroprotectants, antacids, and prokinetic medications may also be of benefit [31, 107, 112–116].

Response to treatment is variable [107].

54.9.2 Diabetic Ketoacidosis (DKA)

DKA is a life-threatening complication of diabetes mellitus [32].

Diabetes mellitus is characterized by hyperglycemia with glucosuria [32, 117]. This may result from one of two states [32, 117]:

- Insulin deficiency due to autoimmune destruction of pancreatic β-cells, so-called Type 1 diabetes mellitus
- Peripheral insulin resistance, so-called Type 2 diabetes

DKA is more likely to occur in patients that have undiagnosed, untreated, or poorly regulated Type 1 diabetes mellitus [32].

Patients with DKA present with metabolic acidosis, ketonemia, and ketonuria in addition to hyperglycemia and glucosuria [32].

Ketone bodies develop from changes in metabolism that result when cells' energy requirements are no longer met by glucose [117].

Recall from basic physiology that insulin is necessary for cells to be able to take up glucose from the bloodstream [117]. Exceptions to this rule are erythrocytes, hepatocytes, renal cortex cells, and cells of the brain [117].

If insulin is deficient and/or if cells are resistant to its effects, then the signal for glucose to enter into insulin-dependent tissues is lost [117].

Glucose-starved cells must tap alternate energy sources [117, 118]. One accessible source of energy is fat [117, 118].

Patients with diabetes mellitus are forced to break down fat via lipolysis and β-oxidation to create energy for glucose-starved tissues [117, 118].

Ketones are the byproducts of lipid metabolism [117, 118]. Specifically, three ketones are formed when fat is converted into energy [117, 118]:

- Acetone
- Acetoacetate
- β-hydroxybutyrate

These ketones are strong acids that lower the pH of the bloodstream [118].

One of these ketones, acetone, is detectable by some clinicians as a characteristic scent that is tied to the breath of patients with DKA [32].

Affected patients also classically present for vomiting [32, 52]. Vomiting is frequently paired with the following clinical signs and/or physical examination findings [32, 52]:

- Dehydration secondary to vomiting
- Dullness, depression, or obtundation
- Hypothermia
- Icterus
- Lethargy
- Hepatomegaly
- Muscle wasting
- Plantigrade stance in both pelvic limbs
- PD
- Polyphagia (PP)
- PU
- Weight loss

Secondary infections are common [32]. So, too, are the following electrolyte imbalances, which perpetuate whole body weakness and malaise [32, 51]:

- Hypochloremia
- Hypokalemia
- Hyponatremia
- Hypophosphatemia

Hyponatremia, in particular, exacerbates neurological dysfunction [51]. Patients with hyponatremia may become mentally dull or depressed, obtunded or stuporous [51]. Severe cases may elicit seizure activity [51].

Patients with DKA are critical. They benefit from aggressive intravenous fluid therapy to address dehydration, with careful attention to the rate at which electrolyte levels are restored [51]. Regular insulin is also administered via continuous rate infusion (CRI) or as time-spaced injections to lower circulating concentrations of glucose and ketones as metabolic acidosis is reversed.

Refer to an internal medicine resource for guidance as to the proper protocols for insulin dosing and administration.

54.9.3 Gastrointestinal Lymphoma

Alimentary tract neoplasia is relatively common in cats. Of the various tumor types that target this region of the body, gastrointestinal lymphoma is most common [119–123].

Affected cats are more likely to be older and male [119]. The majority are negative for feline immunodeficiency virus (FIV) and feline leukemia virus (FeLV) [119].

When disease is low grade based upon histological classification, cats may only present for weight loss or decreased appetite [119, 120]. Hypoproteinemia, which is attributed to hypoalbuminemia, is common due to small bowel involvement [119]. Cats may also have a history of intermittent vomiting or diarrhea; however, the progression is slow [120, 122–125].

High-grade disease is more likely to be associated with the stomach than the small bowel [119]. Affected patients present acutely, with vomiting [120]. An abdominal mass may be palpable [123]. Intestinal obstructions are not uncommon [123]. Intestines may also perforate [123].

Clinically, gastrointestinal lymphoma is difficult to differentiate from lymphocytic-plasmacytic IBD [119].

Histopathologic examination of tissue samples obtained through surgical biopsy or endoscopy is required for a definitive diagnosis [119, 120].

Patient response to treatment for low-grade gastrointestinal lymphoma is promising and typically involves prednisolone and/or chlorambucil [120]. Remission is achieved in 69–75% of patients [119–121].

54.9.4 Inflammatory Bowel Disease (IBD)

IBD represents a conglomeration of conditions that are characterized by chronic gastroenteritis in both dogs and cats [33]. The exact etiology is unclear [33]. It seems likely that affected patients have an aberrant response to gut antigens at the level of the gastrointestinal mucosa [33, 126].

Clinical signs are often cyclical, with bouts of apparent remission [33].

Clinical signs are often extremely variable between patients, which may present for any number of the following [33]:

- Chronic diarrhea
  - Small bowel diarrhea
    - Weight loss
  - Large bowel diarrhea
    - Hematochezia, that is, fresh blood in the stool
    - Mucoid stool
    - Tenesmus, that is, straining to defecate
- Chronic vomiting
- Diminished appetite
- Weight loss

Palpably thickened loops of bowel are often present on physical examination [33]. Affected patients may also exhibit abdominal discomfort on deep palpation [33].

Much like bilious vomiting syndrome, IBD is a diagnosis of exclusion [33]. Care must be taken to rule out other causes of gastrointestinal mucosal inflammation, including the following [33]:

- Adverse food reaction
  - Food allergy
  - Food intolerance
- Alimentary tract neoplasia
- Infectious gastroenteritis
- Lymphangiectasia

Surgical or endoscopic, mucosal biopsy is required for a definitive diagnosis [33].

IBD is subsequently classified based upon which cellular infiltrate is most abundant [33]. Lymphocytic-plasmacytic IBD predominates among affected cats and dogs [33].

Treatment of IBD typically targets the diet, to improve digestibility and limit antigenic stimulation of the gut [33]. Immunosuppressive doses of corticosteroids are often indicated to induce remission [33, 38, 127–133]. Metronidazole is also routinely prescribed to reduce inflammation and curb bouts of diarrhea [33, 38, 127–129, 131, 134–136].

54.9.5 Hepatic Lipidosis

Hepatic lipidosis is a primarily feline syndrome in which excessive accumulations of intracellular triglycerides overwhelm hepatocytcs [32, 33, 49, 137, 138]. This metabolic derangement may be idiopathic or may result from a secondary disease process, including the following [49, 137, 139]:

- Cholangiohepatitis***
- Diabetes mellitus
- IBD***
- Pancreatitis***
  Toxicosis
  - Aflatoxins
  - Bacterial toxins

Starred conditions in the aforementioned list are most likely to induce hepatic lipidosis [137].

Other predisposing factors include the following [32, 49, 137]:

- Low-calorie or protein-restricted diets
- History of anorexia
  - May be due to a change in diet, for instance, to one that the cat considers unpalatable
  - Often stress-induced
- History of rapid weight loss
- Obesity

Increased mobilization of peripheral fats shifts metabolism in favor of β-oxidation of fatty acids, which generates acetyl-CoA [117, 140–143]. Acetyl-CoA is oxidized in the citric acid cycle to generate energy [117, 140–143].

If hepatocytes are overwhelmed by triglycerides waiting to be converted into energy sources, they become distended [32, 137]. Export of hepatocellular triglyceride is compromised, and so-called "fatty liver" results [32, 137]. A "fatty liver" is the colloquial name for hepatic lipidosis. Hepatic lipidosis results in progressive liver dysfunction [32, 137, 139, 144].

From a physiological perspective, "fatty liver" causes cholestasis [32, 137].

From a clinical perspective, cholestasis causes icterus [32, 137].

Patients with hepatic lipidosis typically present for vomiting and anorexia [32, 137]. On physical examination, they are dehydrated and icteric [32, 137]. Dehydration may result in malaise, lethargy, and apparent weakness [32, 137]. Hepatomegaly is common [32, 33].

Severe disease results in hepatic encephalopathy [32, 137, 145]. Hepatic encephalopathy refers to a conglomeration of neurological clinical signs that stem from liver dysfunction [146]. It is caused by the accumulation of toxins, particularly ammonia [146]. Ammonia is removed, in healthy patients, by functional hepatocytes, which convert it into amino acids or urea. Urea is then eliminated from the body in urine by the kidneys.

When the liver fails, blood ammonia concentrations increase. Ammonia is able to cross the blood–brain barrier and disrupt neuronal function and neurotransmission [146].

At the microscopic level, ammonia causes astrocyte swelling [146]. This may result in cerebral edema [146].

Cerebral edema leads to episodic behavioral and neurological disturbances in patients. Clinical signs of hepatic encephalopathy include one or more of the following [32, 137, 146]:

- Abnormal mentation
  - Dull
  - Depressed
  - Obtunded
  - Stuporous
  - Comatose
- Ataxia
- Attacking inanimate objects
- Blindness
- Circling
- Disorientation
- Head pressing
- Pacing
- Ptyalism
- Seizures
- Staring into space
- Unprovoked aggression
- Wandering

Ammonia is difficult to measure clinically [32, 137, 146].

Presumptive diagnosis of hepatic encephalopathy is based upon clinical signs and laboratory evidence of liver dysfunction.

Patients with hepatic lipidosis, for example, tend to have elevations of alanine aminotransferase (ALT), serum alkaline phosphatase (ALKP, ALP, or ALK PHOS), and total bilirubin [32, 33]. In addition, blood urea nitrogen (BUN) is typically low [32]. Potassium (K+) may be low if there is potassium wasting at the level of the kidneys due to tubule triglyceride accumulation [32]. Hypokalemic patients exhibit weakness in the form of cervical ventroflexion [32].

Ultrasonographic evidence of hepatic hyperechogenicity, combined with hepatomegaly, is supportive of a diagnosis of hepatic lipidosis [32, 33]. The diagnosis is ultimately confirmed via hepatic aspirate or biopsy. Hepatocellular vacuolation will be evident [32, 33].

Treatment emphasizes nutrition, that is, meeting caloric needs and reversing anorexia [32, 33]. The placement of feeding tubes for long-term care and support is indicated, and will allow for the delivery of calorie-dense, high-protein meals [32, 33].

Prognosis is good with aggressive medical therapy; however, resolution takes weeks to months, rather than days [32, 33].

Recovery tends to be complicated and prolonged in patients with concurrent pancreatitis [33, 147].

54.9.6 Hypoadrenocorticism

Hypoadrenocorticism, so-called Addison's disease, is a relatively uncommon endocrinopathy in dogs [148–150]. It is rarely seen in cats [32].

Hypoadrenocorticism is also referred to as the "great pretender" because its presentation can be so varied and include so many different clinical signs [148, 151, 152].

Hypoadrenocorticism results from the destruction of 85–90% of the adrenal cortex, specifically the outermost zona glomerulosa and/or the middle layer, the zona fasciculata [148].

The zona glomerulosa is responsible for producing mineralocorticoids, primarily aldosterone [143, 148, 153, 154]. Aldosterone works predominantly on the cortical collecting duct of the kidneys to enhance sodium and chloride reabsorption at the expense of potassium. In other words, in health, potassium is excreted, as sodium and chloride are retained [148]. Water follows sodium and chloride. Therefore, aldosterone impacts whole body water balance in addition to electrolyte homeostasis [148].

The zona fasciculata is responsible for producing glucocorticoids, primarily cortisol [143, 148, 153, 154]. Cortisol's functions are extraordinarily diverse, and its impact is far-reaching [143, 148, 153, 155]. Cortisol is perhaps best known as a stress hormone [148]. As such, its primary roles include the following [143, 148, 150, 152, 153, 155]:

- Maintenance of
  - Blood pressure
  - Endothelial integrity
  - Vascular permeability
  - Vascular tone
  - Vascular volume
  - Water balance
- Promotion of lipolysis and gluconeogenesis in the fasting animal
- Regulation of the immune system
- Stimulation of erythropoiesis
- Suppression of inflammatory responses

Classic hypoadrenocorticism results from mineralocorticoid and glucocorticoid deficiency. Destruction of the adrenal cortex is thought to be immune-mediated [148, 150, 156].

Affected patients are typically young-to-middle-aged dogs, with overrepresentation by females in some, but not all, breeds [32, 148, 150, 156].

Breeds that appear to develop hypoadrenocorticism with greater frequency include the following [32, 148, 150, 156]:

- Bassett Hounds
- Bearded Collies
- Great Danes
- Nova Scotia Duck Tolling Retrievers
- Portuguese Water Dogs
- Rottweilers
- Soft-Coated Wheaten Terriers
- Springer Spaniels
- Standard Poodles
- West Highland White Terriers

Affected dogs tend to present with episodic bouts of gastrointestinal upset [148, 150, 157, 158]. A history of waxing and waning malaise, vomiting, and/or diarrhea is common.

Other commonly reported clinical signs include the following [148, 150, 152, 157, 158]:

- Collapse
- Depression
- Lethargy
- Muscle cramps
- PU/PD
- Shaking and/or shivering
- Tremors
- Weakness
- Weight loss

Due to fluid loss via the gastrointestinal tract, most patients are dehydrated on physical examination [148, 150, 157, 158]. Patients may also present in varying degrees of shock [148, 150, 157, 158]. If hyperkalemia is severe, they may also be bradycardic [148, 150, 157, 158]. Bradycardia in a dog that presents in shock should raise the index of suspicion that the patient in question has classic or typical hypoadrenocorticism [148, 150, 157, 158].

Hyperkalemia, hyponatremia, and hypochloremia are reflective of mineralocorticoid deficiency [148, 150, 157, 158]. Normal patients should have a sodium to potassium ratio between 27:1 and 40:1 [148–150, 156]. Addisonian patients with mineralocorticoid deficiency have a ratio that is less than 27:1 [148–150, 156]. Some patients' ratios will be less than 20:1 [148–150, 156].

The absence of a stress leukogram is suggestive of glucocorticoid deficiency [148, 150, 152, 157, 158]. Dehydrated patients will also be azotemic [148, 150, 157, 158].

Atypical Addisonians will have normal electrolytes and evidence only of glucocorticoid deficiency [148]. These patients represent the minority [148].

An ACTH test confirms the diagnosis of hypoadrenocorticism [148–150, 156, 159, 160].

Treatment of critical patients is aimed at managing the acute Addisonian crisis [150, 156, 159, 161]. This constitutes fluid therapy to correct hypovolemic shock [150,

156, 159, 161]. Aggressive fluid therapy will in and of itself reduce hyperkalemia [150, 156, 159, 161]. However, in the face of life-threatening bradycardia, additional measures may be required. These include the administration of regular insulin, followed by a dextrose bolus [150, 156, 159, 161]. Calcium gluconate may also be administered as a cardioprotective agent to temporarily counter hyperkalemic effects on the heart [150, 156, 159, 161].

After the Addisonian crisis has resolved, patients require lifelong support. Those with classic hypoadrenocorticism

need mineralocorticoid and glucocorticoid replacement. The former is often provided in the form of injectable desoxycorticosterone pivalate (DOCP), which is sold under the veterinary trade name, Percorten-V.

Injections of Percorten-V are administered subcutaneously or intramuscularly approximately every 25 days. Refer to an internal medicine and/or emergency textbook for a discussion of dose, which is beyond the scope of this chapter. Dose alterations are, in large part, dependent upon follow-up bloodwork and the results of the physical examination [150, 159].

References

1 King, L.G. and Donaldson, M.T. (1994). Acute vomiting. *Vet. Clin. North Am. Small Anim. Pract.* 24 (6): 1189–1206.

2 Twedt, D.C. (1983). Differential diagnosis and therapy of vomiting. *Vet. Clin. North Am. Small Anim. Pract.* 13 (3): 503–520.

3 Argenzio, R.A. (2004). Gastrointestinal motility. In: *Dukes' Physiology of Domestic Animals*, 12e (ed. H.H. Dukes and W.O. Reece), 391–404. Ithaca: Comstock Pub. Associates.

4 Tams, T.R. (2017). Diagnosing of acute and chronic vomiting in dogs and cats. Virginia Veterinary Medical Association [Internet]. https://vvma.org/resources/2017%20VVC%20Notes/Tams-Vomiting%20in%20Dogs%20and%20Cats%20-%20Diagnosis.pdf.

5 McGrotty, Y. (2010). Medical management of acute and chronic vomiting in dogs and cats. *In Pract.* 32 (10): 478–483.

6 Tams, T.R. (2009). Diagnosis and management of acute and chronic vomiting in dogs and cats. DVM 360 [Internet]. http://veterinarycalendar.dvm360.com/diagnosis-and-management-acute-and-chronic-vomiting-dogs-and-cats-proceedings.

7 Encarnacion, H.J., Parra, J., Mears, E., and Sadler, V. (2009). Vomiting. *Compendium* 31 (3): 122–131.

8 Batchelor, D.J., Devauchelle, P., Elliott, J. et al. (2013). Mechanisms, causes, investigation and management of vomiting disorders in cats: a literature review. *J. Feline Med. Surg.* 15 (4): 237–265.

9 Armstrong, P.J. (2013). GI Intervention: Approach to diagnosis and therapy of the vomiting patient. *Today's Veterinary Practice* (March/April): 18–27.

10 Devauchelle, P., Elliott, J., and Elwood, C. (2012). Approach to the management of vomiting in cats. Medisch Centrum voor Dieren [Internet]. https://www.mcvoordieren.nl/userfiles/3/file/publicaties/richtlijnbrakenkat.pdf.

11 Elwood, C., Devauchelle, P., Elliott, J. et al. (2010). Emesis in dogs: a review. *J. Small Anim. Pract.* 51 (1): 4–22.

12 Feldman, M. (1989). Nausea and vomiting. In: *Gastrointestinal Disease: Pathophysiology, Diagnosis, and Management. 1*, 4e (ed. M.H. Sleisenger and J.S. Fordtran), 222–238. Philadelphia: WB Saunders.

13 Fuchs, S. and Jaffe, D. (1990). Vomiting. *Pediatr. Emerg. Care* 6: 164–170.

14 Rossmeisl, J.H. Jr. (2010). Vestibular disease in dogs and cats. *Vet. Clin. North Am. Small Anim. Pract.* 40 (1): 81–100.

15 DeLahunta, A., Glass, E., and Kent, M. (2015). *Veterinary Neuroanatomy and Clinical Neurology*, 4e. St. Louis, MO: Elsevier.

16 Angelaki, D.E. and Cullen, K.E. (2008). Vestibular system: the many facets of a multimodal sense. *Annu. Rev. Neurosci.* 31: 125–150.

17 Brandt, T. and Strupp, M. (2005). General vestibular testing. *Clin. Neurophysiol.* 116 (2): 406–426.

18 Thomas, W.B. (2000). Vestibular dysfunction. *Vet. Clin. North Am. Small Anim. Pract.* 30 (1): 227–249, viii.

19 Troxel, M.T., Drobatz, K.J., and Vite, C.H. (2005). Signs of neurologic dysfunction in dogs with central versus peripheral vestibular disease. *J. Am. Vet. Med. Assoc.* 227 (4): 570–574.

20 Evans, H.E. and DeLahunta, A. (2004). *Guide to the Dissection of the Dog*, 6e, xiv, 378 p. St. Louis, Mo: Saunders.

21 Evans, H.E. and Miller, M.E. (2013). *Miller's Anatomy of the Dog*, 4e, xix, 850 p. St. Louis, Missouri: Elsevier.

22 Rylander, H. (2012). Vestibular syndrome: What's causing the head tilt and other neurologic signs? DVM360 [Internet]. http://veterinarymedicine.dvm360.com/vestibular-syndrome-whats-causing-head-tilt-and-other-neurologic-signs.

23 Gallagher, A. (2012). Regurgitation or vomiting? *NAVC Clinician's Brief* (June): 33–35.

24 Sherding, R.G. (2011). Regurgitation, dysphagia, and esophageal dysmotility. DVM 360 [Internet]. http://veterinarycalendar.dvm360.com/regurgitation-dysphagia-and-esophageal-dysmotility-proceedings.

25 Sherding, R.G. (2011). Esophagitis and esophageal stricture. DVM 360 [Internet]. http://veterinarycalendar. dvm360.com/esophagitis-and-esophageal-stricture-proceedings.

26 Englar, R.E. (2017). *Performing the Small Animal Physical Examination*. Hoboken, NJ: Wiley.

27 DiBartola, S.P. and Bateman, S. (2006). Introduction to fluid therapy. In: *Fluid, Electrolyte, and Acid-Base Disorders in Small Animal Practice*, 3e (ed. S.P. DiBartola), 325–344. Saunders/Elsevier: St. Louis, Mo.

28 Bissett, S. (2012). Esophagitis. *NAVC Clinician's Brief* (June): 23–26.

29 Strombeck, D.R. and Guilford, W.G. (1990). *Small Animal Gastroenterology*, 2e, 744 p. Davis, Calif: Stonegate Pub. Co.

30 Tams, T.R. (ed.) (2001). Disorders causing vomiting in cats. Atlantic Coast Veterinary Conference.

31 Tams, T.R. (2003). *Handbook of Small Animal Gastroenterology*, 2e, xiv, 486 p. St. Louis, Mo: Saunders.

32 Tilley, L.P. and Smith, F.W.K. (2004). *The 5-Minute Veterinary Consult: Canine and Feline*, 3e, lviii, 1487 p. Baltimore, MD: Lippincott Williams & Wilkins.

33 Jergens, A.E. (1997). Gastrointestinal disease and its management. *Vet. Clin. North Am. Small Anim. Pract.* 27 (6): 1373–1402.

34 Webb, C. and Twedt, D.C. (2003). Canine gastritis. *Vet. Clin. North Am. Small Anim. Pract.* 33 (5): 969–985, v–vi.

35 Hall, J.A. and Washabau, R.J. (1999). Diagnosis and treatment of gastric motility disorders. *Vet. Clin. N. Am. Small* 29 (2): 377–395.

36 Hall, J.A., Twedt, D.C., and Burrows, C.F. (1990). Gastric-Motility in Dogs.2. Disorders of Gastric-Motility. *Compend. Contin. Educ. Pract. Vet.* 12 (10): 1373–1391.

37 Guilford, W.G. and Strombeck, D.R. (eds.) (1996). Chronic gastric diseases. In: *Strombeck's Small Animal Gastroenterology*, 3e, 275. Philadelphia: W.B.: Saunders.

38 Jergens, A.E., Moore, F.M., Haynes, J.S., and Miles, K.G. (1992). Idiopathic inflammatory bowel disease in dogs and cats: 84 cases (1987–1990). *J. Am. Vet. Med. Assoc.* 201 (10): 1603–1608.

39 Schantz, P.M. (2007). Zoonotic parasitic infections contracted from dogs and cats: How frequent are they? DVM 360 [Internet]. http://veterinarymedicine.dvm360. com/zoonotic-parasitic-infections-contracted-dogs-and-cats-how-frequent-are-they.

40 Bowman, D.D. and Georgi, J.R. (2009). *Georgis' parasitology for Veterinarians*, 9e, ix, 451 p. St. Louis, Mo: Saunders/Elsevier.

41 Magne, M.L. (2006). Selected topics in pediatric gastroenterology. *Vet. Clin. North Am. Small Anim. Pract.* 36 (3): 533–548, vi.

42 Wheeler, S.L. (1988). Emergency management of the diabetic patient. *Semin. Vet. Med. Surg.* 3 (4): 265–273.

43 Morgan, R.V., Moore, F.M., Pearce, L.K., and Rossi, T. (1991). Clinical and laboratory findings in small companion animals with lead poisoning: 347 cases (1977–1986). *J. Am. Vet. Med. Assoc.* 199 (1): 93–97.

44 Kock, M.D. (1979). Peritonitis. *Compend. Contin. Educ. Pract. Vet.* 1: 295–303.

45 Grauer, G.F. and Thrall, M.A. (1982). Ethylene-glycol (antifreeze) poisoning in the dog and cat. *J. Am. Anim. Hosp. Assoc.* 18 (3): 492–497.

46 Fitzgerald, K.T. (2010). Lily toxicity in the cat. *Top. Companion Anim. Med.* 25 (4): 213–217.

47 Gulledge, L., Boos, D., and Wachsstock, R. (1997). Acute renal failure in a cat secondary to tiger lily (Lilium tigrinum) toxicity. *Feline Pract.* 25 (5–6): 38–39.

48 Rumbeiha, W.K., Francis, J.A., Fitzgerald, S.D. et al. (2004). A comprehensive study of easter lily poisoning in cats. *J. Vet. Diagn. Investig.* 16 (6): 527–541.

49 Zawie, D.A. and Garvey, M.S. (1984). Feline hepatic-disease. *Vet. Clin. N. Am. Small* 14 (6): 1201–1230.

50 Davies, J.A., Fransson, B.A., Davis, A.M. et al. (2015). Incidence of and risk factors for postoperative regurgitation and vomiting in dogs: 244 cases (2000–2012). *J. Am. Vet. Med. Assoc.* 246 (3): 327–335.

51 Vera, C.P. and Bissett, S. (2010). Hyponatremia. *NAVC Clinician's Brief* (February): 49–53.

52 Huang, A. (2011). Canined iabetic ketoacidosis. *NAVC Clinician's Brief* (April): 68–70.

53 Durkan, S. (2008). Approach to the acute abdomen. DVM 360 [Internet]. http://veterinarycalendar.dvm360. com/approach-acute-abdomen-proceedings?id=&sk=& date=&pageID=2.

54 Pachtinger, G. (2013). Acute abdomen in dogs & cats: Step-by-step approach to patient care. *Today's Veterinary Practice* (September/October): 14–19.

55 Mazzaferro, E.M. (2003). Triage and approach to the acute abdomen. *Clin. Tech. Small Anim. Pract.* 18 (1): 1–6.

56 Brockman, D.J., Washabau, R.J., and Drobatz, K.J. (1995). Canine gastric dilatation/volvulus syndrome in a veterinary critical care unit: 295 cases (1986–1992). *J. Am. Vet. Med. Assoc.* 207 (4): 460–464.

57 Glickman, L.T., Glickman, N.W., Perez, C.M. et al. (1994). Analysis of risk factors for gastric dilatation and dilatation-volvulus in dogs. *J. Am. Vet. Med. Assoc.* 204 (9): 1465–1471.

58 Glickman, L.T., Glickman, N.W., Schellenberg, D.B. et al. (2000). Non-dietary risk factors for gastric dilatation-volvulus in large and giant breed dogs. *J. Am. Vet. Med. Assoc.* 217 (10): 1492–1499.

59 Glickman, L.T., Glickman, N.W., Schellenberg, D.B. et al. (2000). Incidence of and breed-related risk factors for gastric dilatation-volvulus in dogs. *J. Am. Vet. Med. Assoc.* 216 (1): 40–45.

60 Hosgood, G. (1994). Gastric dilatation-volvulus in dogs. *J. Am. Vet. Med. Assoc.* 204 (11): 1742–1747.

61 Sullivan, M. and Yool, D.A. (1998). Gastric disease in the dog and cat. *Vet. J.* 156 (2): 91–106.

62 Schaible, R.H., Ziech, J., Glickman, N.W. et al. (1997). Predisposition to gastric dilatation-volvulus in relation to genetics of thoracic conformation in Irish setters. *J. Am. Anim. Hosp. Assoc.* 33 (5): 379–383.

63 McCaw, D.L. and Hoskins, J.D. (2006). Canine viral enteritis. In: *Infectious Diseases of the Dog and Cat*, 3e (ed. C.E. Greene), 63–73. St. Louis, Mo.: Saunders/Elsevier.

64 Glickman, L.T., Domanski, L.M., Patronek, G.J., and Visintainer, F. (1985). Breed-related risk factors for canine parvovirus enteritis. *J. Am. Vet. Med. Assoc.* 187 (6): 589–594.

65 Hogg, A.H. (1947). Prostatic disease in the dog; clinical manifestations and treatment. *Vet. Rec.* 59 (5): 47–53.

66 Hornbuckle, W.E., MacCoy, D.M., Allan, G.S., and Gunther, R. (1978). Prostatic disease in the dog. *Cornell Vet.* 68 (Suppl 7): 284–305.

67 Biddle, D. and Macintire, D.K. (2000). Obstetrical emergencies. *Clin. Tech. Small Anim. Pract.* 15 (2): 88–93.

68 Gaschen, F. (ed.) (2006). Large intestinal diarrhea – causes and treatment. WSAVA World Congress.

69 Peterson, M.E. (1984). Feline hyperthyroidism. *Vet. Clin. North Am. Small Anim. Pract.* 14 (4): 809–826.

70 Gilbert, R.O. (1992). Diagnosis and treatment of pyometra in bitches and queens. *Compend. Contin. Educ. Pract. Vet.* 14 (6): 777–785.

71 Rusbridge, C. (2005). Neurological diseases of the Cavalier King Charles spaniel. *J. Small Anim. Pract.* 46 (6): 265–272.

72 Ryan, T.M., Platt, S.R., Llabres-Diaz, F.J. et al. (2008). Detection of spinal cord compression in dogs with cervical intervertebral disc disease by magnetic resonance imaging. *Vet. Rec.* 163 (1): 11–15.

73 Brisson, B.A. (2010). Intervertebral disc disease in dogs. *Vet. Clin. N. Am. Small* 40 (5): 829–858.

74 Denny, H.R. (1978). The surgical treatment of cervical disc protrusions in the dog: a review of 40 cases. *J. Small Anim. Pract.* 19 (5): 251–257.

75 Morgan, P.W., Parent, J., and Holmberg, D.L. (1993). Cervical pain secondary to intervertebral disc disease in dogs – radiographic findings and surgical implications. *Prog. Vet. Neurol.* 4 (3): 76–80.

76 Rothuizen, J., Schrauwen, E., LFH, T., and Verhaert, L. (2009). Digestive tract. In: *Medical History and Physical Examination in Companion Animals*, 2e (ed. A. Rijnberk and F.J. Sluijs), 86–100. Edinburgh; New York: Saunders/Elsevier.

77 Walters, P.C. (2000). Approach to the acute abdomen. *Clin. Tech. Small Anim. Pract.* 15 (2): 63–69.

78 Rijnberk, A. and van Sluijs, F.S. (2009). *Medical History and Physical Examination in Companion Animals*, 333. Elsevier Limited: The Netherlands.

79 Heeren, V., Edwards, L., and Mazzaferro, E.M. (2004). Acute abdomen: diagnosis. *Compend. Contin. Educ. Pract. Vet.* 26 (5): 350–363.

80 Ettinger, S.J., Feldman, E.C., and Côté, E. (2017). *Textbook of Veterinary Internal Medicine: Diseases of the Dog and the Cat*, 8e, 2 volumes (lviii, 2181, I–90 p.). St. Louis, Missouri: Elsevier.

81 Côté, E. (2015). *Clinical Veterinary Advisor. Dogs and Cats*, 3e, xxxvii, 1642 p. St. Louis, Missouri: Elsevier Mosby.

82 Cave, N. (2013). Gastrointestinal gas: eructation, borborygmus, and flatulence. In: *Canine and Feline Gastroenterology* (ed. R. Washabau and M.J. Day), 124–128. St. Louis, MO: Saunders.

83 Papazoglou, L.G., Patsikas, M.N., and Rallis, T. (2003). Intestinal foreign bodies in dogs and cats. *Compend. Contin. Educ. Pract. Vet.* 25 (11): 830–+.

84 Saxon, W.D. (1994). The acute abdomen. *Vet. Clin. North Am. Small Anim. Pract.* 24 (6): 1207–1224.

85 Guilford, W.G. and Strombeck, D.R. (1996). Intestinal obstruction, pseudo-obstruction, and foreign bodies. In: *Strombeck's Small Animal Gastroenterology* (ed. W.B. Guilford, S.A. Center and D.R. Strombeck), 487–502. Philadelphia: WB Saunders.

86 Morris, I.R., Darby, C.F., Hammond, P., and Taylor, I. (1983). Changes in small bowel myoelectrical activity following laparotomy. *Br. J. Surg.* 70 (9): 547–548.

87 Tello, L.H. (ed.) (2009). *Feline as Emergency Patient: Trauma*. Sao Paulo, Brazil: WSAVA.

88 Schaer, M. (2008). Icterus. *NAVC Clinician's Brief* (September): 8.

89 Hubbard, K., Skelly, B.J., McKelvie, J., and Wood, J.L. (2007). Risk of vomiting and diarrhoea in dogs. *Vet. Rec.* 161 (22): 755–757.

90 Lawrence, Y. and Lidbury, J. (2015). Symptomatic management of primary acute gastroenteritis. *Today's Veterinary Practice* (November/December): 46–52.

91 Twedt, D.C. (2007). Managing the vomiting dog. *NAVC Clinician's Brief* (November).

92 Dye, T. (2003). The acute abdomen: a surgeon's approach to diagnosis and treatment. *Clin. Tech. Small Anim. Pract.* 18 (1): 53–65.

93 Boag, A. and Hughes, D. (2004). Emergency management of the acute abdomen in dogs and cats 1. Investigation and initial stabilisation. *In Practice* 26 (9): 476–483.

94 Thrall, D.E. (1998). *Textbook of Veterinary Diagnostic Radiology*. Philadelphia: WB Saunders.

95 Bischoff, M.G. (2003). Radiographic techniques and interpretation of the acute abdomen. *Clin. Tech. Small Anim. Pract.* 18 (1): 7–19.

96 Cruz-Arambulo, R. and Wrigley, R. (2003). Ultrasonography of the acute abdomen. *Clin. Tech. Small Anim. Pract.* 18 (1): 20–31.

97 Nyland, T.G., Matoon, J.S., and Herrgesel, E.J. (2002). Liver. In: *Small Animal Diagnostic Ultrasound* (ed. T.G. Nyland and J.S. Matoon), 144–157. Philadelphia: WB Saunders.

98 Hess, R.S., Saunders, H.M., Van Winkle, T.J. et al. (1998). Clinical, clinicopathologic, radiographic, and ultrasonographic abnormalities in dogs with fatal acute pancreatitis: 70 cases (1986–1995). *J. Am. Vet. Med. Assoc.* 213 (5): 665–670.

99 Nyland, T.G., Matoon, J.S., and Herrgesel, E.J. (2002). Urinary tract. In: *Small Animal Diagnostic Ultrasound* (ed. T.G. Nyland and J.S. Matoon), 158–195. Philadelphia: WB Saunders.

100 Grooters, A.M. and Biller, D.S. (1995). Ultrasonographic findings in renal disease. In: *Current Veterinary Therapy XII: Small Animal Practice* (ed. J.D. Bonagura and R.W. Kirk), 933–937. Philadelphia: WB Saunders.

101 Finn, S.T. and Wrigley, R. (1989). Ultrasonography and ultrasound-guided biopsy of the canine prostate. In: *Current Veterinary Therapy X: Small Animal Practice* (ed. R.W. Kirk and J.D. Bonagura), 1227–1239. Philadelphia: WB Saunders.

102 Matton, J.S. and Nyland, T.G. (2002). Ovaries and uterus. In: *Small Animal Diagnostic Ultrasound* (ed. T.G. Nyland and J.S. Matoon), 231–249. Philadelphia: WB Saunders.

103 Peter, A.T. and Jakovljevic, S. (1992). Real-Time ultrasonography of the small animal reproductive-organs. *Compend. Contin. Educ. Pract. Vet.* 14 (6): 739–744.

104 Poffenbarger, E.M. and Feeney, D.A. (1986). Use of gray-scale ultrasonography in the diagnosis of reproductive disease in the bitch: 18 cases (1981–1984). *J. Am. Vet. Med. Assoc.* 189 (1): 90–95.

105 Lamb, C.R. (1990). Abdominal ultrasonography in small animals – intestinal-tract and mesentery, kidneys, adrenal-Glands, uterus and prostate. *J. Small Anim. Pract.* 31 (6): 295–304.

106 Felkai, C., Voros, K., and Fenyves, B. (1995). Lesions of the renal pelvis and proximal ureter in various nephro-urological conditions – an ultrasonographic study. *Vet. Radiol. Ultrasound* 36 (5): 397–401.

107 Ferguson, L., Wennogle, S.A., and Webb, C.B. (2016). Bilious vomiting syndrome in dogs: retrospective study of 20 cases (2002–2012). *J. Am. Anim. Hosp. Assoc.* 52 (3): 157–161.

108 Eagon, J.C., Miedema, B.W., and Kelly, K.A. (1992). Postgastrectomy syndromes. *Surg. Clin. North Am.* 72 (2): 445–465.

109 Li, X.B., Lu, H., Chen, H.M. et al. (2008). Role of bile reflux and Helicobacter pylori infection on inflammation of gastric remnant after distal gastrectomy. *J. Dig. Dis.* 9 (4): 208–212.

110 Duane, W.C. and Wiegand, D.M. (1980). Mechanism by which bile salt disrupts the gastric mucosal barrier in the dog. *J. Clin. Invest.* 66 (5): 1044–1049.

111 Ritchie, W.P. Jr. (1986). Alkaline reflux gastritis. Late results on a controlled trial of diagnosis and treatment. *Ann. Surg.* 203 (5): 537–544.

112 Washabau, R.J. and Hall, J.A. (1995). Cisapride. *J. Am. Vet. Med. Assoc.* 207 (10): 1285–1288.

113 Washabau, R.J. and Hall, J.A. (1997). Gastrointestinal prokinetic therapy: Serotonergic drugs. *Compend. Contin. Educ. Pract. Vet.* 19 (4): 473–480.

114 Tanaka, T., Mizumoto, A., Mochiki, E. et al. (1998). Effects of EM574 and cisapride on gastric contractile and emptying activity in normal and drug-induced gastroparesis in dogs. *J. Pharmacol. Exp. Ther.* 287 (2): 712–719.

115 Tanaka, T., Mizumoto, A., Mochiki, E. et al. (1999). Effect of EM574 on postprandial pancreaticobiliary secretion, gastric motor activity, and emptying in conscious dogs. *Dig. Dis. Sci.* 44 (6): 1100–1106.

116 Sato, F., Marui, S., Inatomi, N. et al. (2000). EM574, an erythromycin derivative, improves delayed gastric emptying of semi-solid meals in conscious dogs (vol 395,pg 165, 2000). *Eur. J. Pharmacol.* 404 (3): 397.

117 Goff, J.P. (2004). Disorders of carbohydrate and fat metabolism. In: *Dukes' Physiology of Domestic Animals*, 12e (ed. H.H. Dukes and W.O. Reece). Ithaca: Comstock Pub. Associates.

118 Beitz, D.C. (2004). Lipid metabolism. In: *Dukes' Physiology of Domestic Animals*, 12e (ed. H.H. Dukes and W.O. Reece). Ithaca: Comstock Pub. Associates.

119 Matz, M.E. (2007). Chronic vomiting in a cat. *NAVC Clinician's Brief* (January): 29–31.

120 Mitchell, K.D. (2010). Managing feline gastrointestinal lymphoma. DVM 360 [Internet]. http://veterinarycalendar.dvm360.com/managing-feline-gastrointestinal-lymphoma-proceedings.

121 Lingard, A.E., Briscoe, K., Beatty, J.A. et al. (2009). Low-grade alimentary lymphoma: clinicopathological findings and response to treatment in 17 cases. *J. Feline Med. Surg.* 11 (8): 692–700.

122 Richter, K.P. (2003). Feline gastrointestinal lymphoma. *Vet. Clin. North Am. Small Anim. Pract.* 33 (5): 1083–1098, vii.

123 Wilson, H.M. (2008). Feline alimentary lymphoma: demystifying the enigma. *Top. Companion Anim. Med.* 23 (4): 177–184.

124 Kiselow, M.A., Rassnick, K.M., McDonough, S.P. et al. (2008). Outcome of cats with low-grade lymphocytic lymphoma: 41 cases (1995–2005). *J. Am. Vet. Med. Assoc.* 232 (3): 405–410.

125 Evans, S.E., Bonczynski, J.J., Broussard, J.D. et al. (2006). Comparison of endoscopic and full-thickness biopsy specimens for diagnosis of inflammatory bowel disease and alimentary tract lymphoma in cats. *J. Am. Vet. Med. Assoc.* 229 (9): 1447–1450.

126 Strombeck, D.R. and Guilford, W.G. (1990). Idiopathic inflammatory bowel diseases. In: *Small Animal Gastroenterology* (ed. D.R. Strombeck and W.G. Guilford), 357. Davis: Stonegate Publishing.

127 Jergens, A.E. (2015). Which drugs are used to manage feline inflammatory bowel disease? *Veterinary Team Brief/Plumbs Therapeutic Brief* (September).

128 Jergens, A.E. (2012). Feline idiopathic inflammatory bowel disease: what we know and what remains to be unraveled. *J. Feline Med. Surg.* 14 (7): 445–458.

129 Jergens, A.E., Crandell, J., Morrison, J.A. et al. (2010). Comparison of oral prednisone and prednisone combined with metronidazole for induction therapy of canine inflammatory bowel disease: a randomized-controlled trial. *J. Vet. Intern. Med.* 24 (2): 269–277.

130 Jergens, A.E., Crandell, J.M., Evans, R. et al. (2010). A clinical index for disease activity in cats with chronic enteropathy. *J. Vet. Intern. Med.* 24 (5): 1027–1033.

131 Jergens, A.E. and Simpson, K.W. (2012). Inflammatory bowel disease in veterinary medicine. *Front. Biosci. (Elite Ed.)* 4: 1404–1419.

132 Dennis, J.S., Kruger, J.M., and Mullaney, T.P. (1992). Lymphocytic/plasmacytic gastroenteritis in cats: 14 cases (1985–1990). *J. Am. Vet. Med. Assoc.* 200 (11): 1712–1718.

133 Dennis, J.S., Kruger, J.M., and Mullaney, T.P. (1993). Lymphocytic/plasmacytic colitis in cats: 14 cases (1985–1990). *J. Am. Vet. Med. Assoc.* 202 (2): 313–318.

134 Isaacs, K.L. and Sartor, R.B. (2004). Treatment of inflammatory bowel disease with antibiotics. *Gastroenterol. Clin. N. Am.* 33 (2): 335–345, x.

135 Arndt, H., Palitzsch, K.D., Grisham, M.B., and Granger, D.N. (1994). Metronidazole inhibits leukocyte-endothelial cell adhesion in rat mesenteric venules. *Gastroenterology* 106 (5): 1271–1276.

136 Sartor, R.B. (2004). Therapeutic manipulation of the enteric microflora in inflammatory bowel diseases: antibiotics, probiotics, and prebiotics. *Gastroenterology* 126 (6): 1620–1633.

137 Jergens, A.E. (2006). The yellow cat or cat with elevated liver enzymes. In: *Problem-Based Feline Medicine* (ed. J. Rand), 421–442. Edinburgh; New York: Saunders.

138 Kelly, W.R. (1993). The liver and biliary system. In: *Pathology of Domestic Animals* (ed. J. KVF, P.C. Kennedy and N. Palmer), 319. New York: Academic Press.

139 Hardy, R.M. (1983). Diseases of the liver. In: *Textbook of Veterinary Internal Medicine* (ed. S. Ettinger), 1372–1434. Philadelphia: W. B Saunders Co.

140 Bundy, P.K. and Rosenberg, L.E. (1980). *Metabolic Control and Disease*. Philadelphia: W.B. Saunders Co.

141 Alpers, D.H. and Isselbacher, K.J. (1975). Fatty liver: biochemical and clinical aspects. In: *Diseases of the Liver* (ed. L. Schiff), 815–832. Philadelphia: J.B. Lippincott Co.

142 Favarger, P. (1963). The liver and lipid metabolism. In: *The Lilver* (ed. C.H. Rouiller), 549–604. New York: Academic Press.

143 Hall, J.E. and Guyton, A.C. (2011). *Guyton and Hall Textbook of Medical Physiology*, 12e, xix, 1091 p. Philadelphia, Pa: Saunders/Elsevier.

144 Hardy, R.M. (ed.) Diagnosis of hepatic disease. American Animal Hospital Association; 1978.

145 Quesnel, A.D. and Parent, J.M. (2006). The cat with seizures, circling and/or changed behavior. In: *Problem-based Feline Medicine* (ed. J. Rand), 795–820. Edinburgh; New York: Saunders.

146 Center, S.A. (2018). Hepatic encephalopathy in small animals. Merck Veterinary Manual [Internet]. https://www.merckvetmanual.com/digestive-system/hepatic-disease-in-small-animals/hepatic-encephalopathy-in-small-animals.

147 Akol, K.G., Washabau, R.J., Saunders, H.M., and Hendrick, M.J. (1993). Acute pancreatitis in cats with hepatic lipidosis. *J. Vet. Intern. Med.* 7 (4): 205–209.

148 Klein, S.C. and Peterson, M.E. (2010). Canine hypoadrenocorticism: part I. *Can. Vet. J.* 51 (1): 63–69.

149 Reusch, C.E. (2000). Hypoadrenocorticism. In: *Textbook of Veterinary Internal Medicine* (ed. S. Ettinger and E.C. Feldman), 1488–1499. Philadelphia: WB Saunders.

150 Feldman, E.C. and Nelson, R.W. (2004). *Canine and Feline Endocrinology and Reproduction*. St. Louis, MO: WB Saunders.

151 Podell, M. (1990). Canine hypoadrenocorticism. Diagnostic dilemmas associated with the "great pretender". *Probl. Vet. Med.* 2 (4): 717–737.

152 Gaydos, G.A. and DeClue, A.E. (2008). Updates on hypoadrenocorticism. DVM 360 [Internet]. http://veterinarymedicine.dvm360.com/print/318327?page=full.

153 Ganong, W.F. (2003). *Review of Medical Physiology*. New York: Lange Medical Books.

154 LaPerle, K.M.D. and Capen, C.C. (2007). Endocrine system. In: *Pathological Basis of Veterinary Disease* (ed. M.D. McGavin and J.F. Zachary), 693–741. St. Louis, MO: Mosby.

155 Kemppainen, R.J. and Behrend, E.N. (1997). Adrenal physiology. *Vet. Clin. North Am. Small Anim. Pract.* 27 (2): 173–186.

156 Kintzer, P.P. and Peterson, M.E. (1997). Primary and secondary canine hypoadrenocorticism. *Vet. Clin. North Am. Small Anim. Pract.* 27 (2): 349–357.

157 Greco, D.S. (2007). Hypoadrenocorticism in small animals. *Clin. Tech. Small Anim. Pract.* 22 (1): 32–35.

158 Peterson, M.E., Kintzer, P.P., and Kass, P.H. (1996). Pretreatment clinical and laboratory findings in dogs with hypoadrenocorticism: 225 cases (1979–1993). *J. Am. Vet. Med. Assoc.* 208 (1): 85–91.

159 Klein, S.C. and Peterson, M.E. (2010). Canine hypoadrenocorticism: part II. *Can. Vet. J.* 51 (2): 179–184.

160 Roth, L. and Tyler, R.D. (1999). Evaluation of low sodium:potassium ratios in dogs. *J. Vet. Diagn. Investig.* 11 (1): 60–64.

161 Panciera, D.L. (2006). Fluid therapy in endocrine and metabolic disorders. In: *Fluid, Electrolyte, and Acid-base Disorders* (ed. S.P. DiBartola), 478–489. St. Louis: Elsevier.

Part Seven

The Urogenital System

55

Abnormalities Associated with Testicular Palpation

55.1 Introduction to External Male Reproductive Anatomy

The following reproductive structures are readily observed and/or are palpable on physical examination of the male dog and cat:

- Penis
- Prepuce
- Two scrotal testes

The penis, including normal versus abnormal structure and function, will be discussed in Chapters 57 and 58. The emphasis of this chapter is on palpable testicular anatomy.

The male gonads, the testes, are oval-like structures that are housed within a sac-like enclosure, the scrotum [1–3]. In health, the testes are positioned obliquely, with a long axis that runs dorsocaudally [3].

The scrotum is immediately ventral to the anus in cats, and is easiest to see when standing behind the cat, looking at the cat's caudal end, with its tail up [1]. In a sense, the feline scrotum is tacked to the perineum. The feline scrotum tends to be densely furred [1] (see Figures 55.1a–d).

The canine scrotum is more pendulous than the cat's and hangs between the upper thighs of the two pelvic limbs [1]. The canine scrotum is therefore inguinal as opposed to perineal, and is roughly two-thirds of the distance from the anus to the preputial tip [1, 3]. The canine scrotum tends to be loosely furred and thin-skinned [1]. It may or may not be pigmented (see Figures 55.2a, b).

In health, both testes are palpable through the scrotum [1–3]. Testes should be palpated for their [1, 2]

- Presence
- Shape
- Size
- Texture or consistency.

Normal testicles are palpably non-tender [1]. Their surface is smooth, and their consistency is homogenously firm, yet compressible, like a shell-less hardboiled egg or a semi-ripe plum.

Testicular size varies depending upon breed and, therefore, size of the patient [1, 3]. Intact tomcats typically have testicles that approximate 1 cm in diameter as compared to dogs, which may range from 1.5 to 3 cm or more [1, 3].

The epididymis is a tubular structure that connects each testis to the vas deferens, the conduit through which sperm pass into the urethra [3]. The epididymis is palpable along the dorsolateral surface of each canine testis, and the craniolateral surface of each feline testis (see Figure 55.3).

The epididymis consists of a head, body, and tail. The tail of the epididymis is particularly prominent. It is located at the caudalmost pole of the canine testis, and dorsally in the cat [1–3].

As a whole, the epididymis is firmer than the testis itself [1, 3]. The epididymis, including its tail, should feel somewhat rubbery [1]. Like the testis, it, too, should not be painful on gentle palpation [1, 3].

55.2 Failure of Testicular Descent

Canine and feline testes do not originate from the scrotum [1–3]. In embryonic life, the testes develop within the abdomen, near the caudal pole of each kidney [2–4].

The testes must migrate from this intra-abdominal location to the scrotum through the inguinal canal before the canal closes, between four and six months of age [1–8]. The inguinal canal is a passageway through the abdominal wall that is located in the groin [3].

Migration of the testes through the inguinal canal is facilitated by the gubernaculum, a fold of peritoneum that spans from the caudal pole of each testis to the scrotum [2–4].

As the gubernaculum enlarges during the first phase of testicular migration, it dilates the inguinal canal, paving the way for testicular descent [2, 4]. Enlargement of the

(a)　　　　　　　　(b)

(c)　　　　　　　　(d)

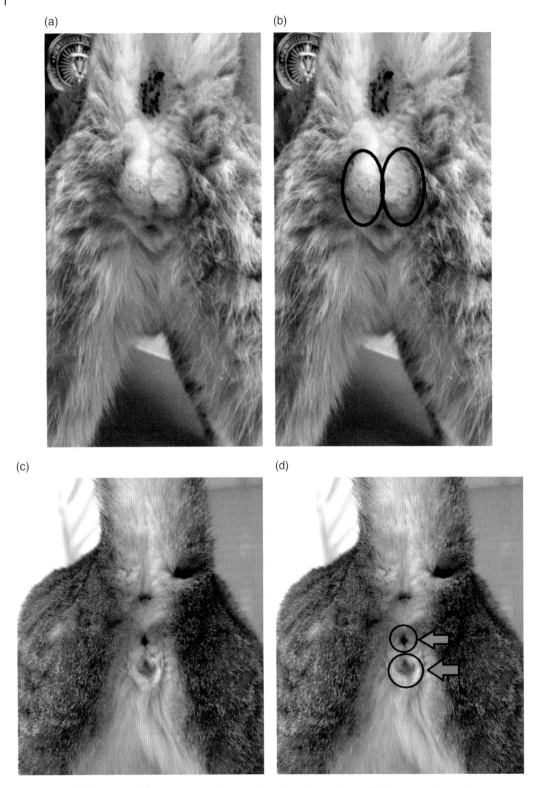

Figure 55.1 (a) Rear view of intact male cat. Note the location of the testes within the scrotal sac, which is seated ventral to the anus, but dorsal to the preputial opening. The feline scrotum is tightly adhered to the perineum. (b) Same view of the tomcat depicted in Figure 55.1a. The testes have been outlined in black. (c) Rear view of castrated male cat. This cat was neutered early in life. Note the empty space between the anus and the preputial opening. *Source:* Courtesy of the Media Resources Department at Midwestern University. (d) Same view of the castrated male cat depicted in Figure 55.1c. The preputial opening has been circled in black and highlighted with an orange arrow. The blue arrow is pointing to the space dorsal to the preputial opening. This is where the scrotal sac would be were the patient an intact male cat. *Source:* Courtesy of the Media Resources Department at Midwestern University.

(a)

(b)

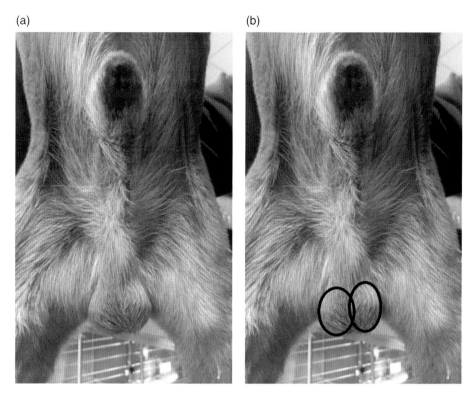

Figure 55.2 (a) Ventral view of intact male dog. Note the inguinal location of the testes within the scrotal sac. The canine scrotum is pendulous, and hangs between the inner thighs of the dog. (b). Same view of the intact male dog depicted in Figure 55.2a. Note the inguinal location of the testes within the scrotal sac. The canine scrotum is pendulous, and hangs between the inner thighs of the dog.

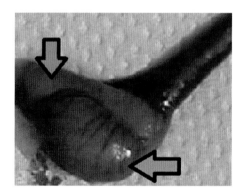

Figure 55.3 Excised canine testis, immediately following orchiectomy. The testis is identified by the blue arrow; the epididymis is identified by the orange arrow.

gubernaculum distal to the inguinal canal also exerts traction upon the intra-abdominal gubernaculum [4]. This action effectively pulls each testis distally toward the groin [4]. Abdominal muscle contraction may also play a role in testicular descent [4].

During the final phase of testicular migration, the gubernaculum shrinks down in the scrotal sac, after drawing the testes through the canal and into the scrotum [4, 9–11].

At birth, the gubernaculum is often palpable within the scrotum, and it may be mistaken for scrotal testicles [2, 4]. In reality, most kittens and puppies lack scrotal testes at birth [2, 4].

Many testes make it through the inguinal canal and into the scrotum between three and 10 days of age [2]. However, testes may continue to pass in and out of the scrotum through the open inguinal canal until 10–14 weeks old [2, 4].

Puppies also have a strong cremaster muscle, which functions to pull each testis tightly against the abdominal wall [3]. The purpose of this action is protective, that is, to guard the testes from cold ambient temperatures [3, 4]. However, this makes it more difficult for the clinician to find testes that are in fact scrotal, yet have been hiked up high within the scrotal sac [12]. Stress and fear exacerbate the cremaster reflex [4].

At four to six months of age, the inguinal canal closes [13, 14]. At that point, canine and feline testes should be scrotal [2, 9, 13–17]. If they are not, the patient is said to be cryptorchid [2, 8, 9, 13–17]. Failure of testicular descent to the scrotum, cryptorchidism, is a common presentation among companion animal patients [1–5, 7, 18–23].

Patients may be unilaterally or bilaterally cryptorchid. If one or both testicles are not scrotal, then

(a)

(b)

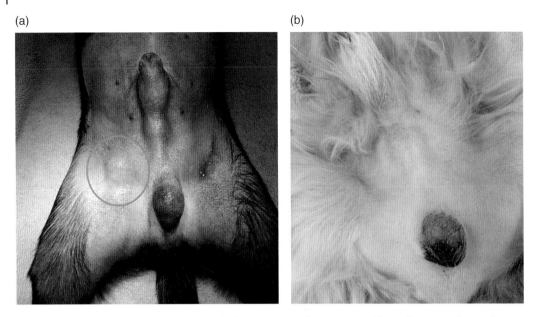

Figure 55.4 (a). Right-sided inguinal cryptorchid canine patient being prepped for orchiectomy. *Source:* Courtesy of Shannon Carey, DVM. (b) Right-sided abdominal cryptorchid canine patient. *Source:* Courtesy of Frank Isom, DVM.

they are either abdominal or inguinal [4–6, 24–26] (see Figures 55.4a, b).

Cryptorchidism occurs with greater frequency in dogs than cats. The incidence in canine patients ranges between 3.3 and 6.8% as compared to 1.3–3.8% in cats [6, 17, 27–29].

Unilateral, right-sided, inguinal cryptorchidism is the most common presentation in dogs, followed by unilateral, right-sided, abdominal cryptorchidism [4, 6, 30, 31].

When cats present as being cryptorchid, the majority have unilateral, inguinal involvement [6, 28, 32].

Historically, pedigreed pets have been overrepresented [4, 33].

In a study of 240 cryptorchid dogs, 77.5% were purebreds. In particular, the following canine breeds appear to be at increased risk for development of cryptorchidism [6, 20, 34–38]:

- Boxer
- Chihuahua
- Cocker Spaniel
- English Bulldog
- German Shepherd
- Maltese
- Miniature Dachshund
- Old English Sheepdog
- Pekingese
- Pomeranian
- Poodle
- Shetland Sheepdog
- Yorkshire Terrier

Small-breed dogs in particular appear to be at increased risk [5, 6, 20, 36, 37, 39].

Among cats, Persians and Ragdolls are overrepresented in the veterinary medical literature [13, 27, 28, 32].

When cryptorchidism occurs, the affected testicle is capable of producing testosterone via functional interstitial or Leydig cells. However, spermatogenesis is impaired because the testes are exposed to core body temperature, which degenerates the germinal epithelium. The net result is impaired testicular size and texture: the cryptorchid testis is smaller and softer than expected [4, 30, 34] (see Figure 55.5).

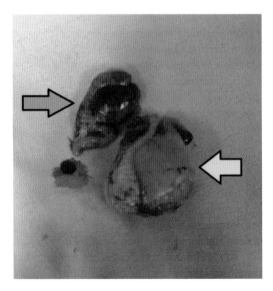

Figure 55.5 Size comparison of the cryptorchid testis (blue arrow) versus the normal, scrotal testis (light orange arrow), post-orchiectomy. Note the small size of the cryptorchid testis. *Source:* Courtesy of Shannon Carey, DVM.

Bilaterally abdominal cryptorchid patients are infertile [3, 4, 20, 40]. Unilaterally cryptorchid patients appear to have reduced fertility [3, 4]. Although most cryptorchid patients can achieve erection, they may not ejaculate [4, 23, 40]. Of those that do, ejaculates may or may not contain live sperm [4, 40]. When they do, progressive motility of sperm is often impaired [4, 40].

Hormonal attempts to correct testicular descent are ineffective in the dog and should be discouraged by the veterinary team because the patient carries a heritable trait [4, 32, 34].

Because cryptorchidism is inherited, cryptorchid dogs should not be bred [2, 4].

It is also advisable that affected patients undergo bilateral orchiectomy [2, 4, 6, 41]. The cryptorchid testis is at increased risk of testicular cancer [4–6, 18, 20, 31, 36, 37, 41, 42]. In fact, the rate of testicular cancer in cryptorchid dogs is 13.6 times greater than in non-cryptorchid dogs [41].

The chance that a cryptorchid dog will develop a Sertoli cell tumor is five times greater than the general population; the chance that a cryptorchid dog will develop a seminoma is three times greater [34].

In addition, the retained testis is more likely to experience torsion [4, 20, 30, 36, 43, 44].

In addition to cancer, cryptorchidism is often associated with other congenital defects, including the following [4]:

- Hernias
  - Inguinal
  - Umbilical
- Patellar subluxation
- Penile-preputial defects, for example, hypospadias, a condition in which the urethral opening is abnormally located, rather than at the tip of the penis

Cryptorchid dogs with an inguinal hernia have a 4.7 times greater risk of developing testicular neoplasia [41].

55.3 Testicular Tumors

Tumors may occur anywhere throughout the reproductive tract. However, the testes are the most common site of primary reproductive neoplasia in the male dog [41, 42, 45–48].

Three types of testicular tumors predominate in the dog [45, 47, 49–53]:

- Interstitial or Leydig cell
- Seminoma
- Sertoli cell

Note that dogs may have more than one type of primary testicular tumor within the same testicle [41, 54–58].

Recent studies suggest that Sertoli cell tumors are less prevalent than the other two tumor types [31, 41, 57–61]. However, the rate of occurrence of Sertoli cell tumors and seminomas increases dramatically in cryptorchid patients [31, 41, 45, 62].

Cryptorchid patients are also more likely to have right-sided testicular tumors [45, 48, 58, 63]. This probably stems from the fact that the right testicle is retained more often than the left [45, 48, 58, 63].

Testicular tumors also occur with greater frequency in the following canine breeds [45, 57]:

- Afghan Hound
- Bouvier de Flandres
- Collie
- Flat-Coated Retriever
- Leonbergers
- Maltese
- Rottweiler
- Shetland Sheepdog

55.3.1 Interstitial or Leydig Cell Tumors

Interstitial or Leydig cell tumors tend to be soft, cystic, and yellow-orange on cross section [45, 64].

These tumors rarely metastasize, and affected patients are rarely clinical at time of presentation [45, 49, 50].

Because Leydig cell tumors are more commonly found in descended than undescended testicles, they are typically first detected as incidental findings – testicular masses – on the physical exam [45, 50, 65].

Affected dogs may develop high concentrations of testosterone in association with Leydig cell tumors [49]. This may result in one or more of the following sequelae [39, 49, 50, 53, 66]:

- Perianal adenoma
- Perianal gland hyperplasia
- Perineal hernia
- Prostatomegaly

55.3.2 Seminomas

Seminomas tend to be soft and ivory white on cross section [45, 64].

Fewer than 15% metastasize to regional lymph nodes or, rarely, to distant sites [39, 45, 49, 50, 65, 67–69].

Like Leydig cell tumors, seminomas more commonly arise in descended testicles than cryptorchid ones [50]. Therefore, they tend to be identified on physical examination as testicular swellings or masses [45].

Note that it is not possible by means of palpation alone to differentiate between Leydig cell tumors and seminomas.

55.3.3 Sertoli Cell Tumors

Sertoli cell tumors tend to be firm, white-to-gray, and lobulated on palpation [45, 64]. They also may feel greasy on cross section [45, 64].

Like seminomas, fewer than 15% metastasize [45]. When they do, metastasis typically involves regional lymph nodes, in addition to both kidneys, pancreas, lungs, and the spleen [39, 49].

More than 50% of Sertoli cell tumors are estrogen-producing [45, 70, 71].

As a result of endogenous estrogen, affected patients may present with significant feminization, which is evident on physical examination [45, 49, 58, 70, 72–76].

Clinical findings that are suggestive of hyperestrogenism include the following [45, 49, 58, 70, 71, 77–79]:

- Atrophy of the non-neoplastic testicle
- Bilaterally symmetrical flank alopecia with hyperpigmentation (see Figure 55.6)
- Galactorrhea, or milk production
- Gynecomastia, or enlargement of the mammary glands
- Pendulous prepuce

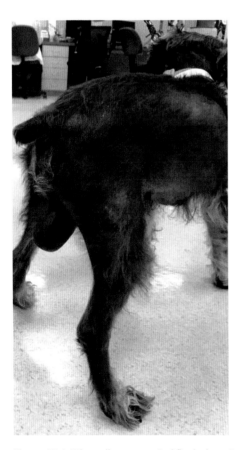

Figure 55.6 Bilaterally symmetrical flank alopecia in a canine patient with testicular neoplasia. *Source:* Courtesy of Beki Cohen Regan, DVM, DACVIM (Oncology).

- Penile atrophy
- Sexual attraction of other males
- Thinning of the epidermis

Hyperestrogenism is also likely to result in blood dyscrasias. After a transient increase in granulopoiesis, the following clinicopathologic abnormalities are expected [45, 49, 75, 80]:

- Neutropenia
- Nonregenerative anemia
- Thrombocytopenia

These changes result from the adverse effect of excessive estrogen on the bone marrow [45, 75, 80]. Hyperestrogenism causes bone marrow suppression [45, 75, 80]. This may be irreversible [45, 75, 80].

55.3.4 Diagnostic Work-up for Canine Testicular Tumors

Patients with Sertoli cell tumors may present with signs of paraneoplastic syndrome, as outlined above. Patients with other testicular tumor types are more often asymptomatic in the absence of metastasis [45].

The index of suspicion is raised when one or both testicles palpate as being enlarged and/or when a mass is detected [45]. Testicular asymmetry is common when there is unilateral involvement: the neoplastic testicle enlarges, and the unaffected testicle atrophies [45].

Any intact male dog should have a testicular exam annually [45]. As dogs age, the risk of testicular neoplasia increases [45].

A dog with a palpable testicular mass should undergo staging. Staging includes the following [45]:

- Complete blood count (CBC)
  - Hemogram
  - Leukogram
- Chemistry panel
- Imaging
  - Abdominal ultrasonography to assess:
    - ○ Liver
    - ○ Prostate
    - ○ Regional lymph nodes
    - ○ Spleen
  - Testicular imaging [81–83]
    - ○ Ultrasound-guided fine-needle aspiration
  - Three-view thoracic radiographs
- Urinalysis

Note that the utility of testicular ultrasound is limited in that it cannot identify tumor type [45]. However, it can differentiate neoplasia from testicular torsion, orchitis, and epididymitis [45, 81–83].

Castration is advisable as a form of excisional biopsy, with histopathologic examination of the excised testis [45].

Although few are clinically detected at the time of initial presentation, up to 50% of dogs have contralateral testicular tumors. Therefore, bilateral orchiectomy is considered standard of care, even if only one testis appears to be involved [45, 63].

If one or both testes are abdominally cryptorchid, then exploratory laparotomy is necessary for excision [45]. Regional lymph nodes may be sampled at the time of surgery, if indicated [45].

Dogs with feminization secondary to testicular neoplasia will spontaneously resolve, 1–3 months following castration, provided that there are no hormonally active areas of metastasis [45, 73, 84, 85]. Recurrence of feminization is a poor prognostic indicator [73]. It suggests that metastasis is present, despite having been undetected [45].

Dogs with bone marrow suppression have a guarded prognosis [45]. If irreversible, the patient is at increased risk of hemorrhage as well as infection secondary to pronounced neutropenia [45, 75, 80].

Metastatic testicular neoplasia requires adjunct therapy following castration [45]. Consult an oncology textbook to review options for chemotherapy, radiation therapy, and other novel approaches to case management.

55.3.5 Feline Testicular Tumors

Testicular tumors are uncommon in feline patients [45, 86–92]. Sporadic case reports suggest that cats may develop the same testicular tumors that dogs do, but at a reduced rate [45].

Because of the paucity of literature, little is known about the progression of testicular cancer in the cat or the feline response to treatment [45]. Until the biologic behavior of testicular tumors is established in these patients, principles of care and case management must be extrapolated from canine practice.

55.4 Testicular Torsion

Testicular torsion is an acutely painful condition in which the spermatic cord twists, occluding the blood supply to the affected testis [93–96].

Cryptorchid testes are at greater risk of torsion than non-cryptorchid testes [4, 20, 30, 36, 43, 44, 93, 97, 98].

When testicular torsion occurs in young dogs, it is most likely due to a retained, intra-abdominal testis, whereas older canine patients are more likely to experience torsion secondary to testicular neoplasia [94, 99].

Affected patients present acutely with a variety of clinical signs, including the following [94–96]:

- Abdominal tenderness
- Anorexia
- Dysuria
- Emesis
- Lethargy
- Pelvic limb lameness
- Ptyalism
- Pyrexia

Abdominal palpation typically confirms pain and/or an abdominal mass [94–96]. Abdominal radiographs may also detect a mass effect caudal to the ipsilateral kidney [94, 95]. Other than a retained testis, the mass effect at this location could represent sublumbar lymph nodes, colon, rectum, or ureter [95].

Ultrasonography is a valuable tool in that it provides more detail concerning the mass [95]. An experienced ultrasonographer can readily identify the mass as being testicular in origin [95].

A diagnosis of testicular torsion is prioritized when the patient is young and palpation confirms cryptorchidism [95].

Alternatively, the retained testis could be abscessed [95]. Testicular hematoma, granuloma, or neoplasia is also possible [95]. Testicular neoplasia is prioritized as a differential in older patients [94, 99].

Testicular torsion is managed by surgically excising the retained testis through either laparotomy or laparoscopy [94–96, 100, 101].

References

1 de Gier, J. and van Sluijs, F.J. (2009). Male reproductive tract. In: *Medical History and Physical Examination in Companion Animals*, 2e (ed. A. Rijnberk and S. FJv), 117–122. Edinburgh; New York: Saunders/Elsevier.

2 Englar, R.E. (2017). *Performing the Small Animal Physical Examination*. Hoboken, NJ: Wiley.

3 Evans, H.E. and Christensen, G.C. (1993). The urogenital system. In: *Miller's Anatomy of the Dog*, 3e (ed. H.E.

Evans and M.E. Miller), 494–558. Philadelphia: W.B. Saunders.

4 Romagnoli, S.E. (1991). Canine cryptorchidism. *Vet. Clin. North Am. Small Anim. Pract.* 21 (3): 533–544.

5 Veronesi, M.C., Riccardi, E., Rota, A., and Grieco, V. (2009). Characteristics of cryptic/ectopic and contralateral scrotal testes in dogs between 1 and 2 years of age. *Theriogenology* 72 (7): 969–977.

6 Yates, D., Hayes, G., Heffernan, M., and Beynon, R. (2003). Incidence of cryptorchidism in dogs and cats. *Vet. Rec.* 152 (16): 502–504.

7 Amann, R.P. and Veeramachaneni, D.N. (2007). Cryptorchidism in common eutherian mammals. *Reproduction* 133 (3): 541–561.

8 Bushby, P.A. (2010). Cryptorchid surgery and simple ophthalmic procedures. DVM 360 [Internet]. http://veterinarycalendar.dvm360.com/cryptorchid-surgery-and-simple-ophthalmic-procedures-proceedings.

9 Baumans, V., Dijkstra, G., and Wensing, C.J. (1981). Testicular descent in the dog. *Anat. Histol. Embryol.* 10 (2): 97–110.

10 Baumans, V., Dijkstra, G., and Wensing, C.J. (1982). The effect of orchidectomy on gubernacular outgrowth and regression in the dog. *Int. J. Androl.* 5 (4): 387–400.

11 Baumans, V., Dijkstra, G., and Wensing, C.J. (1983). The role of a non-androgenic testicular factor in the process of testicular descent in the dog. *Int. J. Androl.* 6 (6): 541–552.

12 Christiansen, I. (1984). *Reproduction in the Dog and Cat*. London: Bailliere Tindall.

13 Kutzler, M.A. and Peterson, M.E. (eds.) (2011). The reproductive tract. In: *Small Animal Pediatrics: The First 12 Months of Life*, 405–417. St. Louis: Elsevier Saunders.

14 Christensen, B.W. (2012). Disorders of sexual development in dogs and cats. *Vet. Clin. North Am. Small Anim. Pract.* 42 (3): 515–526, vi.

15 Peter, A.T. (2001). The reproductive system. In: *Veterinary Pediatrics: Dogs and Cats from Birth to Six Months*, 3e (ed. J.D. Hoskins), 463–475. Philadelphia: Saunders.

16 Rhoades, J.D. and Foley, C.W. (1977). Cryptorchidism and intersexuality. *Vet. Clin. North Am.* 7 (4): 789–794.

17 Meyers-Wallen, V.N. (2012). Gonadal and sex differentiation abnormalities of dogs and cats. *Sex. Dev.* 6 (1–3): 46–60.

18 Wolff, A. (1981). Castration, cryptorchidism, and cryptorchidectomy in dogs and cats. *Vet. Med. Small Anim. Clin.* 76 (12): 1739–1741.

19 Osterhoff, D.R. (1978). Canine cryptorchidism. *J. Am. Vet. Med. Assoc.* 172: 333.

20 Birchard, S.J. and Nappier, M. (2008). Cryptorchidism. *Compend. Contin. Educ. Dent.* 30 (6): 325–336, quiz 36–7.

21 Hannan, M.A., Kawate, N., Kubo, Y. et al. (2015). Expression analyses of insulin-like peptide 3, RXFP2, LH receptor, and 3beta-hydroxysteroid dehydrogenase in testes of normal and cryptorchid dogs. *Theriogenology* 84 (7): 1176–1184.

22 Pathirana, I.N., Yamasaki, H., Kawate, N. et al. (2012). Plasma insulin-like peptide 3 and testosterone concentrations in male dogs: changes with age and effects of cryptorchidism. *Theriogenology* 77 (3): 550–557.

23 Davidson, A.P. (2014). Canine cryptorchidism. *NAVC Clinician's Brief* (January): 102–104.

24 D'Cruz, A.J. and Das, K. (2004). Undescended testes. *Indian J. Pediatr.* 71 (12): 1111–1115.

25 Docimo, S.G., Silver, R.I., and Cromie, W. (2000). The undescended testicle: diagnosis and management. *Am. Fam. Physician* 62 (9): 2037–2044, 47–48.

26 Schindler, A.M., Diaz, P., Cuendet, A., and Sizonenko, P.C. (1987). Cryptorchidism: a morphological study of 670 biopsies. *Helv. Paediatr. Acta* 42 (2–3): 145–158.

27 Millis, D.L., Hauptman, J.G., and Johnson, C.A. (1992). Cryptorchidism and monorchism in cats: 25 cases (1980-1989). *J. Am. Vet. Med. Assoc.* 200 (8): 1128–1130.

28 Richardson, E.F. and Mullen, H. (1993). Cryptorchidism in cats. *Compend. Contin. Educ. Pract. Vet.* 15 (10): 1342–1345.

29 Wallace, J.L. and Levy, J.K. (2006). Population characteristics of feral cats admitted to seven trap-neuter-return programs in the United States. *J. Feline Med. Surg.* 8 (4): 279–284.

30 Foster, R.A. (2012). Common lesions in the male reproductive tract of cats and dogs. *Vet. Clin. North Am. Small Anim. Pract.* 42 (3): 527–545, vii.

31 Reif, J.S. and Brodey, R.S. (1969). The relationship between cryptorchidism and canine testicular neoplasia. *J. Am. Vet. Med. Assoc.* 155 (12): 2005–2010.

32 Little, S.E. (2012). Male reproduction. In: *The Cat: Clinical Medicine and Management* (ed. S.E. Little). St. Louis: Saunders Elsevier.

33 Cox, V.S., Wallace, L.J., and Jessen, C.R. (1978). An anatomic and genetic study of canine cryptorchidism. *Teratology* 18 (2): 233–240.

34 Kutzler, M.A. (2011). The reproductive tract. In: *Small Animal Pediatrics: The First 12 Months of Life* (ed. M.E. Peterson and M.A. Kutzler), 405–417. St. Louis, Mo: Saunders/Elsevier.

35 Pullig, T. (1953). Cryptorchidism in cocker spaniels. *J. Hered.* 44 (6): 250.

36 Hayes, H.M., Wilson, G.P., and Pendergrass, T.W. (1985). Canine cryptorchidism and subsequent testicular neoplasia: case-control study with epidemiologic update. *Teratology* 32: 51.

37 Pendergrass, T.W. (1975). Cryptorchidism and related defects in dogs: epidemiologic comparison with man. *Teratology* 12: 51.

38 Graves, T.K. (2006). Diseases of the testes and scrotum. In: *Saunders Manual of Small Animal Practice* (ed. S.J. Birchard and R.G. Sherding), 963. St. Louis: Elsevier.

39 Johnston, S.D., Root Kustritz, M.V., and Olson, P.N.S. (2001). *Disorders of Canine Testes and Epididymes. Canine and Feline Theriogenology*, 312–332. WB Saunders.

40 Kawakami, E., Tsutsui, T., Yamada, Y., and Yamauchi, M. (1984). Cryptorchidism in the dog: occurrence of cryptorchidism and semen quality in the cryptorchid dog. *Nippon Juigaku Zasshi* 46 (3): 303–308.

41 Hayes, H.M. Jr. and Pendergrass, T.W. (1976). Canine testicular tumors: epidemiologic features of 410 dogs. *Int. J. Cancer* 18 (4): 482–487.

42 Hohsteter, M., Artukovic, B., Severin, K. et al. (2014). Canine testicular tumors: two types of seminomas can be differentiated by immunohistochemistry. *BMC Vet. Res.* 10: 169.

43 Pearson, H. and Kelly, D.F. (1975). Testicular torsion in the dog: a review of 13 cases. *Vet. Rec.* 97 (11): 200–204.

44 Pendergrass, T.W. and Hayes, H.M. (1975). Cryptorchidism and related defects in dogs: epidemiologic comparisons with man. *Teratology* 12: 51–56.

45 Lawrence, J.A. and Saba, C.F. (2013). Tumors of the male reproductive system. In: *Withrow & MacEwen's Small Animal Clinical Oncology*, 5e (ed. S.J. Withrow, D.M. Vail and R.L. Page), 557–571. St. Louis, Missouri: Elsevier.

46 Cotchin, E. (1960). Testicular neoplasms in dogs. *J. Comp. Pathol.* 70: 232–248.

47 von Bomhard, D., Pukkavesa, C., and Haenichen, T. (1978). The ultrastructure of testicular tumours in the dog: I. germinal cells and seminomas. *J. Comp. Pathol.* 88 (1): 49–57.

48 Liao, A.T., Chu, P.Y., Yeh, L.S. et al. (2009). A 12-year retrospective study of canine testicular tumors. *J. Vet. Med. Sci.* 71 (7): 919–923.

49 Paepe, D., Hebbelinck, L., Kitshoff, A., and Vandenabeele, S. (2016). Feminization and severe pancytopenia caused by testicular neoplasia in a cryptorchid dog. *Vlaams Diergen. Tijds.* 85 (4): 197–205.

50 Lopate, C. (2010). Clinical approach to conditions of the male. In: *BSAVA Manual of Canine and Feline Reproduction and Neonatology. Gloucester* (ed. G.C.W. England and A. Von Heimendahl), 191–211. British Small Animal Veterinary Association.

51 Kim, O. and Kim, K.S. (2005). Seminoma with hyperesterogenemia in a Yorkshire Terrier. *J. Vet. Med. Sci.* 67 (1): 121–123.

52 Kang, S.C., Yang, H.S., Jung, J.Y. et al. (2011). Malignant Sertoli cell tumor in shuh tzu dog. *Korean J. Vet. Res.* 51: 171–175.

53 Grieco, V., Riccardi, E., Greppi, G.F. et al. (2008). Canine testicular tumours: a study on 232 dogs. *J. Comp. Pathol.* 138 (2–3): 86–89.

54 Peters, M.A.J., de Rooij, D.G., Teerds, K.J. et al. (2000). Spermatogenesis and testicular tumours in ageing dogs. *J. Reprod. Fertil.* 120 (2): 443–452.

55 Scully, R.E. and Coffin, D.L. (1952). Canine testicular tumors – with special reference to their histogenesis, comparative morphology, and endocrinology. *Cancer* 5 (3): 592–605.

56 Kennedy, P.C., Cullen, J.M., and Edwards, J.F. (eds.) (1998). *Histological Classifications of Tumors of the Genital System of Domestic Animals*, World Health Organization International Histological Classification of Tumors of Domestic Animals. American Registry of Pathology.

57 Nodtvedt, A., Gamlem, H., Gunnes, G. et al. (2011). Breed differences in the proportional morbidity of testicular tumours and distribution of histopathologic types in a population-based canine cancer registry. *Vet. Comp. Oncol.* 9 (1): 45–54.

58 Lipowitz, A.J., Schwartz, A., Wilson, G.P., and Ebert, J.W. (1973). Testicular neoplasms and concomitant clinical changes in the dog. *J. Am. Vet. Med. Assoc.* 163 (12): 1364–1368.

59 Weaver, A.D. (1983). Survey with follow-up of 67 dogs with testicular sertoli cell tumours. *Vet. Rec.* 113 (5): 105–107.

60 Priester, W.A. and McKay, F.W. The occurrence of tumors in domestic animals. *Natl. Cancer Inst. Monogr.* 1980 (54): 1–210.

61 Sapierzynski, R., Malicka, E., Bielecki, W. et al. (2007). Tumors of the urogenital system in dogs and cats. Retrospective review of 138 cases. *Pol. J. Vet. Sci.* 10 (2): 97–103.

62 Ortega-Pacheco, A., Rodriguez-Buenfil, J.C., Segura-Correa, J.C. et al. (2006). Pathological conditions of the reproductive organs of male stray dogs in the tropics: prevalence, risk factors, morphological findings and testosterone concentrations. *Reprod. Domest. Anim.* 41 (5): 429–437.

63 Reif, J.S., Maguire, T.G., Kenney, R.M., and Brodey, R.S. (1979). A cohort study of canine testicular neoplasia. *J. Am. Vet. Med. Assoc.* 175 (7): 719–723.

64 McEntee, M.C. (2002). Reproductive oncology. *Clin Tech Small Anim Pract.* 17 (3): 133–149.

65 Slatter, D.H. (1985). *Textbook of Small Animal Surgery.* Philadelphia: W.B. Saunders.

66 Sanpera, N., Masot, N., Janer, M. et al. (2002). Oestrogen-induced bone marrow aplasia in a dog with a Sertoli cell tumour. *J. Small Anim. Pract.* 43 (8): 365–369.

67 Ciaputa, R., Nowak, M., Kielbowicz, M. et al. (2012). Seminoma, Sertolioma, and Leydigoma in dogs: clinical and morphological correlations. *Bull. Vet. Inst. Pulawy* 56 (3): 361–367.

68 Gawlik-Jakubczak, T. and Krajka, K. (2004). A case of non-seminomatous testis tumor. *Przegl. Lek.* 61 (5): 528–530.

69 Restucci, B., Maiolino, P., Paciello, O. et al. (2003). Evaluation of angiogenesis in canine seminomas by quantitative immunohistochemistry. *J. Comp. Pathol.* 128 (4): 252–259.

70 Hoskins, J.D. (2004). Testicular cancer remains easily preventable disease. DVM 360 [Internet]. http://veterinarynews.dvm360.com/testicular-cancer-remains-easily-preventable-disease.

71 Huggins, C. and Moulder, P.V. (1945). Estrogen production by Sertoli cell tumors of the testis. *Cancer Res.* 5 (9): 510–514.

72 Weaver, A.D. (1983). Survey with follow-up of 67 dogs with testicular Sertoli-cell tumors. *Vet. Rec.* 113 (5): 105–107.

73 Brodey, R.S. and Martin, J.E. (1958). Sertoli cell neoplasms in the dog; the clinicopathological and endocrinological findings in thirtyseven dogs. *J. Am. Vet. Med. Assoc.* 133 (5): 249–257.

74 Mischke, R., Meurer, D., Hoppen, H.O. et al. (2002). Blood plasma concentrations of oestradiol-17 beta, testosterone and testosterone/oestradiol ratio in dogs with neoplastic and degenerative testicular diseases. *Res. Vet. Sci.* 73 (3): 267–272.

75 Morgan, R.V. (1982). Blood Dyscrasias associated with testicular-tumors in the dog. *J. Am. Anim. Hosp. Assoc.* 18 (6): 970–975.

76 Peters, M.A.J., de Jong, F.H., Teerds, K.J. et al. (2000). Ageing, testicular tumours and the pituitary-testis axis in dogs. *J. Endocrinol.* 166 (1): 153–161.

77 Zuckerman, S. and Groome, J.R. (1937). The etiology of benign enlargement of the prostate in the dog. *J. Pathol. Bacteriol.* 44: 113–124.

78 Zuckerman, S. and McKeown, T. (1938). The canine prostate in relation to normal and abnormal testicular changes. *J. Pathol. Bacteriol.* 46: 7–19.

79 Greulich, W.W. and Burford, T.H. (1936). Testicular tumors associated with mammary, prostatic, and other changes in cryptorchid dogs. *Am. J. Cancer* 28: 496–511.

80 Sherding, R.G., Wilson, G.P. 3rd, and Kociba, G.J. (1981). Bone marrow hypoplasia in eight dogs with Sertoli cell tumor. *J. Am. Vet. Med. Assoc.* 178 (5): 497–501.

81 Johnston, G.R., Feeney, D.A., Johnston, S.D., and O'Brien, T.D. (1991). Ultrasonographic features of testicular neoplasia in dogs: 16 cases (1980–1988). *J. Am. Vet. Med. Assoc.* 198 (10): 1779–1784.

82 Pugh, C.R. and Konde, L.J. (1991). Sonographic evaluation of canine testicular and scrotal abnormalities – a review of 26 case-histories. *Vet. Radiol.* 32 (5): 243–250.

83 Eilts, B.E., Pechman, R.D., Hedlund, C.S., and Kreeger, J.M. (1988). Use of ultrasonography to diagnose Sertoli-cell neoplasia and cryptorchidism in a dog. *J. Am. Vet. Med. Assoc.* 192 (4): 533–534.

84 Hogenesch, H., Whiteley, H.E., Vicini, D.S., and Helper, L.C. (1987). Seminoma with metastases in the eyes and the brain in a dog. *Vet. Pathol.* 24 (3): 278–280.

85 Gopinath, D., Draffan, D., Philbey, A.W., and Bell, R. (2009). Use of intralesional oestradiol concentration to identify a functional pulmonary metastasis of canine sertoli cell tumour. *J. Small Anim. Pract.* 50 (4): 198–200.

86 Rosen, D.K. and Carpenter, J.L. (1993). Functional ectopic interstitial cell tumor in a castrated male cat. *J. Am. Vet. Med. Assoc.* 202 (11): 1865–1866.

87 Cotchin, E. (1984). Neoplasia. In: *Diseases of the Cat and their Management* (ed. G.T. Wilkinson). Oxford: Blackwell.

88 Miller, M.A., Hartnett, S.E., and Ramos-Vara, J.A. (2007). Interstitial cell tumor and Sertoli cell tumor in the testis of a cat. *Vet. Pathol.* 44 (3): 394–397.

89 Miyoshi, N., Yasuda, N., Kamimura, Y. et al. (2001). Teratoma in a feline unilateral cryptorchid testis. *Vet. Pathol.* 38 (6): 729–730.

90 Ferreira-da-Silva, J. (2002). Teratoma in a feline unilateral cryptorchid testis. *Vet. Pathol.* 39: 516.

91 Benazzi, C., Sarli, G., and Brunetti, B. (2004). Sertoli cell tumour in a cat. *J. Vet. Med. A Physiol. Pathol. Clin. Med.* 51 (3): 124–126.

92 Meier, H. (1956). Sertoli-cell tumor in the cat: report of two cases. *North Am. Vet.* 37: 979.

93 Quartuccio, M., Marino, G., Garufi, G. et al. (2012). Sertoli cell tumors associated with feminizing syndrome and spermatic cord torsion in two cryptorchid dogs. *J. Vet. Sci.* 13 (2): 207–209.

94 Carr, J.G., Heng, H.G., Ruth, J., and Freeman, L. (2015). Laparoscopic treatment of testicular torsion in a puppy. *J. Am. Anim. Hosp. Assoc.* 51 (2): 97–100.

95 Boza, S., de Membiela, F., Navarro, A. et al. (2011). What is your diagnosis? Testicular torsion. *J. Am. Vet. Med. Assoc.* 238 (1): 37–38.

96 Mostachio, G.Q., Apparicio, M., Vicente, W.R. et al. (2007). Intraabdominal torsion of a neoplastic testicle and prostatic cyst in a cryptorchid dog. *Schweiz. Arch. Tierheilkd.* 149 (9): 408–412.

97 Laing, E.J., Harari, J., and Smith, C.W. (1983). Spermatic cord torsion and Sertoli cell tumor in a dog. *J. Am. Vet. Med. Assoc.* 183 (8): 879–881.

98 Metzger, F.L., Hattel, A.L., and White, D.G. (1993). Hematuria, Hyperestrogenemia, and Hyperprogesteronemia due to a Sertoli-cell tumor in a bilaterally Cryptorchid dog. *Cancer Pract.* 18 (3): 32–35.

99 Hecht, S., King, R., Tidwell, A.S., and Gorman, S.C. (2004). Ultrasound diagnosis: intra-abdominal torsion of a non-neoplastic testicle in a cryptorchid dog. *Vet. Radiol. Ultrasound* 45 (1): 58–61.

100 Lee, K.F., Tang, Y.C., and Leong, H.T. (2001). Emergency laparoscopic orchidectomy for torsion of intra-abdominal testis: a case report. *J. R. Coll. Surg. Edinb.* 46 (2): 110–112.

101 Porpiglia, F., Destefanis, P., Fiori, C. et al. (2001). Laparoscopic diagnosis and management of acute intra-abdominal testicular torsion. *J. Urol.* 166 (2): 600–601.

56

Bilateral Pre-Scrotal Swellings in the Canine Patient

56.1 Introduction to Penile Anatomy

The penis is the copulatory organ of the male dog [1–3].

The canine penis consists of three parts [2–4]:

- The crura, or the roots
- The corpus, or the body
- The glans penis

The crura are the most proximal aspects of the penis [2, 3]. They represent the attachments of the penis to the right and left ischial tuberosities [2–4].

The bulb of the penis is a blood-filled structure that sits between the crura near the ischiatic arch. It blends into the corpus spongiosum distally, and together, both tissues cushion the urethra, which is dorsal [2, 3].

The crura join distal to the bulb to form the body of the penis, the corpus [2–4]. The corpus is composed of two distinct cavernous bodies, one per crus, separated from one another by a septum [2, 3].

The os penis, or baculum, is a penile bone that is present in both the dog and the cat [2–4]. The caudal aspect of this bone attaches to the end of the corpus and extends into the glans penis [2, 3]. The bone tapers proximally to a cartilaginous tip [2, 3]. The purpose of the os penis is to provide structural rigidity [2–4].

Along the ventral aspect of the os penis is a urethral groove [2–4]. The urethra tracks along this groove through the glans penis [2, 3]. The groove is widest at the base of the os penis and narrows appreciably toward its tip [2, 3].

The glans penis is the most distal part of the penis [2, 3, 5]. In its flaccid state, the glans penis is sheathed by a fold of skin, the prepuce, which lies between the upper thighs, along the ventral-most aspect of the caudal abdomen [1–4].

During arousal, columns of erectile tissue within the penis engorge with blood [1–3, 6–9]. This expands the length of the penis, in anticipation of copulation, causing the glans penis to become unsheathed [1–3] (see Figure 56.1).

Note that the canine penis is a vascular structure, which accommodates this elongation [2, 3]. This is in stark contrast to the fibroelastic penis of the bull, boar, and ram, which relies upon the sigmoid flexure to extend penile length to achieve intromission rather than engorgement of the penis with blood [1].

The glans penis of the dog consists of a base, the barrel-shaped bulbus glandis, and the pars longa glandis [2, 3]. Both structures appear as one in the non-erect patient [2]. However, during erection, the bulbus glandis expands with blood to form a prominent ring-like structure at the penile base [7]. Sometimes this swelling is referred to as the "knot" (see Figure 56.2).

This so-called knot allows mating dogs to form the characteristic copulatory tie, which transiently locks the male inside of the female during intromission [2, 3, 10]. The tie prevents separation during mating. During the tie, the male turns around so that he is facing away from the female: they are essentially standing rear-to-rear. This requires the erect penis to rotate 180° just distal to the bulbus glandis [7]. The os penis functions to maintain patency of the urethral opening during this twist [7].

Ejaculation consists of three fractions, the second of which is sperm-rich [7]. The final fraction consists of prostatic fluid to flush the contents of the male reproductive tract into the female [7].

Dogs remain tied together for minutes to over an hour, until detumescence dislodges the bulbus glandis [7, 11].

56.2 Pre-Scrotal Swellings Secondary to Bulbus Glandis Engorgement

Although the bulbus glandis most notably swells in anticipation of sexual activity, the bulbus glandis may also swell in response to generalized excitement. For this reason, swelling of the bulbus glandis may occur in neutered as well as intact male dogs. Swelling of the bulbus glandis often occurs post-orchiectomy, presumably due to manipulation of this region of the body during surgery.

Common Clinical Presentations in Dogs and Cats, First Edition. Ryane E. Englar.

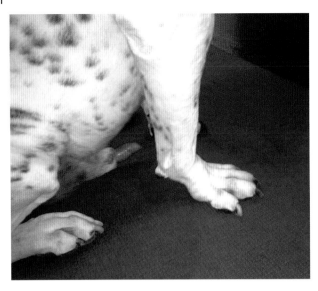

Figure 56.1 This patient's penis has become unsheathed due to excitement. *Source:* Courtesy of Pamela Mueller, DVM.

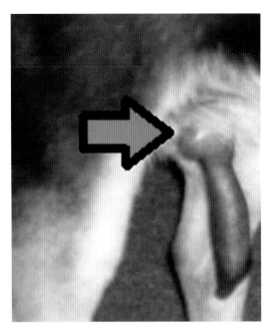

Figure 56.2 Erect canine penis. Note the appreciable swelling at the base of the glans penis. This swelling is the bulbus glandis, engorged with blood.

(a)   (b)

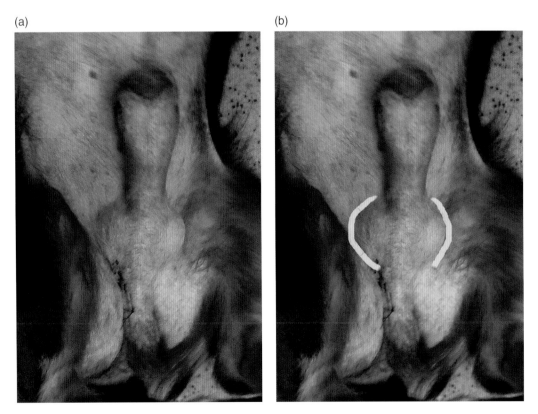

Figure 56.3 (a) Canine patient, post orchiectomy. Note that there are bilateral pre-scrotal swellings. These represent an engorged bulbus glandis. (b). Same patient as depicted in (a). The swellings have been outlined in yellow-orange.

When the bulbus glandis swells in a non-erect dog, the glans penis remains hidden within the preputial sheath, and the observer will notice two discrete swellings under the skin (see Figures 56.3a, b).

When these lumps appear shortly after orchiectomy, clients may become alarmed. In the author's experience, the inexperienced owner may mistake these swellings as testicles and even question if the dog was in fact neutered. It is important to reassure clients that these swellings represent normal canine anatomy and that they should subside when the dog's excitement does.

On the other hand, persistent swelling and/or pain associated with an engorged bulbus glandis is not normal and should be evaluated.

56.3 Canine Transmissible Venereal Tumor (TVT) and Involvement of the Bulbus Glandis

Canine transmissible venereal tumors (TVT) are uncommonly seen in North America, Northern Europe, and Central Europe, but are enzootic throughout most of the world [12].

Recall from Chapter 14, Section 14.5 that TVTs are particularly prevalent in tropical and subtropical regions, including Puerto Rico, Papua New Guinea, and Central and South America [12, 13].

Although TVTs were discussed in Chapter 14 from the standpoint of their potential to invade the skin, these tumors are found predominantly on external genitalia [14–19].

Recall that TVT is spread when tumor cells are deposited on damaged epithelial surfaces [12, 14]. Mating is abrasive to genital surfaces [12, 14].

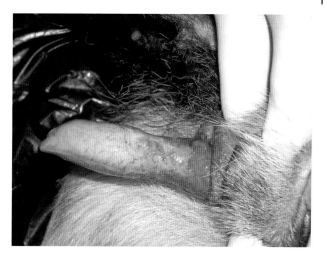

Figure 56.4 Transmissible venereal tumors (TVT) involving the base of a canine penis. *Source:* Courtesy of Laura Polerecky, LVT.

Young, sexually mature, and sexually active dogs are most at risk for development of TVTs, and in males, lesions concentrate most often at the bulbus glandis [12, 14] (see Figure 56.4).

Refer to Chapter 14 for a discussion about diagnosing TVT.

For the purpose of this chapter, be aware that neoplasia involving the bulbus glandis is possible. Any mass-like growth at the bulbus glandis or along the shaft of the penis requires further investigation.

TVT may be more or less likely, depending upon geography, meaning the patient's country of residence, as well as the classic appearance of lesions.

TVTs often develop fronds or are multilobulated [12]. The surfaces of the tumor are likely to be irritated. Ulcerations, hemorrhage, and secondary infection are common [12].

References

1 Englar, R.E. (2017). *Performing the Small Animal Physical Examination*. Hoboken, NJ: Wiley.

2 Evans, H.E. and Christensen, G.C. (1993). The urogenital system. In: *Miller's Anatomy of the Dog*, 3e (ed. H.E. Evans and M.E. Miller), 494–554. Philadelphia: W.B. Saunders.

3 Dyce, K.M., Sack, W.O., and Wensing, C.J.G. (eds.) (1996). The urogenital apparatus. In: *Textbook of Veterinary Anatomy*, 2e, xiii, 856 p. Philadelphia: Saunders.

4 Coomer, A.R. (2013). Male reproductive and penile surgery. World Congress Proceedings [Internet]. https://www.vin.com/apputil/content/defaultadv1.aspx?pId=11372&meta=generic&catId=35320&id=5709894&ind=282&objTypeID=17.

5 Hart, B.L. and Kitchell, R.L. (1965). External morphology of the erect glans penis of the dog. *Anat. Rec.* 152 (2): 193–198.

6 Goericke-Pesch, S., Holscher, C., Failing, K., and Wehrend, A. (2013). Functional anatomy and ultrasound examination of the canine penis. *Theriogenology* 80 (1): 24–33.

7 Kutzler, M.A. (2005). Semen collection in the dog. *Theriogenology* 64 (3): 747–754.

8 Dorr, L.D. and Brody, M.J. (1967). Hemodynamic mechanisms of erection in the canine penis. *Am. J. Phys.* 213 (6): 1526–1531.

9 Christensen, G.C. (1954). Angioarchitecture of the canine penis and the process of erection. *Am. J. Anat.* 95 (2): 227–261.

10 Hart, B.L. (1972). The action of extrinsic penile muscles during copulation in the male dog. *Anat. Rec.* 173 (1): 1–5.

11 Beach, F.A. (1970). Coital behavior in dogs. VI. Long-term effects of castration upon mating in the male. *J. Comp. Physiol. Psychol.* 70 (3): 1–32.

12 Ganguly, B., Das, U., and Das, A.K. (2016). Canine transmissible venereal tumour: a review. *Vet. Comp. Oncol.* 14 (1): 1–12.

13 Rust, J.H. (1949). Transmissible lymphosarcoma in the dog. *J. Am. Vet. Med. Assoc.* 114 (862): 10–14.

14 Vermooten, M.I. (1987). Canine transmissible venereal tumor (TVT): a review. *J. S. Afr. Vet. Assoc.* 58 (3): 147–150.

15 Weir, E.C., Pond, M.J., Duncan, J.R., and Polzin, D.J. (1978). Extra-genital occurrence of transmissible venereal tumor in dog – literature-review and case-reports. *J. Am. Anim. Hosp. Assoc.* 14 (4): 532–536.

16 van Rensburg, I.B. and Petrick, S.W. (1980). Extragenital malignant transmissible venereal tumour in a bitch. *J. S. Afr. Vet. Assoc.* 51 (3): 199–201.

17 Holmes, J.M. (1981). A 125IUdR technique for measuring the cell loss from subcutaneously growing canine transmissible venereal tumours. *Res. Vet. Sci.* 31 (3): 306–311.

18 Higgins, D.A. (1966). Observations on the canine transmissible venereal tumour as seen in the Bahamas. *Vet. Rec.* 79 (3): 67–71.

19 Duncan, J.R. and Prasse, K.W. (1979). Cytology of canine cutaneous round cell tumors. Mast cell tumor, histiocytoma, lymphosarcoma and transmissible venereal tumor. *Vet. Pathol.* 16 (6): 673–679.

57

Spines Along the Feline Penis

57.1   Introduction to Feline Penile Anatomy

The anatomy of the canine penis was introduced in Chapter 56. The feline penis is similar to the dog's in that it is hidden from sight when in its non-erect state. Erection causes the feline penis to be unsheathed from the prepuce.

Unlike the dog, in which the penis is carried between the upper thighs, the feline penis is housed within the perineum. Recall from Chapter 55 that the feline scrotum is ventral to the anus. The preputial opening, in turn, is ventral to the scrotum (see Figures 57.1a, b).

The non-erect feline penis is directed caudally [1]. It is therefore evaluated best when observing the patient from the rear. In this position, the urethra is seated dorsal to the os penis [2].

As the feline penis develops an erection, it changes its orientation to point cranially between the tomcat's thighs, despite the fact that it does not gain significantly in terms of length [1]. This allows the tomcat to mount the queen and achieve intromission in the usual fashion [1].

The tomcat penis is very short compared to the pars longa glandis of the dog, and its shape is rather conical [1].

57.2   Penile Spines

A second important distinguishing feature between tomcats and male dogs is that the glans of the former species is speckled with 120–150 caudally directed keratinized papillae [1–6] (see Figure 57.2).

These keratinized papillae are also called penile spines [1–3, 6]. These spines serve a purpose. They scrape the queen's reproductive tract during copulation [1–3]. This action is thought to stimulate ovulation [1–3]. Queens are induced ovulators: they do not release oocytes without sexual stimulation [5, 7, 8]. The chance of ovulation also increases if copulation occurs more than once [5].

Unlike dogs, intromission in cats is brief [4]. This is attributed to presumed discomfort secondary to vaginal stimulation by the penile spines. Tomcats dismount in haste to avoid being injured by the queen, who is likely to strike out [4].

Penile spines are testosterone-dependent [3, 4, 6]. Testosterone is required for their development and maintenance [3, 4, 6].

Penile spines develop as early as two to three months of age and are fully present by six to seven months of age [3, 4, 6].

Within 24 hours of castration, testosterone levels drop to 0–1.7 nmol/l [4]. This reduction to basal levels will trigger regression of the penile spines [3, 4]. Regression is not immediate [6]. It may take up to six weeks after castration for the papillae to disappear [6–8].

57.3   Clinical Relevance of Penile Spines

Stray cats may present to the clinic for evaluation by good Samaritans who wish to adopt them. If an adult male lacks scrotal testes on physical examination, then it is important for the clinician to discern whether the patient previously underwent orchiectomy or is instead bilaterally cryptorchid [3].

If the adult male was castrated six weeks or more prior to presentation, then one would expect for the surface of his penis to be smooth, when unsheathed from the prepuce.

If, on the other hand, the adult male is bilaterally cryptorchid, then his abnormally located testicles will still produce enough testosterone to maintain the papillae. In this case, he should have penile spines [3, 9].

Common Clinical Presentations in Dogs and Cats, First Edition. Ryane E. Englar.
© 2019 John Wiley & Sons, Inc. Published 2019 by John Wiley & Sons, Inc.

(a)

(b)

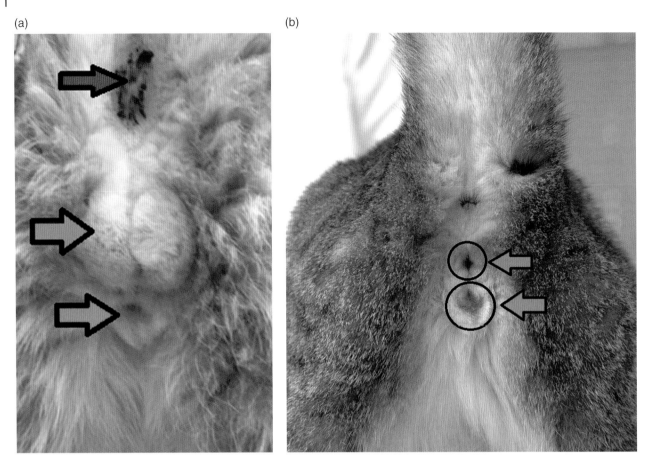

Figure 57.1 (a) Perineal anatomy of the tomcat. The purple arrow indicates the anus. The blue arrow indicates the scrotum. The orange arrow indicates the preputial opening. *Source:* Courtesy of the Media Resources Department at Midwestern University. (b) Perineal anatomy of the neutered male cat. The preputial opening has been circled in black and highlighted with an orange arrow. The blue arrow is pointing to the space dorsal to the preputial opening. This is where the scrotal sac would be were the patient an intact male cat. *Source:* Courtesy of the Media Resources Department at Midwestern University.

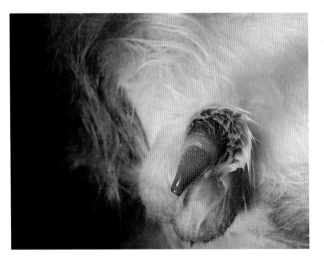

Figure 57.2 Close-up of the glans of the penis in a tomcat. Note the presence of penile spines that is unique to the cat, as compared to the dog. *Source:* Courtesy of Joseph Onello, DVM.

This approach to examining the penis provides an inexpensive way to determine sexual status [3].

Note that testosterone assays may be used for confirmatory testing [3]. Baseline serum testosterone is compared to the testosterone level that results from the administration of gonadotropin-releasing hormone (GnRH) [3].

References

1 Hudson, L.C. and Hamilton, W.P. (1993). *Atlas of Feline Anatomy for Veterinarians* xii, 287 p. p. Philadelphia, PA: Saunders.

2 Schatten, H. and Constantinescu, G.M. (2007). *Comparative Reproductive Biology*, 1e xiii, 402 p. p. Ames, Iowa: Blackwell Pub.

3 Englar, R.E. (2017). *Performing the Small Animal Physical Examination*. Hoboken, NJ: Wiley.

4 August, J.R. (2010). *Consultations in Feline Internal Medicine*. St. Louis, MO: Saunders.

5 Ettinger, S.J., Feldman, E.C., and Côté, E. (2017). *Textbook of Veterinary Internal Medicine: Diseases of the Dog and the Cat*, 8e 2 volumes (lviii, 2181, I-90 pages) p. St. Louis, Missouri: Elsevier.

6 Aronson, L.R. and Cooper, M.L. (1967). Penile spines of the domestic cat: their endocrine-behavior relations. *Anat. Rec.* 157 (1): 71–78.

7 Little, S.E. (2012). Male reproduction. In: *The Cat: Clinical Medicine and Management*. St. Louis: Saunders Elsevier.

8 Dyce, K.M., Sack, W.O., and Wensing, C.J.G. (1996). *Textbook of Veterinary Anatomy*, 2e xiii, 856 p. p. Philadelphia: Saunders.

9 Côté, E. (2015). *Clinical Veterinary Advisor. Dogs and Cats*, 3e xxxvii, 1642 pages p. St. Louis, Missouri: Elsevier Mosby.

58

Abnormal Presentations Involving the Prepuce and the Penis

58.1 Introduction to Pathological Conditions Involving the External Male Genitalia

Preputial and penile anatomy was introduced in Chapter 56. Pathology may affect either structure, and may be congenital or acquired.

Congenital conditions that involve external male genitalia do not occur often in clinical practice [1]. However, when they do, there is typically preputial involvement [1, 2]. For example, the preputial opening may be too small for the penis to extend through [1]. This so-called phimosis or preputial stenosis may cause urine to accumulate within the sheath [1]. The resultant irritation, balanoposthitis, may cause secondary infection [1].

Paraphimosis is a related condition: the penis is initially able to protrude through the opening, but has difficulty returning to its position within the sheath [2]. Paraphimosis may be congenital or acquired, and will be discussed in detail below.

Acquired conditions that involve external male genitalia include three broad categories [1]:

- Neoplasia involving the prepuce and/or penis
- Priapism, that is, persistent erection
- Traumatic injury to the prepuce and/or penis

Neoplasia of the penis was reviewed in brief in Chapter 56, Section 56.3. Recall that canine transmissible venereal tumors (TVT) develop most often on external genitalia [3–8]. In males, the primary location for TVT development is the bulbus glandis [3, 9]. However, TVT can also track up the shaft of the penis (see Figure 58.1).

In addition to having a grossly visible mass, patients with TVT may present for the following [10]:

- Dysuria
- Enlargement of the prepuce
- Excessive licking of the penis
- Hematuria

- Preputial discharge
  - Hemorrhagic
  - Mucopurulent
  - Serosanguinous
- Stranguria
- Urethral obstruction

Note that TVTs are not the only penile tumor that has been recognized in the dog [10, 11]. Mast cell tumor (MCT), melanoma, osteoma, lymphosarcoma, chondrosarcoma, osteosarcoma of the os penis, squamous cell carcinoma (SCC) and transitional cell carcinoma (TCC) of the urethra are uncommon, but possible [1, 11–19].

Priapism and traumatic injury occur more often than neoplasia as acquired pathology of external male genitalia [1]. Therefore, these will be emphasized below.

58.2 Hypospadias as a Congenital Anomaly

Hypospadias is characterized by abnormal development of the urethra [1, 2, 20–26]. Specifically, the tubular structure of the penile urethra is incompletely formed because the urogenital folds do not fuse, as they ought to, during fetal development [21, 22, 25–30].

Hypospadias can occur in both sexes; however, it more typically involves the penile urethra [1, 2].

In males, the normal urethra opens at the tip of the penis [1, 2]. By contrast, patients with hypospadias have an abnormally located urethral orifice [1, 2, 20, 21, 28, 31]. The malpositioned orifice may be along the ventrum of the penis, which is the most common of clinical presentations [1, 2].

Alternatively, the urethral orifice may open up at any point along the glans, penile shaft, scrotal, inguinal, and/or perineal regions [1, 2, 20, 21, 25, 27, 28, 32–34] (see Figure 58.2).

Perineal hypospadias may also be called sub-anal hypospadias because the urethral orifice is nearer to the

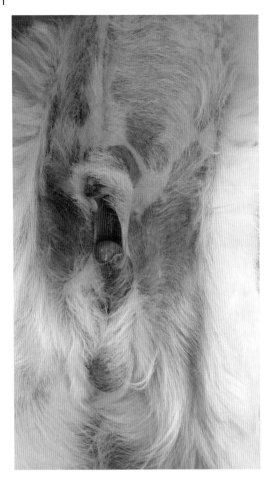

Figure 58.1 Hypospadias in a canine patient, involving the ventral ischial region. This clinical presentation is severe. Note how the non-fused prepuce has resulted in extreme exposure of the penis. *Source:* Courtesy of Adam Riley.

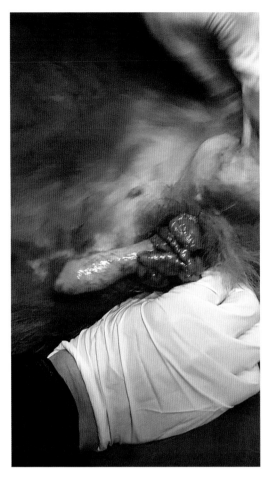

Figure 58.2 Multi-lobed TVT that extends from the base of the penis to the shaft. *Source:* Courtesy of Hannah Butler.

anus than is usual [20]. In these clinical scenarios, secondary cystitis and urinary incontinence are possible [35]. Anal mucosa may also join with urethral mucosa, increasing the risk for ascending urinary tract infections (UTIs) [20].

Patients that are affected by hypospadias are likely to have a deformed or underdeveloped penis [1, 2, 21, 25, 33]. For instance, the penis may exhibit ventral or caudoventral deviation [21, 36].

Patients with hypospadias are also likely to have concurrent congenital defects, including the following [20, 21, 25, 28, 29, 31, 33, 36–41]:

- Cryptorchidism
- Delayed testicular descent
- Hermaphroditism
- Hydrocephalus
- Persistent frenulum
  - The glans penis remains connected to the preputial mucosa.

- This connection prevents the penis from extruding from the prepuce.
- Prostatic agenesis
- Renal aplasia
- Testicular agenesis
- Umbilical hernia

Patients may present for grossly visible deviations from the anatomical norm [20, 21, 25, 33, 34].

Patients with mild hypospadias may present for the following [21, 25, 28, 42]:

- Abnormal urine stream
- Balanitis, inflammation of the glans penis
- Balanoposthitis, inflammation of the glans penis and the prepuce
- Excessive grooming of the prepuce
- Pollakiuria
- Stranguria
- Urine scald dermatitis

Urethral strictures are possible in advanced cases of hypospadias [43].

Hypospadias is inherited in Boston Terriers [1, 2, 21, 25, 33, 40]. Genetic factors are suspected in other breeds as well [20, 21, 31, 32].

Teratogens, decreased exposure to fetal androgen, and/or increased exposure to environmental estrogens may also contribute to the development of hypospadias [1, 21, 33, 44]. However, this has yet to be proven in dogs and cats [1, 21, 25, 31, 33, 44].

When a patient presents with hypospadias, a thorough examination of the reproductive tract is necessary to rule out concurrent issues [25].

Mild hypospadias does not require surgical management [25, 45]. If the urethral orifice opens somewhere on the glands other than at the tip, it may or may not be noticeable, and at most, it may cause a deviated stream of urine.

Surgical intervention is indicated when concurrent defects complicate the presenting complaint and/or if an exceptionally wide preputial opening is present [45].

Phallectomy is often necessary when the penis is both exposed and nonfunctional [22, 26, 28, 29, 45].

58.3 Paraphimosis as Congenital or Acquired Pathology

Paraphimosis was introduced in Section 58.1 as a condition in which the non-erect penis cannot retract back into the prepuce after being extruded from its sheath [2, 12, 13, 46–49].

Patients are typically young at time of presentation [13]. They may be intact or castrated males [46]. Historically, small-breed dogs are overrepresented [13]. However, any breed can be affected.

The etiology of paraphimosis may be idiopathic [2, 46, 50]. Alternatively, it may result from the following [2, 10, 12, 13, 15, 24, 27, 46–48, 51–56]:

- Acquired narrowing of the preputial opening
  - Foreign body
    o Foxtails
    o Long fur:
      - The patient mates as expected;
      - In the process of mating, preputial fur creates a ring around the preputial opening and/or the base of the penis;
      - When the patient dismounts and the glans undergoes detumescence, the penis is unable to retract back into its sheath;
      - The penis becomes strangulated by the fur ring;
      - The penis swells.
  - Scarring from past trauma
- Arousal without an erection

- Balanoposthitis
- Congenitally abnormal, narrowed preputial opening
- Exposure to a female in estrus
- Excessive licking at the prepuce and/or penis by the patient
- Fractured os penis
- Increased sexual activity
- Ineffective preputial muscles
- Masturbation
- Neoplasia
  - TVT
- Neuropathology
- Swelling of the penis
  - Neoplastic
  - Traumatic

When the penis is trapped outside of the sheath for an extended period of time, it becomes dry and irritated [13, 46, 47].

If the extruded penis becomes entrapped because of a preputial fur ring or a narrower-than-ordinary preputial opening, then the tissue will also become ischemic [13, 46]. The exposed penile is more likely to sustain trauma, including self-maiming [12].

The entrapped penis becomes edematous [13, 57]. Blood flow to and from penile tissues is compromised, causing circulatory stasis [13]. In severe cases, the penis undergoes necrosis [46] (see Figure 58.3).

Phallectomy, that is, amputation of the penis, is the only way to manage the patient when penile tissue becomes necrotic [10, 12, 15, 46–49, 56, 58]. A concurrent scrotal urethrostomy allows the patient to urinate without a penis [48].

Milder cases can be managed more conservatively, by lubricating the shaft of the penis with water-soluble gel in an attempt to digitally replace it within the sheath [13, 46, 57]. Hygroscopic agents may be particularly useful to apply topically because they draw water out of the penis [12, 13]. This reduces penile girth to facilitate replacement of the penis within the sheath [12]. These include mannitol, over-the-counter sugar, honey, various salts, and 50% dextrose [12, 13, 48, 59]. Following manual replacement, the patient may benefit from anti-inflammatory medications and a temporary purse-string suture at the opening of the prepuce [15, 48, 53, 56].

Narrowed preputial openings require surgical correction to minimize recurrence [10].

The prepuce can also be surgically advanced and/or the preputial muscles can be surgically shortened to facilitate sheathing of the penis by the prepuce [10, 24, 47, 48, 51]. Note that advancement of the prepuce is only effective when penile exposure is minimal [10]. On average, the prepuce cannot be advanced beyond one to one-and-a-half centimeters [10].

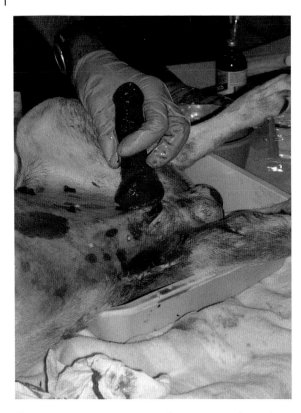

Figure 58.3 Emergency case involving protracted paraphimosis. Note the development of blackened regions along the shaft of this canine penis. The blackened discoloration is indicative of necrosis. The affected tissue is no longer vital. *Source:* Courtesy of Laura Polerecky, LVT.

More recently, surgeons have experimented with phallopexy [10]. The penile shaft is permanently adhered to the adjacent preputial mucosa [10]. This permanent tacking prevents the penis from being extruded.

58.4 Priapism as an Acquired Condition Involving the Penis

Priapism is a state of prolonged erection, beyond that which is ordinary for sexual arousal and intromission [59–62]. Erections that last more than four hours and are painful are reflective of priapism [59, 60, 62–65].

Priapism rarely occurs in companion animal patients [59–63, 66, 67]. When it does, it is the result of the following [1, 10, 12, 46, 59–62, 68–72]:
- Lower urinary tract disease
  - Urethritis
  - UTI
- Overstimulation of parasympathetic pathways via the pelvic nerve
  - Infectious neuropathy

  - Canine distemper virus (CDV)
  - Rabies
    - Rabies-associated priapism has been documented in humans only [73, 74]
  - Mechanical compression of the pelvic nerve
    - Constipation
    - Obstipation
    - Sublumbar mass
  - Pharmacologic agents
    - Acepromazine
    - Amphetamine
    - Sildenafil
  - Spinal cord trauma
- Penile trauma that was sustained during mating Reduced venous outflow from the penis
  - Pelvic mass that occludes circulation
    - Abscess
    - Tumor
  - Penile thromboembolism
  - Post-orchiectomy in cats [62, 67, 75]
- Vasculitis
  - Feline infectious peritonitis (FIP) [61, 62]

Priapism may be confused with paraphimosis [63, 76]. However, they are grossly distinguishable from one another. The penis is flaccid in cases of paraphimosis, as compared to priapism, in which the penis is erect and firm [59, 60].

Patients with priapism are exceptionally uncomfortable [46, 68]. Patients may also present for dysuria and/or stranguria [46, 68].

Few cases appear in the veterinary medicine literature [54, 62, 63, 67, 69, 72, 75–77]. Of those involving cats, the Siamese breed is overrepresented [62].

Many of the same dangers that are associated with case presentations involving paraphimosis apply to priapism. Penile exposure compromises the viability of the tissue, as does the compromised blood supply [59, 60].

Conservative management may be attempted in the same manner as was directed at cases involving paraphimosis: lubrication, to rehydrate the glans and the use of hyperosmotic agents to reduce the edema [12, 13, 46, 48, 57, 59, 67, 78].

In humans, intracavernosal injections of phenylephrine may provide some benefit in terms of restoring blood flow [63]. These may be attempted in veterinary patients [63]. However, the appropriate dose in dogs and cats has not yet been determined [63].

Unfortunately, by the time many patients present to the clinic, ischemic damage is advanced and the patient is beyond the point at which early therapeutic intervention can be initiated. Phallectomy and canine scrotal or feline perineal urethrostomy are often indicated [63].

58.5 Penile Trauma

The male reproductive tract is traumatized more frequently than the female, in large part because it is exteriorized [79].

Trauma to the male reproductive tract may involve the following [10, 79]:

- Os penis
- Penis
- Scrotum

Lacerations of the penile tip are sutured, as are scrotal lacerations, provided that they are minor [79]. Unfortunately, the scrotum presents a challenging region of the body to treat for infection, even if a drain is placed [79]. Scrotal ablation is indicated for significant and/or contaminated wounds [79].

Recall from Chapter 56, Section 56.1 that the os penis, or baculum, is a penile bone that is present in both the dog and the cat [12, 80, 81]. This bone extends into the glans penis, where it tapers proximally to a cartilaginous tip [80, 81]. The purpose of the os penis is to provide structural rigidity [12, 80, 81].

The os penis is visible radiographically (see Figure 58.4).

Because the os penis is a bone, it may be fractured as a result of penile trauma [10, 79]. For example, dogs may sustain a kick to the groin. They may damage the inguinal region when jumping fences. They may be injured during mating, or they may be hit by cars.

The os penis has a close association with the urethra. Recall from Chapter 56, Section 56.1 that there is a groove along the ventral aspect of the os penis, along which the urethra tracks [12, 80, 81]. The groove is widest at the base of the os penis and narrows appreciably toward its tip [80, 81].

If the os penis fractures, it may disrupt the penile urethra [10, 79].

Compression of the urethra may result in urethral occlusion and urinary outflow obstruction [10, 79].

Patients may present for one or more of the following clinical signs:

- Anuria, oliguria, and/or frequent attempts to urinate with minimal production
- Hematuria
- Painful external genitalia
- Swollen prepuce

Physical examination will confirm penile swelling and discomfort. Palpation of the penis may also elicit crepitus.

The fractured os penis may or may not require surgical intervention. If fragments are few and well aligned, and a urinary catheter can be passed without difficulty, then the patient can self-heal [79]. However, comminuted fractures with misalignment require surgical correction and/or removal [79]. If the penile urethra is damaged beyond repair and/or if a stricture has rendered the penile urethra dysfunctional, then a permanent urethrostomy is indicated [79].

In addition to fracture, the os penis may experience avulsion from the penis due to shearing forces, as may occur when hit by a car (see Figures 58.5a–c).

Avulsion injuries compromise blood flow to the tissues and can be quite extensive. Phallectomy is often indicated.

Figure 58.4 Left lateral abdominal radiograph of a canine patient that had presented for acute abdomen, unrelated to the urinary tract. Note that the os penis is visible on radiographic examination. *Source:* Courtesy of Daniel Foy, MS, DVM, DACVIM, DACVECC.

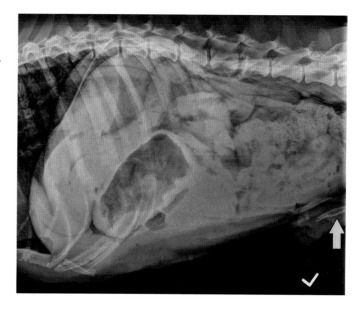

(a)

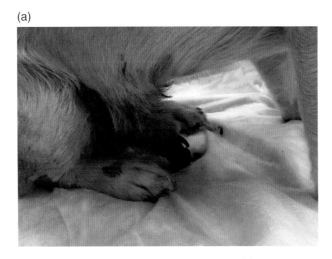

(b)   (c)

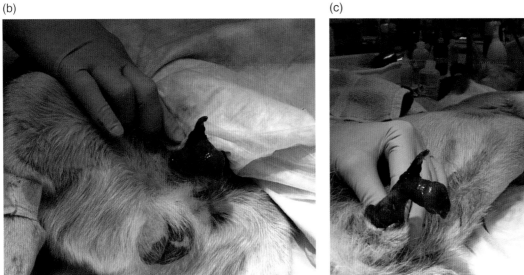

Figure 58.5 (a) Traumatic avulsion of the os penis in a canine patient that was hit by a car. *Source:* Courtesy of Erin M. Miracle. (b) Intraoperative examination of the same patient depicted in Figure 58.5a. *Source:* Courtesy of Erin M. Miracle. (c) Alternate intraoperative view of the same patient that was depicted in Figure 58.5a. *Source:* Courtesy of Erin M. Miracle.

References

1 Graves, T.K. (2006). Diseases of the penis and prepuce. In: *Saunders Manual of Small Animal Practice*, 3e (ed. S.J. Birchard and R.G. Sherding), 97. St. Louis, Mo.: Saunders Elsevier.

2 Boothe, H.W. (2008). Diseases of the external male genitalia. In: *Handbook of Small Animal Practice*, 5e (ed. R.V. Morgan), 587–592. Saunders/Elsevier: St. Louis, Mo.

3 Vermooten, M.I. (1987). Canine transmissible venereal tumor (TVT): a review. *J. S. Afr. Vet. Assoc.* 58 (3): 147–150.

4 Weir, E.C., Pond, M.J., Duncan, J.R., and Polzin, D.J. (1978). Extra-genital occurrence of transmissible venereal tumor in dog – literature-review and case-reports. *J. Am. Anim. Hosp. Assoc.* 14 (4): 532–536.

5 van Rensburg, I.B. and Petrick, S.W. (1980). Extragenital malignant transmissible venereal tumour in a bitch. *J. S. Afr. Vet. Assoc.* 51 (3): 199–201.

6 Holmes, J.M. (1981). A 125IUdR technique for measuring the cell loss from subcutaneously growing canine transmissible venereal tumours. *Res. Vet. Sci.* 31 (3): 306–311.

7 Higgins, D.A. (1966). Observations on the canine transmissible venereal tumour as seen in the Bahamas. *Vet. Rec.* 79 (3): 67–71.

8 Duncan, J.R. and Prasse, K.W. (1979). Cytology of canine cutaneous round cell tumors. Mast cell tumor, histiocytoma, lymphosarcoma and transmissible venereal tumor. *Vet. Pathol.* 16 (6): 673–679.

9 Ganguly, B., Das, U., and Das, A.K. (2016). Canine transmissible venereal tumour: a review. *Vet. Comp. Oncol.* 14 (1): 1–12.

10 Papazoglou, L.G. (2004). Diseases and surgery of the canine penis and prepuce. World Congress Proceedings [Internet]. https://www.vin.com/apputil/content/defaultadv1.aspx?pId=11181&meta=generic&catId=30097&id=3852322&print=1.

11 Lawrence, J.A. and Saba, C.F. (2013). Tumors of the male reproductive system. In: *Withrow & MacEwen's Small Animal Clinical Oncology*, 5e (ed. S.J. Withrow, D.M. Vail and R.L. Page), 557–571. St. Louis, Missouri: Elsevier.

12 Coomer, A.R. (2013). Male reproductive and penile surgery. World Congress Proceedings [Internet]. https://www.vin.com/apputil/content/defaultadv1.aspx?pId=11372&meta=generic&catId=35320&id=5709894&ind=282&objTypeID=17.

13 Pavletic, M.M. (2005). Management of canine paraphimosis. Hungarovet [Internet]. (September):[6–10 pp.]. http://www.hungarovet.com/wp-content/uploads/2008/07/management-of-canine-paraphimosis-2005.pdf.

14 Michels, G.M., Knapp, D.W., David, M. et al. (2001). Penile prolapse and urethral obstruction secondary to lymphosarcoma of the penis in a dog. *J. Am. Anim. Hosp. Assoc.* 37 (5): 474–477.

15 Ndiritu, C.G. (1979). Lesions of the canine penis and prepuce. *Mod. Vet. Pract.* 80: 712–715.

16 Patnaik, A.K., Matthiesen, D.T., and Zawie, D.A. (1988). 2 cases of canine penile neoplasm – squamous-cell carcinoma and mesenchymal chondrosarcoma. *J. Am. Anim. Hosp. Assoc.* 24 (4): 403–406.

17 Bleier, T., Lewitschek, H.P., and Reinacher, M. (2003). Canine osteosarcoma of the penile bone. *J. Vet. Med. A Physiol. Pathol. Clin. Med.* 50 (8): 397–398.

18 Patnaik, A.K. (1990). Canine extraskeletal osteosarcoma and chondrosarcoma: a clinicopathologic study of 14 cases. *Vet. Pathol.* 27 (1): 46–55.

19 Webb, J.A., Liptak, J.M., Hewitt, S.A., and Vince, A.R. (2009). Multilobular osteochondrosarcoma of the os penis in a dog. *Can. Vet. J.* 50 (1): 81–84.

20 Pavletic, M.M. (2007). Reconstruction of the urethra by use of an inverse tubed bipedicled flap in a dog with hypospadias. *J. Am. Vet. Med. Assoc.* 231 (1): 71–73.

21 Adelsberger, M.E. and Smeak, D.D. (2009). Repair of extensive perineal hypospadias in a Boston Terrier using tubularized incised plate urethroplasty. *Can. Vet. J.* 50 (9): 937–942.

22 Hobson, H.P. (1998). Penis and prepuce. In: *Current Techniques in Small Animal Surgery* (ed. M.J. Bojrab, G.W. Ellison and B. Slocum), 527–537. Philadelphia: Lea & Febiger.

23 Smith, C.W. (1993). Surgical diseases of the urethra. In: *Textbook of Small Animal Surgery* (ed. D. Slatter), 1462–1463. Philadelphia: WB Saunders.

24 Fossum, S.J. (1997). Surgery of the reproductive and genital systems. In: *Small Animal Surgery* (ed. S.J. Fossum), 565–572. St. Louis: Mosby.

25 Jurka, P., Galanty, M., Zielinska, P. et al. (2009). Hypospadias in six dogs. *Vet. Rec.* 164 (11): 331–333.

26 Ndikuwera, J. (2005). A case of hypospadias in a dog. *Ir. Vet. J.* 58 (9): 504–506.

27 Boothe, H.W. (2002). Penis, prepuce, and scrotum. In: *Textbook of Small Animal Surgery* (ed. D. Slatter), 1531–1542. Philadelphia: WB Saunders.

28 Hedlund, C.S. (2002). Surgery of the male reproductive tract. In: *Small Animal Surgery* (ed. S.J. Fossum), 662–664. St. Louis: Mosby.

29 Hobson, H.P. (1993). Surgical pathophysiology of the penis. In: *Disease Mechanisms in Small Animal Surgery* (ed. M.J. Bojrab, D.D. Smeak and M.S. Bloomberg), 554–555. Philadelphia: Lea & Febiger.

30 Bleedom, J.A. and Bjorling, D.E. (2012). Urethra. In: *Veterinary Surgery: Small Animal* (ed. K.M. Tobias and S.A. Johnston), 1993–2010. St. Louis: Elsevier.

31 Hayes, H.M. Jr. and Wilson, G.P. (1986). Hospital incidence of hypospadias in dogs in North America. *Vet. Rec.* 118 (22): 605–607.

32 Ader, P.L. and Hobson, H.P. (1978). Hypospadias – review of veterinary literature and a report of 3 cases in dog. *J. Am. Anim. Hosp. Assoc.* 14 (6): 721–727.

33 Guimaraes, L.D., Bourguignon, E., Santos, L.C. et al. (2013). Canine perineal hypospadias. *Arq. Bras. Med. Vet. Zoo.* 65 (6): 1647–1650.

34 Neihaus, S.A. and Goring, R.L. (2011). Clinical snapshot: abnormal genitalia in a pit bull. *Compendium* 33 (11).

35 Archibald, J. (1974). *Canine Surgery*. Santa Barbara, California: American Veterinary Publications.

36 Croshaw, J.E. Jr. and Brodey, R.S. (1960). Failure of preputial closure in a dog. *J. Am. Vet. Med. Assoc.* 136: 450–452.

37 Switonski, M., Payan-Carreira, R., Bartz, M. et al. (2012). Hypospadias in a male (78,XY; SRY-positive) dog and sex reversal female (78,XX; SRY-negative) dogs: clinical, histological and genetic studies. *Sex. Dev.* 6 (1–3): 128–134.

38 Cassata, R., Iannuzzi, A., Parma, P. et al. (2008). Clinical, cytogenetic and molecular evaluation in a dog with bilateral cryptorchidism and hypospadias. *Cytogenet. Genome Res.* 120 (1–2): 140–143.

39 Mcfarland, L. and Deniz, E. (1961). Unilateral renal agenesis with ipsilateral cryptorchidism and perineal hypospadias in a dog. *J. Am. Vet. Med. Assoc.* 139 (10): 1099–1100.

40 Hardy, R.M. and Kustritz, M.V. (2005). Theriogenology question of the month. Hypospadias. *J. Am. Vet. Med. Assoc.* 227 (6): 887–888.

41 Rezaei, M., Azizi, S., Akhtardanesh, B. et al. (2016). Hypospadias and testicular agenesis in two German shepherd puppies. *Iran. J. Vet. Surg.* 11 (1): 51–55.

42 Rawlings, C.A. (1984). Correction of congenital defects of the urogenital system. *Vet. Clin. North Am. Small Anim. Pract.* 14 (1): 49–60.

43 Vnuk, D., Bottegaro, N.B., Slunjski, L. et al. (2014). Prepubic urethrostomy opening within a prepuce in a dog: a case report. *Vet. Med-Czech.* 59 (2): 107–111.

44 Baskin, L.S. (2000). Hypospadias and urethral development. *J. Urol.* 163 (3): 951–956.

45 Galanty, A., Jurka, P., and Zielinska, P. (2008). Surgical treatment of hypospadias. Techniques and results in six dogs. *Pol. J. Vet. Sci.* 11 (3): 235–243.

46 Kustritz, M.V.R. (2001). Disorders of the canine penis. *Vet. Clin. North Am-Small.* 31 (2): 247.

47 Papazoglou, L.G. (2001). Idiopathic chronic penile protrusion in the dog: a report of six cases. *J. Small Anim. Pract.* 42 (10): 510–513.

48 Somerville, M.E. and Anderson, S.M. (2001). Phallopexy for treatment of paraphimosis in the dog. *J. Am. Anim. Hosp. Assoc.* 37 (4): 397–400.

49 Wasik, S.M. and Wallace, A.M. (2014). Combined preputial advancement and phallopexy as a revision technique for treating paraphimosis in a dog. *Aust. Vet. J.* 92 (11): 433–436.

50 Fowler, J.D. (1998). Preputial reconstruction. In: *Current Techniques in Small Animal Surgery* (ed. M.J. Bojrab), 534–537. Baltimore: Williams & Wilkins.

51 Chaffee, V.W. and Knecht, C.D. (1975). Canine paraphimosis: sequel to inefficient preputial muscles. *Vet. Med. Small Anim. Clin.* 70 (12): 1418–1420.

52 Johnston, D.E. (1965). Repairing lesions of the canine penis and prepuce. *Mod. Vet. Pract.* 46: 39.

53 Elkins, A.D. (1984). Canine Paraphimosis of unknown etiology – a case-report. *Vet. Med. Small Anim. Clin.* 79 (5): 638–639.

54 Johnston, S.E. (1989). Disorders of the external genitalia of the male. In: *Textbook of Veterinary Internal Medicine* (ed. S.J. Ettinger), 1881–1889. Philadelphia: W.B. Saunders.

55 Feldman, E.C. and Nelson, R.W. (1996). *Disorders of the Penis and Prepuce*. Philadelphia: W.B. Saunders.

56 Soderbergh, S.F. (1994). Diseases of the penis and prepuce. In: *Saunders Manual of Small Animal Practice* (ed. S.J. Birchard and R.G. Sherding), 886–891. Philadelphia: W.B. Saunders.

57 Nelson, R.W. and Couto, C.G. (2014). *Small Animal Internal Medicine*, 5e, xxix, 1473 p. St. Louis, MO: Elsevier/Mosby.

58 Hobson, H.P. (1990). Surgical procedures of the penis. In: *Current Techniques in Small Animal Surgery* (ed. M.J. Bojrab), 423–430. Philadelphia: Lea and Febinger.

59 Tilley, L.P. and Smith, F.W.K. (2004). *The 5-Minute Veterinary Consult: Canine and Feline*, 3e, lviii, 1487 p. Baltimore, MD: Lippincott Williams & Wilkins.

60 Côté, E. (2015). *Clinical Veterinary Advisor. Dogs and Cats*, 3e, xxxvii, 1642 p. St. Louis, Missouri: Elsevier Mosby.

61 Rota, A., Paltrinieri, S., Jussich, S. et al. (2008). Priapism in a castrated cat associated with feline infectious peritonitis. *J. Feline Med. Surg.* 10 (2): 181–184.

62 Gunn-Moore, D.A., Brown, P.J., Holt, P.E., and Gruffydd-Jones, T.J. (1995). Priapism in seven cats. *J. Small Anim. Pract.* 36 (6): 262–266.

63 Lavely, J.A. (2009). Priapism in dogs. *Top. Companion Anim. Med.* 24 (2): 49–54.

64 Burnett, A.L. and Bivalacqua, T.J. (2007). Priapism: current principles and practice. *Urol. Clin. North Am.* 34 (4): 631–642, viii.

65 Yuan, J., Desouza, R., Westney, O.L., and Wang, R. (2008). Insights of priapism mechanism and rationale treatment for recurrent priapism. *Asian J. Androl.* 10 (1): 88–101.

66 Silverstein, D. and Hopper, K. (2009). *Small Animal Critical Care Medicine*. St. Louis, MO: Saunders.

67 Swalec, K.M. and Smeak, D.D. (1989). Priapism after castration in a cat. *J. Am. Vet. Med. Assoc.* 195 (7): 963–964.

68 Winter, C.C. and Mcdowell, G. (1988). Experience with 105 patients with priapism – update review of all aspects. *J. Urol.* 140 (5): 980–983.

69 Guilford, W.G., Shaw, D.P., O'Brien, D.P., and Maxwell, V.D. (1990). Fecal incontinence, urinary incontinence, and priapism associated with multifocal distemper encephalomyelitis in a dog. *J. Am. Vet. Med. Assoc.* 197 (1): 90–92.

70 Bivalacqua, T.J. and Burnett, A.L. (2006). Priapism: new concepts in the pathophysiology and new treatment strategies. *Curr. Urol. Rep.* 7 (6): 497–502.

71 Rochat, M.C. (2001). Priapism: a review. *Theriogenology* 56 (5): 713–722.

72 Johnston, D.E. and Archibald, J. (1974). Male genital system. In: *Canine Surgery* (ed. J. Archibald), 703–749. California: American Veterinary Publications.

73 Depani, S. and Molyneux, E.M. (2012). Case report: an unusual case of priapism. *Malawi Med. J.* 24 (1): 17–18.

74 Dutta, J.K. (1994). Rabies presenting with priapism. *J. Assoc. Physicians India* 42 (5): 430.

75 Orima, H., Tsutsui, T., Waki, T. et al. (1989). Surgical treatment of priapism observed in a dog and a cat. *Nihon. Juigaku. Zasshi.* 51 (6): 1227–1229.

76 Kustritz, M.V.R. and Olson, P.N. (1999). Theriogenology question of the month. *J. Am. Vet. Med. Assoc.* 214 (10): 1483–1484.

77 Rogers, L., Lopez, A., and Gillis, A. (2002). Priapism secondary to penile metastasis in a dog. *Can. Vet. J.* 43 (7): 547–549.

78 Pearson, H. and Weaver, B.M. (1978). Priapism after sedation, neuroleptanalgesia and anaesthesia in the horse. *Equine Vet. J.* 10 (2): 85–90.

79 Bjorling, D.E. (1984). Traumatic injuries of the urogenital system. *Vet. Clin. North Am. Small Anim. Pract.* 14 (1): 61–76.

80 Dycc, K.M., Sack, W.O., and Wensing, C.J.G. (eds.) (1996). The urogenital apparatus. In: *Textbook of Veterinary Anatomy*, 2e, xiii, 856 p. Philadelphia: Saunders.

81 Evans, H.E. and Christensen, G.C. (1993). The urogenital system. In: *Miller's Anatomy of the Dog*, 3e (ed. H.E. Evans and M.E. Miller), 494–554. Philadelphia: W.B. Saunders.

59

Preputial Discharge

59.1 Introduction to Smegma as Normal Preputial Discharge

Smegma is a normal sebaceous secretion that accumulates within the preputial sheath [1–3]. It represents a mixture of sloughed epithelial cells, neutrophils, other inflammatory cells, and mucoid glycoproteins [2].

Note that smegma is not sterile [2, 4]. In addition to containing the aforementioned populations of cells, it also contains bacteria [2]. The following microbes are believed to constitute normal preputial flora [2, 5]:

- *Escherichia coli*
- *Klebsiella*
- *Mycoplasma*
- *Proteus*
- *Pseudomonas*
- *Staphylococcus*
- *Streptococcus*
- *Ureaplasma*

Of these microbes, *E. coli* is the most common isolate on aerobic culture [6].

In the author's experience, smegma is common in dogs, but not in cats [1].

Among dogs, smegma varies in terms of color and amount.

Smegma may be translucent and colorless, or it may be cloudy-white to yellow-green [1] (see Figure 59.1a, b).

Smegma accumulates at the preputial opening and may adhere to preputial fur. Clients may find it aesthetically displeasing, particularly in patients in which smegma is copious.

Smegma is usually an incidental finding on physical examination. In the absence of other clinical signs related to the urogenital tract, smegma is considered normal [2].

Intact, sexually mature, and brachycephalic dogs have increased amounts of smegma [5].

Preputial discharge may also increase with age [5]. This is thought to be due to decreased grooming among aged patients, which allows smegma to accumulate [5].

59.2 Abnormal Preputial Discharge and Associated Clinical Signs

Although preputial discharge can be normal there are circumstances in which it is pathologic [1].

Patients with pathologic preputial discharge are often irritated. They groom the groin excessively and lick at the prepuce incessantly. This behavior may be apparent in the examination room and mirror what the client has observed in the home environment.

In addition, there may be discomfort associated with these actions. Patients may whine or cry as they lick at the prepuce.

Affected patients may also be resentful of the clinician handling the prepuce during physical examination [1, 7–9].

Whenever clients report an increase in preputial discharge or an increase in the behaviors noted above, close inspection of the groin is indicated to evaluate the patient for the following [1, 9]:

- Abnormal preputial anatomy
  - Hypospadias (see Chapter 58, Section 58.2)
  - Persistent frenulum, an abnormal adhesion between the glans penis and preputial mucosa
- Balanitis, inflammation of the glans penis
- Balanoposthitis, inflammation of the glans penis and the prepuce
- Narrowed preputial opening (see Chapter 58, Section 58.3)
- Penile masses (see Chapter 58, Section 58.1)

It is tempting to restrict the examination to the prepuce and penis. However, it is important to note that pathologic preputial discharge may result from a deeper condition.

In particular, pathologic preputial discharge may stem from the following [10–12]:

- Lower urinary tract disease
  - Associated with urinary calculi
  - Associated with coagulopathy

Common Clinical Presentations in Dogs and Cats, First Edition. Ryane E. Englar.
© 2019 John Wiley & Sons, Inc. Published 2019 by John Wiley & Sons, Inc.

(a)   (b)

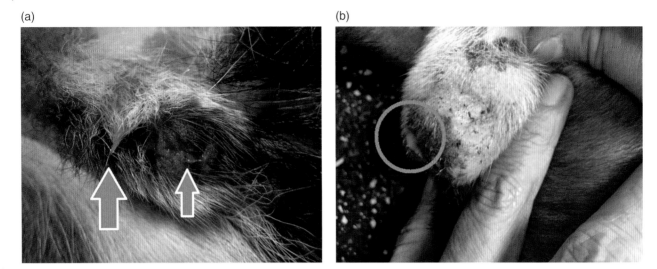

Figure 59.1 (a) Inspection of the canine prepuce. Note the presence of mucoid discharge at the prepuce. This same discharge is also adhered to the adjacent fur. This is normal. (b) Inspection of the canine prepuce. Note the presence of mucopurulent discharge at the preputial opening. This is normal.

- Urethritis
- Urinary tract infection (UTI)
- Prostatic disease
  - Prostatic abscess
  - Prostatic cyst
  - Prostatic neoplasia
    - Prostatic adenocarcinoma
    - Transitional cell carcinoma (TCC)
- Prostatitis
  - Bacterial prostatitis
    - *E. coli*
    - *Proteus*
    - *Pseudomonas*
    - *Staphylococcus*
    - *Streptococcus*
- Upper urinary tract disease
  - Renal hematuria
    - Associated with urinary calculi
    - Associated with coagulopathy
    - Associated with renal cysts
    - Idiopathic
    - Infectious
    - Neoplastic
    - Associated with pyelonephritis
    - Toxin-induced

A comprehensive physical examination is an essential part of case management for all patients with preputial discharge. A comprehensive patient evaluation includes a rectal examination [9].

The rectal examination emphasizes palpation of the following structures [9, 13]:

- The pelvic diaphragm, that is, the muscles and bones that define the rectal canal
- The prostate, located along the ventral floor of the pelvis in male patients
- The sublumbar lymph nodes, located dorsally
- The urethra, palpable along the ventral floor of the pelvis
- The left and right anal sacs

In cases of preputial discharge, it is particularly important to assess the prostate gland. The prostate gland is the primary accessory sex gland in the dog [9]. It is palpable per rectum in both intact and castrated males [7, 8].

The prostate is a bi-lobed structure that is caudal to the neck of the urinary bladder [9]. A palpable, dorsal midline sulcus divides the right side from the left [9].

Palpation over both lobes of the prostate should not elicit pain in healthy dogs [7–9].

Dogs with prostatic disease may have pain on palpation [9]. Consider, for example, dogs with prostatitis. On rectal palpation, the prostate of affected dogs will be uncomfortable to the touch [9]. These dogs may also have palpably enlarged sublumbar lymph nodes [9, 10].

Dogs with prostatitis may have abnormal preputial discharge [2]. Affected patients also tend to be systemically ill. Historically, they may be lethargic and anorexic. On examination, they may be febrile.

Prostatic disease is more likely to occur in intact, middle-aged to older dogs [11].

In cases of preputial discharge, it is equally important to assess the health of the urinary tract. Lower urinary tract disease, including UTIs, may cause abnormal discharge [1, 2]. These patients may present for dysuria, stranguria, pollakiuria, and inappropriate urination or house soiling.

History taking provides invaluable data that, together with the physical examination, paints a complete portrait of the patient's overall health.

59.3 Balanitis and Balanoposthitis

As outlined in Section 59.2, there are many causes of preputial discharge in the dog. Of these, balanitis and balanoposthitis are most common [3, 4].

Both may result from a penile injury or preputial foreign bodies, such as foxtails, seeds, or straw [3]. It is thought that these pathological conditions disrupt the normal microflora of the preputial cavity [2, 6]. The resident bacteria either overgrow or allow for nonresident bacteria to take up residence [2, 5, 6, 14, 15]. For example, *Brucella canis* is an opportunistic invader [1].

Balanitis and balanoposthitis often lead to secondary bacterial infections [2]. However, they may also occur secondary to viral infections or neoplastic disease [2, 3, 16].

Two viruses in particular have been associated with balanitis and balanoposthitis: canine herpesvirus and canine calicivirus [2, 15–19].

Atopic dermatitis may also incite balanitis or balanoposthitis, particularly if the patient is pruritic and causing self-trauma [2, 6].

Regardless of etiology, balanitis and balanoposthitis can vary dramatically in terms of severity [2].

Mild balanoposthitis is characterized by a small amount of mucopurulent preputial discharge [4]. Clients may report that the patient has "pus" dripping from the prepuce.

Upon inspection, the glans of the penis and the prepuce may appear red and inflamed. The patient may lick at the groin intermittently, but does not appear to be systemically ill in mild cases.

This presentation is most likely to occur in sexually mature dogs and has a good prognosis. It is likely to clear on its own, without systemic therapy. However, preputial hygiene may need to be addressed with the veterinary client to lessen the chance of reoccurrence [4].

Balanoposthitis is more likely to be moderate to severe when one or more of the following conditions are involved [4]:

- Foreign body
- Neoplasia
- Paraphimosis
- Phimosis
- Trauma
- Urolithiasis
- UTI

Patients seem to be particularly uncomfortable when a traumatic injury or foreign body is involved [4].

Lacerations, abrasive injuries, or abscesses may lead to systemic signs of illness [2]. Affected dogs are likely to be lethargic, anorexic, and/or febrile [1].

These patients benefit from a diagnostic work-up to establish and remove the inciting factor [2, 3].

Cytology of the preputial cavity or penile tip may provide clues; however, recall that neither of these structures is sterile in the male dog.

A baseline complete blood count (CBC), chemistry panel, and urinalysis provide a starting point in terms of assessing the patient's overall health [5].

Imaging of the urinary bladder, urethra, and prostate may be beneficial for cases in which urinary or prostatic disease is suspected [5].

Urine culture of a sample obtained by cystocentesis is advised and may be compared with a sample from a prostatic aspirate or wash [5] (see Figures 59.2a, b).

Cultures must be interpreted in light of what constitutes the normal flora of the male reproductive tract.

When cultures are positive for cystitis or prostatitis in patients that have systemic signs of illness, antibiotics are indicated [2]. Antibiotic selection should be based upon culture and susceptibility results.

In addition, the preputial cavity may benefit from cleansing with mild antiseptic agents or warm sterile saline lavage [2]. This may require sedation, depending upon the patient's comfort level and tolerance [3].

Treatment is essential for maintaining reproductive health, particularly among stud dogs. If untreated, adhesions may develop between the prepuce and the penis [2, 3]. This may cause reluctance to breed, on account of pain, or inability to achieve intromission [2].

59.4 Bloody Preputial Discharge and Hematuria

Although preputial discharge may become bloody with balanitis and balanoposthitis, hemorrhage is more likely to be associated with the following conditions [2]:

- Coagulopathy
  - Anticoagulant rodenticide ingestion
  - Clotting factor deficiencies
  - Disseminated intravascular coagulation (DIC)
  - Thrombocytopenia
- Prostatitis
- Trauma
  - Penile
  - Preputial
- Urethritis
- Urinary calculi

(a)

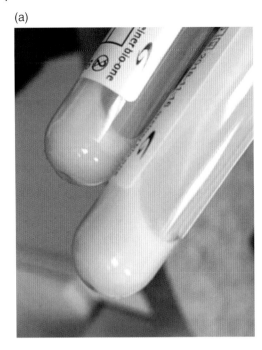

(b)

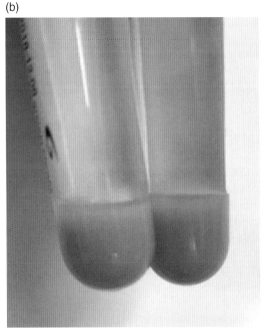

Figure 59.2 (a) Canine urine obtained by cystocentesis. The urine was positive on culture for *E. coli*. (b) Canine urine. This patient was subsequently diagnosed with a prostatic abscess.

- Cystic
- Renal
- Ureteral
- Urethral

History taking and a comprehensive physical examination are essential first steps when a patient presents for bloody preputial discharge.

A diagnostic investigation is also necessary to establish the source of the blood.

Baseline diagnostic tests include a CBC, chemistry profile, and urinalysis with culture [2]. Depending upon patient presentation, a coagulation panel and abdominal imaging may also be indicated [2].

Although it may be tempting to consider that the blood is of preputial or penile origin, it is important to recognize that blood may also originate anywhere within the patient's urinary tract, including the urinary bladder and the kidneys.

Monitoring the patient's stream during urination may facilitate localization [2]. For example, if blood develops in the urine stream early on, then the primary problem is likely to involve the penis, prepuce, or urethra [2].

By contrast, if blood develops near the end of the urine stream, then it is likely to originate in the urinary bladder or the prostate [2].

Renal hematuria, on the other hand, tends to cause discoloration of the urine stream throughout micturition [2].

References

1 Côté, E. (2015). *Clinical Veterinary Advisor. Dogs and Cats*, 3e, xxxvii, 1642 p. St. Louis, Missouri: Elsevier Mosby.

2 Feldman, E.C., Nelson, R.W., Reusch, C., and Scott-Moncrieff, J.C.R. (2015). *Canine & feline endocrinology*, 4e, xi, 669 p. St. Louis, Missouri: Elsevier Saunders.

3 Tobias, K.M. and Johnston, S.A. (2012). *Veterinary Surgery: Small Animal*. St. Louis, MO: Elsevier.

4 Davidson, A.P. (2018). Balanoposthitis in small animals. Merck Veterinary Manual [Internet]. https://www.merckvetmanual.com/reproductive-system/ reproductive-diseases-of-the-male-small-animal/ balanoposthitis-in-small-animals.

5 Lopate, C. (2015). Penile discharge in dogs. *NAVC Clinician's Brief* (May): 22–23.

6 Kustritz, M.V.R. (2001). Disorders of the canine penis. *Vet. Clin. North Am. Small Anim. Pract.* 31 (2): 247–258.

7 van Dongen, A.M. and L'Eplattenier, H.F. (2009). Kidneys and urinary tract. In: *Medical History and Physical Examination in Companion Animals*, 2e (ed. A. Rijnberk and F.J. van Sluijs). St. Louis: Saunders Elsevier.

8 de Gier, J. and van Sluijs, F.J. (2009). Male reproductive tract. In: *Medical History and Physical Examination in Companion Animals*, 2e (ed. A. Rijnberk and S. FJv), 117–122. Edinburgh; New York: Saunders/Elsevier.

9 Englar, R.E. (2017). *Performing the Small Animal Physical Examination*. Hoboken, NJ: Wiley.

10 Davidson, A.P. (2014). Prostatic disease. *NAVC Clinician's Brief* (January): 81–85.

11 Dugas, B., Brunker, J., and Rizzi, T.E. (2008). Prostate cytology. *NAVC Clinician's Brief* (February): 23–24.

12 Bowles, M. (2008). The diagnostic approach to hematuria. DVM 360 [Internet]. http://veterinarymedicine.dvm360.com/diagnostic-approach-hematuria?id=&sk=&date=&pageID=6.

13 Rothuizen, J., Schrauwen, E., Theyse, L.F.H., and Verhaert, L. (2009). Digestive tract. In: *Medical History and Physical Examination in Companion Animals*, 2e (ed. A. Rijnberk and S. FJv), 86–100. Edinburgh; New York: Saunders/Elsevier.

14 Doig, P.A., Ruhnke, H.L., and Bosu, W.T. (1981). The genital mycoplasma and Ureaplasma flora of healthy and diseased dogs. *Can. J. Comp. Med.* 45 (3): 233–238.

15 Poste, G. and King, N. (1971). Isolation of a herpesvirus from the canine genital tract: association with infertility, abortion and stillbirths. *Vet. Rec.* 88 (9): 229–233.

16 Anvik, J.O. (1991). Clinical considerations of canine Herpesvirus-infection. *Vet Med* 86 (4): 394–403.

17 Crandall, R.A. (1988). Isolation and characterization of caliciviruses from dogs with vesicular genital disease. *Arch. Virol.* 98: 65.

18 Hashimoto, A. and Hirai, K. (1986). Canine herpesvirus infection. In: *Current Therapy in Theriogenology* (ed. D.A. Morror), 516. Philadelphia: WB Saunders.

19 Hill, H. and Mare, C.J. (1974). Genital disease in dogs caused by canine herpesvirus. *Am. J. Vet. Res.* 35 (5): 669–672.

60

Ambiguous External Genitalia

60.1 Introduction to Sexual Differentiation in Dogs and Cats

Sexual differentiation in dogs and cats begins long before birth [1–4].

The act of fertilization determines chromosomal sex [2–4]:

- The female genotype is conferred upon those that receive two X chromosomes, one from each parent.
- The male genotype is conferred upon those that receive an X chromosome from the maternal parent and a Y chromosome from the paternal parent.

Although XX and XY zygotes are unique based upon their chromosomes, they initially develop into embryos that are sexually indistinct [2, 3]. The female blueprint is the default [2, 3]. At this early stage of development, both the XX and XY zygotes resemble the female phenotype [2]. It is only after activation of the SRY gene on the Y chromosome of XY zygotes that males differentiate themselves from females by transforming the gonads into testes [2–5].

The presence of the testes initiates the development of phenotypic sex. [2–4] Sertoli cells within the testes produce Mullerian inhibiting substance (MIS) [3, 6, 7]. MIS binds to the Mullerian ducts and facilitates their regression [2, 3]. At the same time, Leydig cells within the testes produce testosterone [2, 3]. Testosterone binds to the Wolffian ducts, facilitating their transformation into the vas deferentia and epididymides [2, 3].

Testosterone also binds to receptors in the precursors of genital tissues, after it has been converted into dihydrotestosterone (DHT) by 5-α-reductase [2, 3]. This causes the urogenital sinus to form the male urethra and prostate [2, 3]. The penis forms from the genital tubercle, and the scrotum forms from the genital swellings [2, 3].

At this point in development, the testes are held in place by cranial and caudal ligaments [2]. With the assistance of insulin-like growth factor 3, testosterone causes regression of the cranial ligaments [2]. The caudal ligaments develop into the gubernaculum [2].

Recall from Chapter 55, Section 55.2 that the gubernaculum plays an important role in testicular descent. The testes must migrate from their intra-abdominal location to the scrotum through the inguinal canal before the canal closures, between four and six months of age [8–15]. The inguinal canal is a passageway through the abdominal wall that is located in the groin [10].

Most kittens and puppies lack scrotal testes at birth [9, 12].

Many testes make it through the inguinal canal and into the scrotum between 3 and 10 days of age [9]. However, testes may continue to pass in and out of the scrotum through the open inguinal canal until 10–14 weeks old [9, 12].

By contrast, the female genotype lacks testes [2, 3]. In the absence of testicular secretions, such as MIS, the Mullerian duct system persists [2, 3]. The oviducts, uterus, and cranial vagina form from this ductwork [2, 3].

In the absence of DHT, the external genitalia that develop are inherently female. The urogenital sinus, genital tubercle, and genital swellings are transformed into the vestibule, caudal vagina, clitoris, and vulva [2].

The ovaries stay tethered to their intra-abdominal position by both the cranial and caudal ligaments [2]. As a result, both ovaries remain as neighbors to the adjacent kidneys [2].

60.2 Introduction to Sexual Differentiation Disorders in Dogs and Cats

The development of sexual phenotypes, which allows for sexual differentiation, is dependent upon complex choreography as outlined above [4]. If any step fails to take place, its absence will impact the rest of the process [2–4, 16].

For ease of consideration, these failures of development can be grouped into the following categories [2, 3]:

- Chromosomal sex abnormalities
- Gonadal sex abnormalities
- Phenotypic sex abnormalities

Common Clinical Presentations in Dogs and Cats, First Edition. Ryane E. Englar.
© 2019 John Wiley & Sons, Inc. Published 2019 by John Wiley & Sons, Inc.

60.2.1 Chromosomal Sex Abnormalities

Chromosomal sex abnormalities are characterized as having an abnormal number of sex chromosomes [2, 3].

A normal cat, for example, will have a karyotype of 38, XX or 38, XY [3]. Contrast this with a cat that has a chromosomal sex anomaly and the karyotype of 39, XXY. This cat has an extra sex chromosome.

A normal dog will have a karyotype of 78, XX or 78, XY [3]. Contrast this with a dog that has a chromosomal sex anomaly and the karyotype of 79, XXY. This dog has an extra sex chromosome.

The XXY configuration, known as Klinefelter's syndrome among human patients, triggers the development of testes, due to activation of the SRY gene on the Y chromosome [1–3, 17–20]. The testes, in turn, produce testosterone, which shapes the reproductive tract such that it is phenotypically male [2]. However, these males are often sterile because of the adverse impact of the extra X chromosome on spermatogenesis [2, 3].

Male tortoiseshell or calico cats are XXY [3]. The tortoiseshell or calico pattern is typically restricted to females because either requires two X chromosomes [3]. For a male cat to have this coat color pattern, he has to be XXY [3].

60.2.2 Gonadal Sex Abnormalities

Gonadal sex abnormalities occur when there is disagreement between the chromosomal and gonadal sex [1–3]. The patient is said to be sex reversed. [1, 2, 21] Consider, for example, an XX male or an XY female [1, 2].

XY females have not been described in cats or dogs [1].

However, XX tomcats and XX male dogs do appear in the veterinary medical literature [1, 2].

Specifically, XX male dogs have been identified in the following canine breeds [1, 2, 22–26]:

- Bassett Hounds
- Beagles
- Chinese Pugs
- Cocker Spaniels
- Doberman Pinschers
- German Shorthaired Pointers
- Kerry Blue Terriers
- Norwegian Elk Hounds
- Pomeranians
- Soft-Coated Wheaton Terriers
- Weimaraners

XX male dogs may be called "true hermaphrodites"; that is, they have both testicular and ovarian tissue within the same gonad, the so-called ovotestis [1, 2, 21, 27–30]. Alternatively, true hermaphrodites may have one ovary and one testicle [1, 2].

Having both sets of gonadal tissue is often just one of several abnormalities that are associated with the internal reproductive tract [1, 2].

In addition, true hermaphrodites may have sexually ambiguous external genitalia [1, 2]. For example, the female phenotype often predominates with variations of male anatomy [1, 2]. An affected patient may present for what appears to be an enlarged clitoris [1, 2, 31–34] (see Figures 60.1a, b).

Radiographically, the patient may also have an os penis [1, 31–34].

(a) (b)

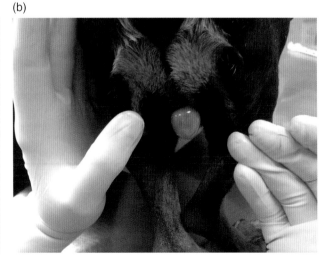

Figure 60.1 (a) This French bulldog patient is considered to be a true hermaphrodite. Note the concurrent presence of a vulva and small penis. *Source:* Courtesy of Frank Isom, DVM. (b) Canine patient, as viewed from the rear. Note the presence of a prominent clitoris in this true hermaphrodite. *Source:* Courtesy of Dr. Stephanie Harris.

Affected patients are sometimes referred to as being intersex, to denote that they have sexually ambiguous external genitalia [1, 2].

XX true hermaphrodites may experience estrous cycles [1, 2]. Although it is uncommon, they can produce offspring [1, 2, 26].

Definitive diagnosis is confirmed by a combination of patient karyotype and histopathology to confirm the presence of at least one ovotestis [1, 2].

Note that not all XX male dogs are true hermaphrodites [1, 2]. Some have what is referred to as XX male syndrome; that is, they only have testes as opposed to ovotestes [1, 2].

Dogs with XX male syndrome tend to be bilaterally cryptorchid [1]. In addition, their external genitalia often possesses abnormal features that include a [1]

- Displaced prepuce
- Hypoplastic, or underdeveloped penis
- Hypospadias
- Penile curvature.

As opposed to XX true hermaphrodites, patients that are affected by XX male syndrome are sterile [1].

60.2.3 Phenotypic Sex Abnormalities

Some patients have good alignment between chromosomal and gonadal sex. [2] The XX females have classically female reproductive tracts, with the female gonad, the ovary [2]. The XY males have classically male reproductive tracts, with the male gonad, the testis [2].

Despite this alignment, the sexual phenotype that is displayed is opposite of that which is expected [2, 3]. This is called pseudohermaphroditism, and it represents a type of phenotypic sex abnormality [2].

Consider, for example, female pseudohermaphrodites. These patients present with sexually ambiguous external genitalia [2]. Females may look like XX true hermaphrodites on the outside, meaning that they exhibit clitoromegaly [2]. Alternatively, female pseudohermaphrodites may appear even more masculinized, with nearly normal male genitalia [1, 2].

In canine medicine, the administration of steroids to the pregnant dam has been known to result in female pseudohermaphrodites [1, 2, 32, 35–37]. Female embryos are masculinized in the womb because they are exposed to androgens or progestogens [2].

Pseudohermaphrodites may also be male [2]. These patients have a male karyotype and testes [2]. However, their Mullerian ducts fail to regress. This causes affected dogs to develop a uterus, oviducts, and the cranial vagina, in addition to the epididymides, vasa deferentia, and the prostate [2].

Outwardly, male patients may appear normal, which is a concern because they can reproduce [2]. Pseudohermaphroditism is heritable in Miniature Schnauzers in the United States, Bassett Hounds in Europe, and, potentially, in the United States–bred Persian cat [2].

Alternatively, male pseudohermaphrodites may be cryptorchid [2]. It is theorized that uterine attachment to one or both testes in affected patients interferes with testicular descent [2].

Male pseudohermaphrodites may also have what appears to be female external genitalia, that is, either a vulva or an enlarged clitoris [1].

Based upon gross appearance, pseudohermaphrodites cannot be distinguished from true hermaphrodites. Karyotyping is indicated, along with histologic evaluation of the gonads to establish that female pseudohermaphrodites truly have ovaries and that male pseudohermaphrodites truly have testes [1].

References

1 Romagnoli, S. and Schlafer, D.H. (2006). Disorders of sexual differentiation in puppies and kittens: a diagnostic and clinical approach. *Vet. Clin. North Am. Small Anim. Pract.* 36 (3): 573–606, vii.

2 Meyers-Wallen, V. (2007). Inherited disorders of sexual development in dogs and cats. Tufts' Canine and Feline Breeding and Genetics Conference [Internet]. https://www.vin.com/apputil/content/defaultadv1.aspx?pId=11243&meta=Generic&catId=31943&id=3861254.

3 Christensen, B.W. (2012). Disorders of sexual development in dogs and cats. *Vet. Clin. North Am. Small Anim. Pract.* 42 (3): 515–526, vi.

4 Buijtels, J.J., de Gier, J., Kooistra, H.S. et al. (2012). Disorders of sexual development and associated changes in the pituitary-gonadal axis in dogs. *Theriogenology* 78 (7): 1618–1626.

5 Tibary, A. (2018). Intersex conditions. Merck Veterinary Manual [Internet]. https://www.merckvetmanual.com/reproductive-system/congenital-and-inherited-anomalies-of-the-reproductive-system/intersex-conditions.

6 Meyers-Wallen, V.N. (1993). Genetics of sexual differentiation and anomalies in dogs and cats. *J. Reprod. Fertil. Suppl.* 47: 441–452.

7 Meyers-Wallen, V.N. (2012). Gonadal and sex differentiation abnormalities of dogs and cats. *Sex. Dev.* 6 (1–3): 46–60.

8 de Gier, J. and van Sluijs, F.J. (2009). Male reproductive tract. In: *Medical history and physical examination in*

companion animals, 2e (ed. A. Rijnberk and S. FJv), 117–122. Edinburgh; New York: Saunders/Elsevier.

9 Englar, R.E. (2017). *Performing the small animal physical examination*. Hoboken, NJ: Wiley.

10 Evans, H.E. and Christensen, G.C. (1993). The urogenital system. In: *Miller's anatomy of the dog*, 3e (ed. H.E. Evans and M.E. Miller), 494–558. Philadelphia: W.B. Saunders.

11 Veronesi, M.C., Riccardi, E., Rota, A., and Grieco, V. (2009). Characteristics of cryptic/ectopic and contralateral scrotal testes in dogs between 1 and 2 years of age. *Theriogenology* 72 (7): 969–977.

12 Romagnoli, S.E. (1991). Canine cryptorchidism. *Vet. Clin. North Am. Small Anim. Pract.* 21 (3): 533–544.

13 Yates, D., Hayes, G., Heffernan, M., and Beynon, R. (2003). Incidence of cryptorchidism in dogs and cats. *Vet. Rec.* 152 (16): 502–504.

14 Amann, R.P. and Veeramachaneni, D.N. (2007). Cryptorchidism in common eutherian mammals. *Reproduction* 133 (3): 541–561.

15 Bushby, P.A. (2010). Cryptorchid surgery and simple ophthalmic procedures. DVM 360 [Internet]. http://veterinarycalendar.dvm360.com/cryptorchid-surgery-and-simple-ophthalmic-procedures-proceedings.

16 Torad, F.A. and Hassan, E.A. (2016). Surgical correction of female pseudohermaphroditism in five pit bull dogs. *Asian J. Anim. Sci.* 10 (1): 77–84.

17 Centerwall, W.R. and Benirschke, K. (1975). An animal model for the XXY Klinefelter's syndrome in man: tortoiseshell and calico male cats. *Am. J. Vet. Res.* 36 (9): 1275–1280.

18 Clough, E., Pyle, R.L., Hare, W.C. et al. (1970). An XXY sex-chromosome constitution in a dog with testicular hypoplasia and congenital heart disease. *Cytogenetics* 9 (1): 71–77.

19 Nie, G.J., Johnston, S.D., Hayden, D.W. et al. (1998). Theriogenology question of the month. Azoospermia associated with 79,XXY chromosome complement (canine Klinefelter's syndrome). *J. Am. Vet. Med. Assoc.* 212 (10): 1545–1547.

20 Reimann-Berg, N., Murua Escobar, H., Nolte, I., and Bullerdiek, J. (2008). Testicular tumor in an XXY dog. *Cancer Genet. Cytogenet.* 183 (2): 114–116.

21 Feldman, E.C., Nelson, R.W., Reusch, C., and Scott-Moncrieff, J.C.R. (2015). *Canine & feline endocrinology*, 4e, xi, 669 p. St. Louis, Missouri: Elsevier Saunders.

22 Meyers-Wallen, V.N. and Patterson, D.F. (1989). Sexual differentiation and inherited disorders of sexual development in the dog. *J. Reprod. Fertil. Suppl.* 39: 57–64.

23 Meyers-Wallen, V. and Patterson, D.F. (1989). Disorders of sexual development in dogs and cats. In: *Current veterinary therapy, small animal practice XIII* (ed. R.W. Kirk), 1261–1269. Philadelphia: WB Saunders.

24 Meyers-Wallen, V.N., Bowman, L., Acland, G.M. et al. (1995). Sry-negative XX sex reversal in the German shorthaired pointer dog. *J. Hered.* 86 (5): 369–374.

25 Meyers-Wallen, V.N., Palmer, V.L., Acland, G.M., and Hershfield, B. (1995). Sry-negative XX sex reversal in the American cocker spaniel dog. *Mol. Reprod. Dev.* 41 (3): 300–305.

26 Meyers-Wallen, V. (2000). CVT update: inherited disorders of the reproductive tract in dogs and cats. In: *Kirk's current veterinary therapy: small animal practice XIII* (ed. J.D. Bonagura), 904–909. Philadelphia: WB Saunders.

27 Kim, K.S. and Kim, O. (2006). A hermaphrodite dog with bilateral ovotestes and pyometra. *J. Vet. Sci.* 7 (1): 87–88.

28 Gurel, A., Yildirim, F., Sennazli, G. et al. (2014). Hermaphroditism in two dogs – pathological and cytogenetic studies: a case report. *Vet. Med. Czech.* 59 (1): 51–54.

29 Schlafer, D.H., Valentine, B., Fahnestock, G. et al. (2011). A case of SRY-positive 38,XY true hermaphroditism (XY sex reversal) in a cat. *Vet. Pathol.* 48 (4): 817–822.

30 Bredal, W.P., Thoresen, S.I., Kvellestad, A., and Lindblad, K. (1997). Male pseudohermaphroditism in a cat. *J. Small Anim. Pract.* 38 (1): 21–24.

31 Walker, R.G. (1961). Hermaphroditism in a bitch: a case report. *Vet. Rec.* 73: 670–671.

32 Allen, W.E., Daker, M.G., and Hancock, J.L. (1981). Three intersexual dogs. *Vet. Rec.* 109 (21): 468–471.

33 Fitzgerald, A.L. and Murphy, D.A. (1990). Bilateral ovotestes in an intersex, mixed breed dog. *Lab. Anim. Sci.* 40 (6): 647–650.

34 Randolph, J.F., Center, S.A., Mcentee, M., and Goldberg, E.H. (1988). H-Y Antigen-Positive Xx true bilateral hermaphroditism in a German shorthaired pointer. *J. Am. Anim. Hosp. Assoc.* 24 (4): 417–420.

35 Curtis, E.M. and Grant, R.P. (1964). Masculinization of female pups by progestogens. *J. Am. Vet. Med. Assoc.* 144: 395–398.

36 Jackson, D.A., Osborne, C.A., Brasmer, T.H., and Jessen, C.R. (1978). Nonneurogenic urinary incontinence in a canine female pseudohermaphrodite. *J. Am. Vet. Med. Assoc.* 172 (8): 926–930.

37 Olson, P.N., Seim, H.B., Park, R.D. et al. (1989). Female pseudohermaphroditism in three sibling greyhounds. *J. Am. Vet. Med. Assoc.* 194 (12): 1747–1749.

61

Vulvovaginal Discharge

61.1 Introduction to the Female Reproductive Tract

From proximal to distal, the female reproductive tract consists of the following [1, 2]:

- Ovaries
- Oviducts, or uterine tubes
- Uterus
- Cervical canal
- Cervix
- Vagina
- Vestibule
- Vulva***
- Urethra***
- Fossa clitoridis***
- Clitoris***

Only the starred structures above comprise the female external genitalia [1].

The majority of the female reproductive tract of both the dog and cat is internal [1, 2].

Of these internal structures, the normal ovaries are never palpable in the dog [3]. Neither is the non-pregnant uterus [3, 4].

The uterus is palpable during the physiologic state of pregnancy [4, 5].

61.1.1 Dog-Specific Internal Reproductive Anatomy Relevant to Abdominal Palpation

From mating to parturition, the gestation length in a dog ranges from 57 to 72 days, averaging 65 days [6]. Developing fetuses may be detected as discrete uterine swellings upon abdominal palpation between days 21 and 25 of gestation. These swellings progressively increase in size until days 33–35 of pregnancy, at which point uterine confluence makes pregnancy diagnosis by palpation unreliable. It is not until at or after day 45 that pregnancy detection by palpation becomes possible again, due to ossification of the fetuses, which allows for the fetal skeleton to be appreciated on abdominal examination [4, 7].

At or after day 45 of pregnancy, abdominal radiographs can be used to estimate litter size by counting fetal skulls (see Figure 61.1).

Although it is possible to underestimate litter size in large litters, abdominal radiography helps the veterinary team to plan ahead. In cases of fetopelvic disproportion, meaning that fetal skulls exceed the width of the maternal pelvic canal, a cesarean (C-) section may be indicated [7].

61.1.2 Cat-Specific Internal Reproductive Anatomy Relevant to Abdominal Palpation

From mating to parturition, the gestation length in a cat is 56–69 days [8]. Individual spherical balls are palpable as discrete developing fetuses as early as day 14–17 [5, 8]. These so-called "beads on a string" are easiest to feel on abdominal palpation between days 21–25 of gestation, at which point the enlarged uterus is also palpable [4, 5]. From day 35 to 45 of gestation, it may be difficult to appreciate the individual fetuses on abdominal palpation because of placental size: at this point, the placentas are so large that the uterus is palpable as one tubular structure rather than as individual sausage links [5] (see Figures 61.2a–c).

Beyond day 45, it may be possible to palpate individual fetal skeletons, which have ossified. In particular, rib cages and skulls are readily appreciated by the experienced clinician on abdominal palpation [4, 5].

61.2 A Review of the Estrous Cycle

The emphasis of this chapter is on the various discharges that can originate from within the female reproductive tract. Some of these discharges are normal and coincide with specific phases of the estrous cycle, while others are pathologic [1, 3].

Common Clinical Presentations in Dogs and Cats, First Edition. Ryane E. Englar.
© 2019 John Wiley & Sons, Inc. Published 2019 by John Wiley & Sons, Inc.

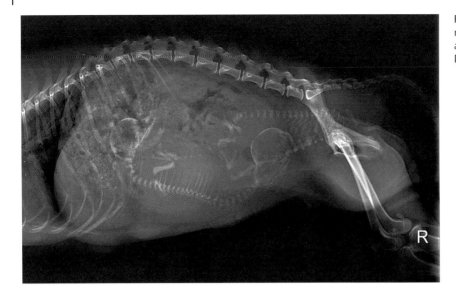

Figure 61.1 Right lateral abdominal radiograph taken prior to whelping to assess litter size. *Source:* Courtesy of Dr. Elizabeth Robbins.

(a)   (b)   (c)

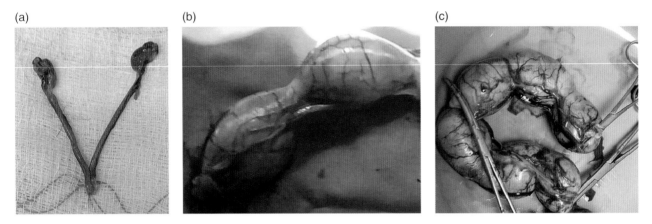

Figure 61.2 (a) Non-pregnant feline uterus removed during elective ovariohysterectomy. *Source:* Courtesy of Alexis Stambaugh, DVM. (b) Feline uterus in early stages of pregnancy, surgically excised via elective ovariohysterectomy. Note the "beads of a string" appearance. The individual fetuses would have been palpable (externally, during physical examination) by an experienced clinician. (c) Feline uterus, between day 35 and 45 of gestation. Note how uterine confluence makes it appear as one giant, tubular structure. At this stage of pregnancy, individual fetal palpation is unlikely. *Source:* Courtesy of Shannon Carey, DVM.

The estrous cycle refers to the physiological changes that recur in the sexually mature female of most mammalian species with the intention of preparing the body for pregnancy [9]. These changes are driven by [9]

- The hypothalamus
  - Gonadotropin-releasing hormone (GnRH)
- The pituitary gland
  - Follicle-stimulating hormone (FSH)
  - Luteinizing hormone (LH)
- The ovaries
  - Estrogen
  - Progesterone.

The estrous cycle is interrupted by pregnancy [9]. Without this physiologic state, the estrous cycle repeats [9].

The estrous cycle has four distinct phases [9, 10]:

- Pro-estrus
- Estrus
- Diestrus
- Anestrus

Pro-estrus is a 3–21 day phase (in dogs) that is characterized by follicular growth within the ovaries [9, 10]. Concurrently, estrogen production by the ovaries promotes the development of the uterine lining, the endometrium [9]. The vaginal epithelium proliferates [9].

Males are sexually attracted to females that are experiencing pro-estrus, but the females are not receptive to males during this time [9, 10].

Estrogen causes water retention [9]. The female reproductive tract becomes edematous. Edema within the vaginal mucosa causes it to take on a smooth, rather than wrinkled appearance.

Estrogen secretion during pro-estrus also causes externally visible changes in the female reproductive tract [9]. The vulva swells [9].

Serosanguinous vulvar discharge may be present [9, 10]. This discharge originates from the uterus [10]. The edematous uterine tissue allows for the passage of erythrocytes through intact capillary walls. This is called diapedesis.

At the microscopic level, estrogen causes a change in vaginal cytology from non-cornified parabasal and intermediate cells to cornified, anuclear cells [10].

Estrogen reaches a peak at the end of pro-estrus [9, 10].

Estrus follows pro-estrus as the phase of sexual receptivity, in which the female tolerates copulation [9, 10]. The female is said to be "in heat." [10] Female tolerance toward the male results from a sharp decline in estrogen [9, 10].

The decrease in estrogen also reverses water retention. The vaginal mucosa is no longer edematous. Water loss causes a wrinkling effect to the vaginal mucosa, which is evident on vaginoscopy.

Estrus lasts, on average, for nine days in the dog [10]. Female receptivity to the male rarely lasts for the duration of estrus [10].

A surge in LH triggers ovulation roughly two days later [2, 9, 10].

Dogs spontaneously ovulate in response to LH, whereas cats require the act of intromission to stimulate the release of oocytes for fertilization [9, 11–13]. Recall from Chapter 57 that the chance of feline ovulation increases if copulation occurs more than once [13].

Following their release from the ovary, oocytes mature over a period of one to three days [10]. Mature oocytes are fertile for two to three days within the female reproductive tract [10].

Diestrus follows estrus as a transitional period in which progesterone becomes the dominant hormone. Progesterone is produced by the corpus luteum, a structure that forms on the surface of the ovary [2].

In most species, the absence of pregnancy terminates diestrus. The corpus luteum regresses, and the female returns to pro-estrus to repeat the estrous cycle [9]. Dogs are unique in that those that do not become pregnant continue through diestrus for its entire length, as if they were carrying a pregnancy [4, 10, 14].

Diestrus in the dog lasts for approximately 60 days, after which the dog enters anestrus [9, 10]. Anestrus is period of sexual quiescence, during which time the uterus repairs itself in preparing to restart the estrous cycle [10].

Diestrus and anestrus collectively make up the interestrus interval, that is, the period between heat cycles [10]. In the dog, the interestrus period averages seven months [10]. For this reason, most patients come into heat twice per year [3]. Basenjis and Tibetan mastiffs are an exception to this rule [3]. They only cycle once per year [4, 14].

61.2.1 The Canine Estrous Cycle and Normal Vulvovaginal Discharge

The canine vulva is small during anestrus (see Figure 61.3).

If the vulvar lips are parted, the mucosa is pink, but lacks sheen. This is because there is minimal to no vulvar discharge during anestrus [10]. If vulvar discharge is present, it is mucoid in the healthy female dog.

During pro-estrus, the canine vulva swells and serosanguinous vulvar discharge develops (see Figures 61.4a, b).

This vulvar discharge arises from the uterus and should not be malodorous [4, 14].

The vulva is still pronounced when the dog reaches estrus [3]. However, despite its size, the vulva softens [3].

If the vulvar lips are parted, the mucosa is edematous. This results in a classic sheen or glossiness to the mucosal appearance.

Vulvar discharge is present at the onset of estrus and is often hemorrhagic [3] (see Figure 61.5).

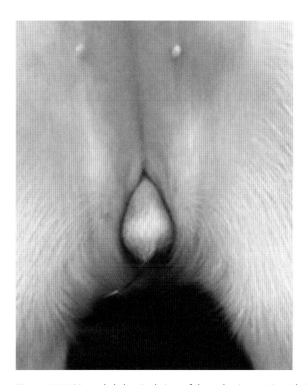

Figure 61.3 Ventral abdominal view of the vulva in a patient that is in anestrus. Note that the vulva is small.

(a)

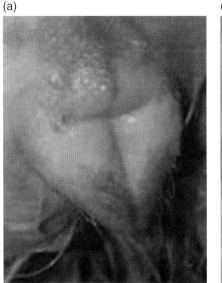

(b)

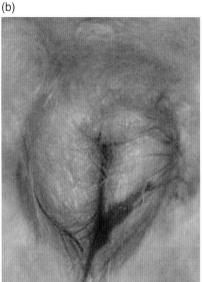

Figure 61.4 (a) Vulvar swelling in a dog in pro-estrus. (b) Serosanguinous vulvar discharge in a dog in pro-estrus.

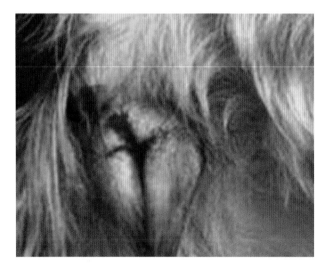

Figure 61.5 Hemorrhagic vulvar discharge in a dog in estrus.

Although vulvar discharge is normal during this phase of the estrous cycle, it is aesthetically unpleasing to many owners of intact females. To avoid staining of furniture and other household items, clients may elect to dress the patient in commercialized canine diapers (see Figure 61.6).

As estrus progresses, vulvar discharge fades, both in terms of amount and color [3]. What was once red discharge becomes light pink or straw-colored [3].

During early diestrus, the patient may have milky, odorless vulvar discharge [3]. However, as diestrus progresses, vulvar discharge should cease [4, 14].

If the patient carries a pregnancy to term, she may develop lochia, that is, postpartum discharge [3]. Lochia is typically blood-tinged, green, or brown, odorless, mucoid discharge [3] (see Figure 61.7).

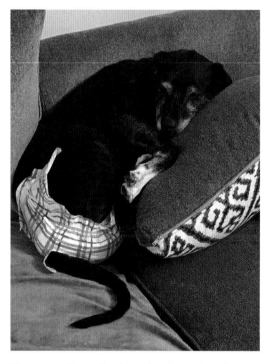

Figure 61.6 Recently adopted canine patient that is in estrus. Note the doggie diaper that has been placed to minimize house soiling by the patient's vulvar discharge. *Source:* Courtesy of Andy and Kristina Burch.

Lochia is considered normal for up to three weeks following the delivery of pups [3].

61.2.2 The Feline Estrous Cycle and Normal Vulvovaginal Discharge

Unlike dogs, cats have minimal vulvar discharge during the estrous cycle [3, 15, 16].

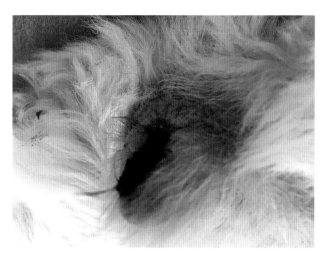

Figure 61.7 Close-up of vulva two days after the successful delivery of pups. Note the presence of lochia, which is normal.

Cats that are in pro-estrus may have a mucoid plug at the vulva [4, 5, 17].

During estrus, cats may or may not have serous to mucoid vulvar discharge [3, 17].

Cats do not typically have hemorrhagic, purulent, or hemopurulent vulvar discharge at any point throughout the estrous cycle [3].

61.3 Causes of Abnormal Vulvovaginal Discharge

Up until now, vulvovaginal discharge has been described as normal during certain phases of the estrous cycle in both dogs and cats.

However, vulvovaginal discharge can also be pathologic.

Pathologic vulvovaginal discharge can originate from anywhere within the genitourinary tract, including the urethra [18].

The most common causes of abnormal vulvovaginal discharge in the dog and cat include the following [15, 17–27]:

- Reproductive tract disease
  - Endometritis
  - Metritis***
  - Mucometra***
  - Neoplasia
  - Ovarian remnant syndrome (ORS) ***
  - Pyometra***
  - Vaginal foreign body***
  - Vaginitis***
- Urinary tract disease
  - Neoplasia
  - Urinary incontinence
  - Urinary tract infection (UTI) (see Chapter 64)

The starred items above (***) will be covered in depth below.

In addition, vulvovaginal discharge may develop as a result of systemic dysfunction, including, but not limited to the following [19]:

- Atopy
- Canine brucellosis
- Canine herpesvirus
- Coagulopathy
- Diabetes mellitus
- Trauma

61.4 Ovarian Remnant Syndrome (ORS)

The ovaries are both removed along with the uterus when canine and feline patients undergo elective ovariohysterectomy. The absence of ovaries prevents subsequent estrous cycles, including the onset of estrus [25].

If, during the procedure a fraction of one or both ovaries is left inside the abdomen, then the patient is likely to still produce female hormones, such as estrogen, and/or even ovulate [25, 28].

This condition is referred to as ORS [25]. It has been described primarily in feline patients that exhibit behavioral signs of estrus despite having been spayed [25]. ORS has also been identified in dogs [29, 30].

Errors in surgical technique may cause ORS [25]. For example, an incision that is too small may prevent adequate visualization of the ovaries, or an obese patient may obscure the surgeon's view [25].

When poor visualization occurs during ovariectomy or ovariohysterectomy, part of one or both ovaries may be entrapped in a ligature [25]. This fragment of ovarian tissue may continue to receive blood, by virtue of omental vasculature [25]. Revascularization allows the tissue to become functional again [25].

ORS is relatively uncommon. However, when it occurs, it is a nuisance for veterinarians and veterinary clients alike.

Cats with ORS are likely to exhibit one or more of the following sexually receptive signs [3, 25, 28–31]:

- Attracting tomcats
- Lordosis
  - Lowered front end
  - Depressed lumbar spine, like a horse with swayback
  - Elevated hindquarters
- Rolling side-to-side
- Tolerating intromission
- Treading with pelvic limbs
- Tucking the tail to one side

Some cats with ORS may develop aggression [25]. Others develop vaginal discharge [25].

Dogs with ORS are likely to exhibit one or more of the following sexually receptive signs:

- Attracting males
- Changes in activity level
- Changes in appetite
- Excessive licking at external genitalia
- Increased flagging of the tail from side-to-side
- Increased urination
- Hemorrhagic vulvovaginal discharge
  Standing heat
  – The dog exerts pressure against your hand if you scratch her at the tail base
- Stands for the male
- Vulvar swelling

Behavioral signs of estrus in a patient that has been spayed is suggestive of ORS [25]. The diagnosis is confirmed by [25, 30, 32]:

- Hormone assays
- Ultrasonography
- Vaginal cytology.

Patients with ORS require exploratory laparotomy to remove the remnant. Until the remnant is removed, the patient will continue to experience the estrous cycle.

61.5 Metritis

Metritis is the appropriate medical terminology for a bacterial uterine infection, following delivery of pups or kittens [27]. Although it may occur in patients that had normal deliveries, it more typically follows cases involving dystocia or retained placentas [27].

Although there are many causes of metritis, the most commonly implicated bacteria include the following [27]:

- β-hemolytic *Streptococcus*
- *Escherichia coli*
- *Pasteurella* spp.

These bacteria create an ascending infection that targets the uterus from the vagina [27]. Most of the bacteria that cause metritis are resident vaginal flora that become opportunistic invaders [23].

Affected patients develop malodorous vulvovaginal discharge [27]. Contrast this with normal lochia, which has no distinct odor [3].

Affected patients are also likely to become febrile [27]. They may go off food and become dehydrated [27]. They may also stop tending to their litter [27]. Distressed kittens or pups that are continuously whining is an indication that the dam may be ill [27].

Vulvovaginal discharge should be cultured in affected patients to determine appropriate antibiotic therapy [27].

If the dam is not intended to be used for breeding in the future, then she should be spayed to remove the source of the infection [27].

If the dam is intended to be bred in the future, then expulsion of uterine contents is of value [27]. During the initial postpartum period, oxytocin may be used for this purpose [27]. However, the uterus is not indefinitely sensitized to its effects [27]. Thereafter, prostaglandin F2α would be the drug of choice [27].

61.6 Mucometra

Mucometra refers to the accumulation of sterile mucus within the uterus [21, 33]. It occurs in both cats and dogs [21, 33].

As the uterus distends with fluid, it may become palpable [21, 33]. Mucometra cannot be distinguished from pyometra based upon palpation alone [33]. However, patients with pyometra are typically clinically ill, whereas those with mucometra are not [33]. Other than a palpable tubular structure on abdominal palpation, the only indication of mucometra may be an apparent inability to conceive [33].

Patients with mucometra tend to have normal serum chemistry panels and complete blood counts (CBCs) other than perhaps a mild, regenerative anemia [33].

61.7 Pyometra

The uterus also becomes palpable during the pathologic state of pyometra [3, 21, 33]. Pyometra is a condition in which purulent material accumulates within the uterus, causing the uterus to distend with pus [3, 33].

In dogs, pyometra is a relatively common uterine disease of the intact female [3]. Most have cycled previously, and present between 2.4 and 7.25 years of age [33–39]. Canine breeds that are overrepresented include the following [3, 33, 40, 41]:

- Airedale Terrier
- Bernese Mountain Dog
- Chow Chow
- Golden Retriever
- Cavalier King Charles Spaniel
- Irish Terrier
- Miniature Schnauzer
- Rough Collie
- Rottweiler
- Saint Bernard

Cats are less often affected than dogs by pyometra [3]. Pyometra occurs in 2.2% of intact queens by the time they reach 13 years of age. Oriental and exotic purebreds, such as the Siamese, Korat, Ocicat, and Bengal, are predisposed and present for pyometra earlier in life than the general feline population [42].

Risk factors for the development of pyometra include the following [33, 37, 39, 43, 44]:

- Being in estrus within the past 12 weeks
- Being nulliparous
- Prior hormonal therapy with estrogens or progestins
- Prior pregnancy termination

The experienced clinician should be able to palpate the tubular, distended uterus on abdominal palpation [3]. Abdominal imaging is helpful to confirm the diagnosis (see Figures 61.8a–d).

There are two main types of pyometras [3]:

- Closed
- Open

In a closed pyometra, the cervix is closed [3]. Uterine contents are therefore retained, meaning that the patient will not present with vulvovaginal discharge [3]. The uterus will continue to distend to the point that uterine rupture is possible [3].

In an open pyometra, the cervix remains open [3]. Uterine contents are free to flow down the female reproductive tract, allowing for vulvovaginal drainage [3]. Sanguinous to mucopurulent discharge will be evident on gross inspection of the vulva [21, 33, 35, 45].

Cytology of this discharge will differentiate pyometra from mucometra [33]. In the case of the former, one would expect to see large populations of degenerate neutrophils and intracellular bacteria [33].

Patients with pyometra are also typically ill, unlike those with mucometra [33].

Systemic signs of illness that are commonly seen in patients with pyometra include the following [33, 39]:

- Anorexia
- Depression
- Diarrhea
- Fever
- Lethargy
- Polydipsia
- Polyuria
- Vomiting

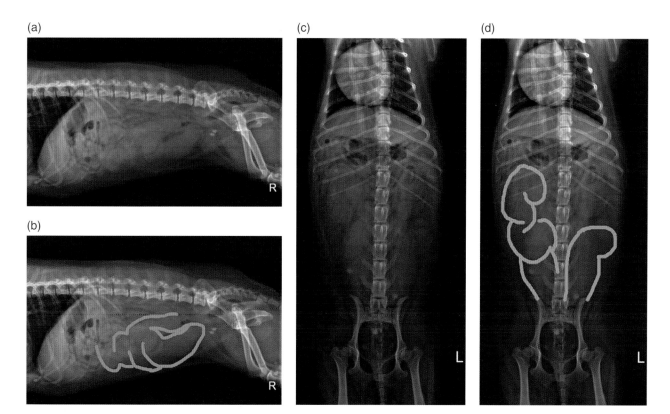

Figure 61.8 (a) Right lateral abdominal radiograph demonstrating canine pyometra. (b) Right lateral abdominal radiograph demonstrating canine pyometra, with the uterus outlined in blue. (c) V/D radiograph demonstrating canine pyometra. (d) V/D radiograph demonstrating canine pyometra, with the uterus outlined in blue.

Patients with closed pyometra present with more signs of systemic illness than those with open pyometra because the purulent material is trapped within the body [33]. These patients may present in shock, due to septicemia. They are also often appreciably dehydrated [33].

Escherichia coli is commonly implicated in cases of pyometra [21, 23, 46].

Other common bacteria include the following [17, 23]:

- *Klebsiella* spp.
- *Proteus* spp.
- *Staphylococcus* spp.
- *Streptococcus* spp.

The treatment of choice for pyometra is ovariohysterectomy [17, 21, 23] (see Figures 61.9a–c).

If the patient is intended to be used for future breeding, then injectable prostaglandin F2α may be administered to those with open pyometras to assist with expulsion of uterine contents [17, 21, 22]. Administration of high-dose prostaglandin F2α is ill advised in those patients with closed pyometras because uterine rupture is likely and would result in peritonitis [21, 23].

61.8 Stump Pyometra

ORS was introduced in Section 61.4.

In addition to causing behavioral estrus, ORS may also result in so-called stump pyometra if uterine tissue has been retained as well as ovarian tissue [3, 17, 23].

Stump pyometra is a rare condition that mirrors pyometra, except that the patient has been spayed [3, 17, 23].

Palpation of a tubular swelling in the caudal abdomen of a recently spayed dog or cat needs to be investigated as a potential stump pyometra until proven otherwise [3, 25, 47].

Note that stump pyometras are not the same as stump granulomas [17]. Stump granulomas are an inflammatory reaction to the suture that was used to ligate the uterine body during ovariohysterectomy [17].

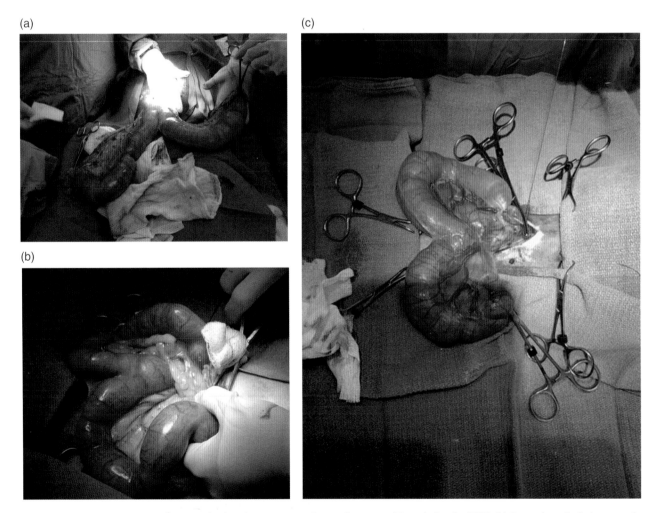

(a)

(b)

(c)

Figure 61.9 (a) Intraoperative photograph of canine pyometra. *Source:* Courtesy of Joseph Onello, DVM. (b) Second surgical photograph of canine pyometra. (c) Intraoperative photograph of feline pyometra. *Source:* Courtesy of Samantha B. Thurman, DVM.

Stump pyometras may also result from the administration of progestogens [25, 31, 48, 49].

61.9 Vaginitis

Vaginitis is defined as inflammation of the vaginal mucosa [15, 19, 24, 50–52]. It can occur in both dogs and cats, intact and neutered [15, 24, 51, 52].

Spayed patients more frequently present for adult-onset vaginitis than intact females [19].

In companion animal patients, vaginitis is rarely a primary condition [15, 51, 53]. More often than not, it is secondary to an underlying issue [15].

There are many causes of vaginitis, including, but not limited to the following [15, 18, 52, 53]:

- Anatomical deviations from the norm
- Foreign body [15, 18, 54–57]
  - Bone fragments from retained fetus
  - Migrating foxtail or grass awn
- Infection
- Neoplasia
- Trauma

Patients with hypoplastic, recessed, or "tucked up" vulvas seem more likely to develop vaginitis (see Figures 61.10a–c).

This conformation also predisposes canine patients to peri-vulvar dermatitis and chronic and/or recurrent UTIs [3] (see Figure 61.11).

These patients may benefit from vulvoplasty [3]. This cosmetic surgery reshapes the vulva so that it is more

(a)

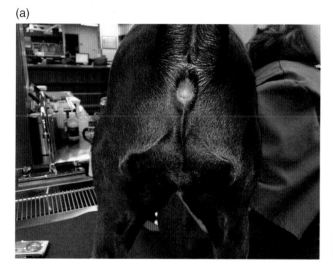

(b)

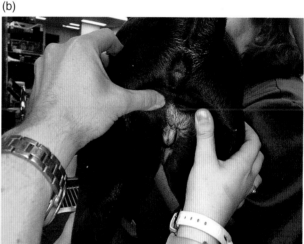

(c)

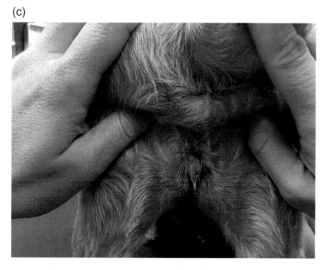

Figure 61.10 (a) Female dog with a recessed or "tucked up" vulva. Note how the vulva is entirely hidden from view. *Source:* Courtesy of Daniel Foy, MS, DVM, DACVIM, DACVECC. (b). Same patient as depicted in Figure 61.10a. Digital manipulation is required to visualize this dog's vulva. *Source:* Courtesy of Daniel Foy, MS, DVM, DACVIM, DACVECC. (c). Second example of a female dog with a recessed or "tucked up" vulva. *Source:* Courtesy of Daniel Foy, MS, DVM, DACVIM, DACVECC.

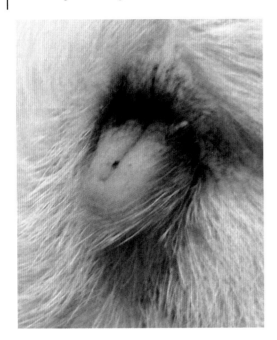

Figure 61.11 Female dog with a recessed or "tucked up" vulva and peri-vulvar dermatitis.

readily exposed to the air, and is therefore less prone to the development of moist dermatitis and/or vaginitis [58].

Overweight patients are also likely to develop excessive peri-vulvar skin folds that lead to persistent moisture and perivascular dermatitis [19]. Vaginitis may result [19].

Patients with vaginitis tend to present with vulvar discharge that ranges from clear to mucoid, purulent to mucopurulent [15, 24]. It is rarely hemorrhagic [15].

Owners may report excessive licking at external genitalia [15, 19, 24, 51–53, 59]. In addition, patients may seem uncomfortable during urination [15, 19]. They may exhibit dysuria or pollakiuria, and/or may cry when voiding [15, 19].

On physical examination, affected patients may exhibit peri-vulvar inflammation or peri-vulvar dermatitis [15].

Juvenile vaginitis may resolve spontaneously [19, 50]. However, adult-onset vaginitis must be evaluated more aggressively [19].

The diagnostic work-up for these patients includes the following [15, 16, 19, 53, 60]:

- CBC and chemistry panel to rule out systemic disease
  - Diabetes mellitus
  - Hyperadrenocorticism
- Digital vaginal examination
  - Vaginal septa or strictures
    - 88% can be detected by digital exam alone [19, 61, 62]
    - The remainder require vaginoscopy
- Urinalysis
- Vaginal cytology
- Vaginal culture
  - Bacterial culture is typically sufficient
    - *Escherichia coli*
    - *Pasteurella multocida*
    - *Proteus mirabilis*
    - *Staphylococcus* spp.
    - *Streptococcus* spp.
  - Fungal vaginitis is rarely observed in North America
- Imaging of the lower urogenital tract
  - Radiography
  - Ultrasonography
- Serologic testing for canine brucellosis in dogs that have been bred

UTIs and vaginitis are often concurrent [19, 24, 63, 64]. Infected urine can set the stage for vaginitis, and vaginitis can cause an ascending UTI due to vaginal flora overgrowth [19, 63].

To rule out a UTI, urine must be collected sterilely, via cystocentesis, to avoid contamination by vaginal contents [19]. Urine can then be cultured to establish bacterial growth and susceptibility to antibiotic therapy.

Vaginal culture can also be performed. However, the results must be interpreted in light of resident flora [19, 20, 65–68].

Canine herpesvirus may cause vesicular lesions along vaginal surfaces as well as other mucosa [19, 69, 70]. Currently available diagnostic tests are not useful [19]. Therefore, canine herpesvirus is a diagnosis of exclusion [19].

References

1 Evans, H.E. and Christensen, G.C. (1993). The urogenital system. In: *Miller's Anatomy of the Dog*, 3e (ed. H.E. Evans and M.E. Miller), 494–558. Philadelphia: W.B. Saunders.

2 Johnson, C.A. (2018). The gonads and genital tract of dogs. Merck Veterinary Manual [Internet]. https://www.merckvetmanual.com/dog-owners/reproductive-disorders-of-dogs/the-gonads-and-genital-tract-of-dogs.

3 Englar, R.E. (2017). *Performing the Small Animal Physical Examination*. Hoboken, NJ: Wiley.

4 Schaefers-Okkens, A.C. and Kooistra, H.S. (2009). Female reproductive tract. In: *Medical History and Physical Examinaiton in Companion Animals* (ed. A. Rijnberk and F.J. van Sluijs), 108–116. St. Louis: Saunders Elsevier.

5 Little, S.E. (ed.) (2012). Female reproduction. In: *The Cat: Clinical Medicine and Management*, 1195–1227. St. Louis: Saunders Elsevier.

6 Concannon, P., Whaley, S., Lein, D., and Wissler, R. (1983). Canine gestation length: variation related to time of mating and fertile life of sperm. *Am. J. Vet. Res.* 44 (10): 1819–1821.

7 Smith, F.O. (2011). Prenatal care of the bitch and queen. In: *Small Animal Pediatrics: the First 12 Months of Life* (ed. M.E. Peterson and M.A. Kutzler), 1–10. St. Louis, Mo: Saunders/Elsevier.

8 Feldman, E.C. and Nelson, R.W. (2004). *Canine and Feline Endocrinology and Reproduction*, 3e, xi, 1089 p. St. Louis, Mo: Saunders.

9 Feldman, E.C., Nelson, R.W., Reusch, C., and Scott-Moncrieff, J.C.R. (2015). *Canine & Feline Endocrinology*, 4e, xi, 669 p. St. Louis, Missouri: Elsevier Saunders.

10 Davidson, A.P. Breeding management of the bitch. UC Davis School of Veterinary Medicine [Internet]. http://www.vetmed.ucdavis.edu/vmth/local_resources/pdfs/repro_pdfs/ceBM.pdf.

11 Little, S.E. (ed.) (2012). Male reproduction. In: *The Cat: Clinical Medicine and Management*, 1184–1194. St. Louis: Saunders Elsevier.

12 Dyce, K.M., Sack, W.O., and Wensing, C.J.G. (1996). *Textbook of Veterinary Anatomy*, 2e, xiii, 856 p. Philadelphia: Saunders.

13 Ettinger, S.J., Feldman, E.C., and Côté, E. (2017). *Textbook of Veterinary Internal Medicine: Diseases of the Dog and the Cat*, 8e, 2 volumes (lviii, 2181, I-90 p.). St. Louis, Missouri: Elsevier.

14 Root Kustritz, M.V. (2010). *Clinical Canine and Feline Reproduction: Evidence-based Answers*, xv, 316 p. Ames, Iowa: Wiley-Blackwell.

15 Nicastro, A. and Walshaw, R. (2007). Chronic vaginitis associated with vaginal foreign bodies in a cat. *J. Am. Anim. Hosp. Assoc.* 43 (6): 352–355.

16 Johnson, C.A. (1989). *Vulvar Discharges. Kirk's Current Veterinary Therapy X: Small Animal Practice*, 1310–1312. Philadelphia: WB Saunders.

17 Pelsue, D. (2001). Pyometra and vaginal discharges. In: *Feline Internal Medicine Secrets* (ed. M.R. Lappin), 295–298. Philadelphia: Hanley & Belfus.

18 Davidson, A.P. (2012). Vulvar discharge in the bitch. *NAVC Clinician's Brief* (January): 70–74.

19 Root Kustritz, M.V. (2008). Vaginitis in dogs: A simple approach to a complex condition. DVM 360 [Internet]. http://veterinarymedicine.dvm360.com/vaginitis-dogs-simple-approach-complex-condition.

20 Memon, M.A. (2018). Vaginitis in small animals. Merck Veterinary Manual [Internet]. https://www.merckvetmanual.com/reproductive-system/reproductive-diseases-of-the-female-small-animal/vaginitis-in-small-animals.

21 Norsworthy, G.D. and Restine, L.M. (2018). *The Feline Patient*, 5e. Hoboken, NJ: Wiley.

22 Nak, D., Nak, Y., and Tuna, B. (2009). Follow-up examinations after medical treatment of pyometra in cats with the progesterone-antagonist aglepristone. *J. Feline Med. Surg.* 11 (6): 499–502.

23 Hollinshead, F. and Krekeler, N. (2016). Pyometra in the queen: to spay or not to spay? *J. Feline Med. Surg.* 18 (1): 21–33.

24 Johnson, C.A. (1991). Diagnosis and treatment of chronic vaginitis in the bitch. *Vet. Clin. North Am. Small Anim. Pract.* 21 (3): 523–531.

25 Demirel, M.A. and Acar, D.B. (2012). Ovarian remnant syndrome and uterine stump pyometra in three queens. *J. Feline Med. Surg.* 14 (12): 913–918.

26 Hagman, R. (2017). Canine pyometra: what is new? *Reprod. Domest. Anim.* 52 (Suppl 2): 288–292.

27 Johnstone, I.P. (2006). The cat with vaginal discharge. In: *Problem-based Feline Medicine* (ed. J. Rand), 1160–1164. Edinburgh; New York: Saunders.

28 Heffelfinger, D.J. (2006). Ovarian remnant in a 2-year-old queen. *Can. Vet. J.* 47 (2): 165–167.

29 Miller, D.M. (1995). Ovarian remnant syndrome in dogs and cats: 46 cases (1988–1992). *J. Vet. Diagn. Investig.* 7 (4): 572–574.

30 Wallace, M.S. (1991). The ovarian remnant syndrome in the bitch and queen. *Vet. Clin. North Am. Small Anim. Pract.* 21 (3): 501–507.

31 Rota, A., Pregel, P., Cannizzo, F.T. et al. (2011). Unusual case of uterine stump pyometra in a cat. *J. Feline Med. Surg.* 13 (6): 448–450.

32 DeNardo, G.A., Becker, K., Brown, N.O., and Dobbins, S. (2001). Ovarian remnant syndrome: revascularization of free-floating ovarian tissue in the feline abdominal cavity. *J. Am. Anim. Hosp. Assoc.* 37 (3): 290–296.

33 Pretzer, S.D. (2008). Clinical presentation of canine pyometra and mucometra: a review. *Theriogenology* 70 (3): 359–363.

34 Johnston, S.D., Root Kustritz, M.V., and Olson, P.S. (2001). Disorders of the canine uterus and uterine tubes (oviducts). In: *Canine and Feline Theriogenology*, 1e (ed. S.D. Johnston, M.V. Root Kustritz and P.S. Olson), 206–224. Philadelphia, PA: Saunders.

35 Feldman, E.C. and Nelson, R.W. (2004). Cystic endometrial hyperplasia/pyometra complex. In: *Canine and Feline Endocrinology and Reproduction* (ed. R. Kersey), 852–867. Philadelphia: WB Saunders Co.

36 Hardy, R.M. and Osborne, C.A. (1974). Canine pyometra: pathogenesis, physiology, diagnosis and treatment of uterine and extra-uterine lesions. *J. Am. Anim. Hosp. Assoc.* 10: 245–268.

37 Dow, C. (1957). The cystic hyperplasia–pyometra complex in the bitch. *Vet. Rec.* 69: 1409–1415.

38 Ewald, B.H. (1961). A survey of the cystic hyperplasia–pyometra complex in the bitch. *Small Anim. Clin.* 1: 383–386.

39 Wheaton, L.G., Johnson, A.L., Parker, A.J., and Kneller, S.K. (1989). Results and complications of surgical-treatment of Pyometra – a review of 80 cases. *J. Am. Anim. Hosp. Assoc.* 25 (5): 563–568.

40 Krook, L., Larsson, S., and Rooney, J.R. (1960). The interrelationship of diabetes mellitus, obesity, and pyometra in the dog. *Am. J. Vet. Res.* 21: 120–127.

41 Smith, F.O. (2006). Canine pyometra. *Theriogenology* 66 (3): 610–612.

42 Hagman, R., Strom Holst, B., Moller, L., and Egenvall, A. (2014). Incidence of pyometra in Swedish insured cats. *Theriogenology* 82 (1): 114–120.

43 Bowen, R.A., Behrendt, M.D., Wheeler, S.L. et al. (1985). Efficacy and toxicity of estrogens commonly used to terminate canine pregnancy. *J. Am. Vet. Med. Assoc.* 186 (8): 783–788.

44 Sutton, D.J., Geary, M.R., and Bergman, J.G.H.E. (1997). Prevention of pregnancy in bitches following unwanted mating: a clinical trial using low dose oestradiol benzoate. *J. Reprod. Fertil.* 239–243.

45 Renton, J.P., Boyd, J.S., and Harvey, M.J. (1993). Observations on the treatment and diagnosis of open pyometra in the bitch (Canis familiaris). *J. Reprod. Fertil. Suppl.* 47: 465–469.

46 Arora, N., Sandford, J., Browning, G.F. et al. (2006). A model for cystic endometrial hyperplasia/pyometra complex in the bitch. *Theriogenology* 66 (6–7): 1530–1536.

47 Johnston, S.D., Kustritz, M.V.R., and Olson, P.N.S. (2001). Disorders of the feline ovaries. In: *Canine and Feline Theriogenology*, 1e (ed. S.D. Johnston, M.V. Root Kustritz and P.S. Olson), 592. Philadelphia, PA: Saunders.

48 Johnston, S.D., Kustritz, M.V.R., and Olson, P.N.S. (2001). Disorders of the feline ovaries. In: *Canine and Feline Theriogenology* (ed. S.D. Johnston, M.V. Root Kustritz and P.N.S. Olson), 453–462. Philadelphia: Saunders.

49 Agudelo, C.F. (2005). Cystic endometrial hyperplasia-pyometra complex in cats. A review. *Vet. Q.* 27 (4): 173–182.

50 Verstegen, J.P. and Onclin, K.J. (2008). Vulvovaginal hemorrhagic discharge in the dog: caudal reproductive tract. *NAVC Clinician's Brief* (December): 11–15.

51 Johnston, S.D., Root Kustritz, M.V., and Olson, P.N.S. (2001). Disorders of the feline vagina, vestibule, and vulva. In: *Canine and Feline Theriogenology* (ed. S.D. Johnston, M.V. Root Kustritz and P.N.S. Olson), 472–473. Philadelphia: Saunders.

52 Feldman, E.C. and Nelson, R.W. (eds.) (2004). Vaginal defects, vaginitis, and vaginal infection. In: *Canine and Feline Endocrinology and Reproduction*, 901–908. St. Louis: WB Saunders.

53 Soderberg, S.F. (1986). Vaginal disorders. *Vet. Clin. North Am. Small Anim. Pract.* 16 (3): 543–559.

54 Dietrich, B.F. (1979). Persistent vaginal discharge in a spayed dog. *Vet. Med. Small Anim. Clin.* 74 (12): 1748–1749.

55 McCabe, J.R. and Steffey, M.A. (2004). What is your diagnosis? Dystocia during a previous parturition. *J. Am. Vet. Med. Assoc.* 224 (8): 1255–1256.

56 Cordery, R. (1997). Unusual foreign body in a cat. *Vet. Rec.* 140 (6): 160.

57 Ratcliffe, J. (1971). Vaginal bleeding in a spayed bitch: a case report. *J. Small Anim. Pract.* 12 (3): 169.

58 Hammel, S.P. and Bjorling, D.E. (2002). Results of vulvoplasty for treatment of recessed vulva in dogs. *J. Am. Anim. Hosp. Assoc.* 38 (1): 79–83.

59 Baker, T. and Davidson, A.P. (2013). CVC highlight: how to handle chronic vaginitis in veterinary patients. DVM 360 [Internet]. http://veterinarymedicine.dvm360.com/cvc-highlight-how-handle-chronic-vaginitis-veterinary-patients.

60 Davidson, A.P. (2001). Frustrating case presentations in canine theriogenology. *Vet. Clin. North Am. Small Anim. Pract.* 31 (2): 411–420.

61 Kyles, A.E., Vaden, S., Hardie, E.M., and Stone, E.A. (1996). Vestibulovaginal stenosis in dogs: 18 cases (1987–1995). *J. Am. Vet. Med. Assoc.* 209 (11): 1889–1893.

62 Root, M.V., Johnston, S.D., and Johnston, G.R. (1995). Vaginal septa in dogs: 15 cases (1983–1992). *J. Am. Vet. Med. Assoc.* 206 (1): 56–58.

63 Freshman, J.L., Reif, J.S., Allen, T.A., and Jones, R.L. (1989). Risk-factors associated with urinary-tract infection in female dogs. *Prev. Vet. Med.* 7 (1): 59–67.

64 Polzin, D.J. and Jeraj, K. (1979). Urethritis, cystitis, and ureteritis. *Vet. Clin. N. Am.* 9 (4): 661–678.

65 Laznicka, A., Huml, O., and Nesnalova, E. (1995). Microflora of genital organs of bitches and its relationship to reproductive disorders. II. Vaginitis. *Veterinarstvi* 45: 210–212.

66 Bjurstrom, L. (1993). Aerobic bacteria occurring in the vagina of bitches with reproductive disorders. *Acta Vet. Scand.* 34 (1): 29–34.

67 Hirsh, D.C. and Wiger, N. (1977). Bacterial-Flora of normal canine vagina compared with that of vaginal exudates. *J. Small Anim. Pract.* 18 (1): 25–30.

68 Jarvinen, A.K. (1981). Urogenital tract infection in the bitch. *Vet. Res. Commun.* 4 (4): 253–269.

69 Hill, H. and Mare, C.J. (1974). Genital disease in dogs caused by canine herpesvirus. *Am. J. Vet. Res.* 35 (5): 669–672.

70 Poste, G. and King, N. (1971). Isolation of a herpesvirus from the canine genital tract: association with infertility, abortion and stillbirths. *Vet. Rec.* 88 (9): 229–233.

62

Abnormal Presentations of the Mammary Glands

62.1 Introduction to the Mammary Chains

Palpation of the mammary chains is a critical component of the comprehensive canine and feline physical examination [1, 2].

Each chain, the left and the right, consists of a row of mammary glands that are oriented along the ventrum in a cranial-to-caudal plane [1–3]. The glands themselves are covered by skin [3].

Beneath the protective covering of skin, each mammary gland is formed by glandular and connective tissues surrounding hollow cavities called alveoli [3]. These cavities are lined by cuboidal cells, which secrete milk when their neighboring myoepithelial cells contract in response to oxytocin. This so-called milk "let down" reflex causes milk to flow from the alveoli into lobules and, ultimately, into ducts. These ducts drain into a centralized nipple or teat [3]. The nipple is what the neonate latches onto and suckles, at the center of each mammary gland [1, 2].

62.1.1 Feline Mammary Chains

Cats typically have four sets of mammary glands for a total of eight glands and their associated nipples [1, 2, 4, 5]. The nipples are obscured by a furred ventral abdomen [2]. The fur must be parted in order to visualize the nipples in a prepubescent female or in a nulliparous cat [2] (see Figures 62.1a, b).

Nipples are much more prominent in queens that have previously delivered one or more litters of kittens, and may not require the clinician to part the fur in order to visualize them (see Figure 62.2).

Note that male cats also have mammary glands [2]. However, these are rudimentary in males, meaning that they are present, but they do not develop secretory tissue [2, 3].

62.1.2 Canine Mammary Chains

Most dogs have five sets of mammary glands for a total of 10 glands and their associated nipples [2, 3]. From cranial to caudal, there are [1–3]

- Two sets of thoracic mammae
- Two sets of abdominal mammae
- One set of inguinal or pubic mammae.

Note that this number is not set in stone; that is, there is significant individual variation between dogs [3]. In actuality, the number of mammary glands in the canine patient ranges from 8 to 12 [3]. Eight glands occur more commonly than twelve [3].

As was true of feline patients, male dogs have rudimentary mammary glands.

Mammary glands will also be present, but underdeveloped, in nulliparous females (see Figures 62.3a, b).

62.1.3 Mammary Chain Evaluation

The left and right mammary chains should be palpated in both cats and dogs, males and females [1, 2]. The tissue should be supple and non-tender to the touch [1].

Normal mammary tissue should be devoid of grossly observable and/or palpable masses [1, 2]. Mammary masses may develop in cats and dogs of either sex [1, 2].

In the lactating female, each gland should be assessed for signs of inflammation, including, but not limited to the following [1, 2]:

- Asymmetrical mammary glands
- Discharge from one or more nipples
- Firmness of one or more glands
- Heat on palpation
- Redness
- Swelling of one or more glands

(a)

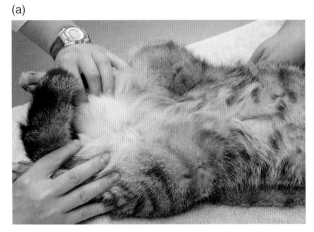

(b)

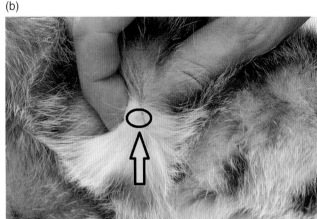

Figure 62.1 (a) The feline patient's furred ventral abdomen obscures the nipples from view. *Source:* Courtesy of the Media Resources Department at Midwestern University. (b) Fur must be parted along the feline patient's ventral abdomen in order to visualize the nipples. *Source:* Courtesy of the Media Resources Department at Midwestern University.

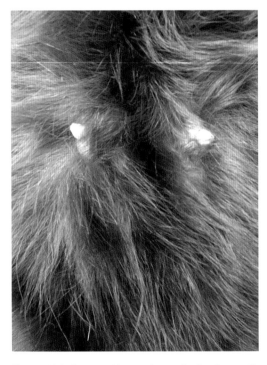

Figure 62.2 Queen with prominent nipples. *Source:* Courtesy of the Media Resources Department at Midwestern University.

Refer to Section 62.2 below for more information about clinical mastitis, that is, inflammation of the mammary gland(s).

Nipples should be counted and examined for surface integrity [2].

The skin immediately surrounding each nipple should also be evaluated for evidence of peri-areolar dermatitis. This could indicate the following [2]:

- Immune-mediated disease
- Neoplasia
- Self-mutilation, as from compulsive grooming (see Figure 62.4)

In the lactating patient, the clinician should express each gland to make sure that the patient is producing milk and to evaluate the milk's consistency [1, 2, 4, 6].

62.2 Mastitis

Mastitis refers to inflammation within mammary tissue [1, 2, 7–13]. It may involve one or more glands, or just a portion of a single gland [7, 14].

Mastitis occurs more commonly in bitches than in queens [7, 9, 14].

Onset is most often during the postpartum period [7, 8, 10, 15, 16]. Dogs are most at risk 6–10 days after whelping [15, 16].

Mastitis may also develop in lactating dogs with pseudopregnancy; however, this presentation is infrequent [7, 10].

Mastitis results from an underlying bacterial infection [7–10, 14, 17–19]. The infection typically ascends the teat canal [9, 13, 17]. It may be precipitated by trauma, for example, pups or kittens vigorously suckling [8, 9, 17] (see Figures 62.5a, b).

Cuts and scrapes on or adjacent to the teat may become a source of infection [8] (see Figure 62.6).

Mastitis may also result from poor hygiene, or unclean surroundings [9, 17].

Mastitis may arise secondary to blood-borne infection [13, 19].

(a)

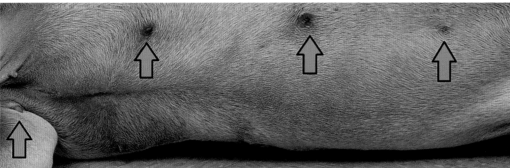

(b)

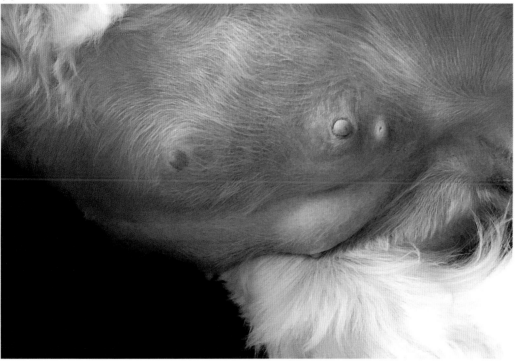

Figure 62.3 (a) Ventral abdomen of a canine patient, demonstrating the position and spacing of the mammary glands in a nulliparous canine patient. Note that the cranial-most set of glands is not captured in this photograph. *Source:* Courtesy of the Media Resources Department at Midwestern University. (b) Ventral abdomen of a canine patient, demonstrating prominent mammary chains in a pregnant bitch seven days prior to whelping. *Source:* Courtesy of Nechama Bloom, DVM.

Patients are predisposed if they delivered a small litter or if pups are removed from the dam [8]. Stress increases the likelihood of developing mastitis [8]. So, too, does metritis [8].

Many bacteria have been implicated in cases of canine and feline mastitis [10]. The most common causative agents among companion animals include the following [8–10, 12, 14, 18, 20, 21]:

- *Escherichia coli*
- *Klebsiella pneumonia*
- *Proteus mirabilis*
- *Staphylococcus* spp.

    – Coagulase-negative *Staphylococci*
    – *Staphylococcus aureus*
    – *Staphylococcus hyicus*
    – *Staphylococcus intermedius*
    – *Staphylococcus pseudintermedius*
- *Streptococcus* spp.
    – *Streptococcus canis*

Patients with subclinical mastitis may have litters with failure to thrive [14]. Tracking birth weight may be the only sign of an issue within the litter [14]. Pups should gain 10% of their birth weight per day [14]. If this rate of gain is not consistent, then bacterial culture

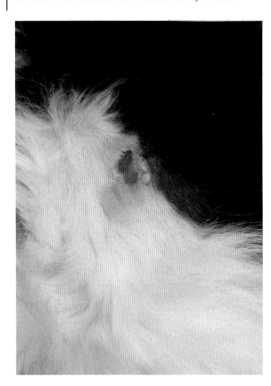

Figure 62.4 Superficial abrasion adjacent to a nipple associated with the left mammary chain of a cat. This lesion was attributed to compulsive grooming by the cat. *Source:* Courtesy of Dr. Elizabeth Robbins.

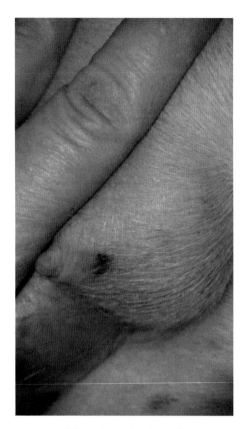

Figure 62.6 Superficial abrasion adjacent to a nipple in a canine patient. This could be a source of mastitis. *Source:* Courtesy of Tara Beugel.

(a)

(b)

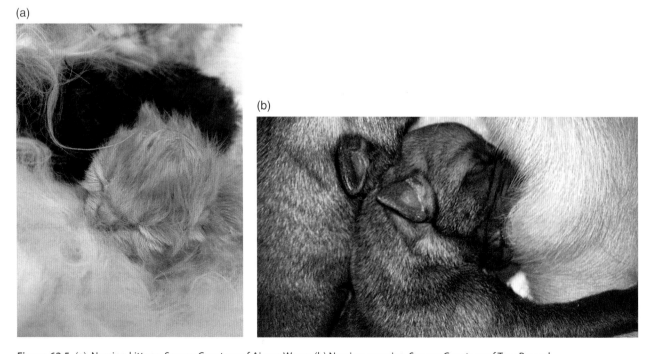

Figure 62.5 (a). Nursing kittens. *Source:* Courtesy of Aimee Wong. (b) Nursing puppies. *Source:* Courtesy of Tara Beugel.

and susceptibility testing of the dam's milk should be considered [14].

More typically, patients develop acute mastitis [14]. On physical examination, these patients will present with one or more swollen, painful glands that are warm to the touch [7, 8, 10] (see Figures 62.7a–c).

Secretions from affected mammary glands are grossly abnormal in terms of color and consistency [8–10]. Color may range from yellow-green to red-brown [8]. Secretions are thicker than expected as compared to normal milk, and may contain clots of blood or flakes of damaged tissue [8].

Progressive mastitis may also reduce the dam's tolerance of nursing and/or her ability to provide milk for her litter [8]. Puppies or kittens that are not allowed to suckle and/or are not receiving adequate nutrition may be excessively vocal [9, 22, 23].

As disease worsens and/or becomes systemic, the dam may also appear to be ill [9, 10]. She may become depressed and lethargic [9]. She may also lose her appetite [9]. It is not uncommon for patients with mastitis to become febrile [9].

If untreated, mastitis may result in intramammary abscesses that rupture open to drain, or necrotic mammary tissue [8, 10]. At this point, puppies and kittens have to be removed from the dam for hand-rearing in order to allow for appropriate wound management and healing [9, 10, 22, 24].

A presumptive diagnosis of mastitis is typically based upon history and physical examination [7–9, 13, 17].

A left shift on complete blood count (CBC) is supportive of systemic involvement [9, 17, 24].

The diagnosis is confirmed through cytological evaluation of the milk [8, 9]. Milk from affected patients will demonstrate microscopic inflammation as well as intracellular bacteria [9, 24].

In addition, culture and susceptibility testing are valuable [8, 9, 24]. A sample is collected either manually, by milking the teat, or via fine-needle aspiration (FNA) [7].

Antibiotic therapy is determined by sensitivity testing [7, 8]. Consideration must be applied to how the treatment plan will impact the neonates [7]. For example, neonates will need to be weaned off of the dam if the following antibiotics are to be used [7–9]:

- Aminoglycosides
- Chloramphenicol
- Tetracycline

These antibiotics are unsafe for puppies and kittens who are nursing, as they will be ingested in the milk [7].

(a)

(b)

(c)

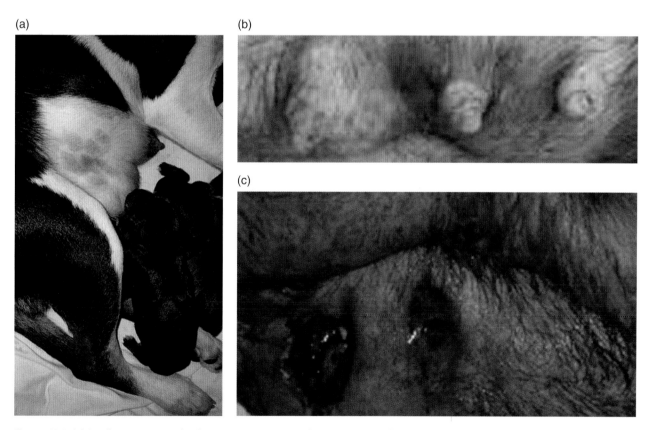

Figure 62.7 (a) Swollen mammary glands in a canine patient with acute mastitis. The dam is still nursing her pups. *Source:* Courtesy of Tara Beugel. (b) Focal mastitis in a canine patient. (c). Ulcerative mastitis.

While cultures are pending, it is appropriate to institute broad-spectrum, bactericidal therapy with cephalexin and/or amoxicillin/clavulanate [7]. Although these antibiotics do concentrate within milk, they are not harmful to neonates [9].

Discomfort of the dam may be reduced by hot-packing the affected gland(s) [7]. This will also encourage drainage [7].

Any abscessed mammary glands benefit from lancing, flushing, and managing as open wounds [7, 9, 14, 22].

62.3 Feline Mammary Fibroepithelial Hyperplasia

Mammary growths are significant concerns in cats because over 80% of tumors in this region are malignant [5, 25–27]. However, it is important to recognize that benign mammary growths do occur in cats, and these can regress or be reversed with treatment [5, 26, 28, 29].

Feline mammary fibroepithelial hyperplasia (FEH) is one such condition that can occur in cats of either sex [5, 26]. Its synonyms include fibroadenomatous changes, mammary hyperplasia, or fibroadenoma complex [26, 28–30].

Affected cats present for sudden onset of swelling of one or more mammary glands [26, 31–35]. Swelling is extreme and progressive [26, 31–35]. Secondary abscesses commonly form, and/or the surface of affected tissue may become ulcerated [26, 31–35].

On clinical presentation, FEH looks strikingly similar to mammary neoplasia [26]. Mammary tissue becomes firm and swollen [26]. Both mammary chains may be involved, or there may be focal involvement only [26]. Non-pregnant patients tend to have an asymmetrical distribution of lesions, as compared to pregnant cats, which tend to present with symmetrical disease [26].

Nipples may be buried within the enlarging affected glands [26]. The skin overlying the affected tissue may become erythematous [26]. Although lesions can grow to become quite pronounced, for example, up to 21 cm, they are not typically painful on palpation [26]. Sizable lesions may restrict mobility [26].

FEH impacts milk production in queens [26]. Ulcerative surfaces will develop if mastitis is concurrent [26]. Ulcerations may also result from excessive grooming or insufficient perfusion of the overstretched skin over affected glands [26].

Mammary tissue proliferation is fueled by progesterone [26, 28–30, 35, 36]. Progesterone may be endogenously produced, as is the case for intact queens or pregnant females [26, 31, 32, 37]. This endogenous progesterone may lead to mammary proliferation one to two weeks after estrus [26].

Alternatively, FEH may occur secondary to exogenous progesterone [26, 31–35, 38]. Cats that receive progestin may develop gynecomastia two to six weeks after hormone therapy [26].

Tomcats that have been treated with delmadinone acetate or cyproterone acetate have also developed FEH [26, 33, 39]. These anti-androgenic substances are prescribed to some cat breeders to reduce the incidence of urine marking [26].

Neutered males that have been treated with megestrol acetate are also at risk [29, 35–37, 40].

Younger intact females appear to be most at risk [26, 35, 41, 42]. Patients have presented as early as six months of age [26, 43–45]. Mammary tumors, on the other hand, tend to present more frequently in middle-aged queens ranging from 10 to 12 years old [26, 27, 46].

In a young cat that develops acute mammary swelling, particularly one that is pregnant, with symmetrical lesions, a diagnosis of FEH is prioritized over mammary neoplasia [26]. History may also prompt consideration of FEH, for example, the cat that was treated with progestins for miliary dermatitis [26].

When a lesion is focal, impacting solely one gland, it becomes more challenging to differentiate from neoplasia [26]. Biopsies are difficult to interpret accurately, particularly because FEH lesions may display cytological atypia and mitotic figures [26, 36, 43].

Hormone assays will reveal high levels of progesterone [5].

Thoracic and abdominal radiographs are beneficial to rule out metastases and calcification, which would indicate neoplastic disease [36].

Response to treatment with the antiprogesterone drug, aglepristone, is confirmatory [33, 36, 45, 47–49]. A positive response is seen as early as three days into treatment [36]. It may take 21–24 days to see complete reversal of FEH [36].

Note that aglepristone is contraindicated during pregnancy as it will induce abortion [26].

One concern about aglepristone is that FEH may recur once the drug is discontinued, particularly if the patient is restarted on progestin treatment [35].

Alternative medical approaches include the use of dopamine agonists, such as cabergoline and bromocriptine [26]. These drugs inhibit prolactin secretion, which has not yet been proven to contribute to the development of FEH [26].

Mastectomy is advisable when all other nonsurgical approaches have been tried without success [26].

62.4 Canine Mammary Gland Neoplasia

Although mammary cancer is a common type of neoplasia among dogs, intact females are most at risk because of hormone exposure [50–56]. Spaying dogs before their first estrus reduces their risk of developing mammary cancer to 0.5% [51, 57]. Spaying dogs before four years of age is still thought to be protective against mammary cancer [51, 58–60]. However, the degree to which protection is offered is reduced with each cycle [51]. It has been suggested that dogs' risk of mammary cancer rises to 8% if spayed after the first heat cycle, but before the second; and to 26% if spayed before cycle three [51, 57].

Dogs that are seven years of age or older are more likely than young dogs to develop mammary cancer [51, 52, 57, 60–63].

Purebreds are likelier to succumb to mammary neoplasia than mixed breeds [51]. Among purebreds, the following breeds appear with frequency in the veterinary medical literature [51–53, 64–66]:

- Brittany Spaniels
- Chihuahuas
- Cocker Spaniels
- Dachshunds
- Dobermans
- English Setters
- English Springer Spaniels
- German Shepherds
- Maltese
- Pointers
- Poodles
- Yorkshire Terriers

Genetics is believed to play a role in canine mammary neoplasia [51]. Certain family lines of dogs have increased risk as compared to others [51]. This has been established among colonies of Beagles [51, 67].

Weight at puberty is an additional risk factor. If patients are underweight at this milestone, then they are less likely to develop mammary cancer [51, 59]. Obese patients, on the other hand, have an increased risk [68, 69]. This mirrors some findings in women that link obesity to breast cancer [51].

When mammary tumors develop in dogs, they tend to involve more than one gland [51, 60, 70–74]. Benign and malignant tumors may occur concurrently [51, 71, 74]. This knowledge gave rise to the theory that mammary tumors in dogs reflect a continuum, in which benign tumors have the potential to transition into malignancy [51]. What provokes this transition remains to be determined: some benign tumors never progress [51].

Most canine mammary tumors affect one or both of the caudal pairs of glands [51, 60, 70, 72, 73] (see Figures 62.8a–c).

Presentations vary tremendously in terms of tumor size, shape, texture, and surface appearance. Tumors may ulcerate and develop secondary bacterial infections (see Figure 62.9).

These patients may be misdiagnosed with mastitis because of the inflammatory appearance [51, 75, 76].

Most dogs at the time of diagnosis are systemically well [51].

Given that benign tumors may transition into malignancy, it is critical that patients be staged. Staging involves, at minimum [51]:

- CBC
- Chemistry profile
- Urinalysis
- Fine-needle aspirate (FNA) of regional lymph nodes
- Three-view thoracic radiographs

Mammary cytology via FNA may be beneficial to rule out dermatopathy, such as a mast cell tumor or a lipoma [51].

The sensitivity and specificity of FNA identification of a mammary malignancy are reported to be 88 and 93%, respectively [51, 77].

Dogs that are suspected to have lymph node involvement also benefit from abdominal ultrasonography [51].

Staging yields a score from one to five, five being indicative of metastasis [51]. The liver, lungs, and bone are the most common distant sites of metastasis [51].

Mammary tumors have a 50/50 chance of being benign in the dog [50, 51]. Benign canine mammary tumors include the following [51, 65]:

- Adenoma
- Duct papilloma
- Ductal adenoma
- Fibroadenoma
- Myoepithelioma

Malignant canine mammary tumors include the following [51, 65, 78, 79]:

- Epithelial tumors
  - Adenocarcinoma
  - Carcinoma
- Mesenchymal tumors
  - Chondrosarcoma
  - Fibrosarcoma
  - Hemangiosarcoma
  - Osteosarcoma

(a)

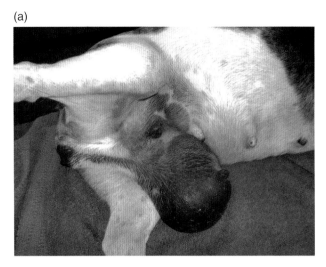

(b)
(c)

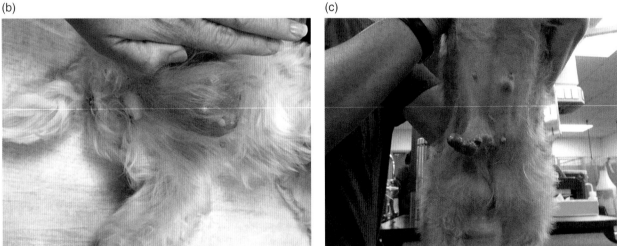

Figure 62.8 (a) Tumor associated with the left caudal mammary chain. *Source:* Courtesy of Patricia Bennett, DVM. (b) Tumor associated with the caudal aspect of the right mammary chain. *Source:* Courtesy of Samantha B. Thurman, DVM. (c) Tumor associated with the right caudal mammary chain. *Source:* Courtesy of Kara Thomas, DVM, CVMA.

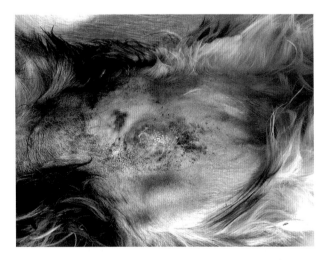

Figure 62.9 Erosive mammary tumor in a canine patient. *Source:* Courtesy of Dr. Stephanie Harris.

Note that malignancies may also be restricted to the nipple [51]. For example, ductal adenoma and carcinoma involve the nipple only [51]. Although rarely seen in clinical practice, these patients present with an enlarged, firm nipple [51].

Poor prognostic factors for canine mammary neoplasia include the following [51, 63, 78, 80, 81]:

- Infiltration into surrounding tissues
- Inflammatory mammary carcinoma
- Local lymph node involvement
- Sarcoma
- Tumors greater than 3.4 cm in diameter
- Ulceration

Wide surgical excision is the treatment of choice for the management of canine mammary neoplasia [51]. Unilateral or bilateral chain mastectomies are not indicated unless there are multiple tumors involving multiple areas of one or both chains [51].

Lumpectomy and/or mastectomy appear to result in a comparable survival time as compared to regional or chain mastectomy when only a single tumor is identified [51].

Dogs with local lymph node involvement may benefit from chemotherapy [51]. There is minimal evidence to suggest that hormonal therapy, for example, estrogen receptor antagonists such as tamoxifen, is beneficial [51].

62.5 Feline Mammary Gland Neoplasia

Mammary cancer occurs less frequently in cats than in dogs [51]. However, when it occurs, it is more likely to be malignant [5, 51, 82, 83]. Between 85 and 93% of mammary masses are cancerous in cats [5, 25].

As compared to clinical presentations of FEH, which favors young cats, feline mammary neoplasia preferentially targets mid-aged to older cats [5, 26, 27, 46, 84]. Most cats are between 10 and 12 years of age at the time of diagnosis [51, 52, 85–88].

Siamese cats are at an increased risk for development of mammary neoplasia and may therefore present at an earlier age [5, 51, 84, 89–91].

Intact cats are seven times more likely than neutered cats to develop mammary cancer [5, 51, 52, 87, 89, 92]. Cats that are spayed before six months of age have a 91% risk reduction [51]. The degree of protection is reduced as the patient ages [5, 51, 92]. Cats that are spayed between 7 and 12 months of age have a risk reduction of 86%, whereas cats that are 13–24 months of age at time of spay have a risk reduction of only 11% [51]. There is no protective benefit from spay relative to mammary neoplasia after two years of age [51].

Treatment with progestins elevates the risk for mammary tumor development [51, 87].

Males develop mammary cancer less frequently than females; however, males that receive progestin therapy are at increased risk [38, 51].

Presentations vary in terms of tumor size, shape, texture, and surface appearance. As is true of those in dogs, feline mammary tumors may ulcerate and develop secondary bacterial infections [5, 51].

Most mammary masses are firm and discrete, and are easily recognized on palpation [51].

Most cats with mammary tumors have more than one at the time of diagnosis [51, 86].

Most feline mammary tumors are aggressive [5, 51]. Local lymph node involvement and invasion of lymphatic vessels are both likely at the time of diagnosis [51].

Metastasis to distant sites is also common [5]. Preferential sites include the lungs, liver, and pleura [5, 93]. Lesson common, but possible sites, include the diaphragm, kidneys, adrenal glands, and skeleton [5, 89, 94, 95].

Mammary masses may also compromise vascular return from the femoral veins [5]. This may result in edematous pelvic limbs and/or associated caudal end discomfort [5].

Given that feline mammary tumors are more likely to be malignant, it is critical that patients be staged. Staging involves the same baseline diagnostic tests as in the dog [5, 51, 84, 96]:

- CBC
- Chemistry profile
- Urinalysis
- FNA of regional lymph nodes
- Three-view thoracic radiographs

Benign feline mammary tumors include the following [5, 51]:

- Adenoma
- Duct papilloma
- Fibroadenoma

Malignant feline mammary tumors include adenocarcinomas and carcinomas [44, 51, 97–102].

Poor prognostic factors for feline mammary neoplasia include the following [5, 51, 96, 103–107]:

- High mitotic index
- Local lymph node involvement
- The breed of cat (Siamese)
- Tumors greater than three centimeters

A more aggressive surgical approach is indicated in cats with mammary neoplasia as compared to dogs [51, 84, 96]. A unilateral chain mastectomy is indicated when there is a single tumor [51]. When multiple tumors are present, a staged bilateral chain mastectomy should be performed [51]. This improves the disease-free interval in cats [90, 104].

Cats with delayed diagnosis, large tumors, or local lymph node involvement require follow-up treatment [51]. Surgery alone is ineffective for this cohort [51]. Chemotherapy protocols have been outlined for the cat with mammary cancer, including a combination of doxorubicin and cyclophosphamide [51, 96, 108, 109]. However, not all studies demonstrate efficacy in this approach [106, 110].

It is unlikely that hormonal therapy is beneficial [51].

References

1 Rutteman, G.R. and Teske, E. (2009). Mammary glands. In: *Medical History and Physical Examination in Companion Animals* (ed. A. Rijnberk and F.J. van Sluijs), 132–134. Philadelphia: Elsevier.

2 Englar, R.E. (2017). *Performing the Small Animal Physical Examination.* Hoboken, NJ: Wiley.

3 Evans, H.E. and Christensen, G.C. (1993). The Urogenital System. In: *Miller's Anatomy of the Dog*, 3e (ed. H.E. Evans and M.E. Miller), 494–558. Philadelphia: W.B. Saunders.

4 Rijnberk, A. and FJv, S. (2009). *Medical History and Physical Examination in Companion Animals*, 2e, viii, 333 p. Edinburgh; New York: Saunders/Elsevier.

5 Gimenez, F., Hecht, S., Craig, L.E., and Legendre, A.M. (2010). Early detection, aggressive therapy: optimizing the management of feline mammary masses. *J. Feline Med. Surg.* 12 (3): 214–224.

6 Johnston, S.D. and Hayden, D.W. (1980). Non-neoplastic disorders of the mammary glands. In: *Current Veterinary Therapy VII* (ed. R.W. Kirk), 1224–1226. Philadelphia: Saunders.

7 Memon, M.A. (2018). Mastitis in small animals. Merck Veterinary Manual [Internet]. https://www.merckvetmanual.com/reproductive-system/reproductive-diseases-of-the-female-small-animal/mastitis-in-small-animals.

8 Orfanou, D.C., Ftenakis, G.C., and Mavrogianni, V.S. (eds.) (2016). Mastitis in lactating bitches. 8th International Symposium on Canine and Feline Reproduction (ISCFR); Paris, France.

9 Wilson, C.R. (2013). Feline gangrenous mastitis. *Can. Vet. J.* 54 (3): 292–294.

10 Ververidis, H.N., Mavrogianni, V.S., Fragkou, I.A. et al. (2007). Experimental staphylococcal mastitis in bitches: Clinical, bacteriological, cytological, haematological and pathological features. *Vet. Microbiol.* 124 (1–2): 95–106.

11 Tilley, L.P. and Smith, F.W.K. (eds.) (2004). Mastitis. In: *The 5-Minute Veterinary Consult: Canine and Feline*, 3e, 812–813. Baltimore, MD: Lippincott Williams & Wilkins.

12 Akgul, O. and Kaya, A. (2016). Microbiological analysis of acute mastitis in a van Cat. *Kafkas Univ. Vet. Fak. Derg.* 22 (1).

13 Vasiu, I., Dabrowski, R., Martinez-Subiela, S. et al. (2017). Milk C-reactive protein in canine mastitis. *Vet. Immunol. Immunopathol.* 186: 41–44.

14 Wiebe, V.J. and Howard, J.P. (2009). Pharmacologic advances in canine and feline reproduction. *Top. Companion Anim. Med.* 24 (2): 71–99.

15 Biddle, D. and Macintirc, D.K. (2000). Obstetrical emergencies. *Clin. Tech. Small Anim. Pract.* 15 (2): 88–93.

16 Wheeler, S.L., Magne, M.L., Kaufman, J. et al. (1984). Postpartum disorders in the bitch. *Compend. Contin. Educ. Pract.* 6 (6): 493.

17 Jutkowitz, L.A. (2005). Reproductive emergencies. *Vet. Clin. North Am. Small Anim. Pract.* 35 (2): 397–420, vii.

18 Vasiu, I., Spinu, M., Niculae, M., Balaci, I., and Brudasca, F.G. (2015). Laboratory methods used for early diagnosis in bitch mastitis. Bulletin UASVM Veterinary Medicine [Internet]. http://journals.usamvcluj.ro/index.php/veterinary/article/view/11026.

19 Kustritz, R.M.V. (ed.) (2010). How do I treat mastitis in a nursing bitch. In: *Clinical Canine and Feline Reproduction: Evidence-based Answers*, 157. Iowa: Wiley-Blackwell.

20 Osbaldiston, G.W. (1978). Bacteriological studies of reproductive disorders of bitches. *J. Am. Anim. Hosp. Assoc.* 14 (3): 363–367.

21 Sager, M. and Remmers, C. (1990). Perinatal mortality in dogs. Clinical, bacteriological and pathological studies. *Tierarztl. Prax.* 18 (4): 415–419.

22 Hopper, K. (ed.) (2003). Pyometra, mastitis, and uterine prolapse. International Veterinary Emergency and Critical Care Symposium; New Orleans, Louisiana.

23 Nelson, R.W. and Couto, C.G. (2009). *Small Animal Internal Medicine*, 4e, xxxii, 1466 p. St. Louis, Mo: Mosby/Elsevier.

24 Traas, A.M. and O'Connor, C. (eds.) (2009). Postpartum emergencies. International Veterinary Emergency and Critical Care Symposium

25 Lana, S.E., Rutteman, G.R., and Withrow, S.J. (2007). Tumors of the mammary gland. In: *Withrow & MacEwen's Small Animal Clinical Oncology*, 4e (ed. S.J. Withrow and D.M. Vail), 629. St. Louis: Saunders.

26 Payan-Carreira, R. (2013). Feline mammary fibroepithelial hyperplasia: A clinical approach. InTech [Internet]. https://www.intechopen.com/books/insights-from-veterinary-medicine/feline-mammary-fibroepithelial-hyperplasia-a-clinical-approach.

27 Murphy, S. (ed.) 2009. Mammary tumours in cats – causes and practical management. European Society of Feline Medicine (ESFM) Symposium; Birmingham, UK.

28 Johnston, S., Root Kustritz, M., and Olson, P. (2001). Disorders of the mammary gland of the queen. In: *Canine and Feline Theriogenology*, 474–485. Philadelphia: W.B. Saunders Comp.

29 Hayden, D.W., Johnston, S.D., Kiang, D.T. et al. (1981). Feline mammary hypertrophy/fibroadenoma complex: clinical and hormonal aspects. *Am. J. Vet. Res.* 42 (10): 1699–1703.

30 Johnson, C. (1994). Diseases of the mammary glands. In: *The Cat: Diseases and Clinical Management* (ed. R. Sherding), 1874–1875. New York: Churchill Livingstone.

31 Loretti, A.P., Ilha, M.R., and Ordas, J. (2005). Martin de las Mulas J. Clinical, pathological and immunohistochemical study of feline mammary fibroepithelial hyperplasia following a single injection of depot medroxyprogesterone acetate. *J. Feline Med. Surg.* 7 (1): 43–52.

32 Loretti, A.P., Ilha, M.R.S., Breitsameter, I., and Faraco, C.S. (2004). Clinical and pathological study of feline mammary fibroadenomatous change associated with depot medroxyprogesterone acetate therapy. *Arq. Bras. Med. Vet. Zoo.* 56 (2): 270–274.

33 Sontas, B.H., Turna, O., Ucmak, M., and Ekici, H. (2008). What is your diagnosis? Feline mammary fibroepithelial hyperplasia. *J. Small Anim. Pract.* 49 (10): 545–547.

34 Rutteman, G.R. and Withrow, S. (2001). Tumours of the mammary gland. In: *Small Animal Clinical Oncology* (ed. S. Withrow and E. MacEwen), 455–477. Philadelphia: W.B. Saunders Comp.

35 Burstyn, U. (2010). Management of mastitis and abscessation of mammary glands secondary to fibroadenomatous hyperplasia in a primiparturient cat. *J. Am. Vet. Med. Assoc.* 236 (3): 326–329.

36 Martin De Las Mulas, J., Millan, Y., Bautista, M.J. et al. (2000). Oestrogen and progesterone receptors in feline fibroadenomatous change: an immunohistochemical study. *Res. Vet. Sci.* 68 (1): 15–21.

37 MacDougall, L.D. (2003). Mammary fibroadenomatous hyperplasia in a young cat attributed to treatment with megestrol acetate. *Can. Vet. J.* 44 (3): 227–229.

38 Skorupski, K.A., Overley, B., Shofer, F.S. et al. (2005). Clinical characteristics of mammary carcinoma in male cats. *J. Vet. Intern. Med.* 19 (1): 52–55.

39 Jelinek, F., Barton, R., Posekana, J., and Hasonova, L. (2007). Gynaecomastia in a tom-cat caused by cyproterone acetate: a case report. *Vet. Med. Czech.* 52 (11): 521–525.

40 Chisolm, H. (1993). Massive mammary enlargement in a cat. *Can. Vet. J.* 34: 315.

41 Griffin, B. (2001). Prolific cats: The estrous cycle. *Compend. Contin. Educ. Pract.* 23 (12): 1049–1055.

42 Gudermuth, D.F., Newton, L., Daels, P., and Concannon, P. (1997). Incidence of spontaneous ovulation in young, group-housed cats based on serum and faecal concentrations of progesterone. *J. Reprod. Fertil. Suppl.* 51: 177–184.

43 Allen, H.L. (1973). Feline mammary hypertrophy. *Vet. Pathol.* 10 (6): 501–508.

44 Hayden, D.W., Barnes, D.M., and Johnson, K.H. (1989). Morphologic changes in the mammary gland of megestrol acetate-treated and untreated cats: a retrospective study. *Vet. Pathol.* 26 (2): 104–113.

45 Wehrend, A., Hospes, R., and Gruber, A.D. (2001). Treatment of feline mammary fibroadenomatous hyperplasia with a progesterone-antagonist. *Vet. Rec.* 148 (11): 346–347.

46 Sorenmo, K.U. (ed.) (2011). Mammary gland tumors in cats: risk factors, clinical presentation, treatments, and outcome. 36th World Small Animal Veterinary Congress; Jeju, Korea.

47 Gorlinger, S., Kooistra, H.S., van den Broek, A., and Okkens, A.C. (2002). Treatment of fibroadenomatous hyperplasia in cats with aglepristone. *J. Vet. Intern. Med.* 16 (6): 710–713.

48 Jurka, P. and Max, A. (2009). Treatment of fibroadenomatosis in 14 cats with aglepristone – changes in blood parameters and follow-up. *Vet. Rec.* 165 (22): 657–660.

49 Leidinger, E., Hooijberg, E., Sick, K. et al. (2011). Fibroepithelial hyperplasia in an entire male cat: cytologic and histopathological features. *Tierarztl. Prax. Ausg. K Klientiere Heimtiere* 39 (3): 198–202.

50 Tilley, L.P. and Smith, F.W.K. (eds.) (2004). Mammary gland tumors – dogs. In: *The 5-Minute Veterinary Consult: Canine and Feline*, 3e, 806–807. Baltimore, MD: Lippincott Williams & Wilkins.

51 Sorenmo, K.U., Worley, D.R., and Goldschmidt, M.H. (2013). *Tumors of the Mammary Gland. Withrow and MacEwen's Small Animal Clinical Oncology*, 5e, 538–556. St. Louis: Elsevier Saunders.

52 Dorn, C.R., Taylor, D.O., Schneider, R. et al. (1968). Survey of animal neoplasms in Alameda and Contra Costa Counties, California. II. Cancer morbidity in dogs and cats from Alameda County. *J. Natl. Cancer Inst.* 40 (2): 307–318.

53 Egenvall, A., Bonnett, B.N., Ohagen, P. et al. (2005). Incidence of and survival after mammary tumors in a population of over 80,000 insured female dogs in Sweden from 1995 to 2002. *Prev. Vet. Med.* 69 (1–2): 109–127.

54 Bronden, L.B., Nielsen, S.S., Toft, N., and Kristensen, A.T. (2010). Data from the Danish veterinary cancer registry on the occurrence and distribution of neoplasms in dogs in Denmark. *Vet. Rec.* 166 (19): 586–590.

55 Dobson, J.M., Samuel, S., Milstein, H. et al. (2002). Canine neoplasia in the UK: estimates of incidence

rates from a population of insured dogs. *J. Small Anim. Pract.* 43 (6): 240–246.

56 Merlo, D.F., Rossi, L., Pellegrino, C. et al. (2008). Cancer incidence in pet dogs: findings of the animal tumor registry of Genoa, Italy. *J. Vet. Intern. Med.* 22 (4): 976–984.

57 Schneider, R., Dorn, C.R., and Taylor, D.O. (1969). Factors influencing canine mammary cancer development and postsurgical survival. *J. Natl. Cancer Inst.* 43 (6): 1249–1261.

58 Misdorp, W. (1988). Canine mammary tumours: protective effect of late ovariectomy and stimulating effect of progestins. *Vet. Q.* 10 (1): 26–33.

59 Sonnenschein, E.G., Glickman, L.T., Goldschmidt, M.H., and McKee, L.J. (1991). Body conformation, diet, and risk of breast cancer in pet dogs: a case-control study. *Am. J. Epidemiol.* 133 (7): 694–703.

60 Taylor, G.N., Shabestari, L., Williams, J. et al. (1976). Mammary neoplasia in a closed beagle colony. *Cancer Res.* 36 (8): 2740–2743.

61 Brodey, R.S., Goldschmidt, M.H., and Roszel, J.R. (1983). Canine Mammary-Gland Neoplasms. *J. Am. Anim. Hosp. Assoc.* 19 (1): 61–90.

62 Priester, W.A. and Mantel, N. (1971). Occurrence of tumors in domestic animals. Data from 12 United States and Canadian colleges of veterinary medicine. *J. Natl. Cancer Inst.* 47 (6): 1333–1344.

63 Kurzman, I.D. and Gilbertson, S.R. (1986). Prognostic factors in canine mammary tumors. *Semin. Vet. Med. Surg.* 1 (1): 25–32.

64 Moe, L. (2001). Population-based incidence of mammary tumours in some dog breeds. *J. Reprod. Fertil. Suppl.* 57: 439–443.

65 Goldschmidt, M., Pena, L., Rasotto, R., and Zappulli, V. (2011). Classification and grading of canine mammary tumors. *Vet. Pathol.* 48 (1): 117–131.

66 Yamagami, T., Kobayashi, T., Takahashi, K., and Sugiyama, M. (1996). Prognosis for canine malignant mammary tumors based on TNM and histologic classification. *J. Vet. Med. Sci.* 58 (11): 1079–1083.

67 Schafer, K.A., Kelly, G., Schrader, R. et al. (1998). A canine model of familial mammary gland neoplasia. *Vet. Pathol.* 35 (3): 168–177.

68 Alenza, D.P., Rutteman, G.R., Pena, L. et al. (1998). Relation between habitual diet and canine mammary tumors in a case-control study. *J. Vet. Intern. Med.* 12 (3): 132–139.

69 Hoskins, J.D. (2008). Prognosis, treatment of canine mammary tumors. DVM 360 [Internet]. http://veterinarynews.dvm360.com/prognosis-treatment-canine-mammary-tumors.

70 Bender, A.P., Dorn, C.R., and Schneider, R. (1984). An epidemiologic-study of canine multiple primary neoplasia involving the female and male reproductive systems. *Prev. Vet. Med.* 2 (5): 715–731.

71 Gilbertson, S.R., Kurzman, I.D., Zachrau, R.E. et al. (1983). Canine mammary epithelial neoplasms: biologic implications of morphologic characteristics assessed in 232 dogs. *Vet. Pathol.* 20 (2): 127–142.

72 Moulton, J.E., Rosenblatt, L.S., and Goldman, M. (1986). Mammary tumors in a colony of beagle dogs. *Vet. Pathol.* 23 (6): 741–749.

73 Benjamin, S.A., Lee, A.C., and Saunders, W.J. (1999). Classification and behavior of canine mammary epithelial neoplasms based on life-span observations in beagles. *Vet. Pathol.* 36 (5): 423–436.

74 Sorenmo, K.U., Kristiansen, V.M., Cofone, M.A. et al. (2009). Canine mammary gland tumours; a histological continuum from benign to malignant; clinical and histopathological evidence. *Vet. Comp. Oncol.* 7 (3): 162–172.

75 Marconato, L., Romanelli, G., Stefanello, D. et al. (2009). Prognostic factors for dogs with mammary inflammatory carcinoma: 43 cases (2003–2008). *J. Am. Vet. Med. Assoc.* 235 (8): 967–972.

76 Perez Alenza, M.D., Tabanera, E., and Pena, L. (2001). Inflammatory mammary carcinoma in dogs: 33 cases (1995–1999). *J. Am. Vet. Med. Assoc.* 219 (8): 1110–1114.

77 Eberle, N., Fork, M., von Babo, V. et al. (2011). Comparison of examination of thoracic radiographs and thoracic computed tomography in dogs with appendicular osteosarcoma. *Vet. Comp. Oncol.* 9 (2): 131–140.

78 Souza, C.H.D., Toledo-Piza, E., Amorin, R. et al. (2009). Inflammatory mammary carcinoma in 12 dogs: Clinical features, cyclooxygenase-2 expression, and response to piroxicam treatment. *Can. Vet. J.* 50 (5): 506–510.

79 Moulton, J.E., Taylor, D.O., Dorn, C.R., and Andersen, A.C. (1970). Canine mammary tumors. *Pathol. Vet.* 7 (4): 289–320.

80 MacEwen, E.G., Harvey, H.J., Patnaik, A.K. et al. (1985). Evaluation of effects of levamisole and surgery on canine mammary cancer. *J. Biol. Response Mod.* 4 (4): 418–426.

81 Hellmen, E., Bergstrom, R., Holmberg, L. et al. (1993). Prognostic factors in canine mammary-tumors – a multivariate study of 202 consecutive cases. *Vet. Pathol.* 30 (1): 20–27.

82 Straw, R.C. (2006). The cat with skin lumps and bumps. In: *Problem-Based Feline Medicine* (ed. J. Rand), 1067–1080. Edinburgh; New York: Saunders.

83 Tilley, L.P. and Smith, F.W.K. (eds.) (2004). Mammary gland tumors – cats. In: *The 5-Minute Veterinary Consult: Canine and Feline*, 3e, 804–805. Baltimore, MD: Lippincott Williams & Wilkins.

84 Silva, M.N., Leite, J.S., Mello, M.F. et al. (2017). Histologic evaluation of Ki-67 and cleaved caspase-3 expression in feline mammary carcinoma. *J Feline Med Surg.* 19 (4): 440–445.

85 Hayden, D.W. and Nielsen, S.W. (1971). Feline mammary tumours. *J. Small Anim. Pract.* 12 (12): 687–698.

86 Hayes, A.A. and Mooney, S. (1985). Feline mammary tumors. *Vet. Clin. North Am. Small Anim. Pract.* 15 (3): 513–520.

87 Misdorp, W., Romijn, A., and Hart, A.A. (1991). Feline mammary tumors: a case-control study of hormonal factors. *Anticancer Res.* 11 (5): 1793–1797.

88 Weijer, K., Head, K.W., Misdorp, W., and Hampe, J.F. (1972). Feline malignant mammary tumors. I. Morphology and biology: some comparisons with human and canine mammary carcinomas. *J. Natl. Cancer Inst.* 49 (6): 1697–1704.

89 Hayes, H.M. Jr., Milne, K.L., and Mandell, C.P. (1981). Epidemiological features of feline mammary carcinoma. *Vet. Rec.* 108 (22): 476–479.

90 Ito, T., Kadosawa, T., Mochizuki, M. et al. (1996). Prognosis of malignant mammary tumor in 53 cats. *J. Vet. Med. Sci.* 58 (8): 723–726.

91 Patnaik, A.K., Liu, S.K., Hurvitz, A.I., and McClelland, A.J. (1975). Nonhematopoietic neoplasms in cats. *J. Natl. Cancer Inst.* 54 (4): 855–860.

92 Overley, B., Shofer, F.S., Goldschmidt, M.H. et al. (2005). Association between ovariohysterectomy and feline mammary carcinoma. *J. Vet. Intern. Med.* 19 (4): 560–563.

93 Hahn, K.A. and Adams, W.H. (1997). Feline mammary neoplasia: biological behavior, diagnosis, and treatment alternatives. *Feline Pract.* 25 (2): 5–11.

94 Novosad, C.A., Bergman, P.J., O'Brien, M.G. et al. (2006). Retrospective evaluation of adjunctive doxorubicin for the treatment of feline mammary gland adenocarcinoma: 67 cases. *J. Am. Anim. Hosp. Assoc.* 42 (2): 110–120.

95 Moulton, J.E. (ed.) (1990). Mammary tumors of the cat. In: *Tumors in Domestic Animals*, 547–552. Berkeley: University of California Press.

96 Morris, J. (2013). Mammary tumours in the cat: size matters, so early intervention saves lives. *J. Feline Med. Surg.* 15 (5): 391–400.

97 Rasotto, R., Caliari, D., Castagnaro, M. et al. (2011). An immunohistochemical study of HER-2 expression in feline mammary tumours. *J. Comp. Pathol.* 144 (2–3): 170–179.

98 Perez-Alenza, M.D., Jimenez, A., Nieto, A.I., and Pena, L. (2004). First description of feline inflammatory mammary carcinoma: clinicopathological and immunohistochemical characteristics of three cases. *Breast Cancer Res.* 6 (4): R300–R307.

99 Seixas, F., Palmeira, C., Pires, M.A., and Lopes, C. (2007). Mammary invasive micropapillary carcinoma in cats: clinicopathologic features and nuclear DNA content. *Vet. Pathol.* 44 (6): 842–848.

100 Seixas, F., Palmeira, C., Pires, M.A., and Lopes, C. (2008). Are complex carcinoma of the feline mammary gland and other invasive mammary carcinoma identical tumours? Comparison of clinicopathologic features, DNA ploidy and follow up. *Res. Vet. Sci.* 84 (3): 428–433.

101 Kamstock, D.A., Fredrickson, R., and Ehrhart, E.J. (2005). Lipid-rich carcinoma of the mammary gland in a cat. *Vet. Pathol.* 42 (3): 360–362.

102 Matsuda, K., Kobayashi, S., Yamashita, M. et al. (2008). Tubulopapillary carcinoma with spindle cell metaplasia of the mammary gland in a cat. *J. Vet. Med. Sci.* 70 (5): 479–481.

103 Weijer, K. and Hart, A.A. (1983). Prognostic factors in feline mammary carcinoma. *J. Natl. Cancer Inst.* 70 (4): 709–716.

104 MacEwen, E.G., Hayes, A.A., Harvey, H.J. et al. (1984). Prognostic factors for feline mammary tumors. *J. Am. Vet. Med. Assoc.* 185 (2): 201–204.

105 Seixas, F., Palmeira, C., Pires, M.A. et al. (2011). Grade is an independent prognostic factor for feline mammary carcinomas: a clinicopathological and survival analysis. *Vet. J.* 187 (1): 65–71.

106 Borrego, J.F., Cartagena, J.C., and Engel, J. (2009). Treatment of feline mammary tumours using chemotherapy, surgery and a COX-2 inhibitor drug (meloxicam): a retrospective study of 23 cases (2002–2007). *Vet. Comp. Oncol.* 7 (4): 213–221.

107 Viste, J.R., Myers, S.L., Singh, B., and Simko, E. (2002). Feline mammary adenocarcinoma: tumor size as a prognostic indicator. *Can. Vet. J.* 43 (1): 33–37.

108 Jeglum, K.A., Deguzman, E., and Young, K.M. (1985). Chemotherapy of advanced mammary adenocarcinoma in 14 cats. *J. Am. Vet. Med. Assoc.* 187 (2): 157–160.

109 Mauldin, G.N., Matus, R.E., Patnaik, A.K. et al. (1988). Efficacy and toxicity of doxorubicin and cyclophosphamide used in the treatment of selected malignant-tumors in 23 cats. *J. Vet. Intern. Med.* 2 (2): 60–65.

110 McNeill, C.J., Sorenmo, K.U., Shofer, F.S. et al. (2009). Evaluation of adjuvant doxorubicin-based chemotherapy for the treatment of feline mammary carcinoma. *J. Vet. Intern. Med.* 23 (1): 123–129.

63

Abnormal Palpation of One or Both Kidneys

63.1 Introduction to the Upper Urinary Tract

The upper urinary tract consists of a left and right kidney as well as a left and right ureter [1, 2].

The kidneys are located within the retroperitoneal space, ventral to the sublumbar musculature [1, 2]. The right kidney sits at the level of the first three lumbar vertebrae and is cranial to the left, which spans the second through the fifth vertebrae [1, 2].

The caudate process of the liver cups the cranial pole of the right kidney [1, 2]. Because of this, the right kidney is somewhat more anchored than the left [1, 2]. However, both kidneys are surprisingly mobile in cats as compared to dogs and should be palpable on abdominal palpation [1–5].

By contrast, canine kidneys are very difficult to appreciate on the physical examination, especially in large and giant breed dogs [1]. It is common for the clinician to feel neither kidney in a normal dog or only the left kidney's caudal pole [1].

When palpating the kidneys, the clinician should gain an appreciation for renal structure, including [1, 2]:

- Shape
- Size
- Symmetry.

The ureters are paired tubular structures that act as conduits for urine to pass from the site of formation, the kidneys, to site of storage, the urinary bladder [1, 2].

Neither the left nor right ureter is palpable [1, 2].

63.2 Normal Renal Features: Shape, Surface Texture, and Size

Normal kidneys are shaped like kidney beans, and they have smooth surfaces, as opposed to being undulated or "lumpy bumpy" [1].

Their palpation should not be painful to the patient [1, 2].

Renal size in cats can be estimated by abdominal palpation, comparing renal length to finger width [1]. The clinician starts by measuring the width of his second through fourth fingers, in centimeters, when they are adjacent to each other, as if wearing mittens. Next, the clinician palpates the patient's kidneys. If, for instance, the clinician notes that the length of the cat's left kidney spans the width of three of his fingers, and he knows in advance how wide his fingers are, he can estimate the length, in centimeters, of that kidney [1].

Renal size estimates are imperfect [1]. For example, renal size may be overestimated in obese patients because of peri-renal fat [4, 5]. However, renal size estimates provide a starting point.

Renal size can also be confirmed by imaging studies [1, 3, 6–18]. Abdominal radiographs allow kidney length to be compared to the length of the body of the second lumbar vertebra (L2). This establishes the patient's renal length to L2 ratio [1, 3]. Normal renal length to L2 ratios in the cat have been cited as 2.0–3.0 [7–11].

By comparison, normal renal length to L2 ratios in the dog, based upon the ventrodorsal (V/D) view, range from 2.54 to 3.45, and from 2.38 to 3.19 on lateral view [1]. Brachycephalic breeds have a greater renal length to L2 ratio than dolichocephalic breeds [18].

Abdominal ultrasonography allows for a direct measurement of renal length and therefore improves accuracy. Renal length in the cat, for instance, is typically between 3.8 and 4.4 cm, but can reach as high as 5.3 cm [6, 8, 12, 14, 15].

The sexual status of the cat appears to play a role in renal size. A study by Shiroma et al. in 1999 demonstrated that neutered cats have a smaller renal length ratio as compared to intact cats [9]. The presence of testosterone stimulates renal hypertrophy [19, 20]. Therefore, tomcats are more likely to have larger-than-anticipated kidneys.

On the other hand, estrogen's impact on renal size is up for debate [1]. Some studies suggest that estrogen enhances renal size; other studies suggest that estrogen diminishes it [21–24].

Common Clinical Presentations in Dogs and Cats, First Edition. Ryane E. Englar.
© 2019 John Wiley & Sons, Inc. Published 2019 by John Wiley & Sons, Inc.

In dogs, there does not appear to be a definitive link between renal length and sexual status [4].

An additional challenge in dogs is determining which renal length constitutes normal because there is marked variation in canine morphology between breeds [25–27].

Rather than evaluating renal length alone to determine if kidneys are under- or oversized in a canine patient, the renal length to aortic luminal diameter (K/Ao) ratio has been suggested, as determined by ultrasonography. Renomegaly is present when the K/Ao ratio is greater than 9.1. By contrast, canine kidneys are undersized when the K/Ao ratio is less than 5.5 [27].

63.3 Common Abnormal Presentations Involving Renal Palpation

Renal palpation may reveal several abnormalities. In companion animal practice, three abnormalities in particular are detected with frequency:

- Enlarged kidneys
- Painful kidneys
- Small kidneys

Note that although changes in renal size alone are not necessarily cause for alarm, they may be an important prompt to investigate the possibility that the patient has underlying, subclinical disease.

63.4 Enlarged Kidneys

Renomegaly is the condition by which one or both kidneys are enlarged [28].

Renomegaly may be detected on palpation or may be an incidental finding on abdominal radiographs [28].

When renomegaly is present, it may indicate one of the following conditions [29, 30]:

- Acute kidney injury (AKI) or acute renal failure (ARF)
- Amyloidosis
- Feline infectious peritonitis (FIP)
- Hydronephrosis
- Infarcts
- Perinephric pseudocyst
- Polycystic kidney disease (PKD)
- Pyelonephritis
- Renal neoplasia

63.4.1 Acute Kidney Injury (AKI) or Acute Renal Failure (ARF)

AKI or ARF are conditions in which there is a sudden dysfunction of one or both kidneys [30]. Initially, this was referred to as ARF in the veterinary literature; however, AKI is a more appropriate reflection of the changes that take place microscopically within the damaged organ [30]. The affected kidneys can no longer regulate water, acid–base, and electrolyte balance [30]. They are also impaired when it comes to excreting waste [30].

Affected patients may present in the early phases of disease as being subclinical, but have an elevated creatinine level on serum biochemistry profile [30]. Other patients may present in anuric renal failure [30]. There is a broad spectrum of presentations that may be seen in clinical practice [30].

AKI is complex because there is not just one etiology [30]. To summarize, the primary causes include the following [30–36]:

- Acromegaly
- Anaphylaxis
- Cardiovascular shock
- Heatstroke
- Infectious disease***
- Sepsis
- Severe dehydration
- Systemic hypotension
- Thromboembolic disease
- Toxicity***
- Urinary tract obstruction (UTO)

The list above includes pre-renal, renal, and post-renal insults that may damage one or both kidneys [30]. The starred items (***) represent common concerns in clinical practice that will be addressed in greater detail here.

63.4.1.1 Toxicities and AKI

Several toxins are known to induce AKI [30]:

- Ethylene glycol
- Grapes and raisins (dogs only)
- Heavy metals
- Lilies (cats only)

History taking is an essential component of the veterinary consultation. It is particularly important when considering potential toxicities that result from patient exposure to and subsequent ingestion of disease-inducing agents.

63.4.1.1.1 Lilies

Lilies within the genera *Lilium* and *Hemerocallis* are nephrotoxic [37, 38]. These include the following [37, 38]:

- Asiatic lilies
- Day lilies
- Easter lilies
- Stargazer lilies
- Tiger lilies

Although Lily of the Valley is cardiotoxic, it is not nephrotoxic, although it is often erroneously lumped into the same group as those above [37].

Other non-nephrotoxic lilies include the peace lily and the rubrum lily [38].

Lily toxicosis was first discovered in 1990 [37]. It has since only been linked to cats [37–43]. Cats are exquisitely sensitive to all parts of the plant [37]. Ingestion of pollen alone or water containing lily pollen is sufficient to induce nephrotoxicity [37].

The pathophysiology of lily toxicosis is unknown [37]. Renal tubular cells die and slough [37]. Initially, affected patients are polyuric [37]. As dehydration sets in, patients will develop oliguria that progresses to anuria [37].

Patients present with palpably swollen kidneys. Patients may also exhibit depression, hypersalivation, decreased appetite, and vomiting as early as two to six hours post-ingestion [37, 38]. Although the gastrointestinal signs will resolve, AKI develops 12–30 hours post ingestion [37]. Anuria may begin as early as 24 hours, but is certainly present by 48 hours [37].

Patients with AKI present with renomegaly and renal pain [37, 38]. They are weak and dehydrated [37]. They are often recumbent [37]. They may also seize [38].

Baseline bloodwork reveals moderate to severe azotemia, meaning that affected patients have elevations in both blood urea nitrogen (BUN) and creatinine on serum biochemistry profile [37]. Unique to lily toxicosis, creatinine appears to increase at a disproportionate rate as compared to BUN [37, 44].

Tubular damage is evident on urinalysis as one or more of the following [37, 38, 41, 42]:

- Cylindruria, casts in the urine
- Glucosuria, sugar spilling into the urine
- Proteinuria, protein spilling into the urine

Casts are made up of gelled protein that has precipitated out into renal tubules. The protein gel forms a mold of the lumen of the tubule before washing out in the urine. Casts are named by their constituent material. In cases of lily toxicosis, tubular epithelial casts predominate [37].

Patients can recover from lily toxicosis; however, the prognosis is guarded if the diagnosis is not made until after they become anuric [37].

63.4.1.1.2 Ethylene Glycol

Ethylene glycol is a component of antifreeze [30]. It is also found in some printer cartridges, paint, and caulk [30]. However, most cases of ethylene glycol toxicosis involve the ingestion of antifreeze [30]. This is because antifreeze typically contains more than 90% ethylene glycol as compared to other products, which may contain 2% or less [30].

Cats are more sensitive to poisoning than dogs [30]. Ingestion of a mere 1.4 ml/kg is toxic to a cat as compared to 4.4–6.6 ml/kg in a dog [30, 45–48].

Ethylene glycol in and of itself does not result in toxicosis; the by-products of its metabolism do [30]. The actions of the enzyme, alcohol dehydrogenase, result in the formation of toxic metabolites. These include the following [30]:

- Glycolaldehyde
- Glycolic acid
- Glyoxylic acid
- Oxalates

Circulating calcium binds with oxalates to form mineralized deposits that effectively plug up the renal tubules [30].

Ethylene glycol presents similarly to lily toxicosis, except that cats that ingest lilies do not tend to exhibit neurological dysfunction [37]. By contrast, dogs, and cats that ingest ethylene glycol do experience ataxia as well as changes in mentation that range from depression to stupor [30].

63.4.1.1.3 Grapes and Raisins

Grape and raisin toxicosis was first reported in 2001 [38]. Dogs residing in the United States and United Kingdom appear to be at increased risk [38, 49–51].

Crushed and fermented grapes are no less toxic than fresh grapes [38]. Red and white varieties have both been implicated [38]. So, too, have organic varieties [38].

To date, no heavy metals or mycotoxins have been implicated [38].

Some dogs, but not all, are exquisitely sensitive to grapes and raisins [38]. Studies report toxicity at 0.41–1.9 oz/kg of body weight [49, 50].

Patient presentation mirrors that of cats with lily toxicosis, in terms of gastrointestinal signs paving the way to renal [38].

ARF develops within 72 h of ingestion [38]. Poor prognostic factors include the development of oliguria or anuria [38].

63.4.1.1.4 Vitamin D Toxicosis

Not all rodenticides contain cholecalciferol, vitamin D_3. Products that do create a hypercalcemic state within the individual that ingested them [38]. Hypercalcemia leads to ARF [38].

Other vitamin-D-containing products that can result in toxicosis include topical creams that contain calcipotriene or calcipotriol [38]. These active ingredients are used in the management of human psoriasis [38]. Oral medications that are used to treat hypoparathyroidism, osteomalacia, and osteoporosis in humans may also result in AKI if inadvertently ingested [38].

Puppies and cats are more sensitive to the nephrotoxic effects of vitamin D toxicosis than adult dogs [38, 52].

Patients that are clinical present as mentioned earlier for other AKI-inducing toxins [38]. Gastrointestinal signs precede urinary signs [38].

Additionally, patients may develop soft tissue mineralization that is anticipated due to a spike in the calcium–phosphorus (Ca–P) product and is detectable on radiographs [38]. Prognosis is poor if the Ca–P exceeds $60 \, mg^2/dL^2$ [38, 53].

63.4.1.1.5 Other Drugs

Drugs can also act as nephrotoxic agents, including the following [30, 38, 54–63]:

- Amphoterin B
- Gentamicin
- Intravenous (IV) contrast agents
- Non-steroidal anti-inflammatory drugs (NSAIDs)
- Polymyxin B

Care must be taken to assess renal function in patients prior to initiating systemic antibiotic therapy with one or more of the aforementioned agents so as not to push a patient with pre-existing renal insufficiency into renal failure.

63.4.1.2 Infectious Diseases and AKI

Several infectious diseases are known to induce AKI in dogs and cats. Of these, the most common are the following [30]:

- Borreliosis (Lyme disease)***
- Leptospirosis***
- Rocky Mountain Spotted Fever (RMSF)

Starred items above (***) will be addressed in detail below.

63.4.1.2.1 Borreliosis

Recall from Chapter 6, Sections 6.5.3 and 6.5.6 that borreliosis is caused by a spirochete, *Borrelia burgdorferi* [64–68]. *B. burgdorferi* is transmitted by several species of ticks: *Ixodes scapularis, Ixodes pacificus,* and *Ixodes dammini* [64–68].

Review the lifecycle of *B. burgdorferi* as it pertains to the pathophysiology of Lyme disease, specifically, how this bacteria shifts its outer surface proteins to elude the host's immune response [68–72].

Recall that the host response to *B. burgdorferi* is highly variable. Lyme disease may be subclinical. More often, it presents as acutely debilitating, cyclical, and/or chronic disease [68].

Dogs and cats do not develop erythema migrans, the classic rash with which infected human patients present [68]. Instead, days to weeks after the initial infection, dogs may develop nonspecific signs of malaise: fever,

lethargy, and lymphadenopathy. These tend to be short-lived [68].

When disease is experimentally induced, infected dogs present with lameness two to six months after infection [73, 74]. Lameness starts at the limb nearest the site of the tick bite, and then appears to spread [73, 74]. Lameness may be intermittent or progressive. It may also appear to jump limb to limb [73, 74].

Certain breeds, such as Golden Retrievers, Labrador Retrievers, and Bernese Mountain Dogs, are predisposed to the development of ARF secondary to Lyme nephritis, a glomerulopathy that is characterized by marked proteinuria. Patients present with azotemia, uremia, and peripheral edema. The disease is often fatal [68, 75, 76].

Cats are also exposed to Borreliosis through tick bites. Little is known about the clinical features of borreliosis in cats because of limited case reports; however, lameness, fever, fatigue, and anorexia have been reported as presenting complaints [66].

63.4.1.2.2 Leptospirosis

Leptospirosis is caused by a spirochete within the genus *Leptospira* [77]. *Leptospira* spp. are further divided into different strains, or serovars [77]. For example, *Leptospira interrogans* has four main serovars that are of clinical importance [77]:

- Bratislava
  - Reservoir hosts: pigs, horses
- Canicola
  - Reservoir host: dogs
- Icterohaemorrhagiae
  - Reservoir host: rats
- Pomona
  - Reservoir hosts: horses, cattle

As a second example, the primary serovar for *Leptospira kirschneri* is grippotyphosa [77]. Grippotyphosa is found within raccoons, foxes, squirrels, mice, rats, voles, cattle, and horses [77].

Leptospira spp. are shed in the urine of infected animals [77]. Infected urine contaminates the environment and perpetuates the life cycle through the infection of new hosts [77]. For example, the ingestion of contaminated water can infect dogs, particularly dogs that swim in lakes or reservoirs [77]. Exposure to wildlife and, by extension, their urine, can also lead to infection [77]. For this reason, both country and city dogs are at risk [77].

Hunting is a risk factor for cats, who may ingest infected prey [77].

Leptospirosis is more prevalent in regions of the world that experience high levels of rainfall [77–80]. Outbreaks notoriously follow wet weather [77]. Within North

America, the peak season is autumn [77, 81–83]. *Leptospira* spp. are inactivated by freezing conditions [77].

Leptospira spp. are distributed worldwide, and the geographical distribution of leptospirosis within the United States is expanding [77, 81, 84–86].

Disease has the potential to occur when spirochetes enter the bloodstream via abraded skin or through penetration of mucous membranes [86]. Urine, soil, water, and food are common sources of infection [77].

Severity of disease depends upon the individual patient [77]. Some patients are subclinical [77]. Others develop only transient illness [77].

Severe infections result in acutely febrile patients with renal and/or hepatic injury [77]. Affected patients are often dehydrated and depressed [77]. They may exhibit peripheral lymphadenopathy and/or peripheral edema [77]. A presentation for acute abdomen is possible. Refer to Chapter 50.

Abdominal pain may be localized to the kidneys or it may be diffuse [77]. Renomegaly is palpable.

When leptospirosis causes renal dysfunction, patients develop oliguria, which may progress to anuria [77].

When leptospirosis causes hepatic dysfunction, patients develop icterus [77]. Recall from Chapter 28, Section 28.2 that icterus is a pigment-associated change in tissue. Tissues become discolored as yellow. In human medicine, this is sometimes referred to as jaundice [1, 87].

Icterus results from the accumulation of bile [88]. It may be grossly visible on inspection of one or more of the following tissues [1]:

- Mucous membranes
- Sclera
- Skin
- Peri-aural or pre-auricular skin (cats) (see Figures 63.1a, b)

Gastrointestinal signs, when present, are usually secondary to ARF [77]. There may also be concurrent pancreatitis or enteritis [77].

Less commonly, leptospirosis may result in uveitis or bleeding disturbances [77]. Hemorrhage may be pinpoint, as in petechiae, or evident in body fluids [77]. Hematuria, hematemesis, melena, epistaxis, and pulmonary hemorrhages have been reported [77, 89–91]. These result from underlying thrombocytopenia [77, 89, 90, 92, 93].

Patients that are pregnant at the time of infection may abort or deliver stillbirths [77].

Refer to an internal medicine or infectious disease textbook to explore the clinicopathologic findings that are associated with leptospirosis.

Vaccinations against canine leptospirosis are available, and are recommended throughout geographical hot beds of leptospirosis within the continental United States.

Note that cats may also develop AKI from leptospirosis [94]. Feline exposure to leptospirosis has been documented in the veterinary medical literature [94–97].

63.4.2 Pyelonephritis

Pyelonephritis refers to inflammation of the kidney(s), specifically the renal pelvis [98–104]. Although it may result from a blood-borne bacterial infection, pyelonephritis more often originates from the distal urinary tract [100, 103, 105, 106]. The ascending infection may be due to any number of bacteria; however, the two most commonly implicated include [99]:

- *Escherichia coli*
- *Staphylococcus* spp.

(a)

(b)

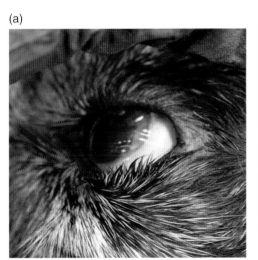
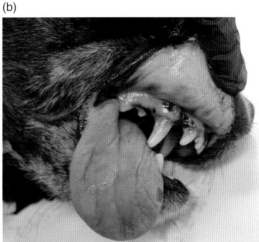

Figure 63.1 (a) Note the icteric sclera in this canine patient. *Source:* Courtesy of Dr. Alexandra Brower. (b) Note the degree to which this patient's mucous membranes and tongue are icteric. *Source:* Courtesy of Dr. Alexandra Brower.

Proteus, Streptococcus, Klebsiella, Enterobacter, and *Pseudomonas* may also contribute, although they are less often isolated from clinical cases [99].

Any patient may develop pyelonephritis. However, patients with any of the following conditions are predisposed [99]:

- ARF
- Ectopic ureter
- Exogenous steroid administration
- History of urinary catheterization
- Metabolic disease
  - Diabetes mellitus
  - Hyperadrenocorticism
- Neoplasia of the urinary tract
- Urine retention
- Urolithiasis
- Renal dysplasia

Many of the pathologies above create favorable conditions for the development of a urinary tract infection (UTI), which, if it ascends, sets the stage for pyelonephritis [99].

Definitive diagnosis of pyelonephritis requires a positive culture of urine collected by pyelocentesis [94]. This is rarely performed in clinical practice [94, 100, 103]. Therefore, the diagnosis is most often presumptive, based upon clinical signs and ultrasonographic detection of a dilated renal pelvis [94]. This is imperfect, but provides a starting point for identifying at-risk patients and developing an approach to case management.

Patients with pyelonephritis may present for nonspecific signs, including the following [99, 100, 103, 106]:

- Acute abdomen
- Decreased appetite
- Diarrhea
- Fever
- Lethargy
- Malaise
- Polydipsia (PD)
- Polyuria (PU)
- Vomiting

One or both kidneys may be affected and palpably enlarged. Pain may be localized to the affected kidney(s) or may be referred to the lumbar spine [99, 100].

The diagnostic work-up for cases in which pyelonephritis is a differential includes the following [99]:

- Complete blood count (CBC)
- Serum biochemistry profile
- Urinalysis
- Urine culture
- Imaging

Baseline bloodwork may be normal, or it may demonstrate neutrophilia with a left shift [99]. This is indicative of inflammation [99].

The serum biochemistry profile may be normal, or it may demonstrate azotemia [99]:

- Pre-renal azotemia in a patient that is clinical for pyelonephritis likely stems from dehydration in an acutely ill patient.
- Renal azotemia may result from chronic pyelonephritis.
- Post-renal azotemia may result from UTO secondary to urolithiasis.

A urinalysis is likely to demonstrate leukocyte casts, which indicate renal inflammation [99].

Urine cultures in dogs with chronic pyelonephritis may be falsely negative. Multiple cultures are often necessary to confirm UTI [99].

The aforementioned tests evaluate renal function. By contrast, imaging of the urinary tract evaluates renal structure. Abdominal radiographs effectively demonstrate radiopaque uroliths that may be contributing to urinary tract dysfunction (see Figures 63.2a–e).

Abdominal ultrasonography provides a way to measure the renal pelvis [99]. Ultrasound may confirm dilation of the renal pelvis and/or the proximal ureter [99].

Excretory urography, pyelograms, may identify obstructed kidneys (see Figures 63.3a, b).

Treatment of acute pyelonephritis is critical not only to patient health, but to the future health of the kidneys. If the infection becomes chronic, renal damage may be permanent [99, 100, 106, 107].

63.4.3 Ureteral Obstruction

Ureteral obstructions are caused by strictures or, more commonly, ureteroliths [30, 108–117]. Of these, calcium oxalates are most often implicated [113].

Obstruction may be unilateral or bilateral [30]. Patients with bilateral obstruction are critical and present in anuric renal failure [30].

Unilateral obstruction may result in many of the nonspecific signs that have been mentioned previously in this chapter [30]:

- Anorexia
- Changes in thirst
  Changes in urination
  - Anuria
  - Oliguria
  - Inappropriate elimination
- Depression
- Lethargy
- Vomiting

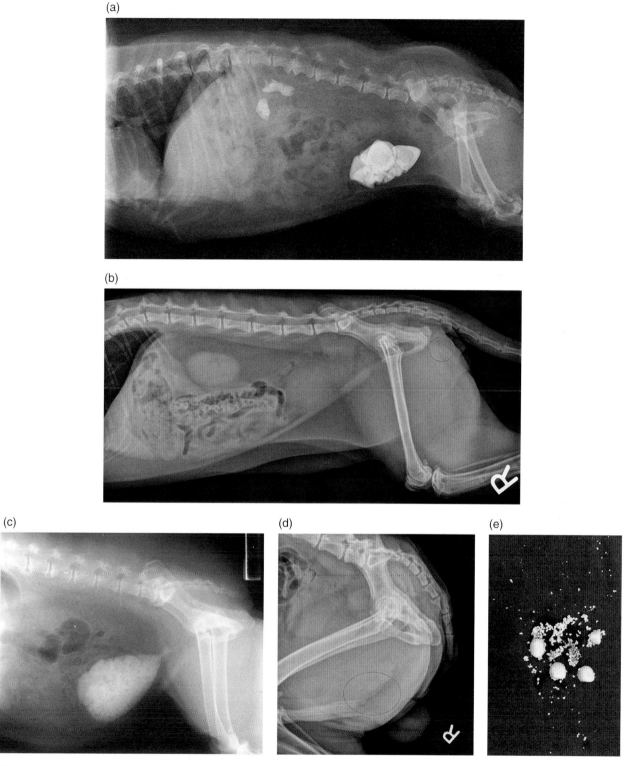

Figure 63.2 (a) Lateral abdominal radiograph, demonstrating an abundance of bladder stones. In addition, note the presence of nephroliths. *Source:* Courtesy of Daniel Foy, MS, DVM, DACVIM, DACVECC. (b) Right lateral abdominal radiograph, demonstrating urethral calculi, circled in orange. *Source:* Courtesy of Daniel Foy, MS, DVM, DACVIM, DACVECC. (c) Lateral abdominal radiograph, demonstrating cystic calculi. *Source:* Courtesy of Daniel Foy, MS, DVM, DACVIM, DACVECC. (d) Right lateral abdominal radiograph, demonstrating urethral calculi, circled in orange. Note their location, proximal to the os penis. This could precipitate urinary tract obstruction (UTO). *Source:* Courtesy of Daniel Foy, MS, DVM, DACVIM, DACVECC. (e) Postsurgical image of uroliths removed by cystotomy. Note the variety of sizes and shapes. These were confirmed to be struvite stones. *Source:* Courtesy of Joseph Onello, DVM.

(a)   (b)

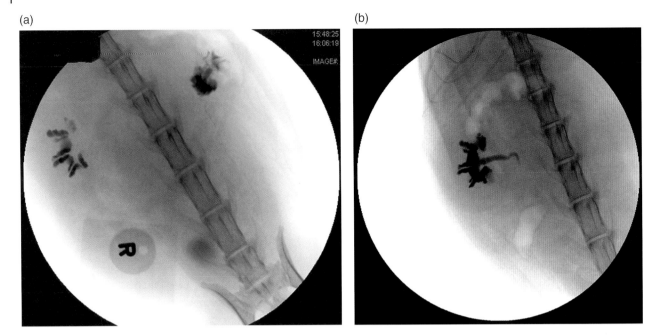

Figure 63.3 (a) Fluoroscopy of the kidneys. The left kidney is obstructed. *Source:* Courtesy of Daniel Foy, MS, DVM, DACVIM, DACVECC. (b) Fluoroscopy to evaluate the structure of the right kidney. *Source:* Courtesy of Daniel Foy, MS, DVM, DACVIM, DACVECC.

Diagnosis cannot be made based upon physical examination alone [30].

Diagnosis requires imaging in the form of radiography, contrast radiography, fluoroscopy, and/or abdominal ultrasonography [30, 113–115].

Case management emphasizes stabilization of the patient first, followed by attempts to alleviate the obstruction [30]. Fluid diuresis may facilitate urolith migration [30]. Continuous rate infusions (CRIs) of mannitol or oral administration of amitriptyline may dilate the ureters [30].

If the obstruction is not alleviated by medical case management, surgical intervention by means of ureterotomy, pyelotomy, and/or ureteral resection may be necessary [30].

63.4.4 Polycystic Kidney Disease (PKD)

PKD is an inherited condition among cats [118–122]. The inheritance pattern is autosomal dominant [118–122]. Persians, Persian-mixes, Himalayans, and Exotic Shorthairs are overrepresented, with up to 45% of some populations being affected [118–128].

Cysts develop within the renal parenchyma of typically both kidneys [122]. They may also develop in the liver of patients that are afflicted with PKD [122].

As renal cysts increase in size and number, they compress the renal parenchyma [122]. Renal failure is expected after a certain degree of functional renal mass is lost [122]. This typically occurs in middle age, usually at around seven years [122].

Prior to this development, patients are subclinical [122]. On physical examination, they exhibit renomegaly [122]. Enlarged kidneys are palpably non-painful, and their surfaces are typically irregular on account of cystic lesions [122, 129].

Diagnosis is via abdominal ultrasonography [119]. Cysts may be present in the cortex and/or the medulla [118, 119, 129]. They are fluid-filled. Therefore, their cores are hypoechoic (see Figure 63.4).

Because PKD has a known inheritance pattern, it can be eliminated by selective breeding [119].

63.4.5 Perinephric Pseudocyst

Perinephric pseudocysts are uncommonly seen in companion animal practice. Grossly, these lesions appear as cysts; however, microscopically they lack an epithelial lining [130].

Perinephric pseudocysts occur in both dogs and cats and are characterized by one or more fluid pockets developing around one or both kidneys [130–133]. Although this pocket may be extracapsular, it more often sits between the renal capsule and the parenchyma [130, 134]. The fluid contained within is most often a transudate or a modified transudate [130].

Male cats may be at increased risk for development of perinephric pseudocysts as compared to females, and most patients are middle-aged at the time of diagnosis [135].

Perinephric pseudocysts may be incidental findings on physical examination. Abdominal palpation reveals apparent renomegaly when in fact it is a perinephric

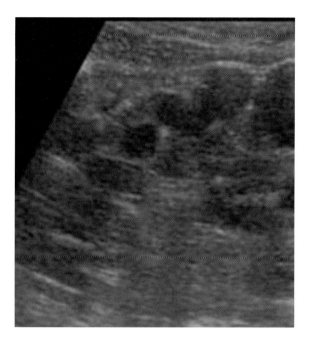

Figure 63.4 Screenshot of feline renal ultrasound. Note the abundance of hypoechoic fluid-filled structures. This Persian cat has PKD.

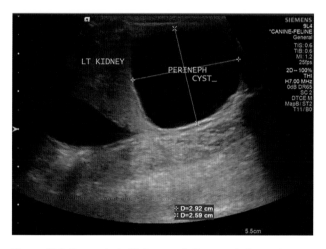

Figure 63.5 Screenshot of feline renal ultrasound, diagnosing a perinephric pseudocyst. *Source:* Courtesy of Daniel Foy, MS, DVM, DACVIM, DACVECC.

pseudocyst rather than the kidney itself that is distorting the renal silhouette [135].

The diagnosis of perinephric pseudocyst is confirmed by abdominal ultrasonography [130, 134] (see Figure 63.5).

Patients with perinephric pseudocysts may present for abdominal distension [130, 135].

Sizable perinephric pseudocysts may rupture, causing abdominal effusion [132].

Surgical resection of the perinephric pseudocyst is the considered the standard case management plan [135]. Incomplete excision will lead to recurrence [135].

63.4.6 Renal Neoplasia

With the exception of renal lymphoma in cats, renal tumors are rarely diagnosed in clinical practice among canine and feline populations [136, 137]. When they arise, primary renal tumors are most commonly carcinomas, transitional cell carcinomas (TCCs), or adenocarcinomas [136–140].

Less common primary renal tumors include fibromas, sarcomas, and nephroblastoma [136, 141].

Renal lymphoma in the cat can be a primary tumor. Alternatively, it may stem from multicentric disease [136, 142, 143].

Few studies track renal neoplasia in companion animal medicine. From the current veterinary medical literature, dogs with primary renal neoplasia are typically middle-aged males [137].

Only 4% of cases involve bilateral disease [137].

Patients present for nonspecific signs [137]:

- Anorexia
- Hematuria
- Lethargy
- Weight loss

Physical examination may detect enlargement of the affected kidney [137]. This is more easily achieved in cats than in dogs due to the increased mobility of both kidneys in the former species.

Renal pain is more likely if the primary tumor is a sarcoma [137].

Abdominal radiographs may detect a mass effect. This can be localized to the affected kidney on ultrasonography.

Fifteen percent of dogs have metastatic lesions on thoracic radiographs at the time of diagnosis [137].

Fine-needle aspiration (FNA) of masses or ultrasound-guided biopsies are possible, but not without risk [137]. Roughly 1 in 10 dogs with a renal mass have TCC [137]. TCCs are known to seed throughout the abdomen if they are given a tract by which to do so [137].

Nephrectomy may be considered to lengthen lifespan; however, these tumors are notoriously aggressive and likely benefit from postoperative chemotherapy [137].

63.5 Small Kidneys

The most common cause of bilaterally symmetrical, small kidneys is chronic kidney disease (CKD) [29, 90, 140]. CKD is defined as structural and/or functional renal impairment for three or more months. [90, 140] CKD is a progressive condition; however, patients may be stable for months to years [140]. Progression may be hastened by concurrent insults to the kidney, such as pre-renal azotemia, as from dehydration, or post-renal azotemia, as from UTO [140].

Historically, CKD has been referred as to renal failure [140]. However, the terminology *renal failure* is misleading because renal failure may be acute, as demonstrated in Section 63.4.

Whereas ARF results in enlarged kidneys, CKD causes shrunken ones [140].

Older, if not elderly, patients are most at risk for developing CKD [90, 140].

Among cats, the following breeds may be predisposed [28, 140]:

- Abyssinian
- Burmese
- Maine Coon
- Russian Blue
- Siamese

As CKD progresses, so, too, does the degree of renal dysfunction [140]. The kidneys play an important regulatory role in the following processes [140, 143]:

- Activation of vitamin D
- Blood pressure
  - Renin production
  - Aldosterone secretion by the associated adrenal glands
- Electrolyte balance
  - Potassium
  - Sodium
- Erythropoietin production
- Excretion of creatinine and phosphorus
- Glomerular filtration
- Hydration
  - Water retention versus excretion
- Metabolic compensation of acid–base status
- Protein retention
- Urine formation
  - Concentration versus dilution

These processes are disrupted in varying degrees as the kidneys become dysfunctional [140].

Patients manifest CKD in different ways; however, there are certain consistencies among clinical presentations. Most patients with CKD demonstrate one or more of the following [28, 90, 140]:

- Decreased appetite
- Gastroenteritis
- Halitosis
- Pallor
- PD
- PU
- Poor body condition
- Reduced muscle mass
- Ulcerative stomatitis
- Weakness

Anorexia and gastroenteritis result from the accumulation of uremic toxins in the bloodstream [28, 90, 140]. This is exacerbated by dehydration, acid–basc disturbances, and electrolyte imbalances [140].

In addition, decreased renal excretion of gastrin results in hypergastrinemia [140]. This reduces stomach pH [140]. Increased gastric acid potentiates gastric ulceration [140].

Gastric ulceration and gastroenteritis are vicious cycles [140]. They further reduce appetite, which potentiates poor nutrition, acid–base, and electrolyte imbalances [140].

On physical examination, many kidneys that are affected by CKD palpate as small and irregular [90, 140]. Size estimates, based upon palpation, can be confirmed by imaging studies [140].

Clinicopathologic findings that are characteristic of CKD include the following [28, 90, 140]:

- Blood gas analysis
  - Metabolic acidosis
- CBC
  - Nonregenerative anemia
- Serum biochemistry profile
  - Azotemia
  - ± Hyperphosphatemia
  - ± Hypocalcemia
  - ± Hypokalemia
    - Contributes to weakness
- Urinalysis
  - Active urine sediment
  - Inappropriately dilute urine
    - Urine specific gravity (USG) < 1.030 in dogs and < 1.035 in cats
  - ± Proteinuria
  - ± Concurrent UTI
- Urine culture
  - Positive in the face of concurrent UTI

In addition, many patients are hypertensive [140].

Patients may be staged in accordance with the International Renal Interest Society (IRIS) (145, 147). Staging is based largely upon the following factors [90, 140]:

- Serum or plasma creatinine concentration
- Urine protein to creatinine ratios (UPCs)

Substages are determined based upon the presence or absence of proteinuria and arterial blood pressure [90, 140].

Case management of CKD is beyond the scope of this textbook. Refer to an internal medicine textbook for details.

However, recognize that the best treatment plan is multifactorial and makes efforts to address the following [28, 90, 140]:

- Blood pH
- Electrolytes
- Hydration
- Nutrition

It is equally important to recognize that cats are not small dogs, and management of CKD must be appropriate for the species that is being treated.

References

1 Englar, R.E. (2017). *Performing the Small Animal Physical Examination*. Hoboken, NJ: Wiley.

2 Evans, H.E. and Christensen, G.C. (1993). The urogenital system. In: *Miller's Anatomy of the Dog*, 3e (ed. H.E. Evans and M.E. Miller), 494–558. Philadelphia: W.B. Saunders.

3 Scherk, M. (2012). The upper urinary tract. In: *The Cat: Clinical Medicine and Management* (ed. S.E. Little), 953–979. St. Louis: Saunders Elsevier.

4 van Dongen, A.M. and L'Eplattenier, H.F. (2009). Kidneys and urinary tract. In: *Medical History and Physical Examination in Companion Animals*, 2e (ed. A. Rijnberk and F.J. van Sluijs), 101–107. St. Louis: Saunders Elsevier.

5 Dyce, K.M., Sack, W.O., and Wensing, C.J.G. (1996). *Textbook of Veterinary Anatomy*, 2e, xiii, 856 p. Philadelphia: Saunders.

6 Barrett, R.B. and Kneller, S.K. (1972). Feline kidney mensuration. *Acta Radiol. Suppl.* 319: 279–280.

7 Lee, R. and Leowijuk, C. (1982). Normal parameters in abdominal radiology of the dog and cat. *J. Small Anim. Pract.* 23 (5): 251–269.

8 Walter, P.A., Feeney, D.A., Johnston, G.R., and Fletcher, T.F. (1987). Feline renal ultrasonography: quantitative analyses of imaged anatomy. *Am. J. Vet. Res.* 48 (4): 596–599.

9 Shiroma, J.T., Gabriel, J.K., Carter, R.L. et al. (1999). Effect of reproductive status on feline renal size. *Vet. Radiol. Ultrasound* 40 (3): 242–245.

10 Owens, J. (1982). The genitourinary system. In: *Radiographic Interpretation for the Small Animal Clinician* (ed. D. Biery), 175. St. Louis: Ralston Purina Co.

11 Biery, D. (1981). Upper urinary tract. In: *Radiographic Diagnosis of Abdominal Disorders in the Dog and Cat* (ed. T. O'Brien), 484–485. Davis: Covel Park Vet. Co.

12 Debruyn, K., Paepe, D., Daminet, S. et al. (2013). Renal dimensions at ultrasonography in healthy ragdoll cats with normal kidney morphology: correlation with age, gender and bodyweight. *J. Feline Med. Surg.* 15 (12): 1046–1051.

13 Barr, F.J. (1990). Evaluation of ultrasound as a method of assessing renal size in the dog. *J. Small Anim. Pract.* 31 (4): 174–179.

14 Yeager, A.E. and Anderson, W.I. (1989). Study of association between histologic features and echogenicity of architecturally normal cat kidneys. *Am. J. Vet. Res.* 50 (6): 860–863.

15 Park, I.C., Lee, H.S., Kim, J.T. et al. (2008). Ultrasonographic evaluation of renal dimension and resistive index in clinically healthy Korean domestic short-hair cats. *J. Vet. Sci.* 9 (4): 415–419.

16 Hoey, S.E., Heder, B.L., Hetzel, S.J., and Waller, K.R. (2016). Use of computed tomography for measurement of kidneys in dogs without renal disease. *Javma-J Am Vet Med A.* 248 (3): 282–287.

17 Finco, D.R., Stiles, N.S., Kneller, S.K. et al. (1971). Radiologic estimation of kidney size of the dog. *J. Am. Vet. Med. Assoc.* 159 (8): 995–1002.

18 Loback, M.A., Sullivan, M., and Mellor, D. (2012). Effect of breed, age, weight and gender on radiographic renal size in the dog. *Vet. Radiol. Ultrasound* 53: 437–441.

19 Selye, H. (1939). The effect of testosterone on the kidney. *J. Urol.* 42 (4): 637–641.

20 Jean-Faucher, C., Berger, M., Gallon, C. et al. (1987). Sex-related differences in renal size in mice: ontogeny and influence of neonatal androgens. *J. Endocrinol.* 115 (2): 241–246.

21 Huang, K.C. and McIntosh, B.J. (1955). Effect of sex hormones on renal transport of p-aminohippuric acid. *Am. J. Phys.* 183 (3): 387–390.

22 Freudenberger, C.B. and Howard, P.M. (1937). Effects of ovariectomy on body growth and organ weights of the young albino rat. *Proc. Soc. Exp. Biol. Med.* 36 (2): 144–148.

23 Selye, H. (1940). Interactions between various steroid hormones. *Can. Med. Assoc. J.* 42 (2): 113–116.

24 Li, J.J., Kirkman, H., and Hunter, R.L. (1969). Sex difference and gonadal hormone influence on Syrian hamster kidney esterase isozymes. *J. Histochem. Cytochem.* 17 (6): 386–393.

25 Barrera, R., Duque, J., Ruiz, P., and Zaragoza, C. (2009). Accuracy of ultrasonographic measurements of kidney dog for clinical use. *Rev. Cient.-Fac. Cienc. V.* 19 (6): 576–583.

26 Barella, G., Lodi, M., Sabbadin, L.A., and Faverzani, S. (2012). A new method for ultrasonographic measurement of kidney size in healthy dogs. *J. Ultrasound* 15 (3): 186–191.

27 Mareschal, A., d'Anjou, M.A., Moreau, M. et al. (2007). Ultrasonographic measurement of kidney-to-aorta ratio as a method of estimating renal size in dogs. *Vet. Radiol. Ultrasound* 48 (5): 434–438.

28 Tilley, L.P. and Smith, F.W.K. (2004). *The 5-minute Veterinary Consult: Canine and Feline*, 3e. Baltimore, MD: Lippincott Williams & Wilkins.

29 Gough, A. and Murphy, K.F. (2015). *Differential Diagnosis in Small Animal Medicine*, 2e. Chichester, West Sussex; Ames, Iowa: Wiley.

30 Balakrishnan, A. and Drobatz, K.J. (2013). Management of urinary tract emergencies in small animals. *Vet. Clin. North Am. Small Anim. Pract.* 43 (4): 843–867.

31 Greco, D.S. (2012). Feline acromegaly. *Top. Companion Anim. Med.* 27 (1): 31–35.

32 Powell, L.L. (2008). Canine heatstroke. *NAVC Clinician's Brief* (August): 13–16.

33 Fitzgerald, K.T. (2010). Lily toxicity in the cat. *Top. Companion Anim. Med.* 25 (4): 213–217.

34 Stokes, J.E. and Forrester, S.D. (2004). New and unusual causes of acute renal failure in dogs and cats. *Vet. Clin. North Am. Small Anim. Pract.* 34 (4): 909–922, vi.

35 Gulledge, L., Boos, D., and Wachsstock, R. (1997). Acute renal failure in a cat secondary to tiger lily (Lilium tigrinum) toxicity. *Feline Pract.* 25 (5–6): 38–39.

36 Hadley, R.M., Richardson, J.A., and SM, G.-B. (2003). A retrospective study of daylily toxicosis in cats. *Vet. Hum. Toxicol.* 45 (1): 38–39.

37 Langston, C.E. (2002). Acute renal failure caused by lily ingestion in six cats. *J. Am. Vet. Med. Assoc.* 220 (1): 49–52, 36.

38 Brady, M.A. and Janovitz, E.B. (2000). Nephrotoxicosis in a cat following ingestion of Asiatic hybrid lily (Lilium sp). *J. Vet. Diagn. Investig.* 12 (6): 566–568.

39 Hall, J.O. (2001). Lily nephrotoxicity. In: *Consultations in Feline Internal Medicine* (ed. J.R. August), 308–310. Philadelphia: W.B. Saunders.

40 Hall, J.O. (2004). Lily toxicity. In: *Clinical Veterinary Toxicology* (ed. K.H. Plumee), 433–435. St. Louis: Mosby.

41 Grauer, G.F. and Thrall, M.A. (1982). Ethylene-Glycol (antifreeze) poisoning in the dog and cat. *J. Am. Anim. Hosp. Assoc.* 18 (3): 492–497.

42 Grauer, G.F., Thrall, M.A., Henre, B.A. et al. (1984). Early clinicopathologic findings in dogs ingesting ethylene-elycol. *Am. J. Vet. Res.* 45 (11): 2299–2303.

43 Claus, M.A., Jandrey, K.E., and Poppenga, R.H. (2011). Propylene glycol intoxication in a dog. *J. Vet. Emerg. Crit. Care (San Antonio)* 21 (6): 679–683.

44 Thrall, M.A., Grauer, G.F., and Mero, K.N. (1984). Clinicopathologic findings in dogs and cats with ethylene-glycol intoxication. *J. Am. Vet. Med. Assoc.* 184 (1): 37–41.

45 Gwaltney-Brant, S., Holding, J.K., Donaldson, C.W. et al. (2001). Renal failure associated with ingestion of grapes or raisins in dogs. *J. Am. Vet. Med. Assoc.* 218 (10): 1555–1556.

46 Campbell, A. and Bates, N. (2003). Raisin poisoning in dogs. *Vet. Rec.* 152 (12): 376.

47 Penny, D., Henderson, S.M., and Brown, P.J. (2003). Raisin poisoning in a dog. *Vet. Rec.* 152 (10): 308.

48 Rumbeiha, W.K., Fitzgerald, S.D., Kruger, J.M. et al. (2000). Use of pamidronate disodium to reduce cholecalciferol-induced toxicosis in dogs. *Am. J. Vet. Res.* 61 (1): 9–13.

49 Murphy, M.J. (2002). Rodenticides. *Vet. Clin. North Am. Small Anim. Pract.* 32 (2): 469–484, viii.

50 Engle, J.E., Abt, A.B., Schneck, D.W., and Schoolwerth, A.C. (1979). Netilmicin and tobramycin. Comparison of nephrotoxicity in dogs. *Investig. Urol.* 17 (2): 98–102.

51 Gookin, J.L., Riviere, J.E., Gilger, B.C., and Papich, M.G. (1999). Acute renal failure in four cats treated with paromomycin. *J. Am. Vet. Med. Assoc.* 215 (12): 1821–1823, 06.

52 Mealey, K.L. and Boothe, D.M. (1994). Nephrotoxicosis associated with topical administration of gentamicin in a cat. *J. Am. Vet. Med. Assoc.* 204 (12): 1919–1921.

53 Reiner, N.E., Bloxham, D.D., and Thompson, W.L. (1978). Nephrotoxicity of gentamicin and tobramycin given once daily or continuously in dogs. *J. Antimicrob. Chemother.* 4 (Suppl A): 85–101.

54 Schultze, R.G., Winters, R.E., and Kauffman, H. (1971). Possible nephrotoxicity of gentamicin. *J. Infect. Dis.* 124 (Suppl): S145–S147.

55 Stubanus, M., Riegger, G.A.J., Kammerl, M.C. et al. (2000). Renal side-effects of cyclo-oxygenase-type-2 inhibitor use. *Lancet* 355 (9205): 753.

56 Villar, D., Buck, W.B., and Gonzalez, J.M. (1998). Ibuprofen, aspirin and acetaminophen toxicosis and treatment in dogs and cats. *Vet. Hum. Toxicol.* 40 (3): 156–162.

57 Silverman, L.R. and Khan, K.N.M. (1999). "Have you seen this?" Nonsteroidal anti-inflammatory drug-induced renal papillary necrosis in a dog. *Toxicol. Pathol.* 27 (2): 244–245.

58 Poortinga, E.W. and Hungerford, L.L. (1998). A case-control study of acute ibuprofen toxicity in dogs. *Prev. Vet. Med.* 35 (2): 115–124.

59 Forrester, S.D. and Troy, G.C. (1999). Renal effects of nonsteroidal antiinflammatory drugs. *Compend. Contin. Educ. Pract.* 21 (10): 910–919.

60 Blagburn, B.L. and Dryden, M.W. (2009). Biology, treatment, and control of flea and tick infestations. *Vet. Clin. N. Am. Small* 39 (6): 1173–1200.

61 Sonenshine, D.E., Lane, R.S., and Nicholson, W.L. (2002). Ticks (Ixodida). In: *Medical and Veterinary Entomology* (ed. G.R. Mullen and L.A. Durden), 517–558. Amsterdam: Academic Press Elsevier Science.

62 Magnarelli, L.A., Anderson, J.F., Levine, H.R., and Levy, S.A. (1990). Tick parasitism and antibodies to Borrelia burgdorferi in cats. *J. Am. Vet. Med. Assoc.* 197 (1): 63–66.

63 Little, S.E., Heise, S.R., Blagburn, B.L. et al. (2010). Lyme borreliosis in dogs and humans in the USA. *Trends Parasitol.* 26 (4): 213–218.

64 Krupka, I. and Straubinger, R.K. (2010). Lyme borreliosis in dogs and cats: background, diagnosis, treatment and prevention of infections with Borrelia burgdorferi sensu stricto. *Vet. Clin. North Am. Small Anim. Pract.* 40 (6): 1103–1119.

65 Grimm, D., Tilly, K., Byram, R. et al. (2004). Outer-surface protein C of the lyme disease spirochete: a protein induced in ticks for infection of mammals. *Proceedings of the National Academy of Sciences of the United States of America* 101 (9): 3142–3147.

66 Ribeiro, J.M., Mather, T.N., Piesman, J., and Spielman, A. (1987). Dissemination and salivary delivery of Lyme disease spirochetes in vector ticks (Acari: Ixodidae). *J. Med. Entomol.* 24 (2): 201–205.

67 Schwan, T.G., Piesman, J., Golde, W.T. et al. (1995). Induction of an outer surface protein on Borrelia burgdorferi during tick feeding. *Proc. Natl. Acad. Sci. U S A* 92 (7): 2909–2913.

68 deSilva, A.M., Telford, S.R., Brunet, L.R. et al. (1996). Borrelia burgdorferi OspA is an arthropod-specific transmission-blocking Lyme disease vaccine. *J. Exp. Med.* 183 (1): 271–275.

69 Straubinger, R.K., Summers, B.A., Chang, Y.F., and Appel, M.J. (1997). Persistence of Borrelia burgdorferi in experimentally infected dogs after antibiotic treatment. *J. Clin. Microbiol.* 35 (1): 111–116.

70 Straubinger, R.K., Straubinger, A.F., Harter, L. et al. (1997). Borrelia burgdorferi migrates into joint capsules and causes an up-regulation of interleukin-8 in synovial membranes of dogs experimentally infected with ticks. *Infect. Immun.* 65 (4): 1273–1285.

71 Grauer, G.F., Burgess, E.C., Cooley, A.J., and Hagee, J.H. (1988). Renal lesions associated with Borrelia-Burgdorferi infection in a dog. *J. Am. Vet. Med. Assoc.* 193 (2): 237–239.

72 Dambach, D.M., Smith, C.A., Lewis, R.M., and VanWinkle, T.J. (1997). Morphologic, immunohistochemical, and ultrastructural characterization of a distinctive renal lesion in dogs putatively associated with Borrelia burgdorferi infection: 49 cases (1987–1992). *Vet. Pathol.* 34 (2): 85–96.

73 Sykes, J.E. (2014). Leptospirosis. In: *Canine and Feline Infectious Diseases* (ed. J.E. Sykes), 474–486. St. Louis: Elsevier Saunders.

74 Adin, C.A. and Cowgill, L.D. (2000). Treatment and outcome of dogs with leptospirosis: 36 cases (1990–1998). *J. Am. Vet. Med. Assoc.* 216 (3): 371–375.

75 Hennebelle, J., Sykes, J.E., and Carpenter, T. (2013;). Spatial and temporal patterns of Leptospira spp. seroreactivity in dogs from northern California. *J. Am. Vet. Med. Assoc.* 242 (7): 941–947.

76 Ward, M.P. (2002). Seasonality of canine leptospirosis in the United States and Canada and its association with rainfall. *Prev. Vet. Med.* 56 (3): 203–213.

77 Prescott, J. (2008). Canine leptospirosis in Canada: a veterinarian's perspective. *CMAJ* 178 (4): 397–398.

78 Raghavan, R., Brenner, K., Higgins, J. et al. (2011). Evaluations of land cover risk factors for canine leptospirosis: 94 cases (2002–2009). *Prev. Vet. Med.* 101 (3–4): 241–249.

79 Gautam, R., Guptill, L.F., Wu, C.C. et al. (2010). Spatial and spatio-temporal clustering of overall and serovar-specific Leptospira microscopic agglutination test (MAT) seropositivity among dogs in the United States from 2000 through 2007. *Prev. Vet. Med.* 96 (1–2): 122–131.

80 Brown, C.A., Roberts, A.W., Miller, M.A. et al. (1996). Leptospira interrogans serovar grippotyphosa infection in dogs. *J. Am. Vet. Med. Assoc.* 209 (7): 1265–1267.

81 Ellis, W.A. (2010). Control of canine leptospirosis in Europe: time for a change? *Vet. Rec.* 167 (16): 602–605.

82 Moore, G.E., Guptill, L.F., Glickman, N.W. et al. (2006). Canine leptospirosis, United States, 2002–2004. *Emerg. Infect. Dis.* 12 (3): 501–503.

83 Boeve, M.H. and Stades, F.C. (2009). Djajadiningrat-Laanen. Eyes. In: *Medical History and Physical Examination in Companion Animals* (ed. A. Rijnberk and F.J. van Sluijs), 175–201. China: Elsevier Limited.

84 Schaer, M. (2008). Icterus. *NAVC Clinician's Brief* (September): 8.

85 Birnbaum, N., Barr, S.C., Center, S.A. et al. (1998). Naturally acquired leptospirosis in 36 dogs: serological and clinicopathological features. *J. Small Anim. Pract.* 39 (5): 231–236.

86 Mastrorilli, C., Dondi, F., Agnoli, C. et al. (2007). Clinicopathologic features and outcome predictors of Leptospira interrogans Australis serogroup infection in dogs: a retrospective study of 20 cases (2001–2004). *J. Vet. Intern. Med.* 21 (1): 3–10.

87 Minke, J.M., Bey, R., Tronel, J.P. et al. (2009). Onset and duration of protective immunity against clinical disease and renal carriage in dogs provided by a bi-valent inactivated leptospirosis vaccine. *Vet. Microbiol.* 137 (1–2): 137–145.

88 Goldstein, R.E., Lin, R.C., Langston, C.E. et al. (2006). Influence of infecting serogroup on clinical features of leptospirosis in dogs. *J. Vet. Intern. Med.* 20 (3): 489–494.

89 Geisen, V., Stengel, C., Brem, S. et al. (2007). Canine leptospirosis infections–clinical signs and outcome with different suspected Leptospira serogroups (42 cases). *J. Small Anim. Pract.* 48 (6): 324–328.

90 Langston, C.E. and Eatroff, A.E. (2015). Acute kidney injury. In: *Small Animal Critical Care Medicine* (ed. D.C. Silverstein and K. Hopper), 483–498. St. Louis, Mo: Saunders/Elsevier.

91 Arbour, J., Blais, M.C., Carioto, L., and Sylvestre, D. (2012). Clinical leptospirosis in three cats (2001–2009). *J. Am. Anim. Hosp. Assoc.* 48 (4): 256–260.

92 Lapointe, C., Plamondon, I., and Dunn, M. (2013). Feline leptospirosis serosurvey from a Quebec referral hospital. *Can. Vet. J.* 54 (5): 497–499.

93 Markovich, J.E., Ross, L., and McCobb, E. (2012). The prevalence of leptospiral antibodies in free roaming cats in Worcester County, Massachusetts. *J. Vet. Intern. Med.* 26 (3): 688–689.

94 Brown, S.A. (2018). Pyelonephritis in small animals. Merck Veterinary Manual [Internet]. https://www.merckvetmanual.com/urinary-system/infectious-diseases-of-the-urinary-system-in-small-animals/pyelonephritis-in-small-animals.

95 Hoskins, J.D. (2002). Clinical diagnosis of pyelonephritis often presumptive. DVM 360 [Internet]. http://veterinarynews.dvm360.com/clinical-diagnosis-pyelonephritis-often-presumptive.

96 Bouillon, J., Snead, E., Caswell, J. et al. (2018). Pyelonephritis in dogs: retrospective study of 47 histologically diagnosed cases (2005–2015). *J. Vet. Intern. Med.* 32 (1): 249–259.

97 Weese, J.S., Blondeau, J.M., Boothe, D. et al. (2011). Antimicrobial use guidelines for treatment of urinary tract disease in dogs and cats: antimicrobial guidelines working group of the international society for companion animal infectious diseases. *Vet. Med. Int.* 2011: 263768.

98 Wettimuny, S.G. (1967). Pyelonephritis in the dog. *J. Comp. Pathol.* 77 (2): 193–197.

99 Parry, N.M.A. (2005). Pyelonephritis. *UK Vet.* 10: 1–5.

100 Harrison, L., Cass, A., Bullock, B. et al. (1973). Experimental pyelonephritis in dogs. Result of urinary infection and vesicoureteral reflux. *Urology* 1 (5): 439–443.

101 Smee, N., Loyd, K., and Grauer, G. (2013). UTIs in small animal patients: part 1: etiology and pathogenesis. *J. Am. Anim. Hosp. Assoc.* 49 (1): 1 7.

102 Olin, S.J. and Bartges, J.W. (2015). Urinary tract infections: treatment/comparative therapeutics. *Vet. Clin. North Am. Small Anim. Pract.* 45 (4): 721–746.

103 Gold, A.C., Jeffs, R.D., and Wilson, R.B. (1968). Experimental pyelonephritis in dogs. *Can. J. Comp. Med.* 32 (2): 450–453.

104 Lane, I. (2008). Acute ureteral obstruction. DVM 360 [Internet]. http://veterinarycalendar.dvm360.com/print/309873?page=full.

105 Cohen, L., Shipov, A., Ranen, E. et al. (2012). Bilateral ureteral obstruction in a cat due to a ureteral transitional cell carcinoma. *Can Vet J.* 53 (5): 535–538.

106 Shipov, A. and Segev, G. (2013). Ureteral obstruction in dogs and cats. *Isr. J. Vet. Med.* 68 (2): 71–77.

107 Kyles, A.E., Stone, E.A., Gookin, J. et al. (1998). Diagnosis and surgical management of obstructive ureteral calculi in cats: 11 cases (1993–1996). *J. Am. Vet. Med. Assoc.* 213 (8): 1150–1156.

108 Moon, M.L. and Dallman, M.A. (1991). Calcium-oxalate ureterolith in a cat. *Vet. Radiol.* 32 (5): 261–263.

109 Kyles, A.E., Hardie, E.M., Wooden, B.G. et al. (2005). Management and outcome of cats with ureteral calculi: 153 cases (1984–2002). *J. Am. Vet. Med. Assoc.* 226 (6): 937–944.

110 Kyles, A.E., Hardie, E.M., Wooden, B.G. et al. (2005). Clinical, clinicopathologic, radiographic, and ultrasonographic abnormalities in cats with ureteral calculi: 163 cases (1984–2002). *J. Am. Vet. Med. Assoc.* 226 (6): 932–936.

111 Adin, C.A., Herrgesell, E.J., Nyland, T.G. et al. (2003). Antegrade pyelography for suspected ureteral obstruction in cats: 11 cases (1995–2001). *J. Am. Vet. Med. Assoc.* 222 (11): 1576–1581.

112 Block, G., Adams, L.G., Widmer, W.R., and Lingeman, J.E. (1996). Use of extracorporeal shock wave lithotripsy for treatment of nephrolithiasis and ureterolithiasis in five dogs. *J. Am. Vet. Med. Assoc.* 208 (4): 531–536.

113 Dupre, G.P., Dee, L.G., and Dee, J.F. (1990). Ureterotomies for treatment of ureterolithiasis in 2 dogs. *J. Am. Anim. Hosp. Assoc.* 26 (5): 500–504.

114 Bosje, J.T. and van den Ingh, T.S. (1998). Polycystic kidney disease in cats. *Vet. Q.* 20 (Suppl 1): S112–S113.

115 Beck, C. and Lavelle, R.B. (2001). Feline polycystic kidney disease in Persian and other cats: a prospective study using ultrasonography. *Aust. Vet. J.* 79 (3): 181–184.

116 Volta, A., Manfredi, S., Gnudi, G. et al. (2010). Polycystic kidney disease in a Chartreux cat. *J. Feline Med. Surg.* 12 (2): 138–140.

117 Barrs, V.R., Gunew, M., Foster, S.F. et al. (2001). Prevalence of autosomal dominant polycystic kidney disease in Persian cats and related-breeds in Sydney and Brisbane. *Aust. Vet. J.* 79 (4): 257–259.

118 Barber, P., Miller, J.B., and Rand, J. (2006). The thin, inappetent cat. In: *Problem-based Feline Medicine* (ed. J. Rand), 333–334. Edinburgh; New York: Saunders.

119 Bear, J.C., Parfrey, P.S., Morgan, J.M. et al. (1992). Autosomal dominant polycystic kidney disease: new information for genetic counselling. *Am. J. Med. Genet.* 43 (3): 548–553.

120 Biller, D.S., DiBartola, S.P., Eaton, K.A. et al. (1996). Inheritance of polycystic kidney disease in Persian cats. *J. Hered.* 87 (1): 1–5.

121 Eaton, K.A., Biller, D.S., DiBartola, S.P. et al. (1997). Autosomal dominant polycystic kidney disease in Persian and Persian-cross cats. *Vet. Pathol.* 34 (2): 117–126.

122 Gabow, P.A. (1993). Autosomal dominant polycystic kidney disease. *N. Engl. J. Med.* 329 (5): 332–342.

123 Gabow, P.A., Johnson, A.M., Kaehny, W.D. et al. (1992). Factors affecting the progression of renal disease in autosomal-dominant polycystic kidney disease. *Kidney Int.* 41 (5): 1311–1319.

124 Vlajkovic, M., Slavkovic, A., Ilic, S. et al. (1998). Evaluation of autosomal dominant polycystic kidney disease by DTPA renal scintigraphy. *Int. Urol. Nephrol.* 30 (6): 799–805.

125 Nyland, T.G., Mattoon, J.S., and Wisner, E.R. (1995). Ultrasonography of the urinary tract and adrenal glands. In: *Veterinary Diagnostic Ultrasound* (ed. T.G. Nyland and J.S. Mattoon), 95–124. Philadelphia: Saunders.

126 Meyerholz, D.K. and Hostetter, S.J. (2005). Unilateral perinephric pseudocyst secondary to hydronephrosis in a C57BL/6J mouse. *Vet. Pathol.* 42 (4): 496–498.

127 Miles, K.G. and Jergens, A.E. (1992). Unilateral perinephric pseudocyst of undetermined origin in a dog. *Vet. Radiol. Ultrasound* 33 (5): 277–281.

128 Orioles, M., Di Bella, A., Merlo, M., and Ter Haar, G. (2014). Ascites resulting from a ruptured perinephric pseudocyst associated with a renal cyst in a dog. *Vet. Rec.* https://doi.org/10.1136/vetreccr-2013-000012.

129 Hill, T.P. and Odesnik, B.J. (2000). Omentalisation of perinephric pseudocysts in a cat. *J. Small Anim. Pract.* 41 (3): 115–118.

130 Beck, J.A., Bellenger, C.R., Lamb, W.A. et al. (2000). Perirenal pseudocysts in 26 cats. *Aust. Vet. J.* 78 (3): 166–171.

131 Morrow, B.L. (2005). Clinical exposures: A perinephric pseudocyst in a cat. DVM 360 [Internet]. http://veterinarymedicine.dvm360.com/clinical-exposures-perinephric-pseudocyst-cat.

132 Borjesson, D.L. and DeJong, K. (2016). Urinary tract. In: *Canine and Feline Cytology* (ed. R.E. Raskin and D.J. Meyer), 284–294. St. Louis: Elsevier.

133 Bryan, J.N., Henry, C.J., Turnquist, S.E. et al. (2006). Primary renal neoplasia of dogs. *J Vet Intern Med.* 20 (5): 1155–1160.

134 Gil da Costa, R.M., Oliveira, J.P., Saraiva, A.L. et al. (2011). Immunohistochemical characterization of 13 canine renal cell carcinomas. *Vet. Pathol.* 48 (2): 427–432.

135 Henry, C.J., Turnquist, S.E., Smith, A. et al. (1999). Primary renal tumours in cats: 19 cases (1992–1998). *J. Feline Med. Surg.* 1 (3): 165–170.

136 Ramos-Vara, J.A., Miller, M.A., Boucher, M. et al. (2003). Immunohistochemical detection of uroplakin III, cytokeratin 7, and cytokeratin 20 in canine urothelial tumors. *Vet. Pathol.* 40 (1): 55–62.

137 Sato, T., Aoki, K., Shibuya, H. et al. (2003). Leiomyosarcoma of the kidney in a dog. *J. Vet. Med. A Physiol. Pathol. Clin. Med.* 50 (7): 366–369.

138 Breshears, M.A., Meinkoth, J.H., Stern, A.W. et al. (2011). Pathology in practice. Renal lymphoma. *J. Am. Vet. Med. Assoc.* 238 (2): 167–169.

139 Snead, E.C. (2005). A case of bilateral renal lymphosarcoma with secondary polycythaemia and paraneoplastic syndromes of hypoglycaemia and uveitis in an English Springer Spaniel. *Vet. Comp. Oncol.* 3 (3): 139–144.

140 Bartges, J.W. (2012). Chronic kidney disease in dogs and cats. *Vet. Clin. North Am. Small Anim. Pract.* 42 (4): 669–692, vi.

141 Langston, C.E. and Eatroff, A.E. (2015). Chronic Kidney disease. In: *Small Animal Critical Care Medicine* (ed. D.C. Silverstein and K. Hopper), 661–666. St. Louis, Mo: Saunders/Elsevier.

142 Polzin, D.J. (2011). Chronic kidney disease in small animals. *Vet. Clin. North Am. Small Anim. Pract.* 41 (1): 15–30.

143 Reece, W.O. (2004). Kidney function in mammals. In: *Dukes' Physiology of Domestic Animals*, 12e (ed. H.H. Dukes and W.O. Reece). Ithaca: Comstock Pub. Associates.

64

Polyuria and Polydipsia

64.1   Introduction to Urine Output

The upper urinary tract was introduced in Chapter 63. Recall that the function of the upper urinary tract is to produce urine by filtering the bloodstream of waste [1]. Urine is formed by the nephrons, the functional units of the kidney [1]. Urine is then conducted from the left and right kidneys, through the left and right ureters, and ultimately to the urinary bladder for storage [1–3].

In health, urine is stored until the patient chooses to empty the urinary bladder through micturition [1]. Micturition is the process of voiding [1]. The initiation of voiding is under conscious control [1]. House-trained dogs, for example, can hold their urinary bladder until they are granted access to the outdoors [1]. In other words, voluntary control overrides the urge to void [1]. However, once voiding has begun, a reflex arc in the brain stem facilitates bladder emptying [1].

Urine storage within the bladder during filling is referred to as continence [1]. Two factors work in concert to maintain continence [1]:

- Keeping a toned external sphincter muscle
- Keeping the neck of the bladder closed

Urine output depends upon many patient-specific factors, including [1]:

- Activity level
- Diet
  - Moisture content
  - Sodium content
- Renal function
  - The ability to concentrate urine
  - The ability to excrete waste
- Thirst and water consumption

In addition, the season, ambient temperature, and humidity determine urine output based upon how much water the patient needs to conserve [1].

In health, urination and thirst are linked processes [1]. If renal function is adequate, a dehydrated patient will

maximally concentrate urine to conserve water, and will be driven to drink [1].

Urine formation is, in essence, a balancing act. If there is too little water in the system, then the body must conserve it. Urine output will decline. On the other hand, if there is too much water in the system, then the excess will be eliminated as urine.

The body relies upon water balance for homeostasis. In addition to the drive to drink, water balance is maintained by the following [1, 4–10]:

- Antidiuretic hormone (ADH) or vasopressin
- Renal tubular function
- Renal medullary hypertonicity

ADH is produced by the hypothalamus [1, 4]. ADH is secreted when plasma osmolality increases [1, 4, 9]. ADH conserves water by reabsorbing it from the distal tubules and collecting ducts of the nephrons [1, 4]. This is made possible through upregulation of aquaporin channels [11]. Aquaporins allow water to flow out of the nephron and back into systemic circulation.

This action reduces urine output [1, 4]. Urine is therefore concentrated in the presence of ADH and functionally responsive kidneys.

Renal function is required to concentrate urine [4]. This requires at least one-third of both kidneys' nephrons to be operational [4]. If more than two-thirds are not, then the ability of the kidneys to concentrate urine is significantly impaired [4].

Renal medullary hypertonicity is also required for water to be passively reabsorbed in the distal tubule and collecting duct [4]. This concentration gradient is established and maintained by the movement of sodium, chloride, and urea out of nephrons' lumens and into the renal medullary interstitium [12].

In the absence of this gradient, osmotic forces are diminished [12]. There is less pull to draw water out of the nephron, and back into the bloodstream [12]. Urine is therefore inadequately concentrated [12]. This state is referred to as medullary washout [4, 12].

Common Clinical Presentations in Dogs and Cats, First Edition. Ryane E. Englar.
© 2019 John Wiley & Sons, Inc. Published 2019 by John Wiley & Sons, Inc.

64.2 Abnormal Urine Output

Urine output varies day to day, between patients and within the same patient. Despite these individual fluctuations, urine production in the average canine or feline patient ranges from 20 to 40 ml/kg/d [12]. Hourly, this equates to roughly 1–2 ml/kg/h [12].

To compensate for this loss of water in urine, dogs consume 50–60 ml/kg/d of water [12]. To the author's knowledge, this amount has not been quantified for cats.

Water consumption will increase in the normal patient if dietary moisture is low or if the ambient temperature is high [12]. Although this is an example of a normal fluctuation in a healthy patient, it is important to recognize that changes in urine output may also be pathological. Urine output may be greater or less than expected [1].

Polyuria is the condition in which urine is overproduced [1, 10, 12]. Polyuria is defined as urine production that exceeds 45 ml/kg/d in the dog and 40 ml/kg/d in the cat [10]. Common causes of polyuria in clinical practice will be reviewed in Section 64.3 below.

Polyuric patients lose excessive amounts of water in the urine. This action is dehydrating. To counter this effect, the body may attempt to remedy the situation. For this reason, polyuric patients often develop compensatory polydipsia. Polydipsia is the medically appropriate term for increased thirst. Polydipsia is defined as drinking more than 90 ml/kg/d in the dog and 45 ml/kg/d in the cat [10].

64.3 Causes of Polyuria

There are many pathological causes of polyuria in companion animals, including, but not limited to the following [4, 8–10, 12–22]:

- Diet
  - High sodium
  - Low protein
- Electrolyte imbalance
  - Hypercalcemia***
  - Hypokalemia
  - Hyponatremia
- Encephalopathy
- Endocrinopathies
  - Acromegaly
  - Central diabetes insipidus (CDI)***
  - Diabetes mellitus***
  - Hyperadrenocorticism (Cushing's disease or Cushing's syndrome)*** (see Chapter 5, Section 5.7 concerning link to cortisol-induced dermatopathy)
  - Hyperthyroidism*** (see Chapter 15, Section 15.4.2.2 concerning link to hypertensive retinopathy)
  - Hypoadrenocorticism*** (Addison's disease)

- Fanconi's syndrome
- Hepatopathy***
- Infectious disease
  - Pyometra*** (see Chapter 61, Section 61.7)
    o *Escherichia coli* endotoxins interfere with the nephron's ability to reabsorb sodium [23].
  Medullary washout
  - Hypoadrenocorticism*** (Addison's disease)
  - Hyperviscosity syndromes
    o Polycythemia
  - Vasculitis
- Neoplasia***
  o Pharmaceutical agents***
  - Anticonvulsants
    o Phenobarbital
    o Phenytoin
    o Primidone
  - Diuretics
  - Glucocorticoids
- Post-obstructive diuresis
- Psychogenic***
- Pyelonephritis***
  Urinary tract pathology
  - Chronic kidney disease (CKD) (see Chapter 63, Section 63.5)***
  - Nephrogenic diabetes insipidus (NDI)***
  - Primary renal glycosuria

There are more topics listed above than can be adequately covered here. The starred items (***) represent those that are most likely to be seen in clinical practice. A number of these conditions have been described in brief below.

For additional details or for conditions not described here, refer to an internal medicine textbook.

64.3.1 Hypercalcemia and Polyuria

Hypercalcemia commonly causes polyuria in dogs [10]. Different mechanisms have been proposed to explain the development of polyuria in response to hypercalcemia, including the following [24–30]:

- Antagonism of ADH
- Downregulation of aquaporin channels
- Hypercalcemia-induced thirst
- Impairment of the sodium-potassium pump in the loop of Henle
- Medullary washout

Consider the sodium-potassium pump, which operates largely to remove sodium from the tubular lumen of the nephron. Sodium moves out of the lumen with potassium; however, potassium ions leak back to re-enter the lumen. This sustains the intraluminal concentration of potassium that is necessary to maintain the pump. However, when there is a high tubular concentration of calcium, the lumen of the nephron is now more positively charged. Because the potassium ion is also positively charged, it is less likely to leak back into the tubular lumen after being pumped across the membrane. There is now less intraluminal potassium to fuel the sodium-potassium pump, so more sodium remains in the tubular lumen. Where sodium goes, water follows, hence the development of polyuria.

In addition to polyuria, hypercalcemic dogs typically experience gastrointestinal disturbances, such as anorexia, vomiting, and constipation [10].

Hypercalcemic cats are less likely to demonstrate clinical signs than dogs [29, 30]. However, those that do may present for lethargy or generalized weakness [10, 29].

Hypercalcemia may be idiopathic [30]. More often, it is secondary to underlying pathology. In clinical practice, hypercalcemia is often the result of renal failure, primary hyperparathyroidism, urolithiasis, hypoadrenocorticism or neoplasia [10, 17, 30, 31].

When hypercalcemia has a neoplastic origin, it is referred to as hypercalcemia of malignancy. The most common causes of hypercalcemia of malignancy in dog and cat are the following [10, 17, 30, 31]:

- Anal sac apocrine gland adenocarcinoma
- Lymphosarcoma
- Multiple myeloma

One concern about rising levels of blood calcium is the potential for the development of soft tissue mineralization if the calcium-phosphorus (Ca–P) exceeds $60 \, mg^2/dL^2$ [32, 33].

64.3.2 Diabetes Mellitus and Polyuria

Diabetes mellitus was introduced in Chapter 54, Section 54.9.2. Recall that diabetes mellitus is a condition in which the patient is hyperglycemic with glucosuria [10, 20, 34]. This results from either insulin deficiency or insulin resistance [10, 14, 20, 34].

Type 1 diabetes mellitus develops when destruction of the insulin-producing pancreatic β-cells leads to true insulin deficiency [20]. This is considered rare in cats, as compared to dogs [20].

Type 2 diabetes mellitus is characterized by the body's inability to make effective use of circulating insulin [20]. This is considered to be common among diabetic cats [20]. Obese cats are particularly at risk for development of Type 2 diabetes mellitus [20, 35].

Other risk factors for cats include the following [20, 35–38]:

- Decreased activity
- Drug administration
  - Glucocorticoids
  - Progestins
- Indoor lifestyle
- Sex (male)

Insulin is needed for uptake of glucose by cells [34]. If insulin is deficient and/or if cells are resistant to its effects, then glucose cannot enter tissues [34]. Most tissues of the body require glucose. Without the ability to take up glucose, cells starve.

In the interim, blood levels of glucose continue to rise.

In health, glucose that is filtered by the kidneys is reabsorbed [14]. This requires glucose to bind to transport proteins in the proximal convoluted tubules [1]. The limiting factor for glucose transport is the number of transport proteins [1]. If these become saturated, as is true of a patient that is hyperglycemic, some glucose will remain behind in the filtrate [1, 14].

Glucose within the tubular lumen sets the stage for osmotic diuresis; that is, water is drawn into the urine to dilute its high concentration of solute [1, 13, 14]. This creates voluminous urine that is rich in glucose.

Hypovolemia is a primary consequence of polyuria [14]. To compensate for water loss in the urine, patients increase their consumption of water. This is a prime example of a situation in which polyuria forces polydipsia [14].

In addition to being polydipsic, patients may initially be polyphagic [10]. This is likely the body's response to signals from starved cells that they are not receiving energy in the form of glucose.

As the disease progresses, patients may become anorexic, lethargic, and depressed [10]. They often lose weight and muscle mass [10].

Some affected cats develop diabetic neuropathy [10]. This is grossly apparent as a plantigrade stance in the pelvic limbs [10]. A normal cat walks as if wearing high heels: only the plantar aspects of the hind paws touch the ground and the tarsi remain elevated. In a diabetic cat, both tarsi are dropped. This appearance is often extreme such that both hocks into contact with the ground. This gives the cat the illusion of walking in flip-flops.

Diabetic ketoacidosis (DKA) is a life-threatening complication of diabetes mellitus [10].

Review Chapter 54, Section 54.9.2 for additional details.

64.3.3 Diabetes Insipidus and Polyuria

Diabetes insipidus is a broad term for any condition in which the patient is both polyuric and polydipsic, and voids urine of low specific gravity without glucosuria [4, 8, 19].

The condition was named because the urine is so dilute that it is said to be insipid, that is, tasteless [4, 10].

Diabetes insipidus can be further characterized as being [4, 8, 10, 19]

- Central
- Nephrogenic.

CDI results from inadequate secretion of ADH [4, 8, 10, 19]. CDI may be congenital or acquired [4]. Neither is common in clinical practice [4].

Acquired CDI may result from the following [4, 8, 10, 19]:

- Cerebral hemorrhage
- Granulomatous disease
  - Histiocytosis
  - Sarcoidosis
- Infarction
- Infectious disease
  - Encephalitis
  - Meningitis
- Neoplasia
- Pituitary surgery
- Thrombosis
- Toxins
  - Snake venom
- Trauma

Recall from Section 64.1 that ADH is produced by the hypothalamus in response to elevations in plasma osmolality increases [1, 4, 9]. The purpose of ADH is to conserve water [1, 4, 9]. It does so by reabsorbing water from the distal tubules and collecting ducts of the nephrons [1, 4]. Increased reabsorption of water reduces urine output [1, 4]. Urine is concentrated in the presence of ADH, so as not to waste water.

If the hypothalamus fails to produce ADH, then the kidneys do not receive the signal to reabsorb water from the distal tubules and collecting ducts. Water is wasted, even in the face of a pressing need to conserve it. Hence, the urine remains dilute, as opposed to concentrated. This sets the stage for hypovolemia and compensatory polydipsia.

NDI occurs more commonly than CDI in companion animals [4, 6, 7, 39–41].

NDI is similar to Type II diabetes mellitus in that both are the result of insensitivity of an organ to a hormone. In Type II diabetes mellitus, patients are insulin-resistant. In NDI, patients lack renal sensitivity to ADH. In other words, ADH is present, but the kidneys fail to respond to it in an effective manner. Renal response may be blunted because of an inherent defect with renal tubular receptors [4]. Alternatively, the kidneys may be unable to respond to ADH because of medullary washout or other factors beyond their control [4–7, 42].

Canine and feline patients rarely present for congenital NDI [4, 6, 43]. More often than not, NDI is acquired. Hypercalcemia is an example of acquired NDI [4]. So, too, is hyperadrenocorticism, outlined in Section 64.3.4 below.

Patients with NDI present with similar histories as those with CDI. Owners may complain of what appears to be compulsive water drinking. Patients may present for urinary accidents, increased litter box use (cats), and/or increased requests to go outdoors to eliminate.

NDI and CDI must be distinguished from psychogenic polydipsia [4, 6, 7, 40, 41, 43]. Psychogenic polydipsia is a behavioral rather than a pathological condition.

64.3.4 Hyperadrenocorticism and Polyuria

Recall from Chapter 5, Section 5.7 that hyperadrenocorticism, or Cushing's syndrome, results from endogenous overproduction or exogenous supplementation of glucocorticoids. Both cause one or more of the following classic changes on physical examination [44, 45]:

- Bilaterally symmetrical truncal alopecia
- Pendulous abdomen
- Potbellied appearance

These patients are often paired with a history of excessive thirst, urination, and appetite. In the medical record, this is often transcribed as "PU/PD/PP" – polyuria, polydipsia, and polyphagia.

Affected patients develop polyuria as the direct result of excessive corticosteroids [46]. Cortisol impairs the ability of the kidney to respond to ADH [46–50]. Concentrations of circulating ADH rise; however, the kidneys are unable to make effective use of it [46].

64.3.5 Hyperthyroidism and Polyuria

Hyperthyroidism, also known as thyrotoxicosis, is the result of endogenous overproduction of thyroxine (T4) and triiodothyronine (T3) by the thyroid gland [3, 51–55]. It is primarily an endocrinopathy of middle-aged to senior cats [51, 56, 57]. It has surpassed diabetes mellitus as the top feline endocrine disease in the United States, Canada, the United Kingdom, Europe, Australia, New Zealand, and Japan, and its incidence is increasing [55, 57–66].

Despite the surge in cases of feline hyperthyroidism, the etiology remains unknown [57]. The following factors may play a role [3]:

- Breed
  - Siamese and Himalayan cats appear to be least at risk [67–69]

- Commercial litter [60, 67, 68]
- Consumption of a canned diet, particularly those containing the following:
  - Fish, liver, and giblets [68, 70]
  - Metal container and a pop-top lid [71–81]
  - Soy isoflavones [82–86]
- Dietary iodine
  - Too little
  - Too much
- Use of topical flea preventative [60, 67, 68]

Soy isoflavones inhibit thyroid peroxidase [84–86] and 5′-iodothyronine-deiodinase [86]. This inhibition may interfere with the synthesis of thyroid hormones.

Metal cans and pop-top lids contain bisphenol A (BPA) [71–73]. This substance is intended to extend shelf life by reducing corrosion [58]. However, during processing and storage, food is contaminated with BPA residue [87, 88]. This is true for human-grade canned foods [73, 87–89] as well as those destined for the pet food industry [89, 90]. BPA is known to act as a thyroid hormone receptor antagonist [71, 74–81].

Much remains to be determined as to the cause(s) of hyperthyroidism. There are many theories, but few have been proven experimentally in cats.

What is known about hyperthyroidism in cats is that the majority of affected patients develop adenomatous hyperplasia of the thyroid as opposed to a functional thyroid carcinoma [3, 51, 91–94].

The resultant thyrotoxicosis promotes catabolism of all body tissues, including lean muscle.

Owner recognition of clinical signs is often delayed because disease progression is gradual. Clients may misinterpret clinical signs of thyrotoxicosis as being normal signs of aging [3, 92].

Over time, patients develop marked sarcopenia, which is grossly observable [3]. They often present for weight loss in spite of a good appetite [3].

Hyperthyroidism alters cardiac excitability [3]. An excess of T4 hypersensitizes the heart to catecholamines by increasing the number of cardiac beta-adrenergic receptors. Cardiac myosin concentration is increased. The resultant tachycardia and increased stroke volume cause the heart to work harder [92, 95]. Heart murmurs and gallop rhythms are common [92, 95, 96].

As the body works harder, it consumes more oxygen and produces more heat [3]. The hyperthyroid cat is intolerant of heat and may develop compensatory polydipsia.

Hyperthyroid cats also experience changes in neuromuscular excitability [3]. They are often weak, with or without tremors [3]. Clients often report nervousness, and an altered mentation [3].

Hyperthyroid cats may also develop polyuria [97, 98]. Polyuria results from a combination of the following [97, 98]:

- Downregulation of aquaporin channels
- Increased blood pressure
- Increased cardiac output
- Increased food intake
  - Increased intake of moisture in food
  - Increased sodium in salt-rich diets
- Increased glomerular filtration rate (GFR)
- Increased renal perfusion
- Increased water intake

64.3.6 Fanconi Syndrome and Polyuria

Fanconi syndrome is a relatively rare condition in which sodium, potassium, glucose, phosphate, bicarbonate, protein, and amino acids are inadequately reabsorbed by the nephrons.

Fanconi syndrome is thought to be inherited [10, 99]. Basenjis are overrepresented [10, 99]. Up to 10% of this breed is affected in the United States [100].

Isolated case reports have also identified Fanconi's syndrome in Irish Wolfhound siblings, Norwegian Elk Hounds, Border Terriers, Yorkshire Terriers, Whippets, Labrador Retrievers, and Shetland Sheepdogs [10, 99].

Fanconi syndrome may be acquired in response to the following [99–113]:

- Chlorambucil
- Copper storage hepatopathy
- Gentamicin
- Primary hypoparathyroidism
- Toxicity
  - Chicken jerky treats
  - Ethylene glycol
  - Lead
    - Batteries
    - Lead shot
    - Lead sinkers
    - Old paint

Patients present for polyuria and polydipsia. Juvenile patients that are affected may also present for reduced rates of growth because of protein wasting in the urine [10].

Clinicopathologic findings include glucosuria in the absence of hyperglycemia, proteinuria, isosthenuria, and cystinuria [10, 99]. One-third of patients may also be hypokalemic due to potassium loss in the urine [10].

Glucose in the urine contributes to osmotic diuresis, hence the development of polyuria.

Metabolic acidosis is common due to loss of bicarbonate in the urine [10].

64.3.7 Primary Renal Glycosuria and Polyuria

Primary renal glycosuria is similar to Fanconi syndrome; however, patients that are affected by the former condition only experience a loss of glucose in the urine. The nephrons are still able to absorb sodium, potassium, phosphate, bicarbonate, protein, and amino acids.

Scottish Terriers, Basenjis, and Norwegian Elkhounds are overrepresented [10, 14].

Affected patients demonstrate glucosuria in the absence of hyperglycemia [10, 14].

64.4 Diagnostic Work-Up for Polyuria

When a patient presents for polyuria, history taking is an important starting point. It is critical to establish that poly-uria truly exists [4]. The client should be asked to describe what s/he considers to be excessive urination and excessive thirst. In other words, what is the client noticing at home?

Are client expectations in line with what is expected of the patient based upon life stage? For example, a three-month-old puppy cannot be expected to hold its urine for a 12-h period overnight. It would be expected for the puppy to house-soil. On the other hand, an adult patient raises a red flag if it is urinating every 2 h now, when previously it had been able to hold its bladder for 8 h consecutively or more.

The owner should be queried about the following:

- Activity level
- Concurrent medications
- Concurrent metabolic or endocrine diseases
- Dietary history
- Environment
  - Indoor
  - Outdoor
    - Ambient temperature
    - Humidity
- Thirst
  - How much water is the patient offered per day?
  - How much water does the patient drink per day?***
  - Does the patient seek out unusual sources of water?
- Urination habits
  - Amount of urine
  - Frequency of urination
  - Other urinary signs
    - Change in urine color
      - Hematuria
    - Change in urine odor
      - Glucosuria
    - Dysuria
    - Hematuria
    - Stranguria

The starred item above (***) should be quantified. Because polyuria and polydipsia often go hand in hand, a polyuric patient should have its water consumption measured [4]. This data may be compared to measurements of urine specific gravity at various points in time [4].

If the patient is drinking more than 90 ml/kg/d (dog) or 45 ml/kg/d (cat), then polydipsia is confirmed, and a work-up is indicated [4, 10]. "Spot-check" measurements of urine specific gravity that are consistently under 1.030 support the need to launch a diagnostic work-up [4].

At minimum, a diagnostic investigation into polyuria and polydipsia includes the following [4, 12]:

- Signalment
- Physical examination
- Complete blood count (CBC)
- Serum biochemistry profile
- Urinalysis
- Urine culture and sensitivity

The signalment helps the clinician to prioritize the list of differential diagnoses. Young patients, for example, are more likely to have hypoadrenocorticism, whereas older patients are at greater risk for hyperthyroidism, hyper-adrenocorticism, and CKD. Cats are more likely than dogs to develop hyperthyroidism. Basenjis are more likely to develop Fanconi syndrome than, say, an English Bulldog.

The physical examination may also provide important clues [12]:

- The canine patient with bilaterally symmetrical truncal alopecia and a potbelly is more likely to have hyperadrenocorticism.
- The feline patient with a palpable thyroid slip is more likely to have hyperthyroidism.
- A patient with peripheral lymphadenopathy may have an infectious disease or lymphoma.
- An intact female patient that was in estrus two months ago and is presenting for mucopurulent vulvar discharge is at greater risk for pyometra.
- A cat with a plantigrade stance should be screened for diabetes mellitus.
- A patient with an enlarged liver may have hyperadren-ocorticism, hepatic neoplasia, or diabetes mellitus.
- A patient with small kidneys may have CKD.
- Bradycardia is supportive of hypoadrenocorticism.
- Cataracts in a canine patient with polyuria and poly-dipsia raise the index of suspicion of diabetes mellitus.
- The non-pregnant uterus is not normally palpable, but will be in cases of pyometra.

There is no substitute for a thorough physical exami-nation [3, 12]. Clues obtained through comprehensive patient evaluation will facilitate diagnostic test selection and narrow differentials to those that are most likely. The author always reminds students to start by looking for horses, rather than zebras.

A CBC may provide additional clues [10, 21, 22]:

- Anemia may reflect anemia of chronic disease, including CKD, endocrinopathies, or neoplasia.
- Neutrophilia may support an underlying infectious process, such as pyelonephritis, or exposure to corticosteroids, as in hyperadrenocorticism.
- Lack of a stress leukogram in an ill patient may support a diagnosis of hypoadrenocorticism.

A chemistry panel may provide additional clues [4, 10]:

- Azotemia may reflect pre-renal dehydration secondary to loss of water in the urine, or it may reflect renal changes that are pathological.
- A low blood urea nitrogen (BUN) is supportive of hepatopathy.
- High liver enzyme activity, especially alkaline phosphatase, is supportive of hyperadrenocorticism, hyperthyroidism, and/or diabetes mellitus.
- Hypercalcemia is supportive of neoplasia, hyperparathyroidism, hypervitaminosis D, and/or hypoadrenocorticism, and should be followed up by evaluating the patient's ionized calcium level.
- Hyperglycemia rules out Fanconi syndrome and primary renal glycosuria.
- Hyperglycemia rules in diabetes mellitus, stress hyperglycemia, and hyperadrenocorticism.
- Hyperkalemia in the face of hyponatremia is supportive of hypoadrenocorticism.
- Hypoalbuminemia suggests protein-losing enteropathy (PLE) or nephropathy (PLN).

A urinalysis may provide additional clues [4, 10, 23]:

- Glucosuria, without hyperglycemia, is supportive of either Fanconi syndrome or primary renal glycosuria.
  - Pyuria and/or bacteriuria may be suggestive of a urinary tract infection (UTI) or pyelonephritis.
  The patient will benefit from a urine culture.
- Urine specific gravity less than 1.008 in an adult dog is likely to be CDI, atypical hyperadrenocorticism, or psychogenic polydipsia.

Submission of urine for culturing is important when urine is dilute as bacteriuria may be easily missed on routine urinalysis [16].

Additional testing may be indicated, including the following [4, 10]:

- ACTH stimulation or dexamethasone suppression tests to evaluate patients for hyperadrenocorticism
- ACTH stimulation test to confirm hypoadrenocorticism
- Lymph node aspirates, when lymph node palpation reveals abnormalities, to evaluate for lymphoma
- Serum T4 levels to confirm hyperthyroidism
- Survey radiographs or abdominal ultrasonography

CDI is much less likely than hyperadrenocorticism and psychogenic polydipsia [4]. Therefore, testing for hyperadrenocorticism should be prioritized before moving onto such diagnostic examinations as the modified water deprivation test or therapeutic trials with an ADH analogue [4].

The water deprivation test, in particular, does not come without risk [4]. A patient with renal insufficiency or pyelonephritis could be harmed in the process [4]. Therefore, it is critical to rule those conditions out prior to proceeding with water deprivation [4].

The purpose of the modified water deprivation test is to discern whether the patient has CDI, NDI, or psychogenic polydipsia [4, 6, 7, 41, 42, 114]. Patients with CDI and NDI cannot concentrate urine even in the face of severe dehydration, in stark contrast to patients with psychogenic polydipsia that are water-restricted [4, 6, 7, 41, 42, 114].

Protocols for the modified water deprivation test and interpretation of test results are beyond the scope of this text. Refer to an internal medicine textbook for additional details. The purpose of this chapter is to introduce the concept as a way to differentiate between disease processes.

An alternate test is the ADH trial [4, 6, 115, 116].

Desmopressin acetate (DDAVP) is a synthetic analogue of ADH that is prescribed for use in humans. Intranasal or oral preparations of DDAVP can be used as a trial. The bottle is rigged such that droplets can be measured and administered intranasally. One droplet equates to 1–4 micrograms of DDAVP. One to four droplets are placed either in the nose or conjunctival sac, twice daily, for five to seven days. If water reduction drops by 50% during the trial, then the patient is likely to have CDI [4, 14, 116].

References

1 Reece, W.O. (2004). Kidney function in mammals. In: *Dukes' Physiology of Domestic Animals*, 12e (ed. H.H. Dukes and W.O. Reece), 73–106. Ithaca: Comstock Pub. Associates.

2 Dyce, K.M., Sack, W.O., and Wensing, C.J.G. (1996). *Textbook of Veterinary Anatomy*, 2e, xiii, 856 p. Philadelphia: Saunders.

3 Englar, R.E. (2017). *Performing the Small Animal Physical Examination*. Hoboken, NJ: Wiley.

4 Nichols, R. (2001). Polyuria and polydipsia - diagnostic approach and problems associated with patient evaluation. *Vet. Clin. N. Am. Small* 31 (5): 833–844.

5 DiBartola, S.P. (2006). Disorders of sodium and water: hypernatremia and hyponatremia. In: *Fluid, Electrolyte,*

and Acid-Base Disorders in Small Animal Practice, 3e (ed. S.P. DiBartola), 47–79. St. Louis, MO: Elsevier.

6 Feldman, E.C. and Melson, R.W. (1996). Water metabolism and diabetes insipidus. In: *Canine and Feline Endocrinology and Reproduction* (ed. E.C. Feldman and R.W. Melson). Philadelphia: WB Saunders.

7 Hardy, R.M. (1982). Disorders of water metabolism. *Vet. Clin. North Am. Small Anim. Pract.* 12 (3): 353–373.

8 Verbalis, J.G. (2003). Disorders of water metabolism. In: *Contemporary Endocrinology: Handbook of Diagnostic Endocrinology* (ed. J.E. Hall and L.K. Nieman), 23–53. Totowa, NJ: Humana Press, Inc.

9 Marks, S.L. and Taboada, J. (1998). Hypernatremia and hypertonic syndromes. *Vet. Clin. North Am. Small Anim. Pract.* 28 (3): 533–543.

10 Tilley, L.P. and Smith, F.W.K. (2004). *The 5-Minute Veterinary Consult: Canine and Feline*, 3e, lviii, 1487 p. Baltimore, MD: Lippincott Williams & Wilkins.

11 Agarwal, S.K. and Gupta, A. (2008). Aquaporins: the renal water channels. *Indian J. Nephrol.* 18 (3): 95–100.

12 Schoeman, J.P. (ed.) (2008). Approach to polyuria and polydipsia in the dog. Proceedings of the 33rd World Small Animal Veterinary Congress; Dublin, Ireland: World Small Animal Veterinary Association (WSAVA).

13 Gordon, J. (2011). Clinical approach to polyuria (Proceedings). DVM 360 [Internet]. http:// veterinarycalendar.dvm360.com/clinical-approach-polyuria-proceedings-0.

14 Feldman, E.C. and Nelson, R.W. (1989). Diagnostic approach to polydipsia and polyuria. *Vet. Clin. North Am. Small Anim. Pract.* 19 (2): 327–341.

15 Osborne, C.A. (2003). The ins and outs of polyuria and polydipsia. DVM 360 [Internet]. http://veterinarynews. dvm360.com/ins-and-outs-polyuria-and-polydipsia.

16 Behrend, E.N. (ed.) 2005. Diagnosis of polyuria/ polydipsia: case-based approach. Proceedings of the North American Veterinary Conference (NAVC); Orlando, Florida.

17 Cone, F. (2009). Polyuria, polydipsia, and hypercalcemia. NAVC Clinician's Brief. (June):46.

18 Nolan, B. and Labato, M.A. (2013). Polyuria and polydipsia in a dog. *NAVC Clinician's Brief* (November): 66–69.

19 Leroy, C., Karrouz, W., Douillard, C. et al. (2013). Diabetes insipidus. *Ann. Endocrinol. (Paris)* 74 (5–6): 496–507.

20 Reusch, C.E. (2015). Feline diabetes mellitus. In: *Canine & feline endocrinology*, 4e (ed. E.C. Feldman, R.W. Nelson, C. Reusch and J.C.R. Scott-Moncrieff), 258–314. St. Louis, Missouri: Elsevier Saunders.

21 de Brito Galvao, J.F., Parker, V., Schenck, P.A., and Chew, D.J. (2017). Update on feline ionized Hypercalcemia. *Vet. Clin. North Am. Small Anim. Pract.* 47 (2): 273–292.

22 de Brito Galvao, J.F., Schenck, P.A., and Chew, D.J. (2017). A quick reference on Hypercalcemia. *Vet. Clin. North Am. Small Anim. Pract.* 47 (2): 241–248.

23 Bruyette, D.S. (2008). Diagnostic approach to polyuria and polydipsia. DVM 360 [Internet]. http:// veterinarycalendar.dvm360.com/diagnostic-approach-polyuria-and-polydipsia-proceedings-0.

24 Levi, M., Peterson, L., and Berl, T. (1983). Mechanism of concentrating defect in hypercalcemia. Role of polydipsia and prostaglandins. *Kidney Int.* 23 (3): 489–497.

25 Suki, W.N., Eknoyan, G., Rector, F.C. Jr., and Seldin, D.W. (1969). The renal diluting and concentrating mechanism in hypercalcemia. *Nephron* 6 (1): 50–61.

26 Vanherweghem, J.L., Ducobu, J., d'Hollander, A., and Toussaint, C. (1976). Effects of hypercalcemia on water and sodium excretion by the isolated dog kidney. *Pflugers Arch.* 363 (1): 75–80.

27 Brunette, M.G., Vary, J., and Carriere, S. (1974). Hyposthenuria in hypercalcemia. A possible role of intrarenal blood-flow (IRBF) redistribution. *Pflugers Arch.* 350 (1): 9–23.

28 Goldfarb, S. and Agus, Z.S. (1984). Mechanism of the polyuria of hypercalcemia. *Am. J. Nephrol.* 4 (2): 69–76.

29 Schenck, P.A., Chew, D.J., and Behrend, E.N. (2005). Update on hypercalcemic disorders. In: *Consultations in Feline Internal Medicine* (ed. J. August), 157–168. St. Louis, MO: Elsevier.

30 Cook, A.K. (2008). Guidelines for evaluating hypercalcemic cats. DVM 360 [Internet]. http:// veterinarymedicine.dvm360.com/guidelines-evaluating-hypercalcemic-cats.

31 Savary, K.C., Price, G.S., and Vaden, S.L. (2000). Hypercalcemia in cats: a retrospective study of 71 cases (1991–1997). *J. Vet. Intern. Med.* 14 (2): 184–189.

32 Stokes, J.E. and Forrester, S.D. (2004). New and unusual causes of acute renal failure in dogs and cats. *Vet. Clin. North Am. Small Anim. Pract.* 34 (4): 909–922, vi.

33 Murphy, M.J. (2002). Rodenticides. *Vet. Clin. North Am. Small Anim. Pract.* 32 (2): 469–484, viii.

34 Goff, J.P. (2004). Disorders of carbohydrate and fat metabolism. In: *Dukes' Physiology of Domestic Animals*, 12e (ed. H.H. Dukes and W.O. Reece), 554–561. Ithaca: Comstock Pub. Associates.

35 Scarlett, J.M. and Donoghue, S. (1998). Associations between body condition and disease in cats. *J. Am. Vet. Med. Assoc.* 212 (11): 1725–1731.

36 Prahl, A., Guptill, L., Glickman, N.W. et al. (2007). Time trends and risk factors for diabetes mellitus in cats presented to veterinary teaching hospitals. *J. Feline Med. Surg.* 9 (5): 351–358.

37 Panciera, D.L., Thomas, C.B., Eicker, S.W., and Atkins, C.E. (1990). Epizootiological patterns of diabetes-mellitus in cats - 333 cases (1980–1986). *J. Am. Vet. Med. Assoc.* 197 (11): 1504–1508.

38 McCann, T.M., Simpson, K.E., Shaw, D.J. et al. (2007). Feline diabetes mellitus in the UK: the prevalence within an insured cat population and a questionnaire-based putative risk factor analysis. *J. Feline Med. Surg.* 9 (4): 289–299.

39 Breitschwerdt, E.B. (1981). Clinical abnormalities of urine concentration and dilution. *Compend. Contin. Educ. Pract. Vet.* 3: 412–414.

40 Robertson, G.L. (1988). Differential diagnosis of polyuria. *Annu. Rev. Med.* 39: 425–442.

41 Swartz-Porsche, D. (1980). Diabetes insipidus. In: *Current Veterinary Therapy VII* (ed. R.W. Kirk), 1005–1011. Philadelphia: WB Saunders.

42 Barsanti, J.A., DiBartola, S.P., and Finco, D.R. (2000). Diagnostic approach to polyuria and polydipsia. In: *Kirk's Current Veterinary Therapy XIII* (ed. J.D. Bonagura), 831–835. Philadelphia: WB Saunders.

43 Grumbaum, E.G. and Moritz, A. (1991). The diagnosis of nephrogenic diabetes insipidus in the dog. *Tierarztl. Prax.* 19: 539.

44 Frank, L.A. (2006). Comparative dermatology–canine endocrine dermatoses. *Clin. Dermatol.* 24 (4): 317–325.

45 Feldman, E.C. and Nelson, R.W. (2004). *Canine and Feline Endocrinology and Reproduction.* St. Louis, Missouri: W.B. Saunders.

46 Joles, J.A., Rijnberk, A., van den Brom, W.E., and Dogterom, J. (1980). Studies on the mechanism of polyuria induced by cortisol excess in the dog. *Vet. Q.* 2 (4): 199–205.

47 Moses, A.M. (1963). Adrenal-Neurohypophysial relationships in the dehydrated rat. *Endocrinology* 73: 230–236.

48 Kleeman, C.R., Czaczkes, J.W., and Cutler, R. (1964). Mechanisms of impaired water excretion in adrenal and pituitary insufficiency. Iv. Antidiuretic hormone in primary and secondary adrenal insufficiency. *J. Clin. Invest.* 43: 1641–1648.

49 Ahmed, A.B., George, B.C., Gonzalez-Auvert, C., and Dingman, J.F. (1967). Increased plasma arginine vasopressin in clinical adrenocortical insufficeincy and its inhibition by glucosteroids. *J. Clin. Invest.* 46 (1): 111–123.

50 Aubry, R.H., Nankin, H.R., Moses, A.M., and Streeten, D.H. (1965). Measurement of the osmotic threshold for vasopressin release in human subjects, and its modification by cortisol. *J. Clin. Endocrinol. Metab.* 25 (11): 1481–1492.

51 Scott-Moncrieff, J.C. (2015). Feline hyperthyroidism. In: *Canine and Feline Endocrinology*, 4e (ed. E.C. Feldman, R.W. Nelson, C. Reusch and J.C.R. Scott-Moncrieff), 136–195. St. Louis: Elsevier Saunders.

52 Peterson, M.E., Kintzer, P.P., Cavanagh, P.G. et al. (1983). Feline hyperthyroidism: pretreatment clinical and laboratory evaluation of 131 cases. *J. Am. Vet. Med. Assoc.* 183 (1): 103–110.

53 Hoenig, M., Goldschmidt, M.H., Ferguson, D.C. et al. (1982). Toxic nodular goitre in the cat. *J. Small Anim. Pract.* 23 (1): 1–12.

54 Peterson, M.E. and Ward, C.R. (2007). Etiopathologic findings of hyperthyroidism in cats. *Vet. Clin. North Am. Small Anim. Pract.* 37 (4): 633–645, v.

55 Baral, R. and Peterson, M.E. (2012). Thyroid gland disorders. In: *The Cat: Clinical Medicine and Management* (ed. S.E. Little), 571–592. Philadelphia: Elsevier Saunders.

56 Peterson, M.E. and Johnson, J.G. (eds.) (1979). *Spontaneous Hyperthyroidism in the Cat. American College of Veterinary Internal Medicine.* Seattle, WA: ACVIM.

57 McLean, J.L., Lobetti, R.G., and Schoeman, J.P. (2014). Worldwide prevalence and risk factors for feline hyperthyroidism: a review. *J. S. Afr. Vet. Assoc.* 85 (1): 1097.

58 Peterson, M. (2012). Hyperthyroidism in cats: what's causing this epidemic of thyroid disease and can we prevent it? *J. Feline Med. Surg.* 14 (11): 804–818.

59 Mooney, C.T. and Peterson, M.E. (2012). Feline hyperthyroidism. In: *Manual of Canine and Feline Endocrinology* (ed. C.T. Mooney and M.E. Peterson), 92–110. Quedgeley, Gloucester: British Small Animal Veterinary Association.

60 Scarlett, J.M. (1994). Epidemiology of thyroid diseases of dogs and cats. *Vet. Clin. North Am. Small Anim. Pract.* 24 (3): 477–486.

61 Gerber, H., Peter, H., Ferguson, D.C., and Peterson, M.E. (1994). Etiopathology of feline toxic nodular goiter. *Vet. Clin. North Am. Small Anim. Pract.* 24 (3): 541–565.

62 Broussard, J.D., Peterson, M.E., and Fox, P.R. (1995). Changes in clinical and laboratory findings in cats with hyperthyroidism from 1983 to 1993. *J. Am. Vet. Med. Assoc.* 206 (3): 302–305.

63 Thoday, K.L. and Mooney, C.T. (1992). Historical, clinical and laboratory features of 126 hyperthyroid cats. *Vet. Rec.* 131 (12): 257–264.

64 Miyamoto, T., Miyata, I., Kurobane, K. et al. (2002). Prevalence of feline hyperthyroidism in Osaka and the Chugoku region. *J. Jpn. Vet. Med. Assoc.* 55: 289–292.

65 Olczak, J., Jones, B.R., Pfeiffer, D.U. et al. (2004). Multivariate analysis of risk factors for feline hyperthyroidism in New Zealand. *N. Z. Vet. J.* 53: 53–58.

66 Sassnau, R. (2006). Epidemiological investigation on the prevalence of feline hyperthyroidism in an urban population in Germany. *Tierarztl. Prax. Ausg. K Klientiere Heimtiere* 34: 450–457.

67 Kass, P.H., Peterson, M.E., Levy, J. et al. (1999). Evaluation of environmental, nutritional, and host factors in cats with hyperthyroidism. *J. Vet. Intern. Med.* 13 (4): 323–329.

68 Wakeling, J., Everard, A., Brodbelt, D. et al. (2009). Risk factors for feline hyperthyroidism in the UK. *J. Small Anim. Pract.* 50 (8): 406–414.

69 De Wet, C.S., Mooney, C.T., Thompson, P.N., and Schoeman, J.P. (2009). Prevalence of and risk factors for feline hyperthyroidism in Hong Kong. *J. Feline Med. Surg.* 11 (4): 315–321.

70 Martin, K.M., Rossing, M.A., Ryland, L.M. et al. (2000). Evaluation of dietary and environmental risk factors for hyperthyroidism in cats. *J. Am. Vet. Med. Assoc.* 217 (6): 853–856.

71 Edinboro, C.H., Scott-Moncrieff, J.C., Janovitz, E. et al. (2004). Epidemiologic study of relationships between consumption of commercial canned food and risk of hyperthyroidism in cats. *J. Am. Vet. Med. Assoc.* 224 (6): 879–886.

72 Tsai, W.T. (2006). Human health risk on environmental exposure to Bisphenol-a: a review. *J. Environ. Sci. Health C Environ. Carcinog. Ecotoxicol. Rev.* 24 (2): 225–255.

73 Noonan, G.O., Ackerman, L.K., and Begley, T.H. (2011). Concentration of bisphenol A in highly consumed canned foods on the U.S. market. *J. Agric. Food Chem.* 59 (13): 7178–7185.

74 Vandenberg, L.N., Maffini, M.V., Sonnenschein, C. et al. (2009). Bisphenol-A and the great divide: a review of controversies in the field of endocrine disruption. *Endocr. Rev.* 30 (1): 75–95.

75 Boas, M., Main, K.M., and Feldt-Rasmussen, U. (2009). Environmental chemicals and thyroid function: an update. *Curr. Opin. Endocrinol., Diabetes Obes.* 16 (5): 385–391.

76 Patrick, L. (2009). Thyroid disruption: mechanism and clinical implications in human health. *Altern. Med. Rev.* 14 (4): 326–346.

77 Diamanti-Kandarakis, E., Bourguignon, J.P., Giudice, L.C. et al. (2009). Endocrine-disrupting chemicals: an Endocrine Society scientific statement. *Endocr. Rev.* 30 (4): 293–342.

78 Meeker, J.D. and Ferguson, K.K. (2011). Relationship between urinary phthalate and bisphenol a concentrations and serum thyroid measures in U.S. adults and adolescents from the National Health and nutrition examination survey (NHANES) 2007–2008. *Environ. Health Perspect.* 119 (10): 1396–1402.

79 Welshons, W.V. and Nagel, S.C. (2006). Vom Saal FS. Large effects from small exposures. III. Endocrine mechanisms mediating effects of bisphenol A at levels of human exposure. *Endocrinology* 147 (6 Suppl): S56–S69.

80 Moriyama, K., Tagami, T., Akamizu, T. et al. (2002). Thyroid hormone action is disrupted by bisphenol A as an antagonist. *J. Clin. Endocrinol. Metab.* 87 (11): 5185–5190.

81 Kitamura, S., Jinno, N., Ohta, S. et al. (2002). Thyroid hormonal activity of the flame retardants tetrabromobisphenol A and tetrachlorobisphenol A. *Biochem. Biophys. Res. Commun.* 293 (1): 554–559.

82 Court, M.H. and Freeman, L.M. (2002). Identification and concentration of soy isoflavones in commercial cat foods. *Am. J. Vet. Res.* 63 (2): 181–185.

83 Bell, K.M., Rutherfurd, S.M., and Hendriks, W.H. (2006). The isoflavone content of commercially-available feline diets in New Zealand. *N. Z. Vet. J.* 54 (3): 103–108.

84 Divi, R.L., Chang, H.C., and Doerge, D.R. (1997). Anti-thyroid isoflavones from soybean: isolation, characterization, and mechanisms of action. *Biochem. Pharmacol.* 54 (10): 1087–1096.

85 Doerge, D.R. and Sheehan, D.M. (2002). Goitrogenic and estrogenic activity of soy isoflavones. *Environ. Health Perspect.* 110 (Suppl 3): 349–353.

86 de Souza Dos Santos, M.C., Goncalves, C.F., Vaisman, M. et al. (eds.) (2011). Impact of flavonoids on thyroid function. *Food Chem. Toxicol.* 49 (10): 2495–2502.

87 Goodson, A., Robin, H., Summerfield, W., and Cooper, I. (2004). Migration of bisphenol A from can coatings–effects of damage, storage conditions and heating. *Food Addit. Contam.* 21 (10): 1015–1026.

88 Cabado, A.G., Aldea, S., Porro, C. et al. (2008). Migration of BADGE (bisphenol A diglycidyl-ether) and BFDGE (bisphenol F diglycidyl-ether) in canned seafood. *Food Chem. Toxicol.* 46 (5): 1674–1680.

89 Schecter, A., Malik, N., Haffner, D. et al. (2010). Bisphenol A (BPA) in U.S. food. *Environ. Sci. Technol.* 44 (24): 9425–9430.

90 Kang, J.H. and Kondo, F. (2002). Determination of bisphenol A in canned pet foods. *Res. Vet. Sci.* 73 (2): 177–182.

91 Turrel, J.M., Feldman, E.C., Nelson, R.W., and Cain, G.R. (1988). Thyroid carcinoma causing hyperthyroidism in cats: 14 cases (1981–1986). *J. Am. Vet. Med. Assoc.* 193 (3): 359–364.

92 Feldman, E.C. and Nelson, R.W. (2004). *Canine and Feline Endocrinology and Reproduction*, 3e, xi, 1089 p. St. Louis, Mo.: Saunders.

93 Hibbert, A., Gruffydd-Jones, T., Barrett, E.L. et al. (2009). Feline thyroid carcinoma: diagnosis and response to high-dose radioactive iodine treatment. *J. Feline Med. Surg.* 11 (2): 116–124.

94 Carpenter, J.L. (1987). Tumors and tumorlike lesions. In: *Diseases of the Cat: Medicine & Surgery* (ed. J. Holzworth), 406. Philadelphia: Saunders.

95 Eiler, H. (2004). Endocrine glands. In: *Dukes' Physiology of Domestic Animals*, 12e, xiv, 999 p. (ed. W.O. Reece). Ithaca: Comstock Pub. Associates.

96 Cote, E., Edwards, N.J., Ettinger, S.J. et al. (2015). Management of incidentally detected heart murmurs in dogs and cats. *J. Vet. Cardiol.* 17 (4): 245–261.

97 Mariani, L.H. and Berns, J.S. (2012). The renal manifestations of thyroid disease. *J. Am. Soc. Nephrol.* 23 (1): 22–26.

98 Wang, W., Li, C., Summer, S.N. et al. (2007). Polyuria of thyrotoxicosis: downregulation of aquaporin water channels and increased solute excretion. *Kidney Int.* 72 (9): 1088–1094.

99 Bommer, N.X., Brownlie, S.E., Morrison, L.R. et al. (2018). Fanconi syndrome in Irish wolfhound siblings. *J. Am. Anim. Hosp. Assoc.* 54 (3): 173–178.

100 Noonan, C.H. and Kay, J.M. (1990). Prevalence and geographic distribution of Fanconi syndrome in basenjis in the United States. *J. Am. Vet. Med. Assoc.* 197 (3): 345–349.

101 Carmichael, N., Lee, J., and Giger, U. (2014). Fanconi syndrome in dog in the UK. *Vet. Rec.* 174 (14): 357–358.

102 King, J.B. (2016). Proximal tubular nephropathy in two dogs diagnosed with lead toxicity. *Aust. Vet. J.* 94 (8): 280–284.

103 Reinert, N.C. and Feldman, D.G. (2016). Acquired Fanconi syndrome in four cats treated with chlorambucil. *J. Feline Med. Surg.* 18 (12): 1034–1040.

104 Sharman, M., Seth, M., Lam, A. et al. (2016). Acquired Fanconi-like syndrome cases associated with dried chicken and duck meat ingestion. *Vet. Rec.* 178 (8): 196.

105 Kim, D.H., Lim, A.Y., Gwag, H.B. et al. (2014). A case of Fanconi syndrome accompanied by crystal depositions in tubular cells in a patient with multiple myeloma. *Kidney Res. Clin. Pract.* 33 (2): 112–115.

106 Bates, N., Sharman, M., Lam, A. et al. (2016). Reporting cases of Fanconi syndrome in dogs in the UK. *Vet. Rec.* 178 (20): 510.

107 Hostutler, R.A., DiBartola, S.P., and Eaton, K.A. (2004). Transient proximal renal tubular acidosis and Fanconi syndrome in a dog. *J. Am. Vet. Med. Assoc.* 224 (10): 1611–1614, 05.

108 Thompson, M.F., Fleeman, L.M., Kessell, A.E. et al. (2013). Acquired proximal renal tubulopathy in dogs exposed to a common dried chicken treat: retrospective study of 108 cases (2007–2009). *Aust. Vet. J.* 91 (9): 368–373.

109 Settles, E.L. and Schmidt, D. (1994). Fanconi syndrome in a Labrador retriever. *J. Vet. Intern. Med.* 8 (6): 390–393.

110 Jamieson, P.M. and Chandler, M.L. (2001). Transient renal tubulopathy in a Labrador retriever. *J. Small Anim. Pract.* 42 (11): 546–549.

111 Freeman, L.M., Breitschwerdt, E.B., Keene, B.W., and Hansen, B. (1994). Fanconi's syndrome in a dog with primary hypoparathyroidism. *J. Vet. Intern. Med.* 8 (5): 349–354.

112 Brown, S.A., Rakich, P.M., Barsanti, J.A. et al. (1986). Fanconi syndrome and acute-renal-failure associated with gentamicin therapy in a dog. *J. Am. Anim. Hosp. Assoc.* 22 (5): 635–640.

113 Appleman, E.H., Cianciolo, R., Mosenco, A.S. et al. (2008). Transient acquired fanconi syndrome associated with copper storage hepatopathy in 3 dogs. *J. Vet. Intern. Med.* 22 (4): 1038–1042.

114 Mulnix, J.A., Rijnberk, A., and Hendriks, H.J. (1976). Evaluation of a modified water-deprivation test for diagnosis of polyuric disorders in dogs. *J. Am. Vet. Med. Assoc.* 169 (12): 1327–1330.

115 Kraus, K.H. (1987). The use of Desmopressin in diagnosis and treatment of diabetes-Insipidus in cats. *Compend. Contin. Educ. Pract.* 9 (7): 752–758.

116 Nichols, R. (2000). Use of DDAVP in the diagnosis and treatment of diabetes insipidus. In: *Current Veterinary Therapy XIII* (ed. J.D. Bonagura), 325–326. Philadelphia: WB Saunders.

65

Acute Presentations of Diminished Urine Output: Urinary Tract Obstruction (UTO)

65.1 Introduction to Diminished Urine Output

Urine output was introduced in Section 64.1. Recall that despite individual variation, urine output for the companion animal patient averages 20–40 ml/kg/d or roughly 1–2 ml/kg/h [1].

Conditions that increase urine output were emphasized in Chapter 64. This chapter concentrates on those conditions in which urine output is less than expected.

The medically appropriate term for diminished urine output is oliguria [2]. By definition, oliguria is urine production at a rate of less than 0.5 ml/kg/h [3, 4].

Anuria is extreme oliguria in which there is less than 0.08 ml/kg/h of urine produced [3]. This is essentially a halt in urination [2].

Oliguria and anuria are medical emergencies, whereas polyuria is not, assuming that the polyuric patient has free access to water and is therefore not water deprived.

65.2 Causes of Diminished Urine Output

When it occurs, oliguria can be physiologic or pathologic.

Physiologic oliguria results from the body's need to conserve water. Dehydration is an example of a state in which physiologic oliguria is beneficial. The rise in plasma osmolality, in combination with diminished circulating fluid volume, triggers the production and release of antidiuretic hormone (ADH) from the hypothalamus [2, 5, 6].

ADH facilitates water reabsorption within the nephron, the functional unit of the kidney [2, 5]. This is made possible by the insertion of aquaporin-2 water channels into the membranes of the distal tubules and collecting ducts [7]. Water now flows down its osmotic gradient, out of the nephron, and back into systemic circulation. Because less water is lost from the body, the urine is said to be concentrated [2, 5]. Urine concentration can only take place in the presence of ADH and functionally responsive kidneys.

The dehydrated patient will likely display one or more of the following signs [3, 8–10]:

- Cool extremities
- Pallor
- Prolonged capillary refill time (CRT)
- Skin tenting
- Tacky mucous membranes
- Weak pulse

Recall from Chapter 54, Section 54.3 that skin tenting is evaluated by grasping a generous fold of skin at the nape of the neck or between the shoulder blades. The skin fold is lifted up gently, but firmly, and is then released [9]. In a euhydrated patient, skin elasticity causes the fold to returns to its normal position almost immediately [9]. In other words, there is not a persistent skin tent.

As the patient dehydrates, skin turgor is progressively lost. The fold of skin is sluggish. The time it takes to return to its original position is delayed. In cases of severe dehydration, the skin remains tented.

The extremely dehydrated patient may also display sunken globes and/or dehydrated corneas [9].

Dehydration is just one clinical scenario that results in physiologic oliguria. Hypotension is a second example. Hypotension causes poor perfusion of the kidneys. Renal hypoperfusion triggers physiologic oliguria in order to raise blood volume and counter hypotension.

It is important to note that, when oliguria is physiologic, it will resolve quickly as soon as the inciting factor is corrected [3]. For instance, as soon as the dehydrated patient is rehydrated, oliguria will reverse itself and normal urine production will resume.

However, oliguria is not always physiologic. There are several clinical scenarios in which oliguria is pathologic. These include the following situations [3, 9, 11, 12]:

- Increased resistance to blood flow at the level of the afferent glomerular vessels
- Loss of nephrons

Common Clinical Presentations in Dogs and Cats, First Edition. Ryane E. Englar.
© 2019 John Wiley & Sons, Inc. Published 2019 by John Wiley & Sons, Inc.

- Macroscopic obstruction of urinary flow
  - Inflammation of the lower urinary tract
    - Urinary bladder
    - Urethra
  - Neoplasia of the urinary bladder or prostate
  - Urethral plug (cats > dogs)
  - Urinary stricture
  - Urolithiasis
- Microscopic obstruction of urinary flow
  - Obstruction of the lumen of nephrons
- Reduced permeability of the glomerulus
  - Rupture of the urinary tract
  - Urethral tear
  - Urinary bladder rupture
- Toxin (see Chapter 63, Section 63.4.1.1)
  - Ethylene glycol
  - Grapes and raisins
  - Lily toxicosis

Oliguria and anuria often denote acute kidney injury (AKI) or acute renal failure (ARF). These patients require immediate attention because AKI can be fatal.

AKI was introduced in Chapter 63, Section 63.4.1. Recall that AKI is a condition in which one or both kidneys is acutely dysfunctional, meaning that regulation of water, acid–base, and electrolyte balance is compromised [13]. So, too, is the excretion of waste through the urinary tract [13].

Refer to Section 63.4.1 for a list of the many causes of AKI [13, 14]. Review common toxicities and infectious diseases that result in AKI. Review the concept of ureteral obstructions. Recall that AKI patients typically present with renomegaly.

Three additional causes of AKI will be discussed below, as they relate to presentations of acute urinary tract obstruction (UTO):

- Feline UTO
- Neoplasia of the lower urinary tract
  - Urethra
  - Urinary bladder
- Urolithiasis

65.3 Clinical Presentations Associated with Diminished Urine Output

Because owners of companion animals are not typically in the habit of measuring urine output, they do not routinely present patients with a chief complaint of oliguria. More often than not, clients report one of more of the following clinical signs:

- Abdominal straining
- "Acute abdomen" (see Chapter 50)

- Dysuria, painful, or difficult urination
- Excessive grooming
  - Perineum of cats and female dogs
  - Prepuce of male dogs
- Extrusion of the penis (males)
- Discoloration of the tip of the penis (males)
  - Purple-blue to black
- Guarding of the abdomen
- Hematuria, or bloody urine
- House soiling
- Increased respiratory rate
  - Likely secondary to pain
- "Marking" behavior (cats)
- Pollakiuria, increased frequency or attempts to urinate
- "Spotting" of the carpet or furniture
- Stranguria, straining to urinate
- Vocalizing during urination

When the patient has a complete obstruction of the urinary tract, clinical signs present acutely. The patient may decompensate rapidly. For example, clients may find their blocked cat laterally recumbent and minimally responsive.

65.4 Urolithiasis and Urinary Tract Obstruction (UTO)

As mentioned earlier, UTO can occur due to urolithiasis. Uroliths may develop at any point throughout the urinary system, including the upper and lower urinary tracts. For example, patients may present with one or more of the following:

- Nephroliths, or kidney stones
- Ureteroliths, or stones in one or both ureters
- Cystoliths, or bladder stones (see Figures 65.1a–g)
- Urethral stones

Note that not all uroliths are obstructive [15]. Many patients are aclinical for cystoliths [15]. Others may present for nonobstructive cystitis, when stones involve the urinary bladder [15]. This is because stones roll around within the lumen of the urinary bladder, scraping against the bladder wall. This may result in microscopic hematuria [15]. Urine does not appear to be bloody; however, more than five erythrocytes per high-power field (hpf) are identified via light microscopy [15].

Alternatively, the patient may have macroscopic hematuria [15]. In the author's experience, this is easiest for clients to detect during the winter months in those climates in which snow is a common groundcover. Dogs that eliminate outdoors will urinate onto snow, which is dyed pink by hematuria, as opposed to urine's normal yellow color.

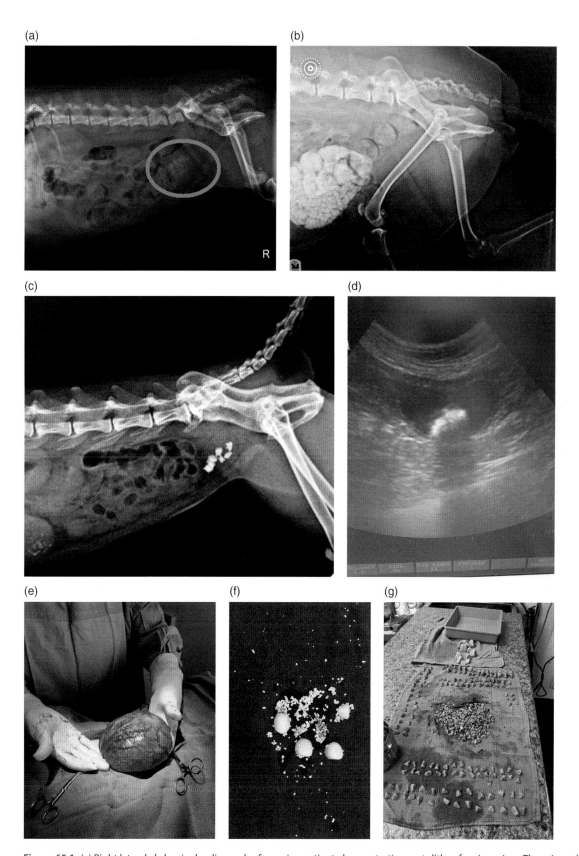

Figure 65.1 (a) Right lateral abdominal radiograph of a canine patient, demonstrating cystoliths of various sizes. The urinary bladder has been circled in orange for ease of identification. (b) Right lateral abdominal radiograph of a canine patient, demonstrating the caudal abdomen. The urinary bladder is filled with cystoliths. *Source:* Courtesy of Samantha Thurman, DVM. (c) Right lateral abdominal radiograph of a feline patient, demonstrating cystoliths of various shapes. (d) Abdominal ultrasonography, demonstrating a single hyperechoic cystolith. Note that fluid, such as urine, is hypoechoic when viewed with ultrasound. This creates effective contrast between the urine and cystolith. (e) Intraoperative photograph. The urinary bladder has been exteriorized through a ventral midline abdominal incision in anticipation of performing a cystotomy to remove bladder stones. *Source:* Courtesy of Samantha Thurman, DVM. (f) Postoperative view of a cystolith collection from a canine patient. These cystoliths were later determined to be struvites. *Source:* Courtesy of Joseph Onello, DVM. (g) Postoperative view of an extensive cystolith collection. *Source:* Courtesy of Samantha Thurman, DVM.

In addition to hematuria, patients with urolithiasis often demonstrate lower urinary tract signs [9, 15]:

- Dysuria
- Pollakiuria
- Stranguria

Patients may posture to urinate, without producing the expected volume of urine. Owners of male dogs may report that the patient's stream is "off."

All patients that present with one or more of the aforementioned complaints require a thorough physical examination. The urinary bladder should be palpated as part of this comprehensive evaluation. In health, the urinary bladder should be palpable in all cats and in dogs that do not tense their abdominal muscles [16].

The urinary bladder is located within the caudal abdominal cavity, between the ventral body wall and the descending colon [9, 16, 17]. The position of the urinary bladder within the abdomen will vary depending upon how distended it is with urine. If the urinary bladder is full, it can extend far cranially [16].

The typical empty urinary bladder feels like a wad of balled up tissue: soft, supple, and non-tender to the touch. As the urinary bladder fills a small amount, it feels like a very small water balloon: fluid surrounded by a stable, yet soft and pliable wall. Even when the bladder is moderately full, it retains that water balloon-like quality; that is, it is compressible [16].

Uroliths are palpable on physical examination in approximately one-fifth of dogs [18]. The larger the uroliths, the more likely they are to be felt. Uroliths may also be palpable in cats.

If there is more than one stone, the stones may roll around and grate against each other [9]. This sensation, too, may be palpable [9].

Because urolithiasis is not detected by physical examination in the majority of patients, abdominal imaging is essential to confirm the diagnosis [15, 19]. Radiopaque uroliths, such as calcium oxalate and silica, will be detected on radiographs [9, 15, 19, 20].

Magnesium ammonium phosphate (struvite) stones are radiopaque, if they contain sufficient amounts of calcium phosphate [21, 22].

Advanced imaging techniques, such as double-contrast cystography, may be necessary to detect radio-lucent uroliths, including urates and cystine [9, 15].

Ultrasonography is another valuable diagnostic tool in that it is capable of diagnosing radiopaque and radiolu-cent stones as well as neoplasia [15].

Note that the type of urolith cannot be diagnosed based upon radiographic size or shape [21, 23]. However, the history and clinicopathologic data from the urinaly-sis may also help the clinician make an educated guess as to the type(s) of stone(s) [9]. For example, struvites are often the result of urinary tract infections (UTIs) [15]. Females less than one year old or greater than ten are most at risk [19, 24–26]. *Staphylococcus, Enterococcus,* and *Proteus* spp. produce the enzyme urease. Urease catalyzes the hydrolysis of urea to produce ammonia [19, 27]. Ammonia makes the urine more alkaline. Alkaline urine promotes the formation of struvites [28].

Calcium oxalate stones, on the other hand, tend to be associated with aciduria and small breeds of dogs, for example, the Miniature Schnauzer, Lhasa Apso, Shih Tzu, Yorkshire Terrier, and Bichon Frise [18, 19, 29].

Prior to 2003, calcium oxalate stones in dogs and cats in the United States were rare by comparison to struvites [9]. By 2003, the occurrence of calcium oxalate equaled that of struvites [9]. Calcium oxalate stones surpassed struvites in 2004 [9]. By 2005, 42% of canine urolith submissions were calcium oxalate [9].

It has been hypothesized that the trend toward acidify-ing diets intended to prevent struviuria has fueled the increase in calcium oxalate stones [18, 30–33].

Dalmatians and English Bulldogs are at increased risk of developing urate stones [34]:

- The chance that a urolith will be urate-based in a Dalmatian is 228.9 times greater than in any other breed, with males being 16.4 times more at risk than females.
- The chance that a urolith will be urate-based in an English Bulldogs is 43 times greater than in any other breed, with males being 14.3 times more at risk than females.

English Bulldogs are also at increased risk of develop-ing cystine stones [34].

Struvite stones within the kidney or urinary bladder may resolve by medical management, aimed at adjusting urinary pH [15]. However, dissolution diets do not appear to work for calcium oxalate stones [15]. Surgical excision or lithotripsy is necessary [15].

Veterinarians must also consider the species and sex of the patient when determining the best approach to case management [15]. Male cats are at increased risk of UTO due to the narrow diameter of their urethra. Therefore, clinicians may be more likely to advocate for surgical excision [15].

65.5 Feline UTO

In addition to urolithiasis, UTO may result from ure-thral plugs [13]. Urethral plugs are protein-rich accu-mulations of inflammatory cells and urinary crystals [35–37]. Plug-associated UTOs are especially common in cats [13, 35, 36, 38, 39].

Male cats are more commonly affected than females because the male urethra is very narrow [13, 38–40].

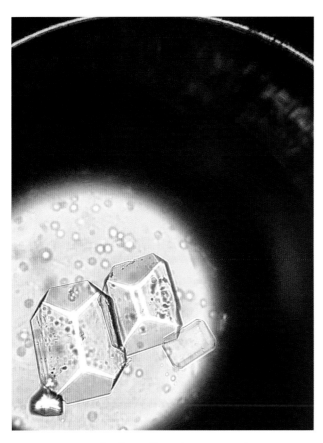

Figure 65.2 Example of crystalluria. Struvite crystals are present in this sample of feline urine, as examined by light microscopy. Note that crystals in and of themselves are not necessarily pathological. However, they may contribute to urinary tract obstruction (UTO). *Source:* Courtesy of Jennifer Lang.

Up to 50% of cases of feline UTO are thought to be idiopathic [13, 41]. However, environmental stress, season, climate, and crystalluria may predispose a patient to UTO [37, 42 46] (see Figure 65.2).

Cats with indoor-only lifestyles are more likely to become obstructed [38]. So, too, are cats that are fed dry diets [38, 42].

Bacterial UTIs may also increase the risk for feline UTO, although the majority of cases do not involve infection [13, 36, 42, 47–49].

Cats with UTO vary widely in terms of clinical presentation [13]. All affected patients are said to be "blocked."

Most blocked cats present for the following [39, 42, 48, 50]:

- Dysuria
- Extruded penis
- Frequent visits to the litter box
- Hematuria
- House soiling
- Lack of urine produced in litter box
- Pollakiuria

- Pulsating prepuce, due to urethral spasms
- Stranguria

Some clients confuse straining to urinate with straining to defecate [50].

Blocked cats also often present for acute onset of anorexia and emesis [38].

Clients may find them in a state of collapse [38, 50].

On physical examination, blocked cats are often hypothermic [38].

The duration and severity of feline UTO dictates patient stability [13]. When obstruction of the urinary tract is complete and/or long-standing, electrolyte and acid–base abnormalities become life-threatening [13].

Azotemia, metabolic acidosis, and hyperkalemia are most commonly identified in critically ill cats with UTO [13, 38, 39, 50].

Hyperkalemia is the direct result of reduced glomerular filtration rate (GFR). When the GFR is adequate, potassium is excreted from the kidneys. When the GFR is compromised, potassium remains in the bloodstream, and concentrations build [39].

The body attempts to compensate by pushing potassium intracellularly [39, 51–53]. This action makes the inside of each cell less negative. This less negative resting potential makes depolarization of each cell more challenging [53]. One adverse effect is difficulty regulating heart rate and rhythm [39, 53].

Mild hyperkalemia causes bradycardia [13, 38].

As potassium levels continue to rise in the bloodstream, patients develop characteristic changes on the electrocardiogram (ECG). These include the following [13, 38]:

- Decreased to flattened P wave amplitude
- Prolonged P-R and Q-T intervals
- So-called "tented," meaning tall, T waves
- Widened QRS complexes

In addition, many blocked cats develop hypocalcemia [39]. Hypocalcemia prolongs the S-T and Q-T intervals [39, 51, 53]. This complicates heart rhythms by prolonging a portion of the action potential, the plateau phase [39].

As a direct result of metabolic disturbances, critically ill patients are likely to develop arrhythmias and weak peripheral pulses [13, 38, 48, 54, 55].

Blocked cats are diagnosed by abdominal palpation [9]. Blocked cats have rock-hard bladders that are firm to the touch [9, 38]. Affected urinary bladders are not compliant, not compressible, and are exceedingly painful. They may spontaneously rupture [9, 40].

Urethral plugs may or may not be evident at the penile tip [38]. Close inspection is important (see Figures 65.3a, b).

(a)

(b)

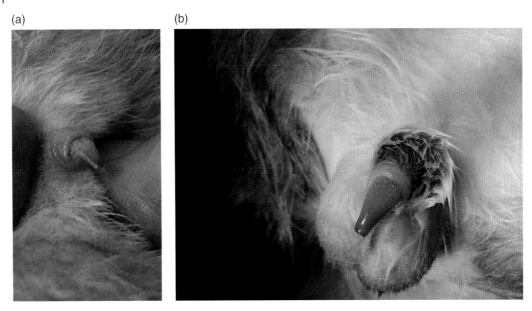

Figure 65.3 (a) Extruded penis from a tomcat. Note the purple discoloration at the penile tip. *Source:* Courtesy of Frank Isom, DVM. (b) Extruded penis from a tomcat. Note the blackish discoloration at the penile tip. *Source:* Courtesy of Joseph Onello, DVM.

Discoloration of the penile tip is common. It may be red due to self-mutilation, or purple-black from ischemic changes [38].

Blocked cats are medical emergencies [13, 38]. Cardiovascular stabilization is a priority, particularly for critically ill cats [13, 38]. Hyperkalemia must be addressed first because this imbalance will prove fatal to the cat before the blockage does [13, 38].

Intravenous (IV) access is vital to case management [13, 38].

Hypovolemic patients benefit from IV fluid therapy [13, 38]. Refer to an internal medicine textbook for additional details.

Obstruction is relieved via one of many commercially available urinary catheters, including the following [13, 38]:

- Tom Cat
- Olive-tipped
- Polyurethane
- Slippery Sam

Refer to an emergency medicine textbook for instructions on proper technique and common complications.

Once the obstruction is relieved, an indwelling red rubber catheter or comparable product is often placed [13, 38].

Post-obstructive diuresis is common [13, 38, 39, 56, 57]. Patients are at risk of worsening hypovolemia if fluid therapy is not aggressive [13]. Ideally, the patient remains in the hospital under observation for monitoring, measurement of ins and outs, and pain management.

The patient is typically not discharged from the hospital until its hydration has been reestablished and it has been observed to urinate on its own, once the urinary catheter has been pulled.

Re-obstruction is possible [37, 39, 41, 58]. Patients that routinely re-obstruct may benefit from perineal urethrostomy (PU) [13].

65.6 Neoplasia of the Lower Urinary Tract

Lower urinary tract neoplasia is relatively uncommon in dogs and cats [59–65]. When it occurs, lower urinary tract neoplasia is almost always malignant [63, 66–69].

The most common malignancy involving the lower urinary tract is transitional cell carcinoma (TCC) [11, 59–63, 65–69].

TCC usually targets the trigone of the urinary bladder [59]. However, it may extend into the urethra and/or prostate [59, 62]. Metastasis may be localized or extend to distant sites, including the liver, lungs, and skeleton [59, 61].

Females appear to be predisposed to TCC [59, 61–63, 67–70]. Certain breeds of dog are also overrepresented in the veterinary medical literature, including the following [59]:

- Beagles
- Miniature Poodles
- Miniature Schnauzers

- Scottish Terriers
- Shetland Sheepdogs
- West Highland White Terriers
- Wire-Haired Fox Terriers

Intact patients, both male and female, are less likely to develop TCC than those that are neutered [59].

The follow risk factors have been proposed [59, 61, 62, 71–74]:

- Exposure to lawn chemicals
- Exposure to pesticides, particularly older-generation flea preventatives
- Obesity

Ingestion of vegetables may be protective against TCC [75].

Patients with TCC often present with many of the same clinical signs that have previously been discussed with regards to urolithiasis and feline UTO [59, 61, 62]:

- Dysuria
- Hematuria
- Pollakiuria
- Stranguria

If metastasis to the skeleeton is present, then the patient may also present with lameness [61].

Secondary UTIs are common [59]. Patients may have previously been treated with apparent success for a UTI only to experience recurrence of clinical signs [59].

On physical examination, a mass may be palpable within the urinary bladder [59]. Thickening of the urethra may be detectable on rectal palpation in those patients with urethral involvement [59].

Ultrasonography will confirm a mass in the urinary bladder [59]. When a mass is detected within the urinary bladder, urine collection via cystocentesis should be avoided [59]. Cystocentesis risks seeding of the abdomen with neoplastic cells [59]. Urine collection should be via free catch or urinary catheterization [59].

Neoplastic cells may exfoliate into the sample of urine; however, they are difficult to differentiate from reactive epithelial cells, which result from urinary tract inflammation [59]. Histologic evaluation is necessary for diagnostic confirmation [59].

To obtain a sample for histopathology, the clinician may consider cystotomy, cystoscopy, or traumatic catheterization [59, 62, 76–78].

Note that TCC is not the only neoplasia to target the lower urinary tract. Other malignancies of the lower urinary tract include the following [59–69, 79–84]:

- Adenocarcinoma
- Fibrosarcoma
- Hemangiosarcoma
- Leiomyosarcoma
- Lymphoma
- Rhabdomyosarcoma
- Squamous cell carcinoma (SCC)
- Undifferentiated carcinoma

Management of urinary tract neoplasia is beyond the scope of this text. Recognize that surgical debulking of masses within the urinary bladder is possible; however, complete resection is typically not [59].

One benefit of surgical excision is that it restores urine flow [59]. Placement of ureteral stents or prepubic cystostomy catheters may be necessary to maintain flow once it has been reestablished, as the tumor is likely to continue to grow [59].

Systemic chemotherapy is often a mainstay of treatment in order to slow rate of tumor growth, thereby extending lifespan [59].

References

1 Schoeman, J.P. (ed.) (2008). Approach to polyuria and polydipsia in the dog. Proceedings of the 33rd World Small Animal Veterinary Congress; Dublin, Ireland: World Small Animal Veterinary Association (WSAVA).

2 Reece, W.O. (2004). Kidney function in mammals. In: *Dukes' Physiology of Domestic Animals*, 12e (ed. H.H. Dukes and W.O. Reece), 73–106. Ithaca: Comstock Pub. Associates.

3 Tilley, L.P. and Smith, F.W.K. (2004). *The 5-Minute Veterinary Consult: Canine and Feline*, 3e, lviii, 1487 p. Baltimore, MD: Lippincott Williams & Wilkins.

4 Senior, D.F. (2017). Acute kidney injury. Veterinary Team Brief [Internet]. https://www.veterinaryteambrief.com/article/acute-kidney-injury.

5 Nichols, R. (2001). Polyuria and polydipsia – diagnostic approach and problems associated with patient evaluation. *Vet. Clin. North Am. Small Anim. Pract.* 31 (5): 833–844.

6 Marks, S.L. and Taboada, J. (1998). Hypernatremia and hypertonic syndromes. *Vet. Clin. North Am. Small Anim. Pract.* 28 (3): 533–543.

7 Agarwal, S.K. and Gupta, A. (2008). Aquaporins: the renal water channels. *Indian J. Nephrol.* 18 (3): 95–100.

8 King, L.G. and Donaldson, M.T. (1994). Acute vomiting. *Vet. Clin. North Am. Small Anim. Pract.* 24 (6): 1189–1206.

9 Englar, R.E. (2017). *Performing the Small Animal Physical Examination*. Hoboken, NJ: Wiley.

10 DiBartola, S.P. and Bateman, S. (2006). Introduction to fluid therapy. In: *Fluid, Electrolyte, and Acid-Base Disorders in Small Animal Practice*, 3e (ed. S.P. DiBartola), 325–344. St. Louis, Mo: Saunders/Elsevier.

11 Fulkerson, C.M. and Knapp, D.W. (2015). Management of transitional cell carcinoma of the urinary bladder in dogs: a review. *Vet. J.* 205 (2): 217–225.

12 Cain, D.T., Battersby, I., and Doyle, R. (2016). Response of dogs with urinary tract obstructions secondary to prostatic carcinomas to the alpha-1 antagonist prazosin. *Vet. Rec.* 178 (4): 96.

13 Balakrishnan, A. and Drobatz, K.J. (2013). Management of urinary tract emergencies in small animals. *Vet. Clin. North Am. Small Anim. Pract.* 43 (4): 843–867.

14 Greco, D.S. (2012). Feline acromegaly. *Top. Companion Anim. Med.* 27 (1): 31–35.

15 Filippich, L.J. (2006). Cat with urinary tract signs. In: *Problem-Based Feline Medicine* (ed. J. Rand), 173–192. Edinburgh; New York: Saunders.

16 van Dongen, A.M. and L'Eplattenier, H.F. (2009). Kidneys and urinary tract. In: *Medical History and Physical Examination in Companion Animals*, 2e (ed. A. Rijnberk and F.J. van Sluijs), 101–107. St. Louis: Saunders Elsevier.

17 van Dongen, A.M. and L'Iplattenier, H.F. (2009). Kidneys and urinary tract. In: *Medical History and Physical Examination in Companion Animals* (ed. A. Rijnberk and F.J. van Sluijs), 101–107. St. Louis: Elsevier Limited.

18 Bartges, J.W., Kirk, C., and Lane, I.F. (2004). Update: management of calcium oxalate uroliths in dogs and cats. *Vet. Clin. North Am. Small Anim. Pract.* 34 (4): 969–987, vii.

19 Bartges, J.W. and Callens, A.J. (2015). Urolithiasis. *Vet. Clin. North Am. Small Anim. Pract.* 45 (4): 747–768.

20 Park, R.D. and Wrigley, R.H. (2002). The urinary bladder. In: *Textbook of Veterinary Diagnostic Radiology*, 4e (ed. D.E. Thrall), 571–592. Philadelphia: Saunders.

21 Feeney, D.A., Weichselbaum, R.C., Jessen, C.R., and Osborne, C.A. (1999). Imaging canine urocystoliths – detection and prediction of mineral content. *Vet. Clin. North Am. Small Anim. Pract.* 29 (1): 59–72.

22 Grauer, G.F. (2014). Ammonium urate urolithiasis. *Clinician's Brief* 51–55.

23 Weichselbaum, R.C., Feeney, D.A., Jessen, C.R. et al. (1998). Evaluation of the morphologic characteristics and prevalence of canine urocystoliths from a regional urolith center. *Am. J. Vet. Res.* 59 (4): 379–387.

24 Okafor, C.C., Pearl, D.L., Lefebvre, S.L. et al. (2013). Risk factors associated with struvite urolithiasis in dogs evaluated at general care veterinary hospitals in the United States. *J. Am. Vet. Med. Assoc.* 243 (12): 1737–1745.

25 Seaman, R. and Bartges, J.W. (2001). Canine struvite urolithiasis. *Comp Cont Educ Pract.* 23 (5): 407–420.

26 Palma, D., Langston, C., Gisselman, K., and McCue, J. (2013). Canine struvite urolithiasis. *Compendium* 35 (8): E1; quiz E.

27 Osborne, C.A., Polzin, D.J., Abdullahi, S.U. et al. (1985). Struvite urolithiasis in animals and man: formation, detection, and dissolution. *Adv. Vet. Sci. Comp. Med.* 29: 1–101.

28 Tarttelin, M.F. (1987). Feline struvite urolithiasis: factors affecting urine pH may be more important than magnesium levels in food. *Vet. Rec.* 121 (10): 227–230.

29 Lekcharoensuk, C., Lulich, J.P., Osborne, C.A. et al. (2000). Patient and environmental factors associated with calcium oxalate urolithiasis in dogs. *J. Am. Vet. Med. Assoc.* 217 (4): 515–519.

30 Osborne, C.A., Lulich, J.P., Kruger, J.M. et al. (2009). Analysis of 451,891 canine Uroliths, feline Uroliths, and feline urethral plugs from 1981 to 2007: perspectives from the Minnesota Urolith center. *Vet. Clin. North Am. Small Anim. Pract.* 39 (1): 183–197.

31 Osborne, C.A., Clinton, C.W., Bamman, L.K. et al. (1986). Prevalence of canine Uroliths – Minnesota-Urolith-center. *Vet. Clin. North Am. Small Anim. Pract.* 16 (1): 27–44.

32 Osborne, C.A., Lulich, J.P., Polzin, D.J. et al. (1999). Analysis of 77,000 canine uroliths – perspectives from the Minnesota Urolith center. *Vet Clin North Am. Small Anim. Pract.* 29 (1): 17–38.

33 Lulich, J.P., Osborne, C.A., and Bartges, J. (1999). Canine lower urinary tract disorders. In: *Textbook of Veterinary Internal Medicine: Diseases of the Dog and Cat*, 5e (ed. S.J. Ettinger and E.C. Feldman), 1747–1783. Philadelphia: W.B. Saunders.

34 Bartges, J.W., Osborne, C.A., Lulich, J.P. et al. (1994). Prevalence of cystine and urate uroliths in bulldogs and urate uroliths in dalmatians. *J. Am. Vet. Med. Assoc.* 204 (12): 1914–1918.

35 Gerber, B., Boretti, F.S., Kley, S. et al. (2005). Evaluation of clinical signs and causes of lower urinary tract disease in European cats. *J. Small Anim. Pract.* 46 (12): 571–577.

36 Kruger, J.M., Osborne, C.A., Goyal, S.M. et al. (1991). Clinical-evaluation of cats with lower urinary-tract disease. *J. Am. Vet. Med. Assoc.* 199 (2): 211–216.

37 Sumner, J.P. and Rishniw, M. (2017). Urethral obstruction in male cats in some northern United States shows regional seasonality. *Vet. J.* 220: 72–74.

38 George, C.M. and Grauer, G.F. (2016). Feline urethral obstruction: diagnosis and management. *Today's Veterinary Practice* (July/August): 36–46.

39 Thomovsky, E.J. (2011). Managing the common comorbidities of feline urethral obstruction. DVM 360 [Internet]. http://veterinarymedicine.dvm360.com/managing-common-comorbidities-feline-urethral-obstruction.

40 Little, S.E. (2012). The lower urinary tract. In: *The Cat: Clinical Medicine and Management*, 980–1013. St. Louis: Saunders.

41 Gerber, B., Eichenberger, S., and Reusch, C.E. (2008). Guarded long-term prognosis in male cats with urethral obstruction. *J. Feline Med. Surg.* 10 (1): 16–23.

42 Segev, G., Livne, H., Ranen, E., and Lavy, E. (2011). Urethral obstruction in cats: predisposing factors, clinical, clinicopathological characteristics and prognosis. *J. Feline Med. Surg.* 13 (2): 101–108.

43 Lund, H.S., Saevik, B.K., Finstad, O.W. et al. (2016). Risk factors for idiopathic cystitis in Norwegian cats: a matched case-control study. *J. Feline Med. Surg.* 18 (6): 483–491.

44 Forrester, S.D. and Towell, T.L. (2015). Feline idiopathic cystitis. *Vet. Clin. North Am. Small Anim. Pract.* 45 (4): 783–806.

45 Defauw, P.A., Van de Maele, I., Duchateau, L. et al. (2011). Risk factors and clinical presentation of cats with feline idiopathic cystitis. *J. Feline Med. Surg.* 13 (12): 967–975.

46 Cooper, E.S. (2015). Controversies in the management of feline urethral obstruction. *J. Vet. Emerg. Crit. Care (San Antonio)* 25 (1): 130–137.

47 Kruger, J.M., Osborne, C.A., and Lulich, J.P. (2008). Changing paradigms of feline idiopathic cystitis. *Vet. Clin. North Am. Small Anim. Pract.* 39: 15–40.

48 Lee, J.A. and Drobatz, K.J. (2003). Characterization of the clinical characteristics, electrolytes, acid-base, and renal parameters in male cats with urethral obstruction. *J. Vet. Emerg. Crit. Car.* 13 (4): 227–233.

49 Lekcharoensuk, C., Osborne, C.A., and Lulich, J.P. (2001). Epidemiologic study of risk factors for lower urinary tract diseases in cats. *J. Am. Vet. Med. Assoc.* 218 (9): 1429–1435.

50 Sabino, C.V. (2017). Urethral obstruction in cats. *Veterinary Team Brief* (April): 37–41.

51 DiBartola, S.P. and de Morais, H.A. (2006). Disorders of potassium: hypokalemia and hyperkalemia. In: *Fluid, Electroyte, and Acid Base Disorders in Small Animal Medicine* (ed. S.P. DiBartola), 91–121. St. Louis, MO: Elsevier.

52 Giebisch, G. and Windhager, E. (2005). Transport of potassium. In: *Medical Physiology: A Cellular and Molecular Approach* (ed. W.F. Boron and E.L. Boupaep), 814–827. Philadelphia: Elsevier.

53 Tag, T.L. and Day, T.K. (2008). Electrocardiographic assessment of hyperkalemia in dogs and cats. *J. Vet. Emerg. Crit. Care* 18 (1): 61–67.

54 Bass, M., Howard, J., Gerber, B., and Messmer, M. (2005). Retrospective study of indications for and outcome of perineal urethrostomy in cats. *J. Small Anim. Pract.* 46 (5): 227–231.

55 Lee, J.A. and Drobatz, K.J. (2006). Historical and physical parameters as predictors of severe hyperkalemia in male cats with urethral obstruction. *J. Vet. Emerg. Crit. Care* 16 (2): 104–111.

56 Francis, B.J., Wells, R.J., Rao, S., and Hackett, T.B. (2010). Retrospective study to characterize post-obstructive diuresis in cats with urethral obstruction. *J. Feline Med. Surg.* 12 (8): 606–608.

57 Baum, N., Anhalt, M., and Carlton, C.E. (1974). Post obstructive diuresis. *J. Urol.* 114: 53–56.

58 Ruda, L. and Heiene, R. (2012). Short- and long-term outcome after perineal urethrostomy in 86 cats with feline lower urinary tract disease. *J. Small Anim. Pract.* 53 (12): 693–698.

59 Knapp, D.W. and McMillan, S.K. (2013). Tumors of the urinary system. In: *Withrow and MacEwen's Small Animal Clinical Oncology*, 5e (ed. S.J. Withrow, D.M. Vail and R.L. Page), 572–582. St. Louis: Elsevier.

60 Valli, V.E., Norris, A., Jacobs, R.M. et al. (1995). Pathology of canine bladder and urethral cancer and correlation with tumour progression and survival. *J. Comp. Pathol.* 113 (2): 113–130.

61 Mutsaers, A.J., Widmer, W.R., and Knapp, D.W. (2003). Canine transitional cell carcinoma. *J. Vet. Intern. Med.* 17 (2): 136–144.

62 Knapp, D.W., Glickman, N.W., Denicola, D.B. et al. (2000). Naturally-occurring canine transitional cell carcinoma of the urinary bladder a relevant model of human invasive bladder cancer. *Urol. Oncol.* 5 (2): 47–59.

63 Norris, A.M., Laing, E.J., Valli, V.E. et al. (1992). Canine bladder and urethral tumors: a retrospective study of 115 cases (1980–1985). *J. Vet. Intern. Med.* 6 (3): 145–153.

64 Nikula, K.J., Benjamin, S.A., Angleton, G.M., and Lee, A.C. (1989). Transitional cell carcinomas of the urinary tract in a colony of beagle dogs. *Vet. Pathol.* 26 (6): 455–461.

65 Capasso, A., Raiano, V., Sontuoso, A. et al. (2015). Fibrosarcoma of the urinary bladder in a cat. *JFMS Open Rep.* 1 (1): 2055116915585019.

66 Osborne, C.A., Low, D.G., Perman, V., and Barnes, D.M. (1968). Neoplasms of the canine and feline urinary bladder: incidence, etiologic factors, occurrence and pathologic features. *Am. J. Vet. Res.* 29 (10): 2041–2055.

67 Strafuss, A.C. and Dean, M.J. (1975). Neoplasms of the canine urinary bladder. *J. Am. Vet. Med. Assoc.* 166 (12): 1161–1163.

68 Tarvin, G., Patnaik, A., and Greene, R. (1978). Primary urethral tumors in dogs. *J. Am. Vet. Med. Assoc.* 172 (8): 931–933.

69 Wilson, G.P., Hayes, H.M., and Casey, H.W. (1979). Canine urethral cancer. *J. Am. Anim. Hosp. Assoc.* 15 (6): 741–744.

70 Caywood, D.D., Osborne, C.A., and Johnston, G.R. (1980). Neoplasms of the canine and feline urinary tract. In: *Current Veterinary Therapy VII* (ed. R.W. Kirk), 1203–1212. Philadelphia: WB Saunders.

71 Glickman, L.T., Raghavan, M., Knapp, D.W. et al. (2004). Herbicide exposure and the risk of transitional cell carcinoma of the urinary bladder in Scottish terriers. *J. Am. Vet. Med. Assoc.* 224 (8): 1290–1297.

72 Glickman, L.T., Schofer, F.S., McKee, L.J. et al. (1989). Epidemiologic study of insecticide exposures, obesity, and risk of bladder cancer in household dogs. *J. Toxicol. Environ. Health* 28 (4): 407–414.

73 Bryan, J.N., Keeler, M.R., Henry, C.J. et al. (2007). A population study of neutering status as a risk factor for canine prostate cancer. *Prostate* 67 (11): 1174–1181.

74 Raghavan, M., Knapp, D.W., Dawson, M.H. et al. (2004). Topical flea and tick pesticides and the risk of transitional cell carcinoma of the urinary bladder in Scottish terriers. *J. Am. Vet. Med. Assoc.* 225 (3): 389–394.

75 Raghavan, M., Knapp, D.W., Bonney, P.L. et al. (2005). Evaluation of the effect of dietary vegetable consumption on reducing risk of transitional cell carcinoma of the urinary bladder in Scottish terriers. *J. Am. Vet. Med. Assoc.* 227 (1): 94–100.

76 Childress, M.O., Adams, L.G., Ramos-Vara, J.A. et al. (2011). Results of biopsy via transurethral cystoscopy and cystotomy for diagnosis of transitional cell carcinoma of the urinary bladder and urethra in dogs: 92 cases (2003–2008). *J. Am. Vet. Med. Assoc.* 239 (3): 350–356.

77 Messer, J.S., Chew, D.J., and McLoughlin, M.A. (2005). Cystoscopy: techniques and clinical applications. *Clin. Tech. Small Anim. Pract.* 20 (1): 52–64.

78 Holak, P., Nowicki, M., Adamiak, Z., and Kasprowicz, A. (2007). Applicability of endoscopic examination as a diagnostic approach in urinary tract ailments in dogs. *Pol. J. Vet. Sci.* 10 (4): 233–238.

79 Liptak, J.M., Dernell, W.S., and Withrow, S.J. (2004). Haemangiosarcoma of the urinary bladder in a dog. *Aust. Vet. J.* 82 (4): 215–217.

80 Heng, H.G., Lowry, J.E., Boston, S. et al. (2006). Smooth muscle neoplasia of the urinary bladder wall in three dogs. *Vet. Radiol. Ultrasound* 47 (1): 83–86.

81 Benigni, L., Lamb, C.R., Corzo-Menendez, N. et al. (2006). Lymphoma affecting the urinary bladder in three dogs and a cat. *Vet. Radiol. Ultrasound* 47 (6): 592–596.

82 Bae, I.H., Kim, Y., Pakhrin, B. et al. (2007). Genitourinary rhabdomyosarcoma with systemic metastasis in a young dog. *Vet. Pathol.* 44 (4): 518–520.

83 Kessler, M., Kandel-Tschiederer, B., Pfleghaar, S., and Tassani-Prell, M. (2008). Primary malignant lymphoma of the urinary bladder in a dog: longterm remission following treatment with radiation and chemotherapy. *Schweiz. Arch. Tierheilkd.* 150 (11): 565–569.

84 Gelberg, H.B. (2010). Urinary bladder mass in a dog. *Vet. Pathol.* 47 (1): 181–184.

66

Grossly Abnormal Urine

66.1 Introduction to Visible Characteristics of Urine

Normal urine varies in terms of shade of yellow, based upon its degree of concentration [1, 2].

The first urine sample of the morning is typically more concentrated, such that it is a stronger shade of yellow, as compared to a sample that is taken later in the day [2] (see Figure 66.1a). Urine can also be made more dilute by drinking large quantities of water or by the administration of intravenous (IV) fluid therapy (see Figure 66.1b).

Normal urine is yellow because it contains partially oxidized urobilinogen [1, 2]. Urobilinogen is excreted by the kidney as a by-product of bilirubin metabolism [1].

Abnormal urine color may result from pathology. Colors that appear routinely in clinical practice as a result of underlying disease include the following [2]:

- Brown, as in myoglobinuria
  - Myoglobin is present in muscle.
  - Rhabdomyolysis results in myoglobinuria.
- Cream or muddy, as in macroscopic pyuria, leukocyte-containing urine
  - Leukocytes may be present in urine secondary to urinary tract infections (UTIs) or prostatic abscesses.
  - Leukocytes may also be present in cases of sterile cystitis, secondary to inflammation of the lower urinary tract.
- Orange
  - Orange discoloration of the urine may indicate significantly concentrated urine, as occurs during extreme cases of dehydration.
  - Orange discoloration of the urine may also indicate bilirubinuria secondary to hepatic or biliary dysfunction.
- Red, as in macroscopic hematuria, blood-containing urine
  - Erythrocytes may be present in urine secondary to UTIs.
  - Erythrocytes may result from urolithiasis causing abrasive injury to the lining of the lower urinary tract.
  - Erythrocytes may also be present in cases of sterile cystitis, secondary to inflammation of the lower urinary tract (see Figures 66.2a–e).

Normal canine and feline urine should be relatively translucent [1, 2]. Opacities may develop when urine contains excessive amounts of the following [1, 2]:

- Fat droplets
- Mucus
- Precipitates
  - Carbonates
  - Phosphates
  - Urates
- Prostatic fluid
- Sperm (see Figure 66.3)

Turbidity of urine may also result from pathology. For example, the presence of erythrocytes in urine, hematuria, and the presence of leukocytes in urine, pyuria, may make urine less translucent (see Figures 66.4a, b).

Urine samples should also be examined microscopically. Urine samples may not outwardly appear to contain blood or pus; however, they may show evidence of microscopic hematuria or pyuria (see Figures 66.5a, b).

Microscopic assessment of the urine can also reveal the presence of the following:

- Bacteria
  - Cocci
  - Rods
- Casts
- Fat droplets
- Urinary crystals (see Figures 66.6a–c)

Be aware of the potential for urine contamination [2]. For example, free-catch samples are likely to contain debris [2] (see Figure 66.7).

Common Clinical Presentations in Dogs and Cats, First Edition. Ryane E. Englar.
© 2019 John Wiley & Sons, Inc. Published 2019 by John Wiley & Sons, Inc.

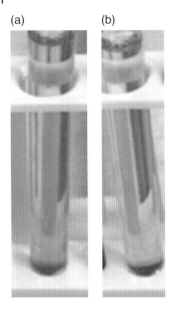

Figure 66.1 (a) First morning catch. Note how concentrated the urine is. (b) As a direct comparison to (a), note that this urine sample is dilute. This patient was receiving intravenous (IV) fluid therapy.

Debris may include bacteria that are commensal organisms from the perineum. Debris may also include bacteria from the environment.

Refer to a clinical pathology textbook to review specific details about urinalysis sediment preparation and examination.

The purpose of this chapter is not to be comprehensive, but to provide a broad overview of one of the most common causes of grossly abnormal urine on visual inspection in clinical practice: hematuria [2].

66.2 Causes of Hematuria

There are many causes of hematuria, including the following [2–17]:

- Bleeding disorders***
  - Coagulopathy
  - Thrombocytopenia
- Estrus (see Chapter 61, Section 61.2)
- Glomerulopathy
- Heatstroke (see Chapter 38, Section 38.4.5.2)
- Infection
  - Kidney (see Chapter 63, Section 63.4.2)
  - Uterus
    - Pyometra*** (see Chapter 61, Section 61.7)
  - UTI***
  - Vagina
- Inflammation
  - Cystitis***

- Idiopathic
  - Feline idiopathic cystitis***
  - Infectious
- Metritis
- Prostatitis (see Chapter 59, Section 59.2)
- Pyelonephritis (see Chapter 63, Section 63.4.2)
- Urethritis
- Vaginitis (see Chapter 61, Section 61.9)
- Neoplasia
  - Kidney
  - Penis (see Chapter 56, Section 56.3)
  - Prepuce
  - Urethra***
  - Urinary bladder*** (see Chapter 65, Section 65.6)
  - Uterus
  - Vagina
  - Vulva
- Prostatic cyst or abscess
- Urethral tear
- Urolithiasis***
- Trauma

Items that are starred above (***) are common clinical presentations in companion animal practice.

UTI and feline idiopathic cystitis (FIC) will be discussed in greater depth below.

66.3 Urinary Tract Infections

UTIs typically result from ascension of skin and gastrointestinal tract flora through the lower urinary tract [12–14]. When one or more of these bacterial species takes up residence and colonizes the urinary tract, a UTI is established.

In female cats and dogs, as compared to males, the distance between the anus and the opening to the urinary tract is small [7]. In addition, the urethra is short and wide [7]. This increases the risk of colonization with bacteria from the digestive tract [7].

To protect against UTIs, the body has a number of inherent defense mechanisms. These include the following [6, 7, 18–20]:

- Commensal flora
- Glycosaminoglycan layer
- Tissue folds along the length of the proximal urethra for bacteria trapping
- Unidirectional flow of urine
- Urine composition
  - High levels of urea
  - High levels of organic acids
- Urine concentration
  - High osmolality

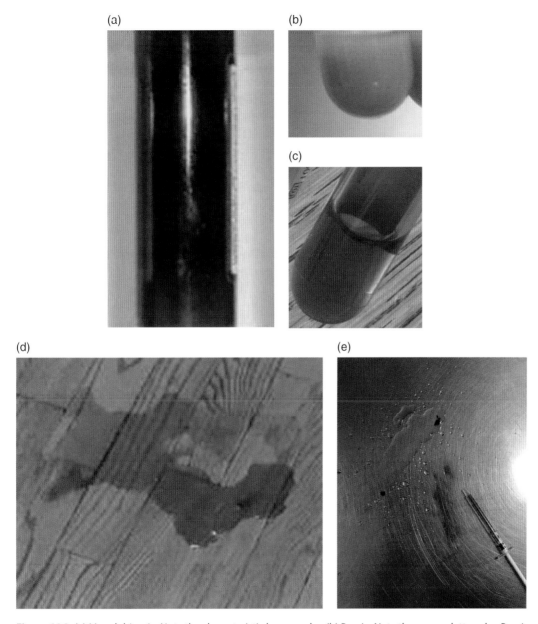

Figure 66.2 (a) Myoglobinuria. Note the characteristic brown color. (b) Pyuria. Note the creamy latte color. Pyuria may also appear cloudy white. (c) Bilirubinuria. Note the characteristic orange color. (d) Macroscopic hematuria on a household floor. *Source:* Courtesy of Ballroom Dance School Manhattan. (e) Macroscopic hematuria on a stainless steel table. Note the presence of a blood clot within the urine itself. *Source:* Courtesy of Brynn Zittle.

Feline urine is especially concentrated [7]. It is not uncommon for cats to have a urine specific gravity (USG) of greater than 1.045 [7, 20].

In light of the defense mechanisms outlined above, UTIs affects cats less often than dogs [7, 21].

In both species, the following risk factors increase the likelihood of UTI development [7, 12–14, 16, 17, 22–24]:

- Abnormal urinary tract anatomy
  - Ectopic ureter
  - Recessed vulva

- Bladder atony
- Bladder mucosa abnormalities
- Endocrinopathy
  - Diabetes mellitus
  - Hyperadrenocorticism
  - Hyperthyroidism
  - Hypoadrenocorticism
- Glycosuria
- Immunosuppression
- Indwelling urinary catheters
  - Associated with urethral irritation

- Neoplasia of the urinary tract
- Perivulvar dermatitis
- Pharmacologic therapy
  - Chemotherapy
  - Corticosteroids
- Prostatitis
- Recent antibiotic therapy
- Urinary surgery
  - Perineal urethrostomy
    ○ May cause urethral incompetence

Canine bacterial UTIs are relatively common in clinical practice [13]. Fourteen percent of dogs develop at least one UTI throughout life [13, 25]. Four percent of dogs may develop persistent and/or recurrent UTIs [13, 25–27].

Recall from Chapter 65, Section 65.4 that canine UTIs are often associated with struvite stone formation, particularly in young females [28–31]. *Staphylococcus, Enterococcus,* and *Proteus* spp. produce the enzyme urease [29, 32]. Urease catalyzes the hydrolysis of urea to produce ammonia [29, 32]. Ammonia makes the urine more alkaline. Alkaline urine promotes the formation of struvites [33].

By contrast, feline UTIs are less often linked to urolithiasis. Age is a risk factor for cats. Cats are more likely

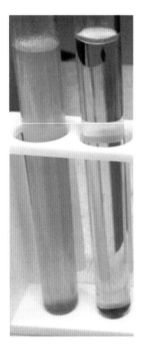

Figure 66.3 Two urine samples. The sample on the left is turbid. This gives the urine a cloudy appearance as compared to the sample on the right, which is translucent.

(a)

(b)

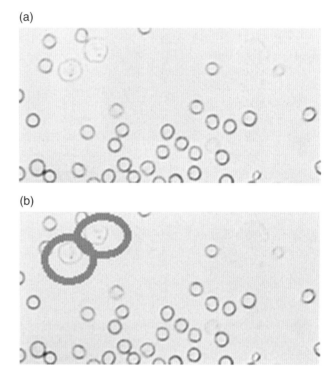

Figure 66.5 (a) Microscopic confirmation of the presence of erythrocytes and leukocytes in an unstained urine sample, as viewed under light microscopy. The leukocytes are approximately twice the size of erythrocytes. (b) Same photograph as in (a); however, the two leukocytes have been outlined in orange. The other cells on the unstained slide are erythrocytes.

(a)   (b)

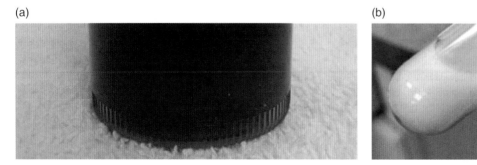

Figure 66.4 (a) Macroscopic hematuria. Note how the presence of erythrocytes in this urine sample has changed not only the color of the urine, but its translucency. The urine is now more turbid. (b) Macroscopic pyuria. Note how the presence of leukocytes in this urine sample has changed not only the color of the urine, but its translucency. The urine is now more turbid.

(a)   (b)   (c)

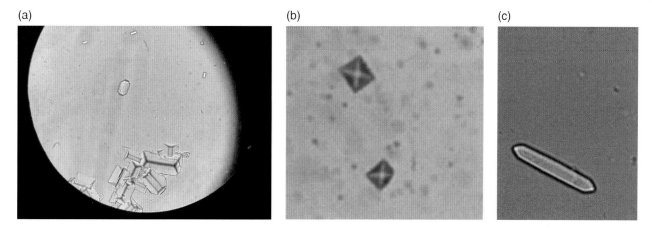

Figure 66.6 (a) Struvituria. *Source:* Courtesy of Kelli L. Crisfulli, RVT. (b) Calcium oxalate dihydrate crystals. (c) Isolated calcium oxalate monohydrate crystal.

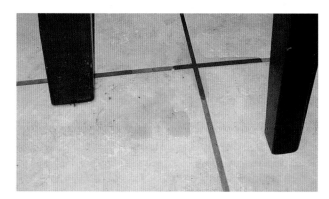

Figure 66.7 Urinary accident on a household floor. This could constitute a free-catch sample. Note that the results from a microscopic examination of this sample must be taken with a grain of salt. The sample is likely to contain bacteria, among other debris. It would be difficult to discern if the bacteria are from the patient's urinary tract, as in the case of a true urinary tract infection (UTI), or if they are environmental contaminants. *Source:* Courtesy of Tara Beugel.

to develop bacterial cystitis when they are older than 10 years of age [22]. Prior to then, UTIs represent less than 2% of lower urinary tract disease in the cat [22].

Cats with chronic renal failure (CRF), otherwise known as chronic kidney disease (CKD), are also more likely to have UTIs [22]. The dilute nature of the urine predisposes this subset of the population to UTIs [22]. Dilute urine also presents a challenge for the diagnostician: UTIs may go undetected on routine urinalysis and often require a culture for diagnosis [22].

Age is also a risk factor for development of UTI in dogs [13]. Older dogs are most at risk [13, 34–37]. Of these, females are overrepresented [13, 34–37].

UTIs may be subclinical, in both dogs and cats [7, 13].

When patients are symptomatic, they present with signs of lower urinary tract disease, including the following [6, 7, 13, 22]:

- Dysuria
- Hematuria
- House soiling/urinating outside of the litter box
- Pollakiuria
- Stranguria

Most UTIs are bacterial and are caused by aerobes [22]. The most common bacterial isolates in both dogs are cats include the following [7, 13, 14, 21, 22, 26, 27, 34, 37]:

- *Enterococcus* spp.
  - *Enterococcus faecalis*
- *Escherichia coli*
- *Streptococcus* spp.

Other species that are routinely cultured include the following [7, 14, 22, 34, 38, 39]:

- *Enterobacter*
- *Klebsiella*
- *Pasteurella*
- *Proteus*
- *Pseudomonas*
- *Staphylococcus* spp.
  - *Staphylococcus aureus*
  - *Staphylococcus bovis*
  - *Staphylococcus intermedius*

Mycoplasma and *Ureaplasma* species are occasionally involved, but require special culture media for growth [22]. *Corynebacterium urealyticum*, in cats, can also be difficult to grow *in vitro* [7].

Although fungal and viral cystitis are possible, they are rare [14]. Immunocompromised patients are most at risk and may succumb to fungal UTI with either *Aspergillus fumigatus* or *Candida albicans* [14, 22, 40–42]. Fungal elements may be identified on urine sediment examination, or fungal culture may be necessary [14].

66.4 Diagnostic Work-Up for UTIs

Urinalysis and culture with sensitivity testing are the primary diagnostic tools for detection of bacterial UTI [22].

Urinalysis may be performed on samples that were collected by the following [2]:

- "Free catch"; that is, catching what the patient voided
- Cystocentesis
- Urinary catheterization

Recognize that free-catch samples are likely to contain debris and bacterial contaminants, which may lead one to infer that a UTI is present when it is not [2].

Urinalysis should be performed within 30 min of sample collection [2]. If samples cannot be evaluated within this time frame, then they ought to be refrigerated until analysis is possible [2]. Prior to analysis, they will need to be brought back to room temperature in order to improve test accuracy [2].

Urinalysis consists of the following [2, 7]:

- Gross observation of the urine
- Dipstick analysis [2, 43–45]
- Examination of the urine sediment using light microscopy
- USG

A brief review of each component will be discussed at this time. Refer to a clinical pathology textbook for additional details. An exhaustive review of urinalysis is beyond the scope of this text.

Gross observation of the urine includes visual assessment of the following [2, 7]:

- Clarity of urine
  - Translucency
  - Turbidity
- Color of urine
- Volume of urine collected

Dipstick analysis evaluates urine for the following [2, 7]:

- Bilirubin
  - Low levels (trace levels to +1) in concentrated dog urine, particularly males, is normal.
  - It is never normal to see bilirubinuria in cats [43].
- Glucose
  - When glucose exceeds 180–220 mg/dl in the dog and 260–280 mg/dl in the cat, glucose will spill into the urine [46].
  - Glycosuria may be due to stress hyperglycemia, particularly in cats.
  - Glycosuria may also be due to true pathology, such as diabetes mellitus or renal tubular disease.
- Heme, or occult blood
  - Detects heme protein in the urine
    - Intact erythrocytes
    - Hemoglobin
    - Myoglobin
  - Note that a false positive reaction can occur if cystocentesis resulted in microscopic hematuria
- Ketones
  - Dipsticks detect acetoacetate >>> acetone.
  - Dipsticks do not detect β-hydroxybutyrate.
- pH
  - Largely dependent upon the patient's diet
    - Meat-based diets will cause aciduria.
    - Plant-based diets will cause alkalinuria.
      - Other causes of alkalinuria include
        - Post-prandial alkaline tide
        - Urease-containing bacterial UTI
  - In general, canine and feline urinary pH ranges from 5.0 to 7.5
- Protein
  - Albumin is the primary protein that is detected
  - Proteinuria may be physiologic:
    - Exercise
    - Fever
    - Seizure activity
    - Stress
  - Proteinuria may be pathologic:
    - Congestive heart failure
    - Glomerular disease
    - Hemorrhage
    - Lower urinary tract inflammation
    - Upper urinary tract inflammation
  - False negatives are common if urine is dilute or acidic
  - False positives are common if urine is concentrated or alkaline.
  - False positives may be more likely to occur in cats.
- Readings for bilirubin and ketones may be inaccurate if urine is discolored.
- The following measurements are unreliable in dogs and cats:
  - Leukocyte esterase
  - Nitrate
  - Urobilinogen

Examination of the urine sediment using light microscopy provides additional details:

- Amorphous debris
- Bacteria
- Epithelial cells
- Erythrocytes
- Fat droplets
- Leukocytes
- Urinary casts
- Urinary crystals
- Yeast

USG must be considered in light of the patient's

- Blood urea nitrogen (BUN) and creatinine
- Fluid therapy
- Hydration status.

When a patient has a UTI, common findings on urinalysis include the following [22]:

- Macroscopic or microscopic hematuria
- Macroscopic or microscopic pyuria
- Proteinuria

Both proteinuria and pyuria indicate lower urinary tract inflammation, and are supportive of a diagnosis of cystitis [22].

The presence of intracellular bacteria is confirmatory for UTI; however, bacteria can be missed on sediment examination.

Urine culture is beneficial in terms of providing a definitive diagnosis [7].

Antibiotic therapy should be selected based upon culture and sensitivity results [14, 15, 22]. Although response to therapy is encouraging, it is important to repeat urinalysis and bacterial culture to guide treatment decisions, including when to stop therapy [22].

Refer to an internal medicine textbook for more information as to the typical duration of treatment.

Abdominal imaging should be performed to rule out concurrent urolithiasis.

66.5 Feline Idiopathic Cystitis

FIC, also referred to as feline urologic syndrome (FUS), is the most common cause of feline lower urinary tract disease (FLUTD) [8, 9, 22, 24, 47–50].

FIC is characterized as a self-limiting, but recurring syndrome of sterile, hemorrhagic cystitis [8, 22, 47, 51–54].

Risk factors for FIC are thought to include the following [9, 22]:

- Inactivity
- Indoor lifestyle
- Conflict between members of the household
- Long coated cats
- Multi-cat household
- Purebred cats
- Obesity
- Stress

FIC appears to mirror a similar syndrome in humans, interstitial cystitis. Humans with interstitial cystitis have abnormal bladder structure and/or innervation [22]. The urinary bladder is essentially overstimulated, and there is increased sympathetic outflow [22].

This condition is painful [22]. The inflammatory response may be perpetuated by the increased concentrations of mast cells as well as increased permeability of the bladder wall [8, 22, 55–60].

Patients typically present with a history of the following [8, 22]:

- Dysuria
- Hematuria
- House soiling
- Pollakiuria
- Stranguria

Voided urine may contain frank blood or blood clots [22].

Patients may vocalize during urination [22]. Patients may posture often to urinate, without producing large quantities of urine [22]. To an outside observer, the patient may appear to be "blocked." Refer to Chapter 65, Section 65.5 for a discussion of feline urinary tract obstruction (UTO).

Recall that blocked cats are diagnosed by abdominal palpation [61]. Blocked cats have rock-hard bladders that are firm to the touch [61, 62]. These bladders are not compliant or compressible. Affected cats are exceedingly painful. Blocked bladders are at risk of spontaneous rupture [61, 63].

By contrast, cats with FIC have small, contracted urinary bladders [22]. Their bladders are too painful to fill, hence the frequency with which affected patients attempt urination [22].

Diagnosis of FIC is by exclusion [22]. The astute clinician may suspect it based upon history and physical examination. However, the clinician must rule out UTI, urolithiasis, and urinary neoplasia before giving the patient a label of FIC.

On urinalysis, hematuria predominates over pyuria in cases of FIC [22]. Despite the presence of cystitis, it would be unusual to see more than five leukocytes per high-powered field (HPF) in a cat with FIC [22]. The urine is sterile; that is, no bacteria is identified on sediment analysis of the urine, and a culture is negative for bacterial growth [22].

Urinary crystals are rarely present [22]. If they are, they are typically a reflection of urinary pH as opposed to instigators of disease.

Abdominal radiographs are negative for urolithiasis [22]. If contrast radiography is used, it may highlight a thickened bladder wall. This thickening may also be detected on ultrasonography; however, it is difficult to confirm because the urinary bladders of FIC cats are small. Therefore, the wall appears thicker than one might normally expect.

Behavioral causes of inappropriate urination are effectively ruled out because these do not cause hematuria [22].

Patients are managed supportively with analgesia [22]. Clinical signs are self-limiting, but their resolution can be expedited by taking measures to improve patient comfort [22]. Some patients may benefit from antispasmodic drugs and/or amitriptyline for its anti-inflammatory and analgesic properties [22].

Strategies to reduce stress and improve household management may also facilitate recovery [22].

References

1 Reece, W.O. (2004). Kidney function in mammals. In: *Dukes' Physiology of Domestic Animals*. 12 (ed. H.H. Dukes and W.O. Reece), 73–106. Ithaca: Comstock Pub. Associates.

2 Grauer, G.F. and Pohlman, L.M. (2016). Urinalysis interpretation. *NAVC Clinician's Brief* (March): 93–101.

3 Daniel, G. and Labato, M.A. (2017). Hematuria in dogs. *NAVC Clinician's Brief* (November): 32–33.

4 Rebar, A.H. (2008). Hematuria in a dog. *NAVC Clinician's Brief*.

5 Galemore, E. and Labato, M.A. (2016). Recurrent hematuria in a dog. *NAVC Clinician's Brief* (December): 86–89.

6 Bartges, J. and Burns, K.M. (2017). Lower urinary tract signs in a cat. *NAVC Clinician's Brief* (September): 35–39.

7 Litster, A., Thompson, M., Moss, S., and Trott, D. (2011). Feline bacterial urinary tract infections: an update on an evolving clinical problem. *Vet. J.* 187 (1): 18–22.

8 Kruger, J.M., Osborne, C.A., and Lulich, J.P. (2008). Changing paradigms of feline idiopathic cystitis. *Vet. Clin. North Am. Small Anim. Pract.* 39: 15–40.

9 Defauw, P.A., Van de Maele, I., Duchateau, L. et al. (2011). Risk factors and clinical presentation of cats with feline idiopathic cystitis. *J. Feline Med. Surg.* 13 (12): 967–975.

10 Callens, A. and Bartges, J. (2016). Update on feline urolithiasis. In: *August's Consultations in Feline Internal Medicine* (ed. S.E. Little), 499–508. St. Louis: Elsevier, Inc.

11 White, J.D., Norris, J.M., Bosward, K.L. et al. (2008). Persistent haematuria and proteinuria due to glomerular disease in related Abyssinian cats. *J. Feline Med. Surg.* 10 (3): 219–229.

12 Dowling, P.M. (2018). Bacterial urinary tract infections. Merck Veterinary Manual [Internet]. https://www.merckvetmanual.com/pharmacology/systemic-pharmacotherapeutics-of-the-urinary-system/bacterial-urinary-tract-infections.

13 Thompson, M.F., Litster, A.L., Platell, J.L., and Trott, D.J. (2011). Canine bacterial urinary tract infections: new developments in old pathogens. *Vet. J.* 190 (1): 22–27.

14 Olin, S.J. and Bartges, J.W. (2015). Urinary tract infections: treatment/comparative therapeutics. *Vet. Clin. North Am. Small Anim. Pract.* 45 (4): 721–746.

15 Jessen, L.R., Sorensen, T.M., Bjornvad, C.R. et al. (2015). Effect of antibiotic treatment in canine and feline urinary tract infections: a systematic review. *Vet. J.* 203 (3): 270–277.

16 Ogeer-Gyles, J., Mathews, K., Weese, J.S. et al. (2006). Evaluation of catheter-associated urinary tract infections and multi-drug-resistant *Escherichia coli* isolates from the urine of dogs with indwelling urinary catheters. *J. Am. Vet. Med. Assoc.* 229 (10): 1584–1590.

17 Adams, L.G. (2010). Diagnosing and managing recurrent urinary tract infections. DVM 360 [Internet]. http://veterinarycalendar.dvm360.com/diagnosing-and-managing-recurrent-urinary-tract-infections-proceedings.

18 Blanco, L.J. and Bartges, J.W. (2001). Understanding and eradicating bacterial urinary tract infections. *Vet. Med.* 96 (10): 776–790.

19 Bartges, J.W. (2005). Bacterial urinary tract infections – simple and complicated. *Vet. Med.* 100 (3): 224–+.

20 Lees, G.E. and Rogers, K.S. (1986). Treatment of urinary tract infections in dogs and cats. *J. Am. Vet. Med. Assoc.* 189 (6): 648–652.

21 Bartges, J. and Barsanti, J.A. (2000). Bacterial urinary tract infections in cats. In: *Current Veterinary Therapy XIII* (ed. J.D. Bonagura), 880–882. Philaldelphia: WB Saunders Co.

22 Filippich, L.J. (2006). Cat with urinary tract signs. In: *Problem-Based Feline Medicine* (ed. J. Rand), 173–192. Edinburgh; New York: Saunders.

23 Gregory, C.R. and Vasseur, P.B. (1983). Long-term examination of cats with perineal urethrostomy. *Vet. Surg.* 12 (4): 210–212.

24 Lekcharoensuk, C., Osborne, C.A., and Lulich, J.P. (2001). Epidemiologic study of risk factors for lower urinary tract diseases in cats. *J. Am. Vet. Med. Assoc.* 218 (9): 1429–1435.

25 Ling, G.V. (1984). Therapeutic strategies involving antimicrobial treatment of the canine urinary tract. *J. Am. Vet. Med. Assoc.* 185 (10): 1162–1164.

26 Norris, C.R., Williams, B.J., Ling, G.V. et al. (2000). Recurrent and persistent urinary tract infections in dogs: 383 cases (1969–1995). *J. Am. Anim. Hosp. Assoc.* 36 (6): 484–492.

27 Seguin, M.A., Vaden, S.L., Altier, C. et al. (2003). Persistent urinary tract infections and reinfections in 100 dogs (1989–1999). *J. Vet. Intern. Med.* 17 (5): 622–631.

28 Okafor, C.C., Pearl, D.L., Lefebvre, S.L. et al. (2013). Risk factors associated with struvite urolithiasis in dogs evaluated at general care veterinary hospitals in the United States. *J. Am. Vet. Med. A* 243 (12): 1737–1745.

29 Bartges, J.W. and Callens, A.J. (2015). Urolithiasis. *Vet. Clin. North Am. Small Anim. Pract.* 45 (4): 747–768.

30 Seaman, R. and Bartges, J.W. (2001). Canine struvite urolithiasis. *Compend. Contin. Educ. Pract. Vet.* 23 (5): 407–429.

31 Palma, D., Langston, C., Gisselman, K., and McCue, J. (2013). Canine struvite urolithiasis. *Compendium* 35 (8): E1; quiz E.

32 Osborne, C.A., Polzin, D.J., Abdullahi, S.U. et al. (1985). Struvite urolithiasis in animals and man: formation, detection, and dissolution. *Adv. Vet. Sci. Comp. Med.* 29: 1–101.

33 Tarttelin, M.F. (1987). Feline struvite urolithiasis: factors affecting urine pH may be more important than magnesium levels in food. *Vet. Rec.* 121 (10): 227–230.

34 Ling, G.V., Norris, C.R., Franti, C.E. et al. (2001). Interrelations of organism prevalence, specimen collection method, and host age, sex, and breed among 8,354 canine urinary tract infections (1969–1995). *J. Vet. Intern. Med.* 15 (4): 341–347.

35 Kivisto, A.K., Vasenius, H., and Sandholm, M. (1977). Canine Bacteriuria. *J. Small Anim. Pract.* 18: 707–712.

36 Bush, B.M. (1978). The incidence of significant bacteriuria in the dog. *Tijdschr. Diergeneeskd.* 103 (14): 750–757.

37 Cohn, L.A., Gary, A.T., Fales, W.H., and Madsen, R.W. (2003). Trends in fluoroquinolone resistance of bacteria isolated from canine urinary tracts. *J. Vet. Diagn. Investig.* 15 (4): 338–343.

38 Litster, A., Moss, S.M., Honnery, M. et al. (2007). Prevalence of bacterial species in cats with clinical signs of lower urinary tract disease: recognition of Staphylococcus felis as a possible feline urinary tract pathogen. *Vet. Microbiol.* 121 (1–2): 182–188.

39 Barsanti, J.A. (2012). Genitourinary infections. In: *Infectious Diseases of the Dog and Cat* (ed. C.E. Greene), 1013–1031. St. Louis, MO: Elsevier Saunders.

40 Pressler, B.M. (2011). Urinary tract infections – fungal. In: *Nephrology and Urology of Small Animals* (ed. D.J. Polzin and J. Bartges), 717–724. Ames, IA: Blackwell Publishing.

41 Pressler, B.M., Vaden, S.L., Lane, I.F. et al. (2003). *Candida* spp. urinary tract infections in 13 dogs and seven cats: predisposing factors, treatment, and outcome. *J. Am. Anim. Hosp. Assoc.* 39 (3): 263–270.

42 Jin, Y. and Lin, D. (2005). Fungal urinary tract infections in the dog and cat: a retrospective study (2001–2004). *J. Am. Anim. Hosp. Assoc.* 41 (6): 373–381.

43 Wamsley, H. and Alleman, R. (2017). Complete urinalysis. In: *BSAVA Manual of Canine and Feline Nephrology and Urology*, 3e (ed. J. Elliott, G.F. Grauer and J.L. Westropp), 60–83. Quedgeley, UK: British Small Animal Veterinary Association.

44 Lefebvre, H.P. (2011). Renal function testing. In: (ed. J. Bartges and D.J. Polzin), 91–96. Ames, IA: Wiley-Blackwell.

45 Fry, M.M. (2011). Urinalysis. In: *Nephrology and Urology of Small Animals* (ed. J. Bartges and D.J. Polzin), 91–96. Ames, IA: Wiley-Blackwell.

46 Osborne, C.A., Stevens, J.B., and Lulich, J.P. (1995). A clinician's analysis of urinalysis. In: *Canine and Feline Nephrology and Urology* (ed. C.A. Osborne and D.R. Finco), 136–205. Baltimore, MD: Williams & Wilkins.

47 Kruger, J.M., Osborne, C.A., Goyal, S.M. et al. (1991). Clinical-evaluation of cats with lower urinary-tract disease. *J. Am. Vet. Med. Assoc.* 199 (2): 211–216.

48 Buffington, C.A., Chew, D.J., Kendall, M.S. et al. (1997). Clinical evaluation of cats with nonobstructive urinary tract diseases. *J. Am. Vet. Med. Assoc.* 210 (1): 46–50.

49 Osborne, C.A., Kruger, J.M., and Lulich, J.P. (1996). Feline lower urinary tract disorders. Definition of terms and concepts. *Vet. Clin. North Am. Small Anim. Pract.* 26 (2): 169–179.

50 Gerber, B., Eichenberger, S., and Reusch, C.E. (2008). Guarded long-term prognosis in male cats with urethral obstruction. *J. Feline Med. Surg.* 10 (1): 16–23.

51 Barsanti, J.A., Finco, D.R., Shotts, E.B. et al. (1982). Feline urologic syndrome – further investigation into etiology. *J. Am. Anim. Hosp. Assoc.* 18 (3): 391–395.

52 Kruger, J.M., Conway, T.S., Kaneene, J.B. et al. (2003). Randomized controlled trial of the efficacy of short-term amitriptyline administration for treatment of acute, nonobstructive, idiopathic lower urinary tract disease in cats. *J. Am. Vet. Med. Assoc.* 222 (6): 749–758.

53 Markwell, P.J., Buffington, C.A.T., Chew, D.J. et al. (1999). Clinical evaluation of commercially available urinary acidification diets in the management of idiopathic cystitis in cats. *J. Am. Vet. Med. Assoc.* 214 (3): 361–365.

54 Gunn-Moore, D.A. and Shenoy, C.M. (2004). Oral glucosamine and the management of feline idiopathic cystitis. *J. Feline Med. Surg.* 6 (4): 219–225.

55 Westropp, J.L., Kass, P.H., and Buffington, C.A.T. (2006). Evaluation of the effects of stress in cats with idiopathic cystitis. *Am. J. Vet. Res.* 67 (4): 731–736.

56 Lavelle, J.P., Meyers, S.A., Ruiz, W.G. et al. (2000). Urothelial pathophysiological changes in feline interstitial cystitis: a human model. *Am. J. Physiol. Renal Physiol.* 278 (4): F540–F553.

57 Gao, X., Buffington, C.A., and Au, J.L. (1994). Effect of interstitial cystitis on drug absorption from urinary bladder. *J. Pharmacol. Exp. Ther.* 271 (2): 818–823.

58 Buffington, C.A., Blaisdell, J.L., Binns, S.P. Jr., and Woodworth, B.E. (1996). Decreased urine glycosaminoglycan excretion in cats with interstitial cystitis. *J. Urol.* 155 (5): 1801–1804.

59 Buffington, C.A., Chew, D.J., and Woodworth, B.E. (1997). Animal model of human disease: feline interstitial cystitis. *Comp. Pathol. Bull.* 29: 3–4.

60 Buffington, C.A. and Chew, D.J. (1993). Presence of mast cells in submucosa and detrusor of cats with idiopathic lower urinary tract disease. *J. Vet. Intern. Med.* 7: 126.

61 Englar, R.E. (2017). *Performing the Small Animal Physical Examination*. Hoboken, NJ: Wiley.

62 George, C.M. and Grauer, G.F. (2016). Feline urethral obstruction: diagnosis and management. *Today's Veterinary Practice* (July/August): 36–46.

63 Little, S.E. (2012). The lower urinary tract. In: *The Cat: Clinical Medicine and Management*, 980–1013. St. Louis.

Part Eight

The Musculoskeletal and Nervous Systems

67

Cervical Ventroflexion

67.1 Introduction to the Concept of Posture

A patient's posture refers to the way in which the body holds itself in space. [1] Posture involves the distribution of weight between the limbs [1]. Posture is equally impacted by the way in which the head, neck, trunk, and tail are positioned [1, 2].

Normal, upright posture requires skeletal stability, muscular tone, and coordinated, functional innervation to drive muscular actions [3]. Muscular tone implies some degree of tension, that is, the tendency to resist passive movement [4]. Some degree of muscular tone is required, even at rest, to support the body against gravity [4]. Note that tone is not static and varies between muscle groups [5]. Flexors and extensors, for example, often have opposing tone [5].

Abnormal posture may be due to skeletal, muscular, and/or neurological dysfunction [3, 4].

Posture may also be altered by behavior [6].

For example, consider the classic posture of a tense cat [6]:

- Crouched body position
- Erect, forward-facing ears
- Hind limbs tucked up underneath of the body
- Lateral or forward-facing whiskers
- Tail twitching

Contrast that with the overtly fearful cat [6]:

- Ears flattened
- Hunched
- Leaning backward
- Tail wrapped around body
- Whiskers drawn back

In both clinical scenarios that have been described above, the patient's posture is characteristically abnormal, yet lacks true structural or functional disease.

This chapter emphasizes abnormal posture that results from underlying pathology. Specifically, the focus of this chapter is on cervical ventroflexion.

67.2 Introduction to Cervical Ventroflexion

Cervical ventroflexion refers to a state in which the patient's head tucks in toward the chest. This can be an intentional movement. However, it more typically occurs secondary to generalized weakness *in cats* [2, 7–9]. The nose of the affected cat tips ventrally and the chin droops to the level of the thoracic inlet [7–9]. The patient tends to stare straight ahead despite the angle of the head being dropped so as to stay aware of its surroundings [8, 9].

The inexperienced clinician may mistake this presentation for a fearful posture. However, the fearful cat's nose does not typically point toward the ground [7]. Instead, its nose remains forward despite the head tucking in close to the body [7].

In addition to cervical ventroflexion, affected cats may display the following signs that are suggestive of generalized weakness [2, 8]:

- Protrusion of the dorsal scapulae during weight bearing
  - Sometimes this is referred to as "winging" of the scapulae
- Reluctance to move
- Stiff gait in the thoracic limbs when the patient does ambulate
- Wide-based, crouched stance

67.3 Causes of Cervical Ventroflexion in the Cat

Cervical ventroflexion is not a common presentation; however, when it occurs in cats, causes of neuromuscular weakness must be considered [8]. These include the following [2, 8–30]:

- Feline primary hyperaldosteronism
- Hereditary myopathies
- Hypernatremia

Common Clinical Presentations in Dogs and Cats, First Edition. Ryane E. Englar.
© 2019 John Wiley & Sons, Inc. Published 2019 by John Wiley & Sons, Inc.

- Hyperthyroidism***
- Hypocalcemia
- Hypokalemia***
- Idiopathic myositis
- Myasthenia gravis
- Organophosphate toxicosis
- Portosystemic encephalopathy
- Thiamine (vitamin B1) deficiency***

Pathologies that are starred above (***) are most commonly associated with cervical ventroflexion in clinical practice. The others are relatively uncommon.

67.4 Hereditary Myopathies

Hereditary myopathies are rare in companion animal practice. They represent an assortment of genetic defects that impair muscular stability or contraction [31]. Affected patients may have mutations in one or more proteins that are integral to muscular structure or function. Alternatively, affected patients may have faulty transmission of signals from nerves to muscles.

Hereditary myopathies may be autosomal or sex-linked. The former is most common. Hereditary myopathies may be dominant or recessive. Inheritance patterns are specific to the disease, and different diseases target different pet populations. What is consistent among presentations for hereditary myopathies is that most patients present with clinical signs at an early age.

Affected patients tend to have focal or generalized weakness [31]. This often manifests as cervical ventroflexion, which is visually apparent. Note that cervical ventroflexion is not the only clinical sign in affected patients; it is just the most obvious one to the observant client or clinician.

67.4.1 Muscular Dystrophy

Sporadic reports of muscular dystrophy in both dogs and cats appear in the veterinary medical literature [10, 32–37].

Muscular dystrophy is a catchall term for a diverse group of inheritable, non-inflammatory conditions that involve the degeneration of skeletal and/or cardiac muscle over time [10, 38–41]. Muscle fibers undergo fibrosis, with limited potential for regeneration [38–40]. Immunohistochemical analysis and molecular diagnostics are required to definitively distinguish between types of muscular dystrophy [38, 42, 43]. However, these are beyond the scope of this text.

The most understood form of muscular dystrophy in companion animal patients resembles Duchenne muscular dystrophy (DMD) in humans [41]. DMD is an X-linked condition that is characterized by a deficiency in the structural protein dystrophin [10, 38, 44, 45].

In health, dystrophin is responsible for maintaining the integrity of muscle. Without dystrophin, muscles are fragile and easily damaged. They also are not supported during muscular contraction [46]. Over time, muscles become fibrotic and dysfunctional. This manifests in patients as stiff, stilted gaits, and progressive weakness.

Early age of onset is characteristic for case presentations of muscular dystrophy. Most dogs are less than six months of age when signs develop [8, 41, 47–50].

Golden Retrievers were the first canine breed to be diagnosed with X-linked muscular dystrophy [32, 38, 51]. This condition has since been documented in other breeds of dog, including the following [38, 41, 45, 49–59]:

- Brittany Spaniel
- German Shorthaired Pointer
- Irish Terrier
- Japanese Spitz
- Labrador Retriever
- Miniature Schnauzer
- Norfolk Terrier
- Old English Sheepdog
- Pembroke Welsh Corgi
- Rat Terrier
- Weimaraner

Cats are less often diagnosed with muscular dystrophy than dogs [60]. Isolated cases have been reported in North America as well as in Belgium, France, the Netherlands, and Switzerland [60–63].

Both cats and dogs with muscular dystrophy are likely to present with cervical ventroflexion. However, because muscular dystrophy does not limit itself to the region of the neck, affected patients will present with other signs.

In addition to cervical ventroflexion, dogs with muscular dystrophy may demonstrate one or more of the following changes [38, 41, 51, 57, 64, 65]:

- Atrophy of major muscle groups
- Cervical spasms
- Contracture of major muscle groups
- Dysphagia
- Exercise intolerance
- Generalized weakness
- Hypertrophy of cervical muscles, throat-associated muscles, and the tongue
- Inspiratory stridor
- Ptyalism
- Respiratory difficulty
- Regurgitation
- Short-strided gait

Cats with muscular dystrophy also typically present with a conglomeration of signs, in addition to cervical ventroflexion. Although we do not typically think of cats as exercising, affected patients are intolerant of prolonged exertion. Clients may report diminished play behavior or reduced duration of play.

Affected cats may also demonstrate an unusual gait. Carpenter et al. described a characteristic swaying gait [61]. Others have described a stiff, "bunny-hopping" gait [8].

Mobility is impaired in both dogs and cats with muscular dystrophy. Patients may have difficulty running or jumping. These deficits worsen as they age.

67.4.2 Devon Rex and Sphynx "Spasticity Syndromes"

So-called "spasticity syndromes" have been described in the veterinary literature, first in Devon Rex cats and, subsequently, in Sphynx [27]. These syndromes have since been diagnosed as a form of muscular dystrophy, characterized by deficiency of α-dystroglycan [10, 20, 22, 27].

Breeders report signs as early as three to seven weeks of age [20, 27].

Cervical ventroflexion is visually apparent [20]. Ventroflexion is exaggerated by stress, excitement, locomotion, and posturing to eliminate [20, 27]. Kittens, for example, may appear normal at the start of micturition. However, as voiding progresses, their heads droop because of weakness associated with the nuchal musculature. Unable to counter the force of gravity, the head dips unless it lands on something else for support, like the rim of the litter box [20].

Other signs of Devon Rex and Sphynx hereditary myopathy include the following [8, 10, 20, 27]:

- Dysphagia
- Generalized muscle weakness
- Head bobbing
- High-stepping, choppy gait
- Fatigue, that is, shaking or tremoring with prolonged muscular contraction
  - May progress to collapse
- Partial trismus, or lockjaw
- "Winging" of the scapulae

Affected patients often develop esophageal dysfunction, including megaesophagus [8]. These patients are likely to exhibit regurgitation, which may precipitate aspiration pneumonia [27]. Refer to Chapters 52 and 54 for a review of regurgitation as compared to vomiting.

67.4.3 Periodic Hypokalemic Polymyopathy in Burmese and Related Cats

A hereditary myopathy has also been described in Burmese, Bombay, and Tonkinese cats [2, 21, 66]. Affected cats are thought to have a mutation of the WNK4 gene, which codes for an enzyme in distal nephrons of the kidneys [21]. Because this enzyme is involved in sodium/potassium exchange, a mutation is likely to contribute to potassium wasting [21].

Hypokalemia is not persistent in these cats. However, periodic hypokalemia promotes episodes of weakness [2, 9, 21].

Affected kittens demonstrate signs of disease as early as two months of age, and most demonstrate signs by six to ten months [2, 21, 67–70].

Episodic weakness most often manifests as bouts of cervical ventroflexion [21, 71]. Affected cats may be described as having a swan-like neck because of the way in which the chin tucks into the sternum [21].

Because cervical musculature is weak, the head does not stay fixed during locomotion, and so it may bob in space. Sometimes this is described by clients as "nodding" [21].

To compensate for this altered head position and to expand their visual field, which cervical ventroflexion has compromised, affected cats may sit up on their haunches like meerkats [21]. Sometimes this is called "squirreling" or "periscoping" [10, 21].

Affected cats may also use an outstretched forelimb as an object on which to rest the drooping head [21, 71, 72].

Unrelated to cervical ventroflexion, affected patients may exhibit carpal knuckling and/or dropped hocks [2].

Some cats may exhibit weakness in one or more limbs; for others, the appendicular skeleton is unaffected [21].

Unlike muscular dystrophy, this condition is treatable with oral replacement therapy to correct deficiencies in serum potassium [21]. Replacing the deficit will resolve signs in some patients; in others, it will lessen the frequency and severity of episodes [21].

For more information on how low potassium contributes to myopathy, refer to the following section, Section 67.5.

67.5 Hypokalemic Myopathy

Potassium is an important cation for mammalian physiology [11]. Its intracellular concentrations are responsible for generating cells' resting membrane potential [11]. When patients are deficient in potassium cells are hyperpolarized, that is, they become less excitable [11]. The impact is especially detrimental to skeletal and cardiac muscles [11, 73–75].

The normal reference range for potassium in adult cats and dogs varies depending upon sample type and methodology [11]. However, in general, potassium should range from 4.0 to 5.5 mEq/l in the healthy, normal patient [11, 12, 73, 76].

When serum potassium drops below 3.0 mEq/l, patients are likely to experience muscle weakness and, potentially, cardiac arrhythmias [11, 12, 73, 75–78]. Generalized weakness most often manifests as cervical ventroflexion in cats [11, 12]. However, dogs, too, may develop cervical ventroflexion secondary to severe hypokalemia [14].

Other signs of hypokalemia include a broad-based stance and a hypermetric gait [11].

Patients with hypokalemia may become anorexic [11].

Hypokalemia most often results from renal disease [11]. Polyuric patients waste potassium. For this reason, diabetes mellitus, hyperadrenocorticism, and hyperthyroidism can induce hypokalemia.

Other causes of hypokalemia in companion animal patients include the following [11, 17]:

- Gastrointestinal losses
  - Vomiting
  - Diarrhea
- Pharmacologic therapy
  - Loop and thiazide diuretics increase renal excretion of potassium
  - Urine acidifiers, such as ammonium chloride, promote acidosis, which increases renal potassium excretion
- Primary hyperaldosteronism (see Section 67.7 below)
- Post-obstructive diuresis
- Vegetarian diet

Diagnosis of hypokalemia is via blood chemistry [11]. Potassium levels can be corrected parenterally or orally [12, 21, 23, 66, 71, 72, 77, 79, 80]. However, the underlying cause of hypokalemia must be addressed.

67.6 Thiamine (Vitamin B1) Deficiency

Thiamine is an essential nutrient, meaning that it cannot be synthesized by the body [16]. It must be ingested in the diet and absorbed in the small intestine [13]. As a coenzyme, it plays a key role in the metabolism of carbohydrates [13, 16, 81–83].

Thiamine-rich foods include the following [83]:

- Eggs
- Grains
- Legumes
- Liver
- Milk
- Poultry
- Red meat
- Vegetables

Thiamine deficiency may result from the following [13, 19, 83–86]:

- Diets that are rich in sulfites, which inactivate thiamine

- Raw diets that are rich in thiaminases, enzymes that preferentially break down thiamine
  - Herring
  - Mackerel
- Excessive heat processing
- Extended food storage
- Inadequate intake in the diet
- Increased renal excretion, secondary to the use of diuretics
- Malabsorption syndrome: an inability of the gut to absorb thiamine

Cats are especially sensitive to thiamine deficiency, and require more dietary thiamine than dogs [13].

In the absence of thiamine, carbohydrate metabolism is impaired [13]. This is particularly detrimental to those tissues, such as the brain, that require glucose as an energy source [13]. Neurological dysfunction is common. Patients may present for one or more of the following signs [13, 16, 18, 83]:

- Altered mentation
- Anisocoria
- Ataxia
- Blindness
- Cervical ventroflexion
- Decreased menace response
- Diminished pupillary light reflexes (PLRs)
- Disorientation
- Incoordination
- Mydriasis
- Paresis, paraparesis, or tetraparesis
- Rigidity
- Seizures
- "Star-gazing" expression
- Tremors
  - Body
  - Head
- Vestibular signs
  - Head tilt
  - Positional nystagmus

Clinical signs vary immensely in terms of severity [18].

Gastrointestinal signs, such as anorexia and vomiting, often precede neurological dysfunction [18, 87].

Cervical ventroflexion is a common sequelae of thiamine deficiency. Note, however, that the head and neck of affected patients tend to be more rigidly placed as opposed to the flaccid weakness that has been described for hereditary myopathies [19, 88].

A presumptive diagnosis of thiamine deficiency is typically based upon the following [19]:

- Dietary history
- Physical examination findings
- Response to thiamine supplementation

Affected patients typically respond rapidly to parenteral supplementation with thiamine hydrochloride [19]. It is common to see improvement in 24–48 h [19, 83]. However, treatment must be extended for at least a month as corrections are made to the diet [19].

Patient outcomes improve when treatment is expedited [18, 83, 89].

67.7 Feline Primary Hyperaldosteronism

Feline primary hyperaldosteronism is sometimes referred to as Conn's disease [26]. This condition has been recognized in people since the 1950s, and was first diagnosed in the cat in 1983 [26, 90, 91]. In both humans and cats, it is characterized by excessive blood levels of aldosterone [26].

Aldosterone is produced by the adrenal cortex, specifically within the zona glomerulosa [26, 92]. In health, its secretion is regulated by the renin-angiotensin-aldosterone system (RAAS) [26, 92, 93]. RAAS is stimulated when renal blood flow is reduced. The decline in renal blood flow is detected by macula densa cells in the distal tubules of the nephrons. Specifically, these cells detect a drop in sodium and chloride delivery [26, 93].

In response to reduced renal blood flow, juxtaglomerular cells of the kidney activate prorenin to renin. Renin converts angiotensinogen to angiotensin 1 [26, 93]. Angiotensin 1 is then converted by angiotensin-converting enzyme (ACE) into angiotensin 2 [26, 93]. Angiotensin 2 promotes vasoconstriction to improve renal blood flow [26, 93]. In addition, angiotensin 2 causes secretion of aldosterone [26, 93].

Aldosterone promotes the reabsorption of sodium and water [25, 92]. To maintain electrolyte balance, potassium is lost in the urine.

The net result is blood volume expansion and a concurrent rise in blood pressure [92, 93].

Patients with primary hyperaldosteronism overproduce aldosterone [26]. Persistent aldosterone promotes systemic hypertension.

Recall the following from Chapter 15, Section 15.4.2.2:

- Hypertension in cats is characterized as having persistently elevated, systolic blood pressure at greater than 160–170 mmHg and/or elevated diastolic pressures greater than 100 mmHg [94–99].
- Hypertension in dogs is characterized as having persistency elevated, systolic pressures of 180–200 mmHg and/or elevated diastolic pressures greater than 100 mmHg [96, 100, 101].

Persistent aldosterone also promotes potassium wasting in the urine [26]. Affected patients may become profoundly hypokalemic [25, 26].

As was discussed in Sections 67.4.3 and 67.5, hypokalemia causes muscular weakness [25]. This may be regional or generalized. Weakness typically manifests as cervical ventroflexion [24–26]. Stiffness associated with the forelimbs has also been described [26, 92].

In addition, patients will likely present with signs related to systemic hypertension [26]. Recall from Chapter 15, Section 15.4.2.2 that persistently elevated blood pressure impacts the arterial system and by extension the eyes, kidneys, heart, and brain [94]. These so-called target organs are critically impacted by hypertension before other tissues in the body because they depend upon a rich arterial supply [94].

Retinopathy, with associated blindness, is a common sequela of systemic hypertension [25, 97, 98, 102]. In the early stages of disease, hypertensive retinopathy may be characterized by retinal edema [94]. As hypertension persists, retinal hemorrhages may be observed during fundoscopy [94, 97, 98, 103–105] (refer to Chapter 15, Figures 15.7a, b).

Retinal detachment represents the most significant ocular change that is associated with hypertensive retinopathy. Retinal detachment occurs when disease is advanced and/or hypertension is extreme (refer to Chapter 15, Figures 15.8a, b).

Patients with one or both retinas detached present with blindness [26, 91, 92, 106].

In addition to hypertensive retinopathy, patients with primary hyperaldosteronism may also present with myocardial hypertrophy or renal dysfunction [25, 26].

A diagnosis of primary hyperaldosteronism may be suspected in patients that have hypertension, hypokalemia, and increased serum aldosterone concentration [26]. In the normal patient, hypokalemia should inhibit aldosterone secretion, rather than promote it [26]. Therefore, a patient with both low potassium and high aldosterone is a red flag [26].

Demonstration of an enlarged adrenal gland via abdominal ultrasonography is supportive of the diagnosis [25, 26].

Patients may be managed medically or surgically [26]. Both avenues of case management are beyond the scope of this text. However, in brief, medical management involves the administration of an aldosterone antagonist, such as spironolactone, along with potassium supplementation and antihypertensive agents [26]. Adrenalectomy is considered the preferred option when there is unilateral disease, with a cure likely [25, 26]. Adrenalectomy is complicated if there is tumor invasion into the caudal vena cava [26].

Note that primary hyperaldosteronism has also been reported in dogs, but its occurrence is even rarer than it is in cats [92, 107, 108].

67.8 Myasthenia Gravis

Myasthenia gravis is a condition in which the affected patient experiences dysfunction at the level of the acetylcholine receptors on the postsynaptic membrane [2]. Although both congenital and acquired forms have been recognized in companion animal patients, the latter are more typically seen in clinical practice [2]. In the acquired form, patients develop autoantibodies against their own acetylcholine receptors [2]. This prevents acetylcholine from binding to its receptor [2]. Neuromuscular paresis results [2].

Patients may have focal or generalized disease. The generalized form is characterized by progressive weakness and intolerance to exercise [2, 29]. When the patient is rested, it regains strength, but this is short-lived and the patient again succumbs to weakness [29].

Pelvic limb lameness is particularly prominent in dogs with myasthenia gravis [29]. Cats, on the other hand, will typically present with cervical ventroflexion as a sign of generalized weakness [2].

Among cats, Somali and Abyssinian breeds are overrepresented [2].

A positive response to the administration of acetylcholinesterase inhibitors, edrophonium chloride or neostigmine, is supportive of a diagnosis [2]. A definitive diagnosis requires the presence of anti-acetylcholine receptor antibodies in the serum; however, false negatives are possible [2].

Lifelong treatment with pyridostigmine bromide or a comparable product is indicated [2].

Patients with myasthenia gravis may be more likely to develop polymyositis, polyneuritis, or neoplastic changes of the thymus [2, 29].

67.9 Causes of Cervical Ventroflexion Other than Generalized Weakness

Cervical ventroflexion is most often, in cats, a sign of generalized weakness [2, 7–9]. However, it may also result from unrelated disease that causes one or more changes to the vertebral column. Consider, for example, case presentations that involve hypervitaminosis A, a condition that is sometimes referred to as deforming cervical spondylosis [2].

Much like thiamine, vitamin A is an essential nutrient. However, unlike thiamine, which is not typically stored in the body, vitamin A is fat soluble and is capable of being held by the body in reserve. Specifically, excess vitamin A is stored within the liver [109].

Hypervitaminosis A is typically the result of diets that are rich in raw avian, porcine, and/or ruminant liver [109–113].

Hypervitaminosis A leads to extensive changes to the feline skeletal system [109, 112–117]. The cervicothoracic spine becomes riddled with bony exostoses and osteophytes [109, 113–115]. These proliferative lesions may also involve the sternum and costal cartilages [118].

New bone deposition causes vertebrae to fuse, including the atlantoaxial joint [2]. This inhibits motion of the spine and, in particular, causes the neck to ventroflex rigidly [110]. Neck palpation may be uncomfortable because of restricted movement [2].

Less common sites of bone formation include the joints of the appendicular skeleton, especially the shoulder, elbow, and pelvis [110].

In severe cases, compression of the brachial plexus may cause neurological deficits, including thoracic limb paresis or paralysis [109, 110]. Limb reflexes and deep pain sensation may be absent [109].

A presumptive diagnosis is made based upon dietary history, physical examination, and radiographic findings [110]. The diagnosis is confirmed by an elevation in serum vitamin A concentration [110].

References

1 van Nes, J.J., Meij, B.P., and van Ham, L. (2009). Nervous system. In: *Medical History and Physical Examination in Companion Animals* (ed. A. Rijnberk and F.J. van Sluijs), 160–174. St. Louis: Elsevier.

2 Nghiem, P., Platt, S., and Schatzberg, S. (2009). The weak cat. Practical approach and common neurological differentials. *J. Feline Med. Surg.* 11 (5): 373–383.

3 Ford, R.B. and Mazzaferro, E.M. (2012). *Kirk & Bistner's Handbook of Veterinary Procedures and Emergency*

Treatment, 9e, 295–380. St. Louis, Mo.: Elsevier/Saunders.Patient Evaluation and Organ System Examination

4 Fahn, S. (2007). Hypokinesia and hyperkinesia. In: *Textbook of Clinical Neurology*, 3e (ed. C.G. Goetz), 289–306. Philadelphia: Saunders.

5 McGee, S. (2018). Examination of the motor system: approach to weakness. In: *Evidence-Based Physical Diagnosis*, 4e (ed. S. McGee), 551–568. Philadelphia: Elsevier.

6 Colleran, E.J. (2015). Feline posture. A visual dictionary. DVM 360 [Internet]. http://veterinarymedicine.dvm360.com/feline-posture-visual-dictionary.

7 Taylor, A.R. and Kerwin, S.C. (2018). Clinical evaluation of the feline neurologic patient. *Vet. Clin. North Am. Small Anim. Pract.* 48 (1): 1–10.

8 LeCouteur, R.A. (ed.) (2006). Feline neuromuscular disorders. World Small Animal Veterinary Association World Congress Proceedings.

9 Colleran, E.J. (2018). Cervical ventroflexion. In: *The Feline Patient*, 5e (ed. G.D. Norsworthy and L.M. Restine), 80–81. Hoboken, NJ: Wiley.

10 Martin, P.T., Shelton, G.D., Dickinson, P.J. et al. (2008). Muscular dystrophy associated with alpha-dystroglycan deficiency in Sphynx and Devon Rex cats. *Neuromuscul. Disord.* 18 (12): 942–952.

11 Kogika, M.M. and de Morais, H.A. (2017). A quick reference on hypokalemia. *Vet. Clin. North Am. Small Anim. Pract.* 47 (2): 229–234.

12 DiBartola, S.P. (2010). Disorders of potassium. DVM 360 [Internet]. http://veterinarycalendar.dvm360.com/disorders-potassium-proceedings.

13 Garcia, J.L. (2014). Journal scan: Food for thought: thiamine deficiency in dogs and cats. DVM 360 [Internet]. http://veterinarymedicine.dvm360.com/journal-scan-food-thought-thiamine-deficiency-dogs-and-cats.

14 Allen, A.E., Buckley, G.J., and Schaer, M. (2016). Successful treatment of severe hypokalemia in a dog with acute kidney injury caused by leptospirosis. *J. Vet. Emerg. Crit. Care. (San Antonio).* 26 (6): 837–843.

15 Feldman, E.C., Nelson, R.W., Reusch, C., and Scott-Moncrieff, J.C.R. (2015). *Canine & Feline Endocrinology*, 4e, xi, 669 p. St. Louis, Missouri: Elsevier Saunders.

16 Moon, S.J., Kang, M.H., and Park, H.M. (2013). Clinical signs, MRI features, and outcomes of two cats with thiamine deficiency secondary to diet change. *J. Vet. Sci.* 14 (4): 499–502.

17 Englar, R.E. (2017). *Performing the Small Animal Physical Examination.* Hoboken, NJ: Wiley.

18 Palus, V., Penderis, J., Jakovljevic, S., and Cherubini, G.B. (2010). Thiamine deficiency in a cat: resolution of MRI abnormalities following thiamine supplementation. *J. Feline Med. Surg.* 12 (10): 807–810.

19 Schaer, M. (2006). Thiamine deficiency. *NAVC Clinician's Brief* (August): 21.

20 Malik, R., Mepstead, K., Yang, F., and Harper, C. (1993). Hereditary myopathy of Devon Rex Cats. *J. Small Anim. Pract.* 34 (11): 539–546.

21 Malik, R., Musca, F.J., Gunew, M.N. et al. (2015). Periodic hypokalaemic polymyopathy in Burmese and closely related cats: a review including the latest genetic data. *J. Feline Med. Surg.* 17 (5): 417–426.

22 August, J.R. (2010). *Consultations in Feline Internal Medicine.* St. Louis: Saunders.

23 Ettinger, S.J. and Feldman, E.C. (2010). *Textbook of Veterinary Internal Medicine: Diseases of the Dog and the Cat*, 7e. St. Louis, Mo: Elsevier Saunders.

24 Bento, D.D., Zahn, F.S., and Duarte, L.C. (2016). Feline primary hyperaldosteronism: an emerging endocrine disease. *Cienc. Rural*, Santa Maria 46 (4): 686–693.

25 Schaer, M. (2011). Hyperaldosteronism in cats. *NAVC Clinician's Brief.* (November): 59–61.

26 Schulman, R.L. (2010). Feline primary hyperaldosteronism. *Vet. Clin. North Am. Small Anim. Pract.* 40 (2): 353–359.

27 Bell, J., Cavanagh, K., Tilley, L., and Smith, F.W.K. (2010). *Veterinary Medical Guide to Dog and Cat Breeds.* Jackson, WY: Teton NewMedia.

28 Côté, E. (2015). *Clinical Veterinary Advisor. Dogs and Cats*, 3e, xxxvii, 1642 p. St. Louis, Missouri: Elsevier Mosby.

29 Dewey, C.W. (2008). *A Practical Guide to Canine and Feline Neurology*, 2e, xiv, 706 p., 7 p. of plates p. Ames, Iowa: Wiley-Blackwell.

30 Silverstein, D.C. and Hopper, K. (2009). *Small Animal Critical Care Medicine.* xxvi, 954 p., 16 p. of plates p. St. Louis, Mo: Saunders/Elsevier.

31 Cardamone, M., Darras, B.T., and Ryan, M.M. (2008). Inherited myopathies and muscular dystrophies. *Semin. Neurol.* 28 (2): 250–259.

32 Cooper, B.J., Winand, N.J., Stedman, H. et al. (1988). The homologue of the Duchenne locus is defective in X-linked muscular dystrophy of dogs. *Nature* 334 (6178): 154–156.

33 Howell, J.M., Fletcher, S., Kakulas, B.A. et al. (1997). Use of the dog model for Duchenne muscular dystrophy in gene therapy trials. *Neuromuscul. Disord.* 7 (5): 325–328.

34 Sharp, N.J., Kornegay, J.N., Van Camp, S.D. et al. (1992). An error in dystrophin mRNA processing in golden retriever muscular dystrophy, an animal homologue of Duchenne muscular dystrophy. *Genomics* 13 (1): 115–121.

35 O'Brien, D.P., Johnson, G.C., Liu, L.A. et al. (2001). Laminin alpha 2 (merosin)-deficient muscular dystrophy and demyelinating neuropathy in two cats. *J. Neurol. Sci.* 189 (1–2): 37–43.

36 Gashen, F.P., Hoffman, E.P., Gorospe, J.R. et al. (1992). Dystrophin deficiency causes lethal muscle hypertrophy in cats. *J. Neurol. Sci.* 110: 149–159.

37 Kornegay, J.N. (2017). The golden retriever model of Duchenne muscular dystrophy. *Skelet. Muscle* 7 (1): 9.

38 Bergman, R.L., Inzana, K.D., Monroe, W.E. et al. (2002). Dystrophin-deficient muscular dystrophy in a Labrador retriever. *J. Am. Anim. Hosp. Assoc.* 38 (3): 255–261.

39 Braund, K.G. (1997). Degenerative causes of myopathies in dogs and cats. *Vet. Med-Us.* 92 (7): 608–617.

40 Shelton, G.D. and Cardinet, G.H. (1987). Pathophysiologic basis of canine muscle disorders. *J. Vet. Intern. Med.* 1 (1): 36–44.

41 Baltzer, W.I., Calise, D.V., Levine, J.M. et al. (2007). Dystrophin-deficient muscular dystrophy in a Weimaraner. *J. Am. Anim. Hosp. Assoc.* 43 (4): 227–232.

42 Bornemann, A. and Anderson, L.V. (2000). Diagnostic protein expression in human muscle biopsies. *Brain Pathol.* 10 (2): 193–214.

43 Cohn, R.D. and Campbell, K.P. (2000). Molecular basis of muscular dystrophies. *Muscle Nerve* 23 (10): 1456–1471.

44 Emery, A.E. (1991). Population frequencies of inherited neuromuscular diseases – a world survey. *Neuromuscul. Disord.* 1 (1): 19–29.

45 Beltran, E., Shelton, G.D., Guo, L.T. et al. (2015). Dystrophin-deficient muscular dystrophy in a Norfolk terrier. *J. Small Anim. Pract.* 56 (5): 351–354.

46 Barresi, R. and Campbell, K.P. (2006). Dystroglycan: from biosynthesis to pathogenesis of human disease. *J. Cell Sci.* 119 (Pt 2): 199–207.

47 Kornegay, J.N. (1986). Golden retriever myopathy. In: *Current Veterinary Therapy IX: Small Animal Practice* (ed. J.D. Bonagura), 792–794. Philadelphia: WB Saunders.

48 Valentine, B.A., Cooper, B.J., Cummings, J.F., and Delahunta, A. (1986). Progressive muscular-dystrophy in a Golden Retriever dog – light-microscope and ultrastructural features at 4 and 8 months. *Acta Neuropathol.* 71 (3–4): 301–310.

49 Wentink, G.H., Vanderli, J., AEFH, M. et al. (1972). Myopathy with a possible recessive X-linked inheritance in a litter of Irish terriers. *Vet. Pathol.* 9 (5): 328–349.

50 Presthus, J. and Nordstoga, K. (1993). Congenital myopathy in a litter of Samoyed dogs. *Prog. Vet. Neurol.* 4 (2): 37–40.

51 Kornegay, J.N., Tuler, S.M., Miller, D.M., and Levesque, D.C. (1988). Muscular dystrophy in a litter of golden retriever dogs. *Muscle Nerve* 11 (10): 1056–1064.

52 Schatzberg, S.J., Olby, N.J., Breen, M. et al. (1999). Molecular analysis of a spontaneous dystrophin 'knockout' dog. *Neuromuscul. Disord.* 9 (5): 289–295.

53 Wetterman, C.A., Harkin, K.R., Cash, W.C. et al. (2000). Hypertrophic muscular dystrophy in a young dog. *J. Am. Vet. Med. Assoc.* 216 (6): 878–881, 64.

54 VanHam, L.M.L., Roels, S.L.M.F., and Hoorens, J.K. (1995). Congenital dystrophy-like myopathy in a brittany spaniel puppy. *Prog. Vet. Neurol.* 6 (4): 135–138.

55 Paola, J., Podell, M., and Shelton, G.D. (1993). Muscular dystrophy in a miniature schnauzer. *Prog. Vet. Neurol.* 4: 14–18.

56 Woods, P. and Sharp, N.J. (eds.) (1998). Muscular dystrophy in Pembroke corgis and other dogs. 16th ACVIM Forum.

57 DeVanna, J.C., Kornegay, J.N., Bogan, D.J. et al. (2014). Respiratory dysfunction in unsedated dogs with golden retriever muscular dystrophy. *Neuromuscul. Disord.* 24 (1): 63–73.

58 Acosta, A.R., Van Wie, E., Stoughton, W.B. et al. (2016). Use of the six-minute walk test to characterize golden retriever muscular dystrophy. *Neuromuscul. Disord.* 26 (12): 865–872.

59 Cosford, K.L., Taylor, S.M., Thompson, L., and Shelton, G.D. (2008). A possible new inherited myopathy in a young Labrador retriever. *Can. Vet. J.* 49 (4): 393–397.

60 Blunden, A.S. and Gower, S. (2011). Hypertrophic feline muscular dystrophy: diagnostic overview and a novel immunohistochemical diagnostic method using formalin-fixed tissue. *Vet. Rec.* 168 (19).

61 Carpenter, J.L., Hoffman, E.P., Romanul, F.C.A. et al. (1989). Feline muscular-dystrophy with dystrophin deficiency. *Am. J. Pathol.* 135 (5): 909–919.

62 Chetboul, V., Blot, S., Sampedrano, C.C. et al. (2006). Tissue Doppler imaging for detection of radial and longitudinal myocardial dysfunction in a family of cats affected by dystrophin-deficient hypertrophic muscular dystrophy. *J. Vet. Intern. Med.* 20 (3): 640–647.

63 Gaschen, F., Haugh, P.G., and Swendrowski, M.A. (1994). Hypertrophic feline muscular dystrophy – a unique clinical expression of dystrophin deficiency. *Feline Pract.* 22: 23–26.

64 Valentine, B.A., Cooper, B.J., de Lahunta, A. et al. (1988). Canine X-linked muscular dystrophy. An animal model of Duchenne muscular dystrophy: clinical studies. *J. Neurol. Sci.* 88 (1–3): 69–81.

65 Shelton, G.D. and Engvall, E. (2005). Canine and feline models of human inherited muscle diseases. *Neuromuscul. Disord.* 15 (2): 127–138.

66 Blaxter, A., Lievesley, P., Gruffydd-Jones, T., and Wotton, P. (1986). Periodic muscle weakness in Burmese kittens. *Vet. Rec.* 118 (22): 619–620.

67 Mason, K. (1988). A Hereditary-Disease in Burmese cats manifested as an episodic weakness with head nodding and neck ventroflexion. *J. Am. Anim. Hosp. Assoc.* 24 (2): 147–151.

68 Musca, F.J.M., Malik, R., and Menrath, V.H. (eds.) (2010). Hypokalaemic polymyopathy of Burmese cats – retrospective analysis of cases, new clinical observations and a call for cases for genomic studies. Annual Meeting of the Australian College of Veterinary Scientists, Small Animal Medicine Chapter.

69 Jones, B.R., Swinney, G.W., and Alley, M.R. (1988). Hypokalaemic myopathy in Burmese kittens. *N. Z. Vet. J.* 36 (3): 150–151.

70 Stolze, M., Lund, C., Kresken, J.G., and Saerg, K.J. (2001). Periodic hypokalemic polymyopathy in the Burmese cat. *Kleintierpraxis* 46 (8): 517–518.

71 Gaschen, F., Jaggy, A., and Jones, B. (2004). Congenital diseases of feline muscle and neuromuscular junction. *J. Feline Med. Surg.* 6 (6): 355–366.

72 Jones, B.R. and Gruffydd-Jones, T.J. (1990). Hypokalemia in the cat. *Cornell Vet.* 80 (1): 13–16.

73 DiBartola, S.P. and de Morais, H.A. (2012). Disorders of potassium: hypokalemia and hyperkalemia. In: *Fluid, Electrolyte, and Acid-Base Disorders* (ed. S.P. DiBartola), 92–119. St. Louis: Elsevier.

74 Sahni, V., Gmurcyk, A., and Rosa, R.M. (2013). Extrarenal potassium metabolism. In: *Seldin and Giebisch's the Kidney.* 1, 5e (ed. R.J. Alpem, O.W. Moe and M. Caplan), 1629–1657. San Diego: Elsevier.

75 Kemel, K.S., Halperin, M.L., and Steigerwalt, S.P. (1996). Disorders of potassium balance. In: *Brenner & Rector's the Kidney.* 1, 5e (ed. B.M. Brenner), 999–1037. Philadelphia: W.B. Saunders Company.

76 DiBartola, S.P., Green, R.A., and de Morais, H.A. (2004). Electrolyte and acid base abnormalities. In: *Small Animal Clinical Diagnosis by Laboratory Methods* (ed. M.D. Willard and H. Tvedten), 117–134. St. Louis: WB Saunders.

77 Dow, S.W., Fettman, M.J., Curtis, C.R., and LeCouteur, R.A. (1989). Hypokalemia in cats: 186 cases (1984–1987). *J. Am. Vet. Med. Assoc.* 194 (11): 1604–1608.

78 Chew, D.J., DiBartola, S.P., and Schenck, P.A. (2011). *Chronic Renal Failure. Canine and Feline Nephrology and Urology*, 145–196. St. Louis: Elsevier Saunders.

79 Dow, S.W., Fettman, M.J., LeCouteur, R.A., and Hamar, D.W. (1987). Potassium depletion in cats: renal and dietary influences. *J. Am. Vet. Med. Assoc.* 191 (12): 1569–1575.

80 Dow, S.W., LeCouteur, R.A., Fettman, M.J., and Spurgeon, T.L. (1987). Potassium depletion in cats: hypokalemic polymyopathy. *J. Am. Vet. Med. Assoc.* 191 (12): 1563–1568.

81 Dreyfus, P.M. and Victor, M. (1961). Effects of thiamine deficiency on the central nervous system. *Am. J. Clin. Nutr.* 9: 414–425.

82 Singh, M., Thompson, M., Sullivan, N., and Child, G. (2005). Thiamine deficiency in dogs due to the feeding of sulphite preserved meat. *Aust. Vet. J.* 83 (7): 412–417.

83 Chang, Y.P., Chiu, P.Y., Lin, C.T. et al. (2017). Outbreak of thiamine deficiency in cats associated with the feeding of defective dry food. *J. Feline Med. Surg.* 19 (4): 336–343.

84 Davidson, M.G. (1992). Thiamin deficiency in a colony of cats. *Vet. Rec.* 130 (5): 94–97.

85 Kimura, M., Itokawa, Y., and Fujiwara, M. (1990). Cooking losses of thiamin in food and its nutritional significance. *J. Nutr. Sci. Vitaminol.* 36 (4): S17–S24.

86 Markovich, J.E., Heinze, C.R., and Freeman, L.M. (2013). Thiamine deficiency in dogs and cats. *J. Am. Vet. Med. Assoc.* 243 (5): 649–656.

87 Loew, F.M., Martin, C.L., Dunlop, R.H. et al. (1970). Naturally-occurring and experimental thiamine deficiency in cats receiving commerrcial cat food. *Can. Vet. J.* 11: 109–113.

88 Gunn-Moore (2006). The cat with neck ventroflexion. In: *Problem-Based Feline Medicine* (ed. J. Rand) xiv, 1479 p. Edinburgh; New York: Saunders.

89 De Lahunta, A. and Glass, E. (2009). Visual system. In: *Veterinary Neuroanatomy and Clinical Neurology* (ed. A.E.G. De Lahunta), 389–432. St. Louis: Saunders Elsevier.

90 Conn, J.W. and Louis, L.H. (1955). Primary aldosteronism: a new clinical entity. *Trans. Assoc. Am. Phys.* 68: 215–231; discussion, 231–233.

91 Eger, C.E., Robinson, W.F., and Huxtable, C.R. (1983). Primary aldosteronism (Conns-syndrome) in a cat – a case-report and review of comparative aspects. *J. Small Anim. Pract.* 24 (5): 293–307.

92 Ash, R.A., Harvey, A.M., and Tasker, S. (2005). Primary hyperaldosteronism in the cat: a series of 13 cases. *J. Feline Med. Surg.* 7 (3): 173–182.

93 Feldman, E.C. and Nelson, R.W. (2003). Renal hormones and atrial natriuretic hormone. In: *Canine and Feline Endocrinology and Reproduction* (ed. E.C. Feldman), 746–749. Pennsylvania: Elsevier Saunders.

94 Maggio, F., DeFrancesco, T.C., Atkins, C.E. et al. (2000). Ocular lesions associated with systemic hypertension in cats: 69 cases (1985–1998). *J. Am. Vet. Med. Assoc.* 217 (5): 695–702.

95 Samsom, J., Rogers, K., and Wood, J.L. (2004). Blood pressure assessment in healthy cats and cats with hypertensive retinopathy. *Am. J. Vet. Res.* 65 (2): 245–252.

96 Henik, R.A. (1997). Systemic hypertension and its management. *Vet. Clin. North Am. Small Anim. Pract.* 27 (6): 1355–1372.

97 Littman, M.P. (1994). Spontaneous systemic hypertension in 24 cats. *J. Vet. Intern. Med.* 8 (2): 79–86.

98 Morgan, R.V. (1986). Systemic hypertension in four cats: ocular and medical findings. *J. Am. Anim. Hosp. Assoc.* 22: 615–621.

99 Stiles, J., Polzin, D.J., and Bistner, S.I. (1994). The prevalence of retinopathy in cats with systemic hypertension and chronic-renal-failure or hyperthyroidism. *J. Am. Anim. Hosp. Assoc.* 30 (6): 564–572.

100 Remillard, R.L., Ross, J.N., and Eddy, J.B. (1991). Variance of indirect blood pressure measurements and prevalence of hypertension in clinically normal dogs. *Am. J. Vet. Res.* 52 (4): 561–565.

101 Ritchie, C.M., Sheridan, B., Fraser, R. et al. (1990). Studies on the pathogenesis of hypertension in Cushing's disease and acromegaly. *Q. J. Med.* 76 (280): 855–867.

102 Littman, M.P. (2000). Hypertension. In: *Textbook of Veterinary Internal Medicine*, 5e (ed. S.J. Ettinger), 179–182. Philadelphia: W.B. Saunders.

103 Snyder, P.S. (1998). Amlodipine: a randomized, blinded clinical trial in 9 cats with systemic hypertension. *J. Vet. Intern. Med.* 12 (3): 157–162.

104 Turner, J.L., Brogdon, J.D., Lees, G.E., and Greco, D.S. (1990). Idiopathic hypertension in a cat with secondary hypertensive retinopathy associated with a high-salt diet. *J. Am. Anim. Hosp. Assoc.* 26 (6): 647–651.

105 Sansom, J., Barnett, K.C., Dunn, K.A. et al. (1994). Ocular-disease associated with hypertension in 16 cats. *J. Small Anim. Pract.* 35 (12): 604–611.

106 Flood, S.M., Randolph, J.F., Gelzer, A.R., and Refsal, K. (1999). Primary hyperaldosteronism in two cats. *J. Am. Anim. Hosp. Assoc.* 35 (5): 411–416.

107 Breitschwerdt, E.B., Meuten, D.J., Greenfield, C.L. et al. (1985). Idiopathic hyperaldosteronism in a dog. *J. Am. Vet. Med. Assoc.* 187 (8): 841–845.

108 Rijnberk, A., Kooistra, H.S., van Vonderen, I.K. et al. (2001). Aldosteronoma in a dog with polyuria as the leading symptom. *Domest. Anim. Endocrinol.* 20 (3): 227–240.

109 Guerra, J.M., Daniel, A.G., Aloia, T.P. et al. (2014). Hypervitaminosis A-induced hepatic fibrosis in a cat. *J. Feline Med. Surg.* 16 (3): 243–248.

110 Polizopoulou, Z.S., Kazakos, G., Patsikas, M.N., and Roubies, N. (2005). Hypervitaminosis A in the cat: a case report and review of the literature. *J. Feline Med. Surg.* 7 (6): 363–368.

111 Morgan, J.P. (1997). Radiographic and myelographic diagnosis of spinal disease. In: *Consultations in Feline Internal Medicine* (ed. J.R. August), 425–428. Philadelphia: WB Saunders.

112 Seawright, A.A. and English, P.B. (1964). Deforming cervical spondylosis in the cat. *J. Pathol. Bacteriol.* 88: 503–509.

113 Buffington, C.A. (1994). Nutritional diseases and nutritional therapy. In: *The Cat: Diseases and Clinical Management* (ed. R.G. Sherding), 161–190. New York: Churchill-Livingstone.

114 Bennett, D. and May, C. (1994). Joint diseases of dogs and cats. In: *Textbook of Veterinary Internal Medicine* (ed. S.J. Ettinger and E.C. Feldman), 2032–2077. Philadelphia: WB Saunders.

115 Hayes, K.C. (1982). Nutritional problems in cats: taurine deficiency and vitamin A excess. *Can. Vet. J.* 23 (1): 2–5.

116 Franch, J., Pastor, J., Franch, B. et al. (2000). Back-scattered electron imaging of a non-vertebral case of hypervitaminosis A in a cat. *J. Feline Med. Surg.* 2 (1): 49–56.

117 Seawright, A.A., English, P.B., and Gartner, R.J. (1970). Hypervitaminosis A of the cat. *Adv. Vet. Sci. Comp. Med.* 14: 1–27.

118 Goldman, A.L. (1992). Hypervitaminosis A in a cat. *J. Am. Vet. Med. Assoc.* 200 (12): 1970–1972.

68

Forelimb Lameness

68.1 Introduction to Forelimb Anatomy

The skeleton is the foundation upon which the body is built [1]. It has two primary components: the axial skeleton and the appendicular skeleton [1]. The former can be thought of as the trunk of the patient, that is, the skull, the rib cage, and the vertebral column [1]. By contrast, the appendicular skeleton consists of the limbs [1]. These extensions of the trunk provide for locomotion, the ability to move from one point in space to another [1]. Such movement requires coordinated efforts between the musculoskeletal and nervous systems in order to initiate and maintain a proper gait.

The forelimbs are paired structures of the appendicular skeleton that attach to the trunk by means of the thoracic girdle [2, 3]. The thoracic girdle includes the scapulae and the clavicles [2, 3].

The humerus is distal to the thoracic girdle. This bone comprises the brachium or upper arm [2, 3].

The radius and ulna are distal to the humerus. These bones collectively make up the antebrachium or forearm [2, 3].

Distal to the forearm is the carpus, or wrist, followed by the metacarpal bones and the phalanges [2, 3].

Each segment of the forelimb has a purpose and an expected range of motion. Motion is made possible via tendons, which attach skeletal muscle to bone [1]. The origin of the muscle is fixed in space, as opposed to the muscle's insertion, which moves upon contraction.

Extrinsic muscles attach the limb to the axial skeleton. As such, they are capable of moving the limb as one structural unit. For example, they may advance or retract the forelimb. By contrast, intrinsic muscles originate and insert upon the appendicular skeleton, allowing for movement to occur across one or more joints.

The coordination of muscular actions provides for a purposeful gait that is structurally sound. In health, both thoracic limbs are equally and fully weight bearing.

68.2 Introduction to and Relevance of Lameness to Clinical Practice

Lameness is a clinical sign that is characterized by a disturbance in gait. This impacts the patient's ability to move through space.

When lameness occurs, it may involve one or more limbs. It may be acute or chronic, traumatic or atraumatic. The patient may be partially weight bearing or not at all weight bearing. Lameness may be static or progressive. It may worsen after periods of rest or periods of exercise.

There is immense variation in clinical presentation. Some patients are also more stoic than others and may effectively mask the degree to which they are lame.

Lameness is a common clinical presentation among canine patients [4, 5].

Feline lameness is also a clinical concern; however, it is less often reported by clients [6–10]. Cat owners are more likely to report changes in activity level or in their cat's ability to jump [6]. In the senior patient, these changes are often attributed to aging and may therefore not be identified as a true "problem."

Clients are more likely to identify and report lameness if cats are overweight or obese [9, 11].

68.3 The Role of Signalment and History Taking in Diagnosing Forelimb Lameness

When a canine or feline patient presents for forelimb lameness, the list of differential diagnoses is extensive [12]. Musculoskeletal causes of forelimb lameness are prioritized over neurological causes based upon their respective incidences, but both are important considerations [13].

Signalment is an important starting point because potential causes of lameness in a juvenile versus adult patient are strikingly distinct, with the exception of traumatic fractures [4, 5, 14–19]. The patient's age, in many ways, alters the way in which a clinician prioritizes his differentials. For example, infectious arthritis, secondary to calicivirus, is most likely to occur in 6–12-week-old kittens [17]. By contrast, a senior cat would be more likely to have arthritis secondary to degenerative joint disease (DJD).

The patient's breed is also important. For example, German Shepherd Dogs, Bassett Hounds, Golden Retrievers, Bernese Mountain Dogs, and Labrador Retrievers are more likely to develop elbow dysplasia than other breeds [15, 17]. Elbow dysplasia would therefore be prioritized as a differential diagnosis in a German Shepherd Dog with forelimb lameness and pain isolated to the elbow joint.

The importance of history taking can never be understated [5].

It is important to ask the following of any client that presents a patient for lameness [20–22]:

- When was the lameness first noticed?
- What, if anything, was observed that may have triggered the lameness?
- How, if at all, has the lameness progressed?
- Is the patient's lameness a new finding?
- Is the patient's lameness a new finding or a recurrent one?
  - If recurrent, how, if at all, has the lameness changed?
- Which limb(s) appear(s) to be affected?
- Is there shifting leg lameness? In other words, does the lame limb appear to switch from one to another?
- Is the patient bearing weight on the affected limb(s)?
  - A patient that is non-weight bearing may hold up the affected limb(s).
  - The patient may also reproducibly lean against the examination room wall to take pressure off the affected limb(s).
- Is the lameness persistent or does it come and go?
- Is the lameness better or worse after periods of inactivity?
- Is the lameness better or worse with continued movement?
- Is the lameness better or worse at faster gaits?
- Does the patient exhibit difficulty or discomfort when standing up or sitting down?

Cat owners, in particular, should be prompted to discuss grooming behavior or changes in coat quality [22]. Cats with underlying musculoskeletal disease may mask lameness, but present with unkempt coats. Musculoskeletal pain may prohibit the patient from maintaining good hygiene [6, 22].

Historical questions about the patient's lifestyle and home environment are equally important. An outdoor, unsupervised cat may be more likely to have sustained traumatic injury to one or more limbs. Multi-pet households and exposure to children are also relevant to case management.

Geography and travel history may make certain differentials more or less likely. For example, fungal diseases tend to be geographically regional. Patients that either reside in or have traveled to these areas are at increased risk of exposure.

68.4 The Role of Observation and the Physical Examination in Diagnosing Forelimb Lameness

Observational and palpation skills are key to accuracy in lameness diagnoses.

Cats often present a challenge in the clinic setting because they are not easily convinced to demonstrate their gait [22, 23]. It is much easier to coax a dog to trot than the cat [22].

Cats may be encouraged to walk in the examination room if they are allowed the opportunity to come out of the carrier on their own. History taking provides this opportunity for them to acclimate to the examination room. If they do make an appearance, they may be observed from afar. A fearful cat may hunch or freeze, but if and when it becomes more comfortable, it may ambulate.

A cat that is ambulating in the examination room may be placed at the opposite end of the room from its carrier or owner. This placement may motivate the cat to walk across the room, providing a glimpse of its gait to the astute observer.

A food-motivated cat may also be encouraged to walk from one end of the room to another by providing a trail of treats.

Laser pointers may also entice a young or adolescent cat to exhibit play behavior, which may be sufficient for the clinician to analyze the gait.

Owners may also volunteer audiovisual footage taken from their own video-recording devices to document abnormal gait within the home environment [6, 9].

Dogs are more easily walked than cats for direct observation of gait [23].

The purpose of gait analysis is to identify which limb(s) is/are involved and to what degree. Owners are not always certain on presentation which limb(s) represent(s) problem areas.

When considering gait analysis relative to the forelimbs, there are two classic gait abnormalities for the clinician to watch out for [5, 6]:

- Unilateral forelimb lameness may cause the patient to have a head bob when bearing weight on the painful limb.

- Bilateral forelimb lameness may cause the patient to abbreviate its stride by taking short, choppy steps.

If the patient is visibly lame, grading the lameness is helpful in outlining progression of disease [20, 24, 25]. There is no universal, standard scoring system for lameness in companion animal patients.

The author makes use of the following scoring system for dogs [22]:

- Grade 1
  - Shifts weight off affected leg when at rest or standing, but no evidence of lameness when in motion.
- Grade 2
  - Mild lameness is only evident at a trot.
- Grade 3
  - Mild to moderate lameness any time the patient is in motion, including at a walk.
- Grade 4
  - Moderate to severe lameness any time the patient is in motion.
  - The patient attempts to carry the affected limb when in motion.
  - The patient may attempt to place the limb when standing, but is only partially weight bearing.
- Grade 5
  - Non-weight bearing in the affected limb.

It is important that each practice adopt its own scale based upon user preference so that team members can be consistent in their assessment of lameness.

A comprehensive physical examination should be performed on every patient that presents for lameness. This includes a heavy emphasis on the musculoskeletal system; however, all body systems should be considered. A lame dog or cat may suffer from systemic illness that will not be identified unless the veterinarian examines the entire patient [5, 23].

With regard to the thoracic limb, each component should be palpated superficially, followed by deep palpation and range of motion through joints. It is common to begin this portion of the examination with the patient standing.

Standing palpation assesses for the following [6, 23]:

- Symmetry between the forelimbs in terms of bone contour: specifically, palpation concentrates on feeling for continuity of bone: are fractures grossly or palpably apparent?
- Symmetry between the forelimbs in terms of muscle mass: specifically, palpation concentrates on feeling for the supraspinatus, infraspinatus, triceps, antebrachial flexors and antebrachial extensors
- Symmetry between the forelimbs in terms of joints: specifically, palpation concentrates on the presence or

absence of joint effusion, and the presence or absence of heat at each joint

Standing palpation then transitions into palpation in lateral recumbency to appreciate the range of motion through the forelimb joints.

If one forelimb is known to be sensitive, then the author tends to examine that limb last [21, 22].

Refer to *Performing the Small Animal Physical Examination* for an exhaustive review of the orthopedic exam. A recap of the key structures of interest on palpation will be provided here.

Both scapulae are palpable as large, flat bones of the shoulder [2, 20]. Their lateral surfaces are divided by the spine of the scapula, which is palpable in patients with an ideal body condition score. The supraspinatus muscle is dorsal to the spine of the scapula, and the infraspinous muscle sits ventrally. Both should be non-painful to the touch and symmetrical when comparing the left and right forelimbs [2, 20].

The acromion is the widest portion of the spine, located at the cranioventral aspect of each scapula. The acromion is an important landmark for muscle attachment [2, 20]. Another important landmark of the scapula is the supraglenoid tubercle, from which the biceps brachii tendon originates [2] (see Figure 68.1).

The shoulder joint is formed by the articulation of the scapula and the proximal humerus. The greater tubercle of the proximal humerus, which is palpable, is where the supraspinatus muscle inserts [2].

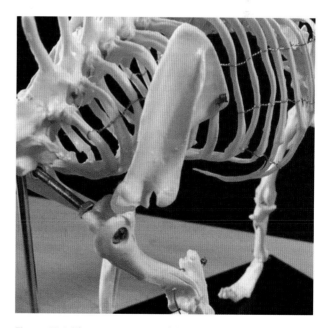

Figure 68.1 Three-quarter view of the left scapula from plastic model of the dog skeleton, with the supraglenoid tubercle outlined in light blue.

The shoulder joint should be assessed for swelling, palpable heat that could indicate active inflammation, crepitus, pain, and range of motion.

The body of the humerus should be palpated for angular limb deformities, swelling, asymmetry between the left and right forelimb, and pain [20].

The medial and lateral epicondyles are palpable at the distal humerus [2].

On the medial aspect of the distal humerus of the cat, but not the dog, there is a supracondylar foramen. Although this structure is not palpable, it should be noted because it allows for the passage of the median nerve and brachial artery. If a fracture were to occur in this location, compression of the nerve and/or artery could result [26].

Distally, the radius and ulna articulate with the humerus to form the elbow joint. The elbow joint is a common site of dysplasia, in young patients, and osteoarthritis, in the aged [26, 27].

The elbow should be assessed for swelling, palpable heat that could indicate active inflammation, crepitus, pain, and tolerance of range of motion.

The radius is the primary weight bearer of the antebrachium. It is shorter than the ulna, which serves primarily as a means of muscle attachment. Proximally, its caudal surface articulates with the ulna; distally, its lateral border articulates with the ulna. Distally, the radius also articulates with the carpus to form the radiocarpal joint [2].

On palpation of the proximal antebrachium, it is possible to appreciate the radial head laterally and the caudally directed protrusion of the ulna, the olecranon. The olecranon plays an important role as a lever for the extensor muscles of the elbow [2].

The radius and ulna crisscross so that on palpation of the distal antebrachium, the radius is now the more medial of the two bones. The styloid process of the distal ulna is palpable laterally, where it articulates with the accessory carpal bone [2].

The carpus has seven bones arranged in two rows.

The distal row of carpal bones articulates with five metacarpal bones. The second through fifth metacarpal bones each bear three phalanges to form the second through fifth digits; the first metacarpal bone, located medially, bears only two phalanges [2].

It is difficult to identify the individual carpal bones through palpation alone with the exception of the accessory carpal bone. Therefore, the clinician's goal in examining the carpus is less to identify individual bones and more to identify any abnormalities such as swelling, heat, crepitus, asymmetry between the left and right forepaw, and pain (see Figure 68.2).

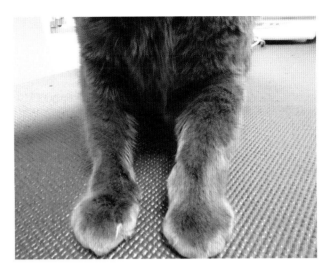

Figure 68.2 Live cat demonstrating grossly visible swelling associated with the left forepaw as compared to the right. *Source:* Courtesy of Dr. Elizabeth Robbins.

The clinician should also assess the range of motion at the carpus.

The individual metacarpal bones can be palpated as well as the digits. In cats, the digits should be manipulated in such a way as to test for the ability to extend and retract the associated claws. However, size is a huge limitation when it comes to examination of the forepaw. Fractures of carpal and metacarpal bones, and phalanges can be missed when evaluated based on the physical exam alone [21]. Radiographs provide clarity that cannot always be appreciated on palpation, and should be encouraged any time pain, swelling, or lameness is localized to the forelimb, particularly the distal forelimb.

68.5 Traumatic Forelimb Lameness

Many cases of limb lameness involve trauma. Traumatic events that may be sustained by the forelimb include, but are not limited to the following [19, 23]:

- Bite wounds
- Chemical injury
- Fractures
- Gunshot wounds
- Luxations
- Self-induced injury
  - Acral lick lesions (refer to Chapter 5, Section 5.16)
- Surgical interventions
  - Onychectomy, or declawing
- Tendon and ligament sprains and strains
- Thermal injury

Bite wounds are common occurrences in clinical practice [9, 23, 28–31]. They often occur along extremities, and they may or may not involve a joint [9, 28, 29, 31, 32].

Bite wounds are often visible immediately following injury (see Figure 68.3).

However, bite wounds may remain hidden beneath fur [9]. If undetected, they may develop into abscesses [9, 23] (see Figure 68.4).

Abscesses are localized accumulations of purulent discharge. They often grow to become quite large and are associated with regional cellulitis [9, 23]. This may be visibly and/or palpably apparent.

How do abscesses form? Recall from Chapter 4, Section 4.2 that small puncture wounds are notorious for sealing over as the body attempts to heal. However, this traps one or more bacterial populations beneath the skin's surface [28, 33]. Bacteria are often a mix of aerobes and anaerobes [33]. The most common bacteria cultured from bite wounds of dogs and cats is *Pasteurella multocida* [34, 35].

The result of bacterial inoculation is a contaminated wound [28, 31, 36]. The wound environment is conducive to bacterial growth [31, 37].

Clipping of the fur may be required to find the puncture wound(s).

If a bite wound, fresh or abscessed, is present on a thoracic limb, it is likely to cause pain and associated

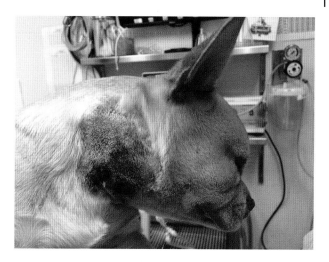

Figure 68.4 Canine patient that sustained bite wounds to the right cervical region. *Source:* Courtesy of Daniel Foy, MS, DVM, DACVIM, DACVECC.

lameness. Lameness may also be exacerbated by localized tissue damage and inflammation.

The patient is likely to have a fever and/or concurrent history of depression [23].

Refer to an emergency medicine and/or surgery textbook for instruction on wound management.

In addition to bite wounds, fractures of all types, including those that involve the forelimb, are common occurrences in companion animal practice [19]. From proximal to distal, forelimb fractures may involve one or more of the following [19, 38–41]:

- Scapula
- Humerus
- Radius
- Ulna
- Carpus
- Metacarpus
- Phalanges

Open fractures, that is, those in which the broken bones pierce through the skin to create an open wound, will be grossly evident.

Closed fractures may evident on palpation or they may require radiographic confirmation (see Figures 68.5a–c).

Diagnostic imaging for confirmation of fractures and surgical planning, when indicated, is essential for case management. However, patient stabilization must take place first [19]. Most patients with forelimb fractures have sustained additional injuries that may be life-threatening [19, 38, 42, 43].

Fractures that involve the growth plate of young dogs and cats are especially concerning [19, 44, 45]. Expedient

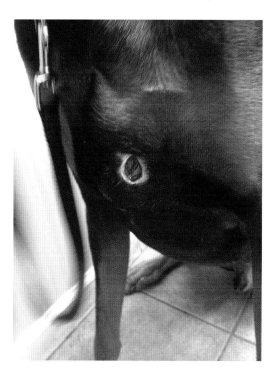

Figure 68.3 Small, right craniolateral thoracic, full thickness laceration in a canine patient. *Source:* Courtesy of Jetta Schirmer.

(a)　　　　　　　　(b)　　　　　　　(c)

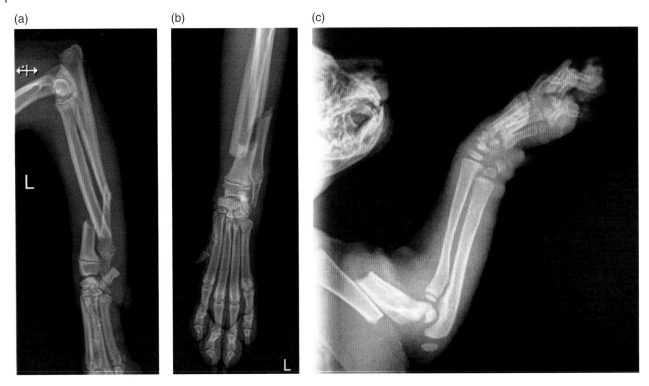

Figure 68.5 (a) Lateral radiographic view of the left antebrachium, demonstrating closed fractures of the radius and ulna. *Source:* Courtesy of Stephanie Shaver, DVM, DACVS-SA and Analucia P. Aliaga. (b) Orthogonal view of the left antebrachium that was depicted in (a), demonstrating closed fractures of the radius and ulna. *Source:* Courtesy of Stephanie Shaver, DVM, DACVS-SA and Analucia P. Aliaga. (c) Radiograph depicting a closed humeral fracture in a five-week-old kitten. *Source:* Courtesy of Genevieve LaFerriere, DVM.

surgical reduction and fracture stabilization optimizes the success rate of repair [19].

68.6 Non-traumatic Forelimb Lameness in the Young Canine Patient

Bite wounds and fractures comprise the majority of traumatic causes of forelimb lameness. However, a large number of non-traumatic conditions may also cause forelimb lameness in the young patient. This topic is too large for the scope of this text. Therefore, the aim will be to cover the most common causes of non-traumatic forelimb lameness. Consult an orthopedic reference for additional details as interest or time allows.

The primary differential diagnoses for juvenile dogs with non-traumatic forelimb lameness include the following [19, 46]:

- Developmental defects
  - Carpal laxity syndrome
  - Elbow dysplasia
  - Shoulder osteochondrosis (OC)
- Infectious disease
  - Osteomyelitis
  - Septic arthritis

- Nutritional and/or metabolic disease
  - Secondary hyperparathyroidism
  - Vitamin D deficiency
- Neoplasia
  - Osteosarcoma
  - Rare, but has been reported as early as six months of age [19]

68.6.1 Canine Elbow Dysplasia

Canine elbow dysplasia is a heritable condition that includes one or more of the following defects [4, 19, 22, 46–51]:

- OC lesions
  - Fragmented medial coronoid process (FMCP)
  - Ununited anconeal process (UAP)
- Incongruity of the elbow joint

FMCP and UAP are two specific types of OC lesions [19]. OC lesions result from the disruption of endochondral ossification [19]. This interruption of bone development causes focal necrosis of epiphyseal cartilage [19]. Cartilage is inappropriately retained, with failure of the matrix to calcify [19]. The concern is that this cartilage is inferior structurally to surrounding tissue [19]. It cannot support normal physiologic loading [19, 52, 53].

When fissures occur in the cartilage, they may create a cartilaginous flap. The presence of a flap transforms the condition, OC, into osteochondritis dissecans (OCD). OCD is a by-product of OC.

If the cartilaginous flap detaches from the underlying bone, it may float around within the joint pouch. Here, it may calcify to form so-called "joint mice". These anomalous structures are evident on radiographs.

Note that OC lesions are not limited to the elbow. However, when they involve the elbow, they most often include the humeral head of male, large or giant breeds of dog [19, 54–62]. In particular, Bernese Mountain dogs, Golden Retrievers, Labrador Retrievers, and Rottweilers are overrepresented [19, 51, 61].

Patients with elbow OC typically present between five and eight months of age [19].

Lameness may involve one or both limbs [19]. Affected patients tend to be weight-bearing lame with lameness aggravated by exertion [19].

Affected patients typically resent elbow flexion and extension [19]. Patient stance may be altered. Clients may observe elbow abduction, which gives the appearance of a bowed limb [19].

On physical examination, affected patients may demonstrate joint effusion between the lateral humeral epicondyle and the olecranon [19]. Sedated radiographs, with multiple views, are necessary to obtain a definitive diagnosis [19, 48, 61, 63, 64].

Elbow OC has the following radiographic characteristics [19, 48, 61, 65]:

- Radiolucent defect(s) and sclerosis of the medial aspect of the humeral condyle
- Roughening of the medial epicondyle
- Osteoarthritic changes
  - Periosteal proliferation of the dorsal anconeal ridge, proximal radius, medial humerus, and medial ulna
  - Sclerosis of the trochlear notch

Clinical signs are expected to worsen with age [19, 51]. Expediting surgical management is key to patient outcomes, and may be performed using arthroscopy [19].

Radiographs of a dysplastic elbow may also reveal UAP and FMCP. They often develop in concert with elbow joint incongruity.

Consider, for example, how a foreshortened ulna may impact the structural stability of the elbow. When the ulna is shorter than normal, the humeral condyle is strapped for space between the anconeal process and the radius. The pressure that it takes to squeeze the humeral condyle into that tight fit is directed onto the anconeal process, which can lead to UAP [66, 67].

UAP most typically affects male, large and giant breed dogs, particularly German Shepherds [49, 68–71]. Diagnosis is via a maximally flexed mediolateral radiographic view [19]. Note that UAP cannot be definitively diagnosed until ossification of the anconeal center and ulna is complete, at or around 20 weeks of age [47, 69].

Consider how a foreshortened radius may impact the structural stability of the elbow. When the radius is shorter than normal, the medial aspect of the humeral condyle and the medial coronoid process are placed under increased pressure. The pressure may be great enough to result in FMCP [66, 72, 73].

Like the other components of elbow dysplasia, FMCP more commonly affects male, large and giant breed dogs, especially Bernese Mountain dogs, Labrador Retrievers, Golden Retrievers, Rottweilers, Newfoundlands, German Shepherd Dogs, and Chow Chows [19, 47, 60, 63, 74, 75]. Patients with radiographic evidence of the fragmented ulna have a definitive diagnosis [19]. Unfortunately, many dogs with FMCP only demonstrate radiographic changes secondary to osteoarthritis [19, 61, 75–79]. Because these changes are present in most patients with any form of elbow dysplasia, these patients would benefit from computed tomography to confirm the diagnosis [19].

Refer to an orthopedic reference for additional details.

68.6.2 Shoulder OC

OC lesions are not limited to the elbow. In the forelimb, the shoulder is also a common site of OC [19].

Dogs that develop shoulder OC typically present between four and eight months of age [19]. Forelimb lameness may be unilateral or bilateral [19]. Dogs with unilateral shoulder OC often progress to bilateral presentations [19, 55, 57, 58].

Shoulder OC causes weight-bearing lameness that is made worse by exercise [19].

Shoulder OC is confirmed by radiographic examination of both shoulders. It is common to see mineralized cartilage as well as radiolucent defects associated with the caudal humeral head [19].

Although nonsurgical case management is possible, surgical excision of detached or abnormal cartilage yields a better prognosis in terms of restoring function [4, 19, 57].

68.6.3 Carpal Laxity Syndrome

A syndrome that involves the carpus has been reported in large and giant breeds puppies, particularly Doberman Pinschers, German Shepherds, and Great Danes [19, 80, 81]. Affected patients have a palmigrade stance due to increased carpal laxity. With controlled exercise, this condition can be reversed [19].

68.6.4 Idiopathic Causes

Non-traumatic forelimb lameness in the young patient may also be idiopathic. Idiopathic causes include panosteitis and hypertrophic osteodystrophy (HOD) [19].

68.6.4.1 Panosteitis

Panosteitis is a relatively common cause of lameness in canine practice, particularly in males, German Shepherds, and Bassett Hounds [15, 19, 82–84]. The marrow of long bones of affected patients undergoes cyclical degeneration [19]. Lameness comes and goes in waves. It may involve one or more limbs. It may also appear to shift limb to limb. Patients may or may not be febrile.

Palpation of affected bone(s) yields pain [15]. Within the forelimb, the distal humerus and proximal ulna are most likely to be affected [15].

Radiographs of panosteitis demonstrate increased opacity of the medullary cavity, which may appear hazy or unusually granular. Proliferation of the periosteum and endosteum may be evident [4, 19].

Treatment is largely supportive and aimed at pain management during flare-ups [15].

Panosteitis is self-limiting. Most cases resolve by 20 months of age [19, 82–84].

Refer to Chapter 70 for more information.

68.6.4.2 Hypertrophic Osteodystrophy

Compared to panosteitis, HOD is a much less common idiopathic cause of forelimb lameness in large and giant breed dogs [4, 19, 63, 85, 86].

Patients that develop HOD suffer from abnormal endochondral ossification that adversely impacts bone neighboring the affected physis [19]. Inflammation, necrosis, and microfracture are anticipated complications that result in swollen, painful metaphyseal areas of affected long bones [19]. The distal radius and ulna are frequent targets. Symmetrical, rather than unilateral, lesions are most likely.

Patients may present with reluctance to move, depression, and fever [19]. Anorexia may stem from generalized malaise [19].

Radiographs of affected long bones are conclusive: they demonstrate a double physeal line due to the presence of an irregular, disease-induced radiolucent line [19, 85, 87].

Like panosteitis, HOD is self-limiting. Treatment is directed at providing supportive care [4, 19]. The prognosis of uncomplicated cases is good [19].

68.7 Forelimb Lameness in the Adult Canine Patient

The primary differential diagnoses for adult dogs with forelimb lameness include the following [18]:

- Arthritis
  - Immune-mediated
  - Infectious
  - Osteoarthritis
- Avulsions
  - Brachial plexus
- Bite wounds
- Cervical spinal cord or nerve root disease
- Fractures
- Infraspinatus contracture
- Neoplasia
- Subluxations
- Tendon tears

68.7.1 Forelimb Fractures of the Adult Canine Patient

Fractures were discussed in brief in Section 68.5. Fractures of the adult canine scapula tend to target the neck or body as opposed to the juvenile patient, who tends to fracture the acromion process or supraglenoid tubercle [18].

In the dog, the most common fracture of the elbow involves the lateral aspect of the humeral condyle [18]. This injury does not require major trauma: jumping out of a vehicle or from the height of a bed is sufficient to shear off the condyle [18].

When the radius and/or ulna are fractured, the middle or distal diaphysis tends to be involved [18].

Carpal fractures are unlikely unless the patient is a racing dog [18]. Carpal hyperextension injuries are more common [18]. Patients that fall from a height may inappropriately extend the carpus beyond its usual 10–15° when landing on one or both front feet [18]. This damages the joint's fibrocartilage and may necessitate arthrodesis [18].

Metacarpal fractures are relatively common.

Fractures of the sesamoids may also occur [18].

Radiographs are an important diagnostic tool any time a fracture is suspected, which could be true of any patient with limb pain and associated lameness [18].

68.7.2 Infraspinatus Contracture in the Adult Canine Patient

Infraspinatus contracture is an unusual condition of unknown etiology [18]. Although it can occur in any breed, hunting dogs appear to be predisposed [18]. This may due to working in an environment in which traumatic injury is more likely [18]. Dogs present with visibly apparent external rotation of the affected forelimb and palpably apparent atrophy of the infraspinatus muscle [18]. Resolution is achieved by surgical management in the form of tenotomy [18].

68.7.3 Biceps Tenosynovitis in the Adult Canine Patient

Inflammation associated with the biceps tendon is increasingly identified as a cause of forelimb lameness in the adult dog [18]. Such injury may be precipitated by a single event or, more typically, is associated with chronic strain in working and performance dogs [18]. Affected patients resent the concurrent actions of extending the elbow while flexing the shoulder [18].

Ultrasonography is diagnostic for biceps-associated disease.

Arthroscopic tenotomy may be indicated. Alternatively, the origin of the biceps tendon may be relocated to the proximal humerus [18]. Both techniques are beyond the scope of this text.

68.7.4 Arthritis of the Forelimb of the Adult Canine Patient

The elbow joint is a common site of osteoarthritis in the dog [88, 89]. It may be related to aging or it may result from joint incongruity or OC, including FMCP and UAP [18]. A history of elbow trauma may precipitate the development of elbow osteoarthritis [18]. Immune-mediated or septic arthritis may also set the stage for osteoarthritis in later life [18].

Arthritis is a diagnosis rather than a clinical sign [18]. The diagnosis is supported by orthopedic examination of the elbow joint [18]. This evaluation may reveal joint thickening and reduced range of motion at the elbow [18]. Grating, clicking, or popping sensations may be palpable when the elbow is flexed and/or extended [18]. These are referred to as crepitus [18]. Crepitus arises from the grinding of bony surfaces against each other when articular cartilage erodes [18].

Radiographic evidence of osteophyte formation is also supportive of arthritis [18].

Arthrocentesis, a "joint tap", is an important diagnostic tool when infectious arthritis is suspected [18].

Osteoarthritis of the carpal joint is also common [18]. In the normal carpus, digital pads should be able to contact the caudal antebrachium when the joint is flexed [18]. As patients age, the periarticular soft tissues may become fibrotic [18]. This reduces the degree to which the arthritic carpus can flex [18]. This restriction may or may not be painful; it may or may not cause forelimb lameness.

Septic arthritis of the carpus is likely when the joint is affected by bite wounds or penetrating foreign bodies [18]. When septic arthritis is suspected, joint cultures are imperative to guide appropriate medical therapy [18].

Immune-mediated arthritis commonly targets the carpus. Joint taps should yield elevated cell counts and large numbers of nondegenerate neutrophils [18].

68.7.5 Neoplasia of the Forelimb of the Adult Canine Patient

Osteosarcoma is a common form of neoplasia that targets skeletal structures, including the forelimbs [90, 91]. Osteosarcoma typically affects sites near the knee and away from the elbow. This implies that the proximal humerus and the distal radius are common sites of osteosarcoma in the forelimb [18]. Osteosarcoma causes extensive limb swelling and associated pain.

Radiographic findings that are supportive of a diagnosis include an aggressive bony lesion that is osteolytic and/or osteoproductive [18] (see Figure 68.6).

Note that osteosarcoma is not the only pathological condition that causes osteolysis. Fungal osteomyelitis can appear strikingly similar and should therefore be included as a differential in certain geographical regions (see Figure 68.7).

Other neoplastic diseases that are capable of causing forelimb lameness include digital squamous cell carcinoma and metastatic disease, as from canine prostatic adenocarcinoma [92, 93].

68.8 Forelimb Lameness in the Cat

The primary differential diagnoses for cats with forelimb lameness include the following [9, 23]:
- Arthritis
  - Immune-mediated
  - Infectious
    - Calicivirus
    - *Escherichia coli*
    - Feline leukemia virus (FeLV)
    - Feline syncytium-forming virus

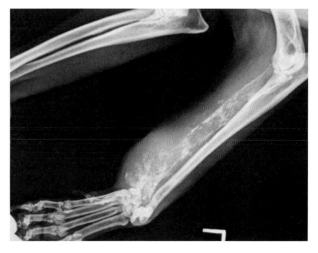

Figure 68.6 Radiographic depiction of an aggressive bony lesion of the distal radius, secondary to osteosarcoma.

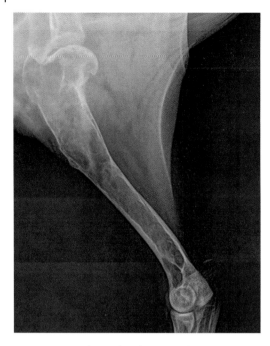

Figure 68.7 Radiographic depiction of an aggressive bony lesion of the proximal humerus, secondary to fungal osteomyelitis.

  o Mycoplasmal arthritis
  o *Pasteurella* spp.
  o *Staphylococcus* spp.
 – Osteoarthritis or DJD
 • Bite wounds
 • Fractures
 • Neoplasia
 • Onychectomy
 • Osteochondrodysplasia

68.8.1 Forelimb Fractures of the Adult Cat

Fractures were discussed in brief in Section 68.5.

Fractures of the adult feline scapula may be difficult to appreciate by palpation alone because of soft tissue swelling [23]. Radiographs are often indicated [23].

Those fractures that involve the body of the scapula may be managed via cage rest [23]. Internal fixation, on the other hand, is indicated when bone fragments are displaced [23]. This is most typically the case for those fractures that involve the neck, glenoid, and/or the suprahamate process, a caudal projection of the acromion is cats only [23]. Scapular surgery is challenging in the feline patient because the scapula is very thin [23]. It is therefore possible to fracture the bone further if it is not handled with caution [23].

Humeral, radial, ulnar, and carpal fractures are uncommonly seen in feline practice [23, 94, 95]. These are more likely to develop in association with high-rise syndrome,

that is, a condition in which a cat inadvertently plummets from a significant height [23, 94, 95].

Radiographs are an important diagnostic tool any time a fracture is suspected, which could be true of any patient with limb pain and associated lameness [18].

68.8.2 Calicivirus and Forelimb Lameness in the Cat

Recall from Chapter 27, Section 27.3.4 and Chapter 33, Section 33.1.1 that feline calicivirus is a common cause of feline conjunctivitis and upper respiratory infection (URI) [96]. Like feline herpesvirus-1 (FHV-1), calicivirus can induce a "chronic snuffler" state [97, 98].

In addition, calicivirus has been linked to the development of transient arthropathy [9]. Kittens with naturally acquired infections may present with hyperesthesia, apparent soreness, and/or stiffness [9].

Vaccination against calicivirus appears to induce arthropathy in some patients [9, 99]. Affected kittens may be stiff-gaited with shifting leg lameness in addition to URI [9]. Oral ulceration and fever may or may not be present [9].

Lameness is thought to be secondary to viremia, given that virus particles have been isolated within the synovium of cats that were experimentally inoculated [9, 99].

68.8.3 Osteochondrodysplasia and Forelimb Lameness in the Scottish Fold Cat

Osteochondrodysplasia is a condition in which bone and cartilage deformities are inherited [23]. A subset of the population of Scottish Fold cats has a dominant gene mutation that codes for cartilage deformities [23, 100]. Because the resultant cartilage lacks structural stability, affected cats have folded ears that bend forward and down. This is aesthetically pleasing to some breeders and cat owners; however, it is not just aural cartilage that is defective. Cartilage defects occur throughout the body, including the joints. Bony exostoses develop, particularly at the distal limbs, causing a painful arthritis [23]. Ultimately, pathological fusion of the affected joints is likely [23]. This is referred to as ankyloses [23, 100].

68.8.4 Lung-Digit Syndrome and Forelimb Lameness in the Cat

Recall from Chapter 3, Section 3.6.3 that primary claw bed and digital neoplasia occur less commonly in the dog as compared to the cat [101, 102]. When regional neoplasia occurs at these locations, it is more likely to be evidence of distant metastasis [101, 103–106].

So-called lung-digit syndrome is often the result of primary bronchial adenocarcinoma or bronchoalveolar carcinoma [103, 104, 107, 108]. Affected cats are often asymptomatic for pulmonary disease [103, 104, 107, 108].

Presentations of lung-digit syndrome vary [106]. Some cases demonstrate relatively minor changes to the nail or nail bed, such as a deviated nail or a claw that will not retract [109]. More commonly, lesions are aggressive, ulcerative, or erosive (see Figure 68.8) [103, 105, 106, 110–112].

Thoracic radiographs should be taken in any cat that presents with a digital, claw, or claw bed mass [106]. There is often a solitary, well-defined, caudal lung lobe lesion [110, 113].

68.8.5 Mammary Adenocarcinoma and Forelimb Lameness in the Cat

Recall from Chapter 62, Section 62.5 that mammary cancer occurs less frequently in cats than dogs, but when it occurs, it is more likely to be malignant [114–117].

Most cats with mammary tumors have more than one at time of diagnosis, and most are aggressive, meaning that there is evidence of local lymph node involvement and invasion of lymphatic vessels [114, 117, 118].

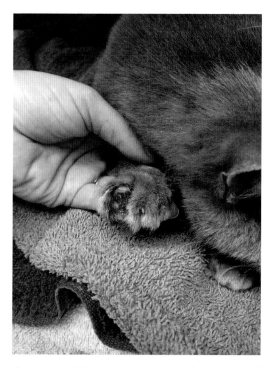

Figure 68.8 Feline patient with erosive lung-digit syndrome that is associated with the forepaw. *Source:* Courtesy of Beki Cohen Regan, DVM, DACVIM (Oncology).

Metastasis to distant sites is common, particularly when mammary masses are adenocarcinomas [117]. Adenocarcinomas preferentially invade the lungs [117, 119]. However, invasion of the bone is also possible [9, 120].

68.9 Neurologic Lameness

Recall from Section 68.1 that movement of the limbs requires coordinated efforts between the musculoskeletal and nervous systems in order to initiate and maintain a proper gait [1]. If the musculoskeletal system is sound, but the patient presents for lameness, then the nervous system may be dysfunctional. Consider, for example, a bulging intervertebral disc or tumor located somewhere between C6 and T2 of the thoracic limb [13]. This may create lameness of neurological, rather than musculoskeletal origin [13].

If musculoskeletal causes of lameness have been ruled out, then the next step is to perform a comprehensive neurological examination.

Gait must be reconsidered to establish if the patient is in fact truly lame or, rather, if the patient has underlying weakness with difficulty supporting its weight [13].

A normal gait should be smooth, strong, and even. Forelimb stride should be roughly equivalent to hind limb stride. Foot placement should be solid, without hesitation, and crisp, meaning that each foot strikes the ground and comes up off the ground without the dorsal surface of the paw knuckling [121].

Subtle gait changes are most easily detected when the patient makes tight turns or sudden movements; however, this is far less easy to reproduce in cats than dogs, who can be guided in their movement by leashes and handlers [121, 122].

When gait changes are noted, the clinician should record which one or more limbs are affected because so doing assists with lesion localization. Paresis is said to occur when there is voluntary movement that is hindered because of underlying weakness. This term may be adjusted to describe the location of apparent weakness as follows [122, 123]:

- Tetraparesis implies that all four limbs are affected.
- Hemiparesis implies that one side of the body is affected.
- Paraparesis implies that both pelvic limbs are affected.
- Monoparesis implies that only one limb is affected.

The clinician should designate which side of the body is affected when the condition is unilateral. For example, the clinician should specify that a patient has right-sided hemiparesis or monoparesis of the left forelimb.

When weakness is present, it may or may not be linked to exertion. Recall from Chapter 67, Section 67.8 that in cases of myasthenia gravis, weakness intensifies as movement continues: the patient starts out strong and then loses momentum [122].

Paresis may also be classified based upon the origin of the underlying problem. In order to generate a gait, the patient must have functional interaction between the upper motor neuron (UMN) system within the central nervous system and the lower motor neuron (LMN) system as the connection piece between the central nervous system and the innervated muscles.

UMN paresis results from inability to generate a gait at the level of the central nervous system. LMN paresis results from difficulty in supporting weight. A patient with UMN paresis will demonstrate a delay in the swing phase of the gait, whereas a patient with LMN paresis will demonstrate abbreviated strides and/or collapse the limb when weight is applied [124].

In addition to the presence and strength of voluntary movement, the quality of the gait should be assessed. The clinician should ask himself if the gait appears to be coordinated. Gait incoordination that is not attributed to weakness is referred to as ataxia [121, 124].

Lesion localization is beyond the scope of this text. However, it is important to recognize that neurological lameness and/or neurological weakness may be present in the absence of orthopedic disease. This serves as a reminder that physical examinations should be comprehensive so that differentials unrelated to the musculoskeletal system are not missed.

Like orthopedic lameness, neurological lameness has many potential causes. When considering the thoracic limb, the most common causes include:

- Acute spinal cord infarction due to fibrocartilaginous embolism
- Brachial plexus avulsion
- Ischemic neuromyopathy
- Radial nerve injury

68.9.1 Fibrocartilaginous Embolic Myelopathy

Fibrocartilaginous embolic myelopathy (FCEM) causes acute, but non-progressive, focal myelopathy that can occur at any location [13, 125, 126]. When an embolus occurs within the spinal segments, C6-T2, it may cause paresis of one or both of the thoracic limbs [13].

Because the spinal cord is not compressed, patients do not appear to be in any pain [13].

Diagnosis is via magnetic resonance imaging (MRI) [13].

Most patients recover function over time, with supportive care and physiotherapy [13].

68.9.2 Brachial Plexus Avulsion

Brachial plexus avulsion is a common traumatic injury in cats [13]. It typically results from high-rise syndrome, that is, falling from a large height, and/or vehicular accidents [13].

The presenting signs vary, patient to patient, depending upon the level of structural damage and its location [13].

When C6-C7 nerve roots are avulsed, the affected limb can still bear weight [13]. However, there is significant restriction to shoulder movement, and the elbow can no longer flex [13]. The patient may no longer have sensation over the dorsal aspect of the paw [13].

When C8-T2 nerve roots are avulsed, innervation to the triceps brachii muscle is compromised [13]. This prevents elbow extension [13]. Without elbow extension, the patient is no longer capable of bearing weight on the affected limb [13]. Both the shoulder and elbow remain flexed [13]. Sensation to the antebrachium may be absent, causing the carpus to knuckle over [13].

If all nerve roots, C6-T2, are avulsed, the affected limb is flaccid and cannot bear weight [13]. The entire limb is also without sensation [13]. This may predispose the patient to self-mutilation, which is thought to occur because of neuropathic pain [13].

68.9.3 Radial Nerve Injury

A radial nerve injury may result from brachial plexus avulsion [13]. Alternatively, it may occur secondary to humeral fractures or fractures of the first rib [13].

When the radial nerve is damaged, carpal extension is prevented.

Nerve function may return in cases of neurapraxia, that is, where nerve transmission was transiently impaired, without overt structural damage. However, prognosis is poor for cases in which the nerve is severed.

68.9.4 Ischemic Neuromyopathy

Ischemic neuromyopathy results from thrombosis of a large vessel. In cats, this most often occurs at the aortic trifurcation secondary to heart disease, particularly hypertrophic cardiomyopathy (HCM) [13, 127–131].

Hyperthyroidism may also predispose cats to aortic thromboembolism (ATE) [13].

Review the pathophysiology underlying ATE in Chapter 39, Section 39.5.1. Recall that many cats that present with ATE have hidden cardiomyopathy, meaning that it has not yet been diagnosed [127, 131–133].

When a thrombus forms at the distal aortic trifurcation, the patient is said to have a "saddle thrombus" [127, 134]. This is the most typical presentation.

However, patients may also experience embolization of the brachial artery [13, 135]. Such patients present acutely with forelimb paresis or paralysis [128, 134].

The condition is intensely painful. Patients are often vocal [128, 134, 136]. They may appear overstimulated or frenzied [134]. They may present with open-mouth breathing [134].

The affected limb is cold to the touch [128]. Paw pads and nail beds are cyanotic [13].

History and presentation are classic for ATE.

Males and the following breeds appear predisposed [13, 128, 136, 137]:

- American Shorthairs
- Burmese
- Maine Coons
- Norwegian Forest cats
- Persians
- Ragdolls
- Siamese

68.10 Summary of Diagnostic Approach to Forelimb Lameness

There are more differential diagnoses for forelimb lameness than have been discussed here. The experienced clinician recognizes the most common causes of forelimb lameness based upon signalment, history taking, and physical examination findings.

If the patient presents for forelimb lameness and has either pain on palpation, pain with hyperextension, or pain with hyperflexion, then a sedated orthopedic examination may be necessary to further localize disease [138].

Whether or not there is a history of trauma, radiographs are an important diagnostic tool to evaluate the patient for fractures, subluxations, or luxations [138].

If, on the other hand, the patient presents without pain on palpation, pain with hyperextension, or pain with hyperflexion, then a neurologic work-up may be indicated [13, 138]. Testing spinal reflexes and postural reactions, such as hopping, wheel-barrowing, and tactile placing, may facilitate lesion localization [13].

For example, the withdrawal reflex tests the following structures within the forelimb [13]:

- Brachial plexus
- C6-T2 spinal cord segments
- Peripheral nerves
  - Axillary
  - Median
  - Musculocutaneous
  - Radial
  - Ulnar

References

1 Singh, B. and Dyce, K.M. (2018). *Dyce, Sack, and Wensing's Textbook of Veterinary Anatomy*, 5e, xv, 854 p. St. Louis, Missouri: Saunders.

2 Evans, H.E. (1993). The skeleton. In: *Miller's Anatomy of the Dog*, 3e (ed. H.E. Evans and M.E. Miller), 122–218. Philadelphia: W.B. Saunders.

3 Gilbert, S.G. (1989). *Pictorial Anatomy of the Cat*, 120 p. Seattle: University of Washington Press.

4 Buback, J. (2012). Evaluating forelimb lameness in juvenile dogs. DVM 360 [Internet]. http://veterinarynews.dvm360.com/ evaluating-forelimb-lameness-juvenile-dogs.

5 Budsberg, S.C. (2010). Lameness exam: what am I missing? DVM 360 [Internet]. http://veterinarycalendar.dvm360.com/ lameness-exam-what-am-i-missing-proceedings.

6 Kerwin, S. (2012). Orthopedic examination in the cat: clinical tips for ruling in/out common musculoskeletal disease. *J. Feline Med. Surg.* 14 (1): 6–12.

7 Hardie, E.M., Roe, S.C., and Martin, F.R. (2002). Radiographic evidence of degenerative joint disease in geriatric cats: 100 cases (1994–1997). *J. Am. Vet. Med. Assoc.* 220 (5): 628–632.

8 Clarke, S.P., Mellor, D., Clements, D.N. et al. (2005). Prevalence of radiographic signs of degenerative joint disease in a hospital population of cats. *Vet. Rec.* 157 (25): 793–799.

9 Leonard, C.A. and Tillson, M. (2001). Feline lameness. *Vet. Clin. North Am. Small Anim. Pract.* 31 (1): 143–163, vii.

10 Lund, E.M., Armstrong, P.J., Kirk, C.A. et al. (1999). Health status and population characteristics of dogs and cats examined at private veterinary practices in the United States. *J. Am. Vet. Med. Assoc.* 214 (9): 1336–1341.

11 Scarlett, J.M. and Donoghue, S. (1998). Associations between body condition and disease in cats. *J. Am. Vet. Med. Assoc.* 212 (11): 1725–1731.

12 Denny, H. and Butterworth, S. (eds.) (2000). Examination and differential diagnosis of forelimb lameness. In: *A Guide to Canine and Feline Orthopaedic Surgery*, 301. Oxford, U.K.: Blackwell Science Limited.

13 Garosi, L. (2012). Neurological lameness in the cat: common causes and clinical approach. *J. Feline Med. Surg.* 14 (1): 85–93.

14 Scott, H. and Witte, P. (2011). Investigation of lameness in dogs: forelimb. *In Pract.* 33: 20–27.

15 Scott, H. (1998). Non-traumatic causes of lameness in the forelimb of the growing dog. *In Pract.* 20 (10): 539–554.

16 Scott, H. and McLaughlin, R. (2006). *Feline Orthopedics*. Taylor & Francis Group.

17 Peterson, M.E. and Kutzler, M. (eds.) (2011). The musculoskeletal system. In: *Small Animal Pediatrics: The First 12 Months of Life*, 451. St. Louis: Saunders.

18 Schulz, K.S. (2001). Forelimb lameness in the adult patient. *Vet. Clin. North Am. Small Anim. Pract.* 31 (1): 85–99, vi.

19 Cook, J.L. (2001). Forelimb lameness in the young patient. *Vet. Clin. North Am. Small Anim. Pract.* 31 (1): 55–83.

20 Hazewinkel, H.A.W., Meij, B.P., Theyse, L.F.H., and van Rijssen, B. (2009). Locomotor system. In: *Medical History and Physical Examination in Companion Animals* (ed. A. Rijnberk and F.J. van Sluijs), 135–159. St. Louis: Saunders Elsevier.

21 Voss, K. and Steffen, F. (2009). Patient assessment. In: *Feline Orthopedic Surgery and Musculoskeletal Disease* (ed. P.M. Montavon, K. Voss and S.J. Langley-Hobbs). St. Louis: Saunders Elsevier.

22 Englar, R.E. (2017). *Performing the Small Animal Physical Examination*. Hoboken, NJ: Wiley.

23 Chandler, J.C. and Beale, B.S. (2002). Feline orthopedics. *Clin. Tech. Small Anim. Pract.* 17 (4): 190–203.

24 Arnoczky, S.P. and Tarvin, G.B. (1981). Physical examination of the musculoskeletal system. *Vet. Clin. North. Am. Small Anim. Pract.* 11 (3): 575–593.

25 P., D., Flo, G., and Brinker, D.C.C. (2006). *Piermattei and Flo's Handbook of Small Animal Orthopedics and Fracture Repair*, 4e. Philadelphia: Saunders.

26 Grierson, J. (2012). Hips, elbows and stifles: common joint diseases in the cat. *J. Feline Med. Surg.* 14 (1): 23–30.

27 Lascelles, B.D. (2010). Feline degenerative joint disease. *Vet. Surg.: VS.* 39 (1): 2–13.

28 Pavletic, M.M. and Trout, N.J. (2006). Bullet, bite, and burn wounds in dogs and cats. *Vet. Clin. North. Am. Small Anim. Pract.* 36 (4): 873–893.

29 Kolata, R.J., Kraut, N.H., and Johnston, D.E. (1974). Patterns of trauma in urban dogs and cats: a study of 1,000 cases. *J. Am. Vet. Med. Assoc.* 164 (5): 499–502.

30 McKiernan, B.C., Adams, W.M., and Huse, D.C. (1984). Thoracic bite wounds and associated internal injury in 11 dogs and 1 cat. *J. Am. Vet. Med. Assoc.* 184 (8): 959–964.

31 Holt, D.E. and Griffin, G. (2000). Bite wounds in dogs and cats. *Vet. Clin. North. Am. Small Anim. Pract.* 30 (3): 669–679, viii.

32 Cowell, A.K. and Penwick, R.C. (1989). Dog bite wounds – a study of 93 cases. *Compend. Contin. Educ. Pract.* 11 (3): 313–320.

33 Brook, I. (2005). Management of human and animal bite wounds: an overview. *Adv. Skin Wound Care* 18 (4): 197–203.

34 Goldstein, E.J. and Richwald, G.A. (1987). Human and animal bite wounds. *Am. Fam. Physician* 36 (1): 101–109.

35 Talan, D.A., Citron, D.M., Abrahamian, F.M. et al. (1999). Bacteriologic analysis of infected dog and cat bites. Emergency Medicine Animal Bite Infection Study Group. *N. Engl. J. Med.* 340 (2): 85–92.

36 Waldron, D.R. and Trevor, P. (1993). Management of superficial skin wounds. In: *Textbook of Small Animal Surgery* (ed. D. Slatter), 269. Philadelphia: WB Saunders.

37 Amalsadvala, T. and Swaim, S.F. (2006). Management of hard-to-heal wounds. *Vet. Clin. North. Am. Small Anim. Pract.* 36 (4): 693–711.

38 Cook, J.L., Cook, C.R., Tomlinson, J.L. et al. (1997). Scapular fractures in dogs: epidemiology, classification, and concurrent injuries in 105 cases (1988–1994). *J. Am. Anim. Hosp. Assoc.* 33 (6): 528–532.

39 Ormrod, A.N. (1966). Limb fractures in the dog and cat. IV. Fractures of the fore limb. *J. Small Anim. Pract.* 7 (2): 155–162.

40 Phillips, I.R. (1979). A survey of bone fractures in the dog and cat. *J. Small Anim. Pract.* 20 (11): 661–674.

41 Turner, T.M. (1995). Fractures of the front limb. In: *Small Animal Orthopedics* (ed. M.L. Olmstead), 195–217. St. Louis: Mosby.

42 Spackman, C.J., Caywood, D.D., Feeney, D.A., and Johnston, G.R. (1984). Thoracic wall and pulmonary trauma in dogs sustaining fractures as a result of motor vehicle accidents. *J. Am. Vet. Med. Assoc.* 185 (9): 975–977.

43 Tamas, P.M., Paddleford, R.R., and Krahwinkel, D.J. (1985). Thoracic trauma in dogs and cats presented for limb fractures. *J. Am. Anim. Hosp. Assoc.* 21 (2): 161–166.

44 Johnson, J.M., Johnson, A.L., and Eurell, J.A. (1994). Histological appearance of naturally occurring canine physeal fractures. *Vet. Surg.* 23 (2): 81–86.

45 Salter, R.B. and Harris, W.R. (1963). Injuries involving the epiphyseal plate. *J. Bone Joint Surg. Am.* 45 (3): 587–622.

46 Michelsen, J. (2013). Canine elbow dysplasia: aetiopathogenesis and current treatment recommendations. *Vet. J.* 196 (1): 12–19.

47 Fox, S.M., Bloomberg, M.S., and Bright, R.M. (1983). Developmental anomalies of the canine elbow. *J. Am. Anim. Hosp. Assoc.* 19 (5): 605–615.

48 Goring, R.L. and Bloomberg, M.S. (1983). Selected developmental abnormalities of the canine elbow – radiographic evaluation and surgical-management. *Compend. Contin. Educ. Pract.* 5 (3): 178–188.

49 Stevens, D.R. and Sande, R.D. (1974). Elbow dysplasia syndrome in dog. *J. Am. Vet. Med. Assoc.* 165 (12): 1065–1069.

50 Zontine, W.J., Weitkamp, R.A., and Lippincott, C.L. (1989). Redefined type of elbow dysplasia involving calcified flexor tendons attached to the medial humeral epicondyle in three dogs. *J. Am. Vet. Med. Assoc.* 194 (8): 1082–1085.

51 Piermattei, D.L. and Flo, G.L. (1997). The elbow joint. In: *Brinker, Piermattei, and Flo's Handbook of Small Animal Orthopedics and Fracture Repair* (ed. W.O. Brinker, D.L. Piermattei and G.L. Flo), 288–320. Philadelphia: WB Saunders.

52 Griffiths, R.C. (1968). Osteochondritis dissecans of the canine shoulder. *J. Am. Vet. Med. Assoc.* 153 (12): 1733–1735.

53 Johnston, S.A. (1998). Osteochondritis dissecans of the humeral head. *Vet. Clin. North Am. Small Anim. Pract.* 28 (1): 33–49.

54 Birkeland, R. (1967). Osteochondritis dissecans in the humeral head of the dog. *Nord. Vet. Med.* 19: 291.

55 Jones, D.G. and Vaughan, L.C. (1970). The surgical treatment of osteochondritis dissecans of the humeral head in dogs. *J. Small Anim. Pract.* 11 (12): 803–812.

56 Whitehair, J.G. and Rudd, R.G. (1990). Osteochondritis Dissecans of the humeral head in dogs. *Compend. Contin Educ. Pract.* 12 (2): 195–204.

57 Rudd, R.G., Whitehair, J.G., and Margolis, J.H. (1990). Results of Management of Osteochondritis-Dissecans of the humeral head in dogs – 44 cases (1982 to 1987). *J. Am. Anim. Hosp. Assoc.* 26 (2): 173–178.

58 Probst, C.W. and Flo, G.L. (1987). Comparison of two caudolateral approaches to the scapulohumeral joint for treatment of osteochondritis dissecans in dogs. *J. Am. Vet. Med. Assoc.* 191 (9): 1101–1105.

59 Person, M.W. (1989). Arthroscopic treatment of osteochondritis dissecans in the canine shoulder. *Vet. Surg.* 18 (3): 175–189.

60 Denny, H.R. and Gibbs, C. (1980). The surgical-treatment of osteochondritis Dissecans and Ununited coronoid process in the canine elbow joint. *J. Small Anim. Pract.* 21 (6): 323–331.

61 Olsson, S.E. (1983). The early diagnosis of fragmented coronoid process and osteochondritis Dissecans of the canine elbow joint. *J. Am. Anim. Hosp. Assoc.* 19 (5): 616–626.

62 Probst, C.W., Flo, G.L., Mcloughlin, M.A., and Decamp, C.E. (1989). A simple medial approach to the canine elbow for treatment of fragmented coronoid process and osteochondritis Dissecans. *J. Am. Anim. Hosp. Assoc.* 25 (3): 331–334.

63 Grondalen, J. (1979). Arthrosis with special reference to the elbow joint of young rapidly growing dogs. II. Occurrence, clinical, and radiographic findings. *Nord. Vet. Med.* 31: 69.

64 Wosar, M.A., Lewis, D.D., Neuwirth, L. et al. (1999). Radiographic evaluation of elbow joints before and after surgery in dogs with possible fragmented medial coronoid process. *J. Am. Vet. Med. Assoc.* 214 (1): 52–58.

65 Kippenes, H. and Johnston, G. (1998). Diagnostic imaging of osteochondrosis. *Vet. Clin. North Am. Small Anim. Pract.* 28 (1): 137–160.

66 Samoy, Y., Van Ryssen, B., Gielen, I. et al. (2006). Review of the literature - elbow incongruity in the dog. *Vet. Comp. Orthopaed.* 19 (1): 1–8.

67 Van Sickle, D.C. (1966). A comparative study of the postnatal elbow development of the greyhound and the German shepherd dog. *J. Am. Vet. Med. Assoc.* 147: 1650.

68 Cawley, A.J. and Archibald, J. (1959). Ununited anconeal process of the dog. *J. Am. Vet. Med. Assoc.* 134: 454.

69 Sjostrom, L. (1998). Ununited anconeal process in the dog. *Vet. Clin. North Am. Small Anim. Pract.* 28 (1): 75–86.

70 Sjostrom, L., Kasstrom, H., and Kallberg, M. (1995). Ununited Anconeal process in the dog – pathogenesis and treatment by osteotomy of the ulna. *Vet. Comp. Orthopaed.* 8 (4): 170–176.

71 Wind, A.P. (1986). Elbow incongruity and developmental elbow diseases in the dog. 1. *J. Am. Anim. Hosp. Assoc.* 22 (6): 711–724.

72 Kirberger, R.M. and Fourie, S.L. (1998). Elbow dysplasia in the dog: pathophysiology, diagnosis and control. *J. S. Afr. Vet. Assoc.* 69 (2): 43–54.

73 Olson, N.C., Brinker, W.O., Carrig, C.B., and Tvedten, H.W. (1981). Asynchronous growth of the canine radius and ulna – surgical-correction following experimental premature closure of the distal radial Physis. *Vet. Surg.* 10 (3): 125–131.

74 Boulay, J.P. (1998). Fragmented medial coronoid process of the ulna in the dog. *Vet. Clin. North Am. Small Anim. Pract.* 28 (1): 51–74.

75 Lewis, D.D., Parker, R.B., and Hager, D.A. (1989). Fragmented medial coronoid process of the canine elbow. *Compend. Contin. Educ. Pract.* 11 (6): 703–734.

76 Berry, C.R. (1992). Evaluation of the canine elbow for fragmented medial coronoid process. *Vet. Radiol. Ultrasoun.* 33 (5): 273–276.

77 Berzon, J.L. (1980). The classification and Management of Epiphyseal Plate Fractures. *J. Am. Anim. Hosp. Assoc.* 16 (5): 651–658.

78 Carpenter, L.G., Schwarz, P.D., Lowry, J.E. et al. (1993). Comparison of radiologic imaging techniques for diagnosis of fragmented medial coronoid process of the cubital joint in dogs. *J. Am. Vet. Med. Assoc.* 203 (1): 78–83.

79 Read, R.A., Armstrong, S.J., Okeefe, J.D., and Eger, C.E. (1990). Fragmentation of the medial coronoid process of the ulna in dogs – a study of 109 cases. *J. Small Anim. Pract.* 31 (7): 330–334.

80 Alexander, J.W. and Earley, T.D. (1984). A carpal laxity syndrome in young dogs. *J. Vet. Orthop.* 3: 22.

81 Shires, P.K., Hulse, D.A., and Kearney, M.T. (1985). Carpal hyperextension in two-month-old pups. *J. Am. Vet. Med. Assoc.* 186 (1): 49–52.

82 Barrett, R.B., Schall, W.D., and Lewis, R.E. (1968). Clinical and radiographic features of canine eosinophilic panosteitis. *J. Am. Anim. Hosp. Assoc.* 4: 94.

83 Bohning, R.H. Jr., Suter, P.F., Hohn, R.B., and Marshall, J. (1970). Clinical and radiologic survey of canine panosteitis. *J. Am. Vet. Med. Assoc.* 156 (7): 870–883.

84 Muir, P., Dubielzig, R.R., and Panosteitis, J.K.A. (1996). *Compend. Contin. Educ. Pract.* 18 (1): 29–33.

85 Alexander, J.W. (1978). Hypertrophic osteodystrophy. *Canine Pract.* 5: 48.

86 Munjar, T.A., Austin, C.C., and Breur, G.J. (1998). Comparison of risk factors for hypertrophic osteodystrophy, craniomandibular osteopathy, and canine distemper virus infection. *Vet. Comp. Orthop. Traumatol.* 11: 37.

87 Grondalen, J. (1976). Metaphyseal osteopathy (hypertrophic osteodystrophy) in growing dogs. A clinical study. *J. Small Anim. Pract.* 17 (11): 721–735.

88 Clements, D.N., Fitzpatrick, N., Carter, S.D., and Day, P.J.R. (2009). Cartilage gene expression correlates with radiographic severity of canine elbow osteoarthritis. *Vet. J.* 179 (2): 211–218.

89 Morgan, J.P., Wind, A., and Davidson, A.P. (1999). Bone dysplasias in the Labrador retriever: a radiographic study. *J. Am. Anim. Hosp. Assoc.* 35 (4): 332–340.

90 Sivacolundhu, R.K., Runge, J.J., Donovan, T.A. et al. (2013). Ulnar osteosarcoma in dogs: 30 cases (1992–2008). *Javma-J. Am. Vet. Med. A.* 243 (1): 96–101.

91 Gasch, E.G., Rivier, P., and Bardet, J.F. (2013). Free proximal cortical ulnar autograft for the treatment of distal radial osteosarcoma in a dog. *Can. Vet. J.* 54 (2): 162–166.

92 Henry, C.J., Brewer, W.G., Whitley, E.M. et al. (2005). Canine digital tumors: a veterinary cooperative oncology group retrospective study of 64 dogs. *J. Vet. Intern. Med.* 19 (5): 720–724.

93 Shafiee, R., Shariat, A., Khalili, S. et al. (2015). Diagnostic investigations of canine prostatitis incidence together with benign prostate hyperplasia, prostate malignancies, and biochemical recurrence in high-risk prostate cancer as a model for human study. *Tumor Biol.* 36 (4): 2437–2445.

94 Hill, F.W. (1977). A survey of bone fractures in the cat. *J. Small Anim. Pract.* 18 (7): 457–463.

95 Whitney, W.O. and Mehlhaff, C.J. (1987). High-rise syndrome in cats. *J. Am. Vet. Med. Assoc.* 191 (11): 1399–1403.

96 Heinrich, C. (2015). Assessing conjunctivitis in cats. Vet Times [Internet]. www.vettimes.co.uk/app/uploads/wp-post-to-pdf-enhanced-cache/1/assessing-conjunctivitis-in-cats.pdf.

97 Henderson, S.M., Bradley, K., Day, M.J. et al. (2004). Investigation of nasal disease in the cat–a retrospective study of 77 cases. *J. Feline Med. Surg.* 6 (4): 245–257.

98 Van Pelt, D.R. and Lappin, M.R. (1994). Pathogenesis and treatment of feline rhinitis. *Vet. Clin. North Am. Small Anim. Pract.* 24 (5): 807–823.

99 Dawson, S., McArdle, F., Bennett, D. et al. (1993). Investigation of vaccine reactions and breakdowns after feline calicivirus vaccination. *Vet. Rec.* 132 (14): 346–350.

100 Malik, R., Allan, G.S., Howlett, C.R. et al. (1999). Osteochondrodysplasia in Scottish fold cats. *Aust. Vet. J.* 77 (2): 85–92.

101 Wobeser, B.K., Kidney, B.A., Powers, B.E. et al. (2007). Diagnoses and clinical outcomes associated with surgically amputated feline digits submitted to multiple veterinary diagnostic laboratories. *Vet. Pathol.* 44 (3): 362–365.

102 Herraez, P., Rodriguez, F., Ramirez, G. et al. (2005). Multiple primary digital apocrine sweat gland carcinosarcoma in a cat. *Vet. Rec.* 157 (12): 356–358.

103 Scarff, D.H. (2004). Nail disease in the dog and cat. *Small Anim. Dermatol.* 9 (7): 1–4.

104 Apple, S. (2015). Senior cat with front paw swelling and pain. *Today's Veterinary Practice* (September/October): 41–44.

105 Gottfried, S.D., Popovitch, C.A., Goldschmidt, M.H., and Schelling, C. (2000). Metastatic digital carcinoma in the cat: a retrospective study of 36 cats (1992–1998). *J. Am. Anim. Hosp. Assoc.* 36 (6): 501–509.

106 Goldfinch, N. and Argyle, D.J. (2012). Feline lung-digit syndrome: unusual metastatic patterns of primary lung tumours in cats. *J. Feline Med. Surg.* 14 (3): 202–208.

107 Maritato, K.C., Schertel, E.R., Kennedy, S.C. et al. (2014). Outcome and prognostic indicators in 20 cats with surgically treated primary lung tumors. *J. Feline Med. Surg.* 16 (12): 979–984.

108 Mehlhaff, C.J. and Mooney, S. (1985). Primary pulmonary neoplasia in the dog and cat. *Vet. Clin. North Am. Small Anim. Pract.* 15 (5): 1061–1067.

109 May, C. and Newsholme, S.J. (1989). Metastasis of feline pulmonary-carcinoma presenting as multiple digital swelling. *J. Small Anim. Pract.* 30 (5): 302–310.

110 Hanselman, B.A. and Hall, J.A. (2004). Digital metastasis from a primary bronchogenic carcinoma. *Can. Vet. J.* 45 (7): 614–616.

111 Jacobs, T.M. and Tomlinson, M.J. (1997). The lung-digit syndrome in a cat. *Feline Pract.* 25 (1): 31–36.

112 van der Linde-Sipman, J.S. and van den Ingh, T.S.G.A.M. (2000). Primary and metastatic carcinomas in the digits of cats. *Vet. Q.* 22 (3): 141–145.

113 Hahn, K.A. and McEntee, M.F. (1997). Primary lung tumors in cats: 86 cases (1979–1994). *J. Am. Vet. Med. Assoc.* 211 (10): 1257–1260.

114 Sorenmo, K.U., Dr, W., and Goldschmidt, M.H. (2013). Tumors of the mammary gland. In: *Withrow and MacEwen's Small Animal Clinical Oncology*, 5e, 538–556. St. Louis: Elsevier Saunders.

115 Straw, R.C. (2006). The cat with skin lumps and bumps. In: *Problem-Based Feline Medicine* (ed. J. Rand), 1067–1080. Edinburgh, New York: Saunders.

116 Tilley, L.P. and Smith, F.W.K. (2004). Mammary gland tumors – cats. In: *The 5-Minute Veterinary Consult: Canine and Feline*, 3e (ed. L.P. Tilley and F.W.K. Smith), 804–805. Baltimore, MD: Lippincott Williams & Wilkins.

117 Gimenez, F., Hecht, S., Craig, L.E., and Legendre, A.M. (2010). Early detection, aggressive therapy: optimizing the management of feline mammary masses. *J. Feline Med. Surg.* 12 (3): 214–224.

118 Hayes, A.A. and Mooney, S. (1985). Feline mammary tumors. *Vet. Clin. North Am. Small Anim. Pract.* 15 (3): 513–520.

119 Hahn, K.A. and Adams, W.H. (1997). Feline mammary neoplasia: biological behavior, diagnosis, and treatment alternatives. *Feline Pract.* 25 (2): 5–11.

120 Waters, D.J., Honeckman, A., Cooley, D.M., and DeNicola, D. (1998). Skeletal metastasis in feline mammary carcinoma: case report and literature review. *J. Am. Anim. Hosp. Assoc.* 34 (2): 103–108.

121 Thomas, W.B. (2000). Initial assessment of patients with neurologic dysfunction. *Vet. Clin. North Am. Small Anim. Pract.* 30 (1): 1–24, v.

122 Averill, D.R. Jr. (1981). The neurologic examination. *Vet. Clin. North Am. Small Anim. Pract.* 11 (3): 511–521.

123 Thomas, W.B. and Dewey, C.W. (2008). Performing the neurologic examination. In: *A Practical Guide to Canine and Feline Neurology*, 2e (ed. C.W. Dewey), 53–74. Ames, Iowa: Wiley-Blackwell.

124 Garosi, L. (2009). Neurological examination of the cat. How to get started. *J. Feline Med. Surg.* 11 (5): 340–348.

125 De Risio, L. and Platt, S.R. (2010). Fibrocartilaginous embolic myelopathy in small animals. *Vet. Clin. North Am. Small Anim. Pract.* 40 (5): 859–869.

126 Mikszewski, J.S., Van Winkle, T.J., and Troxel, M.T. (2006). Fibrocartilaginous embolic myelopathy in five cats. *J. Am. Anim. Hosp. Assoc.* 42 (3): 226–233.

127 Falconer, L. and Atwell, R. (2003). Feline aortic thromboembolism. *Aust. Vet. Pract.* 33 (1): 20–32.

128 Fuentes, V.L. (2012). ARTERIAL THROMBOEMBOLISM risks, realities and a rational first-line approach. *J. Feline Med. Surg.* 14 (7): 459–470.

129 Borgeat, K., Wright, J., Garrod, O. et al. (2014). Arterial thromboembolism in 250 cats in general practice: 2004–2012. *J. Vet. Intern. Med.* 28 (1): 102–108.

130 Smith, S.A., Tobias, A.H., Jacob, K.A. et al. (2003). Arterial thromboembolism in cats: acute crisis in 127 cases (1992–2001) and long-term management with low-dose aspirin in 24 cases. *J. Vet. Intern. Med.* 17 (1): 73–83.

131 Laste, N.J. and Harpster, N.K. (1995). A retrospective study of 100 cases of feline distal aortic thromboembolism: 1977–1993. *J. Am. Anim. Hosp. Assoc.* 31 (6): 492–500.

132 Schoeman, J.P. (1999). Feline distal aortic thromboembolism: a review of 44 cases (1990–1998). *J. Feline Med. Surg.* 1 (4): 221–231.

133 Killingsworth, C.R., Eyster, G.E., Adams, T. et al. (1986). Streptokinase treatment of cats with experimentally induced aortic thrombosis. *Am. J. Vet. Res.* 47 (6): 1351–1359.

134 Smith, S.A. and Tobias, A.H. (2004). Feline arterial thromboembolism: an update. *Vet. Clin. North Am. Small Anim. Pract.* 34 (5): 1245–1271.

135 Moise, N.S. (2007). Presentation and management of thromboembolism in cats. *In Pract.* 29 (1): 2–8.

136 Rishniw, M. (2006). Feline aortic thromboembolism. *NAVC Clinician's Brief* (November): 17–20.

137 Moore, K.E., Morris, N., Dhupa, N. et al. (2000). Retrospective study of streptokinase administration in 46 cats with arterial thromboembolism. *J. Vet. Emerg. Crit. Care* 10: 245–257.

138 Peycke, L.E. (2010). Forelimb lameness & elbow pain. *NAVC Clinician's Brief* (September): 40–41.

69

Pelvic Limb Lameness

69.1 Introduction to Pelvic Limb Anatomy

Recall from Section 68.1 that the appendicular skeleton consists of the limbs of the body [1]. These extensions of the trunk make it possible for patients to move from one point in space to another [1]. Such movement requires coordination between the musculoskeletal and nervous systems to initiate and maintain a proper gait.

The hind limbs are paired structures of the appendicular skeleton that attach to the pelvic girdle. The pelvic girdle includes the ilium, ischium, pubis, and acetabulum [2, 3].

Distal to the pelvis is the femur, which comprises the thigh [2, 3].

The tibia and fibula are distal to the femur. These bones collectively make up the crus, or lower leg [2, 3].

Distal to the lower leg is the tarsus, which is also known as the ankle or hock, followed by the metatarsals and the phalanges [2, 3].

Each segment of the hind limb has a purpose and an expected range of motion. Motion is made possible via tendons, which attach skeletal muscle to bone [1]. The coordination of muscular actions provides for a purposeful gait in which both pelvic limbs are equally and fully weight bearing.

69.2 The Role of Signalment and History Taking in Diagnosing Pelvic Limb Lameness

Pelvic limb lameness is a common presentation in clinical practice [4, 5]. A lame patient has a gait disturbance that affects its ability to move through space.

When a canine or feline patient presents for pelvic limb lameness, the list of differential diagnoses is extensive [6]. It may be difficult to know where to begin the patient work-up for this presenting complaint.

Signalment provides a starting point by helping the clinician to initially focus on those disease processes that are most likely.

Consider, for example, how the patient's age influences the prioritization of differential diagnoses:

- A young cat with hind limb lameness is more likely to have slipped capital femoral epiphysis (SCFE) syndrome than degenerative joint disease (DJD) [7].
- A young dog with hind limb lameness is more likely to have Legg-Calvé-Perthes (LCP) disease than DJD [8].
- An older dog with hind limb lameness is more likely to have DJD or osteosarcoma than osteochondrosis (OC) [8].

These patterns may not initially be apparent to the inexperienced clinician; however, they are more easily recognized with time as the veterinarian develops clinical acumen.

Consider also the impact of breed:

- Small-breed dogs are more likely to develop LCP than large-breed dogs [8].
- Large-breed dogs are more likely to develop hip dysplasia than small-breed dogs [8].

History taking provides additional clues [5].

Recall the following key questions from Chapter 68, Section 68.3 that are important to ask of any client that presents a patient for lameness [9–11]:

- When was the lameness first noticed?
- What, if anything, was observed that may have triggered the lameness?
- How, if at all, has the lameness progressed?
- Is the patient's lameness a new finding or a recurrent one?
  - If recurrent, how, if at all, has the lameness changed?
- Which limb(s) appear(s) to be affected?
- Is there shifting leg lameness? In other words, does the lame limb appear to switch from one to another?

Common Clinical Presentations in Dogs and Cats, First Edition. Ryane E. Englar.
© 2019 John Wiley & Sons, Inc. Published 2019 by John Wiley & Sons, Inc.

- Is the patient bearing weight on the affected limb(s)?
  - A patient that is non-weight bearing may hold up the affected limb(s).
  - The patient may also reproducibly lean against the examination room wall to take pressure off the affected limb(s).
- Is the lameness persistent or does it come and go?
- Is the lameness better or worse after periods of inactivity?
- Is the lameness better or worse with continued movement?
- Is the lameness better or worse at faster gaits?
- Does the patient exhibit difficulty or discomfort when standing up or sitting down?

Remember to discuss grooming behavior or changes in coat quality, particularly in cats [11]. Cats tend to be fastidious groomers, yet those with underlying musculoskeletal disease may not be able to keep up with basic hygiene [11, 12].

Historical questions about patient lifestyle and home environment are also important. An outdoor, unsupervised cat is at potentially greater risk of traumatic injury to one or more limbs.

Geography and travel history may make certain differentials more or less likely. For example, fungal diseases tend to be geographically regional. Patients that reside in, or have traveled to, these areas are at increased risk of exposure.

69.3 The Role of Observation and the Physical Examination in Diagnosing Pelvic Limb Lameness

Observation of the patient's gait may demonstrate hind limb lameness [5, 12]:

- When there is unilateral hind limb lameness, the dog may have a hip hike; that is, the hip of the affected leg elevates when bearing weight on the painful limb.
- When there is bilateral hind limb lameness, the dog may abbreviate its stride by taking short, choppy steps.

If the patient is visibly lame, grading the lameness is helpful to outline the progression of disease [9, 13, 14]. Recall from Chapter 68, Section 68.4 that there is no universal grading system for lameness. For consistency, the author makes use of the following scale:

- Grade 1
  - The patient shifts weight off of the affected leg when at rest or standing, but has no evidence of lameness when in motion.

- Grade 2
  - Mild lameness is only evident at a trot.
- Grade 3
  - Mild to moderate lameness any time the patient is in motion, including at a walk.
- Grade 4
  - Moderate-to-severe lameness any time the patient is in motion.
  - The patient attempts to carry the affected limb when in motion.
  - The patient may attempt to place the limb when standing, but is only partially weight bearing.
- Grade 5
  - Non-weight bearing in the affected limb.

Each practice is encouraged to adopt a scale that meets its own needs, provided that assessment is consistent between team members.

A comprehensive physical examination should be performed on every patient that presents for lameness. This includes a heavy emphasis on the musculoskeletal system; however, all body systems should be considered. A lame dog or cat may suffer from systemic illness that will not be identified unless the veterinarian examines the entire patient [5, 15].

Each component of the pelvic limb should be palpated superficially, followed by deep palpation and range of motion through the joints. It is common to begin this portion of the examination with the patient standing.

Standing palpation assesses for the following [12, 15]:

- Symmetry between the hind limbs in terms of bone contour: specifically, palpation concentrates on feeling for continuity of bone: are fractures grossly or palpably apparent?
- Symmetry between the hind limbs in terms of muscle mass and tendons: specifically, palpation concentrates on the hamstrings, quadriceps, cranial tibial muscles, gastrocnemius, soleus, and the Achilles tendon
- Symmetry between the hind limbs in terms of joints: specifically, palpation concentrates on the presence or absence of joint effusion, and the presence or absence of heat at each joint (see Figure 69.1)

Standing palpation transitions into palpation in lateral recumbency to appreciate the range of motion through each joint. If one pelvic limb is known to be sensitive, then the author tends to examine that limb last [10, 11].

Refer to *Performing the Small Animal Physical Examination* for an exhaustive review of the orthopedic exam. A recap of the key structures of interest on palpation will be provided here.

When examining the pelvic girdle, the wings of the ilium and the ischiatic tuberosity are palpable [2, 9].

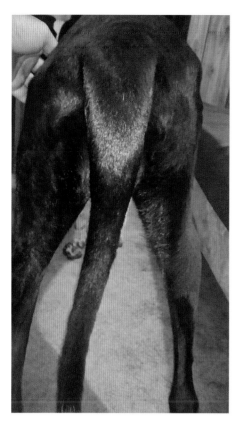

Figure 69.1 Caudal thigh muscle asymmetry in a standing canine patient. Note that the musculature associated with the right hip and caudal thigh is atrophied as compared to the left. *Source:* Courtesy of Hannah Butler.

The coxofemoral joint should be assessed for swelling, palpable heat that could indicate active inflammation, crepitus, pain, and range of motion.

The proximal femur is a key component of the coxofemoral joint. Recall from basic anatomy that the femoral head sits within the pelvic acetabulum. Hyaline cartilage lines the articulating surface of the femoral head except for the fovea capitis, a depression along the medial aspect of the proximal epiphysis. The fovea capitis is the site of attachment of the ligament of the head of the femur. This anchors the femur to the ventral acetabulum. The femoral neck supports the head and joins it to the proximal femoral epiphysis [2, 3, 16].

The proximal femur is exposed to large amounts of tensile and compressive forces during everyday activity.

The greater trochanter of the femur is an attachment site for the middle gluteal, deep gluteal, and piriformis muscles. These muscles initiate hip extension, abduction, and medial rotation of the pelvic limb [2, 3, 16, 17].

The trochanteric fossa is a depression that is located medial to the greater trochanter and is the point of attachment for the internal and external obturator and gemelli muscles to achieve lateral rotation of the hip.

Distal and caudomedial to the femoral neck is the lesser trochanter. Here, the iliopsoas muscle attaches to allow for flexion of the hip [2, 3, 16, 17].

The body of the femur should be palpated for swelling, pain, and asymmetry between the left and right hind limb.

The medial and lateral epicondyles are palpable at the distal femur [2, 3].

The femoral trochlea, located at the cranial surface of the distal femur, between the medial and lateral epicondyles of the femur, is not palpable on physical exam. However, the patella or kneecap articulates with this smooth surface [2].

The patella is palpable as an ossification within the tendon of insertion of the quadriceps femoris muscle, which extends the stifle [2, 9]. To locate the patella, it may be easiest for the clinician to first identify the tibial crest, a prominence at the cranial aspect of the proximal tibia. Proximal to the tibial crest is the tibial tuberosity. The patellar tendon runs from the tibial tuberosity to the patella. So by tracking the patellar tendon from the tibial tuberosity, the clinician should reach the patella.

The patella should be evaluated for tendencies to luxate.

The stifle joint should be evaluated for swelling, palpable heat that could indicate active inflammation, crepitus, pain, and range of motion.

Distal to the stifle, the clinician should consider the crus, which consists of the more cranially positioned tibia and the narrow fibula. The tibia bears the bulk of the weight for the crus. The function of the laterally located fibula is to serve as a site for muscle attachment [2].

Distally, the tibia ends as the medial malleolus. Caudal to the medial malleolus are distinct notches and sulci that provide attachment sites for tarsal flexors [2].

The fibula ends, distally, as the lateral malleolus. Along the medial aspect of the lateral malleolus, there is an articulating surface that allows for the intimate connection involving the trochlea of the tibial tarsal bone or talus [2].

Like the carpus, the tarsus consists of seven bones. However, both the tibia and fibula only articulate with the tibial tarsal bone.

The largest, longest bone of the tarsus is the calcaneus. Proximally, the calcaneus forms a prominent lever, the tuber calcanei, upon which the calcaneal tendon inserts. Distally, it forms a stable joint with the tibial tarsal bone [2].

The distal row of tarsal bones articulates with four metatarsal bones that are identified as being the second through fifth. The second metatarsal bone is the most medial [2].

Each metatarsal bone bears three phalanges to form the second through fifth digits [2].

Given the size of the canine or feline hind paw, it is difficult to identify the individual tarsal bones through palpation, except for the calcaneus. Therefore, the clinician's goal in examining the tarsus is less to identify individual bones and more to identify any abnormalities such as swelling, heat, crepitus, asymmetry between the left and right hind paw, and pain (see Figure 69.2).

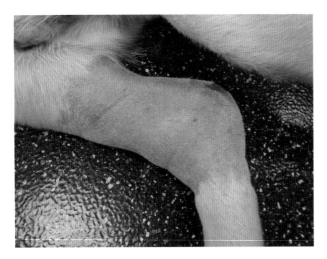

Figure 69.2 Appreciable tarsal swelling in a canine patient. *Source:* Courtesy of Kara Thomas, DVM, CVMA.

Fractures of tarsal, metatarsal bones, and phalanges can easily be missed when evaluated based on the physical exam alone [10]. Radiographs should be prioritized any time pain, swelling, or lameness is localized to the distal hind limb (see Figures 69.3a, b).

69.4 Pelvic Fractures and Coxofemoral Luxations

Trauma to the pelvis commonly results in fractures and is most often due to vehicular injury in dogs [15, 18–20]. Cats may also sustain pelvic fractures secondary to vehicular trauma; however, blunt trauma, bite wounds, and falling are also common causes [15].

Because the pelvis is a box, a single fracture is unlikely. A fracture at one location of the pelvis is likely to translate into a fracture elsewhere. This may potentiate damage to internal organs, resulting in intra-abdominal hemorrhage and/or uroabdomen [21–28].

Nerve damage is also possible. Sacroiliac fractures may result in hind limb dysfunction, urinary retention, and urinary or fecal incontinence [18, 29, 30]. Lack of anal tone and lack of perineal sensation are concerning findings in patients with sacral or sacroiliac fractures [15].

(a)　　　　　　　　　　　　　　(b)

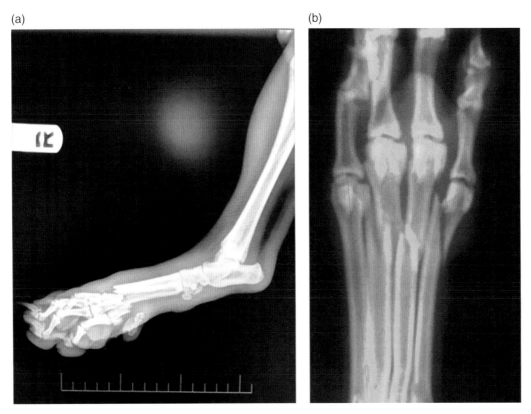

Figure 69.3 (a) Right lateral view of the distal pelvic limb, demonstrating multiple fractures of the metatarsals. (b) Dorsoplantar view demonstrating three fractured metatarsals in a nine-year-old Australian heeler mix. *Source:* Courtesy of Stephanie Perry.

In addition, pelvic fractures may reduce space within the pelvic canal, complicating everyday body functions. For example, pelvic floor fractures may result in constipation or obstipation due to narrowing of the rectal canal [18, 29, 30].

Ilial and acetabular fractures are common sequelae of pelvic trauma [18, 19].

Pelvic fractures may occur with or without coxofemoral luxations. The majority of coxofemoral luxations occur in a craniodorsal direction [31, 32].

Radiographs are diagnostic for both pelvic fractures and coxofemoral luxations (see Figures 69.4a, b).

An experienced clinician may suspect a craniodorsal coxofemoral luxation based upon the physical examination. In a normal dog and cat, the wings of the ilia, ischiatic tuberosities, and greater trochanters should form a triangle that is symmetrical on both the left and right sides (see Figures 69.5a, b).

When there is a craniodorsal coxofemoral luxation, the greater trochanter of the affected limb migrates craniodorsally, thereby disrupting this triangle. This can also be appreciated on radiographic examination [9] (see Figure 69.6).

Another way to assess for craniodorsal coxofemoral luxation is for the clinician to place his thumb between the greater trochanter and the ischiatic tuberosity. Simultaneously, the clinician applies pressure to gently lift both hind limbs up and extend them caudally. Leg length is compared by assessing the location of the right and left calcanei. In cases involving craniodorsal coxofemoral luxation, the affected side will appear to have the shorter leg because the femur has been moved in a craniodorsal direction from its original seat within the acetabulum [9].

Patients with coxofemoral luxations are non-weight bearing on the affected limb [33].

Closed reduction is possible; however, failure is more likely to occur in patients that have pre-existing hip dysplasia [33]. These patients benefit from open reduction, which also allows for repair of concurrent pelvic fractures [33].

(b)

(a)

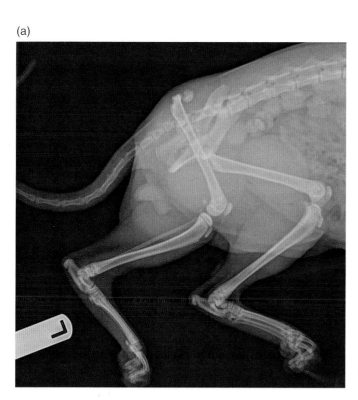
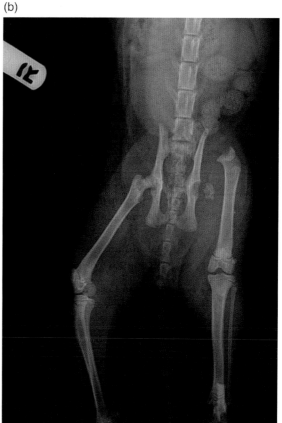

Figure 69.4 (a) Lateral radiograph of a five-month old, intact male, Domestic shorthaired (DSH) kitten that sustained a traumatic, oblique, closed fracture through the left femoral head and neck with craniodorsal displacement of the left femur relative to the coxofemoral joint. (b) Ventrodorsal (V/D) radiograph of the kitten depicted in (a).

(a)

(b)

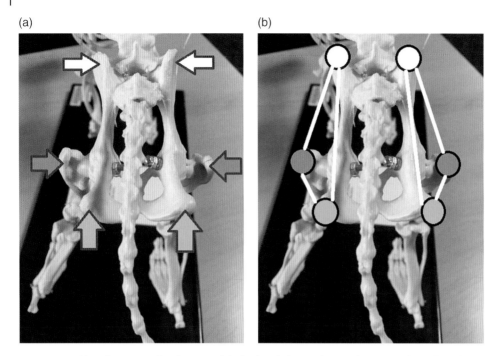

Figure 69.5 (a) End-on-view of a plastic model of a dog skeleton. The emphasis is on the pelvis. The wings of the ilia are identified by white arrows. The ischiatic tuberosities are identified by pink arrows. The greater trochanters are identified by blue arrows. (b) Note the imaginary triangle that is formed by the wings of the ilia (identified by circles filled in with white), the ischiatic tuberosities (identified by circles filled in with pink), and the greater trochanters (identified by circles filled in with blue).

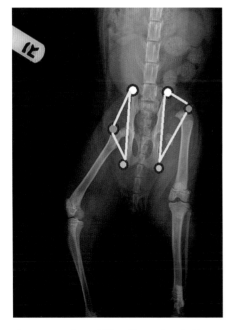

Figure 69.6 Same V/D radiograph as in Figure 69.4b. In this figure, note how the imaginary triangle that is formed by the wings of the ilia (identified by circles filled in with white), the ischiatic tuberosities (identified by circles filled in with pink), and the greater trochanters (identified by circles filled in with blue) has shifted due to craniodorsal coxofemoral luxation of the left femur.

69.5 Distal Pelvic Limb Fractures

Femoral fractures are common traumatic injuries in both dogs and cats [15]. The shaft is the most frequent site of femoral fracture in adults [15].

Fractures of the femoral neck may also occur, particularly in cats [15].

Avulsion fracture of the greater and lesser trochanter have also been reported in both dogs and cats [15, 34].

Physeal fractures may occur in juvenile patients, with distal ones occurring more often than proximal [15]. Refer to Section 69.6 below.

Fractures of the patella are possible, but rare [15].

Tibial fractures occur less often than femoral fractures.

Tarsal and metatarsal fractures are common. They are most often sustained by vehicular trauma; however, they may also occur when patients are inadvertently stepped on or intentionally crushed from bite injuries to the foot [15].

Digital fractures also occur and respond well in most cases to conservative management [15].

Radiographs provide diagnostic confirmation of fractures and assist with case management, particularly when planning surgical repair [15].

69.6 Salter-Harris Growth Plate Fractures and SCFE

Fractures in patients of all ages disrupt bone structure and, potentially, blood supply.

Fractures in juvenile patients may also impact long bone growth, particularly if they involve the growth plate.

Salter and Harris classified traumatic fractures of the growth plate into five types [35]. Type 1 fractures are those in which the epiphysis becomes separated from the metaphysis at the growth plate. Most frequently, these fractures occur through the hypertrophic zone. Type II fractures occur when the fracture is through the growth plate and a corner of the metaphyseal bone. Type III fractures involve the epiphysis and a part of the growth plate; however the metaphysis is not affected. Type IV fractures are those that occur through the epiphysis, through the growth plate, and into the metaphysis. Type V fractures are compressive at the growth plate. Prognosis becomes less favorable between Type I and Type V. Any of these types can adversely affect physeal closure; however, premature closure is nearly guaranteed with Type V fractures [7, 35].

Salter-Harris Type I fractures are the most common type of physeal fracture in small animals, with the proximal femur being the most common site of fracture [35, 36]. Trauma is implicated in the majority of these cases. The result is displacement of the proximal femoral metaphysis from the capital femoral epiphysis through the growth plate. This process or condition is otherwise known as SCFE [37]. Traumatic SCFE in dogs has been reported with some frequency in the literature [38–40].

However, SCFE does not always have to be the result of trauma. In fact, reports of atraumatic SCFE are on the rise in the literature and have included both dogs and cats [7, 37, 41–47].

Juvenile male cats appear to be predisposed [7, 37, 43, 45]. Most are less than two years old at the time of diagnosis [37].

Domestic shorthaired (DSH), Siamese, Siamese mixes, and Maine Coons appear with greater frequency in the veterinary literature than other breeds [37, 43, 45].

Overweight or obese cats are more likely to develop SCFE [37, 45]; so, too, are neutered cats [7, 45, 47–49].

SCFE may be unilateral or bilateral [37, 45]. In bilateral presentations, both femoral heads and necks may be affected concurrently, or a fracture of the contralateral femur can occur separately from the first event [45].

Atraumatic SCFE is thought to reflect a slow, progressive process whereby gradual necrosis of the femoral neck results in a pathological fracture. This progression had previously been referred to in the literature as proximal femoral metaphyseal osteopathy, femoral neck metaphyseal osteopathy, and/or capital physeal dysplasia syndrome. However, all are thought to now be a part of the same process [50].

The pathogenesis of this condition remains unclear. What is understood is that in order for SCFE to develop, atraumatic or otherwise, an open physis is required. As Smith's studies during the 1970s established, normal, healthy, intact cats achieve physeal closure of the femoral head between 30 and 40 weeks (7.5–10 months) of age [51]. Thus, affected cats are thought to have delayed physeal closure or pre-existing morphological abnormalities at or around the physis that predispose them to this condition [46].

Typical presentation of SCFE is lameness associated with one or both pelvic limbs. Severity of the lameness varies from weight-bearing lame to fully non-weight bearing lame. The owner may report perceived stiffness or weakness in the hind end and/or decreased ability to jump [43, 45]. The lameness is often acute in onset, but may progress prior to presentation [47, 52].

Classically there is no known history of trauma, and the majority of the patients reported in the literature maintain indoor-only lifestyles [44, 46].

On physical examination, muscle atrophy of the hip and thigh regions of the affected limb may be subtle but can facilitate localization of disease [45].

A key feature of SCFE is pain on hip flexion and extension [50]. Pain on extension is typically more dramatic than pain on flexion at the hip joint [43]. Palpable crepitus over the hip joint is common as the hip is carried through its range of motion [45].

Palpation over the greater trochanter of the affected limb may also elicit pain [52].

Hind limb reflexes tend to be normal; however, proprioception of the affected limb may be reduced [44].

Orthogonal radiographs of the pelvis and coxofemoral joints facilitate diagnosis. Typically, these regions are imaged via two standard views: a lateral and a ventrodorsal (V/D) view with the limbs in extension. However, the latter view may obscure spontaneous capital physeal fractures because limb extension tightens the collagen fibers of the joint capsule. Such tightening can reduce capital physeal fractures, allowing them to go undetected. Thus, a frog-legged V/D view is encouraged. This decreases tension on the joint capsule and improves visualization of the region of interest [7].

Radiographs are typically performed under heavy sedation or general anesthesia. Radiographic findings classically include loss of definition and loss of bone within the femoral neck, with or without femoral neck sclerosis. If extensive, the femoral neck region begins to take on an "apple-cored" appearance, which is the result of appreciable bone destruction and/or resorption of the proximal femoral metaphysis (see Figure 69.7).

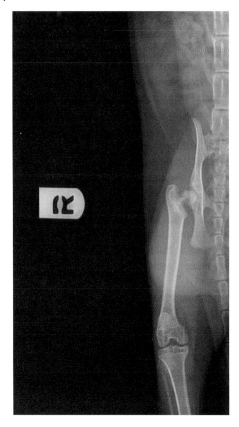

Figure 69.7 Ventrodorsal (V/D) radiograph of an 11-month-old, intact male, DSH – the same kitten that in Figures 69.4a, b, at five months of age, had sustained a traumatic, oblique, closed fracture through the left femoral head and neck with craniodorsal displacement of the left femur relative to the coxofemoral joint. The left femoral head and neck fracture had been surgically repaired. However, note the classic "apple core" appearance of the right femoral neck region. This patient was subsequently diagnosed with right femoral SCFE based upon histopathology.

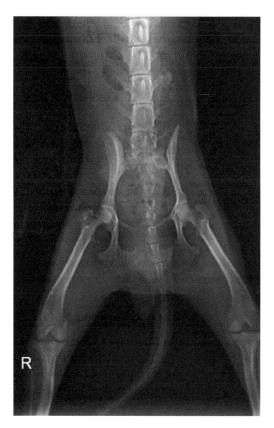

Figure 69.8 Ventrodorsal (V/D) radiograph of canine patient. Note the apple-cored appearance to the right femoral neck. This characteristic feature raises the index of suspicion that this patient has LCP disease.

- Flattened, irregular femoral head
- Moth-eaten appearance to the femoral head
- Shortened, wide femoral neck
- "Apple core" appearance of the femoral neck
- Femoral neck fractures (see Figure 69.8)

Patients most often present with acute lameness following minor injuries, such as a jump or a fall [8]. Examination is likely to reveal non-weight-bearing lameness and a reluctance to walk [8]. The patient is painful over the affected hip, and crepitus may be palpable when establishing range of motion through the coxofemoral joint [8]. Depending upon how long the issue has been brewing, there may be associated muscle atrophy of the affected hip [8].

Case management is most often surgical and involves femoral head and neck excision (FHNE) or femoral head ostectomy (FHO) [8].

The surrounding soft tissue may be encroached upon by spicules of bone [44]. It may be difficult to determine the borders of the femoral head, femoral neck, and the greater trochanter.

Femoral heads may be misshapen or grossly deformed and flattened. In some cases, complete femoral head separation is evident as an irregular, but complete radiolucent line across the femoral neck [43]. If a capital physeal fracture is apparent, there is typically minimal to no displacement [45, 50].

69.7 LCP Disease

LCP disease is a condition that primarily affects small-breed dogs [8, 53]. In LCP disease, the blood supply to the femoral head is compromised [8, 53]. This leads to avascular necrosis of the femoral head [8, 53]. The radiographic appearance is similar to SCFE [8]:

69.8 Hip Dysplasia

Hip dysplasia is an inherited condition in dogs in which there is inadequate coverage of the femoral head by the acetabulum [54–56]. Hip laxity is a significant risk factor for the development of hip dysplasia, as is the breed of dog [57]. Large-breed dogs, including German Shepherds and Labrador Retrievers, are overrepresented; however, selective breeding in under five generations has proved effective in diminishing the percentage of affected patients in both breeds [58].

Patients may present for routine screening for hip dysplasia because they are intended to be breeding stock, or patients may present for routine screening because of a familial history of disease. Alternatively, patients may be symptomatic for hip dysplasia. These present for clinical lameness, apparent stiffness, and/or difficulty with stairs [59].

One or both limbs may be affected. Immature patients often present with an altered, so-called "bunny hopping" gait. Note that this is not pathognomonic for hip dysplasia; it is also appreciated following cranial cruciate ligament rupture (CCLR) [59].

On physical examination, dogs with hip dysplasia are resentful of hip manipulation, particularly full hip extension and abduction. They may struggle in an attempt to resist the clinician's attempts to elicit full range of motion at the coxofemoral joint [59, 60].

Dogs that are suspected of hip dysplasia should be subjected to the Ortolani test, which may require sedation. The Ortolani test is a maneuver that assesses the patient for hip laxity. With the patient in dorsal or lateral recumbency, the stifle and hip are held at 90° of flexion. One hand of the clinician is held at the level of the stifle; the opposite hand is placed over the hip, taking care to have the thumb seated over the greater trochanter. Using the hand on the stifle, the clinician applies a compressive force along the femur; using the opposite hand, the clinician applies a countercompressive force over the hip. No hip laxity should be felt in a non-dysplastic, normal dog at this point. If there is any degree of laxity, the thumb over the greater trochanter will feel the femoral head subluxate.

Next, while maintaining the compressive force along the femur, the stifle is abducted. In a dog with a positive Ortolani test, the clinician will feel a "click" or a "pop" as the femoral head reduces back into the acetabulum, suggesting that there is inadequate coverage of the femoral head [60, 61].

A positive Ortolani sign increases suspicion that the patient has hip dysplasia. However, radiographs are diagnostic for the condition. Radiographs of hip dysplasia depict reduced coverage of the femoral head by the acetabulum (see Figure 69.9).

In an attempt to reduce the perceived subjectivity of scoring of hips for hip dysplasia, several standardized approaches have been developed. These include the following [62]:

- The Orthopedic Foundation for Animals (OFA) approach: A V/D view is examined with the hips in full extension [59].

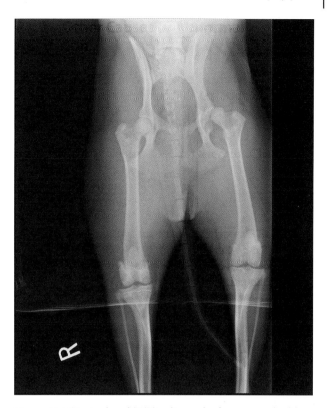

Figure 69.9 Ventrodorsal (V/D) radiograph of a ten-month-old canine patient. Note the reduced coverage of the left femoral head by the acetabulum. This feature is characteristic of canine hip dysplasia. *Source:* Courtesy of Ashley Benson.

- The PennHIP technique [63]: In addition to the hip-extended view, there are distraction and compression views to increase patient data. The theory is that the hip-extended views may mask subtle hip dysplasia because the joint capsule is taut when the hips are hyperextended. The additional two views provide extra details regarding how well the femoral heads are seated within the acetabulum.
- The Norberg angle [64, 65]: This modality has historically been employed more in Europe than in the continental United States. It involves drawing a line connecting the centers of both femoral heads and a line drawn between the craniodorsal rim and the femoral head of the same side. Where the two lines intersect, they create an angle. The greater the angle, the lower the risk for hip laxity

Radiographic interpretation of hip dysplasia is beyond the scope of this text; however, the author finds it important that the veterinary student be aware of hip dysplasia as a condition and recognize that there are various ways by which a diagnosis can be confirmed.

The student clinician should also recognize that radiographic signs do not always correlate with the severity of clinical disease. Mild changes on radiographs may be present in a dog that is clinical for advanced disease. By contrast, severe changes on radiographs may be found in a dog that presents with only subtle signs of disease.

Medical management of hip dysplasia typically includes physical therapy, weight management, and non-steroidal anti-inflammatory drugs (NSAIDs).

Surgical techniques for the management of canine hip dysplasia are beyond the scope of this text; however, they depend upon the patient's age; severity of disease, meaning the amount of osteoarthritis (OA) that is present; and the client's financial considerations [8].

69.9 Stifle Disease and Pelvic Limb Lameness

Stifle disease is a common cause of pelvic limb lameness in both dogs and cats [15]. The three most common clinical presentations result from patellar luxation, cruciate ligament injury, and collateral ligament instability.

69.9.1 Patellar Luxation

Patellar luxation more commonly occurs in dogs than in cats [15, 66–69]. Among cats, the Devon Rex and Abyssinian breeds are predisposed [15, 70, 71].

There are numerous etiologies to explain patellar luxation. Most commonly, it may result from an abnormally shallow patellar groove or a medial deviation of the tibial crest [15].

Patellar luxations can be graded to track their severity and/or progression. In general, the higher the grade of luxation, the more time the patella spends outside of its anatomically correct position [66].

Much like lameness, patellar luxations may be graded using any number of scales. There is no universal system. The author uses the following system to capture grades of patellar luxations in the dog or cat [72]:

- Grade 1: The patella is seated in its correct anatomical position within the patellar groove and does not typically luxate spontaneously, although it can be manually luxated. When it is manually luxated by the clinician and the clinician's pressure is released, the patella returns to its normal anatomical position. There is no impact on flexion and extension of the stifle.
- Grade 2: The patella is typically seated in its correct anatomical position within the patellar groove, but it may luxate spontaneously with flexion of the stifle joint. It may also be manually luxated. Once out of position, the patella may stay luxated until the patient extends at the stifle joint or until the clinician manually reduces the patella.

- Grade 3: The patella is typically out of position, yet can be manually replaced to its normal anatomical location when the patient extends at the stifle.
- Grade 4: The patella is always out of position and cannot be reduced; it is not possible to manually replace it within the patellar groove.

Over time, patellar luxation destabilizes the stifle joint by eroding the joint surfaces. This may incite joint-associated pain with resultant lameness and the development of OA [66, 73].

Patients may develop medial patellar luxation (MPL) or lateral patellar luxation (LPL). Either MPL or LPL can be unilateral or bilateral [69, 72, 74–76].

MPLs occur most commonly in toy and small-breed dogs [69, 77]. Pomeranians, Yorkshire terriers, and Chihuahuas are overrepresented [66, 78]. However, large and giant breeds with MPL have also been reported in the literature [74, 75].

Patients with MPL often have concurrent anatomical anomalies. In addition to having a shallower-than-normal patellar groove, they may have medial displacement of the quadriceps muscle group. As a result, the medial aspect of the distal femoral physis is put under enough pressure to retard growth. At the same time, there is no simultaneous pressure on the lateral aspect of the distal femoral physis such that growth continues normally at this location. The net result is that the distal femur becomes bowed laterally. In mild cases, this may be apparent only on radiographic examination; however, in moderate-to-severe cases, this is grossly visible [72].

When LPLs occur, they are more commonly seen in large and giant breeds [72]. However, MPLs occur with greater frequency than LPLs in large and giant-breed dogs: in a retrospective study evaluating 124 cases of patellar luxation in dogs, 83% of large-breed dogs had a diagnosed MPL compared to 17% with LPL [75]. Toy and small breeds with LPL have also been reported in the literature, albeit rarely: in the aforementioned study, only 2% of small-breed dogs were diagnosed with LPL compared to 98% with MPL [75].

LPL is thought to be due to abnormal, excessive rotation of the proximal femur. The resultant shift in the pull of the quadriceps muscle group laterally forces the patella lateral to the patellar groove [72].

Case management of patellar luxation depends upon the severity of the condition. High-grade patellar luxation often benefits from surgical intervention.

Surgical techniques are beyond the scope of this text; however, trochleoplasty is often employed to deepen the trochlear groove [15].

69.9.2 Cranial Cruciate Ligament Rupture

The stifle joint is stabilized by the cranial and caudal cruciate ligaments [79].

The cranial and caudal cruciate ligaments collectively prevent cranial translocation, movement of the tibia cranial to the femur, during weight bearing [80].

The caudomedial aspect of the lateral femoral condyle is the origin of the cranial cruciate ligament. From the condyle, the cranial cruciate ligament travels craniomedially to insert on the cranial intercondyloid area of the tibia. Think of the cranial cruciate ligament as passing "like a hand in the pants pocket" [9]. Both its craniomedial and caudolateral bands remain taught through extension; however, the caudolateral band relaxes during flexion [79, 80].

The lateral surface of the medial femoral condyle is the origin of the caudal cruciate ligament. From the condyle, the caudal cruciate ligament travels caudodistally to the popliteal notch of the tibia [79, 80].

The cranial and caudal cruciate ligaments cross each other as they course from origin to insertion; the cranial cruciate ligament is ultimately seated lateral to the caudal cruciate ligament [80].

Rupture of the cranial cruciate ligament is more often seen clinically than tears of the caudal cruciate ligament. CCLR also occurs in cats. Historically, it was associated with traumatic injuries in cats such as high-rise syndrome, yet trauma is not always observed. More recent studies suggest that CCLR in the cat may simply be the result of chronic ligament degeneration [81–84].

When rupture of the cranial cruciate ligament occurs, the stifle joint is destabilized. Over time, CCLR causes the abnormal grinding of bone against bone. This results in progressive wear and tear of the articular cartilage as well as the menisci, especially the medial one [84, 85].

In addition, the proximal patella, patellar groove, and mediodorsal tibia tend to develop radiographically diagnosed osteophytes [83].

Patients with CCLR are typically lame, with stifle effusion. They often resent stifle manipulation by the clinician.

When the stifle is put through its range of motion, there may be a palpable click. When present, this "click" has historically been considered indicative of meniscal tearing. However, it is an inconsistent finding at best [81, 86].

When CCLR is suspected, it can be confirmed by the cranial drawer or tibial thrust tests [81, 87, 88].

The cranial drawer test is performed with the patient in lateral recumbency. If the patient's right stifle is suspected of cranial cruciate ligament injury, then the patient should be placed gently in left lateral recumbency so that the right hind limb is available for manipulation. In this example, the tip of the clinician's left index finger will be placed over the patella, and his thumb will be placed over the femoral fabella. This serves to anchor the femur. The clinician then lays his right index finger over the tibial crest and plants his right thumb behind the head of the fibula. This stabilizes the proximal tibia. Holding the femur steady, the clinician then applies a cranially directed force to the tibia with his right hand to attempt cranial translocation of the tibia. If this occurs, then the stifle has been pathologically hyperextended. The patient is said to be positive for cranial drawer, which confirms injury to the cranial cruciate ligament [9, 79] (see Figures 69.10a, b).

The tibial thrust test is also typically performed with the patient in lateral recumbency. The premise of this test is that when the tarsus is flexed while the stifle is extended, an intact cranial cruciate ligament should prevent hyperextension of the stifle. As before, if the patient's right stifle is suspected to have suffered cranial cruciate ligament injury, then the patient should be placed gently

(a)

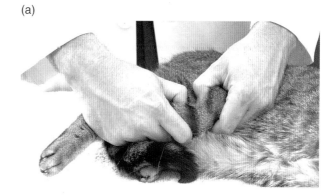

(b)

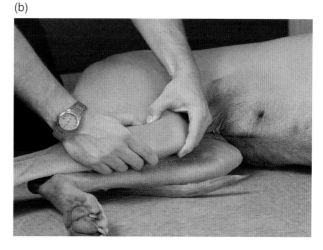

Figure 69.10 (a) Testing for cranial drawer in this feline patient's right stifle. *Source:* Courtesy of the Media Resources Department at Midwestern University. (b) Testing for cranial drawer in this canine patient's right stifle. *Source:* Courtesy of the Media Resources Department at Midwestern University.

(a)

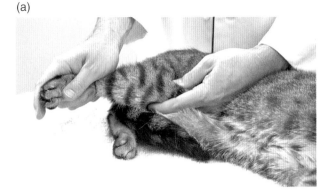

(b)

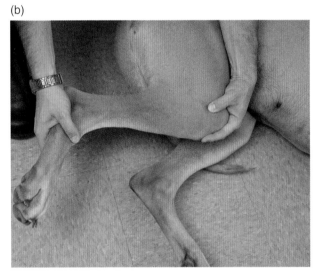

Figure 69.11 (a) Testing for tibial thrust in this feline patient's right stifle. *Source:* Courtesy of the Media Resources Department at Midwestern University. (b) Testing for tibial thrust in this canine patient's right stifle. *Source:* Courtesy of the Media Resources Department at Midwestern University.

in left lateral recumbency so that the right hind limb is available for manipulation. The clinician gently lays his left index finger over patient's patella and tibial crest. He uses the placement of this forefinger to sense for abnormal cranial movement of the tibia as his right hand grasps the right metatarsal region and directs the tarsus into flexion. If cranial cruciate ligament injury is present, then forward motion of the tibia will be appreciated [9, 88] (see Figures 69.11a, b).

69.9.3 Collateral Ligament Instability

In addition to the cruciate ligaments, the stifle joint is stabilized by the medial and lateral collateral ligaments [79].

69.9.3.1 The Medial Collateral Ligament
The medial collateral ligament originates from the medial femoral epicondyle and the medial border of the

tibia. It fuses with the joint capsule and attaches to the medial meniscus. Portions of this ligament selectively tighten throughout stifle flexion and extension to maintain the integrity of the joint [79, 80].

To assess for medial collateral ligament stability, the patient is again placed in lateral recumbency with the limb of interest in the 'up' position and available for manipulation. The limb of interest is held in extension. The clinician grasps the limb's distal femur in one hand and the proximal tibia in the other. With the hand that is on the proximal tibia, the clinician attempts to abduct the tibia relative to the femur.

If the medial collateral ligament is intact, the clinician should not feel displacement of the tibia [9, 89, 90].

69.9.3.2 The Lateral Collateral Ligament
The lateral collateral ligament begins at the lateral femoral epicondyle and inserts on the head of the fibula. During flexion, this ligament is lax to allow for internal rotation of the stifle joint. By contrast, this ligament tightens during extension of the stifle [79, 80].

To assess for lateral collateral ligament stability, the patient remains in lateral recumbency, with the "up" limb held in extension. The clinician grasps the limb's distal femur in one hand and the proximal tibia in the other. With the hand that is on the proximal tibia, the clinician attempts to adduct the tibia relative to the femur.

If the lateral collateral ligament is intact, the clinician should not feel the lateral joint space open up [9, 89, 90].

69.10 Dropped Hocks

Musculoskeletal or neurological disease at the level of one or both tarsi can cause an abnormal stance.

In the normal dog and cat, the tarsus or hock is elevated in space, meaning that it does not come into contact with the ground. In other words, dogs and cats should look like they are walking on "high heels," not as if they are walking flat-footed in "flip-flops" (see Figures 69.12a, b).

It is abnormal for dogs and cats to develop a plantigrade stance, meaning that the ventral aspect of their hind limb, distal to the hock, comes into contact with the surface of the floor.

Cats with this stance should be evaluated for diabetic neuropathy, and dogs should be evaluated for rupture of the common calcaneal tendon [82, 91] (see Figures 69.13a, b).

Both dogs and cats that have dropped hocks may also have an underlying injury to the sciatic nerve [92].

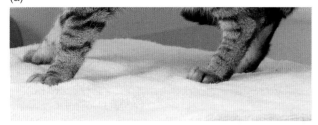

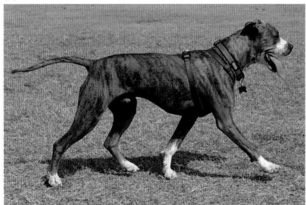

Figure 69.12 (a) Assessing this cat's stance, which is normal. Note that the hocks do not touch the ground. *Source:* Courtesy of the Media Resources Department at Midwestern University.
(b) Assessing this dog's stance, which is normal. Note that the hocks do not touch the ground. *Source:* Courtesy of Analucia Aliaga.

69.11 DJD and Pelvic Limb Lameness

DJD, sometimes referred to as OA, is characterized by progressive changes in one or more components of synovial and/or cartilaginous joints [93]:

- Articular cartilage
- Joint capsule
- Ligaments
- Subchondral bone

When degeneration of synovial joints occurs, there is typically thickening of subchondral bone as well as the joint capsule [93]. In addition, osteophytes form at and around the affected joint(s) [93, 94].

Note that DJD of synovial joints may involve one or both pelvic limbs, and/or one or both thoracic limbs.

When degeneration occurs at the cartilaginous joints of the spinal column, one or more intervertebral discs degenerate, and the spaces between affected discs narrow [93, 95].

DJD is considered non-inflammatory because inflammation requires vascular supply [96]. Because mature articular cartilage is without blood supply, it cannot in and of itself become inflamed [96]. However, tissues surrounding it can [96]. Consider, for example, the surrounding synovial membrane. This is a highly vascular structure and will become inflamed depending upon the degree to which the affected joint is impacted [96–98].

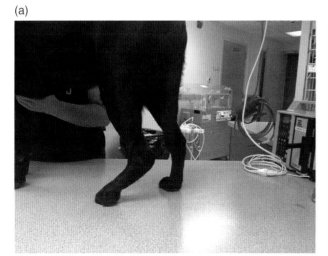

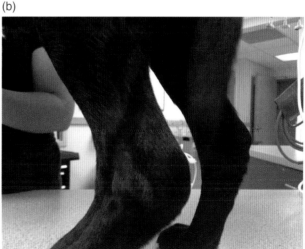

Figure 69.13 (a) Subtle finding of a dropped left hock in a canine patient that was subsequently diagnosed with rupture of the common calcaneal tendon. *Source:* Courtesy of Daniel Foy, MS, DVM, DACVIM, DACVECC. (b) Close-up of dropped and swollen left hock in a canine patient that was subsequently diagnosed with rupture of the common calcaneal tendon. *Source:* Courtesy of Daniel Foy, MS, DVM, DACVIM, DACVECC.

DJD is commonly associated with aging [93, 96, 97, 99]. DJD may also be secondary to the following [93, 96–99]:

- Congenital malformations
  – Joint dysplasia
  – OC
- Endocrinopathy and metabolic disease
- Osteochondrodysplasia of Scottish Folds (see Chapter 68, Section 68.8.3) [100–102]
- Immune-mediated disease
- Infectious disease
  – Bacterial
  – Fungal
  – Mycoplasmal
  – Protozoal
  – Viral
- Trauma

Patients with DJD frequently present for lameness [96]. When DJD involves one or both hind limbs, then patients will present with pelvic limb lameness.

Clients may also report changes in activities or activity level [96]. For example, stair climbing, jumping, ball chasing, or grooming may be difficult [96].

When faced with this type of history, it is important that the clinician not wear blinders. Every senior patient that presents with a change in activity level does not necessarily have DJD that is responsible for the presenting complaint [96]. What this chapter and the previous chapter hope to emphasize is that many conditions produce lameness, including, but not limited to the following [96]:

- Neurologic disease
  – Central nervous system (CNS) disease
  – Intervertebral disc disease (IVDD)
  – Myasthenia gravis
  – Peripheral nerve injury
  – Spinal cord degenerative myelopathy
- Orthopedic disease
  – Fractures
  – Luxations
  – Osteomyelitis
  – Osteosarcoma
  – Other neoplastic disease that involves bone or cartilage
- Soft tissue disease
  – Ligament or tendon injuries
  – Muscle contusions
  – Myositis
  – Neoplasia

Because so many conditions are capable of causing lameness, DJD cannot and should not be assumed. All potential pathologies should be investigated based upon high index of suspicion on account of history and physical examination findings [96]. All limbs should be evaluated, not just the affected one [96].

Joint thickening, crepitus, and reduced range of motion are characteristic of, but not pathognomonic for, DJD [96]. Patients with DJD may be uncomfortable over range-of-motion exercises at the affected joint(s), but pain is not typically severe [96]. Joint effusion may be present, but is rarely extensive in cases of DJD [96].

Radiographs should be taken in any patient that is thought to have articular disease [96]. The following radiographic features support a diagnosis of DJD [96]:

- Calcification
  – Intra-articular
  – Periarticular
- Osteophyte formation
- Subchondral bone sclerosis

Osteophytes are spurs of periarticular bone [96]. Within the pelvic limb, they are most commonly found at the coxofemoral and stifle joints [93, 96].

Sclerosis is most common in chronic cases of DJD [96]. It develops when the bone beneath affected cartilage experiences increased stress [96]. In health, articular cartilage would have borne the brunt of this insult [96]. As cartilage deteriorates, it no longer acts as a shield for underlying bone [96]. The forces are translated to the bone beneath. This causes the affected bone to thicken, which creates a radiodense appearance [96].

Note that radiographic features of DJD do not always correlate with the condition's degree of severity [96, 103]. A patient with what appears to be severe DJD on diagnostic imaging studies may be only mildly clinical for disease, whereas a patient with clinically significant disease may have few radiographic abnormalities [103].

Treatment for DJD is aimed at symptom management [96]. The condition is not curable. The goal is to improve function. This typically includes the following [33, 93, 96, 104–107]:

- Chondroprotective therapy
- Low-impact activity plan
- Pain management
- Weight management

Joint salvage procedures, such as tarsal arthrodesis or FHO, may be indicated [33].

69.12 Neoplasia and Pelvic Limb Lameness

Osteosarcoma is a common form of neoplasia that targets skeletal structures, including the pelvic limbs [33, 108, 109]. Osteosarcoma typically affects sites near the knee and away from the elbow [109]. This implies that the distal femur and the proximal tibia are common sites of osteosarcoma in the hind limb [109].

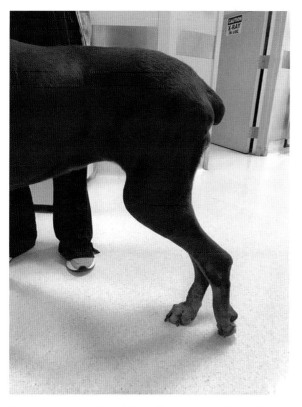

Figure 69.14 Grossly visible swelling associated with the left pelvic limb of a canine patient. This patient was subsequently diagnosed with osteosarcoma of the proximal tibia. *Source:* Courtesy of Beki Cohen Regan, DVM, DACVIM (Oncology).

Osteosarcoma causes extensive limb swelling and associated pain [109] (see Figure 69.14).

Radiographic findings that are supportive of a diagnosis include an aggressive bony lesion that is osteolytic and/or osteoproductive. Refer to Chapter 68, Figure 68.6, which depicts one such lesion at the level of the distal radius.

Osteosarcomas tend to be aggressive [33]. They also tend to metastasize to the lungs in dogs, more so than in cats [33, 108, 109] (see Figures 69.15a–c).

Note that osteosarcoma is not the only pathological condition that causes osteolysis. Fungal osteomyelitis can appear strikingly similar and should therefore be included as a differential in certain geographical regions. Refer to Chapter 68, Figure 68.7.

Other neoplastic diseases that are capable of causing pelvic limb lameness include chondrosarcoma, fibrosarcoma, digital squamous cell carcinoma and metastatic disease, as from canine prostatic adenocarcinoma [33, 110, 111].

69.13 Developmental Diseases and Pelvic Limb Lameness

Hip dysplasia was reviewed in Section 69.8 as a developmental disease that is commonly implicated in the development of pelvic limb lameness in large-breed dogs [58].

However, hip dysplasia is not the only developmental disease with this outcome.

OC, panosteitis, and hypertrophic osteodystrophy (HOD) can also occur in the hind limb [112].

69.13.1 Osteochondrosis

OC results from abnormal endochondral ossification [113]. Review the pathophysiology of this disease process in Chapter 68, Section 68.6.1.

Recall that 4–10-month-old, large-breed, male dogs are predisposed to the development of OC [112]. Although the shoulder is the most frequent site in the dog, OC may also target the femoral condyles and the tarsus, specifically its trochlear ridges [53, 112, 114, 115].

OC lesions may be suspected based upon clinical signs [8]. They are confirmed via diagnostic imaging studies [8].

69.13.2 Panosteitis

Panosteitis is a common cause of lameness in clinical practice. Review the pathophysiology of this disease process in Chapter 68, Section 68.6.4.1.

Recall that young, male, large-breed dogs are predisposed to the development of panosteitis [113, 116–119].

Affected bone(s) are painful on palpation, and lameness is cyclical [119].

Panosteitis may be suspected based upon age, breed, and presentation. Panosteitis is confirmed via diagnostic imaging. Radiographs of panosteitis demonstrate increased opacity of the medullary cavity, which may appear hazy or unusually granular. Proliferation of the periosteum and endosteum may also be evident [4, 113].

Panosteitis is self-limiting [113, 116–118].

Treatment is aimed at managing pain during flare-ups [119].

Refer to Chapter 70 for more information.

69.13.3 Hypertrophic Osteodystrophy

HOD is a developmental disease of large and giant-breed dogs [4, 8, 113, 120–122]. Review the pathophysiology of this disease process in Chapter 68, Section 68.6.4.2.

Patients with HOD develop swollen, painful metaphyseal areas of affected long bones [113]. Lesions are often symmetrical.

Patients tend to be reluctant to move, depressed, and febrile [113].

Radiographs demonstrate a double physeal line that is diagnostic for HOD [113, 120, 123].

Like panosteitis, HOD is self-limiting. Patients tend to do well with supportive care to manage pain [4, 113].

(a)

(b)

(c)

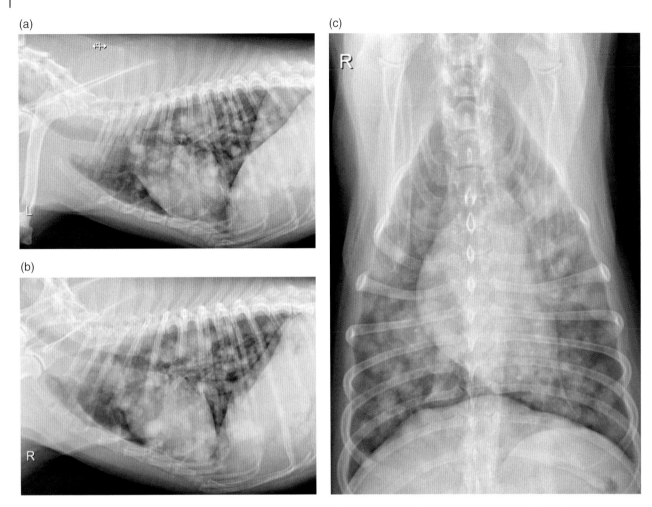

Figure 69.15 (a) Left lateral thoracic radiograph of a canine patient with osteosarcoma, demonstrating innumerable pulmonary metastases. (b) Right lateral thoracic radiograph of the canine patient depicted in (a). (c) Ventrodorsal (V/D) thoracic radiograph of the canine patient depicted in (a).

69.14 Neurologic Causes of Pelvic Limb Lameness

Recall that coordination between the musculoskeletal and nervous systems is required to initiate and maintain a proper gait [1]. If the musculoskeletal system is sound, but the patient presents for lameness, then the nervous system may be dysfunctional. Consider, for example, a bulging intervertebral disc or tumor located somewhere between L4 and S1 [92]. This may create pelvic limb lameness of neurological, rather than musculoskeletal origin [92].

A comprehensive neurological examination should be performed in all lame patients in which musculoskeletal etiologies have been ruled out.

Recall that a neurological examination includes gait analysis. Gait analysis may reveal that voluntary movement is hindered because of underlying weakness.

Review Chapter 68, Section 68.9 for appropriate medical terminology pertaining to so-called paresis, that is, muscular weakness secondary to neuropathology.

In addition to the presence and strength of voluntary movement, the quality of the gait should be assessed. The clinician should ask himself if the gait appears to be coordinated. Gait incoordination that is not due to weakness is referred to as ataxia [124, 125].

Lesion localization is beyond the scope of this text. However, it is important to recognize that neurological lameness and/or neurological weakness may be present in the absence of orthopedic disease. This serves as a reminder to make physical examinations comprehensive so that differentials unrelated to the musculoskeletal system are not missed.

Like orthopedic lameness, neurological lameness has many potential causes. The most common causes for the pelvic limb include [92]:

- Acute spinal cord infarction due to fibrocartilaginous embolism
- Femoral nerve injury
- Ischemic neuromyopathy
- Sciatic nerve injury

69.14.1 Fibrocartilaginous Embolic Myelopathy

Recall from Chapter 68, Section 68.9.1 that fibrocartilaginous embolic myelopathy (FCEM) causes acute, but non-progressive, focal myelopathy [92, 126, 127].

When an embolus occurs within the spinal segments, L4-S1, it may cause non-painful paresis of one or both of the pelvic limbs [92].

Diagnosis is via magnetic resonance imaging (MRI) [92].

Most patients recover function over time, with supportive care and physiotherapy [92].

69.14.2 Ischemic Neuromyopathy

Recall from Chapter 68, Section 68.9.4 that ischemic neuromyopathy results from thrombosis of a large vessel. In cats, this most often occurs at the aortic trifurcation secondary to hypertrophic cardiomyopathy (HCM) [92, 128–132]. The patient that develops a thrombus at this location is said to have a "saddle thrombus" [128, 133].

The condition is painful [129, 133, 134]. The affected limb is cold to the touch [129]. Paw pads and nail beds develop cyanosis [92].

History and presentation are classic for ATE.

69.14.3 Sciatic Nerve Injury

The sciatic nerve may be damaged by femoral or pelvic fractures [92].

Because the quadriceps muscle is still functional, the patient can bear weight on the affected limb [92]. However, the patient typically presents with a dropped hock [92].

In addition, the patient typically loses sensation over the lateral, dorsal, and plantar surfaces of the affected hind paw [92]. This causes the paw to knuckle over, which means that the dorsal aspect curls under to scuff along the floor [92].

69.14.4 Femoral Nerve Injury

The femoral nerve is less often injured than the sciatic nerve [92]. In most instances, the sublumbar musculature offers protection to the femoral nerve [92]. However, if trauma is severe, the femoral nerve can be compressed or even severed [92].

The patient loses its ability to extend the stifle and bear weight on the affected limb [92].

The quadriceps muscle of the affected limb atrophies [92].

Sensation may be lost to the medial limb and medial digit [92].

Knuckling of the affected hind paw is to be expected [92].

69.15 Summary of Diagnostic Approach to Pelvic Limb Lameness

There are more differential diagnoses for pelvic limb lameness than have been discussed here. The experienced clinician recognizes the most common causes of pelvic limb lameness based upon signalment, history taking, and physical examination findings.

If the patient presents for pelvic limb lameness and has either pain on palpation, pain with hyperextension, or pain with hyperflexion, then a sedated orthopedic examination may be necessary to further localize disease [135].

Whether or not there is a history of trauma, radiographs are an important diagnostic tool to evaluate the patient for fractures, subluxations, or luxations [135].

If, on the other hand, the lame patient presents without pain on palpation, then a neurologic work-up may be indicated [92, 135]. Testing spinal reflexes and postural reactions, such as hopping, wheel barrowing, and tactile placing, may facilitate lesion localization [92].

For example, the withdrawal reflex tests the following structures within the pelvic limb [92]:

- Femoral nerve
- L4-S1 spinal cord segments
- Sciatic nerve

References

1 Singh, B. and Dyce, K.M. (2018). *Dyce, Sack, and Wensing's Textbook of Veterinary Anatomy*, 5e, xv, 854 p. St. Louis, Missouri: Saunders.

2 Evans, H.E. (1993). The skeleton. In: *Miller's Anatomy of the Dog*, 3e (ed. H.E. Evans and M.E. Miller), 122–218. Philadelphia: W.B. Saunders.

3 Gilbert, S.G. (1989). *Pictorial Anatomy of the Cat*, 120 p. Seattle: University of Washington Press.

4 Buback, J. (2012). Evaluating forelimb lameness in juvenile dogs. DVM 360 [Internet]. http://veterinarynews. dvm360.com/evaluating-forelimb-lameness-juvenile-dogs.

5 Budsberg, S.C. (2010). Lameness exam: what am I missing? DVM 360 [Internet]. http://veterinarycalendar. dvm360.com/lameness-exam-what-am-i-missing-proceedings.

6 Denny, H. and Butterworth, S. (eds.) (2000). Examination and differential diagnosis of forelimb lameness. In: *A Guide to Canine and Feline Orthopaedic Surgery*, 301. Oxford, U.K.: Blackwell Science Limited.

7 Lafuente, P. (2011). Young, male neutered, obese, lame? Non-traumatic fractures of the femoral head and neck. *J. Feline Med. Surg.* 13 (7): 498–507.

8 McLaughlin, R.M. (2001). Hind limb lameness in the young patient. *Vet. Clin. North Am. Small Anim. Pract.* 31 (1): 101–123.

9 Hazewinkel, H.A.W., Meij, B.P., Theyse, L.F.H., and van Rijssen, B. (2009). Locomotor system. In: *Medical History and Physical Examination in Companion Animals* (ed. A. Rijnberk and F.J. van Sluijs), 135–159. St. Louis: Saunders Elsevier.

10 Voss, K. and Steffen, F. (2009). Patient assessment. In: *Feline Orthopedic Surgery and Musculoskeletal Disease* (ed. P.M. Montavon, K. Voss and S.J. Langley-Hobbs). St. Louis: Saunders Elsevier.

11 Englar, R.E. (2017). *Performing the Small Animal Physical Examination*. Hoboken, NJ: Wiley.

12 Kerwin, S. (2012). Orthopedic examination in the cat: clinical tips for ruling in/out common musculoskeletal disease. *J. Feline Med. Surg.* 14 (1): 6–12.

13 Arnoczky, S.P. and Tarvin, G.B. (1981). Physical examination of the musculoskeletal system. *Vet. Clin. North Am. Small Anim. Pract.* 11 (3): 575–593.

14 Piermattei, D., Flo, G., and DeCamp, C. (2006). *Brinker, Piermattei and Flo's Handbook of Small Animal Orthopedics and Fracture Repair*, 4e. Philadelphia: Saunders.

15 Chandler, J.C. and Beale, B.S. (2002). Feline orthopedics. *Clin. Tech. Small Anim. Pract.* 17 (4): 190–203.

16 Guiot, L.P., Demianiuk, R.M., and Dejardin, L.M. (2012). Fractures of the femur. In: *Veterinary Surgery Small Animal One* (ed. K.M. Tobias and S.A. Johnston), 865–905. St. Louis: Saunders Elsevier.

17 Sebastiani, A.M. and Fishbeck, D.W. (1998). *Mammalian Anatomy: The Cat*. Englewood, CO: Morton Publishing Company.

18 Stieger-Vanegas, S.M., Senthirajah, S.K., Nemanic, S. et al. (2015). Evaluation of the diagnostic accuracy of four-view radiography and conventional computed tomography analysing sacral and pelvic fractures in dogs. *Vet. Comp. Orthop. Traumatol.: VCOT.* 28 (3): 155–163.

19 Harasen, G. (2007). Pelvic fractures. *Can. Vet. J.* 48 (4): 427–428.

20 Draffan, D., Clements, D., Farrell, M. et al. (2009). The role of computed tomography in the classification and management of pelvic fractures. *Vet. Comp. Orthop. Traumatol.: VCOT.* 22 (3): 190–197.

21 Burkhardt, M., Nienaber, U., Pizanis, A. et al. (2012). Acute management and outcome of multiple trauma patients with pelvic disruptions. *Crit. Care* 16 (4): R163.

22 Meeson, R. and Corr, S. (2011). Management of pelvic trauma: neurological damage, urinary tract disruption and pelvic fractures. *J. Feline Med. Surg.* 13 (5): 347–361.

23 Hoffberg, J.E., Koenigshof, A.M., and Guiot, L.P. (2016). Retrospective evaluation of concurrent intra-abdominal injuries in dogs with traumatic pelvic fractures: 83 cases (2008–2013). *J. Vet. Emerg. Crit. Care (San Antonio).* 26 (2): 288–294.

24 Boysen, S.R., Rozanski, E.A., Tidwell, A.S. et al. (2004). Evaluation of a focused assessment with sonography for trauma protocol to detect free abdominal fluid in dogs involved in motor vehicle accidents. *J. Am. Vet. Med. Assoc.* 225 (8): 1198–1204.

25 Simpson, S.A., Syring, R., and Otto, C.M. (2009). Severe blunt trauma in dogs: 235 cases (1997–2003). *J. Vet. Emerg. Crit. Care (San Antonio).* 19 (6): 588–602.

26 Streeter, E.M., Rozanski, E.A., Laforcade-Buress, A. et al. (2009). Evaluation of vehicular trauma in dogs: 239 cases (January–December 2001). *J. Am. Vet. Med. Assoc.* 235 (4): 405–408.

27 Stafford, J.R. and Bartges, J.W. (2013). A clinical review of pathophysiology, diagnosis, and treatment of uroabdomen in the dog and cat. *J. Vet. Emerg. Crit. Care (San Antonio).* 23 (2): 216–229.

28 Kolata, R.J. and Johnston, D.E. (1975). Motor vehicle accidents in urban dogs: a study of 600 cases. *J. Am. Vet. Med. Assoc.* 167 (10): 938–941.

29 Lee, K., Heng, H.G., Jeong, J. et al. (2012). Feasibility of computed tomography in awake dogs with traumatic pelvic fracture. *Vet. Radiol. Ultrasound* 53 (4): 412–416.

30 Anderson, A. and Coughlan, A.R. (1997). Sacral fractures in dogs and cats: a classification scheme and review of 51 cases. *J. Small Anim. Pract.* 38 (9): 404–409.

31 Fry, P.D. (1974). Observations on the surgical treatment of hip dislocation in the dog and cat. *J. Small Anim. Pract.* 15 (11): 661–670.

32 Christopher, S.A. (2011). What is your diagnosis? *J. Am. Vet. Med. Assoc.* 239 (3): 301–302.

33 Roush, J.K. (2001). Hind limb lameness in the mature dog. *Vet. Clin. North Am. Small Anim. Pract.* 31 (1): 125–141, vi.

34 Vidoni, B., Henninger, W., Lorinson, D., and Mayrhofer, E. (2005). Traumatic avulsion fracture of the lesser trochanter in a dog. *Vet. Comp. Orthopaed.* 18 (2): 105–109.

35 Salter, R.B. and Harris, W.R. (1963). Injuries involving the epiphyseal plate. *J. Bone Joint Surg. Am.* 45 (3): 587–622.

36 Milton, J.L. (1993). Fractures of the femur. In: *Textbook of Small Animal Surgery* (ed. D. Slatter), 1806–1817. Philadelphia: WB Saunders.

37 Craig, L.E. (2001). Physeal dysplasia with slipped capital femoral epiphysis in 13 cats. *Vet. Pathol.* 38 (1): 92–97.

38 DeCamp, C.E., Probst, C.W., and Thomas, M.W. (1989). Internal fixation of femoral capital physeal injuries in dogs: 40 cases (1979–1987). *J. Am. Vet. Med. Assoc.* 194 (12): 1750–1754.

39 Gibson, K.L., vanEe, R.T., and Pechman, R.D. (1991). Femoral capital physeal fractures in dogs: 34 cases (1979–1989). *J. Am. Vet. Med. Assoc.* 198 (5): 886–890.

40 Johnson, J.M., Johnson, A.L., and Eurell, J.A. (1994). Histological appearance of naturally occurring canine physeal fractures. *Vet. Surg.* 23 (2): 81–86.

41 Dupuis, J., Breton, L., and Drolet, R. (1997). Bilateral epiphysiolysis of the femoral heads in two dogs. *J. Am. Vet. Med. Assoc.* 210 (8): 1162–1165.

42 Gemmill, T.J., Pink, J., Clarke, S.P., and McKee, W.M. (2012). Total hip replacement for the treatment of atraumatic slipped femoral capital epiphysis in dogs. *J. Small Anim. Pract.* 53 (8): 453–458.

43 Queen, J., Bennett, D., Carmichael, S. et al. (1998). Femoral neck metaphyseal osteopathy in the cat. *Vet. Rec.* 142 (7): 159–162.

44 Ridge, P.A. (2006). What is your diagnosis? Destructive bony lesions of the proximal femoral metaphysis. *J. Small Anim. Pract.* 47 (5): 291–293.

45 McNicholas, W.T. Jr., Wilkens, B.E., Blevins, W.E. et al. (2002). Spontaneous femoral capital physeal fractures in adult cats: 26 cases (1996–2001). *J. Am. Vet. Med. Assoc.* 221 (12): 1731–1736.

46 Burke, J. (2003). Physeal dysplasia with slipped capital femoral epiphysis in a cat. *Can. Vet. J.* 44 (3): 238–239.

47 Forrest, L.J., O'Brien, R.T., and Manlet, P.A. (1999). Feline capital physeal dysplasia syndrome. *Vet. Radiol. Ultrasound.* 40: 672.

48 Beale, B.S. and Cole, G. (2012). Minimally invasive osteosynthesis technique for articular fractures. *Vet. Clin. North Am. Small Anim. Pract.* 42 (5): 1051–1068, viii.

49 Fischer, H.R., Norton, J., Kobluk, C.N. et al. (2004). Surgical reduction and stabilization for repair of femoral capital physeal fractures in cats: 13 cases (1998–2002). *J. Am. Vet. Med. Assoc.* 224 (9): 1478–1482.

50 Chandler, E.A., Gaskell, C.J., and Gaskell, R.M. (2004). *Feline Medicine and Therapeutics*. Ames, IA: Iowa State Press.

51 Smith, R.N. (1969). Fusion of ossification centres in the cat. *J. Small Anim. Pract.* 10 (9): 523–530.

52 Isola, M., Baroni, E., and Zotti, A. (2005). Radiographic features of two cases of feline proximal femoral dysplasia. *J. Small Anim. Pract.* 46 (12): 597–599.

53 Lewis, D.D., Mccarthy, R.J., and Pechman, R.D. (1992). Diagnosis of common developmental orthopedic conditions in canine pediatric-patients. *Compend. Contin. Educ. Pract.* 14 (3): 287–301.

54 Ginja, M.M., Silvestre, A.M., Gonzalo-Orden, J.M., and Ferreira, A.J. (2010). Diagnosis, genetic control and preventive management of canine hip dysplasia: a review. *Vet. J.* 184 (3): 269–276.

55 Maki, K., Janss, L.L., Groen, A.F. et al. (2004). An indication of major genes affecting hip and elbow dysplasia in four Finnish dog populations. *Heredity (Edinb).* 92 (5): 402–408.

56 Janutta, V. and Distl, O. (2006). Inheritance of canine hip dysplasia: review of estimation methods and of heritability estimates and prospects on further developments. *Dtsch. Tierarztl. Wochenschr.* 113 (1): 6–12.

57 Smith, G.K., Popovitch, C.A., Gregor, T.P., and Shofer, F.S. (1995). Evaluation of risk factors for degenerative joint disease associated with hip dysplasia in dogs. *J. Am. Vet. Med. Assoc.* 206 (5): 642–647.

58 Leighton, E.A. (1997). Genetics of canine hip dysplasia. *J. Am. Vet. Med. Assoc.* 210 (10): 1474–1479.

59 Baltzer, W. (2011). Canine hip dysplasia: Part 1. *NAVC Clinician's Brief* (October): 23–26.

60 Innes, J. (2007). Palpating for the Ortolani sign when diagnosing hip dysplasia. *NAVC Clinician's Brief* (January): 71–72.

61 Fox, D.B. (2007). Orthopedic examination of the rear limb in the dog. *NAVC Clinician's Brief* (July): 63–66.

62 Lust, G., Todhunter, R.J., Erb, H.N. et al. (2001). Comparison of three radiographic methods for diagnosis of hip dysplasia in eight-month-old dogs. *J. Am. Vet. Med. Assoc.* 219 (9): 1242–1246.

63 Smith, G.K. (1997). Advances in diagnosing canine hip dysplasia. *J. Am. Vet. Med. Assoc.* 210 (10): 1451–1457.

64 Farese, J.P., Todhunter, R.J., Lust, G. et al. (1998). Dorsolateral subluxation of hip joints in dogs measured in a weight-bearing position with radiography and computed tomography. *Vet. Surg.* 27 (5): 393–405.

65 Comhaire, F.H. and Schoonjans, F.A. (2011). Canine hip dyslasia: the significance of the Norberg angle for healthy breeding. *J. Small Anim. Pract.* 52 (10): 536–542.

66 O'Neill, D.G., Meeson, R.L., Sheridan, A. et al. (2016). The epidemiology of patellar luxation in dogs attending primary-care veterinary practices in England. *Canine Genet. Epidemiol.* 3: 4.

67 Knight, G.C. (1963). Abnormalities and defects in pedigree dogs – III. Tibio-femoral joint deformity and patellar luxation. *J. Small Anim. Pract.* 4 (6): 463–464.

68 Ness, M.G., Abercromby, R.H., May, C. et al. (1996). A survey of orthopaedic conditions in small animal veterinary practice in Britain. *Vet. Comp. Orthopaed.* 9 (2): 43–52.

69 Roush, J.K. (1993). Canine Patellar Luxation. *Vet. Clin. N Am.-Small.* 23 (4): 855–868.

70 Bruce, W.J. (1999). Stifle joint luxation in the cat: treatment using transarticular external skeletal fixation. *J. Small Anim. Pract.* 40 (10): 482–488.

71 Engvall, E. and Bushnell, N. (1990). Patellar luxation in Abyssinian cats. *Feline Pract.* 18 (4): 20–22.

72 Fossum, T.W., Duprey, L.P., and O'Connor, D. (2007). Diseases of the joints. In: *Small Animal Surgery*,

3e (ed. T.W. Fossum, L.P. Duprey and D. O'Connor), 1289–1299. Boston, MA: Elsevier.

73 Dokic, Z., Lorinson, D., Weigel, J.P., and Vezzoni, A. (2015). Patellar groove replacement in patellar luxation with severe femoro-patellar osteoarthritis. *Vet. Comp. Orthopaed.* 28 (2): 124–130.

74 Remedios, A.M., Basher, A.W., Runyon, C.L., and Fries, C.L. (1992). Medial patellar luxation in 16 large dogs. A retrospective study. *Vet. Surg.* 21 (1): 5–9.

75 Hayes, A.G., Boudrieau, R.J., and Hungerford, L.L. (1994). Frequency and distribution of medial and lateral patellar luxation in dogs: 124 cases (1982–1992). *J. Am. Vet. Med. Assoc.* 205 (5): 716–720.

76 Gibbons, S.E., Macias, C., Tonzing, M.A. et al. (2006). Patellar luxation in 70 large breed dogs. *J. Small Anim. Pract.* 47 (1): 3–9.

77 LaFond, E., Breur, G.J., and Austin, C.C. (2002). Breed susceptibility for developmental orthopedic diseases in dogs. *J. Am. Anim. Hosp. Assoc.* 38 (5): 467–477.

78 Priester, W.A. (1972). Sex, size, and breed as risk factors in canine patellar dislocation. *J. Am. Vet. Med. Assoc.* 160 (5): 740–742.

79 Palmer, R. (2005). Diagnosing cranial cruciate ligament pathology. DVM 360 [Internet]. http://veterinary medicine.dvm360.com/diagnosing-cranial-cruciate-ligament-pathology.

80 Evans, H. (1993). Arthrology. In: *Miller's Anatomy of the Dog*, 3e (ed. H.E. Evans and M.E. Miller), 219–257. Philadelphia: W.B. Saunders.

81 Grierson, J. (2012). Hips, elbows and stifles: common joint diseases in the cat. *J. Feline Med. Surg.* 14 (1): 23–30.

82 Harasen, G.L.G. and Little, S.E. (2012). Musculoskeletal Diseases. In: *The Cat: Clinical Medicine and Management* (ed. S.E. Little), 704–733. St. Louis: Saunders Elsevier.

83 Voss, K., Langley-Hobbs, S.J., and Montavon, P.M. (2009). Stifle joint. In: *Feline Orthopedic Surgery and Musculoskeletal Disease* (ed. P.M. Montavon, K. Voss and S.J. Langley-Hobbs), 475–490. St. Louis: Saunders Elsevier.

84 Harasen, G.L. (2005). Feline cranial cruciate rupture: 17 cases and a review of the literature. *Vet. Comp. Orthop. Traumatol.: VCOT.* 18 (4): 254–257.

85 Fossum, T.W., Duprey, L.P., and O'Connor, D. (2007). Diseases of the joints: cranial cruciate ligament rupture. In: *Small Animal Surgery*, 3e (ed. T.W. Fossum, L.P. Duprey and D. O'Connor), 1254–1275. Boston, MA: Elsevier.

86 Scott, H. and McLaughlin, R. (2007). *Feline orthopedics*. London: Manson Publishing, Ltd.

87 Thomson, M. (2006). The cat with lameness. In: *Problem-Based Feline Medicine* (ed. J. Rand). Edinburgh, New York: Saunders.

88 Henderson, R.A. and Milton, J.L. (1978). Tibial compression mechanism – diagnostic aid in stifle injuries. *J. Am. Anim. Hosp. Assoc.* 14 (4): 474–479.

89 Fossum, T.W., Duprey, L.P., and O'Connor, D. (2007). Diseases of the joints: collateral ligament injury. In: *Small Animal Surgery*, 3e (ed. T.W. Fossum, L.P. Duprey and D. O'Connor), 1280–1283. Boston, MA: Elsevier.

90 Millis, D.L. and Mankin, J. (2014). Orthopedic and neurologic evaluation. In: *Canine Rehabilitation & Physical Therapy* (ed. D.L. Millis, D. Levine and R.A. Taylor), 180–192. St. Louis, Mo: Saunders.

91 Feldman, E.C. and Nelson, R.W. (2004). *Canine and Feline Endocrinology and Reproduction*, 3e. St. Louis, Mo: Saunders.

92 Garosi, L. (2012). Neurological lameness in the cat: common causes and clinical approach. *J. Feline Med. Surg.* 14 (1): 85–93.

93 Lascelles, B.D. (2010). Feline degenerative joint disease. *Vet. Surg.* 39 (1): 2–13.

94 Wieland, H.A., Michaelis, M., Kirschbaum, B.J., and Rudolphi, K.A. (2005). Osteoarthritis – an untreatable disease? *Nat. Rev. Drug Discov.* 4 (4): 331–344.

95 Modic, M.T. and Ross, J.S. (2007). Lumbar degenerative disk disease. *Radiology* 245 (1): 43–61.

96 Lipowitz, A.J. and Newton, C.D. (1985). Degenerative joint disease and traumatic arthritis, ch. 87. In: *Textbook of Small Animal Orthopaedics* (ed. C.D. Newton and D.M. Nunamaker). Philadelphia: Lippincott.

97 McDevitt, C., Gilbertson, E., and Muir, H. (1977). An experimental model of osteoarthritis; early morphological and biochemical changes. *J. Bone Joint Surg. (Br.)* 59 (1): 24–35.

98 McDevitt, C.A. and Muir, H. (1976). Biochemical changes in the cartilage of the knee in experimental and natural osteoarthritis in the dog. *J. Bone Joint Surg. (Br.)* 58 (1): 94–101.

99 Pedersen, N.C. and Pool, R. (1978). Canine joint disease. *Vet. Clin. North Am.* 8 (3): 465–493.

100 Mathews, K.G., Koblik, P.D., Knoeckel, M.J. et al. (1995). Resolution of lameness associated with Scottish fold osteodystrophy following bilateral ostectomies and pantarsal arthrodeses: a case report. *J. Am. Anim. Hosp. Assoc.* 31 (4): 280–288.

101 Malik, R., Allan, G.S., Howlett, C.R. et al. (1999). Osteochondrodysplasia in Scottish fold cats. *Aust. Vet. J.* 77 (2): 85–92.

102 Partington, B.P., Williams, J.F., Pechman, R.D., and Beach, R.T. (1996). What is your diagnosis? Scottish fold osteodystrophy. *J. Am. Vet. Med. Assoc.* 209 (7): 1235–1236.

103 Owens, J.M. and Ackerman, N. (1978). Roentgenology of arthritis. *Vet. Clin. North Am.* 8 (3): 453–464.

104 Clarke, S.P. and Bennett, D. (2006). Feline osteoarthritis: a prospective study of 28 cases. *J. Small Anim. Pract.* 47 (8): 439–445.

105 Lascelles, B.D., Hansen, B.D., Roe, S. et al. (2007). Evaluation of client-specific outcome measures and activity monitoring to measure pain relief in cats with osteoarthritis. *J. Vet. Intern. Med.* 21 (3): 410–416.

106 Lascelles, B.D., Henderson, A.J., and Hackett, I.J. (2001). Evaluation of the clinical efficacy of meloxicam in cats with painful locomotor disorders. *J. Small Anim. Pract.* 42 (12): 587–593.

107 Gunew, M.N., Menrath, V.H., and Marshall, R.D. (2008). Long-term safety, efficacy and palatability of oral meloxicam at 0.01–0.03 mg/kg for treatment of osteoarthritic pain in cats. *J. Feline Med. Surg.* 10 (3): 235–241.

108 Goldschmidt, M.H. and Thrall, D.E. (1985). Primary and secondary bone tumors in the cat, ch. 78. In: *Textbook of Small Animal Orthopaedics* (ed. C.D. Newton and D.M. Nunamaker). Philadelphia: Lippincott.

109 Goldschmidt, M.H. and Thrall, D.E. (1985). Malignant bone tumors in the dog, ch. 74. In: *Textbook of Small Animal Orthopaedics* (ed. C.D. Newton and D.M. Nunamaker). Philadelphia: Lippincott.

110 Henry, C.J., Brewer, W.G., Whitley, E.M. et al. (2005). Canine digital tumors: a veterinary cooperative oncology group retrospective study of 64 dogs. *J. Vet. Intern. Med.* 19 (5): 720–724.

111 Shafiee, R., Shariat, A., Khalili, S. et al. (2015). Diagnostic investigations of canine prostatitis incidence together with benign prostate hyperplasia, prostate malignancies, and biochemical recurrence in high-risk prostate cancer as a model for human study. *Tumor Biol.* 36 (4): 2437–2445.

112 McLaughlin, R.M. (2002). Surgical diseases of the feline stifle joint. *Vet. Clin. North Am. Small Anim. Pract.* 32 (4): 963–982.

113 Cook, J.L. (2001). Forelimb lameness in the young patient. *Vet. Clin. North Am. Small Anim. Pract.* 31 (1): 55–83.

114 Wisner, E.R., Berry, C.R., Morgan, J.P. et al. (1990). Osteochondrosis of the lateral trochlear Ridge of the talus in 7 Rottweiler dogs. *Vet. Surg.* 19 (6): 435–439.

115 Montgomery, R.D., Hathcock, J.T., Milton, J.L., and Fitch, R.B. (1994). Osteochondritis-Dissecans of the canine tarsal joint. *Compend. Contin. Educ. Pract.* 16 (7): 835–845.

116 Barrett, R.B., Schall, W.D., and Lewis, R.E. (1968). Clinical and radiographic features of canine eosinophilic panosteitis. *J. Am. Anim. Hosp. Assoc.* 4: 94.

117 Bohning, R.H. Jr., Suter, P.F., Hohn, R.B., and Marshall, J. (1970). Clinical and radiologic survey of canine panosteitis. *J. Am. Vet. Med. Assoc.* 156 (7): 870–883.

118 Muir, P., Dubielzig, R.R., and Johnson, K.A. (1996). Panosteitis. *Compend. Contin. Educ. Pract.* 18 (1): 29–33.

119 Scott, H. (1998). Non-traumatic causes of lameness in the forelimb of the growing dog. *In Pract.* 20 (10): 539–554.

120 Alexander, J.W. (1978). Hypertrophic osteodystrophy. *Canine Pract.* 5: 48.

121 Grondalen, J. (1979). Arthrosis with special reference to the elbow joint of young rapidly growing dogs. II. Occurrence, clinical, and radiographic findings. *Nord. Vet. Med.* 31: 69.

122 Munjar, T.A., Austin, C.C., and Breur, G.J. (1998). Comparison of risk factors for hypertrophic osteodystrophy, craniomandibular osteopathy, and canine distemper virus infection. *Vet. Comp. Orthop. Traumatol.* 11: 37.

123 Grondalen, J. (1976). Metaphyseal osteopathy (hypertrophic osteodystrophy) in growing dogs. A clinical study. *J. Small Anim. Pract.* 17 (11): 721–735.

124 Thomas, W.B. (2000). Initial assessment of patients with neurologic dysfunction. *Vet. Clin. North Am. Small Anim. Pract.* 30 (1): 1–24, v.

125 Garosi, L. (2009). Neurological examination of the cat. How to get started. *J. Feline Med. Surg.* 11 (5): 340–348.

126 De Risio, L. and Platt, S.R. (2010). Fibrocartilaginous embolic myelopathy in small animals. *Vet. Clin. North Am. Small Anim. Pract.* 40 (5): 859–869.

127 Mikszewski, J.S., Van Winkle, T.J., and Troxel, M.T. (2006). Fibrocartilaginous embolic myelopathy in five cats. *J. Am. Anim. Hosp. Assoc.* 42 (3): 226–233.

128 Falconer, L. and Atwell, R. (2003). Feline aortic thromboembolism. *Aust. Vet. Pract.* 33 (1): 20–32.

129 Fuentes, V.L. (2012). ARTERIAL THROMBOEMBOLISM risks, realities and a rational first-line approach. *J. Feline Med. Surg.* 14 (7): 459–470.

130 Borgeat, K., Wright, J., Garrod, O. et al. (2014). Arterial thromboembolism in 250 cats in general practice: 2004–2012. *J. Vet. Intern. Med.* 28 (1): 102–108.

131 Smith, S.A., Tobias, A.H., Jacob, K.A. et al. (2003). Arterial thromboembolism in cats: acute crisis in 127 cases (1992–2001) and long-term management with low-dose aspirin in 24 cases. *J. Vet. Intern. Med.* 17 (1): 73–83.

132 Laste, N.J. and Harpster, N.K. (1995). A retrospective study of 100 cases of feline distal aortic thromboembolism: 1977–1993. *J. Am. Anim. Hosp. Assoc.* 31 (6): 492–500.

133 Smith, S.A. and Tobias, A.H. (2004). Feline arterial thromboembolism: an update. *Vet. Clin. North Am. Small Anim. Pract.* 34 (5): 1245–1271.

134 Rishniw, M. (2006). Feline aortic thromboembolism. *NAVC Clinician's Brief* (November): 17–20.

135 Peycke, L.E. (2010). Forelimb lameness & elbow pain. *NAVC Clinician's Brief* (September): 40–41.

70

Shifting Leg Lameness

70.1 Shifting Leg Lameness as a Clinical Presentation

Chapters 68 and 69 introduced the concepts of forelimb and hind limb lameness, respectively. These may occur in isolation of one another, or they may occur concurrently.

Shifting leg lameness is a distinct form of lameness in which the disturbance in gait appears to jump from one limb to another. A client may schedule an appointment to evaluate the right pelvic limb for lameness only to find that on the day of the consultation, the lameness has shifted to the left front leg. This switch is often disconcerting to the client, who may be adamant about the origin of lameness.

Shifting leg lameness occurs in dogs as well as cats, without any specific timeline. It may come and go in waves. Lameness may also recur in the original limb as it jumps around the patient.

As with any other form of lameness, shifting leg lameness varies in terms of intensity and duration. It frequently progresses without treatment; however, the severity of lameness varies between patients.

70.2 Differential Diagnoses for Shifting Leg Lameness

Although there are many potential causes of shifting leg lameness, the top three differentials in companion animal practice are the following:

- Developmental orthopedic disease
  - Panosteitis
- Immune-mediated arthropathy
- Infectious arthropathy
  - Borreliosis

70.3 Panosteitis

Panosteitis was introduced in Chapter 68, Section 68.6.4.1 and Chapter 69, Section 69.13.2 as both a cause of forelimb and hind limb lameness. However, the lameness that is associated with panosteitis is not necessarily static. Shifting leg lameness has been described as a characteristic of this developmental pathology [1–3]. It is not uncommon for lameness associated with one limb to resolve as other limbs become lame. The process is often cyclical [3]. Each flare-up typically lasts 1–2 weeks, but flares may continue until 18 months of age [2, 4–6].

Panosteitis targets the long bones of young, large-breed dogs. The following breeds are overrepresented [1, 2, 4, 7–9]:

- Doberman Pinschers
- German Shepherds
- Golden Retrievers
- Labrador Retrievers
- Saint Bernards

Bassett Hounds also are at increased risk for development of panosteitis [2, 4].

Males are more likely than females to be affected [2–4, 10, 11].

Textbook cases of panosteitis present between 5 and 12 months of age; however, delayed presentations of up to 5 years old are possible [1, 4, 7, 9].

Recall that the etiology is unknown [2, 3]. What is understood is that osteoblastic and fibroblastic activity increases within the marrow, endosteum, and periosteum of affected patients [2]. This causes the marrow-containing medullary cavity to be replaced by connective tissue [2]. Medullary vessels become congested [2]. Proteinaceous fluid leaks out of these vessels and may stimulate pain receptors [2]. Patients resent palpation of the diaphyses of affected long bones [2].

Common Clinical Presentations in Dogs and Cats, First Edition. Ryane E. Englar.
© 2019 John Wiley & Sons, Inc. Published 2019 by John Wiley & Sons, Inc.

The most common sites to be affected include the [1, 2, 6, 11]:

- Humerus
- Femur
- Radius
- Ulna

In addition to presenting with long bone pain, patients may be anorexic and febrile [1, 6].

The signalment, history, and physical examination findings raise the index of suspicion that panosteitis is likely.

A radiographic diagnosis is made based upon the following findings [2, 3, 11, 12]:

- Hazy or granular appearance of the medullary cavity
- Loss of the trabecular pattern
- Proliferative periosteum and/or endosteum
- Thicker appearance to the cortex

Note that radiographic signs may lag behind the patient's clinical presentation, meaning that diagnostic imaging may not reveal early lesions or mild cases [1, 2, 4, 8]. Even so, diagnostic imaging plays an important role in the clinician's approach to panosteitis because panosteitis may occur concurrently with other developmental orthopedic disease, including osteochondrosis (OC) and hypertrophic osteodystrophy (HOD) [1].

Effective case management for panosteitis involves symptomatic care to reduce pain during flares [1–3, 9]. Maintaining lean body weight and restricting exercise as needed may also benefit the patient by reducing the burden on the skeletal system [2].

70.4 Immune-Mediated Polyarthritis

Immune-mediated polyarthritis (IMPA) refers to a constellation of arthropathies that more commonly occur in dogs than in cats [13, 14].

All forms of disease are characterized by a type III hypersensitivity reaction in which antigen–antibody complexes gather within the affected joint spaces [13, 15–19].

Complement is activated by the presence of these complexes [13]. This sets the stage for an inflammatory response [13]. The release of cytokines creates a vicious cycle [13]. Neutrophils are attracted to the scene by cytokines [13]. Neutrophils release their own cytokines, which, in combination with lysosomal enzymes, damage surrounding tissues [13, 15–19].

Clinical signs are potentiated by this inflammatory response [13].

For classification purposes, IMPA may be erosive or non-erosive [13, 20, 21].

Of the two forms, erosive and non-erosive IMPA, the former is least likely to occur in companion animal practice [13, 20].

70.4.1 Erosive IMPA

Although there are several types of erosive IMPA, the one that is recognized most often in dogs mirrors rheumatoid arthritis (RA) in humans [13, 20].

Middle-aged, toy, and small-breed dogs are predisposed [13, 20, 22].

Patients typically present with one or more painful joints [20]. This may manifest as overt lameness or a generalized reluctance to ambulate [23].

Clients may report depression and lethargy [23]. Patients are often anorexic secondary to systemic malaise [23].

Clients may also report apparent stiffness [17, 21, 23, 24]. This may be described by clients as "walking on eggshells" [17, 21].

This stiffness may be witnessed by the practitioner during clinical observation of the patient's gait [23].

Physical examination typically reveals joint distension at multiple sites [20]. Symmetrical distribution of lesions is common [23].

Disease is cyclical [20]. Clients report episodes that last for several days [20]. Resolution is spontaneous [20].

Over time, disease progression results in more frequent episodes of longer duration [20].

The following criteria facilitate diagnosis of erosive IMPA in the canine patient [13, 17–20, 25, 26]:

- One or more painful joints
- Three or more months of symptoms
- Soft tissue swelling at and around one or more joints
- Deformation of carpal and/or tarsal joints, or any joints distal to these

Patients with erosive IMPA may have mild changes on their hemogram that reflect an ongoing inflammatory process. For instance, they may demonstrate a mild non-regenerative anemia of chronic disease [20, 23].

Neutrophilia may be present, with mild leukocytosis [20].

In addition, mild hypoalbuminemia is common [23].

Serum biochemistry panels often demonstrate mild elevations in alkaline phosphatase [16, 23, 25–30].

Urine cultures may identify systemic infections [23]. Because systemic infections can induce erosive IMPA, this is an important diagnostic tool [23].

Radiographs are an important diagnostic tool in cases in which erosive IMPA is suspected [23]. Radiographic findings that support a diagnosis of early erosive IMPA include the following [20, 23]:

- Joint capsule effusion
- Periarticular changes
  - Soft tissue mineralization
  - Soft tissue swelling

As erosive IMPA progresses, the juxta-articular bone experiences osteoporosis [20, 31, 32]. Cyst-like areas of radiolucency appear in subchondral bone as bone is eroded by disease [20].

Erosion leads to dissolution of articular cartilage [20]. Ultimately, the joint space may collapse as disease progresses [20].

Diagnosis of erosive IMPA is confirmed via arthrocentesis [23, 30]. Because the carpi and tarsi are most commonly affected by IMPA, these joints are often sampled [15–19, 22, 23, 25–30, 32–34].

Use of aseptic technique is critical during joint sampling so as not to introduce infection into one or more joints [23].

Techniques for performing arthrocentesis are beyond the scope of this text.

Normal joints contain small amounts of joint fluid. For example, small-breed dogs may have <0.25 ml available for sampling from a normal joint [23]. When twice that amount is collected, there is a good probability that the sampled joint is diseased [23, 35, 36].

When joints are sampled in health, normal synovial fluid contains fewer than 3000 cells/μl [17, 36]. Of these, the majority are mononuclear [35]. Non-reactive macrophages are commonly observed [35].

Normal joint fluid is viscous [17, 23]. This viscosity is maintained in health by hyaluronic acid [23].

Hyaluronic acid is degraded by inflammatory cells and/or bacteria [23]. This results in decreased viscosity of joint fluid in joints with erosive IMPA. Such joints also may have discolored or turbid synovial fluid due to increased protein and nucleated cell content [23]. Cell counts of joints with erosive IMPA often exceed 5000/μl. Of these, the percentage of neutrophils is greatly increased [23]. Most of these are degenerate [23].

Because degenerate neutrophils may also result from bacterial or fungal infection, it is important to culture synovial fluid to rule out septic arthritis [23]. The presence of intracellular bacteria within neutrophils is suggestive of infectious arthritis [23].

It is possible, although uncommon, to identify infectious agents via cytology of joint fluid [23]. While awaiting culture results, cytological examination should be performed to evaluate for the following [23, 35–37]:

- *Borrelia burgdorferi,* the infectious agent of borreliosis or Lyme disease

- *Mycoplasma* spp.
- *Leishmania*
- Fungal hyphae

If infection is ruled out, treatment of erosive IMPA involves the administration of glucocorticoids at immunosuppressive doses [23]. Additional analgesic and/or immunomodulatory agents may be indicated, depending upon severity of disease and patient response to treatment [23].

70.4.2 Non-Erosive IMPA

Non-erosive IMPA occurs with greater frequency than erosive IMPA in companion animal practice [13, 22, 29, 30]. There are several forms of non-erosive IMPA, including the following [13]:

- Breed-specific polyarthropathies
  - Familial Chinese Shar-Pei fever
  - Juvenile-onset polyarthritis of Akitas
- Drug-induced polyarthritis
- Steroid-responsive meningitis-arteritis
- Systemic lupus erythematosus (SLE)
- Vaccine-induced polyarthritis

The most common cause of canine non-erosive IMPA is idiopathic [13, 16].

70.4.2.1 Drug-Induced Polyarthritis

Several drugs have been linked to the development of polyarthritis, including the following [13, 15, 38–40]:

- Cephalosporin
- Erythromycin
- Erythropoietin
- Lincomycin
- Penicillin
- Phenobarbital
- Sulfonamide

Of those listed above, sulfonamides are most often implicated [13].

Doberman Pinschers appear to be predisposed to sulfonamide-induced polyarthritis [13, 41, 42].

On average, it takes 12 days from the time that sulfonamide therapy is instituted for arthropathy to develop [42]. If the patient had previously been prescribed sulfonamides, then arthropathy may develop sooner, within 1 hour to 10 days of re-exposure [42].

Discontinuation of the medication causes clinical signs to resolve [13].

70.4.2.2 Familial Chinese Shar-Pei Fever

Familial Chinese Shar-Pei fever is an inherited condition that is characterized by an episodic febrile and pro-inflammatory state [13]. Most affected dogs present for their first bout of this disease prior to 18 months of age [13, 43, 44].

Patients experience 24–36 h of high-grade fever [13]. In addition, many present for the following:

- Acute abdomen
- Gastrointestinal distress
  - Diarrhea
  - Vomiting
- Generalized depression and malaise
- Painful back
- Painful joints
- Swollen muzzle

Approximately half the patients have swollen hocks [13, 45, 46].

One concern about this condition is that it leads to elevated levels of acute phase proteins in the bloodstream [13]. These may deposit as amyloid within the kidneys and liver [13]. Multisystemic organ failure is possible [13, 47, 48].

70.4.2.3 Juvenile-Onset Polyarthritis of Akitas
Young Akitas may also develop episodic fever, pain, and swollen joints. Patients may present as early as nine weeks of age [13]. Neck pain, back pain, and peripheral lymphadenopathy are common clinical findings [13]. This condition is believed to be inherited [49]. It has been theorized that vaccinations may trigger development of polyarthritis in this breed; however, this has yet to been established in the veterinary literature [13, 49, 50].

70.4.2.4 Systemic Lupus Erythematosus
SLE was first introduced in Chapter 10, Section 10.1, Chapter 13, Section 13.1.2, and Chapter 32, Section 32.4 as a cause of nasal and footpad hyperkeratosis, seborrhea, and otitis externa.

In addition to these integumentary changes, SLE has also been associated with the following [13, 21]:

- Glomerulonephritis
- Hemolytic anemia
- Leukopenia
- Non-erosive IMPA
- Polymyositis
- Thrombocytopenia

The most common finding of SLE in dogs is non-erosive IMPA [13]. This is manifested most often in dogs as shifting leg lameness [13, 51–54].

Although females are predisposed to SLE in human medicine, both sexes are equally at risk among the canine population [13, 30].

Patients are typically young adults at time of onset [13].

The following breeds are overrepresented [13, 51, 52]:

- Afghan Hounds
- Beagles
- Cocker Spaniels
- Collies
- German Shepherd Dogs
- Irish Setters
- Old English Sheepdogs
- Poodles
- Shetland Sheepdogs

Mixed-breed dogs are also overrepresented [13, 51, 52].

70.4.2.5 Vaccine-Induced Polyarthritis
Polyarthritis may develop in a subset of the population within 30 days of being vaccinated [13, 55]. The inciting injection does not have to be an initial vaccination of a series [13]. It can be a booster [13].

Of those vaccinations that are typically administered in companion animal practice, canine distemper virus (CDV) has been linked to cases of polyarthritis [13].

Synovial fluid collected from these patients demonstrates extreme elevations in cell count, in some cases reaching 72,000 per microliter [55].

Although this is a transient response, it can result in significant joint pain and cyclical fevers [13].

Akitas may be predisposed [13, 50]. However, it is difficult to discern whether affected Akitas truly succumbed to adverse effects of vaccination or simply were presenting with juvenile-onset polyarthritis, which notoriously occurs in puppies that are of vaccination age [13, 50].

70.4.3 Feline Polyarthritis

As compared to the dog, it is uncommon to see IMPA in cats [14]. When IMPA occurs in cats, it is thought to be associated with either feline syncytium-forming virus or feline leukemia virus (FeLV) [14].

Affected cats develop painful swellings in multiple joints [14]. There may be concurrent fever and depression, with or without peripheral lymphadenopathy [14]. Male cats are overrepresented [14, 33, 56–58].

Immunosuppressive therapy with cyclosporine has demonstrated good efficacy in isolated case reports; however, additional research is indicated [14].

70.5 Borreliosis

Borreliosis or Lyme disease was introduced in Chapter 6, Sections 6.5.3 and 6.5.6 as a tick-borne disease, spread by *Ixodes* spp. [59].

Lyme disease was expanded upon in Chapter 63, Section 63.4.1.2.1 in regard to its ability to induce acute kidney injury (AKI) [60].

Recall that borreliosis is caused by *B. burgdorferi*, a spirochete that lives in the midgut of infected ticks [59, 61, 62]. Review the life cycle of this infectious agent in Chapter 6, Section 6.5.6 [61, 63–66].

Erythema migrans, a bull's-eye rash, is a common characteristic of Lyme disease in humans [61]. Because neither dogs nor cats develop this hallmark sign, tick bites in companion animal patients often go unnoticed.

Lyme disease is subclinical in some patients [59, 61, 67].

Others develop symptoms; however, the initial clinical signs in early disease tend to be nonspecific [61, 62, 67]:

- Depression
- Fever
- Lameness
- Lethargy
- Peripheral lymphadenopathy

The aforementioned clinical signs are short-lived and may go unnoticed [61]. They may or may not trigger the diagnostician to test for Lyme disease.

When Lyme disease is suspected, it can be challenging to differentiate actively infected seropositive dogs from those that have had prior exposure [59].

When dogs are infected with Lyme disease, they often have difficulty eliminating *B. burgdorferi* from the body [62, 68]. When this occurs, Lyme disease becomes chronic [61, 62, 68]. Chronic infection with Lyme disease results from persistent inflammatory reactions to the spirochetes, which have developed ways of evading the host's immune system [61].

A common sequela of chronic infection is polyarthritis [61, 68].

Experimentally infected dogs present with lameness two to six months after infection [69, 70]. Lameness starts at the limb nearest the site of the tick bite, and then appears to spread [69, 70]. Lameness may be intermittent or progressive. It may also appear to jump limb to limb [69, 70].

Naturally infected dogs may also develop recurrent bouts of lameness [61]. Affected patients may have reduced activity levels or impaired mobility, especially climbing up or down stairs [61].

Cats are also exposed to Borreliosis through tick bites. Little is known about the clinical features of borreliosis in cats because of limited case reports; however, lameness, fever, fatigue, and anorexia appear to be common presenting complaints [71].

Testing for Lyme disease is beyond the scope of this textbook; however, it is important to consider this condition in any patient that presents with a history of shifting leg lameness [67].

At the same time, other tick-borne diseases should be considered in cases of lameness, including the following [67]:

- Anaplasmosis
- Ehrlichiosis
- Rocky Mountain spotted fever (RMSF)

References

1 Bergh, M.S. (2015). Panosteitis. *NAVC Clinician's Brief* (August): 10–11.

2 Demko, J. and McLaughlin, R. (2005). Developmental orthopedic disease. *Vet. Clin. North Am. Small Anim. Pract.* 35 (5): 1111–1135, v.

3 Cook, J.L. (2001). Forelimb lameness in the young patient. *Vet. Clin. North Am.-Small* 31 (1): 55–83.

4 Bohning, R.H. Jr., Suter, P.F., Hohn, R.B., and Marshall, J. (1970). Clinical and radiologic survey of canine panosteitis. *J. Am. Vet. Med. Assoc.* 156 (7): 870–883.

5 Milton, J.L. (1979). Panosteitis: a review of the literature and 32 cases. *Auburn Vet.* 35 (3): 11–15.

6 Lenehan, T.M., Van Sickle, D.C., and Biery, D.N. (1985). Canine panosteitis. In: *Textbook of Small Animal Orthopaedics* (ed. T.W. Fossum), 591–596. Philadelphia: JB Lippincott.

7 LaFond, E., Breur, G.J., and Austin, C.C. (2002). Breed susceptibility for developmental orthopedic diseases in dogs. *J. Am. Anim. Hosp. Assoc.* 38 (5): 467–477.

8 Barrett, R.B., Schall, W.D., and Lewis, R.E. (1968). Clinical and radiographic features of canine eosinophilic panosteitis. *J. Am. Anim. Hosp. Assoc.* 4: 94–104.

9 Lafuente, P. (2014). Top 5 juvenile orthopedic conditions. *NAVC Clinician's Brief* (August): 11–14.

10 Hulse, D.A. and Johnson, A.L. (eds.) (1997). Other diseases of bones and joints. In: *Small Animal Surgery*, 1009–1030. St. Louis: Mosby-Year Book.

11 Burt, J.K. and Wilson, G.P. 3rd. (1972). A study of eosinophilic panosteitis (enostosis) in German shepherd dogs. *Acta Radiol. Suppl.* 319: 7–13.

12 McLaughlin, R.M. (2001). Hind limb lameness in the young patient. *Vet. Clin. North Am.-Small* 31 (1): 101–123.

13 Johnson, K.C. and Mackin, A. (2012). Canine immune-mediated polyarthritis: part 1: pathophysiology. *J. Am. Anim. Hosp. Assoc.* 48 (1): 12–17.

14 Oohashi, E., Yamada, K., Oohashi, M., and Ueda, J. (2010). Chronic progressive polyarthritis in a female cat. *J. Vet. Med. Sci.* 72 (4): 511–514.

15 Taylor, S.M. (2009). Joint Disorders. In: *Small Animal Internal Medicine* (ed. R.W. Nelson and C.G. Couto), 1119–1141. St. Louis, MO: Mosby Elsevier.

16 Bennett, D. (2010). Immune-mediated and infective arthritis. In: *Textbook of Veterinary Internal Medicine*, 1e (ed. S.J. Ettinger and E.C. Feldman), 743–439. St. Louis: Saunders Elsevier.

17 Kohn, B. (ed.) (2003). Canine immune-mediated polyarthritis. World Small Animal Veterinary Association World Congress.

18 Kohn, B. (ed.) (2007). Canine immune-mediated polyarthritis. FECAVA/CSAVS Congress; Cavtat, Dubrovnik.

19 Kohn, B. (2007). Canine immune-mediated polyarthritis. *Eur. J. Comp. Anim. Pract.* 17 (2): 119–124.

20 Lipowitz, A.J. (1985). Immune-mediated Arthopathies. In: *Textbook of Small Animal Orthopaedics*, xxiv, 1140 p. (ed. C.D. Newton and D.M. Nunamaker). Philadelphia: Lippincott.

21 Kiss, C.M. and Troy, G.C. (2011). Recognizing and treating immune-mediated polyarthritis in dogs. DVM 360 [Internet]. http://veterinarymedicine.dvm360.com/ recognizing-and-treating-immune-mediated- polyarthritis-dogs.

22 Goldstein, R.E. (2010). Swollen joints and lameness. In: *Textbook of Veterinary Internal Medicine. One* (ed. S.J. Ettinger and E.C. Feldman), 130–133. St. Louis: Sanders Elsevier.

23 Johnson, K.C. and Mackin, A. (2012). Canine immune-mediated polyarthritis: part 2: diagnosis and treatment. *J. Am. Anim. Hosp. Assoc.* 48 (2): 71–82.

24 Hoskins, J.D. (2005). Polyarthritis: look for chronic lameness without signs of systemic disease. DVM 360 [Internet]. http://veterinarynews.dvm360.com/ polyarthritis-look-chronic-lameness-without-signs- systemic-disease.

25 Bennett, D. (1987). Immune-based erosive inflammatory joint disease of the dog – canine rheumatoid-Arthritis.2. Pathological investigations. *J. Small Anim. Pract.* 28 (9): 799–819.

26 Bennett, D. (1987). Immune-based erosive inflammatory joint disease of the dog – canine rheumatoid-Arthritis.1. Clinical, radiological and laboratory investigations. *J. Small Anim. Pract.* 28 (9): 779–797.

27 Clements, D.N., Gear, R.N., Tattersall, J. et al. (2004). Type I immune-mediated polyarthritis in dogs: 39 cases (1997–2002). *J. Am. Vet. Med. Assoc.* 224 (8): 1323–1327.

28 Jacques, D., Cauzinille, L., Bouvy, B., and Dupre, G. (2002). A retrospective study of 40 dogs with polyarthritis. *Vet. Surg.* 31 (5): 428–434.

29 Rondeau, M.P., Walton, R.M., Bissett, S. et al. (2005). Suppurative, nonseptic polyarthropathy in dogs. *J. Vet. Intern. Med.* 19 (5): 654–662.

30 Stull, J.W., Evason, M., Carr, A.P., and Waldner, C. (2008). Canine immune-mediated polyarthritis: clinical and laboratory findings in 83 cases in western Canada (1991–2001). *Can. Vet. J.* 49 (12): 1195–1203.

31 Owens, J.M. and Ackerman, N. (1978). Roentgenology of arthritis. *Vet. Clin. North Am.* 8 (3): 453–464.

32 Pedersen, N.C., Weisner, K., Castles, J.J. et al. (1976). Noninfectious canine arthritis: the inflammatory, nonerosive arthritides. *J. Am. Vet. Med. Assoc.* 169 (3): 304–310.

33 Bennett, D. (2005). Immune-mediated and infectious arthritis. In: *Textbook of Veterinary Internal Medicine*, 2e (ed. S.J. Ettinger and E.C. Feldman), 1958–1964. St. Louis: Elsevier Sanders.

34 Shaughnessy, M.L., Sample, S.J., Abicht, C. et al. (2016). Clinical features and pathological joint changes in dogs with erosive immune-mediated polyarthritis: 13 cases (2004–2012). *J. Am. Vet. Med. Assoc.* 249 (10): 1156–1164.

35 Alleman, A.R., DeNicola, D.B., and Wamsley, H.L. (eds.) (2007. Synovial fluid analysis. 79th Annual Western Veterinary Conference; Las Vegas.

36 MacWilliams, P.S. and Friedrichs, K.R. (2003). Laboratory evaluation and interpretation of synovial fluid. *Vet. Clin. North Am. Small Anim. Pract.* 33 (1): 153–178.

37 Yamaguchi, R.A., French, T.W., Simpson, C.F., and Harvey, J.W. (1983). Leishmania-Donovani in the synovial-fluid of a dog with visceral Leishmaniasis. *J. Am. Anim. Hosp. Assoc.* 19 (5): 723–726.

38 Bennett, D. (1987). Immune-based nonerosive inflammatory joint disease of the dog. 1. Canine systemic lupus-Erythematosus. *J. Small Anim. Pract.* 28 (10): 871–889.

39 Bennett, D. (1987). Immune-based nonerosive inflammatory joint disease of the dog. 3. Canine idiopathic polyarthritis. *J. Small Anim. Pract.* 28 (10): 909–928.

40 Bennett, D. and Kelly, D.F. (1987). Immune-based nonerosive inflammatory joint disease of the dog. 2. Polyarthritis polymyositis syndrome. *J. Small Anim. Pract.* 28 (10): 891–908.

41 Cribb, A.E. and Spielberg, S.P. (1990). An Invitro investigation of predisposition to sulfonamide idiosyncratic toxicity in dogs. *Vet. Res. Commun.* 14 (3): 241–252.

42 Giger, U., Werner, L.L., Millichamp, N.J., and Gorman, N.T. (1985). Sulfadiazine-induced allergy in 6 Doberman pinschers. *J. Am. Vet. Med. Assoc.* 186 (5): 479–484.

43 Rivas, A.L., Tintle, L., Kimball, E.S. et al. (1992). A canine febrile disorder associated with elevated interleukin-6. *Clin. Immunol. Immunopathol.* 64 (1): 36–45.

44 Rivas, A.L., Tintle, L., Meyers-Wallen, V. et al. (1993). Inheritance of renal amyloidosis in Chinese Shar-pei dogs. *J. Hered.* 84 (6): 438–442.

45 May, C., Hammill, J., and Bennett, D. (1992). Chinese shar pei fever syndrome: a preliminary report. *Vet. Rec.* 131 (25–26): 586–587.

46 Tellier, L.A. (2001). Immune-mediated vasculitis in a shar-pei with swollen hock syndrome. *Can. Vet. J.* 42 (2): 137–139.

47 Loeven, K.O. (1994). Hepatic amyloidosis in two Chinese Shar Pei dogs. *J. Am. Vet. Med. Assoc.* 204 (8): 1212–1216.

48 Loeven, K.O. (1994). Spontaneous hepatic rupture secondary to amyloidosis in a Chinese Shar-Pei. *J. Am. Anim. Hosp. Assoc.* 30 (6): 577–579.

49 Dougherty, S.A., Center, S.A., Shaw, E.E., and Erb, H.A. (1991). Juvenile-onset polyarthritis syndrome in Akitas. *J. Am. Vet. Med. Assoc.* 198 (5): 849–856.

50 Dodds, W.J. (2001). Vaccination protocols for dogs predisposed to vaccine reactions. *J. Am. Anim. Hosp. Assoc.* 37 (3): 211–214.

51 Marks, S.L. and Henry, C.J. (2000). Diagnosis and treatment of systemic lupus erythematosus. In: *Kirks Current Veterinary Therapy XIII: Small Animal Practice* (ed. J.D. Bonagura), 514–516. Philadelphia: Saunders.

52 Stone, M. (2010). Systemic lupus erythematosus. In: *Textbook of Veterinary Internal Medicine* (ed. S.J. Ettinger and E.C. Feldman), 783–788. St. Louis: Saunders Elsevier.

53 Berent, A.C. and Cerundolo, R. (2005). Systemic lupus erythematosus. *Standards of Care.* 7: 7–12.

54 Scott-Moncrieff, J.C. (2009). Pathogenesis of immune-mediated disorders. In: *Small Animal Internal Medicine* (ed. R.W. Nelson and C.G. Couto), 1422–1423. St. Louis: Mosby Elsevier.

55 Kohn, B., Garner, M., Lubke, S. et al. (2003). Polyarthritis following vaccination in four dogs. *Vet. Comp. Orthopaed.* 16 (1): 6–10.

56 Allan, G.S. (2007). Radiographic signs of joint disease in dogs and cats. In: *Textbook of Veterinary Diagnostic Radiology* (ed. D.E. Thrall), 317–358. St. Louis: Elsevier Saunders.

57 Pedersen, N.C., Pool, R.R., and O'Brien, T. (1980). Feline chronic progressive polyarthritis. *Am. J. Vet. Res.* 41 (4): 522–535.

58 Schulz, K. (2007). Diseases of the joints. In: *Small Animal Surgery*, 3e (ed. T.W. Fossum), 1143–1170. St. Louis: Mosby Elsevier.

59 Little, S.E., Heise, S.R., Blagburn, B.L. et al. (2010). Lyme borreliosis in dogs and humans in the USA. *Trends Parasitol.* 26 (4): 213–218.

60 Balakrishnan, A. and Drobatz, K.J. (2013). Management of urinary tract emergencies in small animals. *Vet. Clin. North Am. Small. Anim. Pract.* 43 (4): 843–867.

61 Krupka, I. and Straubinger, R.K. (2010). Lyme borreliosis in dogs and cats: background, diagnosis, treatment and prevention of infections with Borrelia burgdorferi sensu stricto. *Vet. Clin. North Am. Small Anim. Pract.* 40 (6): 1103–1119.

62 Littman, M.P. (2003). Canine borreliosis. *Vet. Clin. North Am. Small Anim. Pract.* 33 (4): 827–862.

63 Grimm, D., Tilly, K., Byram, R. et al. (2004). Outer-surface protein C of the Lyme disease spirochete: a protein induced in ticks for infection of mammals. *Proc. Natl. Acad. Sci. U. S. A.* 101 (9): 3142–3147.

64 Ribeiro, J.M., Mather, T.N., Piesman, J., and Spielman, A. (1987). Dissemination and salivary delivery of Lyme disease spirochetes in vector ticks (Acari: Ixodidae). *J. Med. Entomol.* 24 (2): 201–205.

65 Schwan, T.G., Piesman, J., Golde, W.T. et al. (1995). Induction of an outer surface protein on Borrelia burgdorferi during tick feeding. *Proc. Natl. Acad. Sci. U. S. A.* 92 (7): 2909–2913.

66 deSilva, A.M., Telford, S.R., Brunet, L.R. et al. (1996). Borrelia burgdorferi OspA is an arthropod-specific transmission-blocking Lyme disease vaccine. *J. Exp. Med.* 183 (1): 271–275.

67 Datz, C. (2007). Lyme disease in dogs. *NAVC Clinician's Brief* (May): 9–12.

68 Greene, C.E. and Straubinger, R.K. (2006). Borreliosis. In: *Infectious Diseases of the Dog and Cat*, 3e (ed. C.E. Greene), 417–435. St. Louis: Elsevier, Inc.

69 Straubinger, R.K., Summers, B.A., Chang, Y.F., and Appel, M.J. (1997). Persistence of Borrelia burgdorferi in experimentally infected dogs after antibiotic treatment. *J. Clin. Microbiol.* 35 (1): 111–116.

70 Straubinger, R.K., Straubinger, A.F., Harter, L. et al. (1997). Borrelia burgdorferi migrates into joint capsules and causes an up-regulation of interleukin-8 in synovial membranes of dogs experimentally infected with ticks. *Infect. Immun.* 65 (4): 1273–1285.

71 Magnarelli, L.A., Anderson, J.F., Levine, H.R., and Levy, S.A. (1990). Tick parasitism and antibodies to Borrelia burgdorferi in cats. *J. Am. Vet. Med. Assoc.* 197 (1): 63–66.

71

Abnormal Mentation

71.1 Introduction to Normal Mentation

The patient's mental status depends upon the function and well-being of the central nervous system (CNS) [1]. Mentation is a function of how the patient interacts with its environment, including the client, and is typically assessed by the clinician within the first few moments of entering the consultation room. Being observant is particularly useful when making this determination, keeping in mind the context in which the patient is being examined.

The patient's response to the environment should be appropriate for that particular environment, with consideration to prior patient history. For example, the adult cat or dog that appears to be sleeping on the examination table, yet has historically been on high alert in the veterinary clinic, is likely to be demonstrating an abnormal mental state.

Note that mentation is different from behavior, although the two are sometimes confused [2]. In terms of behavior, a patient may be described as being docile or aggressive. A patient may also act behaviorally compulsive.

Contrast this with terms that are used to describe a normal patient's mentation: bright, alert, and responsive (BAR) or quiet, alert, and responsive (QAR). These terms depict attentiveness to the patient's surroundings as opposed to emphasizing temperament (see Figures 71.1a, b).

Note that a cat or dog that is described as being BAR may still be aggressive. Normal mentation does not necessarily imply normal or responsible behavior.

In particular, two components manage a patient's mental state [1–3]:

- The cerebrum
- The ascending reticular activating system (ARAS)

The ARAS is not a single entity [1]. Rather, it refers to a cluster of neurons that extend from the medulla of the brainstem to the thalamus, a midline structure that sits between the cerebral cortex and the midbrain [1–4]. The thalamus essentially regulates the flow of information to the cerebral cortex [3–5]. In particular, it transmits details about the following day-to-day inputs [3–5]:

- Behavior
- Consciousness
- Cerebellar coordination of muscular activities
- Sensory information, with the exception of olfaction
  - Exteroception, that is, awareness of stimuli that originate outside of the body
  - Interoception, that is, self-awareness of ongoing body functions within the individual
  - Nociception, that is, the ability to sense pain

Consider, for instance, the special sense of vision. The retina provides information, by way of the thalamic lateral geniculate nucleus, to the visual cortex of the occipital lobe [4, 5].

Consider also the special sense of hearing. The medial geniculate nucleus of the thalamus transmits information about sound to the cerebral cortex for pattern recognition [4, 5].

Information transfer is bidirectional. This allows information to be received and processed by the cerebral cortex, which can then respond accordingly.

The ARAS is concerned with arousal and consciousness [3, 5]. It functions to maintain wakefulness so that the cortex can receive sensory input [3, 5]. When ARAS activity levels dip, sleep is induced [5]. In health, this state can be interrupted by stimulation of the patient by its external environment, and arousal resumes [5].

The ARAS is equally concerned with focus and attention [5]. It is responsible for prioritizing inputs and ignoring those that are extraneous so that a patient can focus on what is essential [5].

To be alert, a patient must have a functional ARAS [5]. To maintain alertness, ARAS must continue to receive, assimilate, and integrate signals from multiple parts of the body [5]. The result is a patient that is aware of itself as well as the external world [5].

Common Clinical Presentations in Dogs and Cats, First Edition. Ryane E. Englar.

(a) (b)

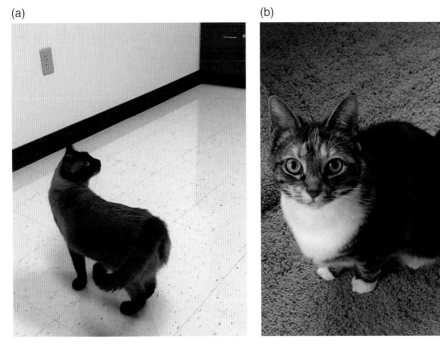

Figure 71.1 (a) This patient is said to be bright, alert, and responsive (BAR) in the examination room. The cat is exploring the space on its own and is aware of the veterinarian's presence. *Source:* Courtesy of Natalie J. Reeser. (b) This patient is said to be BAR within the home environment. The cat is aware of the client's presence and is waiting for instruction. *Source:* Courtesy of Sara D'Addario, DVM.

71.2 Introduction to Abnormal Mentation

Consciousness is not akin to a light switch, with an "off" and an "on." In other words, it is not all-or-none [6–9].

Instead, consciousness represents a sliding scale of awareness [9].

In order of increasing severity, patients may be described as the following [8–10]:

- Depressed
- Obtunded
- Stuporous
- Comatose

Disturbances in consciousness are apparent to the outside observer [5, 9]. One who is observant may notice subtle changes in a patient's mentation before detecting any other signs that might be suggestive of systemic illness.

The clinician is responsible for assessing mentation as part of every clinical examination [1, 9, 11, 12]. However, clients have the advantage of knowing what is considered *normal* for that particular patient [1]. For this reason, clients must be queried carefully concerning the patient's *normal* attitude so that the clinician can conduct an appropriate assessment.

A partnership with the client is particularly helpful when patient behavior in the examination room masks patient mentation. Consider, for instance, the frightened feline patient that tucks up underneath of an examination room chair in an attempt to hide. This patient may outwardly appear to have abnormal mentation, yet may simply be scared. Here, behavioral cues must be examined in the context of the patient's actions to establish if the cat if acting otherwise normally. A frightened, but alert cat, is likely to display the following body posture signals on account of increased sympathetic tone [9]:

- Bilaterally symmetrical, dilated, rounded pupils
- Ear carriage
  - Pinnae may face in opposite directions
  - Pinnae may be backward-facing and/or pinned against the top of the head
- Tucked tail (see Figures 71.2a, c)

History taking is essential: the client should be encouraged to share what s/he considers *normal* or *abnormal* at home versus that which is witnessed in the clinic setting.

Clients may report *abnormal* behavior or changes in behavior without experiencing mentation deficits.

Alternatively, clients may relay details that suggest changes in mental status that may in turn affect patient behavior.

71.2.1 Depression

From a neurologic perspective, depression refers to a slight reduction in the patient's level of consciousness [13]. The patient is aware of its surroundings, but is

(a)

(b)

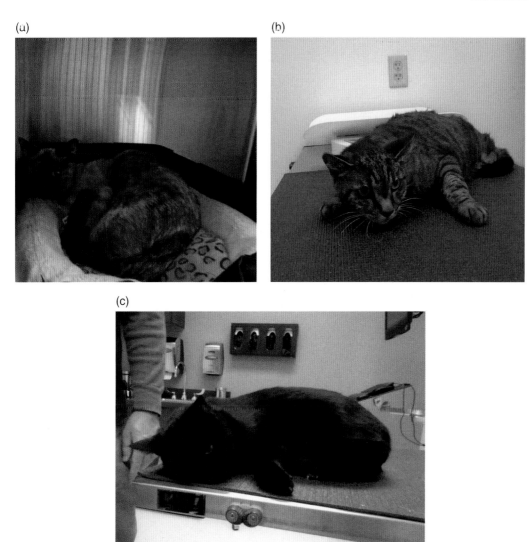

(c)

Figure 71.2 (a) This patient is mentally normal, yet fearful. The cat is tucked into the back of a cage. Note the tail curled around its body and the bilaterally symmetrical, dilated, and round pupils. (b) This patient is mentally normal, yet fearful. Note the cat's hunched posture on the examination room table. The pupils are starting to dilate. (c) This patient is mentally normal, yet fearful. Note how the cat has curled into a ball as if trying to make itself very small and hidden from sight.

somewhat less responsive to external stimuli [9]. Clients may report that the patient is lethargic or otherwise "off" in terms of attitude [9]. The patient may be less inclined to engage in activities. The patient may withdraw from or respond less than usual to interactions.

An example of a depressed patient is one that is febrile [9]. Although fever is a physiologic rather than a neurologic state, it is easy to appreciate how it can lead to depression (see Figure 71.3).

Fever is not the only state that is capable of causing depression. Structural lesions within the CNS may also cause depression [7].

71.2.2 Obtundation

Obtundation refers to a state of mental dullness in which the patient is moderately less attentive to external stimuli [2, 9].

Human patients who are obtunded are described as being confused or delirious [2]. They experience some degree of disorientation and memory loss [2]. They may be unable to complete a thought [2]. These are challenging concepts to apply to the veterinary patient because neither the dog nor cat can articulate this experience [2].

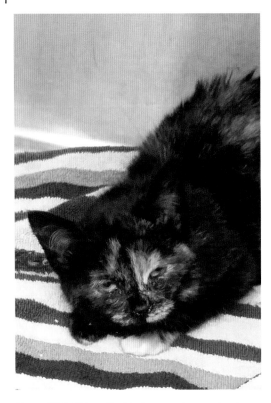

Figure 71.3 This patient is depressed secondary to an upper respiratory infection. The patient's eyes are dull, and the eyelids are droopy. The fur along the topline over the lumbosacral spine is unkempt. This patient has not been grooming well. This patient appears to be unwell.

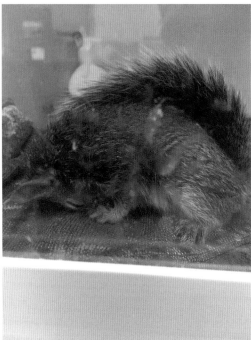

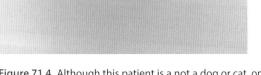

Figure 71.4 Although this patient is a not a dog or cat, one can appreciate that the squirrel in the photograph is stuporous. This squirrel experienced head trauma. Only noxious stimuli could rouse this squirrel. Otherwise, it continued head pressing. *Source:* Courtesy of Ben Turner.

Obtundation is therefore applied to canine and feline patients with some degree of subjectivity. Obtunded patients are less responsive than those that are depressed, but more responsive than those that are stuporous [9].

Consider the action of clapping one's hands to provoke a reaction in the patient. Assuming that hearing is functional, patients will likely react to the sound. The expected reaction may be to raise one's head and/or point the pinnae in the direction of the noise. A depressed patient is likely to react more rapidly than an obtunded patient and with purpose [9].

71.2.3 Stupor

Stupor is a state of being in which the patient only responds to noxious stimuli [2, 9]. Only vigorous or painful sensations are sufficient to rouse the patient from stupor [2, 9] (see Figure 71.4).

71.2.4 Coma

The comatose patient has lost the ability to respond altogether, even to noxious stimuli. Nothing, not even pain, provokes a response [2, 9]. The patient acts as if deeply anesthetized [6–9, 14].

71.3 Causes of Abnormal Mentation

Any disturbance to one or both of the cerebral hemispheres and/or the ARAS can impact mentation [2, 3, 5, 7–9, 13].

Head trauma is responsible for any number of structural lesions that may impair mental status [2, 5, 13]. Head trauma causes primary tissue damage [15]. In addition, tissue damage sets the stage for secondary complications, including the following [15]:

- Edema
- Hemorrhage
- Ischemia

Elevation of intracranial pressure (ICP) is common and potentially life-threatening [15]. As ICP escalates, mentation is impaired.

ICP can also cause brain tissue to herniate [15].

Other structural lesions that may alter mental status include the following [2, 3, 5]:

- Hydrocephalus
- Infectious disease
  - Bacterial
  - Fungal
  - Protozoal
  - Viral
- Neoplasia
- Noninfectious inflammatory disease
  - Granulomatous meningoencephalomyelitis
- Parasitic disease
  - Cuterebriasis (refer to Chapter 6, Section 6.3)
- Vascular accident
  - Infarction

Altered mentation frequently results from metabolic disease, including, but not limited to the following [2]:

- Acid–base imbalance
  - Acidosis
    - Metabolic
    - Respiratory
  - Alkalosis
    - Metabolic
    - Respiratory

- Electrolyte disturbances
  - Calcium
  - Magnesium
  - Potassium
  - Sodium
- Endocrinopathy
  - Diabetes mellitus
  - Hyperthyroidism
  - Hypoadrenocorticism [16]
  - Hypothyroidism
  - Pheochromocytoma
- Hepatopathy
  - Hepatic encephalopathy (HE)
    - Portosystemic shunt (PSS)
- Hypoglycemia
- Uremia

Drug administration may also alter mental status. Consider the following drugs, which are known to impact mentation [2]:

- Anti-convulsants
- Anesthetic agents
- Benzodiazepines
- Cannabis
- Opioids
- Steroids

Non-prescription drugs and illicit substances, such as cocaine and amphetamines, may also alter mentation [2].

Extraneous causes of abnormal mentation include the following [2]:

- Bleeding disorders and associated vascular compromise
- Continuous seizure activity
- Encephalitis
- Hypertension [17]
- Hyperthermia
- Hypotension
- Hypothermia
- Hypovolemia [18]
- Hypoxia
- Meningitis
- Pain
- Post-ictal state
- Sepsis
- Toxicosis
  - Lead

71.4 Diagnostic Approach to Abnormal Mentation

As is evident from Section 71.3 above, the list of differential diagnoses for altered mentation is extensive. Not all differentials can be reviewed here, yet knowing where to begin can be overwhelming for the inexperienced clinician.

Recognition that the patient has abnormal mentation is the first step toward diagnosis. If you as a clinician are not looking for it, then you will not find it.

An assessment of mentation is an important part of every triage and comprehensive physical examination [3, 5, 9, 11, 12]. The role of observation cannot be understated.

Observing the patient interact with its surroundings may reveal obvious deficits in mental status, for example, if the patient struggles to navigate corners or circles when walking [12].

The following questions may facilitate observations [12]:

- Does the patient respond to its name?
- How does the patient interact with the client(s)?
- How does the patient interact with you, the clinician?
- How, if at all, does the patient explore its environment?
- Is the patient responsive to noise, like clapping, hand gestures, or other movement?
- How, if at all, might the patient's behavior be masking mentation?

Note that observations may be subtle. Do not be reluctant to call upon the owner for insight as to what has historically constituted *normal* versus *abnormal* patient behavior.

In addition to observation, history taking is a critical part of the diagnostic plan for a patient with abnormal mentation. Past-pertinent history may reveal important clues that can explain mental deficits. For example, patients with altered mentation that have a history of PSS are likely to be experiencing disease progression. Likewise, patients with chronic kidney disease (CKD) may have progressed to the point of uremic syndrome. Both PSS and CKD can lead to changes in mental status if medical management is ineffective or if the underlying condition intensifies.

In an emergency setting, a history of trauma is often known. For example, the patient that has sustained vehicular injury is likely to have experienced head trauma. Traumatic brain injuries may elevate ICP. These patients are likely to experience altered mentation.

When trauma was not observed, but is suspected, frequent neurologic assessment with serial evaluation of mentation is critical to case management.

Patient stabilization must take a priority in any traumatic case and/or cases in which head trauma is considered probable.

Once the patient is stabilized, patients with altered mentation benefit from having a complete history taken.

A complete history includes the following questions about the change in behavior itself and what, if anything, may have precipitated it:

- What, if anything, has the client noticed at home?
- Is the patient's mental status in the examination room consistent with what the client has noticed at home?
  - If yes, how so?
  - If not, describe what is different at home.
- If the client has noticed mental changes at home, what are they and for how long have they been present?
- Is the change in mental status persistent or episodic?
- If episodic:
  - How frequently do episodes occur?
  - How long do episodes last?
  - Is there a particular time of day when the episodes occur?
    - Morning?
    - Evening?
    - Bedtime?
  - Is there a particular trigger for the episodes?
    - For example, do the episodes occur after eating?
- Are the changes in mentation static or do they appear to be changing?
  - Are they getting better?
  - Are they getting worse?

In addition, the following questions about the patient's health history may be helpful to ask [19]:

- What is the patient's diet?

- A patient that is fed a thiamine-deficient diet (see Chapter 67, Section 67.6) is likely to experience altered mentation [15].
- What is the patient's feeding frequency relative to age?
  - Hypoglycemia is common in toy and small-breed dogs when meals are spaced too far apart. Low blood glucose is likely to impact mentation and may in fact potentiate seizure activity.
- In which region of the country does the patient reside and/or what is the patient's travel history?
  - Fungal diseases may cause CNS signs.
  - The risk of certain fungal diseases varies by region of the country:
    - Actinomycosis
    - Blastomycosis
    - Coccidioidomycosis
    - Cryptococcosis
    - Histoplasmosis
- Has the patient experienced any changes in thirst or urination amount and/or frequency?
  - A patient with undiagnosed diabetes mellitus or renal disease is likely to present for polydipsia (increased thirst) and polyuria (increased urination).
- Has the patient experienced dysuria, stranguria, oliguria, or anuria?
  - A blocked cat, meaning a cat with a urinary tract obstruction (UTO), often presents as either depressed or obtunded [20].
- Has the patient experienced any changes in appetite and weight?
  - A cat with undiagnosed hyperthyroidism is likely to present for weight loss despite increased appetite.
- Has the patient experienced waxing and waning gastrointestinal signs such as bouts of vomiting and diarrhea?
  - A patient with undiagnosed hypoadrenocorticism, or Addison's disease, often presents for recurrent bouts of gastrointestinal upset or distress.
- Does the patient have a seizure history?
- Has the patient experienced any episodes of collapse?
  - Recall from Chapter 40 that collapse describes the loss of postural tone in a patient [21–24]. Without postural tone, the body is unable to maintain itself upright, coordinated, and balanced [25]. The patient, in effect, becomes weak and falls to the ground.
  - Episodes of collapse are either syncopal or related to seizures [21–23, 26, 27]. Both result in loss of consciousness [26].
  - Syncopal episodes are followed by spontaneous recovery [26].
  - In general, seizures last longer than syncopal episodes, and patients are typically slower to recover

[26]. The post-ictal phase that immediately follows a seizure is often characterized by confusion. This may last minutes to hours. Transient changes in mentation are common during this period.

- Does the patient have a history of hydrocephalus?
- Does the patient have a history of hypertension?
- Does the dog have a history of canine distemper virus (CDV)? [28]
- Does the cat have a history of feline infectious peritonitis (FIP)?
- Could the patient have toxoplasmosis or neosporosis?
- Does the patient have a history of neoplasia?
  - Hemangiosarcoma, lymphosarcoma, and mammary carcinoma have the potential to metastasize to the brain [19].
- What, if any, medications are administered to the patient?
- What, if any, over-the-counter products or supplements are administered to the patient?
- Did the patient have access to, or could the patient have ingested, a medication, non-prescription item, or illicit substance?
- Did the patient have access to, or could the patient have ingested, any toxic agent?

Although the questions outlined above are not exhaustive, their answers can effectively rule out a number of differential diagnoses for altered mentation and therefore narrow the list of disease processes to consider.

The patient's vital signs provide an additional layer of information that can help to rule in or rule out differentials [19]:

- Measuring rectal temperature as an indirect assessment of core body temperature will rule out hypothermia or hyperthermia as a cause of altered mentation.
- Measuring systolic blood pressure will rule out hypotension or hypertension as a cause of abnormal mental status.
- Assessing mucous membrane color and capillary refill time (CRT) may provide insight into circulatory status:
  - Pallor may be indicative of anemia.
  - Cyanosis indicates poor oxygenation.
  - Protracted CRT suggests poor perfusion.

In addition to vital signs, the patient's physical examination findings provide additional clues [19]:

- Open wounds confirm trauma.
- Impaired or absent cranial nerve function assists with lesion localization.
  - A midbrain lesion is likely in the absence of cranial nerve III (CN III), the oculomotor nerve. This patient will have an impaired or absent pupillary light reflex (PLR).

- A lesion in the pons and/or medulla is likely if one or more of the following cranial nerves are impaired:
  - Cranial nerve V (CN V), the trigeminal nerve
  - Cranial nerve VI (CN VI), the abducens nerve
  - Cranial nerve VII (CN VII), the facial nerve
  - Cranial nerve VIII (CN VIII), the vestibulocochlear nerve
  - Cranial nerve IX (CN IX), the glossopharyngeal nerve
  - Cranial nerve X (CN X), the vagus nerve
  - Cranial nerve XI (CN XI), the accessory nerve
  - Cranial nerve XII (CN XII), the hypoglossal nerve
- A palpable fluid wave on abdominal palpation is suggestive of ascites. Ascites may result from internal trauma.
- Hemorrhage from any orifice may indicate internal bleeding, as from trauma, or underlying bleeding disorders.
  - Epistaxis refers to a nosebleed.
  - Hematemesis refers to blood in the vomit.
  - Hematochezia refers to fresh blood in the stool.
  - Hematuria refers to blood in the urine.
  - Hemoabdomen refers to blood in the abdominal cavity.
  - Hemothorax refers to blood in the chest cavity.
  - Hyphema refers to blood in the anterior chamber of the eye.
  - Melena refers to digested blood in dark, tarry stool.
- A large, dome-shaped head, with or without an open fontanelle, and with or without ventral or ventrolateral strabismus, is supportive of a diagnosis of hydrocephalus [29].
- A palpably firm, rock-hard, non-compliant, non-compressible, painful urinary bladder in a cat indicates UTO [9, 30].
- Petechial hemorrhages and/or ecchymoses are suggestive of bleeding disorders. Bleeding disorders may result in vascular compromise of any tissue, including the CNS.
- Retinal hemorrhage and/or detachment may be indicative of hypertensive retinopathy.

In addition to physical examination findings, clinicopathologic data assists with the prioritization of differentials [19]:

- Blood smear
  - The presence of basophilic stippling and/or nucleated erythrocytes raises the index of suspicion that the patient has lead toxicosis.
- Complete blood count (CBC)
  - The presence of anemia supports a diagnosis of hypoxemia.
  - An inflammatory leukogram is suggestive of underlying infectious disease.

- An Addisonian patient will lack a stress leukogram despite systemic illness.
- Biochemistry panel
  - Patients with diabetes mellitus have hyperglycemia.
  - Patients with hypoadrenocorticism typically have hyponatremia, hypochloremia, and hyperkalemia.
  - Patients with UTO typically have hyperkalemia.
- Urinalysis
  - Patients with diabetes mellitus have glycosuria.
  - Patients with ethylene glycol toxicosis typically have calcium oxalate crystals.
  - Patients with PSSs may have ammonium biurate crystals.

Arterial blood gases will confirm metabolic and/or respiratory blood gas disturbances, including acidosis and alkalosis. Arterial blood gases will also provide evidence of hypoxemia.

Additional laboratory tests, such as manual platelet counts, prothrombin time (PT), partial thromboplastin time (PTT), buccal mucosal bleeding time, fibrinogen, and fibrin degradation products (FDPs) can provide evidence of coagulopathy.

Imaging is yet another important diagnosis tool. Survey radiographs and/or ultrasonography of the thoracic and abdominal cavities may provide evidence of organ pathology or neoplastic disease. Radiographs of the skull may be useful in confirming fractures in trauma cases; however, computed tomography (CT) and magnetic resonance imaging (MRI) provide superior resolution when assessing the CNS.

Note that there is no "one-size-fits-all" approach to the diagnostic plan for the patient with altered mentation. Each patient that presents for abnormal mentation needs to be managed as an individual, and case management will be unique. However, any of the above modalities provides a solid foundation upon which to manage any patient with altered mentation.

The combined efforts of history taking, vital signs, physical examination, labwork, and diagnostic imaging will effectively narrow the scope of practice to those differentials that are most likely for the patient.

Some, but not all of the differentials for altered mentation, will be reviewed in greater detail below.

71.5 Hypoglycemia as a Cause of Abnormal Mentation

Hypoglycemia is characterized in companion animal patients by a blood glucose level below 50–60 mg/dl [31].

Hypoglycemia is a medical concern because the brain requires glucose as its exclusive energy source [32]. When the CNS is starved for glucose, CNS function is compromised [32]. Neurologic clinical signs are common and include the following [31, 33, 34]:

- Altered mentation
  - Depression
  - Obtundation
  - Stupor
- Apparent confusion
- Drowsiness
- Incoordination
- Lethargy
- Muscle fasciculations and/or tremors
  - Especially facial
- Seizures
- Weakness

Hypoglycemia results from decreased intake, decreased production, or excessive use of glucose [32].

71.5.1 Hypoglycemia in Neonates

Hypoglycemia is common in neonates, particularly toy and small-breed dogs, due to decreased intake, for example, if patients are fasted for longer than they can manage [31, 33, 34]. Neonates are also less proficient at gluconeogenesis, meaning that if they do not take in sufficient glucose in their diet, they may be unable to synthesize enough to meet their needs. Furthermore, they lack sufficient reserves in the form of muscle glycogen and body fat to maintain resting blood glucose levels within the normal range [31].

In addition to small size and body weight, neonatal hypoglycemia may be precipitated by the following physiologic stressors [31, 33, 34]:

- Anemia
- Diarrhea
  - Parvovirus
- Ectoparasitism
- Endoparasitism
  - Coccidiosis
- Pneumonia
- Sepsis
- Temperature extremes
  - Hypothermia

In addition to physiologic stressors, neonatal hypoglycemia may be precipitated by the following external stressors [31, 33, 34]:
- Improper milk replacer
  - Milk replacer that is not formulated for puppies or kittens
- Orphan litter
- Reduced milk production by the dam
- Refusal of the dam to tolerate nursing
- More neonates than teats for nursing

Hypoglycemia is possible in neonatal kittens, although it is less prevalent than in puppies [31, 33]. Persians are overrepresented among hypoglycemic kittens [31].

Refer to an emergency medicine or pediatric textbook to guide treatment of neonatal hypoglycemia.

Note that despite treatment, recurrence of hypoglycemia is possible [31, 33, 34]. Patients that do not respond to medical therapy may have some degree of underlying hepatic dysfunction [33].

71.5.2 Hypoglycemia in Adults

Unlike neonates, adults do have adequate muscle glycogen reserves and the ability to initiate gluconeogenesis when fasting. Therefore, when hypoglycemia occurs in the adult patient, it is usually due to underlying pathology. Although there are several etiologies, the following list is representative of the most common [32]:

- Decreased production of glucose (rare)
  - Hypoadrenocorticism [35]
- Excess of endogenous insulin or insulin-like factors
  - Neoplasia
    - ○ Insulinoma
  - Toxins
    - ○ Xylitol
- Overdose of exogenous insulin [15]
- Overuse of glucose
  - Extreme activity or overexertion
    - ○ Hunting dog
  - Paraneoplastic syndromes
  - Pregnancy
  - Sepsis

71.5.2.1 Insulinoma

An insulinoma is a pancreatic β-cell tumor that produces insulin [32]. Dogs are primarily affected, although rare reports of feline insulinoma appear in the veterinary literature [32, 36–39].

Patients with insulinomas are typically middle-aged to older, and are often large-breed dogs [32]. German Shepherds and Golden Retrievers are overrepresented [40].

Much like neonates with hypoglycemia, affected adults present for the following [15, 32, 41]:

- Depression
- Diarrhea
- Lethargy
- Seizures
- Tremors
- Vomiting
- Weakness

They may also present for collapse [32].

Despite persistent hypoglycemia, signs are frequently episodic [41]. Clinical signs appear to be worsened by one or more of the following [41]:

- Excitement
- Exercise
- Fasting

Diagnosis is confirmed by bloodwork: hypoglycemia in the presence of a normal-to-increased insulin concentration [32, 40].

Patient stabilization during a hypoglycemic crisis is prioritized over identification of the insulinoma [32]. Caution must be taken in patients in whom an insulinoma is suspected because dextrose boluses may cause the tumor to secrete more insulin [32]. This will result in rebound hypoglycemia [32]. Refer to an emergency medicine textbook for tips regarding case management.

Once the patient has been stabilized, surgical excision of the insulinoma will result in the longest survival time [32]. However, surgery is considered palliative rather than curative because metastasis to the regional lymph nodes, liver, duodenum, mesentery, and omentum is common in affected patients [32, 36, 40]. At the time of surgical excision, more than 50% of patients have gross evidence of metastasis [32]. The percentage of cases with microscopic metastasis is thought to be appreciably higher [32].

71.5.2.2 Xylitol

Xylitol is an increasingly popular artificial sweetener that is used in lieu of sugar in human products, such as gum [42, 43]. To match the need for low-glycemic index foods and low-carbohydrate diets, xylitol has been incorporated into many other foods, including candy and baked goods [42, 43]. Xylitol may be found in any number of supplements, including nutritional and diet bars, multivitamins, gummy vitamins, and calcium chews [42, 43]. Because xylitol is protective to dental surfaces, it is also often added to toothpaste and oral rinses [42–44].

Oral xylitol is relatively safe for human consumption: excessive ingestion in humans may cause diarrhea at most [42].

However, when xylitol is ingested by dogs, insulin is released as if the patient had consumed glucose [42, 45, 46]. The resultant hypoglycemia can be severe [38, 42, 46].

Affected patients present with the following [42, 43, 47, 48]:

- Ataxia
- Collapse
- Lethargy
- Pronounced weakness
- Seizure activity
- Vomiting

Patients can be successfully stabilized through their hypoglycemic crisis [42]. However, xylitol ingestion by dogs may also result in fulminant liver failure through mechanisms yet to be established [42–44, 48, 49].

71.6 Hydrocephalus as a Cause of Abnormal Mentation

Hydrocephalus occurs when the ventricular system of the brain becomes distended [29].

In health, cerebrospinal fluid (CSF) is produced by the choroid plexuses, which line the lateral, third, and fourth ventricles [29]. CSF circulates through the ventricles, and is absorbed in the subarachnoid space [29].

Production matches absorption in the normal patient so that there is no buildup of fluid within the ventricular system [29].

When flow is obstructed, hydrocephalus develops [29]. The body may try to compensate for the obstruction by creating alternate routes for CSF flow [29]. However, this takes time [29]. If the obstruction is acute, then the body does not have the opportunity to develop pathways before ICP rises to dangerous levels [29].

Hydrocephalus may be congenital or acquired [29].

Congenital hydrocephalus is most often due to a stenotic mesencephalic aqueduct [29]. This occurs more often in toy and small-breed dogs [29]. In particular, the following breeds are overrepresented [29, 50]:

- Boston Terrier
- Cairn Terrier
- Chihuahua
- English Bulldog
- Lhasa Apso
- Maltese
- Pekingese
- Pomeranian
- Pug
- Yorkshire Terrier

Cats may be affected, too. Affected patients present at several months old, with an appreciably enlarged, dome-shaped head [15, 29]. This is particularly noticeable on the profile view (see Figures 71.5a–d).

Affected patients often also have a persistent open fontanelle [29]. Recall from basic anatomy that the fontanelle is a normal prenatal gap between the frontal and parietal bones [51, 52]. In health, this gap closes before birth or shortly thereafter [51–53]. Failure of the fontanelle to close before birth is a common occurrence in toy breeds of dogs [9].

When dogs present with a persistent gap, the fontanelle is said to be open [9]. Puppies with open fontanelles may be at increased risk of sustaining cerebral trauma [9].

Puppies with open fontanelles also have a higher risk of concurrent congenital hydrocephalus [54]. It is estimated that one-third of dogs with open fontanelles have ventriculomegaly with concurrent neurological signs, and one-third of dogs with open fontanelles have ventriculomegaly without concurrent neurological signs [55, 56].

Ventriculomegaly can be diagnosed via ultrasound of the brain that is performed through the open fontanelle [29, 57–60]. Compared to the paired slit-like anechoic ventricles of a normal puppy, enlarged ventricles are wider and may actually appear to converge [29].

Patients with hydrocephalus, with or without an open fontanelle, may present for episodes of neurological dysfunction [29]. Common clinical signs that are reported include the following [15, 29]:

- Abnormal mentation
- Ataxia
- Blindness
- Circling
- Incoordination
- Seizures

Affected patients also often develop divergent strabismus, or exotropia, as hydrocephalus progresses [29].

Hydrocephalus may also be acquired [29]. Hydrocephalus is acquired when the ventricular system is obstructed by either a mass or inflammatory tissue, as from meningitis or FIP [29, 61–67].

CT and MRI are valuable diagnostic tools for both assessing the ventricular system and identifying space-occupying lesions [29].

71.7 PSS as a Cause of Abnormal Mentation

PSSs were introduced in Chapter 28, Section 28.2.2 as they related to hepatic icterus. PSSs were revisited in Part Six of the text ("Digestive Tract") in Chapter 48, Section 48.3, Chapter 51, Section 51.3, and Chapter 54, Section 54.6 concerning their role in abnormal ingestive behaviors, small bowel diarrhea, and acute vomiting.

A PSS is a condition in which blood bypasses the liver to enter into systemic circulation [68]. Consider how this affects the role that the liver plays in detoxification of the blood. In health, the liver is a functional participant in metabolism. Specifically, the liver functions to receive blood from the intestines, spleen, and pancreas via the portal vein. This incoming blood is detoxified by the liver before it circulates through the rest of the body.

When blood is shunted directly into systemic circulation, toxins have the opportunity to spread throughout the body before they are disarmed. This results in episodic HE. HE is characterized by abnormal mentation

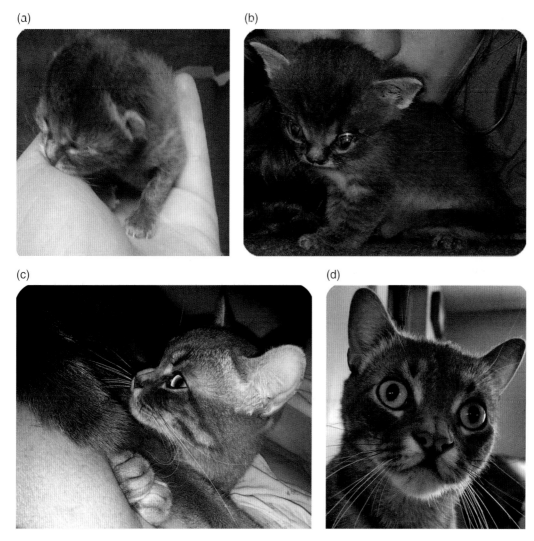

Figure 71.5 (a) Feline neonate with congenital hydrocephalus. Note the dome-shaped head. *Source:* Courtesy of Viola Folsum. (b) Same patient as depicted in Figure 71.5a. This patient has hydrocephalus. Note the prominent ventrolateral strabismus. Courtesy of Viola Folsum. (c) Same patient as depicted in Figures 71.5a, b. Note that the dome-shaped head is still prominent as the patient ages. *Source:* Courtesy of Viola Folsum. (d) Same patient as depicted in Figures 71.5a–c, as an adult. *Source:* Courtesy of Viola Folsum.

[69]. These bouts occur when the cerebral cortex is exposed to toxins from which it ought to have been shielded [69]. Among these toxins, the cerebral cortex is most sensitive to the following [69]:

- Ammonia
- Aromatic amino acids
- Indoles
- Mercaptan
- Short-chain fatty acids

Of those listed above, ammonia is most often implicated in cases of HE [69]. Elevated blood levels of ammonia result in increased delivery of ammonia to the brain [69]. The brain is particularly sensitive to ammonia, but cannot convert it to urea [69]. Instead, neural tissue attempts conversion of ammonia to glutamine [69, 70]. However, this reaction is limited [70].

The brain is easily overwhelmed by the concentrations of ammonia, particularly after a high-protein meal, and succumbs to HE [69, 70].

There is not a single type of PSS that causes HE [19]. PSSs may be extrahepatic or intrahepatic, congenital or acquired [19]. Cats and toy or small-breed dogs tend to develop single extrahepatic shunts, whereas large-breed dogs are more likely to develop single intrahepatic shunts [19].

The majority of PSSs are congenital and primarily affect toy and small-breeds [19]. The following breeds of dog are overrepresented [19]:

- Cairn Terrier
- Maltese
- Miniature Schnauzer
- Yorkshire Terrier

Patients with congenital PSSs may present for the following [19]:

- Altered appetite
- Diarrhea
- Failure to thrive
- Pica
- Stunted growth
- Vomiting

In addition, they frequently demonstrate one or more of the following CNS signs [19]:

- Abnormal behavior
  - Aggression (cats)
- Abnormal mentation
- Ataxia
- Blindness
- Disorientation
- Head pressing
- Incoordination
- Ptyalism (particularly in cats)
- Seizure activity

Clinical signs most often become evident during weaning [19]. After weaning, clinical signs are episodic and accentuated after eating.

Affected patients may also develop urinary tract signs, including, but not limited to the following [19]:

- Crystalluria
  - Ammonium biurate
- Hematuria
- Polydipsia
- Polyuria
- Stranguria

Although PSSs are most often congenital, they can also be acquired [19]. Acquired PSSs most often form in response to portal hypertension [19]. They are the body's attempt to compensate for elevated blood pressure to slow impending liver failure.

Clinical signs that are associated with acquired PSSs mirror those seen in the congenital form [19].

Diagnosis is beyond the scope of this text, but the following clinicopathologic abnormalities are consistent with PSSs:

- CBC
  - Microcytosis
  - Mild nonregenerative anemia
  - Poikilocytosis (cats)
  - Target cells (dogs)
- Biochemistry profile
  - Low blood urea nitrogen (BUN)
  - Low-to-normal creatinine, blood glucose, and cholesterol
  - Variable liver enzyme activity
- Urinalysis

- Crystalluria
  - Ammonium biurate
- Dilute urine

Microhepatica is commonly identified via survey radiography or abdominal ultrasonography of affected dogs [19]. Color-flow Doppler may facilitate identification of PSS [19].

Surgical management of PSS may be indicated; however, patient stabilization with medical management of HE receives priority [19]. Patients are managed via a combination of dietary and pharmacologic therapy, including the following:

- Antibiotic use to alter intestinal flora
- Anticonvulsants as needed
- Lactulose administration
  - Increases stool transit time
  - Traps nitrogen in bacteria
  - Reduces the production of ammonia
  - Reduces the absorption of ammonia
- Protein-restricted diet

71.8 Lead Toxicosis as a Cause of Abnormal Mentation

Lead toxicosis is rare, but underrecognized [71].

Paint and paint dust that results from household renovations are the most common sources of exposure for pets and children alike [71, 72].

The older the house, the higher the risk of lead-containing components [71]. Eighty-seven percent of homes that were built before 1940 are estimated to contain lead paint as compared to 24% of those built between 1960 and 1977 [71].

Lead may also be found in a number of other household items, including pipes, solder, putty, caulk, curtain weights, and ceramic glazes [71].

Outside of the home, lead exposure can occur through ingestion of bone meal supplements, fishing weights, and automobile batteries [71].

Lead enters systemic circulation after ingestion. It is stored in the bone and will leach out into the bloodstream over months to years. Lead may also accumulate in hepatic and renal tissue.

Lead toxicosis in companion animal patients tends to impact the gastrointestinal system, the nervous system, or both [72].

Gastrointestinal signs are nonspecific; however, the following are supportive of lead toxicosis [15, 72, 73]:

- Acute abdomen
- Anorexia
- Constipation or diarrhea
- Vomiting
- Weight loss

Nervous signs are nonspecific; however, the following are supportive of lead toxicosis [15, 72, 73]:

- Ataxia
- Blindness
- Convulsions
- Depression
- Mydriasis
- Seizure-like activity

Because lead interferes with enzymes that are involved in heme synthesis, erythropoiesis is altered in cases of lead toxicosis [19]. Although hematologic changes are not pathognomonic for lead poisoning, they facilitate a diagnosis:

- Anisocytosis
- Basophilic stippling
- Nucleated erythrocytes
- Poikilocytosis
- Polychromasia
- Reticulocytosis

Anemia may or may not be present [19].

Elevations in blood lead levels are diagnostic for lead toxicosis [71].

Consult an emergency medicine or toxicology reference for guidelines as to how to most effectively manage this toxicity.

71.9 Other Causes of Abnormal Mentation

Other causes of abnormal mentation have already been reviewed in other chapters of this text. Consider the following and take the opportunity to review as time or interest allows:

- Acute kidney injury (AKI): Refer to Chapter 63, Section 63.4.1
  - Ethylene glycol
  - Grapes and raisins
  - Lily toxicosis
- Canine hypothyroidism: Refer to Chapter 5, Section 5.7
- Cuterebriasis: Refer to Chapter 6, Section 6.3
- Diabetes mellitus: Refer to Chapter 64, Section 64.3.2
- Feline UTO: Refer to Chapter 65, Section 65.5
- Hypertension
  - Feline primary hyperaldosteronism: Refer to Chapter 67, Section 67.7
  - Hypertensive retinopathy: Refer to Chapter 15, Section 15.4.2.2
- Feline hyperthyroidism: Refer to Chapter 64, Section 64.3.5
- Thiamine deficiency: Refer to Chapter 67, Section 67.6

References

1 Schatzberg, S.J. and Haley, A.C. (2017). Neurologic examination and neuroanatomic diagnosis. In: *Veterinary Surgery: Small Animal Expert Consult* (ed. S.A. Johnston and K.M. Tobias), 347–348. St. Louis: Saunders.

2 Knipe, M.F. (2015). Deteriorating mental status. In: *Small Animal Critical Care Medicine* (ed. D.C. Silverstein and K. Hopper), 419–421. St. Louis, MO: Saunders/Elsevier.

3 MacKay, R.J. (2011). The neurologic examination: the forebrain. DVM 360 [Internet]. http://veterinarycalendar.dvm360.com/neurologic-examination-forebrain-proceedings.

4 Beitz, A.J. and Fletcher, T.F. (1993). The brain. In: *Miller's Anatomy of the Dog*, 3e (ed. H.E. Evans and M.E. Miller), 894–952. Philadelphia: W.B. Saunders.

5 de Lahunta, A., Glass, E.N., and Kent, M. (2015). *Veterinary Neuroanatomy and Clinical Neurology*. St. Louis: Saunders.

6 van Nes, J.J., Meij, B.P., and van Ham, L. (2009). Nervous system. In: *Medical History and Physical Examination in Companion Animals*, 2e (ed. A. Rijnberk and F.J. van Sluijs), 160–174. St. Louis: Saunders Elsevier.

7 Thomas, W.B. (2000). Initial assessment of patients with neurologic dysfunction. *Vet. Clin. North Am. Small Anim. Pract.* 30 (1): 1–24, v.

8 Garosi, L. (2009). Neurological examination of the cat. How to get started. *J. Feline Med. Surg.* 11 (5): 340–348.

9 Englar, R.E. (2017). *Performing the Small Animal Physical Examination*. Hoboken, NJ: Wiley.

10 Thomas, W.B. and Dewey, C.W. (2008). Performing the neurologic examination. In: *A Practical Guide to Canine and Feline Neurology*, 2e (ed. C.W. Dewey), 53–74. Ames, Iowa: Wiley-Blackwell.

11 Defarges, A. (2015). The physical examination. *NAVC Clinician's Brief* (September): 73–80.

12 Nye, C. and Troxel, M. (2017). The neurologic examination. *NAVC Clinician's Brief* (August): 61–69.

13 Platt, S.R. (2015). Coma scales. In: *Small Animal Critical Care Medicine* (ed. D.C. Silverstein and K. Hopper), 422–425. St. Louis, MO: Saunders/Elsevier.

14 Averill, D.R. Jr. (1981). The neurologic examination. *Vet. Clin. North Am. Small Anim. Pract.* 11 (3): 511–521.

15 Bagley, R.S. (2006). The cat with stupor or coma. In: *Problem-Based Feline Medicine* (ed. J. Rand), 821–834. Edinburgh; New York: Saunders.

16 Van Lanen, K. and Sande, A. (2014). Canine hypoadrenocorticism: pathogenesis, diagnosis, and treatment. *Top. Companion Anim. Med.* 29 (4): 88–95.

17 O'Neill, J., Kent, M., Glass, E.N., and Platt, S.R. (2013). Clinicopathologic and MRI characteristics of presumptive hypertensive encephalopathy in two cats and two dogs. *J. Am. Anim. Hosp. Assoc.* 49 (6): 412–420.

18 Davis, H., Jensen, T., Johnson, A. et al. (2013). AAHA/AAFP fluid therapy guidelines for dogs and cats. *J. Am. Anim. Hosp. Assoc.* 49 (3): 149–159.

19 Tilley, L.P. and Smith, F.W.K. (2004). *The 5-Minute Veterinary Consult: Canine and Feline*, 3e. Baltimore, MD: Lippincott Williams & Wilkins.

20 Cooper, E. (2017). Urethral deobstruction in cats. *Veterinary Team Brief* (April): 55–62.

21 Kraus, M.S. (ed.) (2003). *Syncope in Small Breed Dogs*. ACVIM.

22 Thawley, V. and Collapse, S.D. (2012). *NAVC Clinician's Brief* (November): 14–15.

23 Estrada, A. (2017). Differentiating syncope from seizure. *NAVC Clinician's Brief* (July): 50–55.

24 Barnett, L., Martin, M.W., Todd, J. et al. (2011). A retrospective study of 153 cases of undiagnosed collapse, syncope or exercise intolerance: the outcomes. *J. Small Anim. Pract.* 52 (1): 26–31.

25 Gurfinkel, V., Cacciatore, T.W., Cordo, P. et al. (2006). Postural muscle tone in the body axis of healthy humans. *J. Neurophysiol.* 96 (5): 2678–2687.

26 Schwartz, D.S. (ed.) (2009). The syncopal dog. World Small Animal Veterinary Association World Congress Proceedings; Sao Paulo, Brazil.

27 Dutton, E., Dukes-McEwan, J., and Cripps, P.J. (2017). Serum cardiac troponin I in canine syncope and seizures. *J. Vet. Cardiol.* 19 (1): 1–13.

28 Galan, A., Gamito, A., Carletti, B.E. et al. (2014). Uncommon acute neurologic presentation of canine distemper in 4 adult dogs. *Can. Vet. J.* 55 (4): 373–378.

29 Thomas, W.B. (2010). Hydrocephalus in dogs and cats. *Vet. Clin. North Am. Small Anim. Pract.* 40 (1): 143–159.

30 George, C.M. and Grauer, G.F. (2016). Feline urethral obstruction: diagnosis and management. *Today's Veterinary Practice* (July/August): 36–46.

31 Parker, N. (2006). Treating neonatal and pediatric hypoglycemia. Banfield Pet Hospital [Internet]. May/June:[34–42 pp.]. https://www.banfield.com/getmedia/b4c313cc-bf61-49b3-9abc-a131def714e3/2_3-Treating-neonatal-and-pediatric-hypoglycemia.

32 Koenig, A. (2013). Endocrine emergencies in dogs and cats. *Vet. Clin. North Am. Small Anim. Pract.* 43 (4): 869–897.

33 Lewis, H.B. (2006). Hypoglycemia in puppies and kittens. Banfield Pet Hospital [Internet]. May/June: [18–23 pp.]. https://www.banfield.com/getmedia/044861d1-eed8-4e21-9c3c-537a13e6a9bf/2_3-Hypoglycemia-in-puppies-and-kittens.

34 Vroom, M.W. and Slappendel, R.J. (1987). Transient juvenile hypoglycaemia in a Yorkshire terrier and in a Chihuahua. *Vet. Q.* 9 (2): 172–176.

35 Owens, S.L. and Scott-Moncrieff, J.C. (2010). Atypical presentation of hypoglycemia in a dog. *NAVC Clinician's Brief* (June): 22–26.

36 Caywood, D.D., Klausner, J.S., Oleary, T.P. et al. (1988). Pancreatic insulin-secreting neoplasms – clinical, diagnostic, and prognostic features in 73 dogs. *J. Am. Anim. Hosp. Assoc.* 24 (5): 577–584.

37 Dunn, J.K., Bostock, D.E., Herrtage, M.E. et al. (1993). Insulin-secreting tumors of the canine pancreas – clinical and pathological features of 11 cases. *J. Small Anim. Pract.* 34 (7): 325–331.

38 Kruth, S.A., Feldman, E.C., and Kennedy, P.C. (1982). Insulin-secreting islet cell tumors – establishing a diagnosis and the clinical course for 25 dogs. *J. Am. Vet. Med. Assoc.* 181 (1): 54–58.

39 Leifer, C.E., Peterson, M.E., and Matus, R.E. (1986). Insulin-secreting tumor – diagnosis and medical and surgical-management in 55 dogs. *J. Am. Vet. Med. Assoc.* 188 (1): 60–64.

40 Fernandez, N.J., Barton, J., and Spotswood, T. (2009). Hypoglycemia in a dog. *Can. Vet. J.* 50 (4): 423–426.

41 Flory, A.B. (2008). Episodes of weakness and hypoglycemia in a dog. *NAVC Clinician's Brief* (December): 21–22.

42 Murphy, L.A. and Coleman, A.E. (2012). Xylitol toxicosis in dogs. *Vet. Clin. North Am. Small Anim. Pract.* 42 (2): 307–312, vii.

43 Peterson, M.E. (2013). Xylitol. *Top. Companion Anim. Med.* 28 (1): 18–20.

44 Todd, J.A. and Powell, L.L. (2007). Xylitol intoxication associated with fulminant hepatic failure in a dog. *J. Vet. Emerg. Crit. Care* 17 (3): 286–289.

45 Hirata, Y., Fujisawa, M., Sato, H. et al. (1966). Blood glucose and plasma insulin responses to xylitol administrated intravenously in dogs. *Biochem. Biophys. Res. Commun.* 24 (3): 471–475.

46 Kuzuya, T., Kanazawa, Y., and Kosaka, K. (1966). Plasma insulin response to intravenously administered xylitol in dogs. *Metabolism* 15 (12): 1149–1152.

47 Dunayer, E.K. (2004). Hypoglycemia following canine ingestion of xylitol-containing gum. *Vet. Hum. Toxicol.* 46 (2): 87–88.

48 Dunayer, E.K. (2006). New findings on the effects of xylitol ingestion in dogs. Veterinary Medicine [Internet]. (December):[791–7pp.]. https://www.aspcapro.org/sites/pro/files/xylitol.pdf.

49 Dunayer, E.K. and Gwaltney-Brant, S.M. (2006). Acute hepatic failure and coagulopathy associated with xylitol

ingestion in eight dogs. *J. Am. Vet. Med. Assoc.* 229 (7): 1113–1117.

50 Selby, L.A., Hayes, H.M. Jr., and Becker, S.V. (1979). Epizootiologic features of canine hydrocephalus. *Am. J. Vet. Res.* 40 (3): 411–413.

51 Dyce, K.M., Sack, W.O., and Wensing, C.J.G. (1996). Some basic facts and concepts. In: *Textbook of Veterinary Anatomy*, 2e (ed. K.M. Dyce, W.O. Sack and C.J.G. Wensing). Philadelphia: Saunders.

52 Evans, H.E. (1993). Prenatal development. In: *Miller's Anatomy of the Dog*, 3e (ed. H.E. Evans). Philadelphia: W.B. Saunders.

53 Stades, F.C. and Stokhof, A.A. (2009). Health certification. In: *Medical History and Physical Examination in Companion Animals* (ed. A. Rijnberk and F.J. van Sluijs), 245–246. St. Louis: Saunders Elsevier.

54 Przyborowska, P., Adamiak, Z., Jaskolska, M., and Zhalniarovich, Y. (2013). Hydrocephalus in dogs: a review. *Vet. Med. Czech.* 58 (2): 73–80.

55 Root Kustriz, M.V. (2011). History and physical examination of the weanling and adolescent. In: *Small Animal Pediatrics: The First 12 Months of Life* (ed. M.E. Peterson and M.A. Kutzler), 28–33. St. Louis, MO: Saunders/Elsevier.

56 Root Kustriz, M.V. (2011). History and physical examination of the neonate. In: *Small Animal Pediatrics: The First 12 Months of Life* (ed. M.E. Peterson and M.A. Kutzler), 20–27. St. Louis, MO: Saunders/Elsevier.

57 Brown, J.A., Rachlin, J., Rubin, J.M., and Wollmann, R.L. (1984). Ultrasound evaluation of experimental hydrocephalus in dogs. *Surg. Neurol.* 22 (3): 273–276.

58 Esteve-Ratsch, B., Kneissl, S., and Gabler, C. (2001). Comparative evaluation of the ventricles in the Yorkshire terrier and the German shepherd dog using low-field MRI. *Vet. Radiol. Ultrasound* 42 (5): 410–413.

59 Adamiak, Z., Jaskolska, M., and Pomianowski, A. (2012). Low-field magnetic resonance imaging of canine hydrocephalus. *Pak. Vet. J.* 32 (1): 128–130.

60 Partington, B.P. (1995). Physical examination and diagnostic imaging procedures: diagnostic imaging techniques. In: *Veterinary Pediatrics: Dogs and Cats from Birth to Six Months*, 2e (ed. J.D. Hoskins), 7–21. Philadelphia: W.B. Saunders.

61 Vural, S.A., Besalti, O., Ilhan, F. et al. (2006). Ventricular ependymoma in a German shepherd dog. *Vet. J.* 172 (1): 185–187.

62 Zabka, T.S., Lavely, J.A., and Higgins, R.J. (2004). Primary intra-axial leiomyosarcoma with obstructive hydrocephalus in a young dog. *J. Comp. Pathol.* 131 (4): 334–337.

63 Steinberg, H. and Galbreath, E.J. (1998). Cerebellar medulloblastoma with multiple differentiation in a dog. *Vet. Pathol.* 35 (6): 543–546.

64 Pumarola, M. and Vanniel, M.H.F. (1992). Obstructive hydrocephalus produced by parasitic granulomas in a dog. *J. Vet. Med. A* 39 (5): 392–395.

65 Graham, J.C., Okeefe, D.A., Wallig, M.A., and Oluoch, A.O. (1992). Lymphosarcoma causing acquired obstructive hydrocephalus in a dog. *Can. Vet. J.* 33 (10): 669–670.

66 Foley, J.E., Lapointe, J.M., Koblik, P. et al. (1998). Diagnostic features of clinical neurologic feline infectious peritonitis. *J. Vet. Intern. Med.* 12 (6): 415–423.

67 Dewey, C.W. (2002). External hydrocephalus in a dog with suspected bacterial meningoencephalitis. *J. Am. Anim. Hosp. Assoc.* 38 (6): 563–567.

68 Connolly, S.L. (2016). Canine portosystemic shunts: single or multiple tests to make the correct diagnosis? *Vet. J.* 207: 6–7.

69 Nelson, R.W. and Couto, C.G. (2014). *Small Animal Internal Medicine*, 5e. St. Louis, MO: Elsevier/Mosby.

70 Dimski, D.S. (1994). Ammonia metabolism and the urea cycle – function and clinical implications. *J. Vet. Intern. Med.* 8 (2): 73–78.

71 Cima, G. (2017). Lead contamination affects people and probably pets. J. Am. Vet. Med. Assoc. [Internet]. https://www.avma.org/News/JAVMANews/Pages/171015a.aspx.

72 Kowalczyk, D.F. (1976). Lead poisoning in dogs at the University of Pennsylvania veterinary hospital. *J. Am. Vet. Med. Assoc.* 168 (5): 428–432.

73 Mitema, E.S., Oehme, F.W., Penumarthy, L., and Moore, W.E. (1980). Effect of chronic lead exposure on the canine bone marrow. *Am. J. Vet. Res.* 41 (5): 682–685.

72

Head Tilt, Circling, and Other Manifestations of Vestibular Disease

72.1 Introduction to a Deviated Posture: The Head Tilt

Posture was introduced in Chapter 67, Section 67.1 as the way in which the body holds itself in space [1]. Posture describes the positioning of the head, trunk, and tail relative to the weight distribution between the limbs [1, 2].

Recall that a normal, upright posture requires skeletal stability, muscle tone, and muscular innervation to coordinate contractions that counteract gravity [3]. Flexors and extensors, for example, often have opposing tone [4].

Posture is age-dependent.

Consider that an upright position is not possible at birth for kittens or puppies. Neonates are able to raise their heads within hours of parturition; however, they do not have sufficient muscular tone to raise their entire chest and body (see Figures 72.1a–c).

Flexor tone predominates for the first few days of life, creating the classic comma shape that is characteristic of newborns. This allows kittens in particular to be flaccid and portable by the queen, by their scruff [5, 6].

Extensor dominance eventually overtakes flexor tone until eventually the patient is able to coordinate opposing muscular actions simultaneously [7].

By one month of age, the posture of the pediatric patient mirrors that of an adult [8]. The patient is able to sit and stand, keeping head and neck held upright [8]. The left and right sides, when viewed from the front and back, are symmetrical, and the trunk should be held evenly without a lateral tilt [1, 8, 9] (see Figures 72.2a, b).

Abnormal carriage of the head, neck, or trunk may be due to skeletal, muscular, and/or neurological dysfunction [3, 10]. As with all other areas of the physical examination, observational skills are enormously valuable. Deviations from normal posture may be present, but subtle. It is the responsibility of the veterinarian to consider posture in every patient, during every clinical evaluation [8, 11–14].

A head tilt is a specific deviation in posture that may be observed during patient assessment [8, 12–14].

A head tilt is typically defined as a rotation through the median plane of the head [15]. When the head tilts to the left, the chin swings to the right, and the left ear drops lower than the right [15]. When the head tilts to the right, the chin swings to the left, and the right ear drops lower than the left [15]. A head tilt may be subtle or overt, under conscious or unconscious control (see Figures 72.3a–c).

Sometimes a head tilt is referred to as wry neck or torticollis [8]. This is particularly true of those situations in which the neck is twisted, rather than simply deviated [9] (see Figure 72.4).

72.2 Causes of Acute Onset of Head Tilt

An abnormality in head and neck carriage, such as a head tilt, may result from underlying musculoskeletal disease [8]. For instance, abnormal shaping of the vertebral column can lead to scoliosis, a sideways deviation of the spine [1, 8]. This will lead to a persistent change in head and neck position.

For the purposes of this chapter, the author will exclusively consider those patients in which there is an acute head tilt. Acute onset is less likely to be due to developmental musculoskeletal pathology. It is more likely the result of neurological insult or ear canal disease [8].

The following are common differentials for acute onset of head tilt:

- Cerebrovascular accident or stroke [16–18]
- Inflammatory middle or inner ear disease [19, 20] ***
- Neurological insult or traumatic injury [21]
- Vestibular disease [15, 22–25] ***

Those items that are starred above will be the emphasis of this chapter.

Common Clinical Presentations in Dogs and Cats, First Edition. Ryane E. Englar.
© 2019 John Wiley & Sons, Inc. Published 2019 by John Wiley & Sons, Inc.

(a) (b) (c)

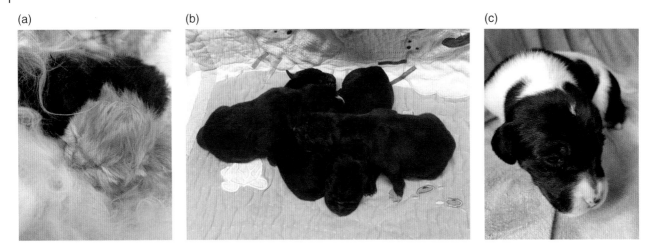

Figure 72.1 (a) Newborn kittens. Note that they are able to raise their heads for nursing, but they lack sufficient tone to lift their entire bodies. *Source:* Courtesy of Aimee Wong. (b). Two-day-old puppies. Note that they, too, are able to raise their heads and rest them upon each other's backs, but they lack sufficient tone to lift their entire bodies. *Source:* Courtesy of Genevieve LaFerriere, DVM. (c) Two-week-old puppy. Note that its ability to lift its head is getting stronger. *Source:* Courtesy of Tara Beugel.

(a) (b)

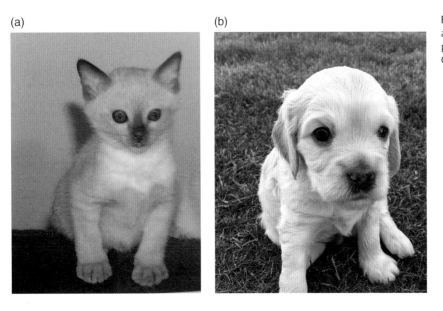

Figure 72.2 (a) Age-appropriate posture in a six-week-old kitten. (b). Age-appropriate posture in a two-month-old puppy. *Source:* Courtesy of Nechama Bloom, DVM.

(a) (b) (c)

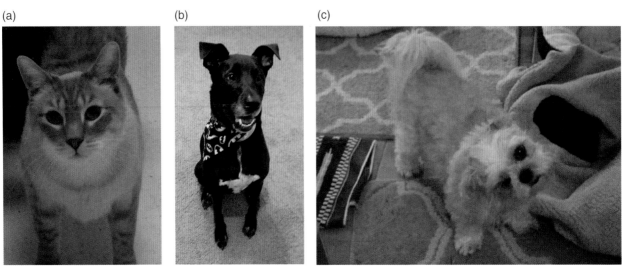

Figure 72.3 (a) Subtle right-sided head tilt in a cat. (b) Subtle left-sided head tilt in a dog. *Source:* Courtesy of Alyssa Show. (c) Overt right-sided head tilt in a dog. *Source:* Courtesy of Mickey Stolarz.

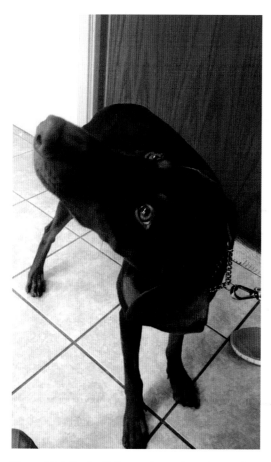

Figure 72.4 Torticollis in a canine patient. *Source:* Courtesy of Tyler Middleton.

72.3 Other Manifestations of Neurological Disease

Note that a head tilt rarely occurs in isolation. Often, it is concurrent with other neurological manifestations of disease, including, but not limited to the following [8, 15, 26]

- Ataxia
- Circling
- Facial nerve paresis or paralysis
- Falling or leaning to one side
- Horner syndrome
- Nystagmus
- Positional strabismus
- Rolling

72.3.1 Ataxia

Ataxia was introduced in Chapter 68, Section 68.9 and Chapter 69, Section 69.14 as an incoordination of gait that is not due to weakness [9, 14].

There are three main categories of ataxia [9, 27, 28].

72.3.2 Cerebellar Ataxia

Cerebellar ataxia is caused by one or more diseases involving the cerebellum.

Because the cerebellum is responsible for gait generation, this type of ataxia is characterized by an abnormal rate, range, or force of movement [28]. The "toy soldier" gait is the classic description for cerebellar ataxia. The affected patient has a stiff, stilted, high-stepping, over-reaching gait, and each step demonstrates exaggerated flexion [28, 29].

72.3.3 Vestibular Ataxia

Vestibular ataxia is caused by one or more disturbances of the vestibular system.

The vestibular system was introduced in Chapter 23, Section 23.4.4 and Chapter 54, Section 54.1. Recall that this system maintains a sense of balance by listening to, coordinating, and responding to various proprioceptive inputs so that the body is in control of its position in space [23, 25, 30–33].

The vestibular system has both central and peripheral components that oversee body posture, head posture, eye position, eye movement, and gait [23, 30, 33].

Vestibular ataxia reflects a true lack of balance [28]. This may be due to peripheral vestibular disease, as in medical conditions that involve the tympanic bulla, or central vestibular disease as occurs when lesions arise at the cerebellopontine angle [34].

When there is unilateral vestibular disease, the patient will lean, drift, or fall toward one side. This may be overt or subtle. The patient may simply lean against the exam room wall to hold himself up. A head tilt may or may not be present [9, 34].

When vestibular disease is bilateral, the patient tends to be reluctant to move and classically presents with exaggerated side-to-side swaying of the head and neck [9, 34].

72.3.4 Proprioceptive or Sensory Ataxia

Proprioceptive or sensory ataxia results from one or more lesions in the peripheral nerve, dorsal root, spinal cord, or brainstem.

Affected patients lose perspective of where their limbs are positioned in space [28]. They often exhibit "knuckling," meaning that they scuff or even stand upon the dorsal aspect of one or more feet (see Figure 72.5).

Knuckling is considered a deficit in conscious proprioception (CP).

Because of CP deficits, they appear clumsy and uncoordinated. Clients may complain that their pet acts drunk.

Affected patients may have concurrent paresis because motor pathways often overlap with proprioceptive ones [9, 34].

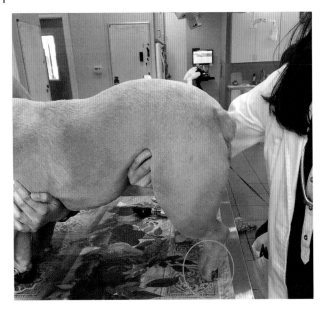

Figure 72.5 This patient is demonstrating abnormal knuckling of the left pelvic limb. *Source:* Courtesy of Shirley Yang, DVM.

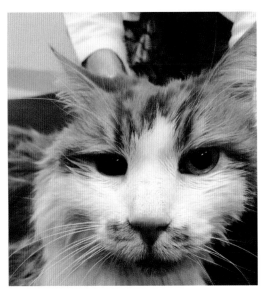

Figure 72.6 This feline patient has ptosis, that is, a droopy right upper eyelid. Note the narrowed right palpebral fissure as compared to the left. This patient was subsequently diagnosed with cryptococcosis. *Source:* Courtesy of Andrew Weisenfeld, DVM.

72.3.5 Circling

Circling is a clinical sign that describes exactly that: the patient appears to walk in circles, repetitively. It is what might occur if a dog were to chase its tail, except that circling is initiated without the tail as a target. Circling is typically to one side. Sometimes, circling is called spinning.

Circling often occurs in combination with a head tilt, as a component of vestibular dysfunction.

The diameter of the circle may facilitate diagnosis [35]. In general, vestibular disease results in tight circles, whereas patients that circle widely are more likely to have a forebrain lesion [35].

72.3.6 Facial Nerve Paresis or Paralysis

The facial nerve (CN VII) is the seventh of 12 cranial nerves [8]. It arises from the medulla oblongata and, along with the eighth cranial nerve, the vestibulocochlear nerve (CN VIII), passes through the internal acoustic meatus [36]. Ultimately, it enters the temporal bone, adjacent to the tympanic bulla [36].

At the level of the stylomastoid foramen, CN VII exits the skull to innervate the following structures [15, 36–38]:

- Eyelids
- Lacrimal gland
- Lip folds
- Muscles of facial expression
- Pinnae
- Rostral tongue
- Salivary glands

- Superficial muscles of the external ear
- Taste buds

Dysfunction of CN VII may result from the following [15, 20, 36, 39–50]:

- Otitis media
- Hypothyroidism
- Trauma

More often than not, CN VII dysfunction is idiopathic [36, 43, 51].

When CN VII is dysfunctional, patients may demonstrate one or more of the following signs [8, 27, 36]:

- Difficulty blinking
  - Decreased to absent menace response on the affected side
  - Decreased to absent palpebral reflex on the affected side
- Ear droop
- Keratoconjunctivitis sicca (KCS), or dry eye
- Lip droop
- Nasal philtrum deviation toward the normal side
- Ptosis, droopiness of the upper eyelid
- Ptyalism, associated with the affected side (see Figure 72.6)

72.3.7 Horner Syndrome

Horner syndrome, otherwise known as Horner's syndrome, was introduced in Chapter 18, Section 18.3.2.4 as a condition that is characterized by sympathetic denervation to the eye [52–54].

(a)

(b)

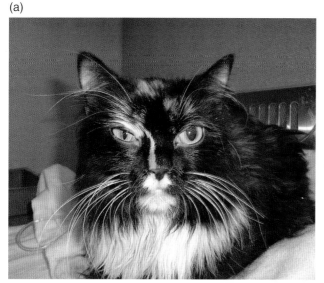
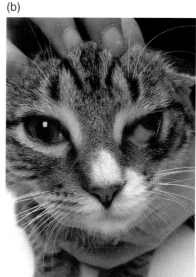

Figure 72.7 (a) Horner syndrome in a feline patient. *Source:* Courtesy of Daniel Foy, MS, DVM, DACVIM, DACVECC. (b) Enophthalmos in a feline patient with Horner syndrome. *Source:* Courtesy of Pamela Mueller, DVM.

This results in the following constellation of clinical signs [55]:

- Enophthalmos
- Miosis, that is, constriction of the affected pupil
- Prominent nictitans membrane
- Ptosis of the affected eye (see Figures 72.7a, b)

Horner syndrome may result from the following [8, 56, 57]:

- Chronic ear disease
  - Otitis interna
  - Otitis media
- Intracranial neoplasia
- Intrathoracic neoplasia
- Trauma
  - Brachial plexus
  - Head and neck
  - Inner ear

Horner syndrome is often idiopathic in the Golden Retriever [56–60].

72.3.8 Nystagmus

Nystagmus was introduced in Chapter 24, Section 24.1 as involuntary, rhythmic oscillations of one or both globes [8, 23, 61, 62].

Recall that oscillations of the globes may be described in terms of their direction [23, 63]:

- Vertical nystagmus involves oscillations that move the pupil in a dorsal-ventral (up/down) plane.

- Horizontal nystagmus involves oscillations that move the pupil in a side-to-side (left/right or right/left) plane.
- Rotary or torsional nystagmus involves oscillations along the globe's cranial-caudal axis.

Recall that nystagmus may also be described in terms of its fluidity [23, 61, 62]:

- Pendular nystagmus is when oscillations are fluid and of equal velocity
- Jerk nystagmus is when oscillations are biphasic: One or both globes move slowly in one direction, only to bounce back rapidly in the opposite direction.

Jerk nystagmus occurs more commonly than pendular nystagmus and is commonly associated with vestibular disease [64].

72.3.9 Positional Strabismus

Strabismus was introduced in Chapter 23, Section 23.2 as a clinical presentation in which one or both eyes deviate from the expected visual axis [8, 65–71].

Recall that there are different types of strabismus:

- Bilateral, or convergent esotropia, in which the globes turn inward, giving the appearance of having crossed eyes [72].
- Exotropia, or divergent strabismus, in which one or both globes turn outward [72].
- Positional, or vestibular, strabismus describes the following clinical scenario [23, 70]:

- When the head and neck are extended, the globes deviate ventrally to ventrolaterally. This causes the sclera to be prominent dorsally.
- When the patient's head returns to a relaxed position, then the strabismus resolves.

Positional strabismus is often associated with vestibular disease [23, 25, 70].

72.4 Neurological Presentations of Ear Disease: Peripheral Vestibular Syndrome

The peripheral vestibular system includes the following anatomical structures [73–75]:

- The middle ear
- Inner ear
  - Saccule
  - Semicircular canals
  - Utricle
- CN VIII

Middle and inner ear disease, otitis media and otitis interna, are the most common causes of peripheral vestibular syndrome [15, 76–78]. There may or may not be concurrent otitis externa, which is a clue that deep-seated ear disease may have precipitated the patient's neurological presentation [79].

Both middle and inner ear disease characteristically have a head tilt that is ipsilateral to the affected ear [15, 26, 80].

In cases of unilateral inner ear disease, the patient may also lean, fall, or circle toward the affected side [15]. This tendency results from decreased extensor tone associated with the ipsilateral limb, and increased extensor tone on the contralateral limb [15, 81, 82].

If there is concurrent nystagmus, the fast phase tends to move in the direction opposite the lesion [23].

Postural reactions are normal, as is CP [23].

Mentation is often normal, although the patient may appear to be somewhat disoriented [26].

When ear disease is bilateral, the patient typically lacks a head tilt [15]. The head characteristically sways from side to side, and the patient may lower its center of gravity toward the ground in a crouched position in an attempt to stabilize itself and preserve its balance [15].

Gross observation of both pinnae and external ear canal openings, as well as otoscopy, should be performed in every patient that presents with vestibular syndrome.

If otitis externa is present, the affected ear canal is likely to be erythematous, tender, and stenotic. Exudate may be grossly evident or visible on otoscopy [79, 83].

Otoscopy may require sedation for patient comfort. Middle and external ear disease can be painful [83, 84]. Patients may resent manipulation of the ears and act head shy [84].

Otoscopy allows for evaluation of the horizontal ear canal. It is not possible to examine the horizontal ear canal without an otoscope [8]. There is an approximately 75° bend between the vertical and horizontal ear canals that leads to the tympanum [8, 85].

Otoscopy also allows for examination of the tympanic membrane or tympanum, that is, the ear drum [8]. The tympanic membrane should be assessed for its integrity. Middle ear disease may cause it to bulge forward, as from buildup of fluid in the middle ear [83, 84]. The tympanic membrane may even rupture [83].

Cytology should be performed on both ears, even if only one appears to be affected, to evaluate for otitis. Bacterial culture and susceptibility profiles are important diagnostic tools to guide therapy.

Diagnostic imaging, such as computed tomography (CT) or magnetic resonance imaging (MRI), allows for detailed examination of the ear canals and bullae, and confirms the diagnosis of otitis media [79, 83] (see Figure 72.8).

Otitis media in dogs is often secondary to otitis externa [83]. It is possible for both bacteria and yeast to reach the bulla of the middle ear by migrating through the tympanum [83]. This material is foreign to the middle ear and incites inflammation [83].

Cats may develop otitis media when retropharyngeal organisms enter the tympanic bulla through the auditory tube [83]. As is true of dogs, the presence of foreign debris within the middle ear sets the stage for inflammatory disease [83]. Increased secretions pressurize the

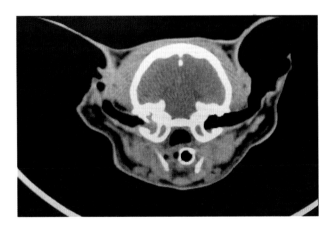

Figure 72.8 Computed tomography (CT) scan of a feline patient with right-sided otitis externa and neurological symptoms that included facial tics. This is confirmatory for bilateral otitis media. The right side appears to have more severe disease than the left. Note the presence of exudate from the bulla to the external meatus.

middle ear, causing the tympanum to bulge forward and potentially rupture [83]. The pressure is what causes middle ear disease to be painful [83].

Oropharyngeal polyps may also trigger the development of otitis media by irritating the lining of the ear [83].

Because of the proximity of CN VII to the tympanic bulla, patients with otitis media may develop ipsilateral facial nerve paresis or paralysis [36, 86].

Patients with otitis media may also develop ipsilateral Horner syndrome due to disruption of the sympathetic nerve fibers that pass through the tympanic bulla [8, 86].

Samples may be collected from the middle ear via myringotomy. As is true for aural swabs, cytology and culture of middle ear samples facilitates diagnostic and treatment planning [23].

The following isolates are commonly cultured from the middle ear in cases of otitis media [23]:

- Bacterial agents
  - *Proteus*
  - *Pseudomonas*
  - *Staphylococcus*
  - *Streptococcus*
- Fungal agents
  - *Candida*
  - *Malassezia*

Multi-drug resistant species of bacteria are increasingly identified, highlighting the importance of antibiotic susceptibility testing [23].

72.5 Less Common Causes of Peripheral Vestibular Syndrome

Peripheral vestibular syndrome is not always the result of middle and/or inner ear disease. Although they occur less frequently in clinical practice, other causes of peripheral vestibular syndrome include the following [15, 76]:

- Aural neoplasia
- Aural and/or oropharyngeal polyps
- Canine hypothyroidism
- Iatrogenic [15, 20, 87–89]
  - Bulla osteotomy
  - Total ear canal ablation
- Idiopathic peripheral vestibular disease
  - Feline idiopathic peripheral vestibular disease
  - Old dog vestibular disease
- Ototoxicity [90]
  - Aminoglycosides
  - Topical chlorhexidine

72.5.1 Aural Neoplasia and Peripheral Vestibular Syndrome

Any component of the ear may become neoplastic [23]. This includes the following anatomic structures:

- Pinna
- External ear canal
- Middle ear
- Inner ear

Peripheral vestibular syndrome results from aural neoplasia when there is compression of any component of the peripheral vestibular system by the tumor(s) [23]. Alternatively, aural neoplasia can incite an inflammatory response within one or more regions of the auditory tract. The inflammation adversely impacts the peripheral vestibular system [23].

Although there are many types of aural neoplasia, the following are most commonly implicated in peripheral vestibular dysfunction [23, 91, 92]:

- Adenocarcinoma
- Adenoma
- Feline lymphoma
- Squamous cell carcinoma (SCC)

SCC of the pinnae, with or without involvement of the nasal planum, is most common in white-coated cats [93–95]. Lesions are erosive and proliferate over time [93].

Other tumors may be grossly evident at the entrance to the external ear canal, or they may be identified within the canal itself, by means of otoscopy [23].

Most are malignant [23, 91, 92].

When suspected, aural masses should be imaged to determine the extensiveness of the lesions. Lytic lesions within the tympanic bulla and/or petrous temporal bone are likely, and are easy to appreciate on either CT or MRI [23].

72.5.2 Hypothyroidism and Peripheral Vestibular Syndrome

Hypothyroidism was introduced in Chapter 5, Section 5.7 as a common cause of endocrine, non-inflammatory hair loss [96]. Recall that hypothyroidism is most typically an acquired condition that results from thyroid atrophy or lymphocytic thyroiditis [96].

The classic textbook vignette for hypothyroidism is a middle-aged to older dog that presents for weight gain without increased daily caloric intake. Its metabolism is said to be sluggish. In addition, the affected patient may be cold- or exercise-intolerant [96]. The patient may be mentally dull.

Because the thyroid plays a significant role in hair growth and replacement, there are several cutaneous manifestations of disease [96, 97]. The most typical patterns of fur loss in the hypothyroid dog include the following [96]:

- "Ring around the collar," in which there is an alopecic patch outlining the neck
- "Rat tail," in which the tail becomes progressively bald

Less commonly, canine hypothyroidism manifests as neurological disease [98, 99]. In particular, CN VII and the fifth cranial nerve, the trigeminal (CN V), are affected [23, 99]. When CN VII is dysfunctional, patients often present with facial nerve paralysis [98]. Although this may resolve with medical management of hypothyroidism, deficits of CN VII may persist [99].

72.5.3 Old Dog Vestibular Disease

Old dog vestibular syndrome is named because of its tendency to target the geriatric canine population; however, it may occur in any age group [23].

Onset of vestibular ataxia, head tilt, and nystagmus is peracute [23].

Clients may be distressed by the severity of symptoms. Affected patients may be quite off-balance, causing them to circle, lean, fall, and/or roll to one side [23].

Anorexia is often seen in association with this neurological presentation, and is likely the result of motion sickness. Emesis may occur in some patients [23].

The etiology of this condition is unknown, and the diagnosis is by exclusion [23].

Treatment emphasizes supportive care and preventative measures to lessen the chance of self-injury by patients as they struggle with coordination and balance [23].

Nausea is medically managed as needed, and benzodiazepines may be administered to reduce patient anxiety [23].

Motion sickness drugs, such as meclizine, and either corticosteroids or non-steroidal anti-inflammatory drugs (NSAIDs) have classically been prescribed [15]. However, evidence-based medicine is lacking to support these clinical decisions [23].

Patient recovery is protracted [23]. Although improvement may occur as early as three to five days after initial presentation, patients typically take several weeks to recover [23]. Even then, patients may have a residual head tilt [23].

72.5.4 Feline Idiopathic Peripheral Vestibular Syndrome

Feline idiopathic peripheral vestibular syndrome presents similarly to old dog vestibular disease, the exception being that it does not preferentially target the geriatric population [23].

Outdoor cats are overrepresented [23, 33, 81, 100]. The condition also appears to be seasonal, with spikes in case presentations during the summer and autumn months [23, 33, 81, 100].

The etiology is also unknown; however, a viral origin has been suspected [23].

72.6 Central Vestibular Syndrome

The central vestibular system is composed of the brainstem, the cerebellum, and two caudal cerebellar peduncles [74, 75]. Within the brainstem, there are eight vestibular nuclei [74, 75]. These communicate, via the medial longitudinal fasciculus and the third, fourth, and sixth cranial nerves, with the spinal cord, the cerebrum, and the extraocular muscles [73–75].

Central vestibular syndrome results from one or more lesions in any of the structures above.

When it occurs, central vestibular syndrome may resemble peripheral vestibular syndrome in the following ways [26]:

- Both presentations involve a head tilt.
- Both presentations may involve nystagmus.
- Both presentations may involve circling.
- Both presentations may involve dysfunction within CN VII.

The head tilt is ipsilateral to the lesion in cases of peripheral vestibular syndrome; the head tilt can be in either direction in cases of central vestibular syndrome [26].

Patients that are affected with central vestibular syndrome may also exhibit dysfunction in the following cranial nerves [26]:

- CN V, the trigeminal nerve
- CN IX, the glossopharyngeal nerve
- CN X, the vagus nerve
- CN XII, the hypoglossal nerve

Patients with central vestibular syndrome are unlikely to develop Horner's syndrome [26].

Central vestibular syndrome frequently causes abnormal mentation [26]. Depression, obtundation, stupor, and coma are possible presentations [26]. Refer to Chapter 71 for a review of mental status and how to differentiate between these states.

If there is concurrent cerebellar dysfunction, then patients with central vestibular syndrome are likely to demonstrate head tremors [26].

Patients with central vestibular syndrome are frequently weak on the side that is ipsilateral to the lesion [26]. They also tend to have proprioceptive deficits, whereas those with peripheral vestibular syndrome do not [26]. Proprioceptive deficits are a reliable distinguishing feature on physical examination between central and peripheral vestibular syndrome [26].

Causes of central vestibular syndrome include the following [23, 26, 81, 90, 98, 101]:

- Aberrant parasitic migration
  - Cuterebriasis
  - *Dirofilaria immitis*
- Canine hypothyroidism
- Infectious disease
  - Bacterial
  - Fungal
    - Aspergillosis
    - Blastomycosis
    - Coccidioidomycosis
    - Cryptococcosis
    - Histoplasmosis
  - Protozoal
    - Neosporosis
    - Toxoplasmosis
  - Rickettsial
    - *Ehrlichia* spp.
    - *Rickettsia ricketsii*
  - Viral
    - Canine distemper virus (CDV)
    - Feline immunodeficiency virus (FIV)
    - Feline infectious peritonitis (FIP)
    - Feline leukemia virus (FeLV)
    - Rabies
- Inflammatory disease
  - Granulomatous meningoencephalitis (GME)
  - Necrotizing leukoencephalitis
    - Yorkshire Terriers
  - Necrotizing meningoencephalitis
    - Chihuahuas
    - Maltese
    - Pugs
- Neoplasia
- Nutritional imbalance
  - Thiamine deficiency (see Chapter 67, Section 67.6)
- Toxicosis
  - Metronidazole
- Vascular accident [16–18]

An exhaustive review of each pathology is beyond the scope of this text. A few examples will be discussed in brief below.

Determining the etiology of central vestibular syndrome typically requires advanced imaging and/or cerebrospinal fluid (CSF) analysis [77].

Note that MRI surpasses the utility of CT when soft tissue resolution is desirable [26, 102].

CSF analysis is particularly useful in the diagnosis of infectious agents; however, caution must be exercised in patients with space-occupying lesions [26].

72.6.1 Intracranial Neoplasia

Intracranial neoplasia may be primary or metastatic.

Among both dogs and cats, meningiomas are the most common type of primary intracranial neoplasia [23, 103].

Other types of primary intracranial neoplasia include the following [23]:

- Choroid plexus tumors
- Gliomas
- Lymphomas
- Oligodendrogliomas

Location of intracranial tumors may vary; however, certain types exhibit regional preferences. For example [23, 103, 104]:

- Meningiomas and choroid plexus tumors tend to develop within the cerebellopontomedullary angle.
- Choroid plexus tumors also tend to prefer the fourth ventricle.
- Gliomas preferentially target the brainstem.

Advanced imaging is essential for diagnosis of space-occupying lesions within the CNS [23]. MRI is preferred over CT because of its superior soft tissue resolution [23, 26, 102]. CT is likely to miss small tumors in the cerebellum, pons, and medulla [23].

The imaging characteristics of each tumor type are beyond the scope of this text; however, they have been defined in the veterinary literature. Consult a diagnostic imaging and/or oncology reference if time and interest allow.

Biopsy is required for definitive diagnosis; however, predictions regarding tumor type and biological behavior can be made based upon tumor location [23].

Extra-axial tumors, such as meningiomas and choroid plexus tumors, have a better prognosis than intra-axial ones, like gliomas [23].

72.6.2 Metronidazole Toxicity

Metronidazole is a commonly administered antibiotic that is used to treat a wide variety of bacterial and parasitic conditions. It is also often prescribed for use in clinical practice as an antidiarrheal agent.

Both cats and dogs can develop dose-dependent neurotoxicity [23]. Although administration of the drug that exceeds 60 mg/kg/day has been reported as toxic in the veterinary literature, there is appreciable individual variation [23, 105–108]. Lower doses are still capable of inducing neurotoxicity, particularly in cats [23].

Forebrain dysfunction is a common consequence of metronidazole-induced neurotoxicity in cats [23]. Cats may present for the following [23, 106, 108]:

- Abnormal mentation
- Blindness
- Seizures

It is thought that high-dose metronidazole interacts with γ-aminobutyric acid receptors [105].

Discontinuation of the drug is essential for recovery, which on average takes one to two weeks [23]. Recovery may be expedited by the administration of diazepam for reasons that remain unclear [105].

References

1 van Nes, J.J., Meij, B.P., and van Ham, L. (2009). Nervous system. In: *Medical History and Physical Examination in Companion Animals*, 2e (ed. A. Rijnberk and F.J. van Sluijs), 160–174. St. Louis: Saunders Elsevier.
2 Nghiem, P., Platt, S., and Schatzberg, S. (2009). The weak cat. Practical approach and common neurological differentials. *J. Feline Med. Surg.* 11 (5): 373–383.
3 Ford, R.B. and Mazzaferro, E.M. (2012). Patient evaluation and organ system examination. In: *Kirk & Bistner's Handbook of Veterinary Procedures and Emergency Treatment*, 9e, 295–380.
4 McGee, S. (2018). Examination of the motor system: approach to weakness. In: *Evidence-Based Physical Diagnosis*, 4e (ed. S. McGee), 551–568. Philadelphia: Elsevier.
5 Kustritz, M.V.R. (2011). History and physical examination of the neonate. In: *Small Animal Pediatrics: The First 12 Months of Life* (ed. M.E. Peterson and M.A. Kutzler). St. Louis, Mo: Saunders/Elsevier.
6 Hoskins, J.D. and Partington, B.P. (2001). Physical examination and diagnostic imaging procedures. In: *Veterinary Pediatrics: Dogs and Cats from Birth to Six Months*, 3e (ed. J.D. Hoskins), 6–7. Philadelphia: Saunders Elsevier.
7 Beaver, B.V. (1980). Neuromuscular development of Felis-Catus. *Lab. Anim.* 14 (3): 197–198.
8 Englar, R.E. (2017). *Performing the Small Animal Physical Examination*. Hoboken, NJ: Wiley.
9 Thomas, W.B. (2000). Initial assessment of patients with neurologic dysfunction. *Vet. Clin. North Am. Small Anim. Pract.* 30 (1): 1–24, v.
10 Fahn, S. (2007). Hypokinesia and Hyperkinesia. In: *Textbook of Clinical Neurology*, 3e (ed. C.G. Goetz), 289–306. Philadelphia: Saunders.
11 Defarges, A. (2015). The physical examination. *NAVC Clinician's Brief* (September): 73–80.
12 Nye, C. and Troxel, M. (2017). The neurologic examination. *NAVC Clinician's Brief* (August): 61–69.
13 Taylor, A.R. and Kerwin, S.C. (2018). Clinical evaluation of the feline neurologic patient. *Vet. Clin. North Am. Small Anim. Pract.* 48 (1): 1–10.
14 Garosi, L. (2009). Neurological examination of the cat. How to get started. *J. Feline Med. Surg.* 11 (5): 340–348.
15 Garosi, L.S., Lowrie, M.L., and Swinbourne, N.F. (2012). Neurological manifestations of ear disease in dogs and cats. *Vet. Clin. North Am. Small Anim. Pract.* 42 (6): 1143–1160.
16 Thomsen, B., Garosi, L., Skerritt, G. et al. (2016). Neurological signs in 23 dogs with suspected rostral cerebellar ischaemic stroke. *Acta Vet. Scand.* 58 (1): 40.
17 Joseph, R.J., Greenlee, P.G., Carrillo, J.M., and Kay, W.J. (1988). Canine cerebrovascular-disease - clinical and pathological findings in 17 cases. *J. Am. Anim. Hosp. Assoc.* 24 (5): 569–576.
18 Wessmann, A., Chandler, K., and Garosi, L. (2009). Ischaemic and haemorrhagic stroke in the dog. *Vet. J.* 180 (3): 290–303.
19 Little, C.J.L., Lane, J.G., Gibbs, C., and Pearson, G.R. (1991). Inflammatory middle-ear disease of the dog - the clinical and pathological features of Cholesteatoma, a complication of otitis-media. *Vet. Rec.* 128 (14): 319–322.
20 Mason, L.K., Harvey, C.E., and Orsher, R.J. (1988). Total ear canal ablation combined with lateral bulla osteotomy for end-stage otitis in dogs. Results in thirty dogs. *Vet. Surg.* 17 (5): 263–268.
21 Boothe, H.W., Hobson, H.P., and McDonald, D.E. (1996). Treatment of traumatic separation of the auricular and annular cartilages without ablation: results in five dogs. *Vet. Surg.* 25 (5): 376–379.
22 Schunk, K.L. (1988). Disorders of the vestibular system. *Vet. Clin. North Am. Small Anim. Pract.* 18 (3): 641–665.
23 Rossmeisl, J.H. Jr. (2010). Vestibular disease in dogs and cats. *Vet. Clin. North Am. Small Anim. Pract.* 40 (1): 81–100.
24 Kornegay, J.N. (1991). Ataxia, head tilt, nystagmus. Vestibular diseases. *Probl. Vet. Med.* 3 (3): 417–425.
25 Troxel, M.T., Drobatz, K.J., and Vite, C.H. (2005). Signs of neurologic dysfunction in dogs with central versus peripheral vestibular disease. *J. Am. Vet. Med. Assoc.* 227 (4): 570–574.

26 Platt, S.R. (2009). Vestibular disease. In: *Small Animal Critical Care Medicine* (ed. D.C. Silverstein and K. Hopper), 452–458. St. Louis, Mo: Saunders/ Elsevier.

27 Thomas, W.B. and Dewey, C.W. (2008). Performing the neurologic examination. In: *A Practical Guide to Canine and Feline Neurology*, 2e (ed. C.W. Dewey), 53–74. Ames, Iowa: Wiley-Blackwell.

28 Casimiro da Costa, R. (ed.) (2009). Ataxia – Recognition and approach. World Small Animal Veterinary Association World Congress Proceedings.

29 Averill, D.R. Jr. (1981). The neurologic examination. *Vet. Clin. North Am. Small Anim. Pract.* 11 (3): 511–521.

30 DeLahunta, A., Glass, E., and Kent, M. (2015). *Veterinary Neuroanatomy and Clinical Neurology*, 4e. St. Louis, MO: Elsevier.

31 Angelaki, D.E. and Cullen, K.E. (2008). Vestibular system: the many facets of a multimodal sense. *Annu. Rev. Neurosci.* 31: 125–150.

32 Brandt, T. and Strupp, M. (2005). General vestibular testing. *Clin. Neurophysiol.* 116 (2): 406–426.

33 Thomas, W.B. (2000). Vestibular dysfunction. *Vet. Clin. North Am. Small Anim. Pract.* 30 (1): 227–249, viii.

34 Parent, J.M. (2006). The cat with a head tilt, vestibular ataxia, or nystagmus. In: *Problem-Based Feline Medicine* (ed. J. Rand), 835–851. Edinburgh; New York: Saunders.

35 Platt, S.R. (2011). Vestibular disease in dogs and cats (Proceedings). DVM 360 [Internet]. http:// veterinarycalendar.dvm360.com/vestibular-disease-dogs-and-cats-proceedings.

36 Troxel, M. (2016). Facial nerve paralysis. *NAVC Clinician's Brief* (May): 95–98.

37 Evans, H.D. and de Lahunta, A. (2013). Facial nerve (cranial nerve VII). In: *Miller's Anatomy of the Dog*, 4e (ed. H.D. Evans and A. de Lahunta), 231–233. St. Louis: Saunders Elsevier.

38 de Lahunta, A., Glass, E.N., and Kent, M. (2015). Neuroanatomy gross description and atlas of transverse sections and magnetic resonance images. In: *Veterinary Neuroanatomy and Clinical Neurology*, 4e (ed. A. de Lahunta, E.N. Glass and M. Kent), 6–44. St. Louis: Saunders Elsevier.

39 Utsugi, S., Saito, M., and Shelton, G.D. (2014). Resolution of polyneuropathy in a hypothyroid dog following thyroid supplementation. *J. Am. Anim. Hosp. Assoc.* 50 (5): 345–349.

40 Vitale, C.L. and Olby, N.J. (2007). Neurologic dysfunction in hypothyroid, hyperlipidemic Labrador retrievers. *J. Vet. Intern. Med.* 21 (6): 1316–1322.

41 McKeown, H.M. (2002). Hypothyroidism in a boxer dog. *Can. Vet. J.* 43 (7): 553–555.

42 Jaggy, A. and Oliver, J.E. (1994). Neurologic manifestations of thyroid disease. *Vet. Clin. North Am. Small Anim. Pract.* 24 (3): 487–494.

43 Braund, K.G., Luttgen, P.J., Sorjonen, D.C., and Redding, R.W. (1979). Idiopathic facial paralysis in the dog. *Vet. Rec.* 105 (13): 297–299.

44 Spivack, R.E., Elkins, A.D., Moore, G.E., and Lantz, G.C. (2013). Postoperative complications following TECA-LBO in the dog and cat. *J. Am. Anim. Hosp. Assoc.* 49 (3): 160–168.

45 Pratschke, K.M. (2003). Inflammatory polyps of the middle ear in 5 dogs. *Vet. Surg.* 32 (3): 292–296.

46 Greci, V., Vernia, E., and Mortellaro, C.M. (2014). Per-endoscopic trans-tympanic traction for the management of feline aural inflammatory polyps: a case review of 37 cats. *J. Feline Med. Surg.* 16 (8): 645–650.

47 Calvo, I., Espadas, I., Hammond, G., and Pratschke, K. (2014). Epineurial repair of an iatrogenic facial nerve neurotmesis after total ear canal ablation and lateral bulla osteotomy in a dog with concurrent cranio-mandibular osteopathy. *J. S. Afr. Vet. Assoc.* 85 (1): 1050.

48 Trevor, P.B. and Martin, R.A. (1993). Tympanic bulla osteotomy for treatment of middle-ear disease in cats: 19 cases (1984–1991). *J. Am. Vet. Med. Assoc.* 202 (1): 123–128.

49 Fraser, A.R., Long, S.N., and le Chevoir, M.A. (2015). Concurrent idiopathic vestibular syndrome and facial nerve paralysis in a cat. *Aust. Vet. J.* 93 (7): 252–254.

50 Bacon, N.J., Gilbert, R.L., Bostock, D.E., and White, R.A. (2003). Total ear canal ablation in the cat: indications, morbidity and long-term survival. *J. Small Anim. Pract.* 44 (10): 430–434.

51 Kern, T.J. and Erb, H.N. (1987). Facial neuropathy in dogs and cats: 95 cases (1975–1985). *J. Am. Vet. Med. Assoc.* 191 (12): 1604–1609.

52 Troxel, M. (2014). Horner syndrome at a glance. *Clinician's Brief* (May): 25.

53 Heller, H.B. and Bentley, E. (2016). The practitioner's guide to neurologic causes of canine anisocoria. Today's Veterinary Practice [Internet]. (January/ February):[77-83 pp.]. http://todaysveterinarypractice. navc.com/wp-content/uploads/2016/05/ TVP_2016-0102_OO-Anisocoria.pdf.

54 Bagley, R.S. (2006). The cat with anisocoria or abnormally dilated or contricted pupils. In: *Problem-Based Feline Medicine* (ed. J. Rand), 870–889. Edinburgh; New York: Saunders.

55 Penderis, J. (2015). Diagnosis of Horner's syndrome in dogs and cats. *In Pract.* 37 (3).

56 Morgan, R.V. and Zanotti, S.W. (1989). Horner's syndrome in dogs and cats: 49 cases (1980–1986). *J. Am. Vet. Med. Assoc.* 194 (8): 1096–1099.

57 Kern, T.J., Aromando, M.C., and Erb, H.N. (1989). Horner's syndrome in dogs and cats: 100 cases (1975–1985). *J. Am. Vet. Med. Assoc.* 195 (3): 369–373.

58 Simpson, K.M., Williams, D.L., and Cherubini, G.B. (2015). Neuropharmacological lesion localization in idiopathic Horner's syndrome in Golden retrievers and dogs of other breeds. *Vet. Ophthalmol.* 18 (1): 1–5.

59 Boydell, P. (1995). Idiopathic Horner's syndrome in the golden retriever. *J. Small Anim. Pract.* 36 (9): 382–384.

60 van Hagen, M.A., Kwakernaak, C.M., Boeve, M.H., and Stades, F.C. (1999). Horner's syndrome in the dog: a retrospective study. *Tijdschr. Diergeneeskd.* 124 (20): 600–602.

61 Côté, E. (2015). *Clinical Veterinary Advisor. Dogs and Cats*, 3e, xxxvii, 1642 p. St. Louis, Missouri: Elsevier Mosby.

62 Tilley, L.P., Smith, F.W.K., and Tilley, L.P. (2007). *Blackwell's Five-Minute Veterinary Consult: Canine and Feline*, 4e. Ames, Iowa: Blackwell.

63 Abramson, C.J. (ed.) (2009). *The Neurological Examination: How to Describe What you See & Know if it Is Normal*. Phoenix, AZ: American Animal Hospital Association.

64 Munana, K. (2013). Head tilt and nystagmus. In: *BSAVA Manual of Canine and Feline Neurology*, 4e (ed. S.R. Platt and N.J. Olby). Quedgeley, Gloucester: British Small Animal Veterinary Association.

65 Tilley, L.P. and Smith, F.W.K. (2016). *Blackwell's Five-Minute Veterinary Consult. Canine and Feline*, 6e, lxix, 1622 p. Ames, Iowa, USA: Wiley.

66 Peterson, M.E. and Kutzler, M.A. (2011). *Small Animal Pediatrics: The First 12 Months of Life*, xvi, 526 p. St. Louis, Mo: Saunders/Elsevier.

67 Delahunta, A. (1997). The neurological examination. *Vet. Q.* 19 (sup1): 6–8.

68 Maggs, D.J., Miller, P.E., Ofri, R., and Slatter, D.H. (2013). *Slatter's Fundamentals of Veterinary Ophthalmology*, 5e, x, 506 p. St. Louis, Mo: Elsevier.

69 Gelatt, K.N. and Plummer, C.E. (2001). *Color Atlas of Veterinary Ophthalmology*. Ames, IA: Wiley-Blackwell.

70 Dewey, C.W. and Da Costa, R.C. (2016). *Practical Guide to Canine and Feline Neurology*, 3e, xi, 672 p. Chichester, West Sussex; Hoboken: Wiley-Blackwell.

71 Mitchell, N. (2006). Feline ophthalmology part I: examination of the eye. *Ir. Vet. J.* 59 (3): 164.

72 Rutstein, R.P. (2011). Care of the patient with strabismus: esotropia and exotropia American Optometric Association [Internet]. https://www.aoa.org/documents/optometrists/CPG-12.pdf.

73 Rylander, H. (2012). Vestibular syndrome: What's causing the head tilt and other neurologic signs? DVM360 [Internet]. http://veterinarymedicine.dvm360.com/vestibular-syndrome-whats-causing-head-tilt-and-other-neurologic-signs.

74 Evans, H.E. and DeLahunta, A. (2004). *Guide to the Dissection of the Dog*, 6e, xiv, 378 p. St. Louis, Mo: Saunders.

75 Evans, H.E. and Miller, M.E. (2013). *Miller's Anatomy of the Dog*, 4e, xix, 850 p. St. Louis, Missouri: Elsevier.

76 Dewey, C.W. (ed.) (2013). Diagnosis and treatment of vestibular disease. World Small Animal Veterinary Association World Congress; Ithaca, NY.

77 Pancotto, T. (2016). Central vs. peripheral vestibular diseases. CVC [Internet]. http://www.thecvc.com/wp-content/uploads/2016/04/CVCVB_2016_neurology.pdf.

78 Kent, M., Platt, S.R., and Schatzberg, S.J. (2010). The neurology of balance: function and dysfunction of the vestibular system in dogs and cats. *Vet. J.* 185 (3): 247–258.

79 Akucewich, L. (2004). Head tilt & nystagmus. *NAVC Clinician's Brief* (April): 49–51.

80 LeCouteur, R.A. (2009). Vestibular disorders of dogs and cats. CVC Proceedings [Internet]. http://veterinarycalendar.dvm360.com/vestibular-disorders-dogs-and-cats-proceedings.

81 de Lahunta, A. and Glass, E.N. (eds.) (2009). Vestibular system: special proprioception. In: *Veterinary Neuroanatomy and Clinical Neurology*, 3e. St. Louis: WB Saunders.

82 de Lahunta, A. and Glass, E.N. (eds.) (2009). Auditory system: special somatic afferent system. In: *Veterinary Neuroanatomy and Clinical Neurology*. St. Louis: WB Saunders.

83 Gotthelf, L.N. (2008). Diagnosis & management of otitis. *NAVC Clinician's Brief* (May): 60–64.

84 Gotthelf, L.N. (2013). Neck stiffness & head tilt in a young spaniel. *NAVC Clinician's Brief* (March): 23–25.

85 Angus, J.C. (2004). Diseases of the ear. In: *Small Animal Dermatology Secrets* (ed. K.L. Campbell), 364–384. Philadelphia: Hanley & Belfus.

86 Paterson, S. (2007). Chronic otitis and surgery. *NAVC Clinician's Brief* (July): 23–26.

87 White, R.A. and Pomeroy, C.J. (1990). Total ear canal ablation and lateral bulla osteotomy in the dog. *J. Small Anim. Pract.* 31: 547–553.

88 Smeak, D.D. and Dehoff, W.D. (1986). Total ear canal ablation: clinical results in the dog and cat. *Vet. Surg.* 15: 161–170.

89 Matthieson, D.T. and Scavelli, T. (1990). Total ear canal ablation and lateral bulla osteotomy in 38 dogs. *J. Am. Anim. Hosp. Assoc.* 26: 257–267.

90 Garosi, L. (2012). Head tilt and nystagmus. In: *Small Animal Neurological Emergencies* (ed. S.R. Platt and L. Garosi), 253–263. Manson.

91 Fan, T.M. and de Lorimier, L.P. (2004). Inflammatory polyps and aural neoplasia. *Vet. Clin. North Am. Small Anim. Pract.* 34 (2): 489–509.

92 London, C.A., Dubilzeig, R.R., Vail, D.M. et al. (1996). Evaluation of dogs and cats with tumors of the ear canal: 145 cases (1978–1992). *J. Am. Vet. Med. Assoc.* 208 (9): 1413–1418.

93 Thomson, M. (2007). Squamous cell carcinoma of the nasal planum in cats and dogs. *Clin. Tech. Small Anim. Pract.* 22 (2): 42–45.

94 Dorn, C.R., Taylor, D.O., and Schneider, R. (1971). Sunlight exposure and risk of developing cutaneous and oral squamous cell carcinomas in white cats. *J. Natl. Cancer Inst.* 46 (5): 1073–1078.

95 Murphy, S. (2013). Cutaneous squamous cell carcinoma in the cat: current understanding and treatment approaches. *J. Feline Med. Surg.* 15 (5): 401–407.

96 Frank, L.A. (2006). Comparative dermatology–canine endocrine dermatoses. *Clin. Dermatol.* 24 (4): 317–325.

97 Baker, K. (1986). Hormonal alopecia in dogs and cats. *In Pract.* 8 (2): 71–78.

98 Higgins, M.A., Rossmeisl, J.H. Jr., and Panciera, D.L. (2006). Hypothyroid-associated central vestibular disease in 10 dogs: 1999–2005. *J. Vet. Intern. Med.* 20 (6): 1363–1369.

99 LeCouteur, R.A. (2009). Vestibular disease in dogs and cats. DVM 360 [Internet]. http://veterinarycalendar.dvm360.com/vestibular-disorders-dogs-and-cats-proceedings.

100 Burke, E.E., Moise, N.S., de Lahunta, A., and Erb, H.N. (1985). Review of idiopathic feline vestibular syndrome in 75 cats. *J. Am. Vet. Med. Assoc.* 187 (9): 941–943.

101 Mununa, K. (2001). Inflammatory disorders of the central nervous system. In: *Consultations in Feline Internal Medicine*, 4e (ed. J.R. August). Philadelphia: Saunders.

102 Tidwell, A.S. and Jones, J.C. (1999). Advanced imaging concepts: a pictorial glossary of CT and MRI technology. *Clin. Tech. Small Anim. Pract.* 14 (2): 65–111.

103 Snyder, J.M., Shofer, F.S., Van Winkle, T.J., and Massicotte, C. (2006). Canine intracranial primary neoplasia: 173 cases (1986–2003). *J. Vet. Intern. Med.* 20 (3): 669–675.

104 Westworth, D.R., Dickinson, P.J., Vernau, W. et al. (2008). Choroid plexus tumors in 56 dogs (1985–2007). *J. Vet. Intern. Med.* 22 (5): 1157–1165.

105 Evans, J., Levesque, D., Knowles, K. et al. (2003). Diazepam as a treatment for metronidazole toxicosis in dogs: a retrospective study of 21 cases. *J. Vet. Intern. Med.* 17 (3): 304–310.

106 Caylor, K.B. and Cassimatis, M.K. (2001). Metronidazole neurotoxicosis in two cats. *J. Am. Anim. Hosp. Assoc.* 37 (3): 258–262.

107 Dow, S.W., LeCouteur, R.A., Poss, M.L., and Beadleston, D. (1989). Central nervous system toxicosis associated with metronidazole treatment of dogs: five cases (1984–1987). *J. Am. Vet. Med. Assoc.* 195 (3): 365–368.

108 Saxon, B. and Magne, M.L. (1993). Reversible central nervous system toxicosis associated with metronidazole therapy in three cats. *Prog. Vet. Neurol.* 4: 25–27.

73

Abnormal Somatic or Spinal Reflexes

73.1 Introduction to the Concept of a Reflex

A reflex is a built-in response to a stimulus [1–3]. Although it can be modulated by the brain, conscious thought is not required to initiate a reflex [3].

There are many types of reflexes and many different ways to categorize them. For the purposes of this chapter, it is easiest to consider reflexes as being either autonomic or somatic [3, 4].

73.1.1 Autonomic Reflexes

Autonomic reflexes exert control over smooth and cardiac muscle, as well as the viscera [4]. Their goal is to maintain homeostasis, a stable internal state [4–6]. For this to occur, certain variables must be confined to an optimal range in spite of external conditions [5].

Many of the variables that are controlled by autonomic reflexes are vital to the maintenance of life [4]:

- Blood pressure
- Core body temperature
- Digestion
- Heart rate
- Micturition
- Peristalsis
- Respiratory rate

Maintaining these variables within their optional ranges requires a minimum of three components [4]:

- Something to measure the variable of interest, that is, a sensor
- Something to change the variable of interest, that is, an effector
- One or more pathways to link the two

Collectively, these components constitute a feedback loop [4, 7–9]. Feedback may be positive or negative [7–10].

- Positive feedback occurs when the body recognizes a change in a variable and acts to amplify it [8, 9].
- Negative feedback occurs when the body recognizes a change and acts to reduce the fluctuation [8, 9].

Many of the body's physiological processes operate via negative feedback [9].

Consider, for example, the baroreceptor reflex that was introduced in Chapter 45, Section 45.4.

Recall that baroreceptors are concentrations of nerve endings within the aortic arch and internal carotid arteries that respond to changes in arterial pressure [11]. Their purpose is to detect stretch within the lumen of blood vessels [11]. Increased stretch is interpreted as elevated blood pressure (BP) [11].

At low pressures, baroreceptors are relatively inactive. When they perceive increased intraluminal stretch, baroreceptors increase their rate of firing [11]. This inhibits sympathetic outflow [11]. There is now less norepinephrine available to bind to cardiovascular targets. This shifts the balance in favor of the parasympathetic pathway [11]. Activation of the parasympathetic nervous system causes reflex bradycardia. This effectively reduces BP, restoring homeostasis [11].

Note that the aforementioned actions are not under conscious control. In this clinical scenario, and many others, the body acts on autopilot. That is the purpose, of a reflex: to make adjustments to physiological processes as needed without requiring conscious input from the patient.

73.1.2 Somatic or Spinal Reflexes

Somatic reflexes exert control over skeletal muscle [4]. They cause involuntary muscle contraction. Because they are mediated by the brainstem and the spinal cord, they are often referred to as spinal reflexes [4, 12, 13]. Spinal reflexes are the focus of this chapter.

Common Clinical Presentations in Dogs and Cats, First Edition. Ryane E. Englar.
© 2019 John Wiley & Sons, Inc. Published 2019 by John Wiley & Sons, Inc.

73.2 The Stretch or Patellar Reflex

The stretch reflex is the simplest spinal reflex because its pathway is monosynaptic, meaning that it involves only involves two neurons: one sensory and one motor [4, 12, 13].

The stretch reflex is initiated when a relaxed muscle is stretched [4, 12, 13]. This stretch activates a sensory neuron, which synapses with a motor neuron to cause muscle contraction [1, 3, 4, 12, 13].

The purpose of this reflex is to maintain posture and muscle length, thereby supporting the body against gravity [4].

Human patients may be most familiar with this classic knee-jerk reflex because it is routinely tested during clinical examination when the plexor, a reflex hammer, is tapped against the patellar tendon. This causes a stretch in the quadriceps femoris. The quadriceps femoris contracts in response, causing the crus to extend at the stifle.

The patellar reflex can also be tested in dogs and cats to evaluate the integrity of the femoral nerve and the associated L4–L6 segments of the spinal cord [3, 14, 15].

The canine patient is typically restrained in lateral recumbency, whereas cats may be more easily tested in dorsal recumbency, between the examiner's thighs [2, 16].

With the patient in lateral recumbency, the clinician uses one hand to support the limb that is "up" by seating this hand under the medial thigh [3, 14]. The stifle of the "up" limb is positioned so that it is partially flexed [3, 14]. The clinician then swings the plexor with his other hand such that it contacts the patellar tendon [3, 14]. The crus responds by extending at the stifle [2, 3, 14, 17–19].

73.3 The Withdrawal or Flexor Reflex

Not all somatic reflexes are basic. Reflex arcs can also be polysynaptic, that is, they require one or more interneurons to connect sensory (afferent) to motor (efferent) signals. An example is the withdrawal or flexor reflex [4].

The withdrawal reflex assesses the integrity of different nerves and spinal segments depending upon whether it is performed on a thoracic or a hind limb [2, 3, 14, 15, 17–19]:

- When performed in the *thoracic* limb, the withdrawal reflex evaluates C6–T2 spinal cord segments as well as the musculocutaneous, axillary, median, ulnar, and radial nerves.
- When performed in the *hind* limb, the withdrawal reflex evaluates L7–S1 segments and the sciatic nerve.

With the patient restrained in lateral recumbency, the clinician pinches interdigital skin or a nail bed on each limb, one limb at a time, with the tested limb held in extension [2, 3, 14, 17–19]:

- When the thoracic limb is tested, the patient should respond by flexing the shoulder, elbow, and carpus to pull the limb away from the clinician.
- When the pelvic limb is tested, the patient should respond by flexing the hip, stifle, and hock to pull the limb away from the clinician.
- The contralateral limb should be unaffected [2, 17–19].

The withdrawal reflex is complex as compared to the stretch reflex. The former requires transmission and integration of more than one signal [4].

73.4 Other Important Somatic or Spinal Reflexes

Although the patellar and withdrawal reflexes are commonly used diagnostic tools in companion animal practice, others may provide additional insight into the neurological status of a patient:

- Panniculus or cutaneous trunci reflex [14, 15, 17, 18, 20–22]:
  - Tests the integrity of the lateral thoracic nerve and C8–T1 spinal segments.
  - The clinician uses a hemostat to pinch the skin lateral to the spine, beginning at the lumbosacral region and moving cranially, one vertebrae at a time, to the level of T2. Both the patient's left lateral and right lateral sides should be tested.
  - In the normal patient, the panniculus reflex results in contraction of the cutaneous trunci muscles. This contraction will be evident as a twitch over the thoracolumbar region.
  - If contraction of the cutaneous trunci muscles is not evident at a discrete cutoff point, then a lesion is likely to be present anywhere from one to four segments cranially.
- Perineal or anal reflex [13, 15, 17]:
  - Assesses anal tone by triggering the anal sphincter to contract.
  - The clinician touches the anal rim with a gloved forefinger:
    - ○ An anus with normal tone will "wink" as the anal sphincters close.
    - ○ Decreased or absent tone is suggestive of a lesion in the S1–S3 segments or dysfunctional anal innervation from branches of the pudendal nerve.

– As the anal sphincter contracts, the perineal reflex should also result in flexion of the tail:
  o Failure of the patient to tail-tuck suggests that there may be a lesion within caudal spinal cord segments.

73.5 The Crossed Extensor Reflex

The crossed extensor reflex is normal in the standing patient: when one limb is flexed, the contralateral limb should extend [13, 15]. This keeps the patient from falling over from an upright position if one limb is lifted off the ground [13, 15].

When a normal patient is laterally recumbent, the crossed extensor reflex is inhibited [13, 15].

If a patient in lateral recumbency exhibits the crossed extensor reflex when testing for the withdrawal reflex, this is considered abnormal [13, 15].

73.6 Less Commonly Tested Somatic or Spinal Reflexes

Less commonly tested reflexes for the thoracic limb include the following [2, 13, 15, 17–19]:

- The biceps reflex:
  – Tests the integrity of the musculocutaneous nerve and C6–C8 spinal cord segments
- The extensor carpi radialis or triceps reflex:
  – Tests the integrity of the radial nerve in the thoracic limb and C7–T1 spinal cord segments

With the exception of the withdrawal reflex, thoracic limb reflexes are particularly difficult to interpret in companion animal patients because many patients that are normal have decreased responses [13].

Less commonly tested reflexes for the pelvic limb include the following [2, 13, 15, 17–19]:

- The cranial tibial reflex:
  – Tests the peroneal branch of the sciatic nerve and L6–L7 spinal cord segments
  – Causes flexion of the hock
- The gastrocnemius reflex:
  – Tests the tibial branch of the sciatic nerve and L7–S1 spinal cord segments

73.7 Describing Spinal Reflexes

In order for spinal reflexes to be intact, all components of their respective pathways must be functional [3].

A single break in the pathway impacts the quality of the reflex [23].

Abnormal reflexes may be exaggerated, weak, or even absent [17, 18, 24].

Characterizing the quality of the reflex helps with neuroanatomic localization [3]. Spinal reflexes are typically graded by the author on a scale from 0 to 4:

- 0: Absent
- 1: Weak or hyporeflexic
- 2: Normal
- 3: Exaggerated or hyperreflexic
- 4: Exaggerated with clonus, meaning that the reflex action repeats multiple times

73.8 The Purpose of Testing for Spinal Reflexes

Neurologic assessment of the patient can be challenging, even for the experienced clinician. However, it is important to keep at it. Spinal reflexes help the clinician to localize lesions.

For example, testing for the patellar, withdrawal, cranial tibial, and perineal reflexes provides the clinician with an assessment of the lumbosacral intumescence, the regional enlargement of the spinal cord that includes segments L4–S3 [25, 26]. This region of the spinal cord contains a large number of neuronal cell bodies that are involved with innervation of the hind limb.

If the patellar, withdrawal, cranial tibial, and/or perineal reflexes are decreased, then a lesion is present between L4–S3 [26]. In other words, evaluation of spinal reflexes effectively localizes the lesion to a range of spinal segments. Although this information does not provide a clinical diagnosis or prognosis, it is valuable because it narrows the scope of pathology to an anatomical region or zone [26]. This assists with case management, particularly diagnostic imaging. Instead of performing computed tomography (CT) or magnetic resonance imaging (MRI) on the entire spine, imaging can be localized to a particular region of interest [26].

If, on the other hand, the patellar, withdrawal, cranial tibial, and/or perineal reflexes are normal to increased, then the lesion is cranial to L4–S3 [26].

73.9 Hyporeflexia

Hyporeflexia is the state of having decreased reflexes.

In veterinary patients, hyporeflexia is most often associated with a reduction in the patellar tendon reflex, or the withdrawal reflex of either the thoracic or the pelvic limb.

When it occurs, hyporeflexia is suggestive of a lower motor neuron (LMN) lesion [26]. Refer to Chapter 74 for examples.

However, hyporeflexia is not always pathologic [27]. In human patients, the strength of the patellar tendon reflex is dependent upon the patient's age and physical activity level [27–31]. This is due to age-dependent changes in skeletal muscle, including muscle atrophy [27, 32–34].

Canine patients also experience age-related hyporeflexia [27]. The patellar tendon reflex is less intense in neurologically normal dogs that are 10 years of age or older [27].

73.10 Hyperreflexia

Hyperreflexia is the state of having increased reflexes.

In veterinary patients, hyperreflexia is most often associated with exaggerated patellar tendon reflexes, or withdrawal reflexes of either the thoracic or the pelvic limb.

When it occurs, hyperreflexia is suggestive of an upper motor neuron (UMN) lesion [26]. Refer to Chapter 74 for examples.

However, hyperreflexia is not always indicative of neuromuscular pathology.

A hyperreflexic patellar reflex is not uncommonly seen in the neurologically healthy, but excited or nervous feline patient.

Hyperreflexia can also result from metabolic dysfunction [35]. For example, some patients with hypocalcemia develop increased reflexes and intense muscle spasms [35]. This is referred to as hypocalcemic tetany, and it results from a hyperexcitable nervous system [35]. Both arms of the nervous system, peripheral and central, are affected.

Patients with hypocalcemia may also demonstrate the following changes [35]:

- Behavioral changes
  - Aggression
  - Fits of growling
- Convulsions
- Episodic rigidity
- Muscle fasciculations
- Seizures
- Splinted abdomens
- Stiff gaits

Hypocalcemia may result from the following [35, 36]:

- Primary hypoparathyroidism
- Puerperal tetany or eclampsia
- Renal disease
- Repeated administration of hypertonic sodium phosphate enemas

73.10.1 Primary Hypoparathyroidism

Primary hypoparathyroidism is uncommonly seen in the dog and rarely in the cat [35–40]. This condition is caused by reduced production of parathyroid hormone (PTH) [35, 37, 38]. In health, PTH maintains homeostasis by helping to keep calcium within a normal physiologic range [35, 37, 38]. In the absence of PTH, patients experience the following [35, 37, 38]:

- Increased renal excretion of calcium
- Less bone resorption
- Less excretion of phosphate by the kidneys
- Reduced absorption of calcium by the intestines
- Reduced serum calcitriol

Collectively, these mechanisms contribute to subnormal serum calcium levels [35, 37, 38].

Primary hypoparathyroidism in dogs is typically the result of immune-mediated disease involving the parathyroid glands [37].

Cats, on the other hand, tend to develop this as an iatrogenic complication: the parathyroid glands are accidentally removed during bilateral thyroidectomy [35, 37–39, 41, 42].

73.10.2 Puerperal Tetany or Eclampsia

Puerperal tetany or eclampsia is sometimes referred to as "milk fever." This condition is most likely to occur in small-breed dogs with large litters [43–45]. It rarely occurs in cats [43–45].

Although the condition can occur at the end of gestation, it more commonly presents in patients two to three weeks after whelping [43–45].

Dogs that received calcium supplementation during pregnancy may be at greater risk of developing eclampsia during the postpartum period [43].

An early sign of eclampsia is panting or restlessness [43]. This progresses to neuromuscular signs of stiffness, muscle spasms, tremors, twitching, and seizing [43].

Patients are hyperreactive to external stimuli [43].

Patients are likely to be hyperreflexive [43].

73.10.3 Chronic Kidney Disease (CKD) and Hypocalcemia

Chronic kidney disease (CKD) was introduced in Chapter 63, Section 63.5 as the most common cause of bilaterally symmetrical, small kidneys [46–48]. Recall that CKD is defined as structural and/or functional renal impairment for three or more months [47, 49]. It is a progressive condition that most commonly targets aged cats [47, 48].

Review Chapter 63, Section 63.5 for common presentations of CKD and to review the appropriate diagnostic investigation for this condition [47, 48, 50].

Uremia secondary to CKD is commonly seen in clinical practice and is what causes malaise in CKD patients. Uremia is worsened by progressive dehydration, acid–base disturbances, and electrolyte imbalances, which are common sequelae of CKD [47, 49, 50].

Hypocalcemia is often associated with CKD. However, the decrease in calcium is typically mild to moderate. This is not usually clinically significant. Marked hypocalcemia is required to produce tetany [36].

References

1 Jennings, D.P. and Bailey, J.G. (2004). Spinal control of posture and movement. In: *Dukes' Physiology of Domestic Animals*, 12e (ed. W.O. Reece), 892–903. Ithaca: Comstock Pub. Associates.

2 Garosi, L. (2009). Neurological examination of the cat. How to get started. *J. Feline Med. Surg.* 11 (5): 340–348.

3 Englar, R.E. (2017). *Performing the Small Animal Physical Examination*. Hoboken, NJ: Wiley.

4 Waterhouse, J. and Campbell, I. (2017). Reflexes: principles and properties. *Anaest. Intens. Care M.* 18 (5): 270–275.

5 Currie, W.B. (1988). *Structure and Function of Domestic Animals*. xiii, 443 p. Boston: Butterworths.

6 Houpt, R.T. (2004). Water and electrolytes. In: *Dukes' Physiology of Domestic Animals*, 12e (ed. H.H. Dukes and W.O. Reece), 12. Ithaca: Comstock Pub. Associates.

7 Norris, D.O. and Carr, J.A. (2013). *Organization of the Mammalian Hypothalamus–Pituitary Axes. Vertebrate Endocrinology*, 93–150. New York: Academic Press.

8 Carroll, R.G. (2007). Endocrine system. In: *Elsevier's Integrated Physiology* (ed. R.G. Carroll), 157–176. Philadelphia: Mosby.

9 Wilkin, T.J. (1997). Molecular and cellular endocrinology. In: *Principles of Medical Biology* (ed. T.J. Wilkin), 1–28. Elsevier.

10 Maeda, K. and Kurata, H. (2018). Long negative feedback loop enhances period tunability of biological oscillators. *J. Theor. Biol.* 440: 21–31.

11 Reece, W.O., Erickson, H.H., Goff, J.P., and Uemura, E.E. (2015). *Dukes' Physiology of Domestic Animals*, 13e, xii, 748 p. Ames, Iowa, USA: Wiley Blackwell.

12 Waldman, S.D. (2009). *The Spinal Reflex Arc. Pain Review*. Philaldelphia: Saunders.

13 Millis, D.L. and Mankin, J. (2014). Orthopedic and neurologic evaluation. In: *Canine Rehabilitation and Physical Therapy*, 2e (ed. D.L. Millis and D. Levine), 180–200. Philadelphia, PA: Elsevier.

14 Nye, C. and Troxel, M. (2017). The neurologic examination. *NAVC Clinician's Brief* (August): 61–69.

15 DeLahunta, A., Glass, E., and Kent, M. (2015). *Veterinary Neuroanatomy and Clinical Neurology*, 4e. St. Louis, MO: Elsevier.

16 Taylor, A.R. and Kerwin, S.C. (2018). Clinical evaluation of the feline neurologic patient. *Vet. Clin. North Am. Small Anim. Pract.* 48 (1): 1–10.

17 Thomas, W.B. and Dewey, C.W. (2008). Performing the neurologic examination. In: *A Practical Guide to Canine and Feline Neurology*, 2e (ed. C.W. Dewey), 53–74. Ames, Iowa: Wiley-Blackwell.

18 Thomas, W.B. (2000). Initial assessment of patients with neurologic dysfunction. *Vet. Clin. North Am. Small Anim. Pract.* 30 (1): 1–24, v.

19 de Lahunta, A. and Glass, E. (2009). The neurologic examination. In: *Veterinary Neuroanatomy and Clinical Neurology* (ed. A. de Lahunta and E. Glass), 487–501. St. Louis: Saunders Elsevier.

20 Gutierrez-Quintana, R., Edgar, J., Wessmann, A. et al. (2012). The cutaneous trunci reflex for localising and grading thoracolumbar spinal cord injuries in dogs. *J. Small Anim. Pract.* 53 (8): 470–475.

21 Holstege, G. and Blok, B.F. (1989). Descending pathways to the cutaneous trunci muscle motoneuronal cell group in the cat. *J. Neurophysiol.* 62 (6): 1260–1269.

22 Muguet-Chanoit, A.C., Olby, N.J., Babb, K.M. et al. (2011). The sensory field and repeatability of the cutaneous trunci muscle reflex of the dog. *Vet. Surg.* 40 (7): 781–785.

23 Averill, D.R. Jr. (1981). The neurologic examination. *Vet. Clin. North Am. Small Anim. Pract.* 11 (3): 511–521.

24 van Nes, J.J., Meij, B.P., and van Ham, L. (2009). Nervous system. In: *Medical History and Physical Examination in Companion Animals*, 2e (ed. A. Rijnberk and F.J. van Sluijs), 160–174. St. Louis: Saunders Elsevier.

25 Kent, M. (2005). Degenerative lumbosacral stenosis in dogs. DVM 360 [Internet]. http://veterinarymedicine.dvm360.com/degenerative-lumbosacral-stenosis-dogs.

26 Zeltzman, P. (2010). Making sense of the neuro exam. *Veterinary Practice News* (February).

27 Levine, J.M., Hillman, R.B., Erb, H.N., and deLahunta, A. (2002). The influence of age on patellar reflex response in the dog. *J. Vet. Intern. Med.* 16 (3): 244–246.

28 Stam, J., Speelman, H.D., and van Crevel, H. (1989). Tendon reflex asymmetry by voluntary mental effort in healthy subjects. *Arch. Neurol.* 46 (1): 70–73.

29 Ryushi, T., Fukunaga, T., Yuasa, K., and Nakajima, H. (1990). The influence of motor unit composition and stature on fractionated patellar reflex times in untrained men. *Eur. J. Appl. Physiol. Occup. Physiol.* 60 (1): 44–48.

30 Larsson, L. (1978). Morphological and functional characteristics of the ageing skeletal muscle in man. A cross-sectional study. *Acta Physiol. Scand. Suppl.* 457: 1–36.

31 Clarkson, P.M. (1978). The relationship of age and level of physical activity with the fractionated components of patellar reflex time. *J. Gerontol.* 33 (5): 650–656.

32 Balagopal, P., Rooyackers, O.E., Adey, D.B. et al. (1997). Effects of aging on in vivo synthesis of skeletal muscle myosin heavy-chain and sarcoplasmic protein in humans. *Am. J. Phys.* 273 (4 Pt 1): E790–E800.

33 Baumgartner, R.N., Stauber, P.M., McHugh, D. et al. (1995). Cross-sectional age differences in body composition in persons 60+ years of age. *J. Gerontol. A Biol. Sci. Med. Sci.* 50 (6): M307–M316.

34 Larsson, L. (1995). Motor units: remodeling in aged animals. *J. Gerontol. A Biol. Sci. Med. Sci.* 50 Spec No: 91–95.

35 Feldman, E.C. and Nelson, R.W. (2004). *Canine and Feline Endocrinology and Reproduction*, 3e. St. Louis, Mo.: Saunders.

36 Peterson, M.E. (2018). Hypocalcemia in dogs and cats. Merck Veterinary Manual [Internet]. https://www.merckvetmanual.com/endocrine-system/the-parathyroid-glands-and-disorders-of-calcium-metabolism/hypocalcemia-in-dogs-and-cats.

37 Brunker, J.D. (2007). Primary hypoparathyroidism in dogs and cats: Physiology, clinical signs, and initial diagnostic tests. DVM 360 [Internet]. http://veterinarymedicine.dvm360.com/primary-hypoparathyroidism-dogs-and-cats-physiology-clinical-signs-and-initial-diagnostic-tests.

38 Feldman, E.C. (2005). Disorders of the parathyroid glands. In: *Textbook of Veterinary Internal Medicine: Diseases of the Dog and Cat* (ed. S.J. Ettinger and E.C. Feldman), 1508–1535. St. Louis, MO: Elsevier Saunders.

39 Bruyette, D.S. and Feldman, E.C. (1988). Primary hypoparathyroidism in the dog. Report of 15 cases and review of 13 previously reported cases. *J. Vet. Intern. Med.* 2 (1): 7–14.

40 Waters, C.B. and Scottmoncrieff, J.C.R. (1992). Hypocalcemia in cats. *Comp. Cont. Educ. Pract.* 14 (4): 497–507.

41 Sherding, R.G., Meuten, D.J., Chew, D.J. et al. (1980). Primary hypoparathyroidism in the dog. *J. Am. Vet. Med. Assoc.* 176 (5): 439–444.

42 Chew, D.J. and Nagode, L.A. (2000). Treatment of hypoparathyroidism. In: *Kirk's Current Veterinary Therapy XIII: Small Animal Practice* (ed. J.D. Bonagura), 340–345. Philadelphia: WB Saunders Co.

43 Hall, J.A. (2018). Puerperal hypocalcemia in small animals. Merck Veterinary Manual [Internet]. https://www.merckvetmanual.com/metabolic-disorders/disorders-of-calcium-metabolism/puerperal-hypocalcemia-in-small-animals.

44 Drobatz, K.J. and Casey, K.K. (2000). Eclampsia in dogs: 31 cases (1995–1998). *J. Am. Vet. Med. Assoc.* 217 (2): 216–219.

45 Aroch, I., Srebro, H., and Shpigel, N.Y. (1999). Serum electrolyte concentrations in bitches with eclampsia. *Vet. Rec.* 145 (11): 318–320.

46 Gough, A. and Murphy, K.F. (2015). *Differential Diagnosis in Small Animal Medicine*, 2e. Chichester, West Sussex; Ames, Iowa: Wiley.

47 Bartges, J.W. (2012). Chronic kidney disease in dogs and cats. *Vet. Clin. North Am. Small Anim. Pract.* 42 (4): 669–692, vi.

48 Langston, C.E. and Eatroff, A.E. (2015). Chronic kidney disease. In: *Small Animal Critical Care Medicine* (ed. D.C. Silverstein and K. Hopper), 661–666. St. Louis, Mo.: Saunders/Elsevier.

49 Polzin, D.J. (2011). Chronic kidney disease in small animals. *Vet. Clin. North Am. Small Anim. Pract.* 41 (1): 15–30.

50 Tilley, L.P. and Smith, F.W.K. (2004). *The 5-Minute Veterinary Consult: Canine and Feline*, 3e. Baltimore, MD: Lippincott Williams & Wilkins.

74

Upper and Lower Motor Neuron Signs and Anatomic Localization of Disease

74.1 Introduction to the Organization of the Nervous System and Neuronal Pathways

The mammalian nervous system is complex [1].

For ease of organization, it is often considered as having two parts [1–4]:

- The central nervous system (CNS)
  - This includes the brain and spinal cord, which are protected by the skull and vertebral column, respectively.
- The peripheral nervous system (PNS)
  - This includes the autonomic and somatic nervous systems.

The CNS can be thought of as the body's control center [1]. It is responsible for receiving, integrating, interpreting, and responding to messages from all other parts of the body [1, 2].

In order to oversee physiologic functions, the CNS requires a network of cells that connect it to the periphery [1]. Neurons are the electrically charged messenger cells of the CNS [1–3]. They transmit information back and forth, between the periphery and the CNS [1–3].

Motor neurons are a specific type of neuron and are responsible for creating connections to effector organs [2].

There are upper motor neurons (UMNs) and lower motor neurons (LMNs) [2, 4]. UMNs originate from the brain and connect it to an appropriate spinal cord segment [2]. UMNs regulate posture and muscle tone, and modulate gait [2, 4]. UMNs are essentially inhibitory [4].

UMNs require intermediaries, LMNs, to transmit electrical signals to muscle fibers and glands [2]. UMN axons may synapse directly onto LMNs or they may synapse onto one or more interneurons that pass the electrical signal onto LMNs [2–4]. Either way, LMNs that receive a signal transmit it to effectors via cranial or spinal nerves [2]. When effectors are muscles, their response is to contract [2].

Neuromuscular dysfunction can result from a break at any point in this pathway [2, 4]. Depending upon which aspect of the pathway is broken, the patient may be said to have UMN or LMN disease [2].

74.2 UMN Dysfunction

UMN dysfunction is characterized by hyperreflexia [4–7]. This is due to loss of inhibition, causing excessive tone [8].

In addition to hyperreflexia, patients with UMN disease may demonstrate one of more of the following clinical signs [4–7]:

- Increased resting muscle tone
- Limb spasticity

Lesions cranial to L4 are likely to cause a so-called UMN bladder. Because there is a loss of inhibition to the bladder, the urethral sphincters are excessively toned. The urinary bladder will fill to the point that it overflows, but it will be difficult to express the urinary bladder.

74.3 LMN Dysfunction

LMN dysfunction is characterized by hyporeflexia [4–7].

In addition to hyporeflexia, patients with LMN disease may demonstrate one of more of the following clinical signs [4–7]:

- Flaccid posture due to loss of muscle tone
- Muscle atrophy
- Weakness

Lesions caudal to L4 are likely to cause a LMN bladder. Because the urethral sphincters lack tone, the urinary bladder will continuously dribble. The urinary bladder is easy to express and will only partially fill.

74.4 Anatomic Localization of Disease

Neuromuscular diseases can be frustrating in clinical practice because many presentations look alike. What facilitates diagnosis is that lesions of certain groups of spinal cord segments or nerves are associated with a characteristic mix of neurologic signs [4, 9, 10]:

- Brain or brainstem
- C1-C5
- C6-T2
- T3-L3
- L4-L6
- L7-S3

74.4.1 Forebrain and Brainstem Lesions

Recall from Chapter 71 that lesions in either of the cerebral hemispheres or within the ascending reticular activating system (ARAS) can alter the patient's mentation. Recall that mentation is a function of how the patient interacts with its environment, including the client. It encompasses awareness and may overlap with behavior [4].

Awareness is a sliding scale [11].

Refer back to Chapter 71, Section 71.1 to review the following descriptors of awareness [4, 10, 11]:

- Depressed
- Obtunded
- Stuporous
- Comatose

In addition to changes in awareness, clients may report one or more of the following forebrain or brainstem-associated clinical signs [4]:

- Aggression
- Compulsive behaviors
  - Circling
  - Head pressing
  - Pacing
- Disorientation
- Unusual or persistent vocalization

74.4.2 C1-C5 Lesions

C1-C5 lesions cause UMN signs in all four limbs [6, 7]. Affected patients will have:

- Exaggerated reflexes
- Increased muscle tone.

74.4.3 C6-T2 Lesions

C6-T2 lesions cause mixed signs [6, 7].

The thoracic limbs demonstrate LMN signs [6, 7]:

- Decreased muscle tone
- Decreased to absent reflexes

The pelvic limbs demonstrate UMN signs [6, 7].

Because the thoracic and pelvic limbs do not share the same presentation, the patient is sometimes said to have a two-engine gait. The appearance of what is going on in the forelimbs is very different from what is going on in the hind limbs.

74.4.4 T3-L3 Lesions

T3-L3 lesions have no impact on the thoracic limbs, which present as being normal in terms of reflexes [6, 7].

T3-L3 lesions cause UMN signs in the pelvic limbs only [6, 7].

74.4.5 L4-L6 Lesions

L4-L6 lesions also have no impact on the thoracic limbs, which present as being normal in terms of reflexes [6, 7].

L4-L6 lesions cause LMN signs in the pelvic limbs only [6, 7].

74.4.6 L7-S3 Lesions

L7-S3 lesions cause LMN signs to the tail and perineum [6, 7].

74.4.7 Revisiting the Purpose of Testing for Spinal Reflexes

Different nerves are associated with each spinal segment cluster.

Where do spinal reflexes fit in? Spinal reflexes help clinicians to test spinal cord segments by assessing the integrity of their associated nerves [4, 9, 10].

Recall the association of nerves and spinal reflexes, as was covered in Chapter 73 [4, 6, 7, 9–16]:

- Biceps reflex: Tests spinal cord segments C6-C8
- Extensor carpi radialis or triceps reflex: Tests spinal cord segments C7-T1
- Panniculus or cutaneous trunci reflex: Tests spinal cord segments C8-T1
- Patellar reflex: Tests spinal cord segments L4-L6
- Perineal reflex: Tests spinal cord segments S1-S3
- Withdrawal reflex
  - Thoracic limb: Tests spinal cord segments C6-T2
  - Pelvic limb: Tests spinal cord segments L4-S2

74.5 Differential Diagnoses for Spinal Cord Disease

When patients present for neuromuscular dysfunction, the list of differential diagnoses to consider is extensive.

Categorizing differentials using the so-called DAMNIT scheme may be helpful for the inexperienced clinician. Depending upon how many letters of each (D, A, M, N, I, and T) are incorporated into the acronym, there are several versions, one of which is outlined below [17, 18]:

- **D**egenerative***
- **D**evelopmental***
- **A**nomalous
- **A**utoimmune
- **M**etabolic
- **M**ental
- **N**utritional
- **N**eoplastic***
- **I**nflammatory***
- **I**nfectious***
- **I**schemic***
- **I**atrogenic
- **I**diopathic
- **T**raumatic***
- **T**oxicity

The categories that are starred above are most typical for presentations involving myelopathy in companion animal practice. Some of these will be touched upon in brief below.

74.5.1 Primary Differentials for C1-C5 Spinal Cord Disease

Primary differentials for diseases that affect C1-C5 include the following [19]:

- Degenerative
  - Intervertebral disc disease (IVDD)
- Developmental, small-breed dogs
  - Atlantoaxial subluxation
- Developmental, large-breed dogs
  - Cervical spondylomyelopathy or Wobbler Syndrome
- Inflammatory or infectious
  - Discospondylitis
  - Meningitis-arteritis
- Neoplastic
  - Meningiomas

Note that atlantoaxial subluxation may also result from trauma. Forceful flexion of the head, for example, may compromise ligamentous support between the first two cervical vertebrae and/or cause fracture of bone [20].

74.5.2 Primary Differentials for C6-T2 Spinal Cord Disease

Primary differentials for diseases that affect C6-T2 include the following [19]:

- Degenerative
  - IVDD
- Developmental, large-breed dogs
  - Cervical spondylomyelopathy
- Inflammatory or infectious
  - Discospondylitis
  - Osteomyelitis
- Ischemic
  - Fibrocartilaginous embolic myelopathy (FCEM)
- Neoplastic
- Traumatic

74.5.3 Primary Differentials for T3-L3 Spinal Cord Disease

Primary differentials for diseases that affect T3-L3 include the following [19]:

- Degenerative
  - Degenerative myelopathy
  - IVDD
- Inflammatory or infectious
  - Discospondylitis
  - Osteomyelitis
- Ischemic
  - FCEM
- Neoplastic
- Traumatic

74.5.4 Primary Differentials for L4-S3 Spinal Cord Disease

Primary differentials for diseases that affect L4-S3 include the following [19]:

- Degenerative
  - IVDD
- Ischemic
  - FCEM
- Neoplastic
- Traumatic

The goal of this chapter is not to introduce every differential, but to increase familiarity with those conditions that are likely to present in clinical practice.

74.6 Atlantoaxial Instability with Subluxation

Atlantoaxial instability with subluxation is a pathological condition of primarily small-breed dogs, especially the following [20–26]:

- Chihuahuas
- Miniature Poodles
- Pekingese
- Pomeranians
- Toy Poodles
- Yorkshire Terriers

Cats and large-breed dogs may be affected; however, these presentations are clinically rare [20, 27, 28].

Recall from basic anatomy that the atlantoaxial joint is formed by the articulation of the first cervical vertebra, the atlas, and the second cervical vertebra, the axis [20]. Stability to this region in the normal patient is in part provided by the dens, a projection of the axis, fitting into the atlas [20]. Additional ligamentous support, by way of the apical ligament of the dens and the paired alar ligaments, is stabilizing [20].

A functional atlantoaxial joint allows for motion of the head in a horizontal plane so that the head can turn left or right [20]. This is in contrast to the motion that is achieved at the atlanto-occipital joint, which concentrates on upward and downward motion of the head that corresponds to cervical extension and flexion.

Abnormal movement of the head and neck at the level of the atlantoaxial joint leads to instability [20]. Patients are affected by atlantoaxial instability to varying degrees; however, all are placed at risk of spinal cord compression [20, 29]. If compression is severe at this level of the spinal cord, respiratory paralysis and death may result [20, 30].

Affected patients are young and present for neck pain [20]. Dogs with atlantoaxial subluxation may be reluctant to engage in cervical ventroflexion [31–35]. Instead,

they may prefer to hold their head and neck parallel to the spine [31–35]. Forcing these patients to ventroflex at the level of the cervical spine is dangerous [20].

In addition to having neck pain, affected patients present with varying degrees of C1-C5 myelopathy, that is, UMN signs to all four limbs. Observation and physical examination findings may reveal one or more of the following changes [20, 23, 29, 36–44]:

- Ataxia
- Increased muscle tone
- Long-strided, spastic gait
- Paresis
- Tetraplegia

Survey radiography of the head and cervical spine provide a definitive diagnosis [20] (see Figure 74.1).

Advanced imaging in the form of computed tomography (CT) or magnetic resonance imaging (MRI) is of value in cases that involve surgical planning [20] (see Figure 74.2).

Surgical reduction of atlantoaxial subluxation is advised in those cases in which neck pain and/or neurological deficits persist in spite of medical management [20].

74.7 Cervical Spondylomyelopathy or Wobbler Syndrome

Whereas atlantoaxial instability with subluxation is most likely to occur in small-breed dogs, cervical spondylomyelopathy is most common among large and giant breeds [45]. In particular, Great Danes, Doberman Pinschers, and Dalmatians are overrepresented [45–52].

The spinal cord of affected patients is compressed, causing neck pain and neurological deficits [45].

Spinal cord lesions may be dynamic, meaning that myelopathy is positional [45, 53–55]. The patient's condition may change for the better or for the worse,

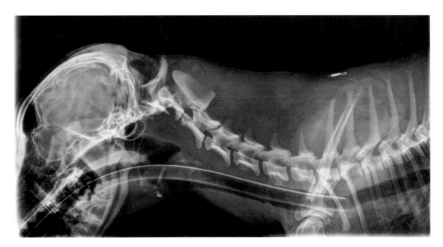

Figure 74.1 This left lateral radiograph is diagnosis for atlantoaxial subluxation in a canine patient. *Source:* Courtesy of Daniel Foy, MS, DVM, DACVIM, DACVECC.

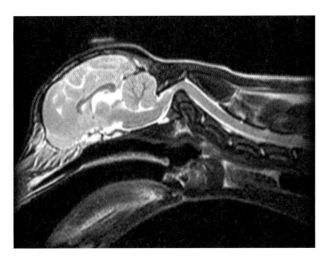

Figure 74.2 Same patient as in Figure 74.1, using magnetic resonance imaging (MRI) as an imaging tool. *Source:* Courtesy of Daniel Foy, MS, DVM, DACVIM, DACVECC.

depending upon how the cervical spine is positioned in space [45, 56].

In middle-aged Doberman Pinschers, spinal cord compression often occurs at the caudal cervical discs [45]. C5-C6 and C6-C7 are most commonly involved [45]. This may be because the caudal cervical spine experiences more torsion than the cranial cervical spine [57].

Congenital vertebral canal stenosis in affected patients exacerbates spinal cord compression, making patients more likely to be symptomatic [45].

Spinal cord compression may also result from vertebral malformations and/or proliferation of the articular facets or the vertebral arch [45, 48, 53, 58, 59]. These presentations are more common among young, giant breeds [45].

In addition to having neck pain, patients with cervical spondylomyelopathy tend to demonstrate one or more of the following signs [45]:

- Proprioceptive ataxia +/− conscious proprioceptive (CP) deficits
  - Cranial cervical lesions should affect all four limbs equally with ataxia.
  - Caudal cervical lesions tend to make ataxia more pronounced in the pelvic limbs than in the thoracic limbs.
- Spastic gait that is sometimes described as "floating"
  - This gait is similar in appearance to hypermetria in that it is stiff; however, it lacks hyperflexion of the thoracic limb joints.
- Tetraparesis
- Toed-in posture, meaning that the digits rotate toward the midline
- "Two-engine" gait, in the presence of caudal cervical lesions, most pronounced at a slow walk

- Short-strides associated with the thoracic limbs
- Long-strides associated with the pelvic limbs
- Wide-based pelvic stance

Spinal radiographs are helpful in terms of ruling out trauma, neoplasia, osteomyelitis, and discospondylitis.

Sclerosis will be evident in those giant-breed dogs with osseous compression.

Myelography, CT, and MRI are superior to spinal radiographs in that these imaging modalities can detect and confirm spinal cord compression [45]. Of these, MRI offers the greatest accuracy [60].

Case management for cervical spondylomyelopathy may be medical or surgical, depending upon patient presentation and severity of disease. A number of decompressive surgical techniques have been described in the veterinary literature.

74.8 Intervertebral Disc Disease (IVDD)

Recall from basic anatomy that intervertebral discs are essentially spacers between all vertebrae except the first and second, and the fused sacrum [61].

Conceptually, discs are a bit like jelly donuts. They have a gelatinous core, the nucleus pulposus, surrounded by an outer ring, the annulus fibrosus [61, 62].

74.8.1 Hansen Type 1 Intervertebral Disc Disease (IVDD)

As dogs and cats age, their intervertebral discs naturally degenerate [61, 63, 64]. Their water content decreases, and they are less able to withstand pressure [65, 66]. This predisposes the aged patient to disc herniation.

The nucleus pulposus is eccentrically located. When it herniates, it does so dorsally, toward the vertebral canal. This disc extrusion is called Hansen Type 1 intervertebral disc disease (IVDD) [61, 62, 67].

Disc degeneration occurs sooner in life in chondrodystrophic breeds. Dachshunds, for example, are estimated to have lost three-quarters of their gelatinous nucleus pulposus by one year of age [64–66, 68–70].

Dachshunds also tend to have discs that calcify as they age. Depending upon the study, up to 90% of dachshunds may develop mineralization with an average of 2.3 calcified discs per dog [64, 66, 71, 72]. In particular, discs between T10 and T13 are most likely to calcify and image radiographically [61, 71–74].

Small- to medium-sized dogs appear to be at an increased risk of developing Hansen Type 1 IVDD, especially chondrodystrophic breeds [61, 75]. The likelihood that a Dachshund will develop IVDD is 12.6 times greater than other breeds [75]. Among small- to medium-sized breeds, the Pekingese, Beagle, and Cocker Spaniel are also predisposed [75]. IVDD preferentially occurs in the cervical spine of the Beagle [76]. The cervical spine is also more likely to be involved when IVDD occurs in geriatric populations [76].

Among the large-breed dogs, Hansen Type 1 IVDD also occurs with greater frequency in Doberman Pinschers, Rottweilers, Dalmatians, and Labrador Retrievers [77–79].

74.8.2   Hansen Type 2 IVDD

The annulus fibrosus can also undergo degeneration as the patient ages. Whereas degeneration of the nucleus pulposus tends to occur along the entire length of the spine, degeneration of the annulus fibrosus tends to be focal. Mineralization rarely occurs, but older, non-chondrodystrophic dogs are most at risk. In these patients, the nucleus pulposus pushes against the weakened annulus fibrosus. The end result is disc protrusion, referred to as Hansen Type II IVDD [61, 64, 66].

74.8.3   Classic Case Presentations of IVDD

IVDD is more common in dogs than cats [80]. In both species, it may occur at any location along the spine. However, it is most likely to occur in the thoracolumbar or cervical regions [75, 76, 81].

74.8.3.1   Thoracolumbar Spine

Thoracolumbar disc disease represents the majority of case presentations for IVDD [75, 76, 81]. Affected patients guard their back because of spinal pain. This may cause them to appear stiff.

Affected patients may also present with paraparesis or paraplegia, and loss of deep pain [61].

They may exhibit knuckling. Recall from Chapter 72, Section 72.3.4 that knuckling refers to scuffing or standing upon the dorsal aspect of one or more feet. This occurs when patients have proprioceptive or sensory ataxia. They lose their perspective of where their limbs are positioned in space [82].

When the thoracolumbar region of the spine is affected by IVDD, T12-T13 and T13-L1 are most often implicated in chondrodystrophic breeds [64, 76, 83–91].

By contrast, T13-L1 and L1-2 predominate, followed by L2-L3, in large-breed dogs [77, 78].

74.8.3.2   Cervical Spine

Cervical disc disease represents up to one-quarter of all case presentations for IVDD [75, 76, 81]. Patients frequently guard their neck because of cervical pain. Patients also tend to present for neurological deficits, including knuckling [32, 92–95].

When considering all dogs, regardless of size, disc disease at C5-C6 [96] and C6-C7 predominates [32].

In small-breed dogs, C3 is the most often reported disc to be affected [32, 76, 79, 93, 94] compared to C6-C7 in large-breed dogs [79].

74.9   Fibrocartilaginous Embolic Myelopathy

FCEM is a condition in which focal blood supply to one or more regions of the spinal cord becomes occluded by material that is thought to originate from an intervertebral disc [97]. When the blood supply is compromised, dependent areas of the spinal cord become ischemic [97].

Onset is peracute [97]. Patient histories vary. Many clients report physical activity at the time of onset. Some clients share that the patient yelped prior to becoming symptomatic [97–99].

Neurologic deficits depend upon the regions affected and the severity of the vascular occlusion; however, lesions are most often asymmetric [97–100].

By 24 hours after onset, clinical signs do not typically progress [97–100]. Clinical signs either remain static, or they improve with time [97–100].

The following regions of the spinal cord appear to be predisposed [97–100]:

- C6-T2
- T3-L3
- L4-S3

Large and giant-breed dogs are overrepresented in the veterinary literature [97].

Small-breed dogs are not immune to FCEM, and in fact, Miniature Schnauzers and chondrodystrophic patients appear to be at heightened risk [98, 99, 101–104].

In dogs, this is not typically a disease of the aged: the median age at presentation is five to six years old [97–100]. However, cats with FCEM tend to be older than seven years of age at the time of onset [105, 106].

Histopathology is the only way to obtain definitive diagnosis. Presumptive diagnosis is based upon the typical presentation.

Coagulation profiles and echocardiography are frequently performed in cases of presumptive FCEM to evaluate for pre-existing conditions that can trigger thromboembolic disease [97]. Cats, in particular, benefit from screening for cardiomyopathy, hyperthyroidism, hypertension, and chronic kidney disease (CKD) [97].

Treatment is aimed at supportive care and keeping the paretic or paraplegic patient safe [97].

FCEM is not thought to be a painful condition.

Physiotherapy is believed to be beneficial. It may reduce the incidence and/or the severity of muscle atrophy and joint contracture [97].

74.10 Canine Degenerative Myelopathy

Canine degenerative myelopathy is a pathological condition that mirrors human amyotrophic lateral sclerosis (ALS) or so-called Lou Gehrig disease [107, 108]. It is characterized by progressive, but non-painful paresis that develops into paraplegia [107].

Canine degenerative myelopathy is typically a disease of the middle-aged patient [107].

Many breeds of dog have been affected by this condition [107]. However, most of the earliest reported cases in the medical literature involve German shepherds, Boxers, and other large breeds [107, 109–111].

Early case reports describe UMN spastic paraparesis with associated pelvic limb ataxia [107].

Clinical signs typically progress from UMN dysfunction in the hind end to LMN paralysis that ultimately extends into the thoracic limbs [107–109, 112–115].

Affected patients may also develop cranial nerve dysfunction, such as dysphagia [107, 108, 112, 114].

Clients may report an abnormal, weakened, or absent bark [107, 108, 112, 114].

The disease is debilitating in terms of mobility, but does not appear to be painful [107].

Quality of life issues arise as affected dogs become incapable of supporting their weight. Clients may struggle to manage mobility, particularly in large-breed patients, and urinary and fecal incontinence may become obstacles to indoor lifestyles [107–109, 112–114].

Definitive diagnosis is obtained, post-mortem, via histopathology [107]. Presumptive diagnosis is based upon the typical presentation and its progression [107].

74.11 Spinal Neoplasia

Spinal neoplasia may be primary or metastatic [116–124].

Spinal neoplasia also varies in terms of location in that tumors may be [116]

- Intramedullary, that is, within the spinal cord itself
- Intradural/extramedullary, that is, outside of the spinal cord, but within the connective tissue that encases the brain and spinal cord, the dura mater
- Extradural, that is, outside of the dura mater.

74.11.1 Extradural Spinal Neoplasia

When spinal neoplasia arises in the dog or cat, it is typically extradural [116]. Primary and secondary bone tumors are common, including the following [116]:

- Chondrosarcoma
- Fibrosarcoma
- Osteosarcoma

Other common types of extradural spinal neoplasia include the following [116, 122, 125, 126]:

- Carcinoma
- Hemangiosarcoma
- Lymphosarcoma
- Multiple myeloma
- Plasma cell tumor

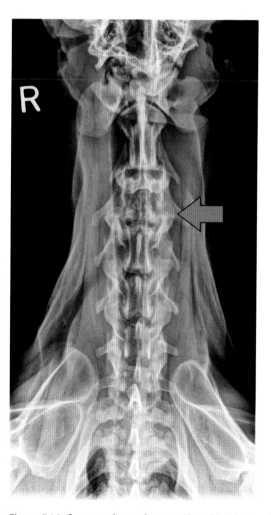

Figure 74.3 Survey radiograph, ventrodorsal (V/D) view. Canine patient with osteolysis at the level of C3. *Source:* Courtesy of Daniel Foy, MS, DVM, DACVIM, DACVECC.

Lymphosarcoma is by far the most common type of spinal neoplasia in cats [125–127]. Cats tend to present for spinal lymphosarcoma at younger ages than might be expected. The tumor is also rarely restricted to the spine [116]. Most cats develop multiple lesions throughout the body [116].

74.11.2 Intradural/Extramedullary Spinal Neoplasia

Meningiomas and nerve sheath tumors are more likely to be intradural/extramedullary [116, 128–134].

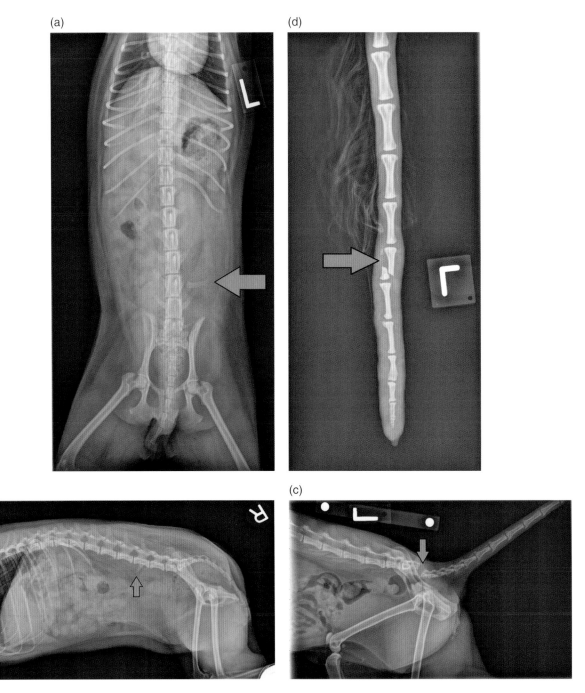

Figure 74.4 (a) Survey radiograph, ventrodorsal (V/D) view. Canine patient with a transverse fracture of L5. *Source:* Courtesy of Daniel Foy, MS, DVM, DACVIM, DACVECC. (b) Orthogonal radiographic view of the patient depicted in Figure 74.4a. *Source:* Courtesy of Daniel Foy, MS, DVM, DACVIM, DACVECC. (c) Survey radiograph, left lateral view. Canine patient with a sacral fracture. *Source:* Courtesy of Daniel Foy, MS, DVM, DACVIM, DACVECC. (d) Survey radiograph, left lateral view. Canine patient with a coccygeal fracture. *Source:* Courtesy of Daniel Foy, MS, DVM, DACVIM, DACVECC.

When meningiomas occur, they preferentially select the cervical spine [116]. Their second choice of location is the lumbar spine [116]. Rarely do they involve the thoracic spine [116].

Peripheral nerves often become involved in cases of spinal neoplasia [116]. When this occurs, patient presentations reflect LMN dysfunction [116]. In particular, patients lose muscular tone and develop extensive atrophy [116]. Reflexes of affected spinal segments are decreased to absent [116].

Nerve sheath tumors are common presentations that involve the PNS [116]. These most typically involve the thoracic limb; however, any nerve in the body can be affected [116]. Nerve sheath tumors are palpable along the length of the nerve and are chronically painful [116].

74.11.3 Intramedullary Spinal Neoplasia

Astrocytomas, oligodendrogliomas, and ependymomas are the most common types of intramedullary tumors [116, 128, 129, 135, 136].

74.11.4 Diagnostic Approach to Spinal Neoplasia

Diagnostic imaging is valuable when evaluating a patient for spinal neoplasia. Survey radiographs may demonstrate osteolysis [116] (see Figure 74.3).

Note that osteolysis is not pathognomonic for spinal neoplasia; however, it is frequently present in aggressive bone diseases such as osteosarcoma.

Osteolysis may be confused with osteomyelitis and/or diskospondylitis [116].

Historically, myelography was used to establish the diagnosis of spinal cord compression [116]. Procedural steps and interpretations of myelograms are beyond the scope of this text. Consult a diagnostic radiology text for details as time and interest allow.

Note that MRI is superior to myelography for evaluation of spinal neoplasia because it is noninvasive [116, 137]. It also provides a detailed description of soft tissue structures that may be involved in neoplastic disease [116, 138].

74.12 Vertebral Fractures

Vertebral fractures are common traumatic injuries in companion animal patients [139]. Vehicular accidents, high-rise syndrome, and gunshot wounds, including air gun pellets, are frequently implicated in the veterinary literature as causing this kind of trauma [139–144].

Less commonly, fractures may occur secondary to osteolytic tumors that weaken one or more vertebrae [139].

Vertebral fractures may occur at any point in the vertebral column, and cause compression, bruising, and/or mechanical trauma of the spinal cord [139] (see Figures 74.4a–d).

Fractures of the cervical region are uncommon except for those involving the axis [139]. When patients run into objects at full speed, the cervical region is forced into flexion under extreme pressure [139]. This increases the risk of fracturing the dens [139].

Fractures rarely occur at the level of the thoracic vertebrae [139]. This may be because this segment of the spine is very rigid [139].

Many fractures occur at the thoracolumbar junction, especially T10-T12 [139, 142, 143].

Lumbar vertebral fractures are also relatively frequent [139].

Cats are more likely than dogs to fracture the sacrococcygeal region [139]. This is often the result of a traction injury. Cats are also likely to get their tails caught, stepped on, or run over [139, 145].

Survey radiographs are diagnostic for vertebral fractures in the majority of cases [139, 146]. Up to 10% of patients have radiographic evidence of more than one vertebral fracture [139, 141, 142].

Although surgical repair is indicated for patients that exhibit severe neurological deficits and are decompensating, most can be managed without going to surgery [139, 140, 144, 147–150].

References

1 Behan, M. (2004). Organization of the nervous system. In: *Dukes' Physiology of Domestic Animals*, 12e (ed. W.O. Reece), 757–769. Ithaca: Comstock Publishing Associates.

2 Molenaar, G.J. (1996). The nervous system. In: *Textbook of Veterinary Anatomy*, 2e (ed. K.M. Dyce, W.O. Sack and C.J.G. Wensing), 259–324. Philadelphia: W.B. Saunders Company.

3 Kitchell, R.L. Introduction to the nervous system. In: *Miller's Anatomy of the Dog*, 3e (ed. H.E. Evans), 758–775. Philadelphia: Saunders.

4 Garosi, L. (2009). Neurological examination of the cat. How to get started. *J. Feline Med. Surg.* 11 (5): 340–348.

5 Schubert, T. (2018). Physical and neurologic examinations. Merck Veterinary Manual [Internet]. https://www.merckvetmanual.com/nervous-system/

nervous-system-introduction/physical-and-neurologic-examinations.

6 Millis, D.L. and Mankin, J. (2014). Orthopedic and neurologic evaluation. In: *Canine Rehabilitation and Physical Therapy*, 2e (ed. D.L. Millis and D. Levine), 180–200. Philadelphia, PA: Elsevier.

7 DeLahunta, A., Glass, E., and Kent, M. (2015). *Veterinary Neuroanatomy and Clinical Neurology*, 4e. St. Louis, MO: Elsevier.

8 Brashear, A. (2005). Spasticity. In: *Animal Models of Movement Disorders* (ed. M. LeDoux), 679–686. London: Elsevier Academic Press.

9 Thomas, W.B. (2000). Initial assessment of patients with neurologic dysfunction. *Vet. Clin. North Am. Small Anim. Pract.* 30 (1): 1–24, v.

10 Thomas, W.B. and Dewey, C.W. (2008). Performing the neurologic examination. In: *A Practical Guide to Canine and Feline Neurology*, 2e (ed. C.W. Dewey), 53–74. Ames, Iowa: Wiley-Blackwell.

11 Englar, R.E. (2017). *Performing the Small Animal Physical Examination*. Hoboken, NJ: Wiley.

12 de Lahunta, A. and Glass, E. (2009). The neurologic examination. In: *Veterinary Neuroanatomy and Clinical Neurology* (ed. A. de Lahunta and E. Glass), 487–501. St. Louis: Saunders Elsevier.

13 Gutierrez-Quintana, R., Edgar, J., Wessmann, A. et al. (2012). The cutaneous trunci reflex for localising and grading thoracolumbar spinal cord injuries in dogs. *J. Small Anim. Pract.* 53 (8): 470–475.

14 Holstege, G. and Blok, B.F. (1989). Descending pathways to the cutaneous trunci muscle motoneuronal cell group in the cat. *J. Neurophysiol.* 62 (6): 1260–1269.

15 Muguet-Chanoit, A.C., Olby, N.J., Babb, K.M. et al. (2011). The sensory field and repeatability of the cutaneous trunci muscle reflex of the dog. *Vet. Surg.* 40 (7): 781–785.

16 Nye, C. and Troxel, M. (2017). The neurologic examination. *NAVC Clinician's Brief* (August): 61–69.

17 Osborne, C.A. (2005). 'DAMN-IT' acronym offers practical diagnostic aid. DVM 360 [Internet]. http://veterinarynews.dvm360.com/damn-it-acronym-offers-practical-diagnostic-aid.

18 Lorenz, M.D., Neer, T.M., and Demars, P.L. (2009). *Small Animal Medical Diagnosis*, 3e, xv, 502 p. Ames, Iowa: Wiley-Blackwell.

19 da Costa, R.C. and Moore, S.A. (2010). Differential diagnosis of spinal diseases. *Vet. Clin. North Am. Small Anim. Pract.* 40: 755–763.

20 Slanina, M.C. (2016). Atlantoaxial instability. *Vet. Clin. North Am. Small Anim. Pract.* 46 (2): 265–275.

21 Denny, H.R., Gibbs, C., and Waterman, A. (1988). Atlantoaxial subluxation in the dog: a review of thirty cases and evaluation of treatment by lag screw fixation. *J. Small Anim. Pract.* 29: 37–47.

22 Dewey, C.W. and da Costa, R.C. (2016). Myelopathies: disorders of the spinal cord. In: *Practical Guide to Canine and Feline Neurology* (ed. C.W. Dewey and R.C. da Costa), 329–405. Ames, IA: Wiley-Blackwell.

23 Havig, M.E., Cornell, K.K., Hawthorne, J.C. et al. (2005). Evaluation of nonsurgical treatment of atlantoaxial subluxation in dogs: 19 cases (1992–2001). *J. Am. Vet. Med. Assoc.* 227 (2): 257–262.

24 Mccarthy, R.J., Lewis, D.D., and Hosgood, G. (1995). Atlantoaxial subluxation in dogs. *Compend. Contin. Educ. Pract.* 17 (2): 215–227.

25 Wheeler, S.J. and NJH, S. (eds.) (1994). Atlantoaxial subluxation. In: *Small Animal Spinal Disorders: Diagnosis and Surgery*, 109–121. London: Mosby-Wolfe.

26 Nanai, B. (2005). Conservative treatment of atlantoaxial subluxation in canine patients. DVM 360 [Internet]. http://veterinarynews.dvm360.com/conservative-treatment-atlantoaxial-subluxation-canine-patients.

27 Jaggy, A., Hutto, V.L., and Roberts, R.E. (1991). Occipitoatlantoaxial malformation with atlantoaxial subluxation in a cat. *J. Small Anim. Pract.* 32: 366–372.

28 Huibregtse, B.A., Smith, C.W., and Fagin, B.D. (1992). A practitioner case-report – atlantoaxial luxation in a Doberman-Pinscher. *Canine Pract.* 17 (5): 7–10.

29 Platt, S.R. and da Costa, R.C. (2012). Cervical spine. In: *Veterinary Surgery* (ed. K.M. Tobias and S.A. Johnston), 410–448. St. Louis: Elsevier/Saunders.

30 Geary, J., Oliver, J., and Hoerlein, B.F. (1967). Atlantoaxial subluxation in the canine. *J. Small Anim. Pract.* 8: 577–582.

31 Rusbridge, C. (2005). Neurological diseases of the Cavalier King Charles spaniel. *J. Small Anim. Pract.* 46 (6): 265–272.

32 Ryan, T.M., Platt, S.R., Llabres-Diaz, F.J. et al. (2008). Detection of spinal cord compression in dogs with cervical intervertebral disc disease by magnetic resonance imaging. *Vet. Rec.* 163 (1): 11–15.

33 Loughin, C.A. and Marino, D.J. (2016). Atlantooccipital overlap and other craniocervical junction abnormalities in dogs. *Vet. Clin. North Am. Small* 46 (2): 243–251.

34 Freeman, A.C., Platt, S.R., Kent, M. et al. (2014). Chiari-like malformation and syringomyelia in American Brussels Griffon dogs. *J. Vet. Intern. Med.* 28 (5): 1551–1559.

35 Linon, E., Geissbuhler, U., Karli, P., and Forterre, F. (2014). Atlantoaxial epidural abscess secondary to grass awn migration in a dog. *Vet. Comp. Orthop.* 27 (2): 155–158.

36 Aikawa, T., Shibata, M., and Fujita, H. (2013). Modified ventral stabilization using positively threaded profile

pins and polymethylmethacrylate for atlantoaxial instability in 49 dogs. *Vet. Surg.* 42 (6): 683–692.

37 Thomas, W.B., Sorjonen, D.C., and Simpson, S.T. (1991). Surgical management of atlantoaxial subluxation in 23 dogs. *Vet. Surg.* 20 (6): 409–412.

38 Platt, S.R., Chambers, J.N., and Cross, A. (2004). A modified ventral fixation for surgical management of atlantoaxial subluxation in 19 dogs. *Vet. Surg.* 33 (4): 349–354.

39 Sanchez-Masian, D., Lujan-Feliu-Pascual, A., Font, C., and Mascort, J. (2014). Dorsal stabilization of atlantoaxial subluxation using non-absorbable sutures in toy breed dogs. *Vet. Comp. Orthop. Traumatol.* 27 (1): 62 67.

40 Shores, A. and Tepper, L.C. (2007). A modified ventral approach to the atlantoaxial junction in the dog. *Vet. Surg.* 36 (8): 765–770.

41 Stalin, C., Gutierrez-Quintana, R., Faller, K. et al. (2015). A review of canine atlantoaxial joint subluxation. *Vet. Comp. Orthop. Traumatol.* 28 (1): 1–8.

42 Jeffery, N.D. (1996). Dorsal cross pinning of the atlantoaxial joint: new surgical technique for atlantoaxial subluxation. *J. Small Anim. Pract.* 37 (1): 26–29.

43 Dickomeit, M., Alves, L., Pekarkova, M. et al. (2011). Use of a 1.5 mm butterfly locking plate for stabilization of atlantoaxial pathology in three toy breed dogs. *Vet. Comp. Orthop. Traumatol.* 24 (3): 246–251.

44 Beaver, D.P., Ellison, G.W., Lewis, D.D. et al. (2000). Risk factors affecting the outcome of surgery for atlantoaxial subluxation in dogs: 46 cases (1978–1998). *J. Am. Vet. Med. Assoc.* 216 (7): 1104–1109.

45 da Costa, R.C. (2010). Cervical spondylomyelopathy (wobbler syndrome) in dogs. *Vet. Clin. North Am. Small Anim. Pract.* 40 (5): 881–913.

46 da Costa, R.C., Parent, J.M., Holmberg, D.L. et al. (2008). Outcome of medical and surgical treatment in dogs with cervical spondylomyelopathy: 104 cases (1988–2004). *J. Am. Vet. Med. Assoc.* 233 (8): 1284–1290.

47 Burbidge, H.M., Pfeiffer, D.U., and Blair, H.T. (1994). Canine wobbler syndrome: a study of the Dobermann pinscher in New Zealand. *N. Z. Vet. J.* 42 (6): 221–228.

48 Denny, H.R., Gibbs, C., and Gaskell, C.J. (1977). Cervical spondylopathy in the dog – a review of thirty-five cases. *J. Small Anim. Pract.* 18 (2): 117–132.

49 McKee, W.M., Butterworth, S.J., and Scott, H.W. (1999). Management of cervical spondylopathy-associated intervertebral, disc protrusions using metal washers in 78 dogs. *J. Small Anim. Pract.* 40 (10): 465–472.

50 Seim, H.B. and Withrow, S.J. (1982). Patho-physiology and diagnosis of caudal cervical spondylo-myelopathy with emphasis on the Doberman-Pinscher. *J. Am. Anim. Hosp. Assoc.* 18 (2): 241–251.

51 Trotter, E.J., Delahunta, A., Geary, J.C., and Brasmer, T.H. (1976). Caudal cervical vertebral malformation malarticulation in Great Danes and Doberman Pinschers. *J. Am. Vet. Med. Assoc.* 168 (10): 917–930.

52 Lewis, D.G. (1989). Cervical spondylomyelopathy (wobbler syndrome) in the dog – a study based on 224 cases. *J. Small Anim. Pract.* 30 (12): 657–665.

53 de Costa, R.C., Echandi, R.L., and Beauchamp, D. (2009). Computed tomographic findings in large and giant breed dogs with cervical spondylomyelopathy: 58 cases. *J. Vet. Intern. Med.* 23 (3): 709.

54 Gray, M.J., Kirberger, R.M., and Spotswood, T.C. (2003). Cervical spondylomyelopathy (wobbler syndrome) in the Boerboel. *J. S. Afr. Vet. Assoc.* 74 (4): 104–110.

55 Levine, D.N. (1997). Pathogenesis of cervical spondylotic myelopathy. *J. Neurol. Neurosurg. Psychiatry* 62 (4): 334–340.

56 White, A.A. 3rd and Panjabi, M.M. (1988). Biomechanical considerations in the surgical management of cervical spondylotic myelopathy. *Spine (Phila Pa 1976)* 13 (7): 856–860.

57 Breit, S. and Kunzel, W. (2002). Shape and orientation of articular facets of cervical vertebrae (C3-C7) in dogs denoting axial rotational ability: an osteological study. *Eur. J. Morphol.* 40 (1): 43–51.

58 Lipsitz, D., Levitski, R.E., Chauvet, A.E., and Berry, W.L. (2001). Magnetic resonance imaging features of cervical stenotic myelopathy in 21 dogs. *Vet. Radiol. Ultrasound* 42 (1): 20–27.

59 da Costa, R.C. and Parent, J.M. (2009). Magnetic resonance imaging findings in 60 dogs with cervical spondylomyelopathy. *J. Vet. Intern. Med.* 13 (3): 181–186.

60 da Costa, R.C., Parent, J.P., and Dobson, H. (2006). Comparison of magnetic resonance imaging and myelography in 18 Doberman pinscher dogs with cervical spondylomyelopathy. *Vet. Radiol. Ultrasound* 47 (6): 523–531.

61 Brisson, B.A. (2010). Intervertebral disc disease in dogs. *Vet. Clin. North Am. Small Anim. Pract.* 40 (5): 829–858.

62 King, A.S. and Smith, R.N. (1955). A comparison of the anatomy of the intervertebral disc in dog and man: with reference to herniation of the nucleus pulposus. *Br. Vet. J.* 3: 135–149.

63 Modic, M.T., Masaryk, T.J., Ross, J.S., and Carter, J.R. (1988). Imaging of degenerative disk disease. *Radiology* 168 (1): 177–186.

64 Hansen, H.J. (1952). A pathologic-anatomical study on disc degeneration in dog, with special reference to the so-called enchondrosis intervertebralis. *Acta Orthop. Scand. Suppl.* 11: 1–117.

65 Ghosh, P., Taylor, T.K., and Braund, K.G. (1977). The variation of the glycosaminoglycans of the canine intervertebral disc with ageing. I. Chondrodystrophoid breed. *Gerontology* 23 (2): 87–98.

66 Hansen, H.J. (1959). Comparative views of the pathology of disk degeneration in animals. *Lab. invest.* (8): 1242–1265.

67 Evans, H.E. and Miller, M.E. (1993). *Miller's Anatomy of the Dog*, 3e, xvi, 1113 p. Philadelphia: W.B. Saunders.

68 Ghosh, P., Taylor, T.K., and Braund, K.G. (1976). A comparative chemical and histological study of the chondrodystrophoid and nonchondrodystrophoid canine intervertebral disc. *Vet. Pathol.* 13: 414–427.

69 Ghosh, P., Taylor, T.K., Braund, K.G., and Larsen, L.H. (1976). The collagenous and non-collagenous protein of the canine intervertebral disc and their variation with age, spinal level and breed. *Gerontology* 22 (3): 124–134.

70 Ghosh, P., Taylor, T.K., and Braund, K.G. (1977). Variation of the glycosaminoglycans of the intervertebral disc with ageing. II. Non-chondrodystrophoid breed. *Gerontology* 23 (2): 99–109.

71 Jensen, V.F. (2001). Asymptomatic radiographic disappearance of calcified intervertebral disc material in the Dachshund. *Vet. Radiol. Ultrasound* 42 (2): 141–148.

72 Jensen, V.F. and Arnbjerg, J. (2001). Development of intervertebral disk calcification in the dachshund: a prospective longitudinal radiographic study. *J. Am. Anim. Hosp. Assoc.* 37 (3): 274–282.

73 Jensen, V.F., Beck, S., Christensen, K.A., and Arnbjerg, J. (2008). Quantification of the association between intervertebral disk calcification and disk herniation in Dachshunds. *J. Am. Vet. Med. Assoc.* 233 (7): 1090–1095.

74 Stigen, O. (1991). Calcification of intervertebral discs in the dachshund. A radiographic study of 327 young dogs. *Acta Vet. Scand.* 32: 197–203.

75 Goggin, J.E., Li, A.S., and Franti, C.E. (1970). Canine intervertebral disk disease: characterization by age, sex, breed, and anatomic site of involvement. *Am. J. Vet. Res.* 31 (9): 1687–1692.

76 Gage, E.D. (1975). Incidence of clinical disc disease in the dog. *J. Am. Anim. Hosp. Assoc.* 11: 135–138.

77 Cudia, S.P. and Duval, J.M. (1997). Thoracolumbar intervertebral disk disease in large, nonchondrodystrophic dogs: a retrospective study. *J. Am. Anim. Hosp. Assoc.* 33 (5): 456–460.

78 Macias, C., McKee, W.M., May, C., and Innes, J.F. (2002). Thoracolumbar disc disease in large dogs: a study of 99 cases. *J. Small Anim. Pract.* 43 (10): 439–446.

79 Cherrone, K.L., Dewey, C.W., Coates, J.R., and Bergman, R.L. (2004). A retrospective comparison of cervical intervertebral disk disease in

nonchondrodystrophic large dogs versus small dogs. *J. Am. Anim. Hosp. Assoc.* 40 (4): 316–320.

80 Marioni-Henry, K. (2010). Feline spinal cord diseases. *Vet. Clin. North Am. Small Anim. Pract.* 40 (5): 1011–1028.

81 Hansen, H.J. (1951). A pathologic-anatomical interpretation of disc degeneration in dogs. *Acta Orthop. Scand. Suppl.* 20: 280–293.

82 Casimiro da Costa, R. (ed.) (2009). Ataxia – recognition and approach. World Small Animal Veterinary Association World Congress Proceedings.

83 Hoerlein, B.F. (1953). Intervertebral disc protrusions in the dog. Incidence and pathological lesions. *Am. J. Vet. Res.* 14: 260–269.

84 Brown, N.O., Helphrey, M.L., and Prata, R.G. (1977). Thoracolumbar disk disease in the dog: a retrospective analysis of 187 cases. *J. Am. Anim. Hosp. Assoc.* 13: 665–672.

85 Knecht, C.D. (1972). Results of surgical treatment for thoracolumbar disc protrusion. *J. Small Anim. Pract.* 13: 449–453.

86 Levine, J.M., Fosgate, A.V., and Rushing, C.R. (2009). Magnetic resonance imaging in dogs with neurological impairment due to acute thoracic and lumbar intervertebral disc herniation. *J. Vet. Intern. Med.* 23: 1220–1226.

87 Brisson, B.A., Moffatt, S.L., Swayne, S.L., and Parent, J.M. (2004). Recurrence of thoracolumbar intervertebral disk extrusion in chondrodystrophic dogs after surgical decompression with or without prophylactic fenestration: 265 cases (1995–1999). *J. Am. Vet. Med. Assoc.* 224 (11): 1808–1814.

88 Tanaka, H., Nakayama, M., and Takase, K. (2004). Usefulness of myelography with multiple views in diagnosis of circumferential location of disc material in dogs with thoracolumber intervertebral disc herniation. *J. Vet. Med. Sci.* 66 (7): 827–833.

89 McKee, W.M. (1992). A comparison of hemilaminectomy (with concomitant disc fenestration) and dorsal laminectomy for the treatment of thoracolumbar disc protrusion in dogs. *Vet. Rec.* 130 (14): 296–300.

90 Gambardella, P.C. (1980). Dorsal decompressive laminectomy for treatment of thoracolumbar disc disease in dogs: a retrospective study of 98 cases. *Vet. Surg.* 9: 24–26.

91 Scott, H.W. (1997). Hemilaminectomy for the treatment of thoracolumbar disc disease in the dog: a follow-up study of 40 cases. *J. Small Anim. Pract.* 38 (11): 488–494.

92 Denny, H.R. (1978). The surgical management of cervical disc protrusions in the dog: a review of 40 cases. *J. Small Anim. Pract.* 19: 251–257.

93 Seim, H.B. and Prata, R.G. (1982). Ventral decompression for the treatment of cervical disk disease in the dog – a review of 54 cases. *J. Am. Anim. Hosp. Assoc.* 18 (2): 233–240.

94 Morgan, P.W., Parent, J., and Holmberg, D.L. (1993). Cervical pain secondary to intervertebral disc disease in dogs – radiographic findings and surgical implications. *Prog. Vet. Neurol.* 4 (3): 76–80.

95 Gill, P.J., Lippincott, C.L., and Anderson, S.M. (1996). Dorsal laminectomy in the treatment of cervical intervertebral disk disease in small dogs: a retrospective study of 30 cases. *J. Am. Anim. Hosp. Assoc.* 32 (1): 77–80.

96 Hillman, R.B., Kengeri, S.S., and Waters, D.J. (2009). Reevaluation of predictive factors for complete recovery in dogs with nonambulatory tetraparesis secondary to cervical disk herniation. *J. Am. Anim. Hosp. Assoc.* 45 (4): 155–163.

97 De Risio, L. and Platt, S.R. (2010). Fibrocartilaginous embolic myelopathy in small animals. *Vet. Clin. North Am. Small Anim. Pract.* 40 (5): 859–869.

98 Gandini, G., Cizinauskas, S., Lang, J. et al. (2003). Fibrocartilaginous embolism in 75 dogs: clinical findings and factors influencing the recovery rate. *J. Small Anim. Pract.* 44 (2): 76–80.

99 Cauzinille, L. and Kornegay, J.N. (1996). Fibrocartilaginous embolism of the spinal cord in dogs: review of 36 histologically confirmed cases and retrospective study of 26 suspected cases. *J. Vet. Intern. Med.* 10 (4): 241–245.

100 De Risio, L., Adams, V., Dennis, R. et al. (2007). Magnetic resonance imaging findings and clinical associations in 52 dogs with suspected ischemic myelopathy. *J. Vet. Intern. Med.* 21 (6): 1290–1298.

101 Gilmore, D.R. and de Lahunta, A. (1986). Necrotizing myelopathy secondary to presumed or confirmed fibrocartilaginous embolism in 24 dogs. *J. Am. Anim. Hosp. Assoc.* 23: 373–376.

102 Abramson, C.J., Garosi, L., Platt, S.R. et al. (2005). Magnetic resonance imaging appearance of suspected ischemic myelopathy in dogs. *Vet. Radiol. Ultrasound* 46 (3): 225–229.

103 Grunenfelder, F.I., Weishaupt, D., Green, R., and Steffen, F. (2005). Magnetic resonance imaging findings in spinal cord infarction in three small breed dogs. *Vet. Radiol. Ultrasound* 46 (2): 91–96.

104 Hawthorne, J.C., Wallace, L.J., Fenner, W.R., and Waters, D.J. (2001). Fibrocartilaginous embolic myelopathy in miniature schnauzers. *J. Am. Anim. Hosp. Assoc.* 37 (4): 374–383.

105 MacKay, A.D., Rusbridge, C., Sparkes, A.H., and Platt, S.R. (2005). MRI characteristics of suspected acute spinal cord infarction in two cats, and a review of the literature. *J. Feline Med. Surg.* 7 (2): 101–107.

106 Mikszewski, J.S., Van Winkle, T.J., and Troxel, M.T. (2006). Fibrocartilaginous embolic myelopathy in five cats. *J. Am. Anim. Hosp. Assoc.* 42 (3): 226–233.

107 Coates, J.R. and Wininger, F.A. (2010). Canine degenerative myelopathy. *Vet. Clin. North Am. Small Anim. Pract.* 40 (5): 929–950.

108 Awano, T., Johnson, G.S., Wade, C.M. et al. (2009). Genome-wide association analysis reveals a SOD1 mutation in canine degenerative myelopathy that resembles amyotrophic lateral sclerosis. *Proc. Natl. Acad. Sci. U. S. A.* 106 (8): 2794–2799.

109 Averill, D.R. Jr. (1973). Degenerative myelopathy in the aging German Shepherd dog: clinical and pathologic findings. *J. Am. Vet. Med. Assoc.* 162 (12): 1045–1051.

110 Braund, K.G. and Vandevelde, M. (1978). German Shepherd dog myelopathy – a morphologic and morphometric study. *Am. J. Vet. Res.* 39 (8): 1309–1315.

111 Griffiths, I.R. and Duncan, I.D. (1975). Chronic degenerative radiculomyelopathy in the dog. *J. Small Anim. Pract.* 16 (8): 461–471.

112 Matthews, N.S. and de Lahunta, A. (1985). Degenerative myelopathy in an adult miniature poodle. *J. Am. Vet. Med. Assoc.* 186 (11): 1213–1215.

113 Kathmann, I., Cizinauskas, S., Doherr, M.G. et al. (2006). Daily controlled physiotherapy increases survival time in dogs with suspected degenerative myelopathy. *J. Vet. Intern. Med.* 20 (4): 927–932.

114 Coates, J.R., March, P.A., Oglesbee, M. et al. (2007). Clinical characterization of a familial degenerative myelopathy in Pembroke Welsh Corgi dogs. *J. Vet. Intern. Med.* 21 (6): 1323–1331.

115 Bichsel, P., Vandevelde, M., Lang, J., and Kull-Hachler, S. (1983). Degenerative myelopathy in a family of Siberian Husky dogs. *J. Am. Vet. Med. Assoc.* 183 (9): 998–1000, 965.

116 Bagley, R.S. (2010). Spinal neoplasms in small animals. *Vet. Clin. North Am. Small Anim. Pract.* 40 (5): 915–927.

117 Lane, S.B. and Kornegay, J.N. (1991). Spinal lymphosarcoma. In: *Consultations in Feline Internal Medicine* (ed. J.R. August), 487. Philadelphia: W.B. Saunders.

118 Woo, G.H., Bak, E.J., Lee, Y.W. et al. (2008). Cervical chondroid chordoma in a Shetland sheep dog. *J. Comp. Pathol.* 138 (4): 218–223.

119 Waters, D.J. and Hayden, D.W. (1990). Intramedullary spinal-cord metastasis in the dog. *J. Vet. Intern. Med.* 4 (4): 207–215.

120 Waters, D.J., Honeckman, A., Cooley, D.M., and DeNicola, D. (1998). Skeletal metastasis in feline mammary carcinoma: case report and literature review. *J. Am. Anim. Hosp. Assoc.* 34 (2): 103–108.

121 Platt, S.R., Sheppard, B.J., Graham, J. et al. (1998). Pheochromocytoma in the vertebral canal of two dogs. *J. Am. Anim. Hosp. Assoc.* 34 (5): 365–371.

122 Macpherson, G.C., Chadwick, B.J., and Robbins, P.D. (1993). Intramedullary spinal-cord metastasis of a primary lung-tumor in a dog. *J. Small Anim. Pract.* 34 (5): 242–246.

123 Jeffery, N.D. and Phillips, S.M. (1995). Surgical treatment of intramedullary spinal cord neoplasia in two dogs. *J. Small Anim. Pract.* 36 (12): 553–557.

124 Cooley, D.M. and Waters, D.J. (1998). Skeletal metastasis as the initial clinical manifestation of metastatic carcinoma in 19 dogs. *J. Vet. Intern. Med.* 12 (4): 288–293.

125 Appel, S.L., Moens, N.M., Abrams-Ogg, A.C. et al. (2008). Multiple myeloma with central nervous system involvement in a cat. *J. Am. Vet. Med. Assoc.* 233 (5): 743–747.

126 Suess, R.P. Jr., Martin, R.A., Shell, L.G. et al. (1990). Vertebral lymphosarcoma in a cat. *J. Am. Vet. Med. Assoc.* 197 (1): 101–103.

127 Aloisio, F., Levine, J.M., and Edwards, J.F. (2008). Immunohistochemical features of a feline spinal cord gemistocytic astrocytoma. *J. Vet. Diagn. Investig.* 20 (6): 836–838.

128 Zaki, F.A., Prata, R.G., Hurvitz, A.I., and Kay, W.J. (1975). Primary tumors of the spinal cord and meninges in six dogs. *J. Am. Vet. Med. Assoc.* 166 (5): 511–517.

129 Rizzo, S.A., Newman, S.J., Hecht, S., and Thomas, W.B. (2008). Malignant mediastinal extra-adrenal paraganglioma with spinal cord invasion in a dog. *J. Vet. Diagn. Investig.* 20 (3): 372–375.

130 Targett, M.P., Dyce, J., and Houlton, J.E.F. (1993). Tumors involving the nerve sheaths of the forelimb in dogs. *J. Small Anim. Pract.* 34 (5): 221–225.

131 Raskin, R.E. (1984). An atypical spinal meningioma in a dog. *Vet. Pathol.* 21 (5): 538–540.

132 Fingeroth, J.M., Prata, R.G., and Patnaik, A.K. (1987). Spinal meningiomas in dogs – 13 cases (1972–1987). *J. Am. Vet. Med. Assoc.* 191 (6): 720–726.

133 Bradley, R.L., Withrow, S.J., and Snyder, S.P. (1982). Nerve sheath tumors in the dog. *J. Am. Anim. Hosp. Assoc.* 18 (6): 915–921.

134 Brehm, D.M., Vite, C.H., Steinberg, H.S. et al. (1995). A retrospective evaluation of 51 cases of peripheral nerve sheath tumors in the dog. *J. Am. Anim. Hosp. Assoc.* 31 (4): 349–359.

135 Gilmore, D.R. (1983). Intraspinal tumors in the dog. *Compend. Contin. Educ. Pract.* 5 (1): 55–64.

136 Huisinga, M., Henrich, M., Frese, K. et al. (2008). Extraventricular neurocytoma of the spinal cord in a dog. *Vet. Pathol.* 45 (1): 63–66.

137 Gavin, P.G. and Bagley, R.S. (2009). *Practical Small Animal MRI*. Ames, IA: Wiley Blackwell.

138 Kippenes, H., Gavin, P.R., Bagley, R.S. et al. (1999). Magnetic resonance imaging features of tumors of the spine and spinal cord in dogs. *Vet. Radiol. Ultrasound* 40 (6): 627–633.

139 Jeffery, N.D. (2010). Vertebral fracture and luxation in small animals. *Vet. Clin. North Am. Small Anim. Pract.* 40 (5): 809–828.

140 Selcer, R.R., Bubb, W.J., and Walker, T.L. (1991). Management of vertebral column fractures in dogs and cats – 211 cases (1977–1985). *J. Am. Vet. Med. Assoc.* 198 (11): 1965–1968.

141 Feeney, D.A. and Oliver, J.E. (1980). Blunt spinal trauma in the dog and cat – insight into radiographic lesions. *J. Am. Anim. Hosp. Assoc.* 16 (6): 885–890.

142 Bruce, C.W., Brisson, B.A., and Gyselinck, K. (2008). Spinal fracture and luxation in dogs and cats – a retrospective evaluation of 95 cases. *Vet. Comp. Orthop.* 21 (3): 280–284.

143 Bali, M.S., Lang, J., Jaggy, A. et al. (2009). Comparative study of vertebral fractures and luxations in dogs and cats. *Vet. Comp. Orthop. Traumatol.* 22 (1): 47–53.

144 Hawthorne, J.C., Blevins, W.E., Wallace, L.J. et al. (1999). Cervical vertebral fractures in 56 dogs: a retrospective study. *J. Am. Anim. Hosp. Assoc.* 35 (2): 135–146.

145 Smeak, D.D. and Olmstead, M.L. (1985). Fracture luxations of the sacrococcygeal area in the cat – a retrospective study of 51 cases. *Vet. Surg.* 14 (4): 319–324.

146 Kinns, J., Mai, W., Seiler, G. et al. (2006). Radiographic sensitivity and negative predictive value for acute canine spinal trauma. *Vet. Radiol. Ultrasound* 47 (6): 563–570.

147 Patterson, R.H. and Smith, G.K. (1992). Backsplinting for treatment of thoracic and lumbar fracture/luxation in the dog: principles of application and case series. *Vet. Comp. Orthop. Traumatol.* 4: 179–187.

148 Bombardeer, C.H., Brown, P.B., Everett, J.J. et al. (1992). Coping with spinal-cord injury – a longitudinal pilot-study. *Rehabil. Psychol.* 37 (3): 216.

149 Bagley, R.S. (2000). Spinal fracture or luxation. *Vet. Clin. North Am. Small Anim. Pract.* 30 (1): 133–153, vi-vii.

150 Carberry, C.A., Flanders, J.A., Dietze, A.E. et al. (1989). Nonsurgical management of thoracic and lumbar spinal fractures and fracture luxations in the dog and cat – a review of 17 cases. *J. Am. Anim. Hosp. Assoc.* 25 (1): 43–54.

75

Diffuse Flaccidity in the Dog

Unusual Presentations Involving Diffuse Lower Motor Neuron Dysfunction

75.1 Diffuse Lower Motor Neuron Disease

The organization of the nervous system was introduced in Chapter 74, Section 74.1. Recall that the central nervous system (CNS) serves as an integration center for messages from the periphery and that an extensive network of neurons serves as the go-betweens [1–5].

Upper motor neurons (UMNs) connect the brain to the spinal cord segments to regulate posture and muscle tone, and modulate gait [1, 4]. UMNs communicate indirectly with effector organs, muscle fibers and glands, via interneurons and lower motor neurons (LMNs) [1, 3, 4]. LMNs signal the musculature to contract [1].

Neuromuscular dysfunction can result from a break at any point in this pathway [1, 4]. Depending upon which aspect of the pathway is broken, the patient may be said to have UMN or LMN disease [1].

Dysfunction may occur at any point along the pathway [5]. When dysfunction occurs at the level of the LMNs, the patient will exhibit hyporeflexia, muscle atrophy, and weakness in those regions of the body that are downstream of the lesion [4, 6–8].

Recall from Chapter 74, Section 74.4 that a lesion between C6 and T2 causes LMN signs to the thoracic limbs, and that a lesion between L4 and L6 will cause LMN signs to the pelvic limbs [6, 7].

What was not discussed in Chapter 74 is that patients may also present with whole-body flaccidity as a result of diffuse LMN disease [5, 9–16].

A patient that is diffusely flaccid will experience a four-legged absence of all stretch reflexes, such as the patellar reflex, and withdrawal reflexes [9]. Refer to Chapter 73, Sections 73.2 and 73.3 to recall these reflexes and how to effectively test them in the companion animal patient.

The affected patient's body will be floppy to handle and manipulate because of reduced-to-absent muscle tone [9].

The patient will exhibit tetraparesis or tetraplegia [9].

Because all musculature has the potential to be impacted, respiratory muscles may themselves be weak [9, 15]. Phrenic and intercostal nerve involvement may result in respiratory paralysis, which is life-threatening, and/or aspiration pneumonia [9, 15–17].

75.2 Causes of Acute Diffuse LMN Disease in the Dog

When diffuse LMN signs develop in the dog, they may result from the following [9, 15]:

- Diffuse neuromuscular disease
- Diffuse spinal cord disease

Diffuse neuromuscular disease is by far more common in the dog than diffuse spinal cord disease [9]. Diffuse disease is caused by dysfunction associated with the following [9]:

- Motor nerve roots
- Motor neurons
- Peripheral motor nerves
- Neuromuscular junction

The most common differentials that are associated with diffuse neuromuscular disease in the dog include the following [5, 9–11, 13–19]:

- Acute idiopathic polyradiculoneuritis
- Botulism
- Coral snake envenomation
- Myasthenia gravis
- Tick paralysis

75.3 Acute Idiopathic Polyradiculoneuritis

Acute idiopathic polyradiculoneuritis is sometimes called coonhound paralysis because the syndrome historically targeted hunting dogs that were exposed to raccoon saliva [5, 9, 14, 16]. Clinical signs developed 7 to 10 days after exposure to raccoons, leading scientists to believe that salivary antigen incited inflammation of the ventral roots and subsequent demyelination [5, 9, 14].

However, dogs that have not been bitten by raccoons and dogs that have in fact had zero raccoon exposure may also develop a similar syndrome [5, 14, 16, 20–25]. This suggests that there are other factors at play, including exposure to viruses, drugs, or even vaccines [5, 22].

The condition mirrors Guillain-Barré syndrome (GBS) in humans [5, 16].

Affected dogs initially develop weakness in both pelvic limbs [5, 9, 14, 16]. Over 24–48 h, paraparesis transforms into paralysis that ascends to both thoracic limbs [5, 9, 14, 16, 26, 27]. Ultimately, the patient is rendered recumbent [5, 9]. If the patient is lifted, generalized lack of muscle tone will be appreciated: limbs hang, and the patient is whole-body limp.

Stretch and withdrawal reflexes are absent in all four legs [5, 9]. However, pain sensation remains intact [5, 9]. Affected dogs will feel a toe pinch and will vocalize [5, 9]. They simply are powerless to move the pinched limb away from the stimulus.

Clients may report a change in quality of the patient's bark [9]. This results from involvement of the recurrent laryngeal nerve [5]. Bark tone and volume may progressively decline to the point of aphonia [5, 9].

Urinary and/or fecal incontinence is rare [5, 9].

Respiratory compromise is the primary concern [5, 9, 16]. In the event of respiratory paralysis, the patient will require mechanical ventilation [5, 16].

Treatment emphasizes supportive care [5, 9]. Patients require turning to alternate the side that is down so as to reduce the chance of pressure sores [5, 9]. Range of motion exercises may reduce rate of muscle atrophy [5, 9].

Intravenous hydration may be necessary, and a urinary catheter may be placed to prevent urine scald due to recumbency-associated soiling [9].

Acute idiopathic polyradiculoneuritis is more often suspected and medically managed than it is definitively diagnosed. Although abnormalities in electrical activity confirm the diagnosis, these do not develop until the patient has been symptomatic for five to seven days [5, 9, 16]. By the time that nerve conduction tests are abnormal on account of diminished conduction velocity, the patient has already been supported by nursing care [9].

Barring the development of respiratory compromise, patient prognosis for a full recovery is good [5, 9, 14]. Spontaneous recovery is expected, but a full recovery is slow [16]. Patients typically turn the corner three weeks after presentation. Beyond that, it is likely to take weeks to months of continued rehabilitation before the patient is back to normal [9, 16].

Physical therapy may expedite recovery [9, 16]. The administration of glucocorticoids hinders it [9, 16]. Although this condition is the result of inflammation,

glucocorticoids do not shorten the disease [9, 16, 23, 28]. They seem to perpetuate weakness on account of pathways not yet discovered [9].

Experimental treatment with human intravenous (IV) immunoglobulin may hasten recovery; however, anaphylaxis and hematuria are possible adverse effects for which patients will need to be monitored [29].

75.4 Botulism

Botulism is a clinical condition that involves the grampositive, anaerobic, spore-forming, neurotoxin-producing bacteria, *Clostridium botulinum* [5, 9, 10, 12, 14, 20]. When dogs ingest type C neurotoxin in contaminated or otherwise spoiled food, they are at risk for developing botulism [5, 9, 10, 12–14, 17, 20, 30].

Type C neurotoxin is absorbed into general circulation by the gut [9, 12]. Using the bloodstream as a vehicle, this toxin travels to presynaptic neurons, where it prevents the release of acetylcholine [9, 12, 14].

Clinical signs may develop within 12 h of ingestion [9]. They may also exhibit delayed onset of up to one week post-ingestion [14].

Like acute idiopathic polyradiculoneuritis, botulism causes ascending flaccid paralysis that begins with pelvic limb weakness [5, 9, 10, 12–14, 31].

The tail wag may be preserved in affected patients for reasons that are not understood [12, 30].

Also, like acute idiopathic polyradiculoneuritis, botulism does not affect nociception [9, 12]. Patients are capable of feeling pain in the limbs and often react with vocalization to toe-pinch tests, despite being unable to retract the limb away from the stimulus.

Mentation is also preserved [30].

Stretch and withdrawal reflexes are absent in all four legs [5, 9, 12].

In addition to absent reflexes, affected patients often develop cranial nerve dysfunction, including the following [9, 12, 13]:

- Fifth cranial nerve, the trigeminal nerve (CN V)
- Seventh cranial nerve, the facial nerve (CN VII)
- Ninth cranial nerve, the glossopharyngeal nerve (CN IX)
- Tenth cranial nerve, the vagus nerve (CN X)

The fifth cranial nerve, CN V, innervates the muscles of mastication [32]. If CN V is dysfunctional, then patients may develop a weak or "dropped" jaw due to atrophy associated with the temporalis or masseter muscles [9, 32].

The loss of the seventh cranial nerve, the facial nerve, results in facial paralysis [9, 13, 32].

CN IX and X coordinate swallowing [32]. Patients with deficits in one or both of these nerves may exhibit dysphagia or regurgitation [32]. They may lack a gag reflex [9, 32].

If innervation to the phrenic or intercostal muscles is compromised, then muscle weakness may include the diaphragm [9]. When it does, respiratory paralysis is a primary concern [9]. Aspiration pneumonia may result from respiratory paralysis, particularly if there is concurrent dysphagia [13].

Patients may exhibit weakened vocalization [12]. Barks may be of decreased intensity or they may be absent altogether.

It is also not uncommon to have patients present with the following changes due to adverse effects upon the autonomic nervous system [9, 12]:

- Bradycardia
- Delayed pupillary light reflexes (PLRs)
- Keratoconjunctivitis sicca, that is, dry eye
- Mydriasis, that is, dilated pupils
- Retained urine and feces

The presence of toxin in food or carrion, or patient body fluids such as serum, feces, or vomitus, is diagnostic for botulism [5, 9, 10].

Although antitoxin is available, it must be administered before the toxin binds to neurons in order to be effective [5, 9]. This is rarely possible in general practice because patient presentation occurs after the patient is symptomatic for neuromuscular dysfunction [5, 9].

Nursing care is the primary mode of case management, keeping in mind many of the same principles that were discussed for cases of acute idiopathic polyradiculoneuritis [5, 9, 12, 14].

Artificial tears may be administered to protect against keratitis and conjunctivitis secondary to keratoconjunctivitis sicca [12].

Patients require feeding tube placement if they cannot swallow on their own [12].

Botulism is short-lived as compared to acute idiopathic polyradiculoneuritis: on average, clinical signs last for less than two weeks [14].

75.5 Coral Snake Envenomation

Venomous snakes are distributed throughout the world [33–35]. Within North America, Elapidae, and Crotalidae are two prevalent families of snakes [33]. The family Crotalidae includes the pit vipers: rattlesnakes, cottonmouths, and copperheads [33]. Elapidae includes the coral snake, cobras, mambas, and tiger snakes [33].

Several species of coral snakes are common in North America [33]:

- The Eastern coral snake, *Micrurus fulvius fulvius*
- The Sonoran coral snake, *Micruroides euryanthus*
- The South Florida coral snake, *Micrurus fulvius barbouri*
- The Texas coral snake, *Micrurus fulvius tenere*

Of those listed above, the Sonoran coral snake does not appear to be harmful [36]. To the author's knowledge, fatalities from this snake have not been reported in the medical or veterinary literature [36].

The coral snake is a brightly colored snake with red, yellow, and black bands [33, 36]. The red and yellow bands are adjacent to one another, as opposed to non-venomous look-alike snakes, in which black bands separate the red from yellow [33, 36]. This visual discrepancy can be remembered by the common saying, "red touches black, friend of Jack; red touches yellow kills a fellow." Note that this saying only holds true in North America [36].

Note that some species of North American coral snakes replace yellow with white [36].

To cause envenomation, coral snakes must sink their fixed front fangs into prey and chew on their tissues [33, 36].

Bites most often occur on the lips, muzzle, and distal limbs [33]. Punctures are small and may be mistaken for scratches [33]. They do not typically cause severe pain, and, unlike rattlesnake envenomation, do not result in severe tissue swelling and/or necrosis [14, 33].

About two-thirds of coral snake bites do not cause envenomation [33, 36, 37]. Those that do result in initial excitation of the autonomic nervous system [33]. This is exhibited in the form of ptyalism and/or emesis [33].

Neurotoxicity often is delayed, and may take up to 18 h post-bite to develop [33, 36–40]. Because the neurotoxin targets the acetylcholine receptor sites, affected patients exhibit diffuse LMN dysfunction [33, 34, 36]. This manifests as the following [33, 37, 41]:

- Lethargy
- Respiratory paralysis
- Tetraparesis or tetraplegia

CNS depression is commonly seen in cases involving elapid bites [36].

Affected patients may also develop hemoglobinuria and cardiac arrhythmias [14, 33, 36, 37, 41].

Cats are not immune to elapid bites, but there are fewer reports of these in the veterinary literature [39]. In addition to aforementioned clinical signs, affected cats may present with hypothermia [36]. Loss of the cutaneous trunci reflex, in addition to loss of stretch and withdrawal reflexes, is typical [36, 39]. Refer to Chapter 73, Section 73.4 to review the cutaneous trunci reflex and how to test for it in companion animal patients.

Treatment is largely supportive [14]. If antivenom is given early on in the disease process, it hastens recovery and improves chances for survival [14]. However, more often than not, patients present after the window during which time treatment with antivenom would be most effective [14].

Consult an emergency reference for details concerning case management.

75.6 Myasthenia Gravis

Myasthenia gravis was introduced in Chapter 67, Section 67.8 as a condition that involves dysfunctional acetylcholine receptors on the postsynaptic membrane [17, 42]. Recall that although a congenital form has been recognized in companion animal patients, acquired myasthenia gravis is more commonly diagnosed in clinical practice [17, 42]. In the acquired form, patients develop autoantibodies against their own acetylcholine receptors [42]. This prevents the binding of acetylcholine [42]. Without acetylcholine, flaccid paralysis ensues [42].

Acquired myasthenia gravis may be focal or generalized [17]. This discussion will focus upon generalized dysfunction [17].

At rest, patients appear to be neurologically normal [14].

Patients are exercise-intolerant [14, 42, 43]. When patients engage in physical activity, they develop progressive weakness [14].

When rested, affected patients regain strength, but this is short-lived. Affected patients again succumb to weakness the next time they are asked to exert themselves [43].

Pelvic limb lameness is particularly prominent in dogs with myasthenia gravis [43]. Cats, on the other hand, will typically present with cervical ventroflexion as a sign of generalized weakness [42].

A positive response to the administration of acetylcholinesterase inhibitors, edrophonium chloride or neostigmine, is supportive of a diagnosis [17, 42]. A definitive diagnosis requires the presence of anti-acetylcholine receptor antibodies in the serum; however, false negatives are possible [17, 42].

Treatment for patients is lifelong. Medical management is possible by means of administering pyridostigmine bromide [42].

Note that patients with myasthenia gravis may be more likely to develop polymyositis, polyneuritis, or neoplasia of the thymus [20, 42, 43].

75.7 Tick Paralysis

Tick paralysis is a clinical response to tick-associated salivary neurotoxin, which blocks acetylcholine release at the neuromuscular junction [5, 9].

Although several species of ticks have been implicated, the following two are the most likely to induce the disease in the United States [9, 11, 18, 19]:

- The American dog tick, *Dermacentor variabilis*
- The Rocky Mountain wood tick, *Dermacentor andersoni*

Within five to nine days of tick attachment, affected dogs present with ascending flaccid paralysis [9, 19].

Stretch and withdrawal reflexes are absent in all four legs [5, 9, 12, 19].

Nociception pathways are intact [19].

Like acute idiopathic polyradiculoneuritis and botulism, respiratory paralysis is possible [5, 9, 12, 18].

The coats of affected patients must be searched thoroughly for evidence of one or more ticks [9]. Ticks may be hidden within the following regions [9]:

- Interdigital spaces
- Perivulvar skin
- Pinnae
- Underneath the tail

Finding one attached tick should not halt the search through the patient's coat [9]. Disease may be caused by more than one tick [9, 19]. It is therefore important to remove them all [9].

Although topical treatments against ticks are an important part of the treatment plan, these products are not instantly effective, which is why a thorough coat search is essential [9].

Within hours of tick removal by hand, affected patients experience improvement in clinical signs [9].

Barring respiratory compromise, patients recover fully within two to three days [5, 9].

Although tick serology can be performed, its role as a diagnostic is limited [9]. When tick serology tests positive, it confirms tick exposure rather than active disease [9].

References

1 Molenaar, G.J. (1996). The nervous system. In: *Textbook of Veterinary Anatomy*, 2e (ed. K.M. Dyce, W.O. Sack and C.J.G. Wensing), 259–324. Philadelphia: W.B. Saunders Company.

2 Behan, M. (2004). Organization of the Nervous System. In: *Dukes' Physiology of Domestic Animals*, 12e (ed. W.O. Reece), 757–769. Ithaca: Comstock Publishing Associates.

3 Kitchell, R.L. Introduction to the nervous system. In: *Miller's Anatomy of the Dog*, 3e (ed. H.E. Evans), 758–775. Philadelphia: Saunders.

4 Garosi, L. (2009). Neurological examination of the cat. How to get started. *J. Feline Med. Surg.* 11 (5): 340–348.

5 Coates, J.R. (2009). The flaccid dog. DVM 360 [Internet]. http://veterinarycalendar.dvm360.com/flaccid-dog-proceedings.

6 DeLahunta, A., Glass, E., and Kent, M. (2015). *Veterinary Neuroanatomy and Clinical Neurology*, 4e. St. Louis, MO: Elsevier.

7 Millis, D.L. and Mankin, J. (2014). Orthopedic and neurologic evaluation. In: *Canine Rehabilitation and Physical Therapy*, 2e (ed. D.L. Millis and D. Levine), 180–200. Philadelphia, PA: Elsevier.

8 Schubert, T. (2018). Physical and neurologic examinations. Merck Veterinary Manual [Internet]. https://www.merckvetmanual.com/nervous-system/nervous-system-introduction/physical-and-neurologic-examinations.

9 Troxel, M. (2014). Diffuse lower motor neuron dysfunction in dogs. *NAVC Clinician's Brief* (January): 75–79.

10 Barsanti, J.A., Walser, M., Hatheway, C.L. et al. (1978). Type C botulism in American foxhounds. *J. Am. Vet. Med. Assoc.* 172 (7): 809–813.

11 Otranto, D., Dantas-Torres, F., Tarallo, V.D. et al. (2012). Apparent tick paralysis by Rhipicephalus sanguineus (Acari: Ixodidae) in dogs. *Vet. Parasitol.* 188 (3–4): 325–329.

12 Bailey, E.M. (2013). Botulism. In: *Small Animal Toxicology*, 3e (ed. M.E. Peterson and P.A. Talcott), 465–469. St. Louis, Mo: Elsevier.

13 Uriarte, A., Thibaud, J.L., and Blot, S. (2010). Botulism in 2 urban dogs. *Can. Vet. J.* 51 (10): 1139–1142.

14 Donahue, S. and Silverstein, D.C. (2015). Chest wall disease. In: *Small Animal Critical Care Medicine* (ed. D.C. Silverstein and K. Hopper), 148–150. St. Louis, Mo: Saunders/Elsevier.

15 Rutter, C.R., Rozanski, E.A., Sharp, C.R. et al. (2011). Outcome and medical management in dogs with lower motor neuron disease undergoing mechanical ventilation: 14 cases (2003–2009). *J. Vet. Emerg. Crit. Care (San Antonio).* 21 (5): 531–541.

16 Cuddon, P.A. (2002). Acquired canine peripheral neuropathies. *Vet. Clin. North Am. Small Anim. Pract.* 32 (1): 207–249.

17 Shelton, G.D. (2002). Myasthenia gravis and disorders of neuromuscular transmission. *Vet. Clin. North Am. Small Anim. Pract.* 32 (1): 189–206, vii.

18 Eppleston, K.R., Kelman, M., and Ward, M.P. (2013). Distribution, seasonality and risk factors for tick paralysis in Australian dogs and cats. *Vet. Parasitol.* 196 (3–4): 460–468.

19 Olson, P. and Carithers, R.W. (1982). Differential diagnosis of conditions mimicking intervertebral disc disease in the canine. *Iowa State Univ. Vet.* 44 (2): 60–65.

20 Lorenza, M.D., Coates, J.R., and Kent, M. (2010). Tetraparesis, hemiparesis, and ataxia, ch. 7. In: *Handbook of Veterinary Neurology* (ed. J.E. Oliver, M.D. Lorenz and J.N. Kornegay), 162–249. St. Louis: Saunders.

21 Bors, M., Valentine, B.A., and de Lahunta, A. (1988). Neuromuscular disease in a dog. *Cornell Vet.* 78 (4): 339–345.

22 Chetboul, V. (1989). Cas clinique: polyradiculonevrite post-vaccinale. *Le Pointe Veterinaire* 21: 83–85.

23 Cuddon, P.A. (2001). Coonhound paralysis (idiopathic polyradiculoneuritis). In: *The 5-Minute Veterinary Consult* (ed. L.P. Tilley and F.W.K. Smith), 588–589. Philadelphia: Lippincott Williams & Wilkins.

24 Harve, R.S. (1979). Acute idiopathic polyradiculoneuritis in a dog. *Vet. Med. Small Anim. Clin.* 74: 675–679.

25 Northington, J.W., Brown, M.J., Farnbach, G.C., and Steinberg, S.A. (1981). Acute idiopathic polyneuropathy in the dog. *J. Am. Vet. Med. Assoc.* 179 (4): 375–379.

26 Summers, B.A., Cummings, J.F., and de Lahunta, A. (1995). *Diseases of the Peripheral Nervous System, Veterinary Neuropathology*, 402–501. St. Louis: Mosby.

27 Cuddon, P.A. (1998). Electrophysiologic assessment of acute polyradiculoneuropathy in dogs: comparison with Guillain-Barre syndrome in people. *J. Vet. Intern. Med.* 12 (4): 294–303.

28 Arnason, B.G.W. and Soliven, B. (1993). Acute inflammatory demyelinating polyradiculoneuropathy. In: *Peripheral Neuropathy* (ed. P.J. Dyck and P.K. Thomas), 1437–1497. Philadelphia: WB Saunder.

29 Hirschvogel, K., Jurina, K., Steinberg, T.A. et al. (2012). Clinical course of acute canine polyradiculoneuritis following treatment with human IV immunoglobulin. *J. Am. Anim. Hosp. Assoc.* 48 (5): 299–309.

30 Manning, A.M. (2001). Standards of care: emergency and critical care medicine. *Vet. Learn. Sys.* 3 (10): 1–6.

31 Arnon, S.S., Schechter, R., Inglesby, T.V. et al. (2001). Botulinum toxin as a biological weapon: medical and public health management. *JAMA* 285 (8): 1059–1070.

32 Englar, R.E. (2017). *Performing the Small Animal Physical Examination*. Hoboken, NJ: Wiley.

33 Gilliam, L.L. and Brunker, J. (2011). North American snake envenomation in the dog and cat. *Vet. Clin. North Am. Small Anim. Pract.* 41 (6): 1239–1259.

34 Heller, J., Mellor, D.J., Hodgson, J.L. et al. (2007). Elapid snake envenomation in dogs in New South Wales: a review. *Aust. Vet. J.* 85 (11): 469–479.

35 Lomonte, B., Rey-Suarez, P., Fernandez, J. et al. (2016). Venoms of Micrurus coral snakes: evolutionary trends in compositional patterns emerging from proteomic analyses. *Toxicon* 122: 7–25.

36 Peterson, M.E. (2006). Snake bite: coral snakes. *Clin. Tech. Small Anim. Pract.* 21 (4): 183–186.

37 Marks, S.L., Mannella, C., and Schaer, M. (1990). Coral Snake envenomation in the dog – report of 4 cases and review of the literature. *J. Am. Anim. Hosp. Assoc.* 26 (6): 629–634.

38 Ellis, M. (1978). Venomous and non-venomous snakes. In: *Dangerous Plants, Snakes, Arthropods, and Marine Life: Toxicity and Treatment* (ed. M. Ellis), 125–142. Hamilton, IL: Drug Intelligence Publications, Inc.

39 Chrisman, C.L., Hopkins, A.L., Ford, S.L., and Meeks, J.C. (1996). Acute, flaccid quadriplegia in three cats with suspected coral snake envenomation. *J. Am. Anim. Hosp. Assoc.* 32 (4): 343–349.

40 Kitchens, C.S. and Van Mierop, L.H. (1987). Envenomation by the eastern coral snake (Micrurus fulvius fulvius). A study of 39 victims. *JAMA* 258 (12): 1615–1618.

41 Kremer, K.A. and Schaer, M. (1995). Coral snake (Micrurus fulvius fulvius) envenomation in five dogs: present and earlier findings. *J. Vet. Emerg. Crit. Care* 5: 9–15.

42 Nghiem, P., Platt, S., and Schatzberg, S. (2009). The weak cat. Practical approach and common neurological differentials. *J. Feline Med. Surg.* 11 (5): 373–383.

43 Dewey, C.W. (2008). *A Practical Guide to Canine and Feline Neurology*, 2e, xiv, 706 p., 7 p. of plates p. Ames, Iowa: Wiley-Blackwell.

76

Unusual Presentations of Spastic Rigidity in the Dog

76.1 Brief Review of Upper Motor Neuron Function

The organizational structure of the nervous system was introduced in Chapter 74, Section 74.1 as a central site of integration, the central nervous system (CNS), connected to the periphery by an extensive network of neurons [1–5].

Upper motor neurons (UMNs) regulate posture and muscle tone, and modulate gait [1, 4]. They originate from the brain and connect it to the appropriate spinal cord segments to effect change in the body [1]. Specifically, UMNs communicate indirectly with effector organs, muscle fibers and glands, via interneurons and lower motor neurons (LMNs) [1, 3, 4].

The spinal cord receives inputs that are either excitatory or inhibitory. UMNs tend to provide the latter [6].

76.2 Introduction to the Clinical Sign Spastic Rigidity or Hypertonia

When there is UMN dysfunction, inhibitory pathways are removed from those signals that modulate input to the spinal cord [6]. This allows for uninhibited firing of those motor neurons that initiate and maintain muscle contraction [6]. Because this firing is no longer under inhibition, there is an increased resting level of muscle activity [6]. Affected muscles are, in a sense, hyperexcitable. This creates an excess of muscle tone, which is called hypertonia [6, 7]. Hypertonia is sometimes referred to as spastic rigidity [6, 7]. Spastic rigidity is characterized by muscles that seem stiff, undergoing wave-like contractions and seemingly uncontrollable spasms [7, 8]. Muscle resistance fights against range of motion, causing it to decrease [7, 8].

Over time, spasticity of the musculature promotes weakness [9]. Muscles that are spastic are shortened and therefore cannot do the work that is expected of them [9]. Without treatment, they may become permanently tight and fixed in space, a condition that is known as contracture [9].

At the same time, loss of inhibition causes stretch reflexes, such as the patellar reflex, to be exaggerated [4, 10–12]. This is called hyperreflexia [4, 10–12].

Recall from Chapter 74, Sections 74.4.2 and 74.4.4 that a lesion between C1 and C5 causes UMN signs in all four limbs and that a lesion between T3 and L3 causes UMN in the pelvic limbs only [11, 12].

What was not discussed in Chapter 74 is that patients may also present with whole-body spasticity as a result of diffuse disease, as from a systemic toxin [13, 14]. Although rare, two case presentations are recognized clinically in companion animal medicine [13, 14]:

- Strychnine
- Tetanus

Tetanus is the result of infection with an environmental toxin, whereas strychnine is man-made [13, 14]. Both can be life-threatening [13, 14].

76.3 Strychnine Toxicosis

Strychnine is a rodenticide that was introduced in Germany during the sixteenth century [14, 15]. Strychnine continues to exist in circulation today as marketable baits for use in the United States to manage ground squirrels, gophers, mice, moles, and rats [14, 16, 17]. In the Southwestern United States, it has been employed as a form of predator control to reduce the population of coyotes [16, 18].

Most strychnine-infused bait is dyed red or green [16].

Strychnine's presence in the environment can inadvertently poison free-roaming dogs and cats [14, 16, 17, 19–25]. It has also been used maliciously to target companion animals that landowners considered nuisances [14]. Dogs appear to be more susceptible to poisoning with strychnine than cats [14]. Even so, ingestion of a few tablespoons of bait in either species is sufficient to cause death [14].

In theory, death can also occur by ingesting strychnine-containing carrion [14]. However, this does not seem to be a common occurrence as compared to direct ingestion of the bait [14].

Strychnine is ingested and absorbed into general circulation via the digestive tract [14]. Its distribution among tissues is widespread, causing diffuse neuromuscular dysfunction [14].

In health, glycine acts as an inhibitory neurotransmitter of motor neurons and interneurons [14].

When a patient ingests strychnine, the chemical prevents the release of glycine [14, 26, 27]. In addition, strychnine prevents circulating glycine from performing its function [14, 26, 27]. In other words, strychnine eliminates the effect of inhibition on cells of the spinal cord [14].

As a result of the actions of strychnine against glycine, neuronal activity is unchecked [14]. Affected patients demonstrate whole-body hypertonia and hyperreflexia [14, 16, 17].

Extensor tone exceeds flexor tone, causing the body to be held in exaggerated hyperextension [14, 16, 17]. Extreme hyperextension of the head, neck, and spine create the classic posture, opisthotonus [14, 16]. Opisthotonus may be episodic or continuous [14].

Affected patients experience convulsions, during which time respiration is impaired [14, 16].

Patients remain aware of their surroundings and in fact their senses may be heightened [14, 16]. They seem photophobic and sensitive to both loud noise and touch [14, 16].

As convulsions continue, patients are likely to become hyperthermic [14].

Death is due to respiratory paralysis [14, 16].

Diagnosis is typically postmortem, but is supported by case history and clinical presentation [14]. Diagnosis can be confirmed by testing the vomitus, liver, bile, or kidneys [14, 20, 22].

Affected patients can survive strychnine poisoning if treatment is initiated early. Medical management emphasizes rapid decontamination [14]. However, many patients present at later stages of disease and are likely to succumb to its effects [14].

Note that the presentation described above is not pathognomonic for strychnine [14]. Clinical signs can mirror tetanus [14]. Clinical signs may also be synonymous with other toxicoses, including the following [14, 20]:

- Amphetamines
- Bromethalin
- Caffeine
- Metaldehyde
- Nicotine
- Pyrethrins and pyrethroids (cats)
- Theobromine

Toxic plants may also cause similar presentations. These include the following [14]:

- Bleeding heart and Dutchman's breeches (*Dicentra* spp.)
- Roquefortine, and other mycotoxins
- Some species of mushrooms
- Water hemlock (*Cicuta* spp.)
- Yew (*Taxus* spp.)

76.4 Tetanus

Tetanus is a clinical condition that involves the grampositive, anaerobic, spore-forming, neurotoxin-producing bacteria, *Clostridium tetani* [13, 28–32]. Spores are worldwide and hardy, meaning that they are able to withstand harsh environmental conditions [13, 28–30]. They are ubiquitous in soil and dust [28].

Spores contain two toxins, tetanolysin, and tetanospasmin [13, 29]. The latter migrates, in retrograde fashion, from peripheral nerves to the CNS [13, 33]. Within the CNS, tetanospasmin prevents the release of glycine and γ-aminobutyric acid (GABA) by binding to inhibitor neurons [13, 33, 34]. Because such binding is irreversible, patients must generate new axonal terminals in order to recover [34, 35]. On average, this takes two weeks to achieve, causing a delay in signs of clinical improvement [13, 34, 36].

Tetanus can be localized or generalized [13]. Which case presentation develops may depend upon the route of inoculation: subcutaneously, intramuscularly, or hematogenously [31]. Wounds are a common route by which toxins gain access to the body [13]. Wounds may result from an injury or they may be surgical [13, 37–39].

Tetanus also thrives in anaerobic environments [28]. Therefore, it may arise from cases involving necrotic tissue, including burn wounds and snake bites [28].

Generalized tetanus is more common than localized tetanus in dogs [13]. Males and German Shepherd dogs may be predisposed [13].

Most dogs are infected via contamination of a wound with soil or feces [28, 30]. Paw and limb wounds, for instance, are common routes by which dogs are exposed to toxin [28, 40].

Case presentations involving generalized tetanus mirror those for strychnine in that severely affected patients are recumbent and exhibit extensor rigidity [13, 33].

Less affected patients may demonstrate a stiff, socalled sawhorse gait in the absence of recumbency [13, 30]. Patients that are ambulatory may be ataxic [13].

Affected patients also tend to exhibit clinical signs that involve the face and oral cavity [13]. Classically, these include the following [13, 30, 40]:

- Dysphagia
- Enophthalmos
- Erect ears
- Protrusion of the nictitans bilaterally
- Ptyalism
- Risus sardonicus, that is, a sardonic grin caused by sustained facial muscle spasms
- Torticollis, that is, unilateral cervical muscle contraction, causing the head to twist to the side
- Trismus, that is, lockjaw
- Worried facial expression (see Figure 76.1)

Cranial nerves tend to be affected before spinal nerves that innervate the extremities [28, 41].

Different species exhibit different sensitivities to tetanospasmin [13, 31]. Horses and humans are much more sensitive than dogs, which are more susceptible than cats [13, 30, 31, 33].

Isolated case reports of cats that have developed localized tetanus appear in the veterinary literature [28, 30]. Affected cats tend to develop spastic rigidity and associated paralysis in one limb [28].

Treatment of tetanus in companion animals involves supportive care as well as medical management of the disease [13]. Antibiotics should be initiated to eliminate

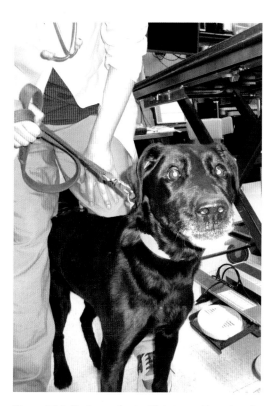

Figure 76.1 Canine patient with tetanus. Note that the sustained facial spasms give this patient the appearance of a persistently worried look. *Source:* Courtesy of Daniel Foy, MS, DVM, DACVIM, DACVECC.

the infectious organism, *C. tetani* [13, 29]. Historically, penicillin has been effective [13, 30]. However, metronidazole may be equally, if not more, effective in patients that have regions of the body with compromised blood supply, such as abscesses [13, 29, 30, 42].

Because muscle spasms are painful, analgesia is a critical component of patient care [13, 30, 34]. The administration of muscle relaxants may also help to provide relief [13, 30, 34]. Specifically, the use of benzodiazepines may be advantageous because they potentiate GABA [13].

Affected patients are likely to be hypersensitive to external stimuli [30]. Quiet, poorly lit rooms may be advised [30, 34].

Patients with open wounds require wound management, including lavage and/or surgical exploration [30]. Pieces of debris may act as a nidus for spores and toxin [30].

Cases of tetanus are complicated by pharyngeal and/or laryngeal spasms, which may lead to aspiration pneumonia [13, 28, 30]. Respiratory muscle spasms may also lead to laryngeal paralysis, respiratory arrest, and/or airway obstruction [13, 28, 30, 33].

Recumbency results in additional complications, such as decubital ulcers [28].

Autonomic dysfunction is common [33, 43–47]. Tetanus-induced autonomic dysfunction may cause urine retention and constipation [28]. Patients may develop hiatal hernias or megaesophagus [28, 29, 48].

As is true of strychnine poisoning, tetanus may cause hyperthermia secondary to extensive, sustained muscular contractions [13, 30]. Hyperthermia in and of itself may be life-threatening [13].

The use of tetanus antitoxin (TAT) may hasten recovery, but because it is derived from horses, it may be associated with hypersensitivity [13, 30]. Treatment is also controversial because of lack of proof that it is effective [13, 28, 30, 33]. The theory behind TAT is that it binds any free or unbound toxin [29]. This means that it would need to be given very early on in the course of disease in order to effect a positive outcome [29].

Diagnosis is typically presumptive, based upon clinical signs [28]. Culture and isolation of *C. tetani* is possible, but the process is protracted. It may take 12 days to see growth, and patients cannot survive for that long without initiating treatment [29]. Isolation also requires special culture media and anaerobic conditions [29].

76.5 Spastic Rigidity and Polioencephalomalacia

Polioencephalomalacia (PEM) is a pathological condition that is characterized by cerebrocortical necrosis [49]. The gray matter of the brain is said to soften. That is, it essentially degenerates.

Recall from basic anatomy that the CNS is composed of two tissue types: gray matter and white matter [50]. Gray matter is composed of neuronal cell bodies, dendrites, and axons [50]. It is the site of synapses [50].

Gray matter has a number of functions, including sensory perception and control over musculature [50].

When gray matter softens, various neuromuscular manifestations of disease result [49].

Most, but not all canine patients, exhibit convulsive fits [49, 51]. Seizures may be episodic or continuous [49].

Most dogs develop spastic rigidity [52]. A wide-based stance may be observed early on in the disease process [52]. Affected patients may become weak in the hind end [52]. Paraparesis often ascends to the point of four-legged involvement, causing lateral recumbency [52]. Convulsions continue in recumbency [52].

Other neurological signs, in dogs, may include the following [49, 52, 53]:

- Ataxia
- Changes in mentation
  - Depression
  - Obtundation
  - Stupor
  - Coma
- Decreased or absent menace response
- Disorientation
- Exophathlmos
- Extensor dominance
- Facial spasms
- Head-pressing
- Head tilt
- Hyperaesthesia
- Hyperreflexia
- Hypertonia
- Nystagmus
- Opisthotonus
- Reported changes in "personality" or behavior
- Sluggish pupillary light reflexes (PLRs)
- Temporal muscle spasms

Clinical signs tend to be progressive [53].

PEM is relatively rare in companion animal patients, and has more often been described in ruminants [54]. When it occurs in companion animals, it is typically the result of the following [49, 52, 54–57]:

- Cyanide poisoning
- Hypoglycemia
- Lead poisoning
- Thiamine deficiency
- Trauma to the cranium

Atypical presentations of canine distemper virus (CDV) can also result in PEM [58].

Thiamine deficiency was introduced in Chapter 67, Section 67.6 as a cause of cervical ventroflexion and blindness in cats. Recall that thiamine cannot be synthesized by the body [59]. It must be ingested in the diet and absorbed in the small intestine [60]. As a coenzyme, it plays a key role in glucose metabolism [53, 59–62].

In the absence of thiamine, carbohydrate metabolism is impaired [60]. This is particularly detrimental to those tissues, such as the brain, that require glucose as an energy source [60]. Neurological dysfunction is common.

Cats require more dietary thiamine than dogs, and therefore reports of deficiency among feline patients are more prevalent in the veterinary literature [60].

Recall from Chapter 67, Section 67.6 that thiamine deficiency may result from the following [60, 62–68]:

- Diets that are rich in sulfites, which inactivate thiamine
- Raw diets that are rich in thiaminases, enzymes that preferentially break down thiamine
  - Herring
  - Mackerel
- Excessive heat processing
- Extended food storage
- Inadequate intake in the diet
- Increased renal excretion, secondary to the use of diuretics
- Malabsorption syndrome: an inability of the gut to absorb thiamine

Like cats, dogs may also be affected by thiamine deficiency. Puppies have greater requirements for thiamine than adult dogs [53]; so, too, do working dogs, pregnant dogs, and seniors [53].

Thiamine deficiency in dogs tends to result from ingestion of meat that has been preserved with sulfites [53]. Sulfites extend shelf life and improve palatability of meat [53]. They also preserve the hearty color of red meat [53, 69].

Affected dogs develop PEM [53]. Without intervention, PEM is fatal [53].

Magnetic resonance imaging (MRI) and cerebrospinal fluid (CSF) analysis may be performed, but results are not specific for thiamine deficiency. A presumptive diagnosis must be made based upon dietary history and clinical signs that are consistent with this pathology [53].

If thiamine supplementation is administered, response to treatment is rapid [53, 68–70]. Many, if not all, of the clinical signs can be reversed when treatment is initiated early. However, patients in which treatment is delayed may have residual effects, including dullness and partial blindness.

References

1 Molenaar, G.J. (1996). The nervous system. In: *Textbook of Veterinary Anatomy*, 2e (ed. K.M. Dyce, W.O. Sack and C.J.G. Wensing), 259–324. Philadelphia: W.B. Saunders Company.

2 Behan, M. (2004). Organization of the nervous system. In: *Dukes' Physiology of Domestic Animals*, 12e (ed. W.O. Reece), 757–769. Ithaca: Comstock Publishing Associates.

3 Kitchell, R.L. Introduction to the nervous system. In: *Miller's Anatomy of the Dog*, 3e (ed. H.E. Evans), 758–775. Philadelphia: Saunders.

4 Garosi, L. (2009). Neurological examination of the cat. How to get started. *J. Feline Med. Surg.* 11 (5): 340–348.

5 Coates, J.R. (2009). The flaccid dog. DVM 360 [Internet]. http://veterinarycalendar.dvm360.com/flaccid-dog-proceedings.

6 Brashear, A. (2005). Spasticity. In: *Animal Models of Movement Disorders* (ed. M. LeDoux), 679–686. London: Elsevier Academic Press.

7 Sheean, G. and McGuire, J.R. (2009). Spastic hypertonia and movement disorders: pathophysiology, clinical presentation, and quantification. *Phys.Med. Rehabil.* 1 (9): 827–833.

8 Alverzo, J.P., Rosenberg, J.H., and Sorensen, C.A. (2009). Nursing care and education for patients with spinal cord injury. In: *Spinal Cord Injuries: Management and Rehabilitation* (ed. S.A. Sisto, E. Druin and M.M. Sliwinski), 37–68. St. Louis: Mosby Elsevier.

9 McGee, S. (2012). Examination of the motor system: approach to weakness. In: *Evidence-Based Physical Diagnosis*, 3e (ed. S. McGee), 550–566. Philadelphia: Saunders.

10 Schubert, T. (2018). Physical and neurologic examinations. Merck Veterinary Manual [Internet]. https://www.merckvetmanual.com/nervous-system/nervous-system-introduction/physical-and-neurologic-examinations.

11 Millis, D.L. and Mankin, J. (2014). Orthopedic and neurologic evaluation. In: *Canine Rehabilitation and Physical Therapy*, 2e (ed. D.L. Millis and D. Levine), 180–200. Philadelphia, PA: Elsevier.

12 DeLahunta, A., Glass, E., and Kent, M. (2015). *Veterinary Neuroanatomy and Clinical Neurology*, 4e. St. Louis, MO: Elsevier.

13 Adamantos, S. and Boag, A. (2007). Thirteen cases of tetanus in dogs. *Vet. Rec.* 161 (9): 298–302.

14 Talcott, P.A. (2013). Strychnine. In: *Small Animal Toxicology*, 3e (ed. M.E. Peterson, P.A. Talcott and M.E. Peterson), 827–831. St. Louis, Mo: Elsevier.

15 Franz, D.N. (1985). Central neurotransmitters. In: *The Pharmacological Basis of Therapeutics* (ed. A.G. Gilman, L.S. Goodman and T.W. Rall). New York: Macmillan.

16 McLean, M.K. (2010). Toxicology brief: epidemiology and management of strychnine poisoning. DVM 360 [Internet]. http://veterinarymedicine.dvm360.com/toxicology-brief-epidemiology-and-management-strychnine-poisoning.

17 Cowan, V.E. and Blakley, B.R. (2015). A retrospective study of canine strychnine poisonings from 1998 to 2013 in Western Canada. *Can. Vet. J.* 56 (6): 587–590.

18 Robinson, W.B. (ed.) (1962). Methods of controlling coyotes, bobcats, and foxes. 1st Vertebrate Pest Conference.

19 Barton, J. and Oehme, F.W. (1981). The incidence and characteristics of animal poisonings seen at Kansas State University from 1975 to 1980. *Vet. Hum. Toxicol.* 23 (2): 101–102.

20 Lowes, N.R., Smith, R.A., and Beck, B.E. (1992). Roquefortine in the stomach contents of dogs suspected of strychnine poisoning in Alberta. *Can. Vet. J.* 33 (8): 535–538.

21 Osweiler, G.D. (1969). Incidence and diagnostic considerations of major small animal toxicoses. *J. Am. Vet. Med. Assoc.* 155 (12): 2011–2015.

22 Blakley, B.R. (1984). Epidemiologic and diagnostic considerations of strychnine poisoning in the dog. *J. Am. Vet. Med. Assoc.* 184 (1): 46–47.

23 Edwards, W.C., Kerr, L.A., and Whaley, M.W. (1981). Strychnine poisoning in dogs: sources and availability. *Vet. Med. Small Anim. Clin.* 76 (6): 823–824.

24 Osweiler, G.D., Carson, T.L.B., and Strychnine, W.B. (1985). *Clinical and Diagnostic Veterinary Toxicology*, 345–348. Duburque, Iowa: Kedall/Hunt Publishing Co.

25 Morgan, S., Martin, T., Edwards, W.C., and Stair, E.L. (1987). Investigating a case of Strychnine poisoning. *Vet. Med.-Us.* 82 (10): 1044.

26 Curtis, D.R., Duggan, A.W., and Johnston, G.A. (1971). The specificity of strychnine as a glycine antagonist in the mammalian spinal cord. *Exp. Brain Res.* 12 (5): 547–565.

27 Curtis, D.R., Hosli, L., and Johnston, G.A. (1968). A pharmacological study of the depression of spinal neurones by glycine and related amino acids. *Exp. Brain Res.* 6 (1): 1–18.

28 Fawcett, A. and Irwin, P. (2014). Diagnosis and treatment of generalised tetanus in dogs. *In Pract.* 36 (November/December): 482–493.

29 Acke, E., Jones, B.R., Breathnach, R. et al. (2004). Tetanus in the dog: review and a case-report of concurrent tetanus with hiatal hernia. *Ir. Vet. J.* 57 (10): 593–597.

30 Bandt, C., Rozanski, E.A., Steinberg, T., and Shaw, S.P. (2007). Retrospective study of tetanus in 20 dogs: 1988–2004. *J. Am. Anim. Hosp. Assoc.* 43 (3): 143–148.

31 Greene, C.E. (ed.) (1998). Tetanus. In: *Infectious Diseases of the Dog and Cat*, 267–273. Philadelphia: WB Saunders.

32 Cook, T.M., Protheroe, R.T., and Handel, J.M. (2001). Tetanus: a review of the literature. *Br. J. Anaesth.* 87 (3): 477–487.

33 Burkitt, J.M., Sturges, B.K., Jandrey, K.E., and Kass, P.H. (2007). Risk factors associated with outcome in dogs with tetanus: 38 cases (1987–2005). *J. Am. Vet. Med. Assoc.* 230 (1): 76–83.

34 Ohio State University College of Veterinary Medicine. (2015). Canine tetanus treatment requires time and care. Update for Veterinarians [Internet]. https://vet.osu.edu/sites/vet.osu.edu/files/legacy/documents/pdf/news/vmc/ovmaVeterinarianUpdate/20150304.pdf.

35 Sanford, J.P. (1995). Tetanus – forgotten but not gone. *N. Engl. J. Med.* 332 (12): 812–813.

36 Bleck, T.P. and Brauner, J.S. (1997). Tetanus. In: *Infections of the Central Nervous System* (ed. W.M. Scheld, R.J. Whitley and D.T. Durack), 629–653. Philadelphia: Lippincourt-Raven.

37 Bagley, R.S., Dougherty, S.A., and Randolph, J.F. (1994). Tetanus subsequent to Ovariohysterectomy in a dog. *Prog. Vet. Neurol.* 5 (2): 63–65.

38 Gansbauer, B., Kramer, S., Meyer-Lindenberg, A., and Nolte, I. (2000). Tetanus following ovariohysterectomy in a dog. *Tierarztl. Prax. K H.* 28 (4): 225–229.

39 Rubin, S., Faulkner, R.T., and Ward, G.E. (1983). Tetanus following Ovariohysterectomy in a dog – a case-report and review. *J. Am. Anim. Hosp. Assoc.* 19 (3): 293–298.

40 Jackson, C.B. and Drobatz, K.J. (2004). Iatrogenic magnesium overdose: 2 case reports. *J. Vet. Emerg. Crit. Care* 14 (2): 115–123.

41 Rhee, P., Nunley, M.K., Demetriades, D. et al. (2005). Tetanus and trauma: a review and recommendations. *J. Trauma* 58 (5): 1082–1088.

42 Ahmadsyah, I. and Salim, A. (1985). Treatment of tetanus: an open study to compare the efficacy of procaine penicillin and metronidazole. *Br. Med. J. (Clin. Res. Ed.)* 291 (6496): 648–650.

43 Benedict, C.R. and Kerr, J.H. (1977). Assessment of sympathetic overactivity in tetanus. *Br. Med. J.* 2 (6090): 806.

44 Hollow, V.M. and Clarke, G.M. (1975). Autonomic manifestations of tetanus. *Anaesth. Intensive Care* 3 (2): 142–147.

45 Kanarek, D.J., Kaufman, B., and Zwi, S. (1973). Severe sympathetic hyperactivity associated with tetanus. *Arch. Intern. Med.* 132 (4): 602–604.

46 Kerr, J.H., Corbett, J.L., Prys-Roberts, C. et al. (1968). Involvement of the sympathetic nervous system in tetanus. Studies on 82 cases. *Lancet* 2 (7562): 236–241.

47 Sutton, D.N., Tremlett, M.R., Woodcock, T.E., and Nielsen, M.S. (1990). Management of autonomic dysfunction in severe tetanus: the use of magnesium sulphate and clonidine. *Intensive Care Med.* 16 (2): 75–80.

48 Dieringer, T.M. and Wolf, A.M. (1991). Esophageal hiatal hernia and megaesophagus complicating tetanus in two dogs. *J. Am. Vet. Med. Assoc.* 199 (1): 87–89.

49 Braund, K.G. and Vandevelde, M. (1979). Polioencephalomalacia in the dog. *Vet. Pathol.* 16 (6): 661–672.

50 Fletcher, T.F. (1993). Spinal cord and meninges. In: *Miller's Anatomy of the Dog*, 3e (ed. H.E. Evans and M.E. Miller), 800–828. Philadelphia: W.B. Saunders.

51 Beresford, H.R., Posner, J.B., and Plum, F. (1969). Changes in brain lactate during induced cerebral seizures. *Arch. Neurol.* 20 (3): 243–248.

52 Read, D.H., Jolly, R.D., and Alley, M.R. (1977). Polioencephalomalacia of dogs with thiamine deficiency. *Vet. Pathol.* 14 (2): 103–112.

53 Singh, M., Thompson, M., Sullivan, N., and Child, G. (2005). Thiamine deficiency in dogs due to the feeding of sulphite preserved meat. *Aust. Vet. J.* 83 (7): 412–417.

54 Levy, M. (2018). Overview of polioencephalomalacia. Merck Veterinary Manual [Internet]. https://www.merckvetmanual.com/nervous-system/polioencephalomalacia/overview-of-polioencephalomalacia.

55 Krook, L. and Kenney, R.M. (1962). Central nervous system lesions in dogs with metastasizing islet cell carcinoma. *Cornell Vet.* 52: 385–415.

56 Hartley, W.J. (1963). Polioencephalomalacia in dogs. *Acta Neuropathol.* 3: 271–281.

57 Haymaker, W., Ginzler, A.M., and Ferguson, R.L. (1952). Residual neuropathological effects of cyanide poisoning; a study of the central nervous system of 23 dogs exposed to cyanide compounds. *Mil. Surg.* 111 (4): 231–246.

58 Amude, A.M., Headley, S.A., Alfieri, A.A. et al. (2011). Atypical necrotizing encephalitis associated with systemic canine distemper virus infection in pups. *J. Vet. Sci.* 12 (4): 409–412.

59 Moon, S.J., Kang, M.H., and Park, H.M. (2013). Clinical signs, MRI features, and outcomes of two cats with thiamine deficiency secondary to diet change. *J. Vet. Sci.* 14 (4): 499–502.

60 Garcia, J.L. (2014). Journal scan: food for thought: thiamine deficiency in dogs and cats. DVM 360 [Internet]. http://veterinarymedicine.dvm360.com/

journal-scan-food-thought-thiamine-deficiency-dogs-and-cats.

61 Dreyfus, P.M. and Victor, M. (1961). Effects of thiamine deficiency on the central nervous system. *Am. J. Clin. Nutr.* 9: 414–425.

62 Chang, Y.P., Chiu, P.Y., Lin, C.T. et al. (2017). Outbreak of thiamine deficiency in cats associated with the feeding of defective dry food. *J. Feline Med. Surg.* 19 (4): 336–343.

63 Schaer, M. (2006). Thiamine deficiency. *NAVC Clinician's Brief* (August): 21.

64 Davidson, M.G. (1992). Thiamin deficiency in a colony of cats. *Vet. Rec.* 130 (5): 94–97.

65 Kimura, M., Itokawa, Y., and Fujiwara, M. (1990). Cooking losses of Thiamin in food and its nutritional significance. *J. Nutr. Sci. Vitaminol.* 36 (4): S17–S24.

66 Markovich, J.E., Heinze, C.R., and Freeman, L.M. (2013). Thiamine deficiency in dogs and cats. *J. Am. Vet. Med. Assoc.* 243 (5): 649–656.

67 Steele, R.J.S. (1997). Thiamine deficiency in a cat assocatied with the preservation of 'pet meat' with Sulphur dioxide. *Aust. Vet. J.* 75: 719–721.

68 Davidson, M.G. (1992). Thiamine deficiency in a colony of cats. *Vet. Rec.* 130: 94–97.

69 Studdert, V.P. and Labuc, R.H. (1991). Thiamin deficiency in cats and dogs associated with feeding meat preserved with Sulphur dioxide. *Aust. Vet. J.* 68: 54–57.

70 Geraci, J.R. (1974). Thiamine deficiency in seals and recommendations for its prevention. *J. Am. Vet. Med. Assoc.* 165 (9): 801–803.

77

Involuntary Movements or Dyskinesias

77.1 Review of Motor Control

Recall from Chapter 74, Section 74.1 that the nervous system consists of a central site of integration, the central nervous system (CNS), and the peripheral nervous system (PNS). These systems communicate with one another via an extensive network of neurons [1–5].

Recall also that movement is initiated and modulated by upper motor neurons (UMNs). UMNs are responsible for signaling effector organs, such as muscle fibers, to contract. These messages reach their target organs by means of interneurons and lower motor neurons (LMNs) [1, 3, 4].

In order for movement to be functional, all components of the patient's motor system must work together. Coordination is essential so that electrical activity translates into motor activity that generates muscle tone, posture, and gait.

Many movements are reflexive, meaning that they occur without conscious thought. Others operate under voluntary control so that self-directed movement guides the patient where it wishes to go.

77.2 Introduction to Paroxysmal Dyskinesias

A variety of movement disorders have been recognized in companion animal patients [6]. These are referred to collectively as dyskinesias, which is translated from Greek to imply *bad movement.*

Paroxysmal dyskinesias refer to a family of movement disorders that are episodic [6]. Some, more than others, may appear to be epileptic [7]. However, unlike epilepsy, paroxysmal dyskinesias do not result in loss of consciousness, autonomic signs, and a postictal phase [6, 7].

Paroxysmal dyskinesias may be primary. These conditions are either inherited or idiopathic.

Secondary paroxysmal dyskinesias may result from an underlying structural lesion within the CNS or may be drug- or diet-induced [8].

Both primary and secondary dyskinesias involve impaired movement or posture due to involuntary muscle contractions, a phenomenon that is referred to as dystonia [7, 9]. Contractions may be either sustained or intermittent [9].

Clinical presentations of dystonia vary, depending upon the condition, but may involve one or more of the following signs [7–10]:

- Athetosis
  - Twisting and writhing movements, which may involve the trunk and/or the extremities
- Chorea
  - Translated from the Greek word for *dance,* to indicate abrupt, jerky movements that appear to flow from one muscle group into the next
  - Often involves the distal limbs and/or the face
  - Ballism or ballismus is a particularly violent type of chorea in which one or more limbs exhibits flailing
- Cramps
  - Sudden, severe, and potentially painful muscle contraction with concurrent immobility until spontaneous resolution occurs
- Fasciculations
  - Subtle flicker of contraction that involves a small percentage of muscle fibers, causing a slight twitch under the skin
- Myokymia
  - Continuous rippling of musculature beneath the skin
- Neuromyotonia
  - Delayed muscle relaxation, causing muscle to exhibit generalized stiffness
- Tremor
  - Involuntary quivering, caused by rhythmic muscle contractions

Common Clinical Presentations in Dogs and Cats, First Edition. Ryane E. Englar.
© 2019 John Wiley & Sons, Inc. Published 2019 by John Wiley & Sons, Inc.

Note that these presentations are not mutually exclusive [8]. For example, chorea may occur with athetosis.

Presentations are incredibly varied between patients. Clinical signs are periodic and sometimes repetitive [7, 11]. Most importantly, they are involuntary, meaning that their occurrence is not under conscious control [7, 11].

Depending upon the underlying condition, clinical signs may be precipitated by one or more of the following [7, 12]:

- Exercise
- Stress
- Sudden movement

In between episodes, patients are normal [7].

Several dyskinesias have been described in companion animal practice.

A genetic foundation has been proven for some dyskinesia [7–9, 13–16]. For example, episodic falling in Cavalier King Charles Spaniels has been linked to a deletion in the brevican gene (BCAN) [7–9, 13]. This mutation has an autosomal recessive mode of inheritance [9, 13, 17].

Others have been associated with diet, for instance, paroxysmal gluten-sensitive dyskinesia, which previously was called canine epileptoid cramping syndrome (CECS) [8].

Dyskinesias are increasingly recognized in companion animals [18]. However, the majority that have been described in the veterinary literature are idiopathic.

This chapter does not intend to be exhaustive. Instead, it will emphasize the most commonly observed dyskinesias in clinical practice.

77.3 Episodic Falling Syndrome of Cavalier King Charles Spaniels

Cavalier King Charles Spaniels may inherit this dyskinesia, which is characterized by episodes of collapse that are often precipitated by exercise, excitement, and stress [7, 9]. At the start of an episode, patients often lower the head and arch the spine [7, 9]. All limbs become very rigid before the patient falls to the ground [7, 19–21]. This rigidity is sometimes referred to as the "deer-stalking" position [7, 9].

When patients collapse, they do so with limbs extended [9]. Extensor rigidity is unmistakable [19–21].

A stiff, stilted, or "bunny-hopping" gait may precede the episode of collapse [9, 15]. Unlike many of the episodes of cardiogenic collapse, or syncope, that were described in Chapter 40, episodic falling syndrome of Cavalier King Charles Spaniels occurs without loss of consciousness [7].

Patients typically present for their first episode by four years of age, although episodes may occur as early as three months old [19].

Episodes are short-lived, lasting seconds to minutes [7, 19–21].

Patient interactions with the owner can abbreviate episodes [19]. The administration of clonazepam and/or acetazolamide may also be effective at reducing signs and/or frequency [7, 16, 22].

Spontaneous remission is possible, but inconsistent [7, 9].

77.4 Scottie Cramp

Scottie cramp is another example of an inherited dyskinesia [23, 24]. It occurs in Scottish Terriers, hence its name [23, 25].

Like episodic falling syndrome of Cavalier King Charles Spaniels, its mode of inheritance is autosomal recessive [9, 23, 24, 26–29].

Patients typically present for their first episode between six weeks of age and eighteen months old [9, 24, 25, 30].

Exercise and excitement are inciting factors [23]. During an episode, signs vary from focal hind limb gait changes to a whole-body cramp [23]. The following changes have been reported, but are inconsistently observed in affected patients [23, 25, 30]:

- Arching of the lumbar spine
- Cervical ventroflexion
- Spastic kicking with the pelvic limbs like a "bucking bronco" [23]
- Tail ventroflexion

Scottie cramp is a misnomer in that episodes do not appear to be painful [30].

Many episodes take place when running [23].

Most patients exhibit extensor rigidity of all four limbs, followed by collapse [23, 30]. Upon collapse, patients curl into a ball [23, 30].

Episodes are longer-lasting than those seen in episodic falling syndrome of Cavalier King Charles Spaniels [23]. It is not uncommon for episodes to last 20 min [23].

Clinical signs can be interrupted by calming excitable behavior [23, 30]. Patients that learn to sit on command when owners notice excitement levels ramping up may be able to limit their signs, reduce episodes, or reduce episode duration [23, 30].

Episodes may also be reduced by instituting fluoxetine and/or fluoxetine with diazepam [23]. However, the combination approach may over-sedate patients or cause unacceptable changes in behavior, such as aggression [23].

Fluoxetine, a selective serotonin reuptake inhibitor (SSRI), is thought to improve clinical signs because Scottie cramp is believed to be associated with lower-than-normal serotonin concentrations within the spinal cord [30].

Clinical signs are non-progressive [25]. In fact, they may improve with age [23].

77.5 Canine Epileptoid Cramping Syndrome

CECS is more appropriately referred to as paroxysmal gluten-sensitive dyskinesia, to distinguish it from the genetic condition, Scottie cramp [8].

CECS or paroxysmal gluten-sensitive dyskinesia is observed in the Border Terrier [9, 31].

Episodes are often prompted by excitement or waking from sleep [9].

Episodes vary in intensity and duration, lasting on average from 2 to 30 min [9].

Owners may recognize an impending episode by observing one or more of the following changes in their dogs [31]:

- Diarrhea
- Eating grass
- Subdued behavior
- Glueing themselves to the client
- Vomiting bile

The episodes themselves are varied in terms of their descriptions [9, 31]:

- Difficulty with ambulating
- Extensor rigidity
- Facial muscle dystonia
  - Often unilateral
- Grimacing facial expression
- Inability to support weight
- Torticollis
- Tremor

Gastrointestinal signs tend to persist during an episode. Borborygmi is common [9, 31].

Clients often describe their dogs as appearing uncomfortable [31]. Many clients felt that they could provide comfort by stroking their dogs, even though doing so did not appear to abbreviate the episode [31].

This condition responds well to dietary change to a gluten-free diet [9]. For this reason, this dyskinesia is thought to reflect underlying gluten sensitivity [9].

77.6 Idiopathic Head Tremor Syndrome

Idiopathic head tremor syndrome (IHTS) is most often reported in Doberman Pinschers, English Bulldogs,

Boxers, and Labrador Retrievers [7, 10, 32–34]. It is thought to be an inherited dyskinesia [7, 10, 32–35].

Dogs are typically less than two years old at time of onset, but they can be middle-aged to seniors [7].

Stress, illness, excitement, and exhaustion are thought to precipitate IHTS in Doberman Pinschers, but this does not appear to be the case in English Bulldogs [7, 10, 33].

Tremors typically consist of "head bobbing," which gives the appearance that the patient is nodding vertically [7]. Tremors may also occur side to side as if head-shaking "no" [7].

Cervical dystonia may or may not be noted during tremor activity [7].

Some patients appear anxious or uncomfortable during episodes [7]. They may bark or yawn in the middle of an episode [7]. Others seem to press their heads against inanimate objects [7].

Tremors may be short-lived or long-lasting [7]. Episodes of up to 3 h have been reported [7]. Episodes may occur multiple times per day [7]. Alternatively, patients may experience cluster episodes every couple of months [7].

Distractions may be helpful in terms of interrupting the episode [7]. The following actions appear to short-circuit the tremor [33]:

- Offering a toy
- Offering a treat
- Tactile stimulation
- Verbal communication

Spontaneous resolution of this dyskinesia is possible and occurs roughly 50% of the time [7, 32].

77.7 Benign, Idiopathic, Rapid, and Postural Tremors

Older dogs may develop tremors that are restricted to the hind limbs [8, 35]. These only switch on during standing, when there is some tension in the pelvic limb muscles [8, 35]. These tremors are therefore postural. They also tend to be bilaterally symmetrical [8]. They do not require treatment [35].

77.8 Intention Tremors

The preceding section considered tremors that occur at rest. However, tremors may also be associated with motion [8]. Consider, for example, intention tremors. Intention tremors are associated with goal-directed movement [8, 10]. This means that a particular action turns on the tremor. Discontinuing the action extinguishes the tremor.

Intention tremors may be idiopathic. However, more commonly they are a type of dyskinesia that results from cerebellar disease, particularly those pathologies that are inflammatory or degenerative [8]. Consider, for instance, feline cerebellar hypoplasia [36–40].

When cerebellar hypoplasia occurs in kittens, it is most often the result of feline panleukopenia. Feline panleukopenia was introduced in Chapter 51, Section 51.5.3. Recall that it is caused by a DNA virus that targets unvaccinated cats and cats less than one year of age [41].

Feline panleukopenia is environmentally stable, and is spread most often by indirect contact [41]. Queens may also transmit the virus in utero [41].

If infection occurs late in gestation, then live kittens will be birthed that have varying degrees of cerebellar hypoplasia [41]. Because the cerebellum is responsible for coordinated, fluid movement, hypoplasia results in variable ataxia and hypermetria, that is, a high-stepping gait [41–43]. Movement is disjointed and jerky [41].

Affected kittens typically have a wide-based stance, as if trying to improve their balance [41].

They are also likely to develop intention tremors [41]. These may be accentuated during bouts of feeding or when getting in and out of the litter box.

77.9 Positive Myoclonus and Canine Distemper Virus

Positive myoclonus is an exaggerated or violent tic, with an extremely intense, albeit brief, muscle contraction that results in a very pronounced jerking of the affected body part [44].

Myoclonus is not always pathological [44]. In humans, physiological myoclonus is associated with two benign actions [44]:

- Hiccups, which are caused by a jerk that targets the diaphragm
- Hypnic jerk or "sleep starts," in which the body unconsciously jolts when falling asleep

Hiccups may also occur in companion animal patients. Clients often report their development in puppies.

Myoclonus may also be drug-induced. It is seen in some patients that are being induced and/or are recovering from anesthetic cocktails [10, 45, 46]. Patients may also develop myoclonus as an adverse reaction to an administered drug, such as intrathecal administration of morphine [47, 48].

The classic textbook case of myoclonus involves a dog that is recovering from encephalitis secondary to canine distemper virus (CDV) [49–51].

CDV was introduced in Chapter 10, Section 10.5 with regard to its involvement in the development of so-called hard pad disease. Recall that hard pad disease refers to footpad hyperkeratosis, a commonly reported finding in dogs with CDV [52–54]. Nasal hyperkeratosis is also prevalent among survivors [52–54].

CDV was re-introduced in Parts Three, Four, and Six of the text as a cause of ocular, respiratory, and digestive clinical signs, including, but not limited to the following:

- Conjunctivitis [55]
- Viral pneumonia in dogs [56]
- Vomiting and diarrhea [57]

In addition, CDV is associated with grossly apparent enamel defects, including diffuse enamel hypoplasia [58–61].

Recall from Chapter 10, Section 10.5 that CDV is a negative-stranded, enveloped RNA virus within the genus Morbillivirus and the family Paramyxoviridae [62]. Although it is most commonly associated with multi-systemic disease in the dog, the principle reservoir host, CDV can also infect other carnivores, including members of the following orders of Carnivora [62–64]:

- Ailuridae, such as the lesser panda
- Felidae, such as the large wild cats
- Herpestidae, such as mongoose and meerkats
- Mustelidae, such as ferrets
- Procyonidae, such as raccoons
- Ursidae, such as bears and the giant panda
- Viverridae, such as civets

CDV is spread via body secretions, primarily respiratory exudates [62]. Puppies are most at risk; however, non-immunized adult dogs may become infected by contact with one or more patients that have already succumbed to CDV [62]. Stress, crowding, and immunosuppression are precipitating factors [62]. Dolichocephalic breeds of dog are overrepresented as compared to brachycephalic breeds [62].

When infected respiratory exudates contact the upper respiratory tract epithelium of a naïve dog, CDV replicates locally before spreading to the tonsils and regional lymph nodes [62]. As the virus replicates within lymphoid tissue, the affected patient develops a fever and leukopenia [62]. This occurs early on in the infection, within three to six days of exposure [62].

Conjunctivitis and a dry cough are commonly seen among patients infected with CDV [62]. Anorexia and depression are nonspecific, but common clinical signs [62].

Within eight or nine days of infection, CDV has spread to the CNS [62].

By day fourteen, patients with adequate immune response are able to clear the virus [62]. Those that cannot clear the virus will experience the spread of CDV throughout the body [62]. Most notably, CDV targets the genitourinary, gastrointestinal, and respiratory tracts [62].

Infection during pregnancy may result in abortions or the birth of failure-to-thrive pups [62].

Patients that survive CDV infection are likely to develop neurological manifestations of disease within a few weeks of recovery [62].

Neurological presentations are varied and may include one or more of the following signs [62, 63]:

- Ataxia
  - Cerebellar ataxia (see Chapter 72, Section 72.3.2)
    - Head bobbing
    - Hypermetric, "toy soldier" gait [42, 43]
      - Exaggerated flexion
      - High-stepping
      - Over-reaching
      - Stiff
      - Stilted
  - Central vestibular disease (refer to Chapter 72, Section 72.6)
  - Abnormal mentation
  - Circling
  - Cranial nerve dysfunction
    - The trigeminal nerve (CN V)
    - The facial nerve (CN VII)
    - The glossopharyngeal nerve (CN IX)
    - The vagus nerve (CN X)
    - The hypoglossal nerve (CN XII)
  - Head tilt
  - Nystagmus
- Blindness
  - Bilateral
  - Unilateral
- Paraparesis
- Proprioceptive deficits
- Retinitis
- Seizures (see Chapter 78)

Seizures may be generalized, but they are often partial, meaning that they are focal [62]. A classic type of partial seizure that occurs in dogs that are recovering from CDV is the "chewing gum" seizure [62]. The patient repetitively experiences twitching of the jaw as if chewing gum.

Myoclonus may be the only neurological manifestation of disease [62]. It is present in approximately 40% of cases involving CDV [63].

CDV-associated myoclonus most often targets the head and the limbs as opposed to the trunk [62]. Myoclonus is most apparent in CDV-infected dogs when they are asleep, although it may occur also while they are awake [62]. It is unclear how myoclonus originates in cases of CDV [62, 63]. It has been theorized that CDV induces a lesion within the basal nucleus that establishes the rhythmic pacing of this dyskinesia [44, 63, 65].

77.10 Fly-Catching Syndrome

Fly-catching syndrome refers to isolated episodes of licking and snapping at the air as if at an imaginary object [66–68]. These episodes may or may not involve swallowing [66].

Although fly-catching syndrome is thought to be a type of dyskinesia, many alternate theories have been suggested to explain this aberrant behavior [66, 69, 70]:

- Dietary allergy to meat-based protein [71]
- Epilepsy [68]
- Gastroesophageal reflux (GER) [72]
- Hallucinatory behavior
- Hyperactivity [73]
- Obsessive–compulsive disorder (OCD) [74]
- Stereotypy [17, 69, 74, 75]
- Visual deficits [73]

Fly-catching syndrome is not unique to one breed, although the following may be predisposed [66]:

- Greater Swiss Mountain Dog
- Cavalier King Charles Spaniel
- Miniature Schnauzer

Episodes may be infrequent, on the order of once per week, or as often as 30 times an hour [66]. There is great variety in terms of presentation and age at onset [66].

Patients do not typically respond to phenobarbital, primidone, or diazepam [17, 66, 67, 70, 71].

Some patients are responsive to trials of fluoxetine [66].

It is likely that there is not one single cause of fly-catching syndrome, but rather, several contributing factors [66].

Dyskinesia cannot be ruled out [66].

References

1 Molenaar, G.J. (1996). The nervous system. In: *Textbook of Veterinary Anatomy*, 2e (ed. K.M. Dyce, W.O. Sack and C.J.G. Wensing), 259–324. Philadelphia: W.B. Saunders Company.

2 Behan, M. (2004). Organization of the Nervous System. In: *Dukes' Physiology of Domestic Animals*, 12e (ed. W.O. Reece), 757–769. Ithaca: Comstock Publishing Associates.

3 Kitchell, R.L. Introduction to the nervous system. In: *Miller's Anatomy of the Dog*, 3e (ed. H.E. Evans), 758–775. Philadelphia: Saunders.

4 Garosi, L. (2009). Neurological examination of the cat. How to get started. *J. Feline Med. Surg.* 11 (5): 340–348.

5 Coates, J.R. (2009). The flaccid dog. DVM 360 [Internet]. http://veterinarycalendar.dvm360.com/flaccid-dog-proceedings.

6 Akin, E. (2017). Classifying paroxysmal dyskinesias. *NAVC Clinician's Brief* (June): 68–69.

7 Urkasemsin, G. and Olby, N.J. (2014). Canine paroxysmal movement disorders. *Vet. Clin. North Am. Small Anim. Pract.* 44 (6): 1091–1102.

8 Lowrie, M. and Garosi, L. (2016). Classification of involuntary movements in dogs: tremors and twitches. *Vet. J.* 214: 109–116.

9 Richter, A., Hamann, M., Wissel, J., and Volk, H.A. (2015). Dystonia and paroxysmal Dyskinesias: under-recognized movement disorders in domestic animals? A comparison with human dystonia/paroxysmal Dyskinesias. *Front. Vet. Sci.* 2: 65.

10 Englar, R. (ed.) (2017). Evaluating the nervous system of the dog. In: *Performing the Small Animal Physical Examination*, 412–431. Hoboken, NJ: Wiley.

11 de LaHunta, A. and Glass, E. (2009). *Veterinary Neuroanatomy and Clinical Neurology*. St. Louis: Sanders Elsevier.

12 Jankovic, J. and Demirkiran, M. (2002). Classification of paroxysmal dyskinesias and ataxias. *Adv. Neurol.* 89: 387–400.

13 Lowrie, M. and Garosi, L. (2017). Classification of involuntary movements in dogs: paroxysmal dyskinesias. *Vet. J.* 220: 65–71.

14 O'Brien, D., Kolicheski, A., Packer, R. et al. (2015). Paroxysmal non-kinesogenic dyskinesia in soft coated wheaten terriers associated with a missense mutation in PIGN and responds to acetazolamide therapy. *J. Vet. Intern. Med.* 29: 1257–1283.

15 Gill, J.L., Tsai, K.L., Krey, C. et al. (2012). A canine BCAN microdeletion associated with episodic falling syndrome. *Neurobiol. Dis.* 45 (1): 130–136.

16 Forman, O.P., Penderis, J., Hartley, C. et al. (2012). Parallel mapping and simultaneous sequencing reveals deletions in BCAN and FAM83H associated with discrete inherited disorders in a domestic dog breed. *PLoS Genet.* 8 (1): e1002462.

17 Rusbridge, C. (2005). Neurological diseases of the cavalier king Charles spaniel. *J. Small Anim. Pract.* 46 (6): 265–272.

18 Lowrie, M. and Garosi, L. (2016). Natural history of canine paroxysmal movement disorders in Labrador retrievers and Jack Russell terriers. *Vet. J.* 213: 33–37.

19 Herrtage, M.E. and Palmer, A.C. (1983). Episodic falling in the cavalier King Charles spaniel. *Vet. Rec.* 112 (19): 458–459.

20 Wright, J.A., Brownlie, S.E., Smyth, J.B. et al. (1986). Muscle hypertonicity in the cavalier King Charles spaniel–myopathic features. *Vet. Rec.* 118 (18): 511–512.

21 Wright, J.A., Smyth, J.B., Brownlie, S.E., and Robins, M. (1987). A myopathy associated with muscle hypertonicity in the cavalier King Charles spaniel. *J. Comp. Pathol.* 97 (5): 559–565.

22 Garosi, L.S., Platt, S.R., and Shelton, G.D. (2002). Hypertonicity in cavalier King Charles spaniels. *J. Vet. Intern. Med.* 16: 330.

23 Urkasemsin, G. and Olby, N.J. (2015). Clinical characteristics of Scottie cramp in 31 cases. *J. Small Anim. Pract.* 56 (4): 276–280.

24 Meyers, K.M., Lund, J.E., Padgett, G., and Dickson, W.M. (1969). Hyperkinetic episodes in Scottish terrier dogs. *J. Am. Vet. Med. Assoc.* 155 (2): 129–133.

25 Shelton, G.D. (2004). Muscle pain, cramps and hypertonicity. *Vet. Clin. North Am. Small.* 34 (6): 1483–1496.

26 de LaHunta, A. and Glass, E. (2009). Upper motor neuron: movement disorders. In: *Veterinary Neuroanatomy and Clinical Neurology* (ed. A. de LaHunta and E. Glass), 217–220. St. Louis: Saunders/Elsevier.

27 Clemmons, R.M., Peters, R.I., and Meyers, K.M. (1980). Scotty cramp: a review of cause, characteristics, diagnosis, and treatment. *Compend. Contin. Educ. Pract. Vet.* 2: 385.

28 Garosi, L. and Harvey, R.J. (2012). Scottie cramp and canine epileptoid cramping syndrome in border terriers. *Vet. Rec.* 170 (7): 186–187.

29 Meyers, K.M., Padgett, G.A., and Dickson, W.M. (1970). The genetic basis of a kinetic disorder of Scottish terrier dogs. *J. Hered.* 61 (5): 189–192.

30 Geiger, K.M. and Klopp, L.S. (2009). Use of a selective serotonin reuptake inhibitor for treatment of episodes of hypertonia and kyphosis in a young adult Scottish terrier. *J. Am. Vet. Med. Assoc.* 235 (2): 168–171.

31 Black, V., Garosi, L., Lowrie, M. et al. (2014). Phenotypic characterisation of canine epileptoid cramping syndrome in the border terrier. *J. Small Anim. Pract.* 55 (2): 102–107.

32 Shell, L.G., Berezowski, J., Rishniw, M. et al. (2015). Clinical and breed characteristics of idiopathic head tremor syndrome in 291 dogs: a retrospective study. *Vet. Med. Int.* 2015: 165463.

33 Wolf, M., Bruehschwein, A., Sauter-Louis, C. et al. (2011). An inherited episodic head tremor syndrome in Doberman pinscher dogs. *Mov. Disord.* 26 (13): 2381–2386.

34 Guevar, J., De Decker, S., Van Ham, L.M. et al. (2014). Idiopathic head tremor in English bulldogs. *Mov. Disord.* 29 (2): 191–194.

35 de Lahunta, A., Glass, E.N., and Kent, M. (2006). Classifying involuntary muscle contractions. *Compend. Contin. Educ. Pract.* 28 (7): 516–530.

36 Lavely, J.A. (2006). Pediatric neurology of the dog and cat. *Vet. Clin. North Am. Small Anim. Pract.* 36 (3): 475–501, v.

37 Bagley, R.S. (2006). The cat with tremor or twitching. In: *Problem-Based Feline Medicine* (ed. J. Rand), 852–869. St. Louis: Saunders Elsevier.

38 Hoskins, J.D. and Shelton, G.D. (2001). The nervous and neuromuscular systems. In: *Veterinary Pediatrics: Dogs and Cats from Birth to Six Months*, 3e (ed. J.D. Hoskins), 425–462. Philadelphia: Saunders.

39 Blythe, L.L. (2011). The neurologic system. In: *Small Animal Pediatrics: The First 12 Months of Life* (ed. M.E. Peterson and M.A. Kutzler), 418–435. St. Louis, Mo.: Saunders/Elsevier.

40 Barone, G. (2012). Neurology. In: *The Cat: Clinical Medicine and Management* (ed. S.E. Little), 734–767. St. Louis: Elsevier Saunders.

41 Greene, C.E. and Addie, D.D. (2006). Feline parvovirus infections. In: *Infectious Diseases of the Dog and Cat*, 3e (ed. C.E. Greene), 78–88. St. Louis, Mo: Saunders/Elsevier.

42 Averill, D.R. Jr. (1981). The neurologic examination. *Vet. Clin. North Am. Small Anim. Pract.* 11 (3): 511–521.

43 Casimiro da Costa, R. (ed.) (2009). Ataxia – Recognition and approach. World Small Animal Veterinary Association World Congress Proceedings.

44 Lowrie, M. and Garosi, L. (2017). Classification of involuntary movements in dogs: myoclonus and Myotonia. *J. Vet. Intern. Med.* 31 (4): 979–987.

45 Ferreira, J.P., Dzikit, T.B., Zeiler, G.E. et al. (2015). Anaesthetic induction and recovery characteristics of a diazepam-ketamine combination compared with propofol in dogs. *J. S. Afr. Vet. Assoc.* 86 (1): 1258.

46 Cattai, A., Rabozzi, R., Natale, V., and Franci, P. (2015). The incidence of spontaneous movements (myoclonus) in dogs undergoing total intravenous anaesthesia with propofol. *Vet. Anaesth. Analg.* 42 (1): 93–98.

47 Iff, I., Valeskini, K., and Mosing, M. (2012). Severe pruritus and myoclonus following intrathecal morphine administration in a dog. *Can. Vet. J.* 53 (9): 983–986.

48 da Cunha, A.F., Carter, J.E., Grafinger, M. et al. (2007). Intrathecal morphine overdose in a dog. *J. Am. Vet. Med. Assoc.* 230 (11): 1665–1668.

49 Thomas, W.B. (2000). Initial assessment of patients with neurologic dysfunction. *Vet. Clin. North Am. Small Anim. Pract.* 30 (1): 1–24, v.

50 Schubert, T., Clemmons, R., Miles, S., and Draper, W. (2013). The use of Botulinum toxin for the treatment of generalized myoclonus in a dog. *J. Am. Anim. Hosp. Assoc.* 49 (2): 122–127.

51 Koutinas, A.F., Polizopoulou, Z.S., Baumgaertner, W. et al. (2002). Relation of clinical signs to pathological changes in 19 cases of canine distemper encephalomyelitis. *J. Comp. Pathol.* 126 (1): 47–56.

52 Martella, V., Elia, G., and Buonavoglia, C. (2008). Canine distemper virus. *Vet. Clin. North Am. Small Anim. Pract.* 38 (4): 787–797, vii–viii.

53 Greene, E.C. and Appel, M.J. (1990). Canine distemper virus. In: *Infectious Diseases of the Dog and Cat* (ed. E.C. Greene), 226–241. Philadelphia: W.B. Saunders.

54 Engelhardt, P., Wyder, M., Zurbriggen, A., and Grone, A. (2005). Canine distemper virus associated proliferation of canine footpad keratinocytes in vitro. *Vet. Microbiol.* 107 (1–2): 1–12.

55 Ofri, R. (2017). Conjunctivitis in dogs. *NAVC Clinician's Brief* (April): 89–93.

56 Palma, D. (2016). Common pulmonary diseases in dogs. *NAVC Clinician's Brief* (October): 77–109.

57 Greene, E.C. and Appel, M.J. (2006). Canine distemper, ch. 3. In: *Infectious Diseases of the Dog and Cat*, 3e (ed. E.C. Greene), 25–41. St. Louis, MO: Elsevier.

58 Boy, S., Crossley, D., and Steenkamp, G. (2016). Developmental structural tooth defects in dogs – experience from veterinary dental referral practice and review of the literature. *Front. Vet. Sci.* 3: 9.

59 Miles, A.E.W., Grigson, C., and Colyer, F. (1990). *Colyer's Variations and Diseases of the Teeth of Animals*. Rev. ed., xvi, 672 p. Cambridge England; New York: Cambridge University Press.

60 Bittegeko, S.B., Arnbjerg, J., Nkya, R., and Tevik, A. (1995). Multiple dental developmental abnormalities following canine distemper infection. *J. Am. Anim. Hosp. Assoc.* 31 (1): 42–45.

61 Dubielzig, R.R. (1979). The effect of canine distemper virus on the ameloblastic layer of the developing tooth. *Vet. Pathol.* 16 (2): 268–270.

62 Greene, C.E. and Appel, M.J. (2006). Canine distemper. In: *Infectious Diseases of the Dog and Cat*, 3e (ed. C.E. Green), 25–41. St. Louis: Elsevier, Inc.

63 Tipold, A., Vandevelde, M., and Jaggy, A. (1992). Neurological manifestations of canine-distemper virus-infection. *J. Small Anim. Pract.* 33 (10): 466–470.

64 Deem, S.L., Spelman, L.H., Yates, R.A., and Montali, R.J. (2000). Canine distemper in terrestrial carnivores: a review. *J. Zoo Wildl. Med.* 31 (4): 441–451.

65 de La Lhunta, A. (1983). *Veterinary Neuroanatomy and Clinical Neurology*, 2e. Philadephia: W.B. Saunders.

66 Wrzosek, M., Plonek, M., Nicpon, J. et al. (2015). Retrospective multicenter evaluation of the "fly-catching syndrome" in 24 dogs: EEG, BAER, MRI, CSF findings and response to antiepileptic and antidepressant treatment. *Epilepsy Behav.* 53: 184–189.

67 Cash, W.C. and Blauch, B.S. (1979). Jaw snapping syndrome in eight dogs. *J. Am. Vet. Med. Assoc.* 175 (7): 709–710.

68 Manteca, X. (1994). Fly snapping syndrome in dogs. *Vet. Q.* 16 (sup1): 49.

69 Lorenz, M.D., Coates, J., and Kent, M. (2012). *Handbook of Veterinary Neurology*. St. Louis: Elsevier Saunders.

70 Thomas, W.B. and Dewey, C.W. (2009). Seizures and narcolepsy. In: *A Practical Guide to Canine and Feline Neurology* (ed. C. Dewey), 237–240. Ames, IA: Wiley-Blackwell.

71 Brown, P.R. (1987). Fly catching in the cavalier King Charles spaniel. *Vet. Rec.* 120 (4): 95.

72 Frank, D., Belanger, M.C., Becuwe-Bonnet, V., and Parent, J. (2012). Prospective medical evaluation of 7 dogs presented with fly biting. *Can. Vet. J.* 53 (12): 1279–1284.

73 Voith, V. (1979). Behavioral problems. In: *Canine Medicine and Therapeutics* (ed. E.A. Chandler, W.B. Singleton, F.G. Startup, et al.), 415. Oxford: Blackwell Scientific.

74 Overall, K.L. and Dunham, A.E. (2002). Clinical features and outcome in dogs and cats with obsessive-compulsive disorder: 126 cases (1989–2000). *J. Am. Vet. Med. Assoc.* 221 (10): 1445–1452.

75 Tynes, V.V. and Sinn, L. (2014). Abnormal repetitive behaviors in dogs and cats: a guide for practitioners. *Vet. Clin. North Am. Small Anim. Pract.* 44 (3): 543–564.

78

Seizures

78.1 Introduction to Seizing as a Clinical Sign

At the most basic level, a seizure is defined as a sudden event or attack [1]. Another name for seizure is ictus [1, 2]. This term appears more frequently in the human medical literature. However, the term post-ictal is used very commonly in veterinary medicine to describe the events that immediately follow ictus.

There are many different types of seizures, just as there are many different causes.

When clinicians use the word *seizure*, they are most often referring to an epileptic seizure. An epileptic seizure is a specific type of event that is characterized by an uncontrolled surge of electrical activity [3–5]. This surge originates from the central nervous system (CNS) and represents an imbalance between excitatory and inhibitory impulses [3–5]. Neuronal hyperactivity predominates [3].

With the exception of status epilepticus, which is a continuous seizure state without recovery between events, epileptic seizures are transient episodes [1, 4, 5].

Epileptic seizures may occur once in a lifetime, or they may reappear at intervals. Intervals may be fixed and predictable, or they may be variable [1].

In humans, epileptic seizures are preceded by what is referred to as an aura [1, 2]. An aura is a subjective experience that indicates to the patient that a seizure is coming [1, 2, 6].

A variety of auras have been described throughout the human medical literature, including the following [1, 2]:

- Auditory cues
  - Buzzing
  - Drumming
- Changes in emotion
  - Aggression
  - Depression
  - Fear
- Gastrointestinal discomfort
  - Abdominal pain
  - Nausea
  - Unusual taste in mouth
- Olfactory cues
  - Perceiving an unusual odor
- Somatosensory cues
  - Electric shocks
  - Numbness
  - Tingling
- Visual cues
  - Flashing or flickering of lights
  - Perceiving spots across the visual field

It is difficult to appreciate whether these sensations occur in epileptic veterinary patients [1]. However, based upon the behaviors that some exhibit just before a seizure occurs, it is likely that affected animals do experience one or more unusual sensations [1, 2, 7, 8]. For example, some animals have been described to spontaneously run just prior to an episode, as if trying to escape it [1]. Others start pacing and/or panting at the start of a seizure as if they are either anxious or seeking attention [9].

Clients have reported that the following behavior changes in some cats appear to precede seizure activity [10]:

- Growling
- Increased affection toward owners
- Increased aggression toward owners
- Restlessness
- Vocalizing

Many seizures are convulsive as a result of heightened motor activity [1]. Motor activity may take one of several forms. Tonic–clonic phases of motor activity are most often described in the veterinary literature [1, 11]:

- Tonic phase
  - Prolonged muscular contraction
  - Causes tightening of one or more muscles or muscle groups
  - This may cause the patient to adopt an unusual posture
  - If both agonist and antagonist muscles are involved, the patient will exhibit a twisting or writhing movement

Common Clinical Presentations in Dogs and Cats, First Edition. Ryane E. Englar.
© 2019 John Wiley & Sons, Inc. Published 2019 by John Wiley & Sons, Inc.

- Clonic phase
  - Follows the tonic phase
  - Is characterized by a jerking action of somatic muscles

Tonic–clonic motor activity is characteristic of so-called grand mal or generalized seizures [1, 2]. See below.

78.1.1 Generalized Seizure Activity

Generalized seizures involve both cerebral hemispheres [1, 2]. This results in whole-body involvement, collapse, and loss of consciousness [9].

The presentation, collapse, was introduced in Section 40.1. Recall that collapse describes the loss of postural tone [12–15]. Without postural tone, the body is unable to maintain itself upright, and falls to the ground [16].

Episodes of collapse may be due to syncope or seizures [12–14, 17, 18]. Recall that syncope and seizures may be difficult to distinguish based upon observation alone [15, 18–20]. Let us review key differences between the two.

In general, syncope is preceded by pelvic limb weakness and/or ataxia [17]. These occur when cerebral perfusion is reduced to the point of losing consciousness [17]. The fainting spell itself is typically brief, one minute or less [17]. Patients are most often flaccid when they collapse [17].

Generalized seizures, on the other hand, have historically been described as having abnormal motor signs, with, or without autonomic activity [2, 13, 17]. Patients typically fall to the side in recumbency, and demonstrate opisthotonus [2]. They have increased tone, particularly in the limbs [2]. Extensor rigidity is common [2].

During tonic–clonic seizures, clients may describe the motor activity in the limbs as paddling [2, 9]. Note that seizures may also be simply tonic, meaning that they involve muscle rigidity, without paddling [2].

Ptyalism is common among those with generalized seizures, and patients may lose control of their urinary bladders or bowels [2, 9].

Patients often exhibit automatism, that is, unconscious behaviors. These are not unique to veterinary patients and may include the following [1]:

- Oral fixations
  - Chewing
  - Grinding teeth
  - Licking
  - Swallowing
- Vocalizations
  - Barking
  - Growling
  - Meowing

Respirations are irregular during a generalized seizure [2]. It is possible for patients to become cyanotic [2].

On average, seizures last longer than syncopal episodes, and patients are typically slower to recover [17].

Immediately following the seizure is a post-ictal period [1, 2]. Its duration varies from minutes to hours [1, 2].

Common post-ictal clinical signs among dogs include the following [1, 2, 4, 7, 21, 22]:

- Ataxia
- Disorientation
- Hunger
- Impaired awareness
- Impaired vision
- Lethargy
- Pacing
- Thirst

78.1.2 Partial Seizure Activity

Seizures may also be partial or focal, meaning that only one part of one cerebral hemisphere is involved [1, 2]. This limits which body parts are involved [9]. For instance, partial seizures may involve the following [1, 2]:

- The neck
- The trunk
- The proximal thoracic limb
  - Any region from the shoulder to the carpus
- The proximal pelvic limb
  - Any region from the hip to the tarsus
- The distal thoracic limb
  - Any region from the metacarpals to the phalanges
- The distal pelvic limb
  - Any region from the metatarsals to the phalanges

As an example of a partial seizure, one limb may contract [2]. Alternatively, the patient may exhibit chewing behavior, due to isolated contractions of the jaw [2]. These types of partial seizures do not involve loss of consciousness [2].

However, there are complex partial seizures in which awareness is impaired [2]. These seizures are sometimes referred to as psychomotor seizures. Patients may exhibit the following [2, 7, 23, 24]:

- Extreme changes in behavior
  - Aggression
  - Exaggerated startle response
  - Fear
- Repetitive motor activities
  - Escape behavior
  - Head pressing
  - Running
  - Vocalizing

Just as generalized seizures can be difficult to distinguish from syncope, partial seizures may be difficult to distinguish from vestibular episodes or dyskinesias [9]. Refer to Chapters 72 and 77 for a review of these clinical presentations.

78.2 Causes of Seizures

There are many causes of seizures. It may help to consider these causes in light of whether they originate from within the brain itself or are extracranial.

78.2.1 Intracranial Causes of Seizures

Intracranial causes of seizures include the following [2, 3, 9, 10, 25–39]:

- Anoxia
- CNS trauma
- Degenerative disease
  - Senile changes associated with aging
  - Thiamine deficiency
- Idiopathic epilepsy
- Infectious disease
  - Bacterial
    o *Escherichia coli*
    o *Staphylococcus* spp.
    o *Streptococcus* spp.
  - Fungal
    o Blastomycosis
    o Coccidioidomycosis
    o Cryptococcosis
  - Parasitic
    o Aberrant migration of *Cuterebra* larvae
    o Aberrant migration of adult *Dirofilaria immitis*
  - Protozoal
    o Neosporosis, caused by *Neospora caninum*
    o Toxoplasmosis, caused by *Toxoplasma gondii*
  - Rickettsial
    o Ehrlichiosis
    o Rocky Mountain Spotted Fever (RMSF)
  - Viral
    o Canine distemper virus (CDV) (see Chapter 77, Section 77.9)
    o Feline immunodeficiency virus (FIV)
    o Feline infectious peritonitis (FIP)
    o Feline leukemia virus (FeLV)
    o Rabies virus
- Neoplasia
- Noninfectious inflammatory disease
  - Meningoencephalomyelitis
    o Granulomatous meningoencephalomyelitis (GME)
  - Necrotizing encephalitis
    o Yorkshire Terriers

- Necrotizing leukoencephalitis (NLE)
- Necrotizing meningoencephalomyelitis (NME)
  o Maltese
- Pug dog encephalitis
- Storage diseases
- Structural diseases
  - Hydrocephalus
  - Lissencephaly
- Vascular accident

78.2.2 Extracranial Causes of Seizures

Extracranial causes of seizures include the following [3, 10, 25, 32]:

- Changes in electrolytes
  - Hyperkalemia
  - Hypocalcemia
- Endocrinopathy
  - Hyperthyroidism
  - Hypothyroidism
- Hypoglycemia
- Metabolic dysfunction
  - Hepatic encephalopathy (HE)
  - Uremia
- Nutritional
  - Thiamine deficiency
- Polycythemia vera
- Portosystemic shunts (PSSs)
- Toxicosis
  - Chocolate
    o Methylxanthines
    o Theobromine
  - Ethylene glycol
  - Heavy metals
    o Arsenic
    o Lead
    o Mercury
  - Metaldehyde
  - Tremorogenic mycotoxins
    o Penitrem A
    o Roquefortine

78.3 The Diagnostic Approach to Seizures

Any time that a patient presents for evaluation of seizure activity, the clinician must ask two questions [2, 4, 40].

First, did the patient truly seize? [2, 4, 40]

As aforementioned, many clinical conditions can mimic seizures [40]. These include, but are not limited to the following [40]:

- Narcolepsy
- Neuromuscular weakness
- Stereotypy
- Syncope
- Tremors
  - Idiopathic
  - Postural
- Vestibular disease

History taking allows for data gathering that can support or refute seizure activity [40]. See Section 78.3.2 below.

If it appears that the patient did seize, then the second question that the clinician must ask of himself is

- What is the cause? [2, 4, 40]

As is evident from Section 78.2, the list of differential diagnoses to consider for seizure activity is extensive. It can be overwhelming for any veterinarian to conduct an exhaustive search through all potential differentials. Furthermore, time and finances are often rate-limiting steps.

It is therefore important to consider the diagnostic approach to seizures in light of which differentials are most likely. That is the most appropriate starting point.

78.3.1 The Signalment

The diagnostic approach to seizures begins with the patient's signalment. The signalment refers to the following demographic characteristics of the patient:

- Age
- Sex
- Sexual status
- Breed
- Species

The signalment is often used to prompt case discussion within the hospital setting. For instance:

- Bailey is a 14-year-old female spayed Tonkinese cat
- Bliss is a four-year-old female spayed British Shorthair cat
- Suzy Q is a two-year-old female intact Shih Tzu dog
- Panda is a six-week-old male intact Chihuahua puppy.

The above features can aid the prioritization of differentials so that the clinician can approach case management from the perspective of the individual patient.

Consider age and breed, for example. Hypoglycemia was introduced in Chapter 71, Section 71.5.1 as a common condition in neonates, particularly toy and small-breed dogs [41–43]. These patients are often unable to endure long periods of fasting without experiencing a drop in blood glucose [41–43]. This dip in glucose

can precipitate seizure activity. Therefore, if a pediatric Chihuahua were to present to the clinic with a history of seizing, age-related hypoglycemia would be a top differential.

Hypoglycemia is less common in kittens, but when it occurs, Persian cats are overrepresented [41, 42]. Therefore, if a neonatal Persian kitten were to present with the same history as the pediatric Chihuahua, then hypoglycemia would be a top differential.

By contrast, a young to middle-aged patient is more likely to have idiopathic epilepsy [3, 25].

A middle-aged to senior patient is more likely to seize secondary to degenerative disease, neoplasia, or vascular compromise [3, 25].

Note that signalment is not a guarantee that the prioritized differential list will be correct, but it is a starting point that factors into consideration that which is most probable.

78.3.2 The Clinical History

History taking also provides invaluable information for any clinical consultation. It is especially important to obtain a comprehensive history from a patient that may have had a seizure.

Unless the patient presents in status epilepticus, most appear clinically normal in terms of appearance, mentation, and neurologic status when they arrive to the clinic for evaluation [18, 44–51]. This is not unlike patients that present for a work-up of presumptive syncope.

Because it is rare to demonstrate clinically abnormal findings in patients with transient episodes, the presumptive diagnosis relies heavily upon patient history [18–20, 44–51].

In addition to standard history-taking questions, the following content areas should be explored [2]:

- Changes in appetite
- Changes in behavior
  - At home
  - Within the examination room
- Changes in gait
- Changes in sleep patterns and wake cycles
- Dietary history, including any recent changes in diet and/or dietary indiscretions
  - What is the current diet?
  - Was there a recent change in diet?
  - What, if anything, is fed as a treat?
  - What, if anything, is fed as a supplement?
  - Have there been any recent dietary indiscretions?
- Familial history of seizures
- Known or potential exposure to toxins, including access to illicit substances

- Prescribed medications, including flea/tick and heartworm preventative, and over-the-counter topical or oral products
- Prior medical health history, including any chronic diseases, such as those known to cause metabolic dysfunction or electrolyte derangement
- Vaccination history
  - Which, if any vaccines, were previously administered?
  - Which, if any vaccine series, have been completed?
  - Is the patient current on vaccines?
  - Has vaccine protection lapsed?

Concerning the event itself, it is important to obtain the following details [2, 40]:

- Client observations
  - What did the client witness?
  - Did the client observe a head tilt or tremor?
  - Did the client observe eye or muzzle twitching that would suggest facial involvement?
  - Can the client describe the patient's mentation during the episode?
    - Was the patient alert and aware?
    - Was the patient unconscious?
  - Was the patient responsive to the client during the episode?
  - Can the client describe the patient's muscle tone during the event?
    - Was the patient flaccid?
    - Was the patient rigid?
  - Did the patient collapse?
  - Did the patient exhibit extensor rigidity?
  - Did the patient exhibit unusual breathing patterns?
  - Did the patient paddle?
  - Did the patient exhibit autonomic signs?
    - Defecation
    - Salivation
    - Urination
    - Vomiting
- Duration
  - How long did the event last?
- First occurrence or repeat episode
  - Is this the first time that this event has occurred, to the best of the client's knowledge?
  - Is this a recurrent episode? If so:
    - How many times has it happened before?
    - How frequently do these episodes occur?
    - Is the interval between episodes predictable?
    - How was this episode similar to past episodes?
    - How, if at all, did this episode differ?
- Precipitating factors
  - What was the patient doing just before the event?
  - Did anything unusual happen prior to the event that could have triggered it?

- Post-episode changes
  - Did the patient appear to be affected after the event ended?
  - Was there a post-ictal period? If so:
    - What behaviors did the client witness?
    - How long did it last?

History may be imperfect. It is, after all, the client's account of what transpired. It is subjective, and it is colored by emotion. It also may change as memory of the event fades.

For this reason, it is challenging to differentiate syncope from seizures based upon observation or recounted history alone [14, 19].

However, without history, the clinician has very little information to move forward with the investigation.

78.3.3   The Physical Examination

Although most patients with a seizure history do not present with physical examination findings that are pathognomonic for the cause of the seizure, the importance of the physical examination cannot be overstated.

The physical examination may reveal signs of systemic disease that could precipitate seizure activity.

Consider, for example, the classic clinical vignette of the hypothyroid dog. Hypothyroidism was introduced in Chapter 5, Section 5.7 as a cause of endocrine-associated, non-inflammatory alopecia.

The hypothyroid canine patient may present as one of the most commonly affected breeds: Doberman Pinschers, Golden Retrievers, Old English Sheepdogs, Irish Setters, and Great Danes [52].

Clients may report increased weight gain without a change in caloric intake.

On physical examination, the hypothyroid canine patient may exhibit changes in the following systems [52–54]:

- Cardiovascular system
  - Bradycardia
- Integumentary system
  - Alopecia over pressure points, such as the elbows and hips
  - Bilaterally symmetrical truncal alopecia
  - "Rat tail"
  - "Ring around the collar"
- Musculoskeletal system
  - Muscle weakness
  - Slow, stiff gait
- Special senses
  - Anterior uveitis
  - Corneal lipid deposits

Of the physical examination findings outlined above, the changes in the integumentary system are most consistent with an endocrinopathy. These findings, in addition to the signalment and the history, paint a picture that is strongly suggestive of hypothyroidism. The clinician should, in this case, conduct a diagnostic investigation to explore whether or not this patient is hypothyroid. If it is, then seizure activity could be explained by endocrinopathy and expected to resolve with medical correction of the hypothyroid state.

In this patient, it is still beneficial and warranted to explore other potential causes of seizures so as not to miss a case diagnosis on account of tunnel vision.

But it is proper to follow the trail of clues that lead to the diagnosis.

Keep in mind that the physical examination of all seizure suspects should be comprehensive. To be complete, the physical examination should include the following components [55]:

- Fundoscopic examination
- Neurologic examination

Because the optic nerves are extensions of the CNS, diseases within the CNS can cause pathology in these structures [55].

Thalamocortical lesions typically cause changes in behavior in addition to seizure activity. Affected patients may also present with the following changes on neurologic examination [10, 55]:

- Blindness
- Circling
- Miotic pupils
- Postural reaction deficits

78.3.4   Clinicopathologic Data

Patients that present with a seizure history benefit from the gathering of clinicopathologic data that may round out the clinical picture and build a case for a diagnosis [2].

At minimum, a complete blood count (CBC) and chemistry panel are warranted in a patient with one or more seizures [2].

A CBC provides insight into the patient's hemogram and leukogram.

Hematologic changes that could explain seizures include the following [2]:

- Basophilic stippling and/or nucleated erythrocytes or red blood cells (RBCs)
  - These changes are suggestive of lead toxicosis.
- Increased numbers of RBCs
  - Polycythemia vera is a myeloproliferative disease in which the bone marrow overproduces RBCs.
- Inflammatory leukogram

- This suggests the presence of inflammatory cytokines, which may indicate ongoing inflammation or an infectious process.

A chemistry panel provides insight into organ function. In particular, renal and hepatic values are of interest, given that both uremia and HE can result in seizure activity.

A chemistry panel also provides insight into key electrolyte levels and serum glucose. Derangements in either may precipitate seizure activity.

Add-on blood tests may be indicated on a case-by-case basis [2]:

- Bile acid testing is of interest in a young animal in which a portosystemic shunt (PSS) is suspected (see Chapter 71, Section 71.7).
- Blood lead levels are important if lead toxicosis is suspected (see Chapter 71, Section 71.8).

78.3.5   Advanced Diagnostics in Patients with Seizure Activity

Most skull radiographs are normal in patients with seizure activity [55]. However, they may be of value in trauma cases. They may also demonstrate osteolytic lesions of tumors that invade bone [55].

Advanced imaging in the form of computed tomography (CT) or magnetic resonance imaging (MRI) is a superior diagnostic tool because these modalities provide details of the brain and spinal cord [27, 55]. Although both typically require referral, they are of value in being able to rule out space-occupying lesions that could trigger seizure activity [2, 55].

Collection of cerebrospinal fluid (CSF) in a patient with unremarkable imaging allows for consideration of infectious encephalitis [2, 55].

Cytology of CSF may provide insight as to the causative agent of disease [10]. For example [10]:

- Eosinophilic pleocytosis is supportive of aberrant parasitic migration.
- Lymphocytic pleocytosis is consistent with a diagnosis of rabies, CNS lymphoma, or toxoplasmosis.
- Mixed cell pleocytosis is suggestive of fungal encephalitis or chronic FIP.
- Neutrophilic pleocytosis is supportive of bacterial encephalitis, particularly when neutrophils are degenerate.

CSF may also be evaluated by culture and infectious disease titers [10]. For example, the following conditions may be tested for using CSF [10, 56–59]:

- Cryptococcosis
- FIP
- Toxoplasmosis

78.4 The Most Common Causes of Seizures in Adult Dogs and Cats

Seizures are a relatively common neurologic complaint in companion animal practice [7, 10, 11, 38, 40, 55, 60–82]. Although their occurrence in cats is less so than in dogs, they are recognized with frequency in both species [10].

It is therefore important for the veterinarian to be aware of the most common causes of seizures in both species from the standpoint of clinical presentations and case management.

78.4.1 Idiopathic Epilepsy

Idiopathic epilepsy, sometimes referred to as genetic epilepsy or primary epilepsy, is a common clinical presentation in adult dogs and cats [2, 10]. These patients do not have a structural lesion within the CNS [2]. They simply possess a focus of neuronal hyperactivity that leads to recurrent seizures [2].

Affected patients are young when they experience their first seizure [2, 10]. Most dogs present between one and five years old [2, 7, 11, 66, 75, 83]. The average cat presents at age three-and-a-half [10].

This condition is believed to be inherited in the following breeds of dog [2, 11, 22, 61, 70, 71, 73, 76, 77, 84–88]:

- Australian Shepherd
- Beagle
- Bernese Mountain Dog
- Dachshund
- Dalmatian
- English Springer Spaniel
- Golden Retriever
- Irish Wolfhound
- Keeshond
- Labrador Retriever
- Shetland Sheepdog
- Standard Poodle
- Vizsla

A genetic link has been suspected in many more breeds [2]. Precipitating factors are well established in people and include the following [2, 89]:

- Illness
- Sleep deprivation
- Stress

It is thought that companion animal patients share similar precipitating factors based upon clinical anecdotes [2].

Reflex epilepsy is possible in both humans and animals [2]. This implies that one or more targets reproducibly cause a seizure [2]. In humans, triggers have been self-reported to include the following [2, 10, 38, 90]:

- Auditory stimulation
  - High-pitched sound
  - Music
- Gustatory stimulation
- Tactile
  - Grooming
- Thermal stimulation
  - Hot bath
- Visual stimulation
  - Flickering lights

The author has experienced a case of reflex epilepsy involving the veterinary clinic. A patient of hers seized every time it entered the front door.

Veterinary patients with idiopathic epilepsy have varied presentations in terms of seizure type and frequency [2]. Historically, it was thought that idiopathic epilepsy involved only tonic–clonic seizures [2, 11]. However, affected patients may also have partial seizures, complex partial seizures, or any combination thereof [2, 11, 21, 22, 75, 83].

Seizure frequency also varies among affected patients [2]. Patients may seize as infrequently as once per year or as often as several times each day [2, 66, 83].

Seizures may be more likely to occur at rest [2, 21].

One isolated seizure of short duration is unlikely to necessitate anti-epileptic therapy [60].

If seizures are infrequent, with long disease-free intervals and/or minor episodes of short duration without the tendency to cluster, daily medication is likely unnecessary [2].

Patients with reflex seizures are also unlikely to require medication [2]. It would be more effective to limit exposure to the inciting agents.

Daily maintenance treatment is advised when seizures become more frequent, longer in terms of duration, or more severe in terms of intensity [2]. Treatment is also advised if seizures begin to layer on top of one another, as this is an indication that episodes may progress to status epilepticus [2].

Each clinician and client has his or her own comfort level in terms of when to initiate maintenance therapy. It has been proposed that maintenance therapy is indicated when [10, 61]

- Patients experience one or more seizures within a week of experiencing traumatic injury
- Patients have more than one seizure each month
- Patients have cluster seizures, that is, more than one seizure within 24 h
- Patients have a seizure that lasts for more than 5 min
- Patients have status epilepticus, that is, continuous seizure activity.

Ideally, daily maintenance treatment would extinguish seizures while being safe to administer to the patient long term [2]. Rarely, however, do patients become seizure-free [2, 61]. A more realistic goal of anti-epileptic therapy is to increase the disease-free interval and/or reduce seizure severity such that quality of life is maximized without risking serious adverse effects [2, 10, 61, 67].

Some patients have epilepsy that is refractory to conventional therapies, such as phenobarbital and potassium bromide [65].

For more information regarding newer treatment options for canine and feline epilepsy, consult an internal medicine, emergency medicine, neurology, and/or pharmacology text.

78.4.2 Intracranial Neoplasia

The incidence of intracranial neoplasia in dogs and cats varies between case reports in the veterinary literature. Some authors document 14.5 cases out of every 100,000 dogs [91, 92]. Others report a higher incidence of nearly 3 % in dogs and 2.2% in cats [37, 91–94].

Older dogs and cats are more likely to develop intracranial neoplasia as compared to younger dogs and cats, which are more likely to develop idiopathic epilepsy [10, 37, 93].

78.4.3 Canine Intracranial Neoplasia

Seizures are the most common clinical sign in dogs with intracranial neoplasia, followed by changes in mentation [93].

Other common signs of intracranial neoplasia include the following [93]:

- Anisocoria
- Blindness
- Circling
- Neck pain
- Regurgitation
- Tremors of the appendages
- Vestibular syndrome

Among dogs, the following breeds may be predisposed to primary brain tumors [93]:

- Boxer
- Doberman Pinscher
- Golden Retriever
- Old English Sheepdog
- Scottish Terrier

Dogs are most likely to develop meningiomas and gliomas [37, 93, 95–100]. The former arise from mesodermal cells; the latter arise from neuroectodermal cells [93, 99].

Meningiomas are slow-growing intracranial tumors [93]. They may be present for a while before they cause clinical signs that are apparent to the client [93, 101, 102].

When clinical signs do develop, they may be so subtle that clients consider them to be the result of normal aging [95]. Subtle changes in mentation, for instance, may be overlooked in a senior pet, and pacing may be chalked up to senility rather than considered to be the result of a space-occupying lesion [93].

Some meningiomas are even discovered on necropsy as incidental findings in patients with no evidence of neurologic dysfunction [93].

On advanced imaging studies, most meningiomas are supratentorial [103–107]. In particular, meningiomas preferentially select the fronto-olfactory region of the brain [103–107]. On occasion, meningiomas will extend through the cribriform plate [103, 104, 108].

Most meningiomas have well-defined borders as depicted by MRI [103–105].

Less common canine intracranial tumors include the following [93, 99]:

- Choroid plexus tumors
- Ependymomas
- Medulloblastomas
- Neuroblastomas
- Undifferentiated sarcomas

Consult an oncology text for information as to the regional distribution of these tumors, their prognosis, and appropriate case management for best patient outcome.

78.4.4 Feline Intracranial Neoplasia

There are fewer retrospective studies concerning feline intracranial neoplasia, so it is difficult to hypothesize about breed predispositions in cats. However, intracranial neoplasia has been documented in the following breeds of cat [37]:

- Abyssinian
- Devon Rex
- Domestic shorthaired (DSH)
- Domestic longhaired (DLH)
- Himalayan
- Maine Coon
- Manx
- Siamese

Many cats with intracranial tumors seize, and roughly one in four cats with intracranial tumors develops abnormal mentation or circling [37, 38, 109, 110]

Other potential clinical signs include ataxia and changes in behavior, specifically an increase in aggression [37].

Clinical signs may also be nonspecific in cats [37]. For instance, many cats with intracranial neoplasia develop lethargy and anorexia [37].

In cats, the most common type of primary intracranial neoplasia is meningioma [38, 109, 110]. A number of cats develop more than one meningioma at the same time [37].

It is not uncommon for cats to develop another tumor type in addition to meningioma, such as lymphoma or pituitary tumors [37]. These are common types of secondary intracranial neoplasia in the cat [38, 109, 110].

Other less common intracranial tumors in cats include the following [33, 38, 110, 111]:

- Ependyoma
- Glioma
- Olfactory neuroblastoma

Consult an oncology text for information as to the regional distribution of these tumors, their prognosis, and appropriate case management for best patient outcome.

Note that FeLV and FIV do not appear to be risk factors for intracranial neoplasia in the cat [37].

78.4.5 Infectious Disease Within the CNS: Blastomycosis

Blastomycosis was introduced in Chapter 9, Section 9.5.1 as a systemic fungal infection, for which the causative agent is *Blastomyces dermatitidis* [112]. Recall that *B. dermatitidis* is endemic to North American soil [112, 113]. Those who reside near the Mississippi, Missouri, and Ohio River valleys are most at risk for contracting disease [112].

Most patients are infected through the inhalation of spores that then establish colonies within the respiratory tract [112]. Infection of the pulmonary tree causes potentially life-threatening respiratory signs: tachypnea, dyspnea, and cyanosis [112].

B. dermatitidis is also capable of hematogenous spread, such that distant sites may be colonized [112].

Disseminated disease causes a multitude of clinical signs that include the following [112, 114–116]:

- Cutaneous lesions
  - Claw bed disease
    Depigmentation of the nasal planum (recall Chapter 9, Figure 9.13)
  - Nodules
  - Papules
  - Paronychia
  - Plaques
- Musculoskeletal dysfunction
  - Lameness
  - Osteolysis

- Periosteal proliferation
- Soft tissue swelling
- Nonspecific malaise, lethargy, anorexia, and protracted weight loss
- Ocular disease
  - Anterior uveitis
  - Chorioretinitis
  - Glaucoma
  - Lens rupture
  - Retinal detachment

CNS involvement is also possible, with gross lesions identifiable on necropsy [116] (see Figures 78.1a, b).

78.4.6 Infectious Disease Within the CNS: Coccidioidomycosis

Coccidioidomycosis, also known as valley fever, is caused by a soil-borne fungus, *Coccidioides* [117]. This agent is exceptionally resistant to arid climates, making it regionally suited to the southwestern United States as well as to Central and South America [117].

When the soil is disturbed either intentionally or indirectly, by rainfall, *Coccidioides* sporulates and releases arthroconidia [117]. Inhalation of arthroconidia leads to infection of susceptible hosts [117]. The infectious dose is small: a few arthroconidia are capable of causing disease [117].

Infection develops within the respiratory tract first [117]. Respiratory signs develop one to three weeks after inhalation [117]. Generalized pneumonia may be severe [117].

Disseminated disease results when the infectious agent extends beyond the hilar lymph nodes [117]. When disease is seeded throughout the body, multiple organ systems and their respective organs may be affected [117]. The following pathologies are possible [117]:

- Cardiac disease
  - Congestive heart failure (CHF)
  - Constrictive pericarditis
- Cutaneous lesions
  - Abscesses
  - Draining tracts, as from sites adjacent to infected bone
- Musculoskeletal dysfunction
  - Lameness
  - Osteolysis
  - Joint infection (rare)
- Nonspecific malaise, lethargy, anorexia, and protracted weight loss
- Ocular disease
  - Blindness
  - Keratitis
  - Uveitis

(a)

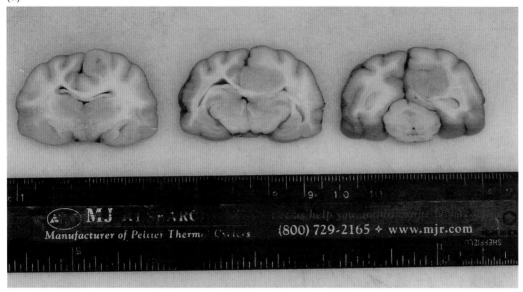

(b)

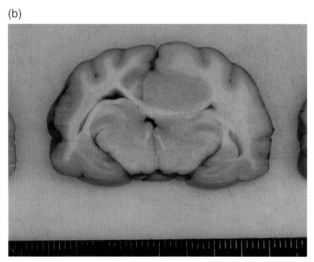

Figure 78.1 (a) Coronal sections of the brain of a feline patient that developed CNS signs secondary to blastomycosis. *Source:* Courtesy of Daniel Foy, MS, DVM, DACVIM, DACVECC. (b) Close-up of coronal section of the brain a feline patient that developed CNS signs secondary to blastomycosis. *Source:* Courtesy of Daniel Foy, MS, DVM, DACVIM, DACVECC.

CNS involvement is also possible. When it occurs, meningeal inflammation is likely to trigger seizure activity [117]. Clients may also report unusual behaviors and apparent incoordination [117].

78.4.7 Infectious Disease Within the CNS: Cryptococcosis

Cryptococcosis was introduced in Chapter 33, Section 33.5.3 as a systemic fungal infection of cats that takes root when spores from a contaminated environment are inhaled [118, 119]. Recall that *Cryptococcus* spp. prefer to grow in soils that are rich in pigeon droppings [118, 120]. Pigeons are also carriers for *Cryptococcus*

neoformans, contributing to the spread of this fungus worldwide [118, 121].

Once the fungus is within the respiratory tract, it can take on one or more forms [118]. The yeast form tends to predominate in mammalian hosts [118, 122, 123].

Most cats are asymptomatic despite harboring this infectious agent [118, 124].

When clinical disease occurs, it is primarily associated with the upper respiratory tract [118, 119]. Affected cats may present with chronic nasal discharge [118].

Recall that affected patients often develop swelling along the bridge of the nose [118]. This is referred to as the Roman nose sign. Skin overlying this swelling often ulcerates and drains [118]. Dyspnea may result from occlusion of the nasal passageways as the muzzle progressively becomes deformed [118, 125].

The ethmoid bone allows for fungal dissemination to the CNS [118, 126]. This is an uncommon clinical presentation in a cat, unless the patient is immunosuppressed [126].

Depending upon the precise location of CNS involvement, cryptococcosis may lead to one or more of the following clinical signs [119]:

- Ataxia
- Blindness
- Circling
- Head pressing
- Head tilt
- Loss of sense of smell
- Personality changes
- Unusual behavior
- Vestibular syndrome

Seizures are also potential sequelae of cryptococcosis that involves the CNS [119].

Cryptococcosis is primarily a feline fungal disease; however, it may also occur in predominantly young adult dogs [118, 127].

Dogs with cryptococcosis tend to have systemic disease that includes CNS dysfunction [128]. Neurological manifestations of disease are similar to clinical presentations in cats. In addition, dogs may exhibit cervical hyperesthesia, paraplegia, or tetraplegia [128].

78.4.8 Infectious Disease Within the CNS: Toxoplasmosis

Toxoplasmosis was introduced in Chapter 24, Section 24.3.3 as systemic disease that results from the infectious coccidian parasite, *T. gondii* [129, 130]. Recall that toxoplasmosis infects cats, dogs, humans, and most other mammals [129]. However, only members of *Felidae* are definitive hosts that excrete oocysts [129, 130].

Infection occurs primarily through one of three routes [129]:

- In utero
- Ingestion of contaminated food or water
- Ingestion of intermediate hosts whose CNS, muscle, and visceral organs contain cysts

Stress, the prolonged administration of glucocorticoids, and concurrent disease, including FeLV and FIV, are risk factors for the development of toxoplasmosis [129].

Toxoplasmosis causes varied clinical presentations in cats, including the following [129]:

- Cardiac
  - Arrhythmias
  - Sudden death

- Gastrointestinal
  - Abdominal pain
  - Diarrhea
  - Vomiting
- Hepatic
  - Icterus
- Musculoskeletal
  - Arthritis
  - Joint pain
  - Myalgia
  - Shifting leg lameness
- Ocular
  - Anisocoria
  - Anterior uveitis
  - Blindness
  - Conjunctivitis
  - Glaucoma
  - Lens luxation
  - Optic neuritis
  - Retinal detachment
- Respiratory
  - Coughing
  - Dyspnea
  - Rhinitis
  - Tachypnea

By comparison, canine toxoplasmosis targets primarily the respiratory, gastrointestinal, and neuromuscular systems [129].

Both cats and dogs with toxoplasmosis may exhibit signs of CNS dysfunction, including seizures [129].

In addition to seizure activity, neurological manifestations of disease may include the following [129–131]:

- Ataxia
- Changes in behavior
- Nystagmus
- Tremors

78.4.9 Inflammatory Disease Within the CNS: GME

GME is a pathological condition in dogs that is characterized by progressive inflammation within the CNS [9, 132–134].

GME may be focal or disseminated [9, 132–134]. In the disseminated form, GME preferentially targets white matter [9, 132–134]. Lesions most often develop with the cerebrum, cerebellum, brainstem, and cervical spinal cord [9, 134].

Histologic examination of lesions reveals perivascular accumulation of inflammatory cells, particularly macrophages and lymphocytes [9, 134]. Occasionally, cellular aggregates are so extensive as to create a macroscopic granulomatous mass [9].

The etiology is unknown. Although infectious agents have been suspected, no legitimate links to GME have been confirmed [9, 134]. Other theories have suggested an immune-mediated component, such as a delayed hypersensitivity reaction [9, 134].

It is likely that the development of GME is multifactorial [9, 134].

Young adult and middle-aged, small-breed dogs are predisposed [9, 134].

Clinical presentations for GME depend upon the location of the lesion (s) [134].

If there is forebrain involvement, meaning the cerebral cortex and thalamus, then seizures are likely [134]. Other clinical signs that are associated with forebrain disease include abnormal mentation, behavioral changes, abnormal movements and postures [134]. Affected patients may circle, pace, wander, or head-press [134]. They may also exhibit the following contralateral deficits [134]:

- Reduced or absent facial sensation
- Reduced or absent menace response
- Reduced or absent postural reactions
- Reduced or absent vision

GME lesions within the hypothalamus may also provoke seizure activity [134]. Given the location of the lesions, these patients may also have difficulty regulating core body temperature and appetite [134]. They may also develop endocrinopathies in addition to changes in mentation and/or behavior [134].

Definitive diagnosis requires a biopsy and is therefore not typically available until postmortem examination [9, 134].

Presumptive diagnoses are made based upon CSF analysis: mononuclear pleocytosis and increased protein are most commonly seen in cases of inflammatory brain disease [9, 134].

MRI may also be of value in differentiating GME from other inflammatory brain diseases [9, 134]. However, it is not always possible to differentiate GME from neoplasia [9, 134].

Although patients may respond to immunosuppressive doses of corticosteroids, the prognosis for dogs with GME is guarded [9, 134].

78.5 The Most Common Causes of Seizures in Pediatric Practice

When patients that are less than a year of age present with a history of seizure activity, both idiopathic epilepsy and intracranial neoplasia are rare [25]. More likely, either the patient has an underlying defect of development, such as hydrocephalus, or the patient has experienced traumatic brain injury [25].

If the cause of the seizure is extracranial, then the top four differentials are prioritized [25]:

- HE, as from a PSS
- Intestinal parasitism
- Neonatal hypoglycemia
- Toxicosis

78.5.1 PSSs, HE, and Seizure Activity

PSSs were reviewed in Chapter 28, Section 28.2.2, Chapter 48, Section 48.3, Chapter 51, Section 51.3, Chapter 54, Section 54.6, and Chapter 71, Section 71.7 as they relate to hepatic icterus, abnormal ingestive behaviors, small bowel diarrhea, acute vomiting, and HE.

Recall that PSSs are congenital or acquired conditions in which blood bypasses the liver to enter into systemic circulation [9, 135]. Because the liver is unable to detoxify blood from the intestines, spleen, and pancreas, toxic substances enter the general circulation [136].

When the cerebral cortex is exposed to noxious substances, such as ammonia, the patient experiences episodes of HE [136]. HE is characterized by the following [3, 136]:

- Abnormal mentation
- Ataxia
  - Particularly common in cats
- Circling
  - Especially in dogs
- Disorientation
- Head pressing
  - Especially in dogs
- Lethargy
- Ptyalism
  - Particularly in cats
- Unusual behavior
  - Aggression, especially in cats
- Wandering

Seizures are common sequelae of episodic HE [3].

The majority of dogs with PSSs have CNS signs as described above, including seizures [9, 137–139].

Refer back to Chapter 71, Section 71.7 for a brief review of diagnosis and management options.

78.5.2 Hydrocephalus

Hydrocephalus was introduced in Chapter 71, Section 71.6 as a pathological condition in which the ventricular system of the brain distends [140]. It occurs when there is an increase in CSF or an obstruction to its flow [9, 140]. If the obstruction is acute, then the body risks life-threatening elevations of intracranial pressure (ICP) [140].

Recall that hydrocephalus may be congenital or acquired [140].

Pediatric patients that develop hydrocephalus most often have a stenotic mesencephalic aqueduct [9, 140, 141]. Toy and small-breed dogs are predisposed [140, 142].

Recall that affected patients develop an enlarged, dome-shaped head [140, 143]. They are likely to have open fontanelles [140]. Many develop divergent strabismus, or exotropia, in which one or both globes deviate outward [144].

Patients may present because of their misshapen calvaria.

Others may present because of the impact that hydrocephalus has on their day-to-day function. Recall that abnormal mentation is frequently observed in patients with hydrocephalus. Clients often report that patients are dull or unusually sleepy [3, 140, 143].

Other common clinical signs include the following [3, 140, 143]:

- Ataxia
- Circling
- Incoordination
- Reduced postural reactions
- Visual deficits

Seizures may result from hydrocephalus [3, 140, 143].

Which clinical signs are seen in each patient depends upon which region of the brain is affected most [9]. Patients may present with primarily cerebral signs [9]. Alternatively, clinical signs may be vestibular or cerebellar [9].

Note that clinical signs are tolerated better when hydrocephalus is gradual as opposed to when patients experience acute obstruction to CSF flow [9].

If ICP rises suddenly, patients present with extreme changes to mentation [3]. They may be stuporous or comatose [3]. Pupils often become fixed and either pinpoint or dilated [3]. Respiration patterns change, and the patient assumes a decerebrate posture: all four limbs are extended in recumbency, often with concurrent head and neck dorsiflexion [145–147]. Brain herniation is not only possible, it is probable [3].

78.5.3 Neonatal Hypoglycemia

Neonatal hypoglycemia was introduced in Chapter 71, Section 71.5.1. Recall that toy and small-breed dogs are predisposed to developing this condition because, as pediatric patients, they are unable to maintain their resting blood glucose levels during protracted fasting [41–43].

The brain requires glucose for energy [148]. When the brain is deprived of this energy source, it becomes dysfunctional [148]. Many of the same clinical signs that develop in hydrocephalic patients are demonstrated in cases of hypoglycemia [41–43]. Patients appear disoriented and dull. Mentation continues to decline as hypoglycemia worsens [41–43]. Ataxia and incoordination are likely [41–43].

Muscle fasciculations, tremors, and seizures are common sequelae [41–43].

78.5.4 Lissencephaly

Lissencephaly is a rare condition in which the gyri and sulci of the brain fail to develop [9]. The result is a continuously smooth cerebral surface [9].

The interior of affected brains is also impacted structurally [9]. The cortex of the cerebrum thickens, and white matter is absent [9, 141, 149]. These changes are confirmed via MRI [9].

Lhasa Apsos are predisposed among dogs [9, 141, 149–151]. Korats are overrepresented among cats [141].

Affected patients present at a young age for unusual behaviors, such as circling, blindness, and seizures [9, 141, 149–151].

78.6 Potential Complications of Seizures

Most seizures are isolated events, from which patients recover spontaneously, without the need for emergency administration of anti-epileptic agents [152]. This bounce-back feature is critical to preserving CNS function [152]. If seizure activity is prolonged, then neuronal damage is likely [152]. This is caused by the excessive release of glutamate, which causes irreversible neuronal injury [152, 153].

In addition to damaging the CNS, protracted seizures create additional areas of interest or foci that may precipitate subsequent seizure activity [152, 154].

Extended seizure activity may also result in one or more of the following pathologic changes [2, 152, 154, 155]:

- Arrhythmias
- Hyperglycemia
- Hypertension
- Hyperthermia

The development of disseminated intravascular coagulation (DIC) is possible and life-threatening. Cardiorespiratory compromise and renal failure are also potential outcomes [152].

Protracted seizure activity may be defined as:

- Increased frequency of seizure activity
- Increased duration of ictus.

Cluster seizures are one form of protracted seizure activity in which the patient experiences more than two seizures during a 24-h period [152].

Some studies have reported that cluster seizures may appear more often in intact than in neutered males [156, 157]. Other reports in the veterinary medical literature have not found any association between sex and cluster seizures [156].

The following breeds may also be predisposed to cluster seizures [88, 156–158]:

- Australian Shepherd
- Border Collie
- Boxer
- German Shepherd

Cluster seizures may lead to the development of status epilepticus [152]. Status epilepticus refers to either [152]:

- Continuous activity in which seizures overlap, without opportunity for recovery in between each attack
- Seizure activity that lasts for more than 5 min

Cluster seizures and status epilepticus are not uncommon among companion animal patients with idiopathic epilepsy [152]. Roughly one-third to two-thirds of epileptic dogs experience either cluster seizures or status epilepticus [2, 152, 157, 159–161].

Status epilepticus is a medical emergency [10, 152]. Patient stabilization takes priority. Intravenous access is essential. The following parameters need to be monitored closely [152]:

- Blood pressure
- Pulse oximetry
- Core body temperature

Diagnostic blood tests, including a CBC and chemistry profile, should be performed to screen for potential causes of protracted seizure activity. Abnormalities such as hypoglycemia and/or hypocalcemia should be addressed immediately [152].

Intravenous administration of diazepam is considered the first line of treatment to halt status epilepticus [2, 10, 152, 162, 163]. When intravenous access is not possible, for instance, if the patient has not yet arrived at the clinic, alternative routes of administration are possible [152]. The administration of diazepam per rectum and/or intranasally has been proposed [152, 164].

If status epilepticus is refractory to injectable diazepam, then diazepam may need to be administered as a continuous rate infusion (CRI). Alternatively, injectable phenobarbital or levetiracetam may be given [152].

A CRI of the anesthetic induction agent, propofol, may be required by patients that are refractory to case management as described [152].

Consult an emergency medicine, internal medicine, neurology, and/or pharmacology text as well as the ACVIM Small Animal Consensus Statement for additional details regarding treatment plans [60].

References

1 Mariani, C.L. (2013). Terminology and classification of seizures and epilepsy in veterinary patients. *Top. Companion Anim. Med.* 28 (2): 34–41.

2 Thomas, W.B. (2010). Idiopathic epilepsy in dogs and cats. *Vet. Clin. North Am. Small Anim. Pract.* 40 (1): 161–179.

3 Tilley, L.P. and Smith, F.W.K. (2004). *The 5-Minute Veterinary Consult: Canine and Feline*, 3e. Baltimore, MD: Lippincott Williams & Wilkins.

4 De Risio, L., Bhatti, S., Munana, K. et al. (2015). International veterinary epilepsy task force consensus proposal: diagnostic approach to epilepsy in dogs. *BMC Vet. Res.* 11: 148.

5 Fisher, R.S., van Emde, B.W., Blume, W. et al. (2005). Epileptic seizures and epilepsy: definitions proposed by the International League Against Epilepsy (ILAE) and the International Bureau for Epilepsy (IBE). *Epilepsia* 46 (4): 470–472.

6 Blume, W.T., Luders, H.O., Mizrahi, E. et al. (2001). Glossary of descriptive terminology for ictal semiology: report of the ILAE task force on classification and terminology. *Epilepsia* 42 (9): 1212–1218.

7 Berendt, M. and Gram, L. (1999). Epilepsy and seizure classification in 63 dogs: a reappraisal of veterinary epilepsy terminology. *J. Vet. Intern. Med.* 13 (1): 14–20.

8 So, N.K. (1993). Epileptic aura. In: *The Treatment of Epilepsy: Principles and Practices* (ed. E. Wyllie), 369. Philadelphia: Lea & Febiger.

9 Lavely, J.A. (2014). Pediatric seizure disorders in dogs and cats. *Vet. Clin. North Am. Small Anim. Pract.* 44 (2): 275–301.

10 Smith Bailey, K. and Dewey, C.W. (2009). The seizuring cat. Diagnostic work-up and therapy. *J. Feline Med. Surg.* 11 (5): 385–394.

11 Chandler, K. (2006). Canine epilepsy: what can we learn from human seizure disorders? *Vet. J.* 172 (2): 207–217.

12 Kraus, M.S. (ed.) (2003). *Syncope in Small Breed Dogs.* ACVIM.

13 Thawley, V. and Silverstein, D. (2012). Collapse. *NAVC Clinician's Brief* (November): 14–15.

14 Estrada, A. (2017). Differentiating syncope from seizure. *NAVC Clinician's Brief* (July): 50–55.

15 Barnett, L., Martin, M.W., Todd, J. et al. (2011). A retrospective study of 153 cases of undiagnosed collapse, syncope or exercise intolerance: the outcomes. *J. Small Anim. Pract.* 52 (1): 26–31.

16 Gurfinkel, V., Cacciatore, T.W., Cordo, P. et al. (2006). Postural muscle tone in the body axis of healthy humans. *J. Neurophysiol.* 96 (5): 2678–2687.

17 Schwartz, D.S. (ed.) (2009). The syncopal dog. World Small Animal Veterinary Association World Congress Proceedings; Sao Paulo, Brazil.

18 Dutton, E., Dukes-McEwan, J., and Cripps, P.J. (2017). Serum cardiac troponin I in canine syncope and seizures. *J. Vet. Cardiol.* 19 (1): 1–13.

19 Penning, V.A., Connolly, D.J., Gajanayake, I. et al. (2009). Seizure-like episodes in 3 cats with intermittent high-grade atrioventricular dysfunction. *J. Vet. Intern. Med.* 23 (1): 200–205.

20 Motta, L. and Dutton, E. (2013). Suspected exercise-induced seizures in a young dog. *J. Small Anim. Pract.* 54 (4): 213–218.

21 Pakozdy, A., Leschnik, M., Tichy, A.G., and Thalhammer, J.G. (2008). Retrospective clinical comparison of idiopathic versus symptomatic epilepsy in 240 dogs with seizures. *Acta Vet. Hung.* 56 (4): 471–483.

22 Patterson, E.E., Armstrong, P.J., O'Brien, D.P. et al. (2005). Clinical description and mode of inheritance of idiopathic epilepsy in English springer spaniels. *J. Am. Vet. Med. Assoc.* 226 (1): 54–58.

23 Dodman, N.H., Knowles, K.E., Shuster, L. et al. (1996). Behavioral changes associated with suspected complex partial seizures in bull terriers. *J. Am. Vet. Med. Assoc.* 208 (5): 688–691.

24 Dodman, N.H., Miczek, K.A., Knowles, K. et al. (1992). Phenobarbital-responsive episodic dyscontrol (rage) in dogs. *J. Am. Vet. Med. Assoc.* 201 (10): 1580–1583.

25 Côté, E. (2013). Seizures. In: *Clinical Veterinary Advisor Dogs and Cats*, 3e (ed. E. Côté), 593–594. St. Louis, Missouri: Elsevier Mosby.

26 Thomas, W.B. (1998). Inflammatory diseases of the central nervous system in dogs. *Clin. Tech. Small Anim. Pract.* 13 (3): 167–178.

27 Lowrie, M. (2016). Infectious and non-infectious inflammatory causes of seizures in dogs and cats. *In Pract.* 38 (3): 99–110.

28 Gaunt, M.C., Taylor, S.M., and Kerr, M.E. (2009). Central nervous system blastomycosis in a dog. *Can. Vet. J.* 50 (9): 959–962.

29 Hecht, S., Adams, W.H., Smith, J.R., and Thomas, W.B. (2011). Clinical and imaging findings in five dogs with intracranial blastomycosis (Blastomyces dermatiditis). *J. Am. Anim. Hosp. Assoc.* 47 (4): 241–249.

30 Bromel, C. and Sykes, J.E. (2005). Epidemiology, diagnosis, and treatment of blastomycosis in dogs and cats. *Clin. Tech. Small Anim. Pract.* 20 (4): 233–239.

31 Irwin, P.J. and Parry, B.W. (1999). Streptococcal meningoencephalitis in a dog. *J. Am. Anim. Hosp. Assoc.* 35 (5): 417–422.

32 Schriefl, S., Steinberg, T.A., Matiasek, K. et al. (2008). Etiologic classification of seizures, signalment, clinical signs, and outcome in cats with seizure disorders: 91 cases (2000–2004). *J. Am. Vet. Med. Assoc.* 233 (10): 1591–1597.

33 Barnes, H.L., Chrisman, C.L., Mariani, C.L. et al. (2004). Clinical signs, underlying cause, and outcome in cats with seizures: 17 cases (1997–2002). *J. Am. Vet. Med. Assoc.* 225 (11): 1723–1726.

34 Singh, M., Foster, D.J., Child, G., and Lamb, W.A. (2005). Inflammatory cerebrospinal fluid analysis in cats: clinical diagnosis and outcome. *J. Feline Med. Surg.* 7 (2): 77–93.

35 Quesnel, A.D., Parent, J.M., McDonell, W. et al. (1997). Diagnostic evaluation of cats with seizure disorders: 30 cases (1991–1993). *J. Am. Vet. Med. Assoc.* 210 (1): 65–71.

36 Rand, J.S., Parent, J., Percy, D., and Jacobs, R. (1994). Clinical, cerebrospinal fluid, and histological data from twenty-seven cats with primary inflammatory disease of the central nervous system. *Can. Vet. J.* 35 (2): 103–110.

37 Troxel, M.T., Vite, C.H., Van Winkle, T.J. et al. (2003). Feline intracranial neoplasia: retrospective review of 160 cases (1985–2001). *J. Vet. Intern. Med.* 17 (6): 850–859.

38 Barnes, H.H. (2018). Feline epilepsy. *Vet. Clin. North Am. Small Anim. Pract.* 48 (1): 31–43.

39 Kline, K.L. (1998). Feline epilepsy. *Clin. Tech. Small Anim. Pract.* 13 (3): 152–158.

40 Moore, S.A. (2013). A clinical and diagnostic approach to the patient with seizures. *Top. Companion Anim. Med.* 28 (2): 46–50.

41 Parker, N. (2006). Treating neonatal and pediatric hypoglycemia. Banfield Pet Hospital [Internet]. May/June:[34–42 pp.]. https://www.banfield.com/getmedia/b4c313cc-bf61-49b3-9abc-a131def714e3/2_3-Treating-neonatal-and-pediatric-hypoglycemia.

42 Lewis, H.B. (2006). Hypoglycemia in puppies and kittens. Banfield Pet Hospital [Internet]. May/June: [18–23 pp.]. https://www.banfield.com/getmedia/044861d1-eed8-4e21-9c3c-537a13e6a9bf/2_3-Hypoglycemia-in-puppies-and-kittens.

43 Vroom, M.W. and Slappendel, R.J. (1987). Transient juvenile hypoglycaemia in a Yorkshire terrier and in a Chihuahua. *Vet. Q.* 9 (2): 172–176.

44 Grubb, B.P., Gerard, G., Roush, K. et al. (1991). Differentiation of convulsive syncope and epilepsy with head-up tilt testing. *Ann. Intern. Med.* 115 (11): 871–876.

45 Linzer, M., Grubb, B.P., Ho, S. et al. (1994). Cardiovascular causes of loss of consciousness in patients with presumed epilepsy: a cause of the increased sudden death rate in people with epilepsy? *Am. J. Med.* 96 (2): 146–154.

46 Scheepers, B., Clough, P., and Pickles, C. (1998). The misdiagnosis of epilepsy: findings of a population study. *Seizure* 7 (5): 403–406.

47 Sheldon, R., Rose, S., Ritchie, D. et al. (2002). Historical criteria that distinguish syncope from seizures. *J. Am. Coll. Cardiol.* 40 (1): 142–148.

48 Smith, D., Defalla, B.A., and Chadwick, D.W. (1999). The misdiagnosis of epilepsy and the management of refractory epilepsy in a specialist clinic. *QJM* 92 (1): 15–23.

49 Zaidi, A., Clough, P., Cooper, P. et al. (2000). Misdiagnosis of epilepsy: many seizure-like attacks have a cardiovascular cause. *J. Am. Coll. Cardiol.* 36 (1): 181–184.

50 Chadwick, D. and Smith, D. (2002). The misdiagnosis of epilepsy. *BMJ* 324 (7336): 495–496.

51 Werz, M.A. (2005). Idiopathic generalized tonic-clonic seizures limited to exercise in a young adult. *Epilepsy Behav.* 6 (1): 98–101.

52 Frank, L.A. (2006). Comparative dermatology–canine endocrine dermatoses. *Clin. Dermatol.* 24 (4): 317–325.

53 Baker, K. (1986). Hormonal alopecia in dogs and cats. *In Pract.* 8 (2): 71–78.

54 Scott-Moncrieff, J.C. (2007). Clinical signs and concurrent diseases of hypothyroidism in dogs and cats. *Vet. Clin. North Am. Small Anim. Pract.* 37 (4): 709–722, vi.

55 Parent, J.M. (1988). Clinical management of canine seizures. *Vet. Clin. North Am. Small Anim. Pract.* 18 (4): 947–964.

56 Foster, S.F., Charles, J.A., Parker, G. et al. (2001). Cerebral cryptococcal granuloma in a cat. *J. Feline Med. Surg.* 3 (1): 39–44.

57 Pfohl, J.C. and Dewey, C.W. (2005). Intracranial *Toxoplasma gondii* granuloma in a cat. *J. Feline Med. Surg.* 7 (6): 369–374.

58 Timmann, D., Cizinauskas, S., Tomek, A. et al. (2008). Retrospective analysis of seizures associated with feline infectious peritonitis in cats. *J. Feline Med. Surg.* 10 (1): 9–15.

59 Dewey, C.W. (2006). Anticonvulsant therapy in dogs and cats. *Vet. Clin. North Am. Small Anim. Pract.* 36 (5): 1107–1127, vii.

60 Podell, M., Volk, H.A., Berendt, M. et al. (2016). 2015 ACVIM small animal consensus statement on seizure management in dogs. *J. Vet. Intern. Med.* 30 (2): 477–490.

61 Munana, K.R. (2013). Update: seizure management in small animal practice. *Vet. Clin. North Am. Small Anim. Pract.* 43 (5): 1127–1147.

62 Schwartz-Porsche, D. (ed.) (1986). Epidemiological, clinical, and pharmacokinetic studies in spontaneously epileptic dogs and cats. Proceedings of the 4th Annual American College of Veterinary Internal Medicine Forum; Washington, D.C.

63 Bunch, S.E. (1986). Anticonvulsant drug therapy in companion animals. In: *Current Veterinary Therapy IX* (ed. R.W. Kirk), 836–844. Philadelphia: WB Saunders Co.

64 Pakozdy, A., Leschnik, M., Sarchahi, A.A. et al. (2010). Clinical comparison of primary versus secondary epilepsy in 125 cats. *J. Feline Med. Surg.* 12 (12): 910–916.

65 Munana, K. (2009). Newer options for medically managing refractory canine epilepsy. DVM 360 [Internet]. http://veterinarymedicine.dvm360.com/ newer-options-medically-managing-refractory-canine-epilepsy.

66 Podell, M., Fenner, W.R., and Powers, J.D. (1995). Seizure classification in dogs from a nonreferral-based population. *J. Am. Vet. Med. Assoc.* 206 (11): 1721–1728.

67 Meland, T. and Carrera-Justiz, S. (2018). A review: emergency management of dogs with suspected epileptic seizures. *Top. Companion Anim. Med.* 33 (1): 17–20.

68 Fluehmann, G., Doherr, M.G., and Jaggy, A. (2006). Canine neurological diseases in a referral hospital population between 1989 and 2000 in Switzerland. *J. Small Anim. Pract.* 47 (10): 582–587.

69 Gesell, F.K., Hoppe, S., Loscher, W., and Tipold, A. (2015). Antiepileptic drug withdrawal in dogs with epilepsy. *Front. Vet. Sci.* 2: 23.

70 Licht, B.G., Licht, M.H., Harper, K.M. et al. (2002). Clinical presentations of naturally occurring canine seizures: similarities to human seizures. *Epilepsy Behav.* 3 (5): 460–470.

71 Cunningham, J.G. and Farnbach, G.C. (1988). Inheritance and idiopathic canine epilepsy. *J. Am. Anim. Hosp. Assoc.* 24 (4): 421–424.

72 Van Meervenne, S.A., Volk, H.A., Matiasek, K., and Van Ham, L.M. (2014). The influence of sex hormones on seizures in dogs and humans. *Vet. J.* 201 (1): 15–20.

73 Casal, M.L., Munuve, R.M., Janis, M.A. et al. (2006). Epilepsy in Irish wolfhounds. *J. Vet. Intern. Med.* 20 (1): 131–135.

74 Gullov, C.H., Toft, N., Baadsager, M.M., and Berendt, M. (2011). Epilepsy in the petit basset griffon Vendeen: prevalence, semiology, and clinical phenotype. *J. Vet. Intern. Med.* 25 (6): 1372–1378.

75 Jaggy, A. and Bernardini, M. (1998). Idiopathic epilepsy in 125 dogs: a long-term study. Clinical and electroencephalographic findings. *J. Small Anim. Pract.* 39 (1): 23–29.

76 Jaggy, A., Faissler, D., Gaillard, C. et al. (1998). Genetic aspects of idiopathic epilepsy in Labrador retrievers. *J. Small Anim. Pract.* 39 (6): 275–280.

77 Kathmann, I., Jaggy, A., Busato, A. et al. (1999). Clinical and genetic investigations of idiopathic epilepsy in the Bernese mountain dog. *J. Small Anim. Pract.* 40 (7): 319–325.

78 Kearsley-Fleet, L., O'Neill, D.G., Volk, H.A. et al. (2013). Prevalence and risk factors for canine epilepsy of unknown origin in the UK. *Vet. Rec.* 172 (13): 338.

79 Thomas, W.B. and Dewey, C.W. (2008). Seizures and narcolepsy. In: *A Practical Guide to Canine and Feline Neurology* (ed. C.W. Dewey), 193. Ames: Wiley Blackwell.

80 Shell, L.G. (1998). Seizures in cats. *Vet. Med.* 93 (6): 541–552.

81 Quesnel, A.D., Parent, J.M., and McDonell, W. (1997). Clinical management and outcome of cats with seizure disorders: 30 cases (1991–1993). *J. Am. Vet. Med. Assoc.* 210 (1): 72–77.

82 Platt, S.R. (2001). Feline seizure control. *J. Am. Anim. Hosp. Assoc.* 37 (6): 515–517.

83 Heynold, Y., Faissler, D., Steffen, F., and Jaggy, A. (1997). Clinical, epidemiological and treatment results of idiopathic epilepsy in 54 labrador retrievers: a long-term study. *J. Small Anim. Pract.* 38 (1): 7–14.

84 Hall, S.J. and Wallace, M.E. (1996). Canine epilepsy: a genetic counselling programme for keeshonds. *Vet. Rec.* 138 (15): 358–360.

85 Bielfelt, S.W., Redman, H.C., and McClellan, R.O. (1971). Sire- and sex-related differences in rates of epileptiform seizures in a purebred beagle dog colony. *Am. J. Vet. Res.* 32 (12): 2039–2048.

86 Morita, T., Shimada, A., Takeuchi, T. et al. (2002). Cliniconeuropathologic findings of familial frontal lobe epilepsy in Shetland sheepdogs. *Can. J. Vet. Res.* 66 (1): 35–41.

87 Srenk, P. and Jaggy, A. (1996). Interictal electroencephalographic findings in a family of golden retrievers with idiopathic epilepsy. *J. Small Anim. Pract.* 37 (7): 317–321.

88 Weissl, J., Hulsmeyer, V., Brauer, C. et al. (2012). Disease progression and treatment response of idiopathic epilepsy in Australian shepherd dogs. *J. Vet. Intern. Med.* 26 (1): 116–125.

89 Haut, S.R., Hall, C.B., Masur, J., and Lipton, R.B. (2007). Seizure occurrence: precipitants and prediction. *Neurology* 69 (20): 1905–1910.

90 Lowrie, M., Bessant, C., Harvey, R.J. et al. (2016). Audiogenic reflex seizures in cats. *J. Feline Med. Surg.* 18 (4): 328–336.

91 Vandevelde, M. (ed.) (1984). Brain tumors in domestic animals: an overview. Proceedings: Brain Tumors in Man and Animals; Research Triangle Park, NC: National Institute of Environmental Sciences.

92 Zaki, F.A. (1977). Spontaneous central nervous system tumors in the dog. *Vet. Clin. North Am.* 7 (1): 153–163.

93 Snyder, J.M., Shofer, F.S., Van Winkle, T.J., and Massicotte, C. (2006). Canine intracranial primary neoplasia: 173 cases (1986–2003). *J. Vet. Intern. Med.* 20 (3): 669–675.

94 Zaki, F.A. and Hurvitz, A.I. (1976). Spontaneous neoplasms of central nervous-system of cat. *J. Small Anim. Pract.* 17 (12): 773–782.

95 LeCouteur, R.A. (1990). Brain tumors of dogs and cats: diagnosis and management. *Vet. Med. Rep.* 2: 332–342.

96 Gavin, P.R., Fike, J.R., and Hoopes, P.J. (1995). Central nervous system tumors. *Semin. Vet. Med. Surg.* 10 (3): 180–189.

97 LeCouteur, R.A. (1999). Current concepts in the diagnosis and treatment of brain tumours in dogs and cats. *J. Small Anim. Pract.* 40 (9): 411–416.

98 Moore, M.P., Bagley, R.S., Harrington, M.L., and Gavin, P.R. (1996). Intracranial tumors. *Vet. Clin. North Am. Small Anim. Pract.* 26 (4): 759–777.

99 Nafe, L.A. (1990). The clinical presentation and diagnosis of intracranial neoplasia. *Semin. Vet. Med. Surg.* 5 (4): 223–231.

100 Patnaik, A.K., Kay, W.J., and Hurvitz, A.I. (1986). Intracranial meningioma: a comparative pathologic study of 28 dogs. *Vet. Pathol.* 23 (4): 369–373.

101 de Lahunta, A. (1983). *Veterinary Neuroanatomy and Clinical Neurology*. Philadelphia: WB Saunders.

102 Foster, E.S., Carrillo, J.M., and Patnaik, A.K. (1988). Clinical signs of tumors affecting the rostral cerebrum in 43 dogs. *J. Vet. Intern. Med.* 2 (2): 71–74.

103 Bentley, R.T. (2015). Magnetic resonance imaging diagnosis of brain tumors in dogs. *Vet. J.* 205 (2): 204–216.

104 Hathcock, J.T. (1996). Low field magnetic resonance imaging characteristics of cranial vault meningiomas in 13 dogs. *Vet. Radiol. Ultrasoun* 37 (4): 257–263.

105 Kraft, S.L., Gavin, P.R., DeHaan, C. et al. (1997). Retrospective review of 50 canine intracranial tumors evaluated by magnetic resonance imaging. *J. Vet. Intern. Med.* 11 (4): 218–225.

106 Motta, L., Mandara, M.T., and Skerritt, G.C. (2012). Canine and feline intracranial meningiomas: an updated review. *Vet. J.* 192 (2): 153–165.

107 Sturges, B.K., Dickinson, P.J., Bollen, A.W. et al. (2008). Magnetic resonance imaging and

histological classification of intracranial meningiomas in 112 dogs. *J. Vet. Intern. Med.* 22 (3): 586–595.

108 McDonnell, J.J., Kalbko, K., Keating, J.H. et al. (2007). Multiple meningiomas in three dogs. *J. Am. Anim. Hosp. Assoc.* 43 (4): 201–208.

109 Cameron, S., Rishniw, M., Miller, A.D. et al. (2015). Characteristics and survival of 121 cats undergoing excision of intracranial Meningiomas (1994–2011). *Vet. Surg.* 44 (6): 772–776.

110 Tomek, A., Cizinauskas, S., Doherr, M. et al. (2006). Intracranial neoplasia in 61 cats: localisation, tumour types and seizure patterns. *J. Feline Med. Surg.* 8 (4): 243–253.

111 DeJesus, A., Cohen, E.B., Galban, E., and Suran, J.N. (2017). Magnetic resonance imaging features of intraventricular ependymomas in five cats. *Vet. Radiol Ultrasound* 58 (3): 326–333.

112 Kerl, M.E. (2003). Update on canine and feline fungal diseases. *Vet. Clin. North Am. Small Anim. Pract.* 33 (4): 721–747.

113 Werner, A. and Blastomycosis, N.F. (2011). *Compend. Contin. Educ. Vet.* 33 (8): E1–E4; quiz E5.

114 Warren, S. (2013). Claw disease in dogs: part 2 - diagnosis and management of specific claw diseases. *Companion Anim.* 18 (5): 226–231.

115 Outerbridge, C.A. (2006). Mycologic disorders of the skin. *Clin. Tech. Small Anim. Pract.* 21 (3): 128–134.

116 Legendre, A.M. (2006). Blastomycosis. In: *Infectious Diseases of the Dog and Cat*, 3e (ed. C.E. Greene), 569–576. St. Louis, Mo.: Saunders/Elsevier.

117 Greene, R.T. (2006). Coccidioidomycosis and Paracoccidioidomycosis. In: *Infectious Diseases of the Dog and Cat*, 4e (ed. C.E. Greene), 598–608. St. Louis, Mo.: Elsevier/Saunders.

118 Pennisi, M.G., Hartmann, K., Lloret, A. et al. (2013). Cryptococcosis in cats: ABCD guidelines on prevention and management. *J. Feline Med. Surg.* 15 (7): 611–618.

119 Malik, R., Krockenberger, M., O'Brien, C.R. et al. (1998). Cryptococcosis. In: *Infectious Diseases of the Dog and Cat*, 2e (ed. C.E. Greene), 584–598. Philadelphia: W.B. Saunders.

120 Duncan, C.G., Stephen, C., and Campbell, J. (2006). Evaluation of risk factors for Cryptococcus gattii infection in dogs and cats. *J. Am. Vet. Med. Assoc.* 228 (3): 377–382.

121 Pal, M. (1989). Cryptococcus neoformans var. neoformans and munia birds. *Mycoses* 32 (5): 250–252.

122 Alspaugh, J.A., Davidson, R.C., and Heitman, J. (2000). Morphogenesis of Cryptococcus neoformans. *Contrib. Microbiol.* 5: 217–238.

123 Lin, X. and Heitman, J. (2006). The biology of the Cryptococcus neoformans species complex. *Annu. Rev. Microbiol.* 60: 69–105.

124 Malik, R., Wigney, D.I., Muir, D.B., and Love, D.N. (1997). Asymptomatic carriage of Cryptococcus neoformans in the nasal cavity of dogs and cats. *J. Med. Vet. Mycol.* 35 (1): 27–31.

125 Malik, R., Martin, P., Wigney, D.I. et al. (1997). Nasopharyngeal cryptococcosis. *Aust. Vet. J.* 75 (7): 483–488.

126 Martins, D.B., Zanette, R.A., Franca, R.T. et al. (2011). Massive cryptococcal disseminated infection in an immunocompetent cat. *Vet. Dermatol.* 22 (2): 232–234.

127 McGill, S., Malik, R., Saul, N. et al. (2009). Cryptococcosis in domestic animals in Western Australia: a retrospective study from 1995–2006. *Med. Mycol.* 47 (6): 625–639.

128 Norton, R. and Burney, D.P. (2012). Cryptococcosis. *NAVC Clinician's Brief* (December): 39–42.

129 Dubey, J.P. and Lappin, M.R. (2006). Toxoplasmosis and Neosporosis. In: *Infectious Diseases of the Dog and Cat*, 3e (ed. C.E. Greene), 755–775. St. Louis, Mo.: Saunders/Elsevier.

130 Czopowicz, M., Szalus-Jordanow, O., and Frymus, T. (2010). Cerebral toxoplasmosis in a cat. *Med. Weter.* 66 (11): 784–786.

131 Spellman, P.G. (1988). Toxoplasmosis in cats. *Vet. Rec.* 122 (13): 311.

132 Tipold, A. and Vandevelde, M. (2006). Neurologic diseases of suspected infectious origin and prion disease. In: *Infectious Diseases of the Dog and Cat* (ed. C.E. Greene), 795–798. Philadelphia: W.B. Saunders.

133 Adamo, P.F., Adams, W.M., and Steinberg, H. (2007). Granulomatous meningoencephalomyelitis in dogs. *Compend. Contin. Educ. Vet.* 29 (11): 678–690.

134 O'Neill, E.J., Merrett, D., and Jones, B. (2005). Granulomatous meningoencephalomyelitis in dogs: a review. *Ir. Vet. J.* 58 (2): 86–92.

135 Connolly, S.L. (2016). Canine portosystemic shunts: single or multiple tests to make the correct diagnosis? *Vet. J.* 207: 6–7.

136 Nelson, R.W. and Couto, C.G. (2014). *Small Animal Internal Medicine*, 5e. St. Louis, MO: Elsevier/Mosby.

137 Tisdall, P.L., Hunt, G.B., Youmans, K.R., and Malik, R. (2000). Neurological dysfunction in dogs following attenuation of congenital extrahepatic portosystemic shunts. *J. Small Anim. Pract.* 41 (12): 539–546.

138 Mehl, M.L., Kyles, A.E., Hardie, E.M. et al. (2005). Evaluation of ameroid ring constrictors for treatment for single extrahepatic portosystemic shunts in dogs: 168 cases (1995–2001). *J. Am. Vet. Med. Assoc.* 226 (12): 2020–2030.

139 Hunt, G.B., Tisdall, P.L., Webb, A. et al. (2000). Congenital portosystemic shunts in toy and miniature poodles. *Aust. Vet. J.* 78 (8): 530–532.

140 Thomas, W.B. (2010). Hydrocephalus in dogs and cats. *Vet. Clin. North Am. Small Anim. Pract.* 40 (1): 143–159.

141 Summers, B.A., Cummings, J.F., and de Lahunta, A. (1995). *Malformations of the Central Nervous System. Veterinary Neuropathology*, 68–94. St. Louis: Mosby.

142 Selby, L.A., Hayes, H.M. Jr., and Becker, S.V. (1979). Epizootiologic features of canine hydrocephalus. *Am. J. Vet. Res.* 40 (3): 411–413.

143 Bagley, R.S. (2006). The cat with stupor or coma. In: *Problem-Based Feline Medicine* (ed. J. Rand), 821–834. Edinburgh; New York: Saunders.

144 Rutstein, R.P. (2011). Care of the patient with strabismus: esotropia and exotropia. American Optometric Association [Internet]. https://www.aoa.org/documents/optometrists/CPG-12.pdf.

145 Thomas, W.B. (2000). Initial assessment of patients with neurologic dysfunction. *Vet. Clin. North Am. Small Anim. Pract.* 30 (1): 1–24, v.

146 Thomas, W.B. and Dewey, C.W. (2008). Performing the neurologic examination. In: *A Practical Guide to Canine and Feline Neurology*, 2e (ed. C.W. Dewey), 53–74. Ames, Iowa: Wiley-Blackwell.

147 Englar, R. (ed.) (2017). Evaluating the nervous system of the dog. In: *Performing the Small Animal Physical Examination*, 412–431. Hoboken, NJ: Wiley.

148 Koenig, A. (2013). Endocrine emergencies in dogs and cats. *Vet. Clin. North Am. Small Anim. Pract.* 43 (4): 869–897.

149 Saito, M., Sharp, N.J., Kortz, G.D. et al. (2002). Magnetic resonance imaging features of lissencephaly in 2 Lhasa Apsos. *Vet. Radiol. Ultrasound* 43 (4): 331–337.

150 Greene, C.E., Vandevelde, M., and Braund, K. (1976). Lissencephaly in two Lhasa Apso dogs. *J. Am. Vet. Med. Assoc.* 169 (4): 405–410.

151 Zaki, F.A. (1976). Lissencephaly in Lhasa Apso dogs. *J. Am. Vet. Med. Assoc.* 169 (11): 1165–1168.

152 Patterson, E.N. (2014). Status epilepticus and cluster seizures. *Vet. Clin. North Am. Small Anim. Pract.* 44 (6): 1103–1112.

153 Huff, J.S. and Fountain, N.B. (2011). Pathophysiology and definitions of seizures and status epilepticus. *Emerg. Med. Clin. North Am.* 29 (1): 1–13.

154 Berg, A.T., Berkovic, S.F., Brodie, M.J. et al. (2010). Revised terminology and concepts for organization of seizures and epilepsies: report of the ILAE commission on classification and terminology, 2005–2009. *Epilepsia* 51 (4): 676–685.

155 Raith, K., Steinberg, T., and Fischer, A. (2010). Continuous electroencephalographic monitoring of status epilepticus in dogs and cats: 10 patients (2004–2005). *J. Vet. Emerg. Crit. Care (San Antonio).* 20 (4): 446–455.

156 Packer, R.M., Shihab, N.K., Torres, B.B., and Volk, H.A. (2016). Risk factors for cluster seizures in canine idiopathic epilepsy. *Res. Vet. Sci.* 105: 136–138.

157 Monteiro, R., Adams, V., Keys, D., and Platt, S.R. (2012). Canine idiopathic epilepsy: prevalence, risk factors and outcome associated with cluster seizures and status epilepticus. *J. Small Anim. Pract.* 53 (9): 526–530.

158 Hulsmeyer, V., Zimmermann, R., Brauer, C. et al. (2010). Epilepsy in border collies: clinical manifestation, outcome, and mode of inheritance. *J. Vet. Intern. Med.* 24 (1): 171–178.

159 Bateman, S.W. and Parent, J.M. (1998). Clinical findings, treatment, and outcome of dogs with status epilepticus or cluster seizures: 156 cases (1990–1995). *J. Am. Anim. Hosp. Assoc.* 215 (10): 1463–1468.

160 Saito, M., Munana, K.R., Sharp, N.J., and Olby, N.J. (2001). Risk factors for development of status epilepticus in dogs with idiopathic epilepsy and effects of status epilepticus on outcome and survival time: 32 cases (1990–1996). *J. Am. Vet. Med. Assoc.* 219 (5): 618–623.

161 Zimmermann, R., Hulsmeyer, V., Sauter-Louis, C., and Fischer, A. (2009). Status epilepticus and epileptic seizures in dogs. *J. Vet. Intern. Med.* 23 (5): 970–976.

162 Podell, M. (1998). Antiepileptic drug therapy. *Clin. Tech. Small Anim. Pract.* 13 (3): 185–192.

163 Platt, S. and Garosi, L. (2012). *Small Animal Neurological Emergencies*. London: Manson Publishing.

164 Podell, M. (1995). The use of diazepam per rectum at home for the acute management of cluster seizures in dogs. *J. Vet. Intern. Med.* 9 (2): 68–74.

Index

Common Clinical Presentations in Dogs and Cats, First Edition. Ryane E. Englar.
© 2019 John Wiley & Sons, Inc. Published 2019 by John Wiley & Sons, Inc.

squamous cell carcinoma (SCC)
25–26, 45, 215, 226, 295, 305, 326,
362, 425, 438, 689–691, 737, 817,
851, 875, 913
testicular 723–725
tuna 689
turbinates 161–162, 278, 431,
436–438, 464
turbulence 505–506, 569–570
turbulent blood flow 536, 569–570
tympanic
bulla 277–278, 909–910, 912–913
cavity 325
membrane 411, 415, 912
tympanum 411, 912–913
type C neurotoxin 942
tyrosinase 135–136, 139–140
tyrosine 84, 142–143, 149
tyrosine kinase inhibitors 84, 142

u

Ukrainian Levkoy (cat) 68
ulcerative stomatitis 792
ulna 843, 846–850, 884
ulnar 852, 855, 922
ultraviolet radiation 390, 404, 425
umbilical hernia 630, 738
Uncinaria stenocephala 658, 700
underbite 684, 689
unilateral chain mastectomy 777
upper
airway obstruction 278, 449, 455,
457, 485, 487, 507, 529
esophageal sphincter 671, 676
motor neuron (UMN) 277, 854,
924, 927–928, 930, 933, 941,
947, 955
respiratory infection (URI) 139,
358, 360, 433, 437, 465, 852, 894
respiratory tract 431, 436, 449,
467, 519, 958, 972
urinary tract 748, 783, 799, 826
upright position 907, 923
urates 632, 814, 821
urea 345, 614, 642, 709, 785, 799,
805, 814, 822, 824, 827, 901–902
Ureaplasma 747, 825
urease 814, 824, 826
uremia 109, 250, 563, 683, 701, 704,
786, 895, 925, 965, 968
uremic syndrome 896
ureter 725, 783, 788, 790, 799,
812, 823
ureteral obstruction 788

ureteroliths 630, 788, 812
urethral
calculi 638, 789
length 822
obstruction 590, 737
orifice 737, 739
plugs 643, 814–815
stones 812
strictures 738
tear 630, 812, 822
urethritis 740, 748–749, 822
urethrostomy 739–741, 816, 824
urinalysis 5, 261, 267, 544, 585, 637,
705–706, 724, 749–750, 766, 775,
777, 785, 788, 792, 804–805, 814,
822, 825–827, 898, 902
urinary
bladder 84, 279, 519, 590, 630,
634, 637–638, 640, 642–643,
748–750, 783, 799, 812–814,
816–817, 822, 827, 897,
927, 964
calculi 630, 632, 749
casts 826
catheterization 788, 817, 826
crystals 643, 814, 821, 826–827
incontinence 73, 248, 279,
738, 761
neoplasia 827
retention 864
stricture 812
tract 8, 87, 115, 273, 547, 590, 630,
634, 642–643, 701, 738, 740–741,
747–748, 750, 761, 783–784,
787–789, 799–800, 805, 811–812,
814–817, 821–827, 896, 902
tract disease 87, 643, 701, 740,
747–749, 761, 825, 827
tract infection (UTI) 634, 701,
738, 748, 761, 766, 788, 792, 805,
814, 817, 821–827
tract obstruction (UTO) 8, 547,
590, 630, 632, 634, 643, 701–703,
705, 784, 788–789, 791, 811–812,
814–817, 827, 896–898, 903
urination 69, 277, 521, 543, 591,
598, 643, 749–750, 762, 766,
788, 799, 802, 804, 811–812,
827, 896, 967
urine
acidifiers 836
composition 822
concentration 811, 822
contamination 821

culture 749, 788, 792, 804–805,
827, 884
marking 774
output 799–800, 802, 811–812,
814–817
production 800, 811
retention 596, 788, 949
sediment 637, 706, 792, 825–826
specific gravity (USG) 696, 792,
804–805, 823
stream 738, 750
uro-
urobilinogen 368, 821, 826
urolithiasis 630, 632, 634,
642, 701, 703, 706, 749, 788,
801, 812, 814, 817, 821–822,
824, 827
urticaria 79, 81, 181, 184–185,
187–189
uterus 136, 481, 643, 753, 755,
757–759, 761–763, 804, 822
utricle 324, 696, 912
uvea 261, 265, 267–268, 314, 337,
393, 396, 398, 404–405
uveal melanoma 265, 314
uveitis
anterior 69, 107, 159, 257, 261,
265–266, 271–272, 274, 287, 314,
341, 349, 362, 967
phacolytic 404, 406
uveodermatologic syndrome 267,
286–287

v

vaccination history 14, 262, 435, 634,
703, 967
vacuolar hepatopathy 80, 130
vagal tone 546–547, 589, 591, 598
vagina 234, 753, 755, 757, 762, 822
vaginal
culture 766
cytology 759, 762, 766
discharge 705, 762
epithelium 758
examination 766
foreign body 761
mucosa 759, 765
septa 766
vaginitis 761, 765–766, 822
vaginoscopy 759, 766
vagosympathetic trunk 277–278
vagus nerve 463, 591, 598, 897, 914,
942, 959
Valley Fever 435, 563, 971